AF668986

Refractive Surgery

Refractive Surgery

Second Edition

Editors

Amar Agarwal
MS FRCS FRCOphth (Lon)

Athiya Agarwal
MD DO FRSH (Lon)

Soosan Jacob
MS FRCS DipNB MNAMS

Dr Agarwal's Group of Eye Hospital's and Eye Research Centre
19, Cathedral Road, Chennai, Tamil Nadu (India)
dragarwal@vsnl.com

Forewords

Daniel Durrie
Charles D Kelman

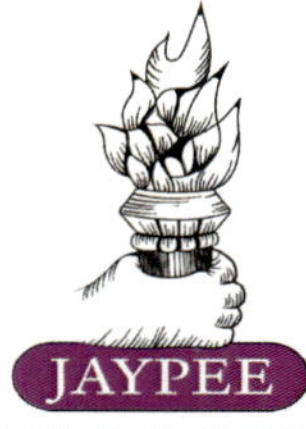

JAYPEE BROTHERS MEDICAL PUBLISHERS
The Health Sciences Publisher
New Delhi | London

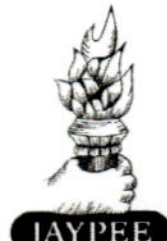
Jaypee Brothers Medical Publishers (P) Ltd

Headquarters
EMCA House
23/23-B, Ansari Road, Daryaganj
New Delhi 110 002, India
Landline: +91-11-23272143, +91-11-23272703
+91-11-23282021, +91-11-23245672
E-mail: jaypee@jaypeebrothers.com

Corporate Office
4838/24, Ansari Road, Daryaganj
New Delhi 110 002, India
Phone: +91-11-43574357
Fax: +91-11-43574314
E-mail: jaypee@jaypeebrothers.com

Overseas Office
J.P. Medical Ltd
83 Victoria Street, London
SW1H 0HW (UK)
Phone: +44 20 3170 8910
E-mail: info@jpmedpub.com

EU GPSR Authorised Representative Logos Europe, 9 rue Nicolas Poussin 17000, La Rochelle, France
Phone: +33 (0) 6 67 93 73 78
E-mail: contact@logoseurope.eu

Website: www.jaypeebrothers.com
Website: www.jaypeedigital.com

Refractive Surgery

First Edition: 2000

Second Edition: **2009, Reprint: 2025 (POD)**

ISBN 978-81-8448-412-0

Printed at: Samrat Offset Pvt. Ltd.

Dedicated to
Three people—
Mr S Rajagopalan
Mr V Suresh
and
Mrs Bhuvana Rajagopalan,
Who have made a difference

Contributors

Adam M Kartz, MD
Charles Retina Institute
6401, Popular Ave, Suite 190
Memphis, Tennessee, USA

Ajay V Kulkarni
LV Prasad Eye Institute
Hyderabad, India

Alaa EL-Danasoury, MD FRCS
Magrabi Eye Hospital
Jeddah, Saudi Arabia

Amar Agarwal, MS FRCS FRCOphth
Dr Agarwal's Group of Eye Hospitals
and Eye Research Centre
19 Cathedral road
Chennai 600 086, Tamil Nadu (India)

Amin Ashrafzadeh, MD
Northern California Eye Physicians
Modesto and Turlock, CA
Assistant Clinical Professor of
Ophthalmology
University of California, Davis, USA.
www.McHenryLASIK.com
DrAsh@McHenryLASIK.com

Arthur Cummings
2A, Weelington Road
Ballsbridge, Dublin 4
Ireland

Arun C Gulani, MD MS
Director
Gulani Vision Institute
4500 Salisbury Rd. Suite 160
Jacksonville, Florida, USA

Athiya Agarwal, MD FRSH DO
Dr Agarwal's Group of Eye Hospitals
and Eye Research Centre
19 Cathedral road
Chennai 600 086, Tamil Nadu (India)

Benjamin F Boyd
Highlights of Ophthalmology
International Technopark
Bldg 207, City of Knowledge
Gailard Highway Clayton
Panama, Rep. of Panama
Tel: 001-507-317-0160

Carmelita Coronel
St. George Correction Vision Center
4145 W Peterson Avenue Suite 200
Chicago, Illinosis, USA

Cristina Simón-Castellvi
Simon Eye Clinic (Barcelona-Spain)

Daniel Wyler, BS
MS Candidate
Georgetown University
1802 21st St N
Arlington, VA 22209, USA
Djw42@georgetown.edu

David P Pinero, PhD
Instituto Oftalmologico De Alicante
Alicante, Spain

Debby Holmes-Higgin, MS
Northwest Corneal Services
6950 SW Hampton, Suite 150
Portland, OR 97223, USA

Demetrio Pita-Salorio
Department of Ophthalmology
Hospital Clinic I Provincial
University of Barcelona
Spain

Dhivya A Kumar, MD
Dr Agarwal's Group of Eye Hospitals
and Eye Research Centre
19 Cathedral road
Chennai 600 086
Tamil Nadu (India)

Dimitrios S Siganos, MD
VLemma Eye Center
Patission Street 88
Athens 104 34, Greece + 30-1-8210808

Donald G Johnson, MD
Vancouver, British Columbia
Canada

Dolores Ortiz, PhD
Instituto Oftalmologico De Alicante
Alicante, Spain

Elizabeth A Davis, MD FACS
Minnesota Eye Consultants, PA
710, East 24th St., Suite 100
Minneapolis, MN 55404, USA
Tel: 001-612-813-3600

Ellen E Anderson Penno
Gimbel Eye Center
450, 4935-40th Avenue, NW
Calgary, Alberta, Canada

Esperanza Sala, OD
Instituto Oftalmologico De Alicante
Alicante, Spain

F Hampton Roy, MD
Hampton Roy Eye Center
9800, Lile Drive, Suite 660
Little Rock, Arkansas, USA

Francesco Carones, MD
Carones Ophthalmology Center,
Via Pietro Mascagni, 20
20122 Milano, Italy
www.carones.com
info@carones.com

Frank Lavery
Wellington Ophthalmic Laser Clinic
2A, Wellington Road
Ballsbridge, Dublin 4, Ireland

Gemma Walsh B Optom
New Vision Clinics, Melbourne
Australia

Gene W Zdenek
Bellaire Eye and Laser Center
Texas
USA

George Kymionis, MD
Vardinoyannion Eye Institute of Crete
University of Crete
Medical School
Dept of Ophthalmology, 71110
Heraklion, Crete, Greece

Gregg Feinerman, MD, FACS
Feinerman Vision Center
Newport Beach, California
Associate Professor, University of California at Irvine

Guillermo Avalos, MD
Guadaljara, Jalisco
Mexico

Guillermo L Simon-Castellvi
Chief Anterior Segment Surgeon
Refractive Surgery Unit
Simon Eye Clinic (Barcelona-Spain)

Helen Boerman, OD
Wang Vision Institute
Nashville, TN, USA
tlschroe@bellsouth.net

Howard V Gimbel
Gimbel Eye Center
Suite 450, 4935-40
Avenue NW
Calgary, Alberta
Canada T3A 2NI

Ioannis Pallikaris, MD, PhD
Vardinogiannion Eye Institute
University of Crete, Greece
vikatsan@med.uoc.gr

Jack C Griffis III
Bellaire Eye and Laser Center
Texas, USA

J Agarwal, FORCE DO FICS
Dr Agarwal's Group of Eye Hospitals and Eye Research Centre
19 Cathedral road
Chennai 600 086
Tamil Nadu (India)

Jaime Javaloy, MD PhD
Instituto Oftalmologico de Alicante
Cabanal 1, 03016, Alicanto, Spain

Jaime R Martiz
26 S, Willow Point Cr
The Woodlands, Tx 77382, USA

Jairo E Hoyos, MD PhD
Chairman of Ophthalmology of the *Instituto Oftalmológico Hoyos*
KM Study Group President
Sabadell - Barcelona – Spain
jairoca@iohoyos.com

Jairo Hoyos-Chacón, MD
Ophthalmologist of the *Instituto Oftalmológico Hoyos*
Sabadell, Barcelona, Spain
jairoca@iohoyos.com

Jes Mortension, MD
University Hospital of Orebro
Sweden
jes.mortensen@orebroll.se

JL Guell, MD PhD
Instituto De Microcirugia
Ocular De Barcelona
Spain

Jonathan Woolfson, MD
TLC The Windsor Laser Center
3200, Deziel Drive
Suite 208, Windsor
Ontario, Canada

Jorge L Alió, MD, PhD
Instituto Oftalmologico De Alicante
Alicante, Spain

José Mª Simon-Castellvi
Chairman
Simon Eye Clinic (Barcelona-Spain)

José María Simón-Tor, MD
Chairman
Glaucoma Senior Consultant
Simon Eye Clinic, Barcelona, Spain

Kent Zocchi
Charles Retina Institute
6401, Popular Ave, Suite 190
Memphis, Tennessee, USA

Kim Nguyen
Feinerman Vision Center
Newport Beach, California

Laura de Benito-Llopis MD, PhD
Vissum Madrid, Santa Hortensia 58
28002 Madrid, Spain

Louis D "Skip" Nichamin
Laurel Eye Clinic
50, Waterford Pike
Box J, Brookville
Pennsylvania, USA

Louis E Probst, MD
Medical Director TLC
The Windsor Laser Center
3200 Deziel Drive
Suite 208, Windsor
Ontario, Canada

Luis W Lu
Eye Physician
ELK County Eye Clinic
765, Johnson Burg Road
St. Marys, PA 15857, USA

Masanao Fujieda, MA
Nidek Ltd, Co, Japan

Massimo Camellin
Health Director
Sekal Microchirurgia Rovigo
Via Dunant 10, Rovigo 45100, Italy
cammas@tin.it www.lasek.it

Melania Cigales, MD
Ophthalmologist of the *Instituto Oftalmológico Hoyos*
Sabadell - Barcelona – Spain
mcigales@teleline.es

Michiel Kritzinger, MD
TLC The Windsor Laser Center
3200, Deziel Drive, Suite 208, Windsor
Ontario, Canada

Miguel A Teus MD, PhD
Vissum Madrid, Santa Hortensia 58,
28002 Madrid, Spain
mteus@vissum.com

Ming Wang, MD, PhD
Wang Vision Institute
Nashville, TN, USA
drwang@wangvisioninstitute.com

Mohamad Rosman, MD, FRCS(Ed), FAMS
Instituto Oftalmologico De Alicante
Alicante, Spain

Mukesh Jain, PhD
Nidek Ltd, Co, Japan

Murali K Aasuri
LV Prasad Eye Institute
Hyderabad, India

M Vazquez
Instituto De Microcirugia Ocular De
Barcelona, Barcelona, Spain

Nicholas C Caro, MD
St George Corrective Vision Center
4145, W Peterson Ave., Chicago
illinois 60646, USA
Tel: 001-773-685, 6559

Noel A Alpins FRACO FRCOphth FACS
University of Melbourne, Australia
alpins@newvisionclinics.com.au

Paul Graczyk
B Graczyk Inc,
Universal™ Surgical Eye Care Products
61, Brookside Drive, Glendale Heights
Illinois, USA

Payman Haft, MD
Bascom Palmer Eye Institute
University of Miami
Miller School of Medicine
Miami, Florida

Peter Keller, PhD
Department of Optometry and
Vision Sciences, University of Australia
Melbourne

Rahul Tiwari, MBBS FERC
Dr Agarwal's Group of Eye Hospitals
and Eye Research Centre
19 Cathedral road
Chennai 600 086, Tamil Nadu (India)

R Bruce Wallace III
4110, Parliament Drive
Alexandria, LA 71303, USA

Rasik B Vajpayee, MD
Professor of Ophthalmology
RP Center of Ophthalmology
AIIMS, Ansari Nagar
New Delhi 110 029, India

Richard Foulkes, MD
Associate Professor at the University of
Illinois, Future Vision Laser Center
Chicago, Illinois

Roberto Pinelli MD
Scientific Director of the Instituto Laser
Microchirurgia Oculare
Crystal Palace, Suite
Via Cefalonia, 70 25124 Brescia, Italy
pinelli@ilmo.it

Roger F Steinert, MD
Professor of Ophthalmology
Professor of Biomedical Engineering
Vice Chairman of Clinical
Ophthalmology
Director of Cornea, Refractive, and
Cataract Surgery
University of California, Irvine
118 Med Surge I, Irvine CA 92697-4375
949-824-0327
Roger Steinert <roger@drsteinert.com>

Ronald J Smith
Clear Sight Now
9033, Wilshire Blvd
Suite 402, Beverly Hills
CA 90211, USA
Tel: 001-310-276-5333

Ronald R Krueger MD
USA

Samuel Boyd MD
Editor in Chief and Executive Vice
President
Highlights of Ophthalmology
Director Laser Section, and
Associate Director
Retina and Vitreous Department
Clinica Boyd - Ophthalmology Center
Panama, Rep. of Panama.
sboyd@thehighlights.com

Sarabel Simon-Castellvi
Simon Eye Clinic (Barcelona-Spain)

Satish Gupta
Maxivision, Alladin Building
Street No. 3, Begumpet
Hyderabad, India

Scott G Hauswirth, OD FAAO
Minnesota Eye Consultants, PA
710, East 24th St., Suite 100
Minneapolis, MN 55404, USA
Tel: 001-612-813-3600

Silvia Pastor, PhD
Cellular Therapy and Tissue
Engineering Lab., Research and
Development Department
VISSUM
Ophthalmology Institute of Alicante
Spain

Sonia Yoo, MD
Bascom Palmer Eye Institute
University of Miami
Miller School of Medicine
Miami, Florida

Soosan Jacob, MS FRCS DipNB MNAMS
Dr Agarwal's Group of Eye Hospitals
and Eye Research Centre
19 Cathedral road
Chennai 600 086, Tamil Nadu (India)

Steve Charles
Charles Retina Institute
6401, Popular Avenue, Suite 190
Memphis, Temessee, USA

T Agarwal, FORCE DO FICS
Dr Agarwal's Group of Eye Hospitals
and Eye Research Centre
19 Cathedral road
Chennai 600 086
Tamil Nadu (India)

Takeshi Ide, MD
Osaka University Medical School
Osaka, Japan

Tammo Ripken, PhD
Laser Zentrum Hannover e.V.
Biomedical Optics Department
Head of Medical Applications Group
Hollerithallee 8
D-30419 Hannover

Tanuj Dada, MD
RP Center of Ophthalmology
AIIMS, Ansari Nagar
New Delhi 110 029, India

Terry E Burris, MD
Northwest Corneal Services
6950 SW Hampton, Suite 150
Portland, OR 97223, USA

Timothy Peters, MD
Clear Advantage Vision Correction
Center, Portsmouth, New Hampshire

Terrence O' Brien
Osaka University Medical School
Osaka, Japan

Tracy S Swartz, OD, MS, FAAO
Wang Vision Institute
Nashville, TN, USA
tlschroe@bellsouth.net

Vanessa Pongo, MD
Fellowship
Instituto Oftalmologico de Alicante
Cabanal 1, 03016
Alicante, Spain

William W Culbertson, MD
Bascom Palmer Eye Institute
University of Miami
Miller School of Medicine
Miami, Florida

Foreword to the Second Edition

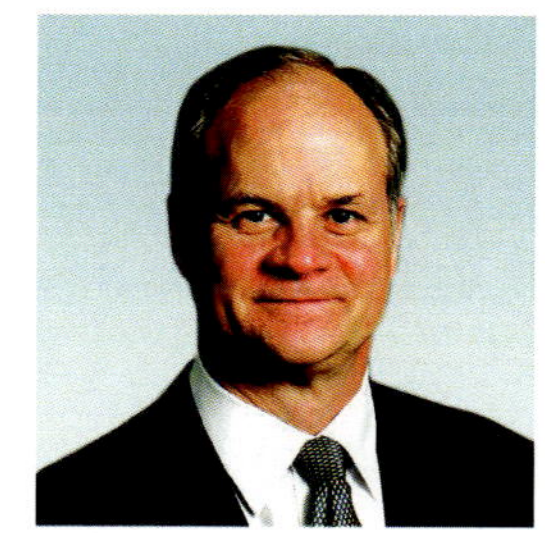

It is my privilege to write the foreword to this very important book *Refractive Surgery*. Prof. Amar Agarwal is an internationally recognized innovator in diagnostic evaluations and surgical techniques, but is also known as an outstanding educator with his contributions of over 40 books, award winning videos, and outstanding presentations.

Reading this book reminded me the tremendous progress we have made during my 30 years of experience in the development of refractive surgery. When I started refractive surgery in 1978, I was fortunate to work with pioneers such as Drs Fyodorov and Barraquer who brought their expertise in "radial keratotomy and keratomileusis" to the United States. For the next two decades, the industry was focused on reshaping the cornea with incisions, excimer lasers and other technologies.

The next major breakthrough was in 1998 with the development of refractive cataract surgery. Advances in lens-based surgical technique and technology, such as those described in the intraocular lens chapters in this book, were driven by improved outcomes. In addition to accurate lens power calculations, considerations such as corneal curvature and lens sphericity lead to advances such as spheric intraocular lenses and bioptic procedures that combine intraocular lens implantation with corneal excimer laser surgery. Contemporary refractive surgeons need to be skilled in both cornea and lens-based refractive procedures for optical optimization. As refractive surgeons, our goals are evolving to meet increasing patient demands such as a full range of excellent uncorrected vision for a lifetime. As this book illustrates, we now have the capability to successfully address both congenital and senile refractive defects.

This text will aid refractive surgeons in understanding the evolution of the subspecialty, in addition to serving as an excellent reference for the development of their knowledge and skills. We are entering into a new age of refractive surgery where diagnostic equipment can evaluate both corneal and lenticular aberrations with increasing accuracy, and these state-of-the-art diagnostic modalities are described in detail in this text. In addition, future refractive surgical applications, such as those described in Pediatric Refractive Surgery, will likely gain popularity as we advance research in this exciting area.

Corneal excimer laser surgery is covered extensively in the book with chapters on sub-Bowman's keratomileusis and advanced surface ablation, as well as femtosecond lasers and microkeratomes. Furthermore, the book is well balanced for its contributions in lens- and corneal-based refractive surgery and clearly outlines the potential benefit of combining these procedures.

When I began refractive surgery in 1978, the goals were simple—to replace thick glasses with thin glasses and provide contact intolerant patients an alternative to glasses. Today, however, my aim is for complete spectacle and contact lens independence. In future, refractive surgeons will use the tools and techniques beautifully outlined in this text to provide not only an alternative for glasses and contact lenses, but possibly a universal replacement for them.

Dr Daniel Durrie, MD
Director of Refractive Surgery and
Clinical Professor of Ophthalmology
University of Kansas Medical Center
Founder and President of Durrie Vision, USA
ddurrie@durrievision.com

Foreword to the First Edition

The promise of non-spectacle vision correction has been a dream for centuries. Contact lenses offered a solution to the cosmetic aspect but placed the cornea at risk if care guidelines were not strictly adhered to. Many patients simply cannot tolerate contact lenses for medical reasons and many are not willing to perform the daily maintenance required.

In 1953, Professor T Sato proposed an *in-situ* method for flattening of the corneal curvature by making a series of external and internal partial thickness incisions. In 1973, SN Fyodorov and V Durnev of Moscow further refined the technique of radial keratotomy using only external partial thickness corneal incisions. This procedure offered promise for a quick and inexpensive *in-situ*-corneal-modifying procedure for myopia, but glare induced by the radial spokes and unpredictable regression caused many ophthalmologists to seek a new approach to the problem.

Over the years, many modalities have been used to reshape the cornea, each having its advantages and drawbacks. In 1963, Jose Barraquer proposed a technique called 'keratomileusis' which required the development of a precision microkeratome for removal of a partial thickness corneal button which was placed on a cryolathe to reshape the patient's own frozen cornea. Krumeich developed a nonfreezing lathing technique in the 1980s. Later Ruiz proposed an *in situ* keratomileusis technique that required a superficial lamellar cut followed by a refractive cut which resulted in further refinement of the precision microkeratome. Today the precision microkeratome is a vital part of the LASIK procedure. Barraquer could never have foreseen in 1963 that the refinements to the microkeratome such as the suction ring and guides would 37 years later be a vital ingredient of today's LASIK procedure.

The same can be said in the case of implants. I am presently developing a foldable anterior chamber refractive implant which appears to have promising results. The concepts of anterior chamber implant design from the 1970s and 1980s are being refined and applied to today's phakic myopic implants. Others are developing foldable posterior chamber implants. These implants along with intracorneal rings offer the surgeon a more reversible procedure for refractive correction. At the present time, phakic implants offer a solution to refractive conditions beyond the capabilities of modern laser surgery.

The future of refractive surgery will no doubt continue to be refined and could be a mix of modalities to achieve the desired result. Dr Agarwal and his associates through the *Refractive Surgery* present an overview of all of today's refractive surgery modalities with a look towards the future.

Charles D Kelman MD
The Eye Center
New York, USA

Preface to the Second Edition

The field of refractive surgery has been changing and churning so ceaselessly that to be abreast, one needs to keep updated on all its developments. In 2000, we brought out the first edition of *Refractive Surgery* which was a best seller. As refractive surgery has been moving so fast it was necessary to bring out the second edition. When we started writing this book, we decided that we would try to incorporate all the latest developments in refractive surgery and also all the tips and tricks which would help you (dear reader) in becoming a better refractive surgeon.

Today the femtosecond lasers have come into vogue, not only for LASIK but also for a variety of other indications such as DALK, DLEK, INTACS and so on. But along with this new development, there is also the issue of complications of femtosecond lasers. The ophthalmologist is totally confused whether to go for the blade microkeratome or the femtolasers. The trick here is to learn how to avoid complications or manage them if they occur, be it with the microkeratome or the femtosecond. So also it is in every aspect of refractive surgery. Whether is it presbyopia treatment, aberropia or lens surgery includng phakic IOLs one is really confused on which technology is the best. The idea of this book is to help solve all these riddles. We aimed to provide all this information in the one book so that you would not need to go hunting around to find out the answers to your questions.

We have selected the best refractive surgeons in the world to help you understand the puzzle termed 'Refractive Surgery'. We are extremely grateful to all the contributors for helping in the preparation of this book. We are also grateful to Shri JP Vij, CMD of M/s Jaypee Brothers Medical Publishers (P) Ltd., New Delhi, who has always been a pillar of support to us. Finally, a very big thank to you (dear reader) for it is your support that makes us bring out books continuously.

Amar Agarwal
Athiya Agarwal
Soosan Jacob

Preface to the First Edition

Whenever a question is posed to us as to why did we take up Ophthalmology as a medical specialty, the first and foremost answer that comes to mind is the imperative need to eradicate darkness from a patient's life and restore sight and light by changing refraction. This decision is strengthened by additional factors that augment the transition—in the shortest possible time, minimal trauma to ocular tissue and least dependence on spectacles. The reward is the happiness that lights up a patient's eye in being able to see nature in its true perspective.

Four to five centuries ago when man started to discover the necessity of eyeglasses, skeptics belittled this notion as a charade propounded by charlatans and quacks. However, Benjamin Franklin's scientific research on the development of bifocals confirmed the necessity and acceptance of eyeglass power. We seem to have traversed a complete circle when we realize that due to excellence in technology and surgical expertize, we may be able to give the human eye a permanent cure sans eyeglass power.

The process of evolution spans many millennia. However, the pressing need to cure the less fortunate of our brethren spurs medical practitioners to extend their horizons of knowledge and expertize in improving the sophisticity of ophthalmic instrumentation—all geared towards eradicating afflictions of the eye.

In the field of ophthalmic science, an important facet is to understand the why's and wherefore's of emmetropia, delving in the daylight that we are not very far from the desired, ultimate goal, even though we are not very close to it. A time will come undoubtedly when no surgical intervention would be necessary in achieving total success to emmetropia.

Eye surgeons from all the five continents, in all manners possible, keep their patients as the pinnacle of their existence. With the world getting to be a smaller place—a global village with communication network fast encompassing the entire earth, it does not take long for technology to spread to all the remote corners of the world. So much so that, dear reader in this very book you see names and places strewn all across the world but threaded through the same necklace of learning and teaching to make refractive technology a distinct possibility.

Through six sections of this book, one may go through the curve of learning the basics with the most wanted tool in refractive technology—*Corneal Topography,* through the era of refractive surgical techniques to the epitome of refractive technologies—*The Excimer Laser.*

The technique to develop worldwide acceptance and patient compatibility is the *LASIK Technique*. A variety of needs have been fulfilled by this technology. A wide panel of eye surgeons practicing the art of LASIK, with many others under their wing, give their valuable experiences through the pages of this book.

In this book, importance is given to another big group, which is the *Phakic IOL*. The most important refractive surgery tool in the world is *Phacoemulsification* and today with No Anesthesia Cataract Surgery this is very important to learn. *Phakonit* and *Laser Phakonit* which remove cataract through a 0.9 mm incision have also changed the ball-game of refractive and cataract surgery.

Finally, the book has one of the most important topics for the next millennium, namely *Presbyopia Correction*. Other important topics are the Intrastromal Corneal Rings and the Holmium Laser. With so many chapters from such a distinguished faculty, we hope you would enjoy reading this book as much as we enjoyed during compiling and writing it.

Editors

Contents

SECTION THREE: ABERROPIA

SECTION FOUR: LASIK, CUSTOMISED LASIK AND FEMTOSECOND LASER

SECTION FIVE: LENS-BASED REFRACTIVE SURGERY

SECTION SIX: COMPLICATIONS

SECTION SEVEN: MISCELLANEOUS

SECTION ONE

Basics, Instrumentation and Preoperative Assessment

1 The History of Refractive Surgery

Ioannis Pallikaris

INTRODUCTION

Based on the letter written by a prominent Roman, there were no instruments to improve vision at the time of the ancient Egyptians, Greeks or Romans. The letter is dated about 100 B.C. in which the Roman complains that he can no longer read for himself, instead he has to rely on his slaves. Lenses made of polished crystal did exist, but were used as "burning glasses" to erase writing from wax tablets; physicians at that time used burning glasses to cauterize wounds according to Pliny.

Around 1000 A.D. the reading stone, a segment of a glass sphere that could be laid against reading material to magnify the letters was first developed. The Venetians developed the first reading stones held in a frame in front of the eyes instead of directly on the reading material. However, it took over 350 years to develop a practical means to keep them on the face. Ribbons and strings were tied about the head for several hundred more years, until a London based optician named Edward Scarlett perfected the use of rigid sidepieces that rested atop the ears in 1730. These spectacles cost as much as $200 in the early 1700's. Benjamin Franklin is credited with creation of the bifocal in the 1780's by cutting two lenses in half and placing one above the other. As glass-making improved, so did the lenses and improvements in frame-making and materials resulted in several styles to choose from. But even at the turn of the 20th century, glass fitting was largely trial and error with the patient responsible for determining the correct lens, often in a rather casual manner.

As early as 1845, Sir John Herschel suggested the idea for contact lenses, but he evidently did nothing about it. The term contact lens originated with Dr. A. Eugen Fick, a Swiss physician, who published the results of experiments with contact lenses in 1887. Early contacts were created by blowing glass in different-sized bubbles and cutting them in half, polishing the edges and placing them in the eyes. Several doctors and optical firms in Europe cooperated in creating practical contact lenses over the decades around the turn of the 20th century. By the early 1940's a variety of materials were available: blown glass, ground glass, molded glass, plastic and glass and all plastics. All of these lenses were large and uncomfortable and couldn't be worn for long. By 1964 over 6 million people in the United States were wearing contact lenses, 65 percent of them were women.

The first experimental study about refractive surgery was performed by Lendeer Jans Lans, an ophthalmology teacher in Holland. In 1896 he published a theoretic work proposing penetrating corneal cuts to correct astigmatism. In 1930 the Japanese ophthalmologist Sato made the first practical attempt to perform such surgery in military pilots. He practiced radial cuts in the cornea to correct effects by up to 6 diopters. This approach proved disasterous as the operated corneas became swollen and cloudy due to destruction of the endothelium (whose function was understood later). The greatest pioneer of radial keratotomy (RK) was Dr. Fyordorov in the former USSR. In the early 1960's he converted the incisions to the front of the cornea, by making cuts 90 percent through the thickness of the cornea. He was able to devise a system of correction for different degrees of near-sightedness by making the cuts longer or shorter. From 1978-80, Drs. Leo Bores, et al, improved RK by devising ways to account for astigmatism. RK reached its peak in the mid-1980's to early 1990's.

In 1963, in the Barraquer ophthalmologic clinic (Bogotá,Colombia) Ignacio Barraquer developed the first proficient technique of refractive surgery, called keratomileusis (from the Greek Kerato: cornea and Mileusis: to sculpt) meaning corneal reshaping. Keratomileusis allowed the correction not only of myopia but also of hyperopia. The early surgeries were done by removing a corneal layer, freezing it so that it can be manually sculpted in the required shape and finally reimplanting the layer (keratomileusis with freezing). In 1986 Dr Swinger improved the surgery (keratomileusis without freezing) but it was still a slightly imprecise technique. In 1958 Arthur Schawlow and Townes, from Bell laboratories published their theory of stimuled emission of shorter wavelengths of light, which gave place to the development of Laser. In 1975 experiments with laser using a mix of argon and FLUOR ended with the invention of the Excimer. This Laser was used for industrial purposes. In 1980, R. Srinivasan, a scientist of IBM who was using the excimer to make microscopic circuits in microchips for informative equipments, discovered that the excimer could also be used to cut organic tissues with high accuracy without significant thermal damage.

In 1983 Stephen Trokel, scientist of Columbia University in collaboration with Srinivasan performed the Photorefractive Keratectomy (PRK) or keratomileusis in situ (without separation of corneal layer) which was more technically exact, but the patients reported it to be very uncomfortable. Also a delay in the healing was observed. The first phototherapeutic keratectomy (a procedure for removing superficial scars from the cornea) in a sighted eye was performed in 1985 by Dr. Theo Seiler in Germany. Dr. Margeurite McDonald accidentally perfomed the first successful photorefractive keratectomy (PRK) in June of 1987. While performing one of the initial studies on patients with blind eyes, one of the subjects miraculously recovered her vision seven weeks after surgery. The patient apparently had a sudden reversal of hysterical blindness, a condition originally described by Freud. She was 20/20 upon the return of her vision and remained so in the years to follow. Dr. McDonald also performed the first PRK on a sighted eye (within an FDA trial) in 1988. Improvements in the excimer laser over the past 15 years have been made in the area treated, the homogeneity of the laser beam itself, and the addition of infrared tracking of the pupil to follow any eye movement during the procedure.

The combination of Ignacio Barraquer work and the introduction of the excimer lasers lead to a new surgical technique. Ioannis Pallikaris, M.D. coined the term LASIK (laser-assisted in-situ keratomileusis), and was the first to create a "flap" of the tissue with the microkeratome, rather than to remove the entire top layer (Fig. 1.1). He conducted the first animal trials of what is now modern LASIK in the late 1980's in his native Greece. Today LASIK is the dominant corneal refractive technique used to correct ammetropias around the world. Improvements in the creation of corneal flap continue with the improved keratome reliability. Today's microkeratomes have the ability to create 90 µm thick flaps with a high degree of repeatability and safety. Flap creation has further improved after the introduction of femptosecond laser technology.

LAMELLAR TECHNIQUES

Keratomileusis in situ

Was the first developed in the 1940's. The procedure involved raising a corneal cap and the removal of corneal tissue from the residual stromal bed. Barraquer's initial technique consisted of performing

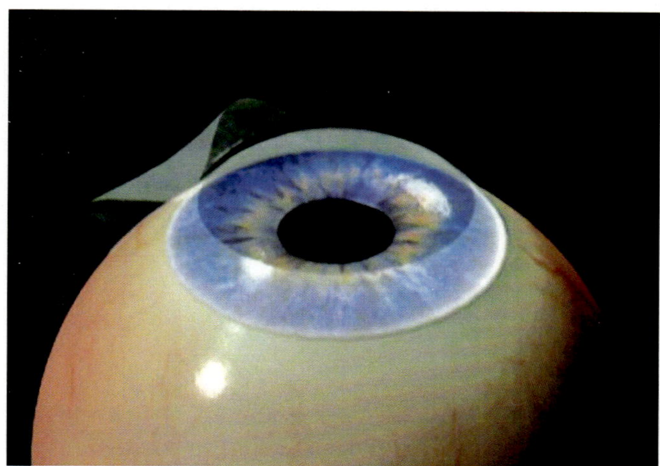

Fig. 1.1: LASIK. Note the flap created (*Courtesy* Dr Agarwal's Eye Hospital, India)

a free hand lamellar dissection of the anterior half of the cornea using a Paufique knife or a keratome. The refractive cut was attempted by removing stroma from the bed with a second pass of the knife or keratome. As a result the anterior corneal curvature was flettened, and therefore the myopic refractive error was reduced.[1] Due to the many technical difficulties of this procedure, which were hard to overcome with the instrumentation available at the time, keratomileusis in situ had to be temporarily abandoned.[1]

Keratophakia

Barraquer did not abandon his efforts to perfect lamellar techniques. His ingenuity and persistence led to the development of keratophakia (KF), which was introduced in 1961.[2] KF resulted to steepening of the central corneal curvature by placing a disk of tissue under the lamellar cap. The disk of tissue at that time was an alloplastic stromal disk harvested from a donor cornea with the use of a microkeratome.

The disk diameter and thickness varied, depending on the initial refractive error and on the attempted correction. KF attracted the attention of the ophthalmic community as a possible solution in the treatment of aphakia after cataract surgery.[3] With the evolution and improvements of IOL technology, the interest in KF subsided, since IOLs demonstrated more accurate refractive results without the technical difficulties of harvesting the donor tissue and performing the lamellar cut.

Freeze Myopic Keratomileusis

In order to overcome the technical difficulties of the manual cut, Barraquer was the first to use the contact lens lathe to sculpture the frozen lamellar corneal cap; as a result freeze keratomileusis was introduced.[2-5] This new technique could be used to correct myopic and hyperopic refractive errors. Barraquer found myopic corrections more successful and thus he focused his research on refining the freeze myopic keratomileusis (MKM) technique. He recognized that the cutting speed as well as the relation between IOP and the diameter of the resection, were factors directly affecting the quality and the depth of the cut.[1] Barraquer's effort for more predictable, reproducible and accurate cuts, led to the development of applanator lenses, suction rings of various diameters and various heights of microkeratome tracks.[4] This work constituted the basis for future microkeratome evolution.

Even though the first reported results concerning freeze MKM were encouraging,[1] freeze MKM had two major disadvantages. The cryolathe was too expensive to obtain and too complex to maintain and the learning curve was too steep, involving high rate if complications such as irregular astigmatism or corneal scarring.[5]

During the time, other techniques were introduced for the correction of refractive errors, such as epikeratophakia,[3,6-11] incisional keratotomy[12-14] and IOL implantation.[15]

Epikeratophakia

Also known as epikeratoplasty, this was introduced by Kaufman and Werblin in 1979.[6] In an effort to avoid the use of cryolathe, the innovators attempted to use preprocessed refractive lenticles. A stromal disk was removed from a donor eye with the use of a microkeratome. The disk was frozen and lathed into a concave or convex lens. The lens was then lyophilized and stored for later use. Epikeratophakia was intended for use in the treatment of aphakia, myopia, hyperopia and keratoconus.[9-11] Its major advantages were simplicity and reversibility. Unfortunately, the initial reports revealed that the technique was neither predictable nor safe.[15] Several modifications were proposed in an effort to improve epikeratophakia.[16,17] Burrato and Ferrari used the BKS system and Altmann used the excimer laser to shape epilenticles without freezing.[18] However, as the difficulties could not be solved, epikeratoplasty was withdrawn from the market and research turned once again towards keratomileusis techniques.

Barraquer Krumeich Swinger (BKS) Technique

Due to complications that were demonstrated when using the epikeratoplasty and freeze MKM, investigations in the direction of developing nonfreezing techniques led to development of the Barraquer Krumeich Swinger (BKS) technique in 1985.[19] BKS included an improved microkeratome, a set of dyes and a suction stand. The microkeratome was used to perform a total lamellar cut. The cap was then placed epithelial side down, on one of the suction dyes for the microkeratome to perform the second refractive cut at the stromal aspect of the cap. The dye was selected depending on the amount of the attempted correction of myopia or hyperopia. The sculptured lamellar disk was finally sutured back to the bed. Despite of their technical difficulty, nonfreezing techniques proved to have a major advantage; rapid and comfortable recovery of the patients. This was attributed to the preservation of fibroblasts and corneal epithelium. However, significant amount of irregular astigmatism could not be avoided.[20]

In 1987, Leo Bores performed the first keratomileusis in situ in the US.[21] Keratomileusis in situ with the use of manual microkeratomes, however, was reported as being not technically safe, precise or predictable and failed to be adopted by a large number of surgeons.[22] Research began in the direction of developing new improved microkeratomes in an effort to improve the reproductibility and accuracy of the in situ technique.[23]

Automated Lamellar Keratoplasty (ALK)

The development of the automated geared microkeratome by Ruiz in 1980's introduced automated lamellar keratoplasty (ALK) in the field of lamellar refractive corneal surgery. The speed of the cut could be controlled by the foot pedal resulting in more even and consistent cuts. The keratome would also automatically reverse at the end of the procedure, without disturbing the lamellar cut. The second, refractive cut was subsequently performed on the bed. The depth of the second cut was adjusted by altering the hight of the suction ring.

ALK was a breakthrough for lamellar surgery. Initially, the corneal cap was sutured back to the stromal bed, but very soon suturing was abandoned as it was proved unnecessary. The total operative time was reduced significantly and the procedure could be safely performed under topical anesthesia. Recovery time also improved. ALK was adopted by many surgeons since it overcame the use of manual microkeratomes.

The first clinical trials on ALK revealed its advantages: (1) Easy to use, (2) Rapid recovery and stability of refraction, and (3) Efficacy in the correction of high myopia. Major disadvantages, however, were the relative high rate of irregular astigmatism (2%) and the poor predictability of the procedure (within 2 diopters).[24] The later was attributed to the imprecision of the depth obtained with the second disk. Research was then focused on improving the accuracy of the second disk resection. It was at that time when thoughts of combining the precision of photorefractive keratectomy (PRK) with ALK came in the forefront.

Trokel et al suggested PRK in 1983.[25] As the use of the 193 nm excimer laser in refractive surgery generated, it was revealed that for myopias greater than 6 diopters, PRK resulted in significant central corneal haze, regression of refractive effect and poor predictability.[26]

Laser in Situ Keratomileusis (LASIK)

LASIK was introduced, designed and developed at the Institute of Vision and Optics (University of Crete, Department of Medicine) in 1988.[27] The term LASIK was used to describe a combination of lamellar refractive corneal surgery and excimer laser photoablation of the cornea under a hinged corneal flap. The idea of raising a corneal flap and removing central tissue from the bed was first described by Pureskin in 1966.[28] He attempted to do the cut manually and cut the in situ part with a trephine.

In LASIK the automated microkeratome is used to create a corneal flap. The refractive second cut is then substituted by the excimer laser, with submicron accuracy of stromal tissue removal. The initial hypothesis was that a flap would assure better fitting of tissue after removing the intrastromal tissue with laser and would not affect the anatomic relations of corneal layers; since the Bowmans layer and also the subepithelial nerve plexus were preserved.

The first animal studies to determine wound healing reactions after LASIK, began in 1987, using a Lamda Physic excimer laser and a specially designed microkeratome which was able to produce a 150 microns thick flap instead of a total cap. It was suggested that stromal ablation could potentially avoid the regression of effect and stromal haze related to PRK, as the ablated area is hidden from the normal healing process of the eye that takes place at the epithelium/stroma interface.[29]

The first papers concerning LASIK were presented in Zurich in August 1989 and published in 1990.[29] The first LASIK on a blind human eye was performed in June 1989, as a part of an unofficial blind eye protocol.

Excimer Laser Intrastromal Keratomileusis

In 1992, Lucio Burrato reported the excimer laser intrastomal keratomileusis, a technique where photoablation was performed under a corneal cap. First results on a large series of human eyes proved that this technique was efficient yet not safe. Complication rates were comparable to that of MKM.[30]

Stephen Slade and Brint were the first to perform LASIK in the US in 1992. During the 1993 AAO meeting, George O Waring gave LASIK the temporary name 'flap and zap' in order to emphasize the alacrity of the procedure. The major advantages of the procedure, appreciated by patients and surgeons alike include: (1) Minimal postoperative discomfort, (2) Early recovery of visual function, (3) Lack of adverse healing phenomena such as haze formation, (4) Increased range of efficacy over PRK in myopia, hyperopia and astigmatism.

LASIK is the most recent step in the evolution of lamellar corneal techniques, initiated by Barraquer 50 years ago. Reports of 10 postoperative LASIK were encouraging, demonstrating good predictability and stability of refractive outcomes.[31,32]

SURFACE TECHNIQUES

Photorefractive Keratectomy (PRK)

After Trokel and Srinivasan demonstrated a new form of laser–tissue interaction, photoablation, in 1983[25] doctor McDonald and co-workers treated the first sighted human eye in 1988. PRK is the sculpting of the de-epithelialized corneal surface to alter refractive power. Due to the wound healing response of the cornea which leads to refractive regression and haze formation especially in high attempted corrections the popularity of PRK faded when LASIK began to be performed in the late 1990s.

PRK Mitomycin C and Epi-LASIK

In last few years the refractive surgery community has a shift to surface treatments in order to avoid complication of LASIK.[33] Furthermore, in order to avoid PRK complications such as corneal haze, new surgical techniques and pharmaceutical aids have been introduced. These advanced surface ablation techniques include Epi-LASIK and PRK with the intraoperative use of MMC.

Nine years after experimental studies on rabbit corneas,[34] the first clinical study of PRK with adjuvant MMC in 2001 demonstrated satisfactory refractive

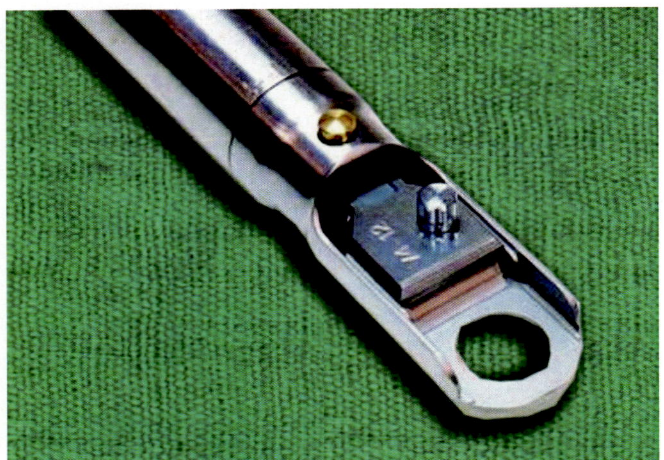

Fig. 1.2: Epilasik separator

outcomes by modulating corneal healing and controlling haze formation.[35] Today the use of MMC during PRK has become common practice, despite the inhibition of haze formation by MMC's cytostatic action, concerns regarding its adverse effects on different ocular tissues and its long term safety have been raised.[36] For instance, the effect of MMC on the endothelial cell density has been controversial. Even though most reports do not demonstrate a significant change in endothelial cell density after PRK with MMC,[37] there has been one report suggesting a significant decrease.[38]

Epipolis laser in situ keratomileusis (Epilasik) refers to an alternative surgical approach for epithelial separation by mechanical means. With this technique, the epithelial separation is performed using an instrument (Fig. 1.2) that was initially designed at the University of Crete and operates in a manner similar to that of a microkeratome.[39] (The epithelial flap after stromal ablation is placed on the corneal surface reducing patient discomfort postoperatively and modulating the wound healing response of the cornea).[40]

SUMMARY

Reviewing the history of refractive surgery is essential for better understanding and future refining of the currently used techniques. Continuing evolution in all fields of refractive surgery is an obligation of all ophthalmologists, since it's the only way to approach the ultimate goal, to offer our patients a better vision both qualitatively and quantitatively.

REFERENCES

1. Barraquer JI. Keratomileusis. Int Surg 1967;48:103-17.
2. Barraquer JI. Method for cutting lamellar grafts in frozen corneas—new orientations for refractive surgery. Arch Soc Am Ophthalmol 1958;1:237.
3. Kaufmann HE. The correction of aphakia. Am J Ophthalmol 1980;89:1-10.
4. Barraquer JI. Results of myopic keratomileusis. J Refract Surg 1987;3:98-101.
5. Littman H. Optic of Barraquer's keratomileusis. Arch Oftal Optom 1966;6:1.
6. Werblin TP, Klyce SD. Epikeratophakia, the correction of aphakia: 1, lathing corneal tissue. Curr Eye Res 1981;1:591-7.
7. Barraquer JI. Modification of refraction by means of intra-corneal inclusions. Int Ophthalmol Clin 1966;6:53-78.
8. Baumgartner SD, Binder PS, Deg JK, et al. Epikeratophakia, clinical and histopathologic evaluation in non human primates. Invst Ophthalmol Vis Sci 1983;24:148.
9. Werblin TP, Kaufmann HE, Friedlander MH, et al. A prospective study of the use of hyperopic epikeratophakia grafts for the correction of aphakia in adults. Ophthalmology 1981;88:1137-40.
10. Kaufmann HE, Werblin TP. Epikeratophakia, a form of lamellar keratoplasty for the treatment of keratoconus. Am J Ophthalmol 1982;93:342-7.
11. Werblin TP, Blaydes JE, Kaufmann HE. Epikeratophakia, the correction of astigmatism: preliminary experimental results. CLAOJ 1983;9:61-3.
12. Bores LD, Myers W, Cowden J. Radial keratotomy, an analysis of the American experience. Am Ophthalmol 1981;13:941-8.
13. Arrowsmith PN, Sanders DR, Marks RG. Visual, refractive and keratometric results of radial keratotomy. Arch Ophthalmol 1983;101:873-81.
14. Deitz MR, Sanders DR, Marks RG. Radial keratotomy, an overview of the Kansas city study. Ophthalmology 1984;91:467-78.
15. Mc Donald MB, Kaufamann HE, Aquavella JV, et al. The nationwide study of epikeratophakia for myopia in adults. Am J Ophthalmol 1987;103:350-65.
16. Slade SG, Strauss GH. Use of tissue adhesive in epikeratophakia. Invest Ophthalmol Vis Sci 1990;31:30.
17. Goosey JD, Prager TC, Marvelli TL, et al. Epikeratophakia without annular keratectomy. Am Ophthalmol 1987;19: 388-91.
18. Altamann J, Grabner C, et al. Corneal lathing using the excimer laser and a computer controlled positioning system: part I, lathing of epikeratoplasty lenticules. Refract Corneal Surg 1991;7:377-84.

19. Swinger CA, Krumeich J, Cassiday D. Planar lamellar refractive keratoplasty. I Refract Surg 1986;2:17-24.
20. Colin J, Mimouni F, Robinet A. The surgical treatment of high myopia—comparison of epikeratoplasty, keratosmileusis and minus power anterior chamber lenses. Refract Corneal Surg 1990;6:245-51.
21. Bores L. Lamellar refractive surgery. In Bores L (Ed): Refract Eye Surgery. Blackwell Publications: Boston 1993;324-92.
22. Arenas-Archila E, Sanchez-Thorin JC, et al. Myopic keratomileusis in situ – a preliminary report. J Cataract Refract Surg 1991;17:424-35.
23. Hofmann RF, Bechara SJ. An independent evaluation of second generation suction microkeratomes. Refract Corneal Surg 1992;8:348-54.
24. Slade SG, Updegraff SA. Complications of automated lamellar keratectomy (comment). Arch Ophthalmol 1995;113(9):1092-3.
25. Trokel S, Shrinisavan R, Braven B. Excimer laser surgery of the cornea. Am J Ophthalmol 1983;94:125.
26. Seiler T, McDonnell PJ. Excimer laser photorefractive keratectomy. Surv Ophthalmol 1995;94:125.
27. Pallikaris I, Papatzanaki M, Stathi EZ, et al. Laser in situ keratomileusis. Laser Surg Med 1990;10:463-8.
28. Pureskin N. Weakening ocular refraction by means of partial stromectomy of the cornea under experimental conditions. Vestn Oftalmol 1967;8:1-7.
29. Pallikaris I, Papatzanaki M, Georgiadis A, et al. A comparative study of neural regeneration following corneal wounds induced by argon fluoride excimer laser and mechanical methods. Lasers Light Ophthalmol 1990;3:89-95.
30. Buratto L, Ferrari M, Rama P. Excimer laser intrastromal keratomileusis. Am J Ophthalmol 1992;113:291-5.
31. Kymionis GD, Tsiklis NS, Astyrakakis NI, et al. Eleven-year follow-up of laser in situ keratomileusis. J Cataract Refract Surg 2007;33:191-6.
32. Alio JL, Muftuoglu O, Ortiz D, et al. Ten-year follow-up of laser in situ keratomileusis for myopia of up to -10 diopters. Am J Ophthalmol 2008;145(1):46-54.
33. Melki SA, Azar DT. LASIK complications: etiology, management, and prevention. Survey of Ophthalmol 2001;46:95-116.
34. Talamo JH, Gollamudi S, Green WR, et al. Modulation of corneal wound healing after excimer laser keratomileusis using topical mitomycin-C and steroids. Arch Ophthalmol 1991;109:1141-6.
35. Majmudar PA, Forstot SL, Nirankari VS, et al. Topical mitomcyin-C for subepithelial fibrosis after corneal surgery. Ophthalmology 2000;107:89-94.
36. Rubinfeld RS, Pfister RR, Stein RM, Foster CS, Martin NF, Stoleru S, et al. Serious complications of topical mitomycin-C after pterigium surgery. Ophthalmology 1992;99:1647-54.
37. Diakonis VF, Pallikaris AI, Kymionis GD, et al. Alterations in endothelial cell density after photorefractive keratectomy with adjuvant mitomycin. Am J Ophthalmol 2007;144(1):99-103.
38. Morales AJ, Zadok D, Mora-Retana R, et al. Intraoperative mitomycin and corneal endothelium after photorefractive keratectomy. Am J Ophthalmol 2006;142(3): 400-4.
39. Pallikaris IG, Katsanevaki VJ, Kalyvianaki MI, et al. Advances in subepithelial excimer refractive surgery techniques: epi-LASIK. Curr Opin Ophthalmol 2003;14: 207-12.
40. Katsanevaki VJ, Kalyvianaki MI, Kavroulaki DS, et al. One year clinical results after Epi LASIK for myopia. Ophthalmology 2007;114(6):1111-7.

2 Corneal Topography and the Orbscan

Amar Agarwal, Athiya Agarwal

INTRODUCTION

Keratometry and corneal topography with placido disks systems were originally invented to measure anterior corneal curvature.[1-3] Computer analysis of the more complete data acquired by the latter has in recent years been increasingly more valuable in the practice of refractive surgery. The problem in the placido disk systems is that one cannot perform a slit scan topography of the cornea. This has been solved by an instrument called the Orbscan that combines both slit scan and placido images to give a very good composite picture for topographic analysis. Bausch and Lomb manufacture this.

PARAXIAL OPTICS

Spectacle correction of sight is designed only to eliminate defocus errors and astigmatism. These are the only optical aberrations that can be handled by the simplest theory of imaging, known as paraxial optics, which excludes all light rays finitely distant from a central ray or power axis. Ignoring the majority of rays entering the pupil, paraxial optics examines only a narrow thread-like region surrounding the power axis. The shape of any smoothly rounded surface within this narrow region is always circular in cross-section. Thus from the paraxial viewpoint, surface shape is toric at most: only its radius may vary with meridional angle. As a toric optical surface has sufficient flexibility to null defocus and astigmatism, only paraxial optics is needed to specify corrective lenses for normal eyes. Paraxial optics is used in keratometers and two-dimensional topographic machines.

RAYTRACE OR GEOMETRIC OPTICS

The initial objective of refractive surgery was to build the necessary paraxial correction in to the cornea. When outcomes are less than perfect, it is not just because defocus correction is inadequate. Typically, other aberrations (astigmatism, spherical aberration, coma, etc) are introduced by the surgery. These may be caused by decentered ablation, asymmetric healing, biomechanical response, poor surgical planning and inadequate or misinformation. To assess the aberrations in the retinal image all the light rays entering the pupil must properly be taken in account using raytrace (or geometric) optics. Paraxial optics and its hypothetical toric surfaces must be abandoned as inadequate, which eliminates the need to measure surface curvature. Raytrace optics does not require surface curvature, but depends on elevation and especially surface slope. The Orbscan uses raytrace or geometric Optics.

ELEVATION

Orbscan measures elevation, which is not possible in other topographic machines. Elevation is especially important because it is the only complete scalar measure of surface shape. Both slope and curvature can be mathematically derived from a single elevation map, but the converse is not necessarily true. As both slope and curvature have different values in different directions, neither can be completely represented by a single map of the surface. Thus, when characterizing the surface of non-spherical test objects used to verify instrument accuracy, elevation is always the gold standard.

Curvature maps in corneal topography (usually misnamed as power or dioptric maps) only display curvature measured in radial directions from the map center. Such a presentation is not shift-invariant, which means its values and topography changes as the center of the map is shifted. In contrast, elevation is shift-invariant. An object shifted with respect to the map center is just shifted in its elevation map. In a meridional curvature view it is also described. This makes elevation maps more intuitively understood, making diagnosis easier.

To summarize:

1. Curvature is not relevant in raytrace optics.
2. Elevation is complete and can be used to derive surface curvature and slope.
3. Elevation is the standard measure of surface shape.
4. Elevation is easy to understand.

The problem we face is that there is a cost in converting elevation to curvature (or slope) and vice versa. To go from elevation to curvature requires mathematical differentiation, which accentuates the high spatial frequency components of the elevation function. As a result, random measurement error or noise in an elevation measurement is significantly multiplied in the curvature result. The inverse operation, mathematical integration used to convert curvature to elevation, accentuates low-frequency error. The Orbscan helps in good mathematical integration. This makes it easy for the ophthalmologist to understand as the machine does all the conversion.

ORBSCAN I AND II

Previously, Orbscan I was used. This had only slit scan topographic system. Then the placido disk was added in Orbscan I. Hence Orbscan II came into the picture.

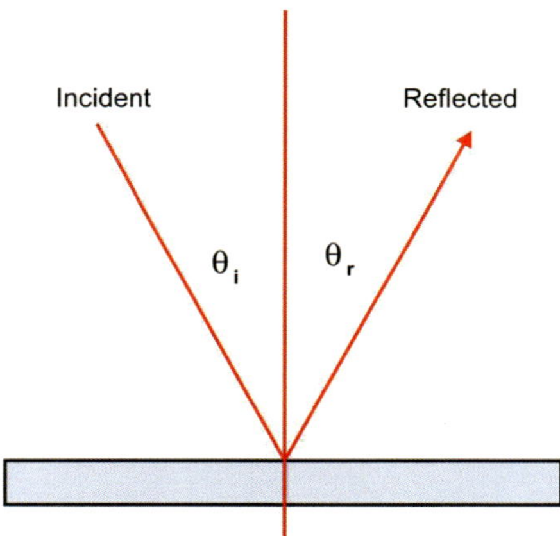

Fig. 2.1: Specular reflection. This is used in keratometers. This is angle dependent

SPECULAR VS BACK-SCATTERED REFLECTION

The keratometer eliminates the anterior curvature of the pre-corneal tear film. It is an estimate because the keratometer only acquires data within a narrow 3 mm diameter annulus. It measures the anterior tear-film because it is based on specular reflection (Fig. 2.1), which occurs primarily at the air-tear interface. As the keratometer has very limited data coverage, abnormal corneas can produce misleading or incorrect results.

Orbscan can calculate a variety of different surface curvatures and on a typical eye, these are all different. Only on a properly aligned and perfectly spherical surface are the various curvatures equal. The tabulated SimK values (magnitudes and associated meridians) are the only ones designed to give keratometer-like measurements. Therefore, it only makes sense to compare keratometry reading with SimK values.

Orbscan uses slit-beams and back-scattered light (Fig. 2.2) to triangulate surface shape. The derived mathematical surface is then raytraced using a basic keratometer model to produce simulated keratometer (SimK) values. So it is the difficulty of calculating curvature from triangulated data, the repeatability of Orbscan I SimK values is usually not as good as a clinical keratometer. But when several readings of the

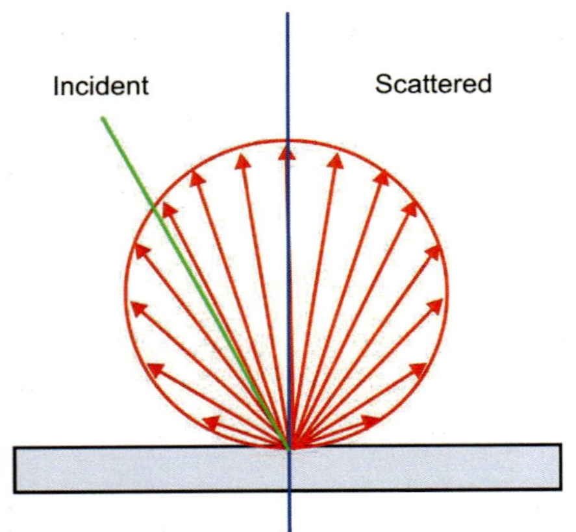

Fig. 2.2: Back-scatter reflection. This is used in Orbscan. This is omni-directional

same eye are averaged, no discernible systematic error is found.

So if one reading is taken and a comparison is made, the difference may be significant enough to make you believe the instrument is not working properly. So when the placido illuminator was added to Orbscan II to increase its anterior curvature accuracy, it also provided reflected data similar to that obtained with a keratometer. This reflective data are now used in SimK analyses, resulting in repeatabilities similar to keratometers and other placido based corneal topography instruments.

Keratometry measures the tear-film, while slit-scan triangulation (Fig. 2.3) as embodied in Orbscan sees through the tear-film and measures the corneal surface directly. Thus an abnormal tear film can produce significant differences in keratometry but not in Orbscan II.

Curvature measures the geometric bending of a surface, and its natural unit is reciprocal length, like inverse millimeters (1/mm). When keratometry was invented this unfamiliar unit was replaced by a dioptric interpretation, making keratometry values equivalent on average (i.e. over the original population) to the paraxial back-vertex power of the cornea. As it has become increasingly more important to distinguish optical from geometric properties, it is now more proper to evaluate keratometry in "keratometric diopters". The keratometric diopter is strictly defined as a geometric unit of curvature with no optical significance. One inverse millimeter equals to 337.5 keratometric diopters.

IMAGING IN THE ORBSCAN

In the Orbscan, the calibrated slit, which falls on the cornea, gives a topographical information, which is captured and analyzed by the video camera (Fig. 2.4). Both slit beam surfaces are determined in camera object space. Object space luminance is determined for each pixel value and framegrabber setting. Forty slit images are acquired in two 0.7 second periods. During acquisition, involuntary saccades typically move the eye by 50 microns. Eye movement is measured from anterior reflections of stationary slit beam and other light sources. Eye tracking data permit saccadic movements to be subtracted from the final topographic surface. Each of the 40 slit images triangulates one slice of the ocular surface

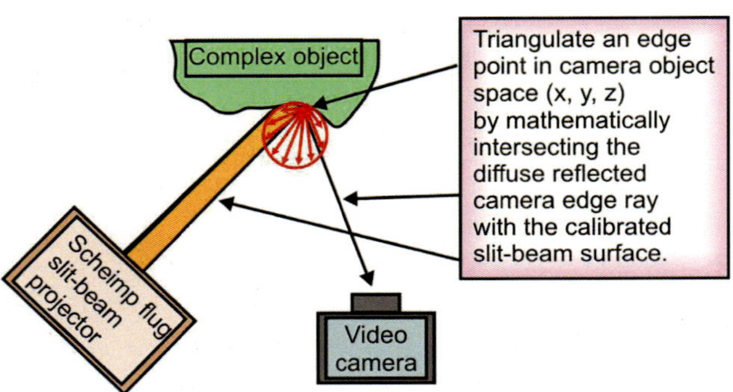

Fig. 2.3: Direct triangulation

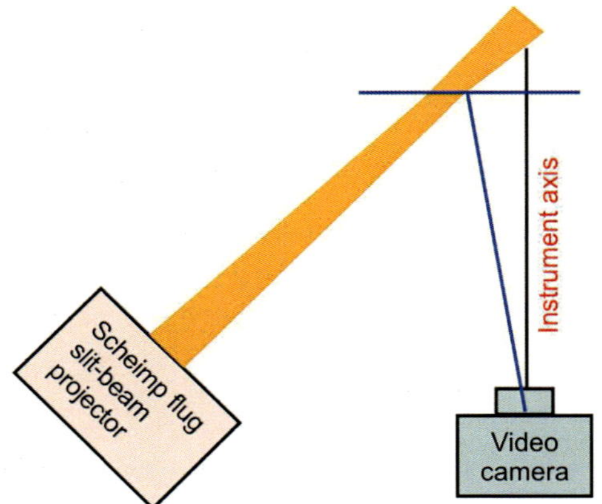

Fig. 2.4: Beam and camera calibration in the Orbscan

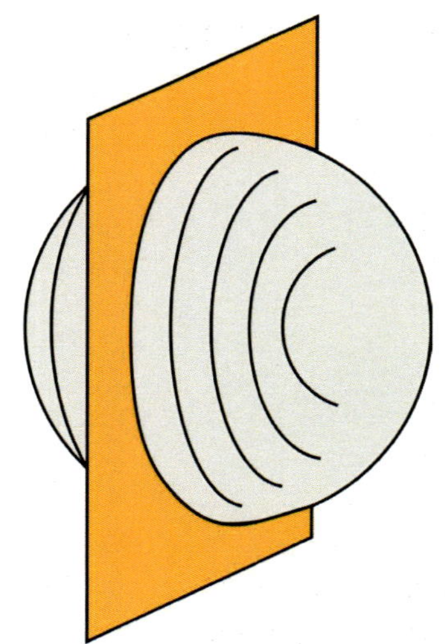

Fig. 2.5: Ocular surface slicing by the Orbscan slit

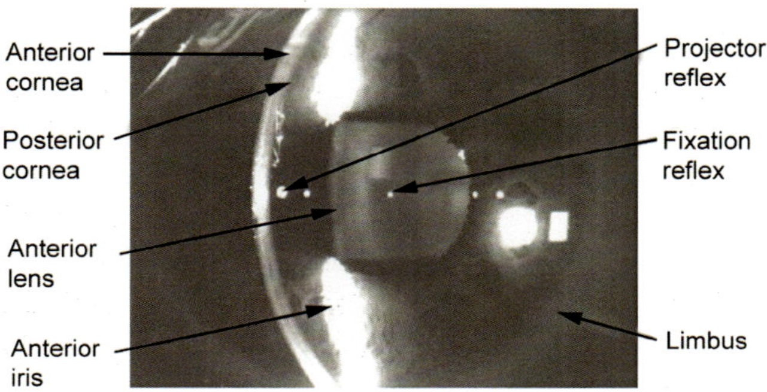

Fig. 2.6: Detailed Orbscan examination

(Fig. 2.5). Before an interpolating surface is constructed, each slice is registered in accordance with measured eye movement. Distance between data slices averages 250 microns in the coarse scan mode (40 slits limbus to limbus). So Orbscan examination consists of a set of mathematical topographic surfaces (x, y), for the anterior and posterior cornea, anterior iris and lens and backscattering coefficient of layers between the topographic surfaces (and over the pupil) (Fig. 2.6).

MAP COLORS CONVENTIONS

Color contour maps have become a standard method for displaying 2D data in corneal and anterior segment topography. Although there are no universally standardized colors, the spectral direction (from blue to red) is always organized in definite and intuitive way.

Blue = low, level, flat, deep, thick or aberrated.

Red = high, steep, sharp, shallow, thin or focused.

ANALYSIS OF THE NORMAL EYE BY THE ORBSCAN MAP

The general quad map in the Orbscan of a normal eye (Fig. 2.7) shows 4 pictures. The upper left is the anterior float, which is the topography of the anterior surface of the cornea. The upper right shows the posterior float, which is the topography of the posterior surface of the cornea. The lower left map shows the keratometric pattern and the lower right map shows the pachymetry (thickness of the cornea). The Orbscan is a three-dimensional slit scan topographic machine. If we were doing topography with a machine, which does not have slit scan imaging facility, we would not be able to see the topography of the posterior surface of the cornea. Now, if the patient had an abnormality in the posterior surface of the cornea, for example as in primary posterior corneal elevation this would not be diagnosed. Then if we perform Lasik on such a patient we would create an iatrogenic keratectasia. The Orbscan helps us to detect the abnormalities on the posterior surface of the cornea.

Another facility, which we can move onto once we have the general quad map, is to put on the normal band scale filter (Fig. 2.8). If we are in suspicion of any abnormality in the general quad map then we put on the normal band scale filter. This highlights the abnormal areas in the cornea in orange to red colors. The normal areas are all shown in green. This is very helpful in generalized screening in preoperative examination of a LASIK patient.

CLINICAL APPLICATIONS

Let us now understand this better in a case of a primary posterior corneal elevation. If we see the General quad map of a primary posterior corneal elevation (Fig. 2.9) we will see the upper left map is normal. The upper right map shows abnormality

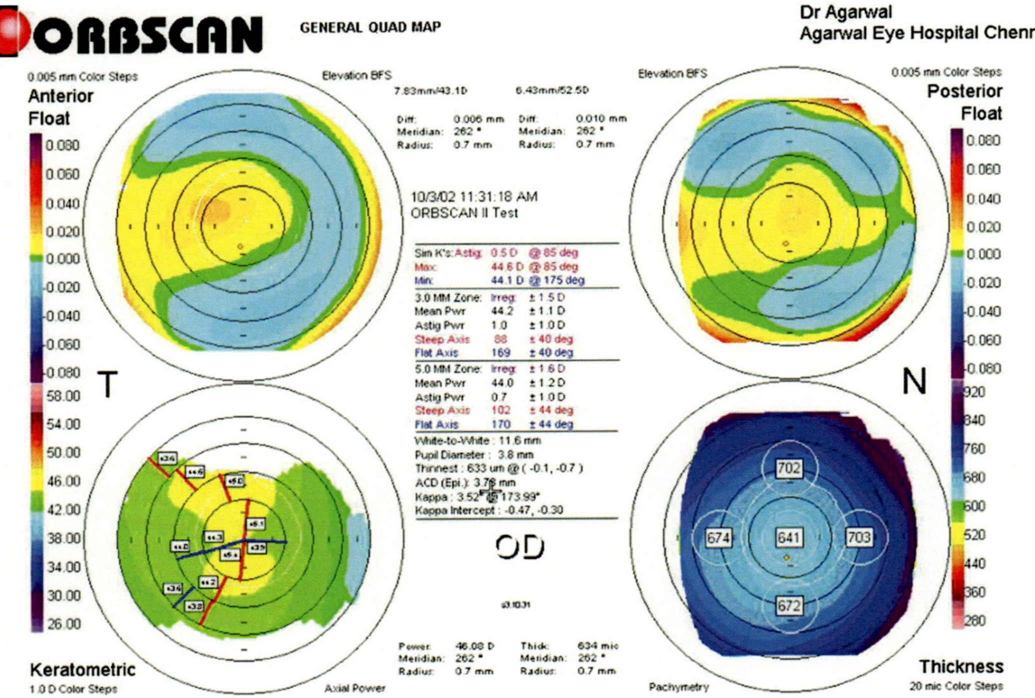

Fig. 2.7: General quad map of a normal eye

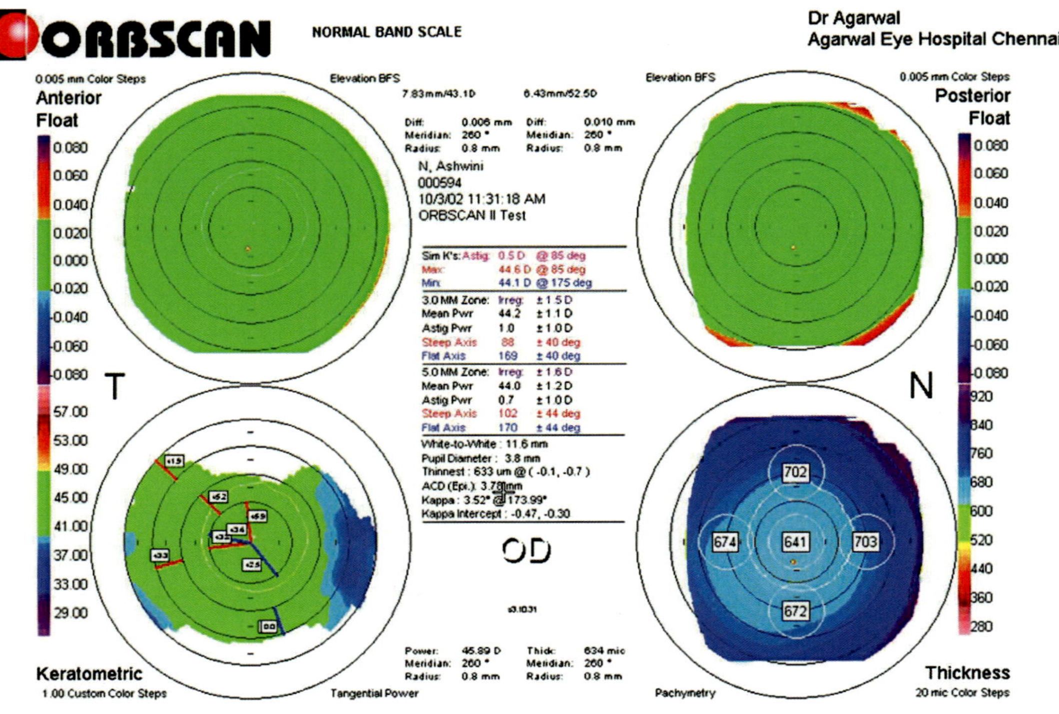

Fig. 2.8: Normal band scale filter on a normal eye

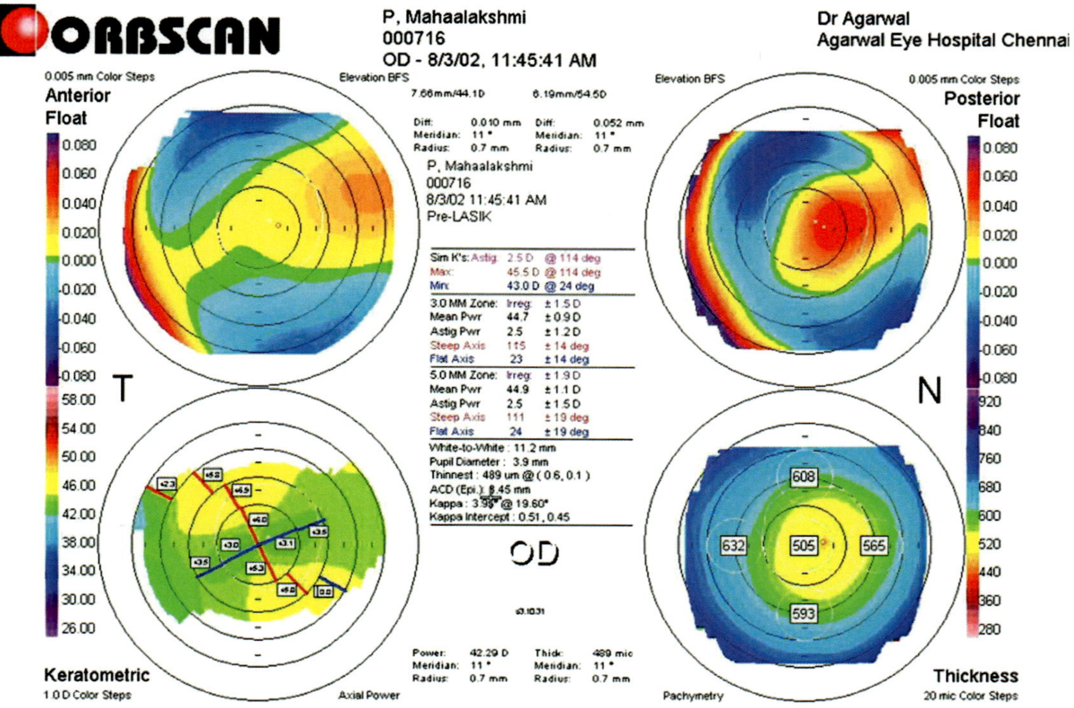

Fig. 2.9: General quad map of a primary posterior corneal elevation. Notice the upper right map has an abnormality whereas the upper left map is normal. This shows the anterior surface of the cornea is normal and the problem is in the posterior surface of the cornea

highlighted in red. This indicates the abnormality in the posterior surface of the cornea. The lower left keratometric map is normal and if we see the lower right map, which is the pachymetry map one will see slightly, thin cornea of 505 microns but still one cannot diagnose the primary posterior corneal elevation only from this reading. Thus we can understand that if not from the upper right map, which denotes the posterior surface of the cornea, one would miss this condition. The Orbscan can only diagnose this.

Now, we can put on the normal band scale filter on (Fig. 2.10) and this will highlight the abnormal areas in red. Notice in Figure 2.10 the upper right map shows a lot of abnormality denoting the primary posterior corneal elevation. One can also take the three-dimensional map of the posterior surface of the cornea (Fig. 2.11) and notice the amount of elevation in respect to the normal reference sphere shown as a black grid. In a case of a keratoconus (Fig. 2.12) all four maps show an abnormality, which confirms the diagnosis.

If we take a LASIK patient's topography we can compare the pre- and the post-LASIK (Fig. 2.13). This helps to understand the pattern and amount of ablation done on the cornea. The picture on the upper right is the preoperative topographic picture and the one on the lower right is the post-Lasik picture. The main picture on the left shows the difference between the pre and post-Lasik topographic patterns. One can detect from this any decentered ablations or any other complication of LASIK surgery.

Corneal topography is extremely important in cataract surgery. *The smaller the size of the incision, lesser the astigmatism and earlier stability of the astigmatism will occur.* One can reduce the astigmatism or increase the astigmatism of a patient after cataract surgery. The simple rule to follow is that *wherever you make an incision that area will flatten and wherever you apply*

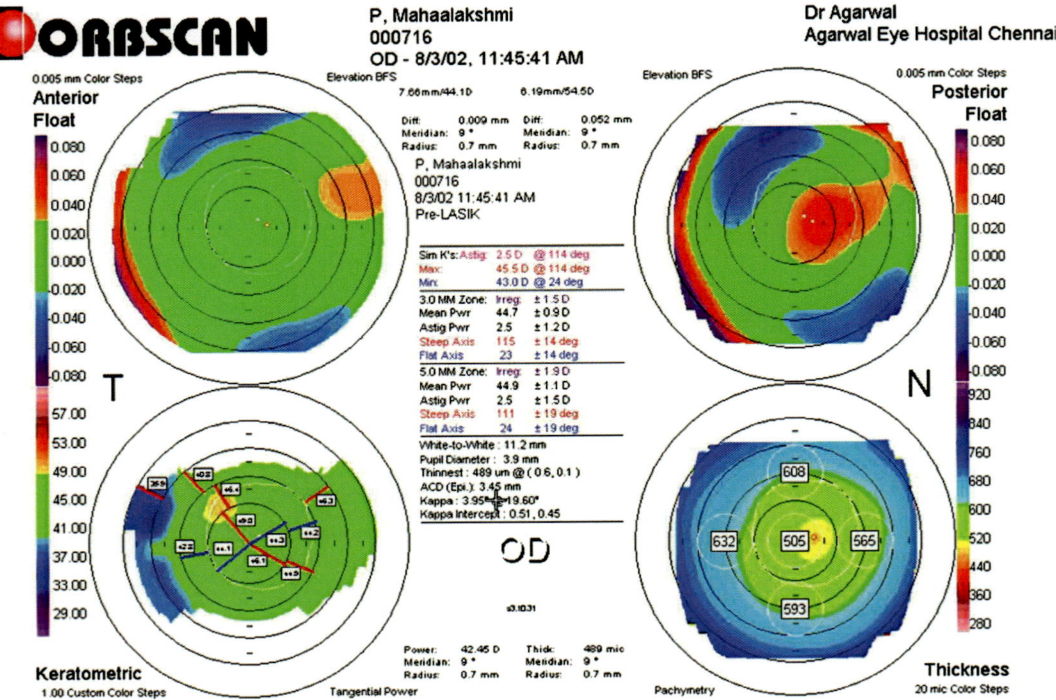

Fig. 2.10: Quad map of a primary posterior corneal elevation with the normal band scale filter. This shows the abnormal areas in red and the normal areas are all green. Notice the abnormailty in the upper right map

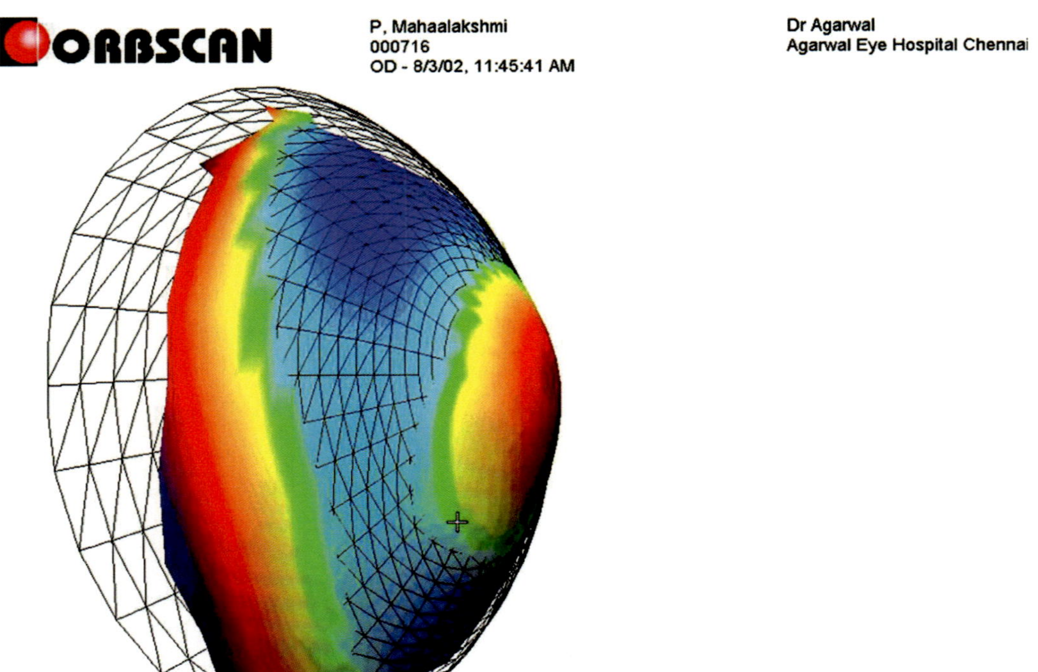

Fig. 2.11: Three-dimensional map of primary posterior corneal elevation. This shows a marked elevation in respect to a normal reference sphere highlighted as a black grid. Notice the red color protrusion on the black grid. This picture is of the posterior surface of the cornea

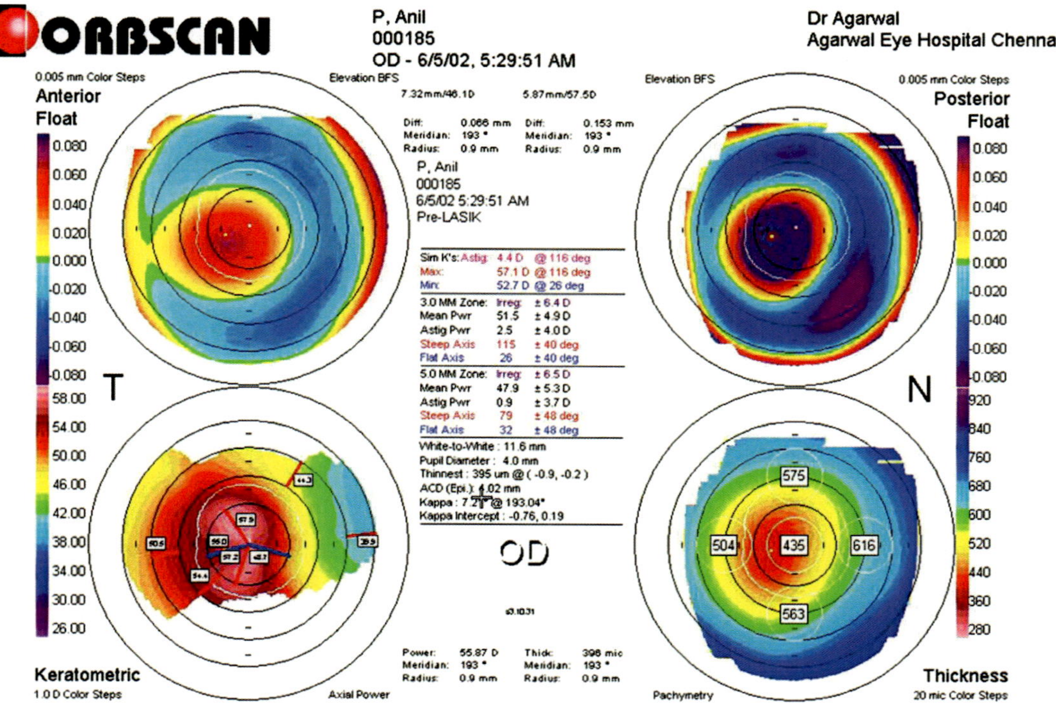

Fig. 2.12: General quad map of a keratoconus patient showing abnormailty in all four maps

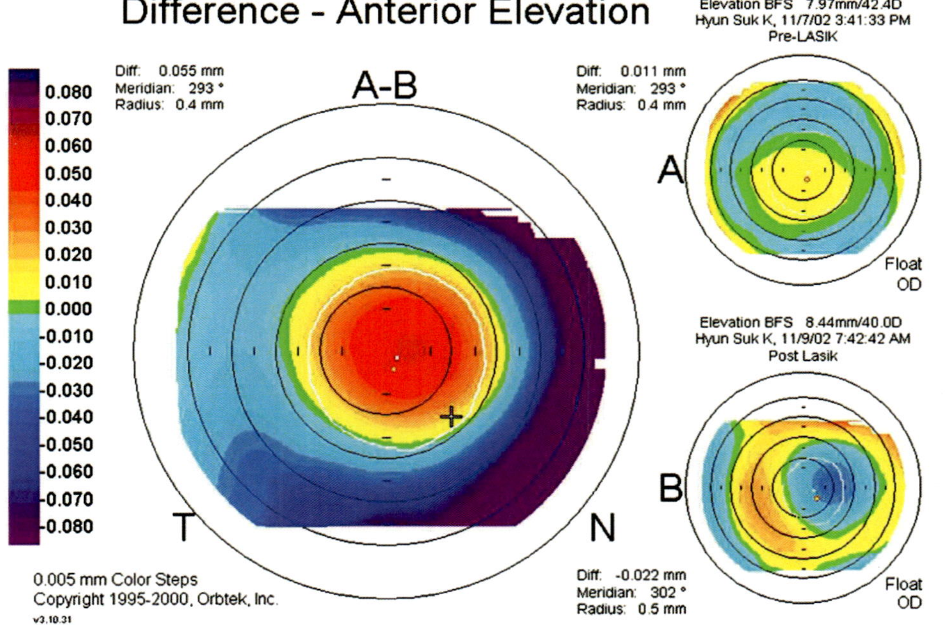

Fig. 2.13: Difference of pre- and post-LASIK

sutures that area will steepen. One can use the Orbscan to analyze the topography before and after cataract surgery. For instance in an extracapsular cataract extraction one can check to see where the astigmatism is most and remove those sutures. In a phaco the astigmatism will be less and in Phakonit where the incision is sub 1.5 mm the astigmatism will be the least.

We can use the Orbscan to determine the anterior chamber depth and also analyze where one should place the incision when one is performing astigmatic keratotomy. The Orbscan can also help in a good fit of the contact lens with a fluorescein pattern.

SUMMARY

The Orbscan has changed the world of topography as it gives us an understanding of a slit scan three-dimensional picture. One can use this in understanding of various conditions.

REFERENCES

1. Agarwal S, Agarwal A, Agarwal A. Four volume Textbook of Ophthalmology; Jaypee; India 2000.
2. Agarwal A. Handbook of Ophthalmology; Slack Inc, USA 2005.
3. Agarwal A. Refractive surgery Nightmares: Conquering Refractive Surgery Catastrophes; Slack Inc, USA 2007.

3 Anterior Keratoconus

Rahul Tiwari, Amar Agarwal, Athiya Agarwal

INTRODUCTION

Keratoconus is characterized by non-inflammatory stromal thinning and anterior protrusion of the cornea. Keratoconus is a slowly progressive condition often presenting in the teen or early twenties with decreased vision or visual distortion. Family history of keratoconus is seen occasionally. Patients with this disorder are poor candidates for refractive surgery because of the possibility of exacerbating keratectasia.[1] The development of corneal ectasia is a well recognized complication of LASIK and attributed to unrecognized preoperative forme fruste Keratoconus.

ORBSCAN

The Orbscan (Bausch and Lomb) corneal topography system uses a scanning optical slit scan that is fundamentally different than the corneal topography that analyses the reflected images from the anterior corneal surface. The high-resolution video camera captures 40 light slits at 45 degrees angle projected through the cornea similarly as seen during slit lamp examination. It has an acquisition time of 4 seconds.[2] The diagnosis of keratoconus is a clinical one and early diagnosis can be difficult on clinical examination alone. Orbscan has become a useful tool for evaluating the disease, and with the advent of its use, morphology and any subtle changes in the topography can be detected in early keratoconus. We always use the Orbscan system to evaluate our potential LASIK candidates preoperatively to rule out anterior keratoconus.

TECHNIQUE

All eyes to undergo LASIK are examined by Orbscan. Eyes are screened using quad maps with the normal band (NB) filter turned on. Four maps included (a) anterior corneal elevation: NB = ± 25 μ of best-fit sphere. (b) Posterior corneal elevation: NB = ± 25 μ of best-fit sphere. (c) Keratometric mean curvature: NB = 40 to 48 D, K. (d) Corneal thickness (pachymetry): NB = 500 to 600 μ. Map features within normal band are colored green. This effectively filters out variation falling within normal band. When abnormalities are seen on the normal band quad map screening, a standard scale quad map is examined. For those cases with anterior keratoconus, we also generate three-dimensional views of anterior and posterior corneal elevation.

The following parameters are considered to detect anterior keratoconus: (a) radii of anterior and posterior curvature of the cornea, (b) posterior best-fit sphere, (c) difference between the thickest corneal pachymetry value in 7 mm zone and thinnest pachymetry value of the cornea, (d) normal band (NB) scale map, (e) elevation on the anterior float of the cornea, (f) elevation on the posterior float of the cornea, (g) location of the cone on the cornea.

ANTERIOR KERATOCONUS

On Orbscan analysis in patients with anterior keratoconus the average ratio of radius of the anterior curvature to the posterior curvature of cornea is 1.25 (range 1.21 to 1.38), average posterior best-fit sphere is –56.98 Dsph (range –52.1 Dsph to –64.5), average difference in pachymetry value between thinnest point on the cornea and thickest point in 7 mm zone on the cornea is 172.7 µm (range 117 µm to 282 µm), average elevation of anterior corneal float is 55.25 µm (range 25 µm to 103 µm), average elevation of posterior corneal float is 113.6 µm (range 41 µm to 167 µm). Figures 3.1 to 3.6 show the various topographic features of an eye with anterior keratoconus. In Figure 3.1 (general quad map) upper left corner map is the anterior float, upper right corner map is posterior float, lower left corner is keratometric map while the lower right is the pachymetry map showing a difference of 282 µm between the thickest pachymetry value in 7 mm zone of cornea (597 µm) and thinnest pachymetry value (315 µm). In Figure 3.2, normal band scale map of anterior surface shows significant elevation on the anterior and posterior float with abnormal keratometric and pachymetry maps. Figure 3.3 is three-dimensional representation of the anterior float with reference sphere 64 µm. Figure 3.4 shows three-dimensional representation of posterior float with reference sphere. Figure 3.5 shows amount of elevation (color coded) of the anterior corneal surface in microns (64 µm). Figure 3.6 shows amount of elevation (color coded) of the posterior corneal surface in microns (167 µm).

DISCUSSION

Topography is valuable for preoperative ophthalmic examination of LASIK candidates. Three-dimensional imaging allows surgeons to look at corneal thickness, as well as the corneal anterior and posterior surface and can predict the shape of cornea after LASIK surgery. Topographic analysis using three dimensional slit scan system allows us to predict which candidates would do well with LASIK and also

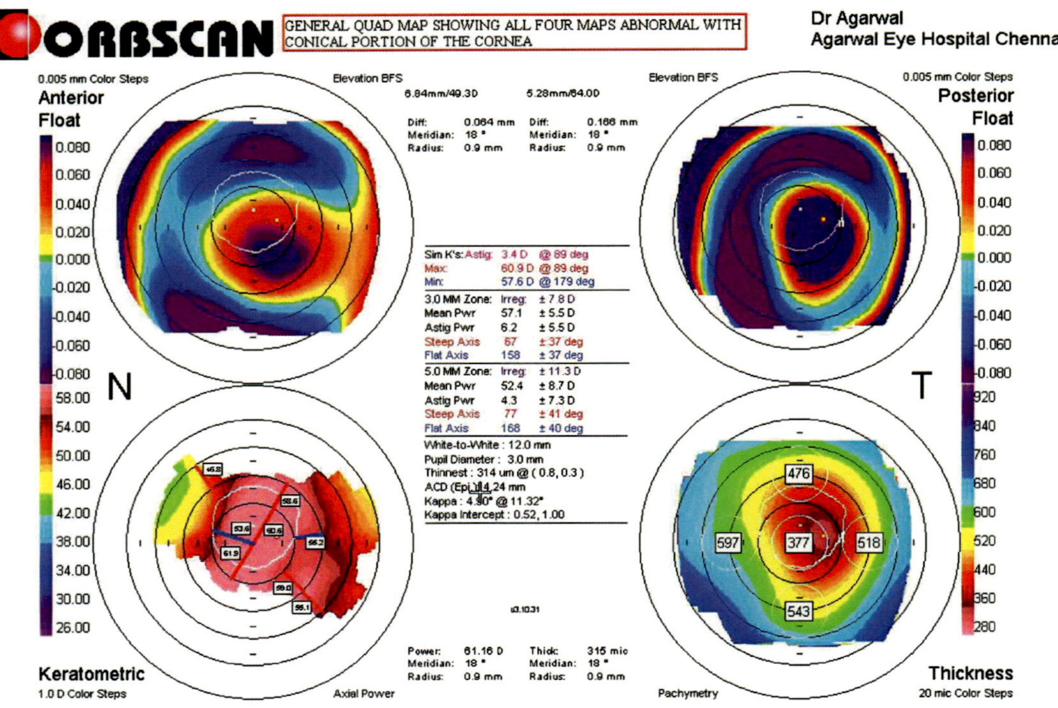

Fig. 3.1: General quad map of an eye with keratoconus

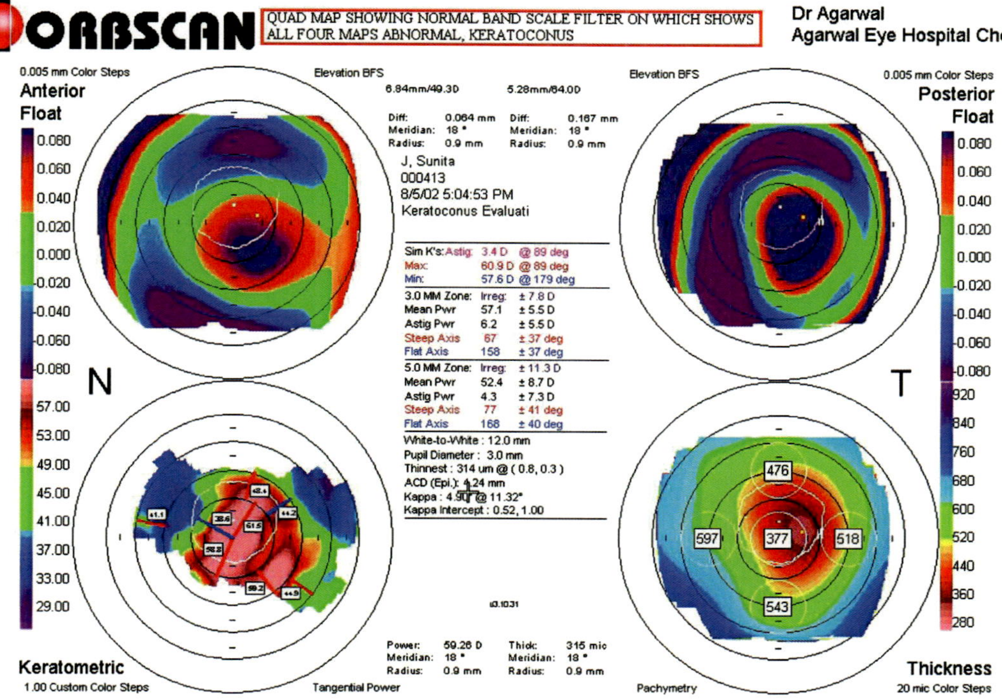

Fig. 3.2: Quad map with normal band scale filter on in the same eye as in Figure 3.1

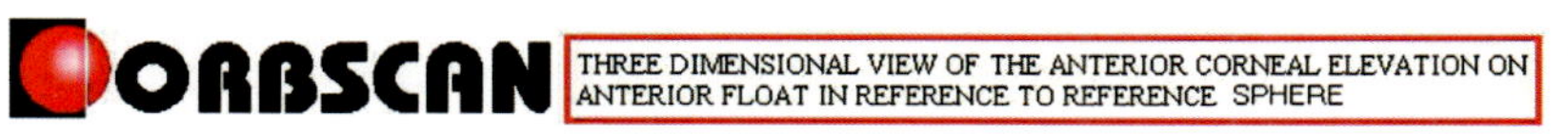

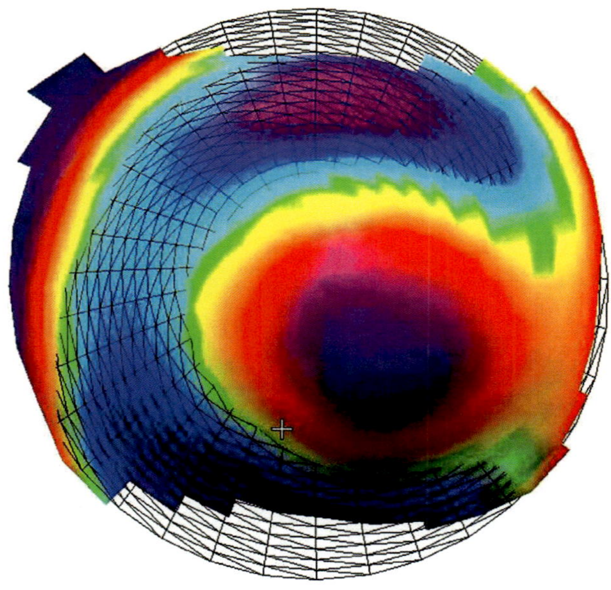

Fig. 3.3: Three-dimensional anterior float

ORBSCAN THREE DIMENSIONAL VIEW OF THE POSTERIOR CORNEAL ELEVATION ON POSTERIOR FLOAT IN REFERENCE TO REFERENCE SPHERE

Dr Agarwal
Agarwal Eye Hospital Chennai

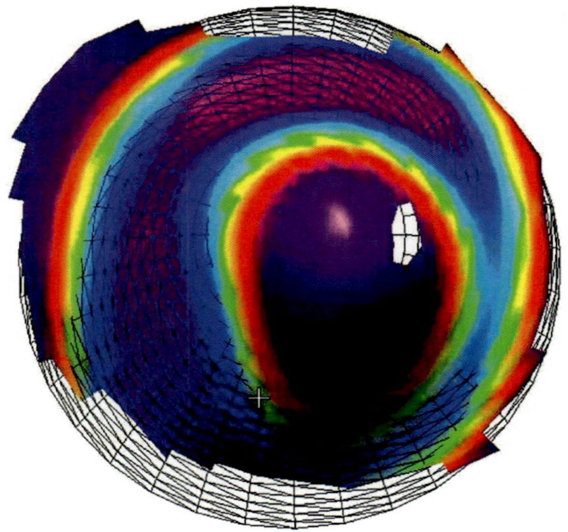

Fig. 3.4: Three-dimensional posterior float

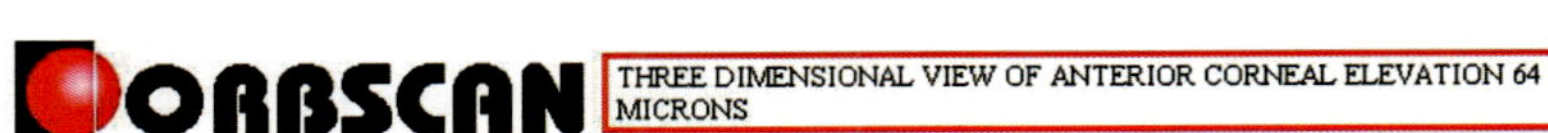

Dr Agarwal
Agarwal Eye Hospital Chennai

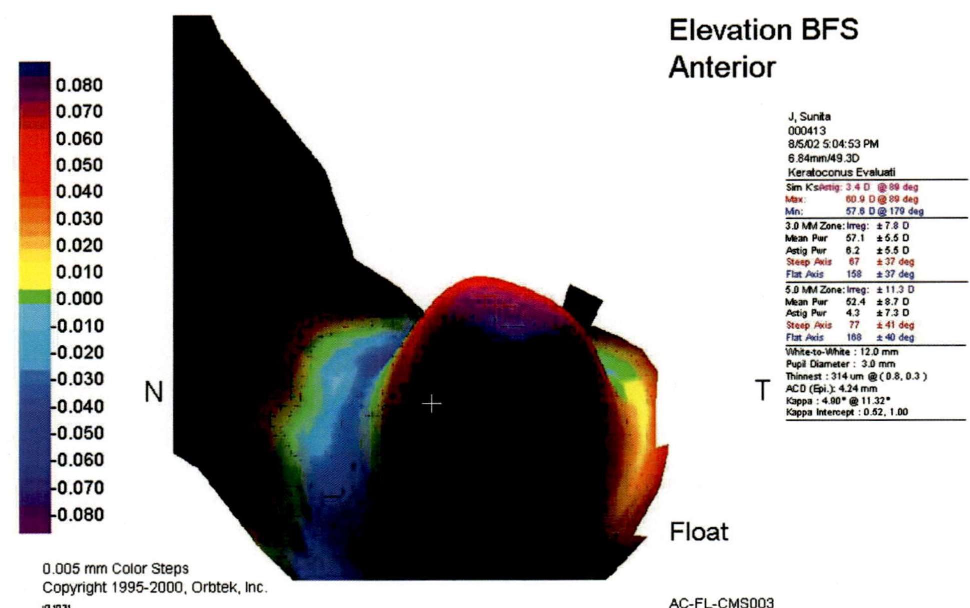

Fig. 3.5: Three-dimensional anterior corneal elevation measured in microns

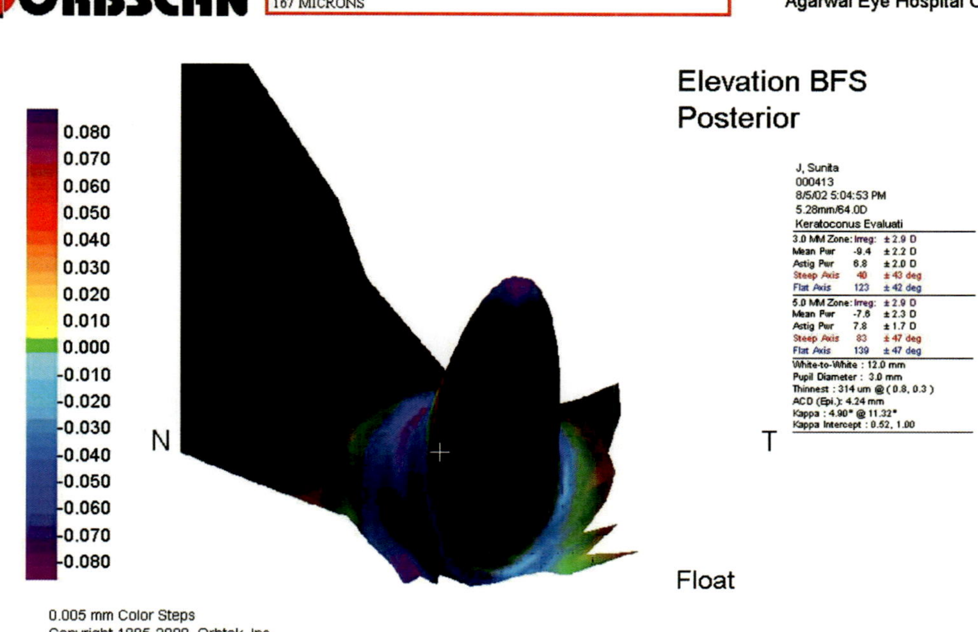

Fig. 3.6: Three-dimensional posterior corneal elevation measured in microns

confers the ability to screen for subtle configurations which may be contraindication to LASIK.[3] It is known that corneal ectasias and keratoconus have posterior corneal elevation as the earliest manifestation. In addition Wang et al have shown that the posterior corneal elevation increases after LASIK, and the increase is correlated with residual corneal bed thickness.[4] We found that patients with positive keratoconus have higher posterior and anterior elevation on Orbscan II topography.

Elevation is not measured directly by Placido based topographers, but certain assumptions allow the construction of elevation maps. Elevation of a point on the corneal surface displays the height of the point on the corneal surface relative to a spherical reference surface. Reference surface is chosen to be a sphere. Best mathematical approximation of the actual corneal surface called best-fit sphere is calculated. Posterior corneal surface topographic changes after LASIK are known. Increased negative keratometric diopters and oblate asphericity of the PCC are common after LASIK leading to mild keratectasia.[5,6] Lamellar refractive surgery reduces the biomechanical strength of cornea that may lead to mechanical instability and keratectasia. Iatrogenic keratectasia represents a complication after LASIK that may limit the range of myopic correction.[7] Corneal ectasia has also been reported after LASIK in cases of forme fruste keratoconus.[8] Posterior corneal bulge may be correlated with residual corneal bed thickness. The risk of keratectasia may be increased if the residual corneal bed is thinner than 250 μm.[9] Age, attempted correction and the optical zone diameter are other parameters that have to be considered to avoid post LASIK ectasia.[10,11]

CONCLUSION

The Orbscan provides reliable, reproducible data of the anterior corneal surface; posterior corneal surface, keratometry, and pachymetry values with three-dimensional presentations and all LASIK candidates must be evaluated by this method preoperatively to detect an "early keratoconus". We suggest that Orbscan II is an important preoperative investigative tool to decide the suitable candidate for lasik and thus avoiding any complication of LASIK surgery and helping the patient out by contact lens or keratoplasty. The following parameters must be analyzed in all lasik candidates to rule out keratoconus: (a) ratio of radii of anterior to posterior curvature of cornea: > 1.21 and < 1.27, (b) posterior best fit sphere: > -52.0 Dsph, (c) difference between thickest corneal pachymetry value at 7 mm zone and thinnest pachymetry value: > 100 µm and (d) posterior corneal elevation > 50 µm.

REFERENCES

1. Seiler T, Quurke AW. Iatrogenic keratectasia after LASIK in a case of forme fruste keratoconus. J Cataract Refract Surg 1998;24:1007-9.
2. Fedor P, Kaufman S. Corneal topography and imaging. eMedicine Journal 2001;2(6).
3. McDermott GK. Topography's benefits for LASIK. Review of Ophthalmology. Editorial, vol no: 9:03 issue.
4. Wang Z, Chen J, Yang B. Posterior corneal surface topographic changes after laser in situ keratomileusis are related to residual corneal bed thickness. Ophthalmology 1999;106:406-9; discussion 409-10.
5. Seitz B, Torres F, Langenbucher A, et al. Posterior corneal curvature changes after myopic laser in situ keratomileusis. Ophthalmology 2001;108(4):666-72.
6. Geggel HS, Talley AR. Delayed onset keratectasia following laser in situ keratomileusis. J Cataract Refract Surg 1999;25(4):582-6.
7. Seiler T, Koufala K, Richter G. Iatrogenic keratectasia after laser in situ keratomileusis. J Refract Surg 1998;14(3):312-7.
8. Seiler T, Quurke AW. Iatrogenic keratectasia after laser in situ keratomileusis in a case of forme fruste keratoconus. J Refract Surg 1998;24(7):1007-9.
9. Wang Z, Chen J, Yang B. Posterior corneal surface topographic changes after laser in situ keratomileusis are related to residual corneal bed thickness. Ophthalmology 1999;106(2):406-9.
10. Pallikaris IG, Kymionis GD, Astyrakakis NI. Corneal ectasia induced by laser in situ keratomileusis. J Cataract Refract Surg 2001;27(11):1796-802.
11. Argento C, Cosentino MJ, Tytium A, et al. Corneal ectasia after laser in situ keratomileusis. J Cataract Refract Surg 2001;27(9):1440-810.

4 Posterior Corneal Changes in Refractive Surgery

Amar Agarwal, Soosan Jacob, Athiya Agarwal

INTRODUCTION

The development of corneal ectasia is a well-recognized complication of LASIK and amongst other contributory factors, unrecognized preoperative forme fruste keratoconus is also an important one. Patients with this disorder are poor candidates for refractive surgery because of the possibility of exacerbating keratectasia. It is known that posterior corneal elevation is an early presenting sign in keratoconus and hence it is imperative to evaluate posterior corneal curvature (PCC) in every LASIK candidate.

TOPOGRAPHY

Topography is valuable for preoperative ophthalmic examination of LASIK candidates. Three-dimensional imaging allows surgeons to look at the corneal thickness, as well as the corneal anterior and posterior surface and it can also predict the shape of the cornea after LASIK surgery. Topographic analysis using three dimensional slit scan system allows us to predict which candidates would do well with LASIK and also confers the ability to screen for subtle configurations which may be a contraindication to LASIK.

ORBSCAN

The Orbscan (Bausch and Lomb) corneal topography system uses a scanning optical slit scan which makes it fundamentally different from the corneal topography that analyses the reflected images from the anterior corneal surface. The high-resolution video camera captures 40 light slits at 45 degrees angle projected through the cornea similarly as seen during slit lamp examination. The slits are projected on to the anterior segment of the eye: the anterior cornea, the posterior cornea, the anterior iris and anterior lens. The data collected from these four surfaces are used to create a topographic map. Each surface point from the diffusely reflected slit beams that overlap in the central 5 mm zone is independently triangulated to x, y, and z coordinates, providing three-dimensional data.

This technique provides more information about the anterior segment of the eye, such as anterior and posterior corneal curvature, elevation maps of the anterior and posterior corneal surface and corneal thickness. It has an acquisition time of 4 seconds.[1] This improves the diagnostic accuracy. It also has passive eye-tracker from frame to frame and 43 frames are taken to ensure accuracy. It is easy to interpret and has good repeatability.

PRIMARY POSTERIOR CORNEAL ELEVATION

The diagnosis of frank keratoconus is a clinical one. Early diagnosis of forme fruste can be difficult on clinical examination alone. Orbscan has become a useful tool for evaluating the disease, and with its advent, abnormalities in posterior corneal surface topography have been identified in keratoconus. Posterior corneal surface data is problematic because it is not a direct measure and there is little published information on normal values for each age group. In the patient with increased posterior corneal elevation in the absence of other changes, it is unknown whether this finding represents a manifestation of early keratoconus. The decision to proceed with refractive surgery is therefore more difficult.

Posterior Corneal Topography

One should always use the Orbscan system to evaluate potential LASIK candidates preoperatively to rule out primary posterior corneal elevations. Eyes are screened using quad maps with the normal band (NB) filter turned on. Four maps include: (a) anterior corneal elevation: NB = ± 25 µ of best-fit sphere, (b) posterior corneal elvevation : NB = ± 25 µ of best fit sphere, (c) keratometric mean curvature: NB = 40 to 48 D, (d) corneal thickness (pachymetry): NB = 500 to 600 µ. Map features within normal band are colored green. This effectively filters out variations falling within the normal band. When abnormalities are seen on normal band quad map screening, a standard scale quad map should be examined. For those cases with posterior corneal elevation, three-dimensional views of posterior corneal elevation can also be generated. In all eyes with posterior corneal elevation, the following parameters are generated: (a) radii of anterior and posterior curvature of the cornea, (b) posterior best fit sphere, (c) difference between the corneal pachymetry value in 7 mm zone and thinnest pachymetry value of the cornea.

Pre-existing Posterior Corneal Abnormalities

Figures 4.1 to 4.6 show the various topographic features of an eye with primary posterior corneal elevation detected during pre-LASIK assessment. In Figure 4.1 (general quad map) upper left corner map is the anterior float, upper right corner map is posterior

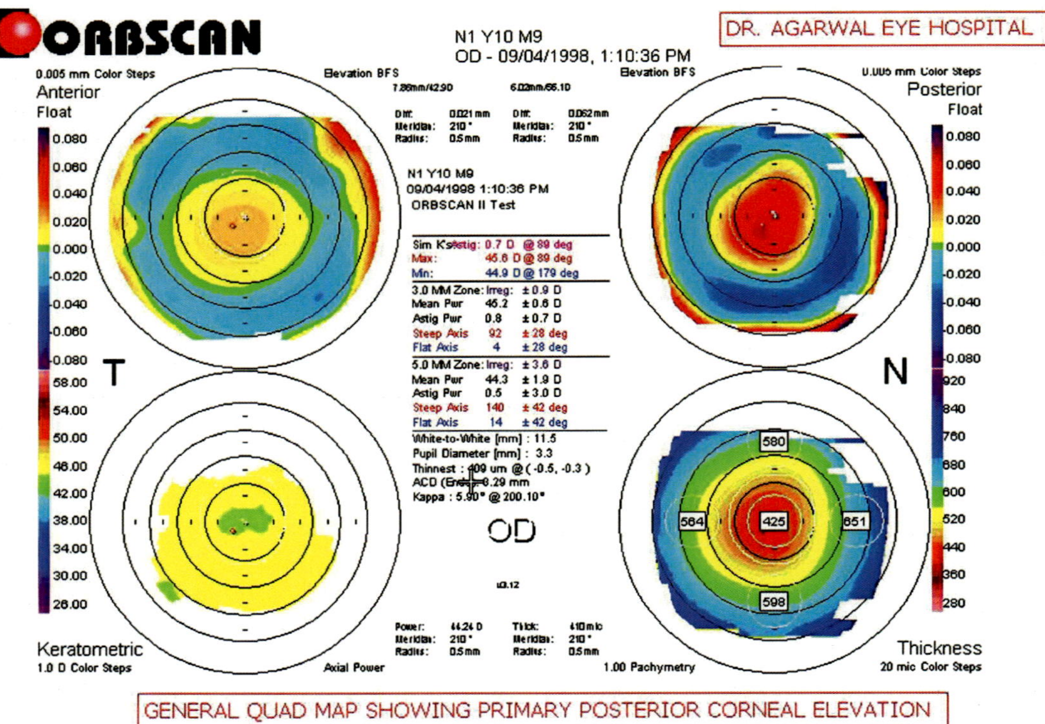

Fig. 4.1: General quad map of an eye with primary posterior corneal elevation. Notice the red areas seen in the top right picture showing the primary posterior corneal elevation

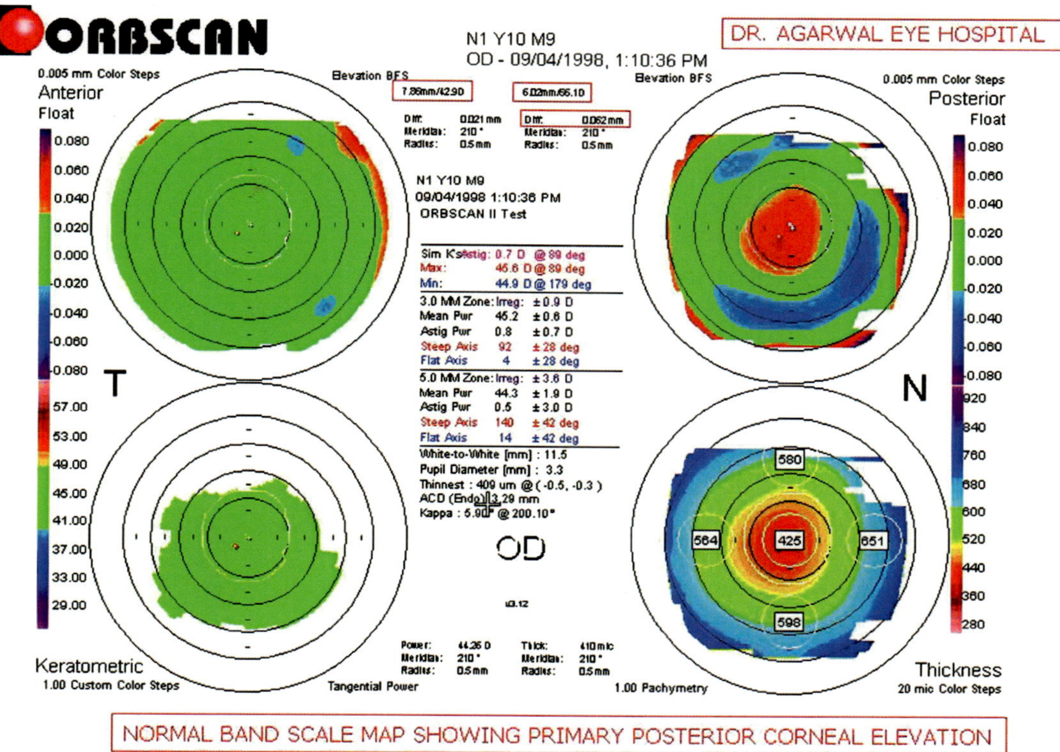

Fig. 4.2: Quad map with normal band scale filter on in the same eye as in Figure 4.1

float, lower left corner is keratometric map while the lower right is the pachymetry map showing a difference of 100 µm between the thickest pachymetry value in 7 mm zone of the cornea and thinnest pachymetry value. In Figure 4.2, normal band scale map of anterior surface shows "with the rule astigmatism" in an otherwise normal anterior surface (shown in green), the posterior float shows significant elevation inferotemporally. In Figure 4.2 only the abnormal areas are shown in red for ease in detection. Figure 4.3 is three-dimensional representation of the maps in Figure 4.2. Figure 4.4 shows three-dimensional representation of anterior corneal surface with reference sphere. Figure 4.5 shows three-dimensional representation of posterior corneal surface showing a significant posterior corneal elevation. Figure 4.6 shows amount of elevation (color coded) of the posterior corneal surface in microns (50 µm).

In the light of the fact that keratoconus may have posterior corneal elevation as the earliest manifestation, preoperative analysis of posterior corneal curvature to detect a posterior corneal bulge is important to avoid post-LASIK keratectasia. The rate of progression of posterior corneal elevation to frank keratoconus is unknown. It is also difficult to specify that exact amount of posterior corneal elevation beyond which it may be unsafe to carry out LASIK. Atypical elevation in the posterior corneal map more than 45 µm should alert us against a post LASIK surprise. Orbscan provides reliable, reproducible data of the posterior corneal surface and all LASIK candidates must be evaluated by this method preoperatively to detect an " early keratoconus".

Elevation is not measured directly by Placido based topographers, but certain assumptions allow the construction of elevation maps. Elevation of a point on the corneal surface displays the height of the point on the corneal surface relative to a spherical reference surface. Reference surface is chosen to be a sphere. Best mathematical approximation of the actual corneal surface called best-fit sphere is calcu-

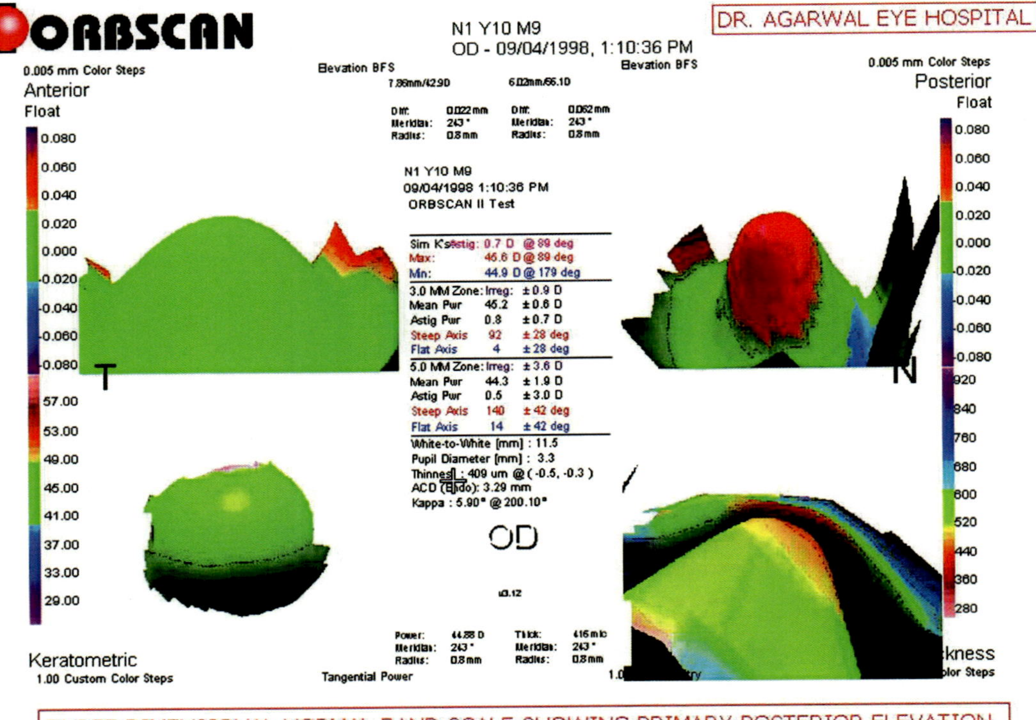

Fig. 4.3: Three-dimensional normal band scale map. In the top right note the red areas which shows the elevation on the posterior cornea. The anterior cornea is normal

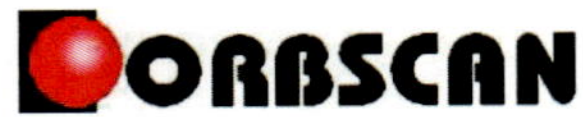

N1 Y10 M9
OD - 09/04/1998, 1:10:36 PM

Dr agarwal
Agarwal Eye Hospital Chenn

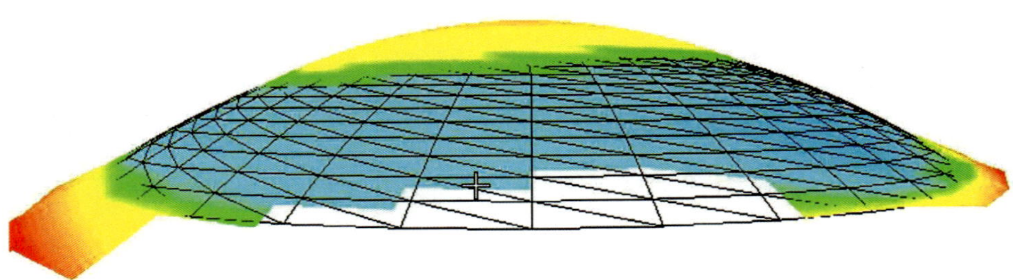

Fig. 4.4: Three-dimensional anterior float. Notice it is normal

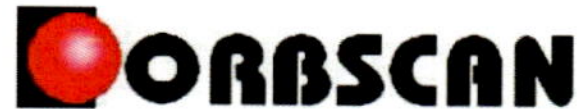

N1 Y10 M9
OD - 09/04/1998, 1:10:36 PM

Dr agarwal
Agarwal Eye Hospital Chenn:

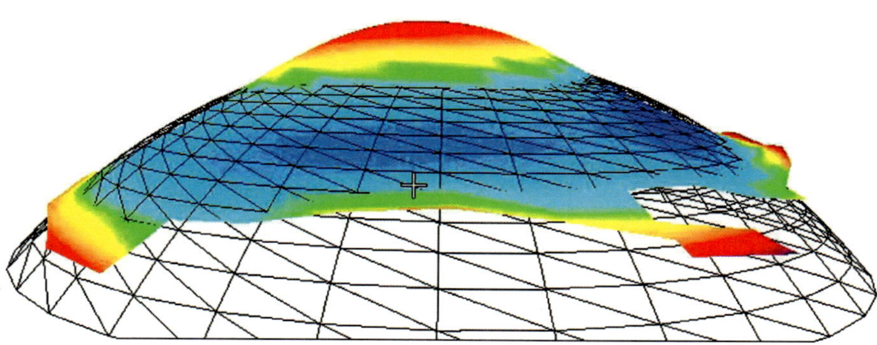

Fig. 4.5: Three-dimensional posterior float. Notice in this there is marked elevation as seen in the red areas

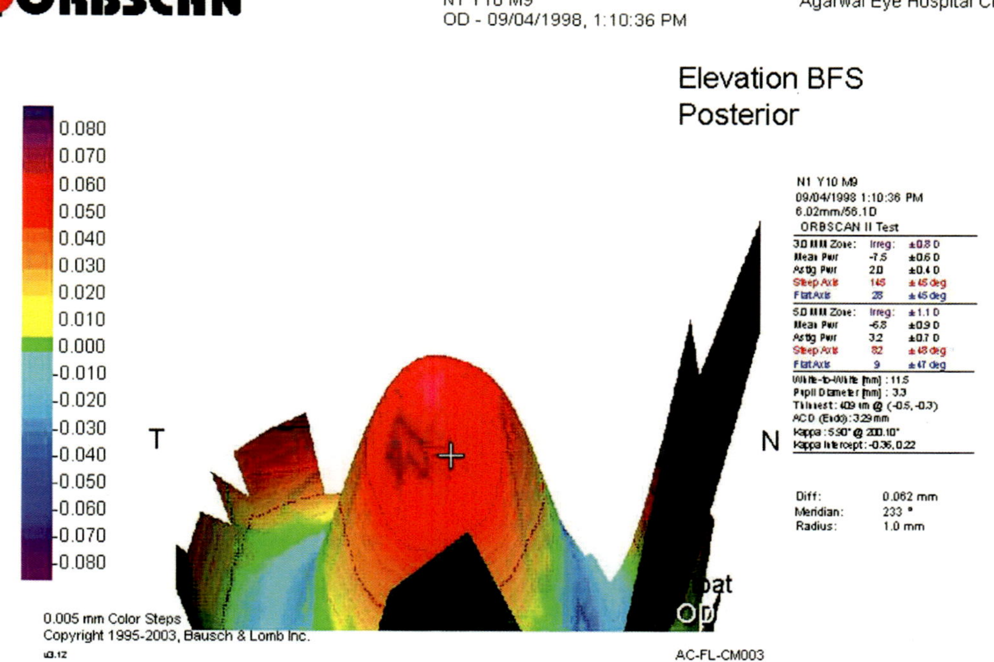

Fig. 4.6: Three-dimensional posterior corneal elevation measured in microns

lated. One of the criteria for defining forme fruste keratoconus is a posterior best fit sphere of > 55.0 D.

Ratio of radii of anterior to posterior curvature of cornea ≥ 1.21 and ≤ 1.27 has been considered as a keratoconus suspect . Average pachymetry difference between thickest and the thinnest point on the cornea in the 7 mm zone should normally be less than 100 μm.

Agarwal Criteria to Diagnose Primary Posterior Corneal Elevation

1. Ratio of the radii of anterior and posterior curvature of the cornea should be more than 1.2 . In Figure 4.2 note the radii of the anterior curvature is 7.86 mm and the radii of the posterior curvature is 6.02 mm. The ratio is 1.3.
2. Posterior best fit sphere should be more than 52 D. In Figure 4.2 note the posterior best fit sphere is 56.1 D
3. Difference between the thickest and thinnest corneal pachymetry value in the 7 mm zone should be more than 100 microns. The thickest pachymetry value as seen in Figure 4.2 is 651 microns and the thinnest value is 409 microns. The difference is 242 microns.
4. The thinnest point on the cornea should correspond with the highest point of elevation of the posterior corneal surface. The thinnest point as seen in Figure 4.2 bottom right picture is seen as a cross. This point or cursor corresponds to the same cross or cursor in Figure 4.2 top right picture which indicates the highest point of elevation on the posterior cornea.
5. Elevation of the posterior corneal surface should be more than 45 microns above the posterior best fit sphere. In Figure 4.2 you will notice it is 0.062 mm or 62 microns.

IATROGENIC KERATECTASIA

Iatrogenic keratectasia may be seen in some patients following ablative refractive surgery (Figs 4.7 and 4.8). The anterior cornea is composed of alternating

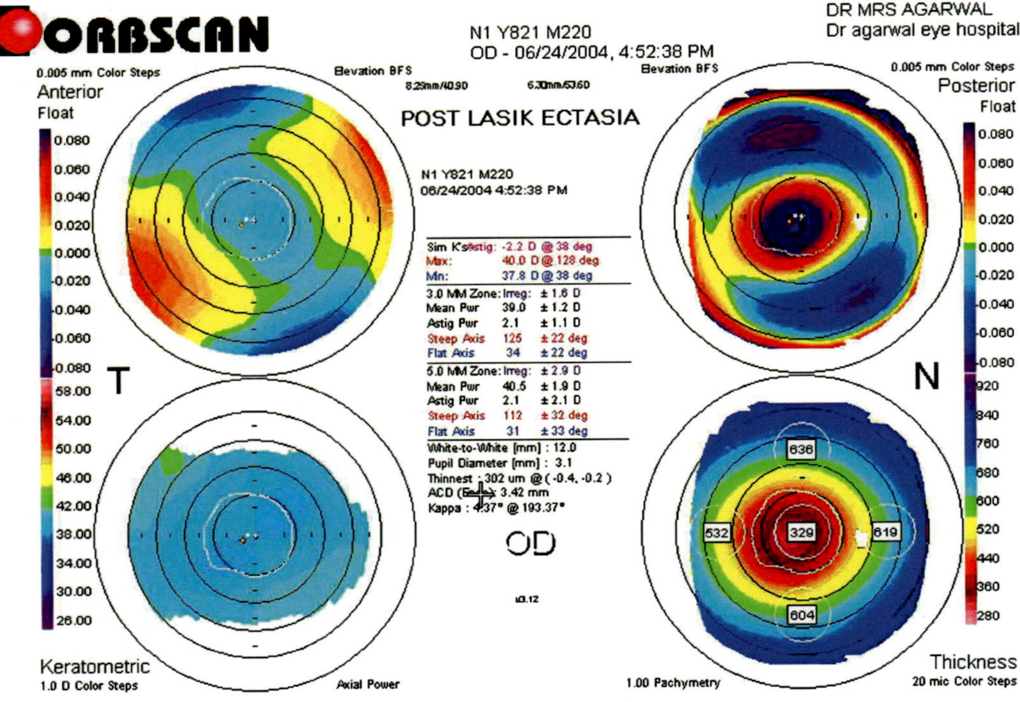

Fig. 4.7: A patient with iatrogenic keratectasia after lasik. Note the upper right hand corner pictures showing the posterior float has thinning and this is also seen in the bottom right picture in which pachymetry reading is 329

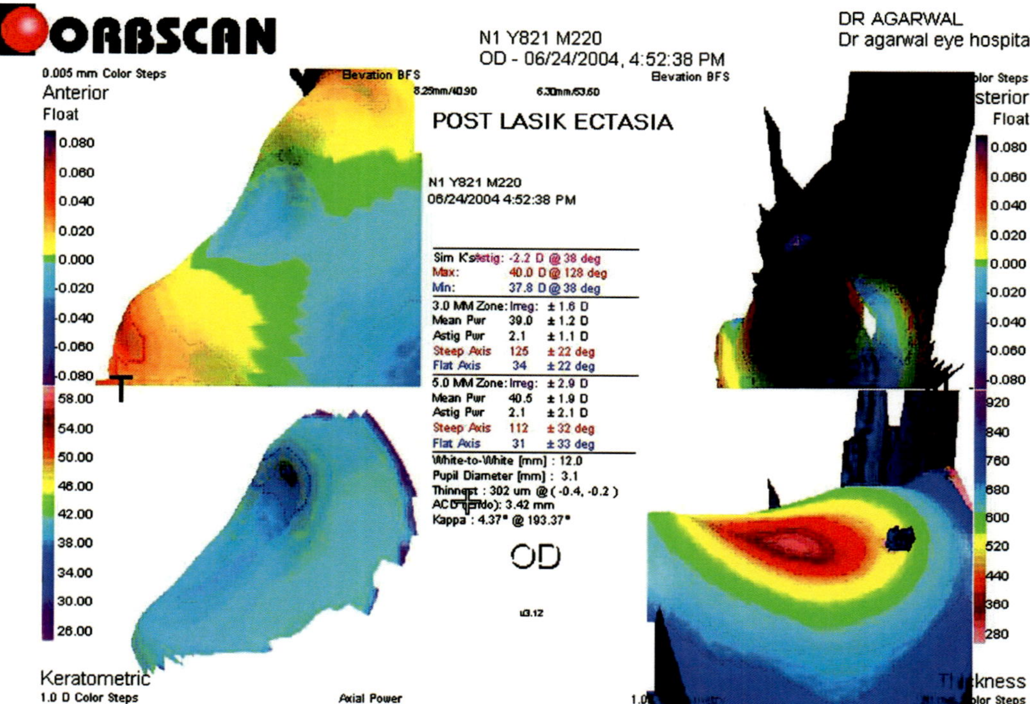

Fig. 4.8: The same patient with iatrogenic keratectasia after lasik in a 3 D pattern. Notice the ectasia seen clearly in the bottom right picture

collagen fibrils and has a more complicated interwoven structure than the deeper stroma and it acts as the major stress-bearing layer. The flap used for LASIK is made in this layer and thus results in a weakening of that strongest layer of the cornea which contributes maximum to the biomechanical stability of the cornea.

The residual bed thickness (RBT) of the cornea is the crucial factor contributing to the biomechanical stability of the cornea after LASIK. The flap as such does not contribute much after its repositioning to the stromal bed. This is easily seen by the fact that the flap can be easily lifted up even up to 1 year after treatment. The decreased RBT as well as the lamellar cut in the cornea both contribute to the decreased biomechanical stability of the cornea. A reduction in the RBT results in a long term increase in the surface parallel stress on the cornea. The intraocular pressure (IOP) can cause further forward bowing and thinning of a structurally compromised cornea. Inadvertent excessive eye rubbing, prone position sleeping, and the normal wear and tear of the cornea may also play a role. The RBT should not be less than 250 mm to avoid subsequent iatrogenic keratectasias.[2–4] Reoperations should be undertaken very carefully in corneae with RBT less than 300 mm. Increasing myopia after every operation is known as "dandelion keratectasia".

The ablation diameter also plays a very important role in LASIK. Postoperative optical distortions are more common with diameters less than 5.5 mm. Use of larger ablation diameters implies a lesser RBT postoperatively. Considering the formula: Ablation depth [mm] = 1/3 . (diameter [mm])^2 × (intended correction diopters [D])), [4,5] it becomes clear that to preserve a sufficient bed thickness, the range of myopic correction is limited and the upper limit of possible myopic correction may be around 12 D.[6]

Detection of a mild keratectasia requires knowledge about the posterior curvature of the cornea. Posterior corneal surface topographic changes after LASIK are known. Increased negative keratometric diopters and oblate asphericity of the PCC, which correlate significantly with the intended correction are common after LASIK leading to mild keratectasia.[6,7] This change in posterior power and the risk of keratectasia was more significant with a RBT of 250 μm or less.[8] The difference in the refractive indices results in a 0.2 D difference at the back surface of the cornea becoming equivalent to a 2.0 D change in the front surface of the cornea.[6] Increase in posterior power and asphericity also correlates with the difference between the intended and achieved correction 3 months after LASIK. This is because factors like drying of the stromal bed may result in an ablation depth more than that intended.[6] Reinstein et al predict that the standard deviation of uncertainty in predicting the RBT preoperatively is around 30 μm. [Invest Ophthalmol Vis Sci 40 (Suppl):S403, 1999]. Age, attempted correction, the optical zone diameter and the flap thickness are other parameters that have to be considered to avoid post-LASIK ectasia.[9,10]

The flap thickness may not be uniform throughout its length. In studies by Seitz et al, it has been shown that the Moris Model One microkeratome and the Supratome cut deeper towards the hinge, whereas the Automated Corneal Shaper and the Hansatome create flaps that are thinner towards the hinge. Thus, accordingly, the area of corneal ectasia may not be in the centre but paracentral, especially if it is also associated with decentered ablation. Flap thickness has also been found to vary considerably, even upto 40 μm, under similar conditions and this may also result in a lesser RBT than intended.[11-17]

It is known that corneal ectasias and keratoconus have posterior corneal elevation as the earliest manifestation.[18] The precise course of progression of posterior corneal elevation to frank keratoconus is not known. Hence it is necessary to study the posterior corneal surface preoperatively in all LASIK candidates.

EFFECT OF POSTERIOR CORNEAL CHANGE ON IOL CALCULATION

IOL power calculation in post-LASIK eyes is different because of the inaccuracy of keratometry, change in anterior and posterior corneal curvatures, altered relation between the two and change in the standardized index of refraction of the cornea. Irregular astigmatism induced by the procedure, decentered ablations and central islands also add to the problem.

Routine keratometry is not accurate in these patients. Corneal refractive surgery changes the asphericity of the cornea and also produces a wide range of powers in the central 5 mm zone of the cornea. LASIK makes the cornea of a myope more oblate so that keratometry values may be taken from the more peripheral steeper area of the cornea, which results in calculation of a lower than required IOL power resulting in a hyperopic "surprise". Hyperopic LASIK makes the cornea more prolate, thus resulting in a myopic "surprise" post cataract surgery.

Post-PRK or LASIK, the relation between the anterior and posterior corneal surface changes. The relative thickness of the various corneal layers, each having a different refractive index also changes and there is a change in the curvature of the posterior corneal surface. All these results in the standardized refractive index of 1.3375 no longer being accurate in these eyes.

At present there is no keratometry, which can accurately measure the anterior and posterior curvatures of the cornea. The Orbscan also makes mathematical assumptions of the posterior surface rather than direct measurements. This is important in the LASIK patient because the procedure alters the relation between the anterior and posterior surfaces of the cornea as well as changes the curvature of the posterior cornea.

Thus direct measurements such as manual and automated keratometry and topography are inherently inaccurate in these patients. The corneal power is therefore calculated by the calculation method, the contact lens overrefraction method and by the CVK method. The flattest K reading obtained by any method is taken for IOL power calculation (the steepest K is taken for hyperopes who had undergone LASIK). One can still aim for 1.00 D of myopia rather than emmetropia to allow for any error, which is almost always in the hyperopic direction in case of pre LASIK myopes. Also, a third or fourth generation IOL calculating formula should be used for such patients.

REFERENCES

1. Fedor P, Kaufman S. Corneal topography and imaging. eMedicine Journal 2001;2(6).
2. Seiler T, Koufala K, Richter G. Iatrogenic keratectasia after laser in situ keratomileusis. J Refract Surg 1998;14(3):312-7.
3. Seiler T, Quurke AW. Iatrogenic keratectasia after laser in situ keratomileusis in a case of forme fruste keratoconus. J Refract Surg 1998;24(7):1007-9.
4. Probost LE, Machat JJ. Mathematics of laser in situ keratomileusis for high myopia. J Cataract refract Surg 1998;24.
5. Mc Donnell PJ. Excimer laser corneal surgery: new strategies and old enemies {review}. Invest Ophthalmol Vis Sci 1995;36;4-8.
6. Seitz B, Torres F, Langenbucher A, et al. Posterior corneal curvature changes after myopic laser in situ keratomileusis. Ophthalmology 2001;108(4):666-72.
7. Geggel HS, Talley AR. Delayed onset keratectasia following laser in situ keratomileusis. J Cataract Refract Surg 1999;25(4):582-6.
8. Wang Z, Chen J, Yang B. Posterior corneal surface topographic changes after laser in situ keratomileusis are related to residual corneal bed thickness. Ophthalmology 1999;106(2):406-9.
9. Pallikaris IG, Kymionis GD. Astyrakakis N I. Corneal ectasia induced by laser in situ keratomileusis. J Cataract Refract Surg 2001;27(11):1796-802.
10. Argento C, Cosentino M J, Tytium A, et al. Corneal ectasia after laser in situ keratomileusis. J Cataract Refract Surg 2001;27(9):1440-8.
11. Binder PS, Moore M, Lambert RW, et al. Comparison of two microkeratome systems. J Refract Surg 1997;13;142-53.
12. Hofmann RF, Bechara SJ. An independent evaluation of second generation suction microkeratomes. Refract Corneal Surg 1992;8:348-54.
13. Schuler A, Jessen K, Hoffmann F. accuracy of the micro-keratome keratectomies in pig eyes. Invest Ophthalmol Vis Sci 1990;31:2022-30.
14. Behrens A, Seitz B, Langenbucher A, et al. Evaluation of corneal flap dimensions and cut quality using a manually guided microkeratome [published erratum appears in J Refract Surg 1999;15:400]. J Refract Surg 1999;15:118-23.
15. Behrens A, Seitz B, Langenbucher A, et al. Evaluation of corneal flap dimensions and cut quality using the Automated Corneal Shaper microkeratome. J Refract Surg 2000;16:83-9.
16. BehrensA, Langenbucher A, Kus MM, et al. Experimental evaluation of two current generation automated microkeratomes: the Hansatomeâ and the Supratomeâ. Am J Ophthalmol. 2000;129:59-67.
17. Jacobs BJ, Deutsch TA, Rubenstein JB. Reproducibility of corneal flap thickness in LASIK. Ophthalmic Surg Lasers 1999;30:350-3.
18. McDermott GK. Topography's benefits for LASIK. Review of Ophthalmology. Editorial, vol no:9:03 issue.

5 Pentacam

Tracy Swartz

INTRODUCTION

The Pentacam Ocular Scanner is a specialized camera which utilizes Scheimpflug imaging to accomplish with a variety of ophthalmic applications. Scheimpflug imaging was patented by Theodor Scheimpflug in 1904 after he discovered that when the planes within a camera intersect rather than being placed in parallel, the depth of focus is extended.

In a typical camera, three imaginary surfaces exist: the film plane, lens plane and sharp image plane. These are parallel to each other such that the image of the object placed in the plane of sharp focus will pass through the lens plane perpendicular to the lens axis and fall on to the film plane. The depth of focus is limited in such a camera.

In a Scheimpflug camera, the three planes are not parallel but intersect in a line, called the "Scheimpflug line". When the lens is tilted such that it intersects the film plane, the plane of sharp focus also passes through the Scheimpflug line, extending the depth of focus. Note that this results in mild image distortion, which is then corrected by the Pentacam system.[1]

A two-dimensional cross-sectional image results, as shown in Figure 5.1. When performing a scan, two cameras are used to capture the image. One centrally located camera detects pupil size and orientation, and controls fixation. The second rotates 180 degrees to capture 25 or 50 images of the anterior segment to the level of the iris, and through the pupil to evaluate the lens. 500 true elevation data points are generated per image to yield up to 25,000 points for each surface. Data points are captured for the center of the cornea, an area that placido disk topographers and slit-scanning devices are unable to evaluate.

Elevation data measured using this technique has several advantages. Because it is independent of axis, orientation and position, it yields a more accurate representation of true corneal shape. Thus, the Pentacam's curvature map, because it is not sensitive to position, is theoretically more accurate. The elevation maps are created using one of three reference bodies: a best fit sphere, an ellipse of revolution, and toric. The best fit sphere calculation approximates the sphere as accurately as possible to the true nature of the cornea. This facilitates comparison between other topographers but is not the best fit for the aspheric cornea.

The ellipsoid of revolution is calculated from the keratometry eccentricity and the mean central radius. This reference shape correlates well with the true shape of the normal cornea.

The toric is based on the central radii and keratometry eccentricity as well. The flat and steep radii are automatically used. The toric is a good estimation for astigmatic corneas. The toric ellipsoid float display best facilitates pattern recognition of abnormalities on the front and back surfaces, such as found in keratoconus.[2] Figures 5.2 to 5.4 show the same astigmatic eye mapped using the three different reference

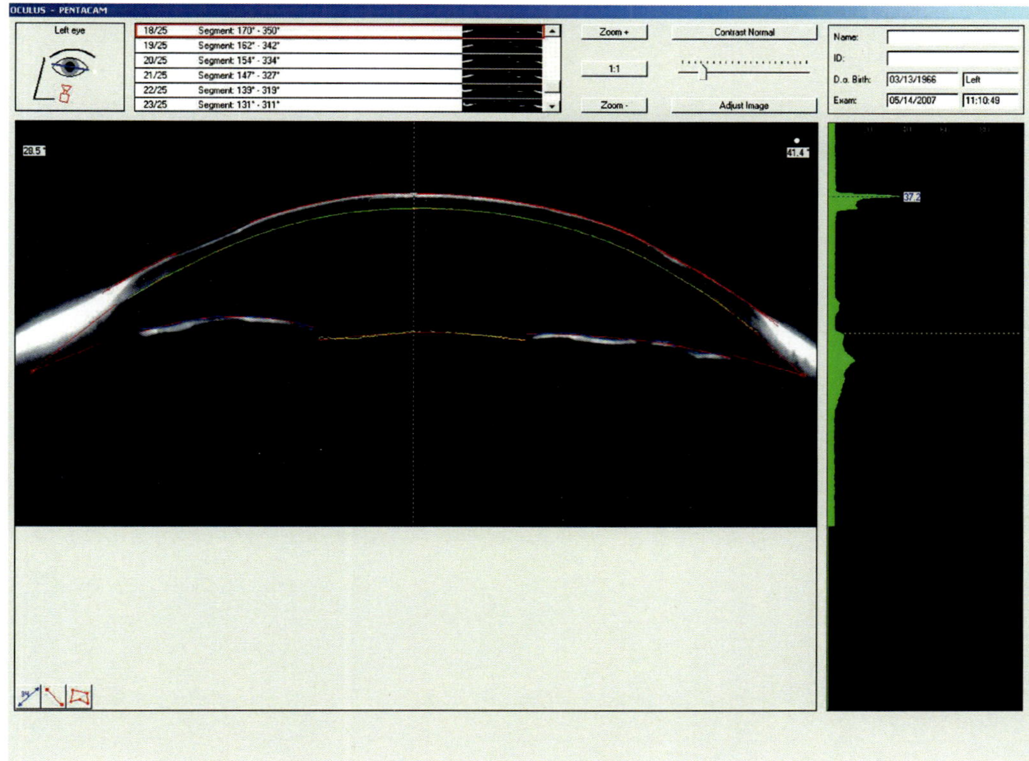

Fig. 5.1: Scheimpflug image of a flap tear. Thinning is seen secondary to loss of tissue where the flap was rotated away from the bed

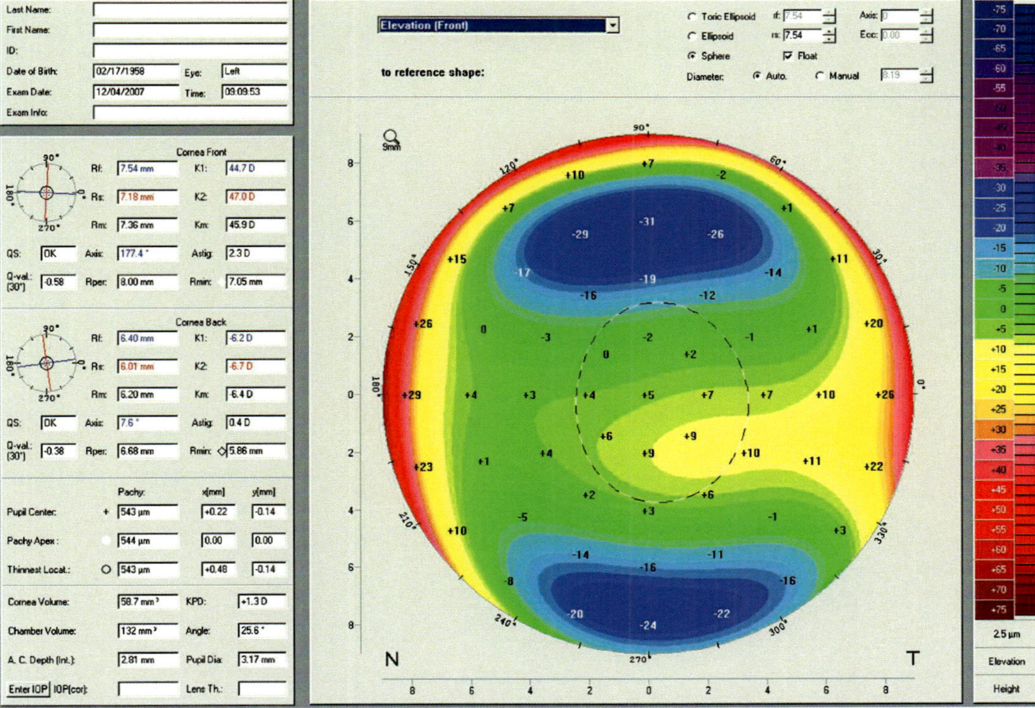

Fig. 5.2: Elevation map using the best fit sphere reference body. The astigmatism appears to be a "saddle" without a significant cone

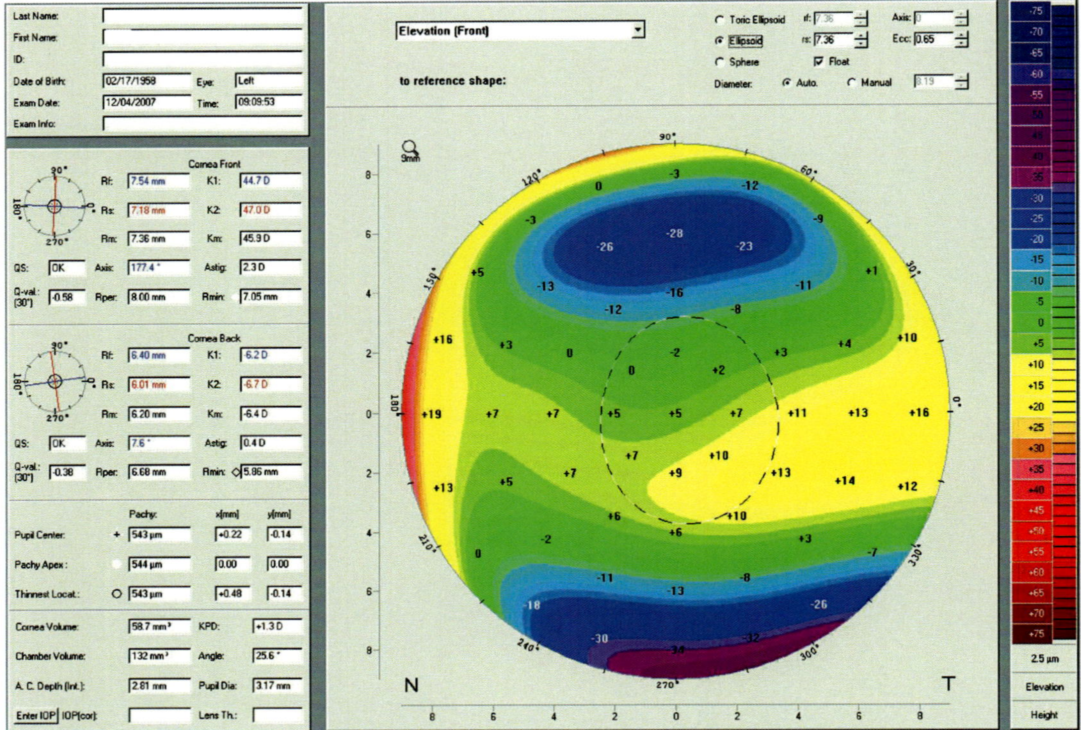

Fig. 5.3: Elevation map using the ellipse reference body

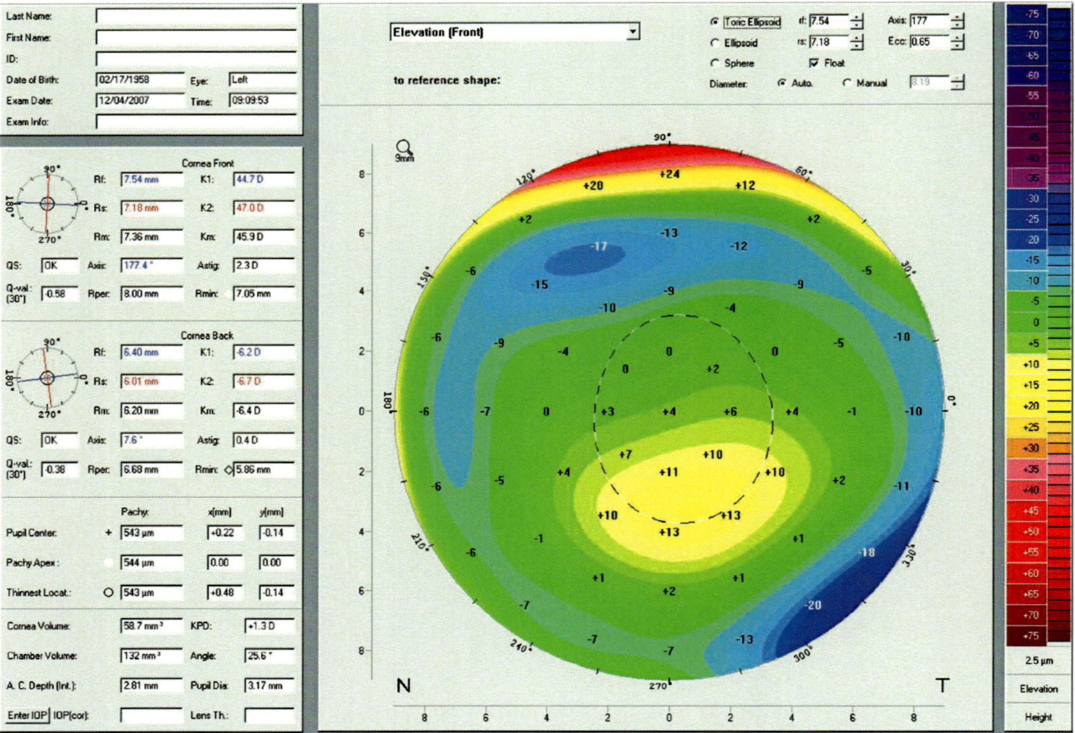

Fig. 5.4: Elevation map using the toric ellipse reference body. Note the cone is best represented using this reference body

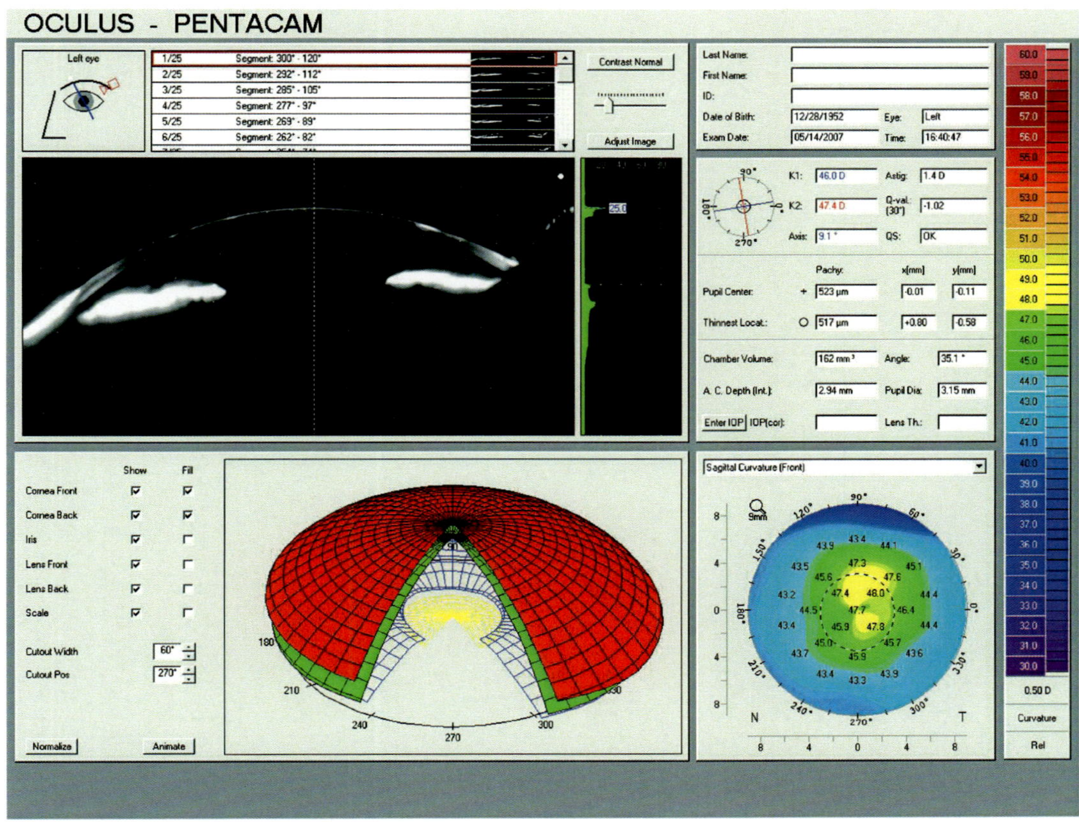

Fig. 5.5: Overview display from a patient with a history of conductive keratoplasty and cataract

bodies. The cone is easily detected using the toric ellipse reference body.

DISPLAYS

The default view presented following data capture is the "Overview display", which includes the Scheimpflug image, three-dimensional model, an additional map, keratometry, pupil, anterior chamber measurements and pachymetry. An example of an overview display in a patient with a history of conductive keratoplasty is shown in Figure 5.5. From here, other displays are typically chosen relative to the reason for scanning: surgical vision correction, keratoconus evaluation, cataract or anterior chamber evaluation, etc.

Topography and Keratometry

The Refractive and Topographic displays for the patient in Figure 5.5 are shown in Figures 5.6 and 5.7. Single maps can also be viewed by selecting the preferred single display. Several indices, listed in Table 5.1, are presented to aid in clinical diagnosis, and system set-up guidelines to facilitate pattern recognition of pathology are listed in Table 5.2. Table 5.3 lists the examination quality measures used to determine if the map is of sufficient quality or needs to be repeated. The "Quality Score", listed as QS on the printout, will be highlighted in yellow for caution and red when the map should be repeated. Note that even with the talented operators, highly irregular corneas may show QS values. Clicking on this value opens the Examination Quality Specification screen which details errors.

The two major meridians, determined using the 3 mm ring and at 90 degrees from each other, are listed as K1 (flat) and K2 (steep), with corresponding radii R1 and R2. The mean radius and mean keratometry are the arithmetic average of the corresponding

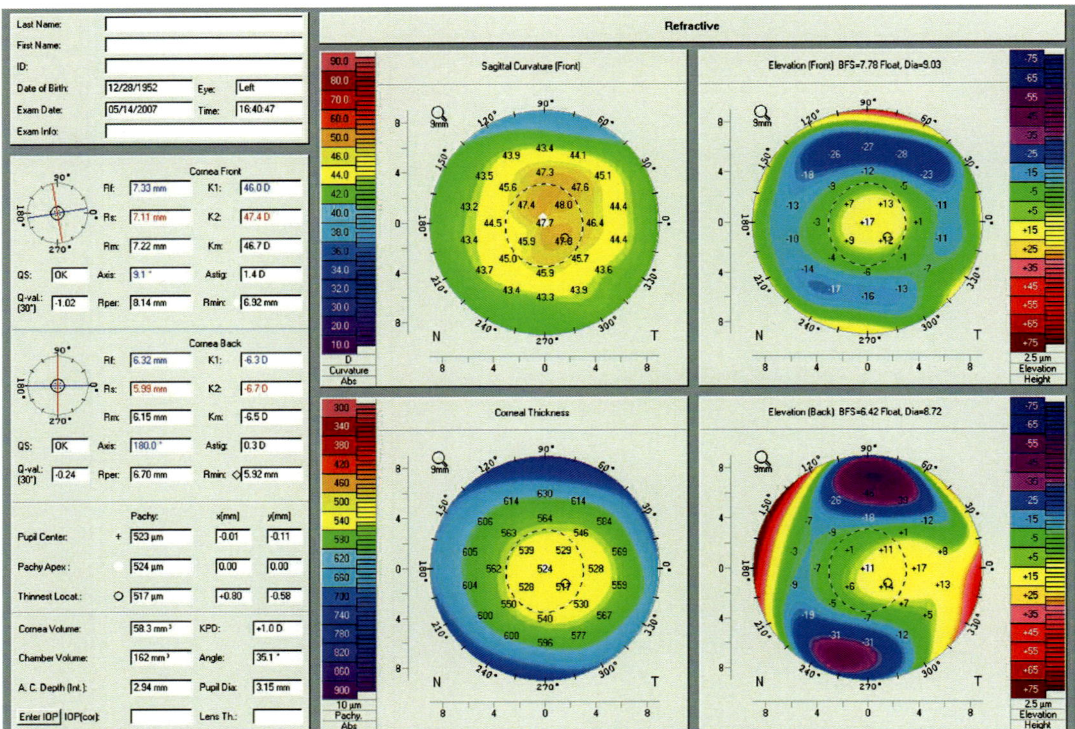

Fig. 5.6: Refractive display for the patient in Figure 5.5. It is commonly used when evaluating patients for elective vision correction

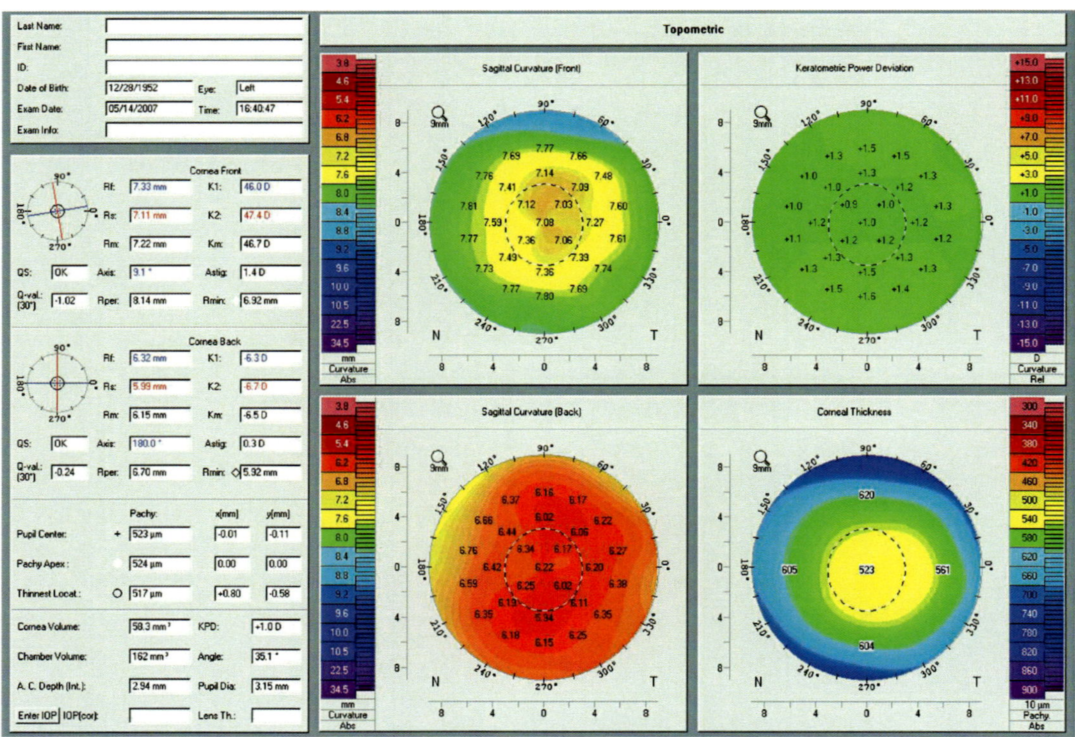

Fig. 5.7: Topometric display for the patient in Figure 5.5. It is most commonly used when fitting contact lenses

Table 5.1: Topographic indices

- ISV = Index of surface variance
  - Gives the deviation of the individual corneal radii from the mean value
  - Elevated with irregular corneas
- IVA = Index of vertical asymmetry
  - Gives the degree of symmetry of the corneal radii with respect to the 180° meridian as axis of reflection.
  - Elevated in cases of oblique axes, KC or limbal ectasias.
- IHA = Index of height asymmetry
  - Degree of symmetry of height data with respect to the horizontal meridian as axis of reflection
  - Analogous to IVA but sometimes more sensitive
- ABR = Aberration coefficient
  - Calculated on basis of Zernicke analysis
  - 0.0 is perfect system, becomes 1.0 or greater with aberrations
- KI = Keratoconus index
  - Elevated in KC
- CKI = Center keratoconus index
  - Elevated in central keratoconus
- RMin = Radii minimum
  - Smallest radius of curvature in entire field measurement
  - Elevated in KC
- IHD = Index of height decentration
  - Calculated from Fourier analysis of height
  - Gives degree of vertical decentration.
  - Steeper in KC

measures. "Astig" describes the central corneal astigmatism. The mean radii of the 7 mm and 9 mm rings are described as the "Rper".

The Q-value describes the corneal shape factor or the eccentricity of the cornea. A value of –0.26 is ideal. Highly prolate corneas with significantly higher negative values may suggest keratoconus or hyperopic treatment. Positive values suggest oblate corneas, such as those with a history of myopic treatment.

The presentation of the now widely accepted "Quad map" includes the sagital curvature, anterior and posterior elevation, and pachymetry maps. When examining the Pentacam quad map to determine candidacy for elective vision correction, the relationship between the maps must be assessed. Since the posterior surface is the first to manifest ectatic changes, inspect this map first. Elevated areas noted on the posterior surface map may correspond to a

Table 5.2: Guidelines for system set up to aid in pattern recognition

- Scans: 25
- Elevation map: Sphere fitted in float, automatic diameter
- Keratometer: Rstp/Rflat, diameter automatic
- Corneal form factor asphericity Q
  - Q < 0, indicates an untreated case
  - Q > 1, indicates a treated cornea (LASIK, PRK, RK)
- Color scale
  - Pachymetry step width normal: 10 μm
  - Topography step width normal: 1D
  - Elevation step with minimum 2.5 μm
- 4 maps refractive: similar to Orbscan quad map layout

Table 5.3: Examination quality measures

- Yellowed comments in the "Quality Score" (QS) box alert the technician to retake the examination due to suspect quality. This may read "Fix!" (Fixation) or "Model!" (severely irregular shape) to indicate the nature of the problem.
- "Analyzed Area" decreases if the eye is not opened widely, and the map should be corrected by instructing patient to open the eye widely. This must be higher than 60 percent for the anterior surface, and 50 percent for the posterior.
- "Valid Data" considers lighting conditions. It should be 95 percent for the anterior surface and 90 percent for the posterior.
- "Lost segments" represents loss of image and subsequently, data. If the number of Scheimpflug images lost due to blinking exceeds three, the image needs to be repeated.
- If the number of continuous segments exceeds two, the scan must be repeated.
- Model evaluation considers the deviation between the corneal height data points and the smooth calculation of the 3D model. The difference must be lower than 10 for the anterior surface and 14 for the posterior surface.
- Alignment (XY) describes the horizontal (X) and vertical (Y) alignment, and must be less than 1000.
- Alignment (Z) describes the distance between the patient's eye and the Pentacam, and must be less than 1000.
- "Eye movement" indicates the stability of the eye during acquisition. High values indicate excessive movement, and value should be less than 150.

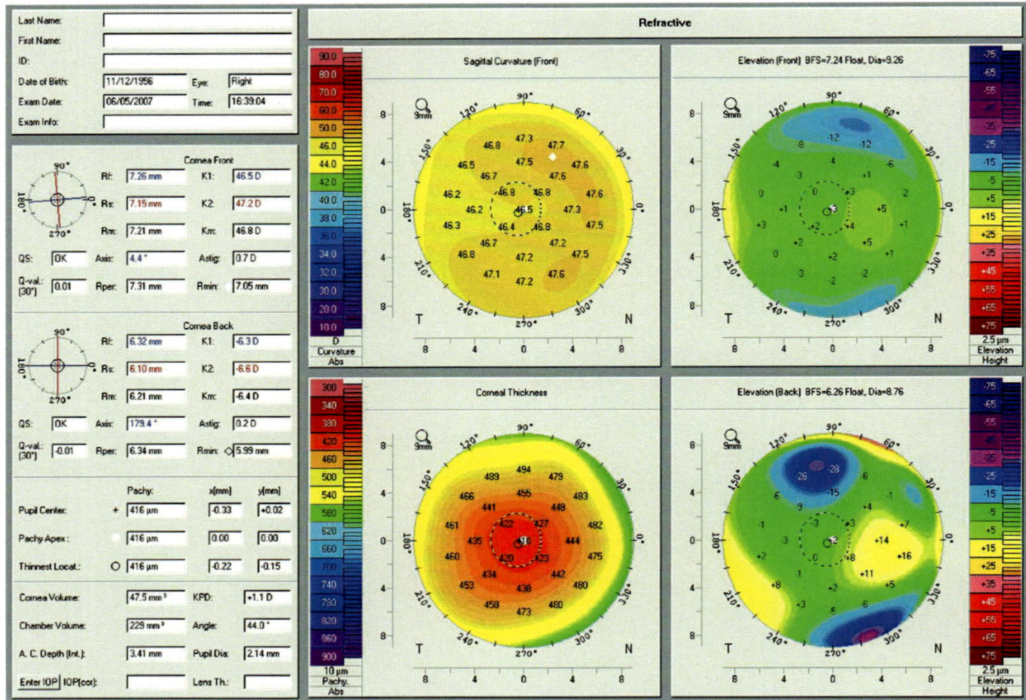

Fig. 5.8: When considering a patient for refractive surgical correction, look at the relationship between the four maps on the refractive display. This illustrates a suspicious "two point touch" where the posterior elevation corresponds to a mild anterior elevation. This patient had low pachymetry, but the pachymetry map was otherwise normal, symmetrical around the center

displaced "thinnest area" on the pachymetry map, elevated area on the anterior elevation map, and irregular astigmatism on the curvature map. Examples are shown in Figures 5.8 to 5.10. Astigmatism often manifests as a "saddle" on the posterior surface as seen in Figure 5.11 and may not be pathological. Checking the elevation map using the toric ellipse is an excellent method to ruling out ectasia in these eyes.

PACHYMETRY

Optical pachymetry is calculated from direct measurement of the anterior and posterior surface elevations. While ultrasound remains the standard for pachymetry measurement, optical pachymetry has been reported to be reproducible and reliable in the literature.[3,4] One advantage of optical pachymetry is display of values over the corneal surface (Fig. 5.12). It is important to inspect the pachymetry values relative to those around it as well as the thinnest value. One study found Pentacam provided measurements that were slightly but systematically lower than the measurements provided by ultrasonic pachymetry in normal corneas,[5] and another found measurements obtained with the Orbscan II (CF) are thinner than those obtained with the Pentacam in normal eyes.[6] Most essentially reported significant agreement with one another, but these methods may not be simply interchangeable.[7-10]

Pachymetry after PRK has been shown to be problematic for slit-scanning devices.[11,12] Corneal thickness was measured using Pentacam, Orbscan II, and ultrasonic pachymetry in unoperated eyes, and in those after myopic PRK. Authors reported following myopic PRK, the Pentacam measurement were comparable to ultrasonic pachymetry, while Orbscan measurements were thinner.[13] Pachymetry after LASIK has been shown to be variable as well.[14,15] Several studies have been published, with reports of

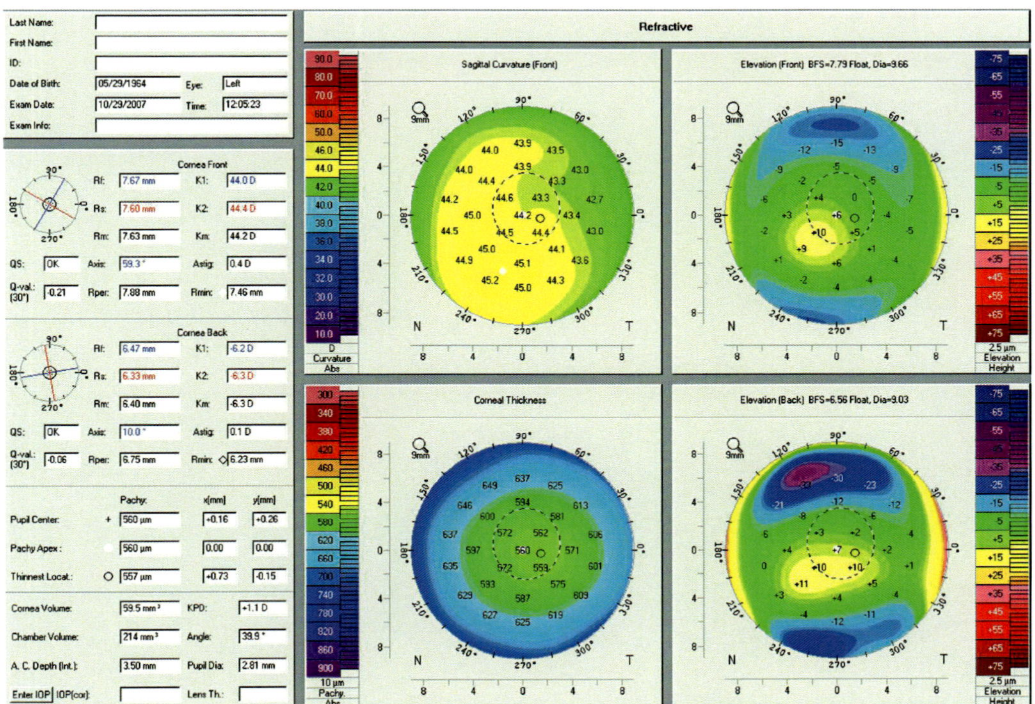

Fig. 5.9: This is an example of a "three point touch" where the elevation on the posterior and anterior surface corresponds to a steep area on the curvature map

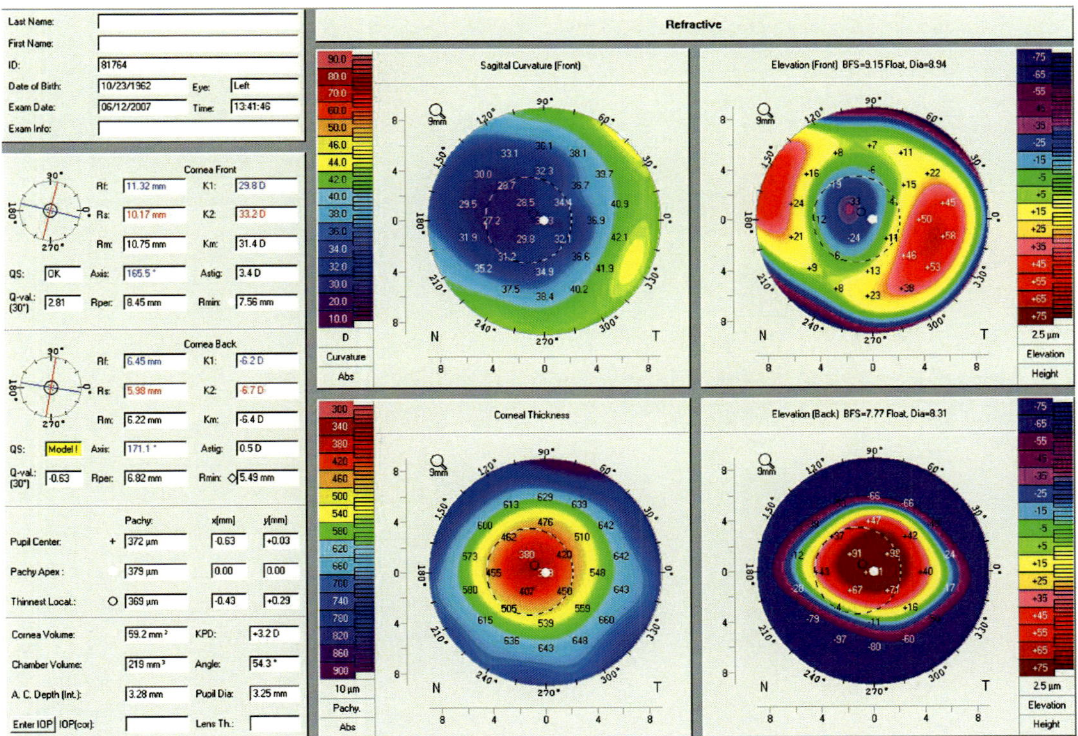

Fig. 5.10: This is an example of a classic ectasia following excimer ablation for high myopia, where all four maps show characteristic signs of ectasia

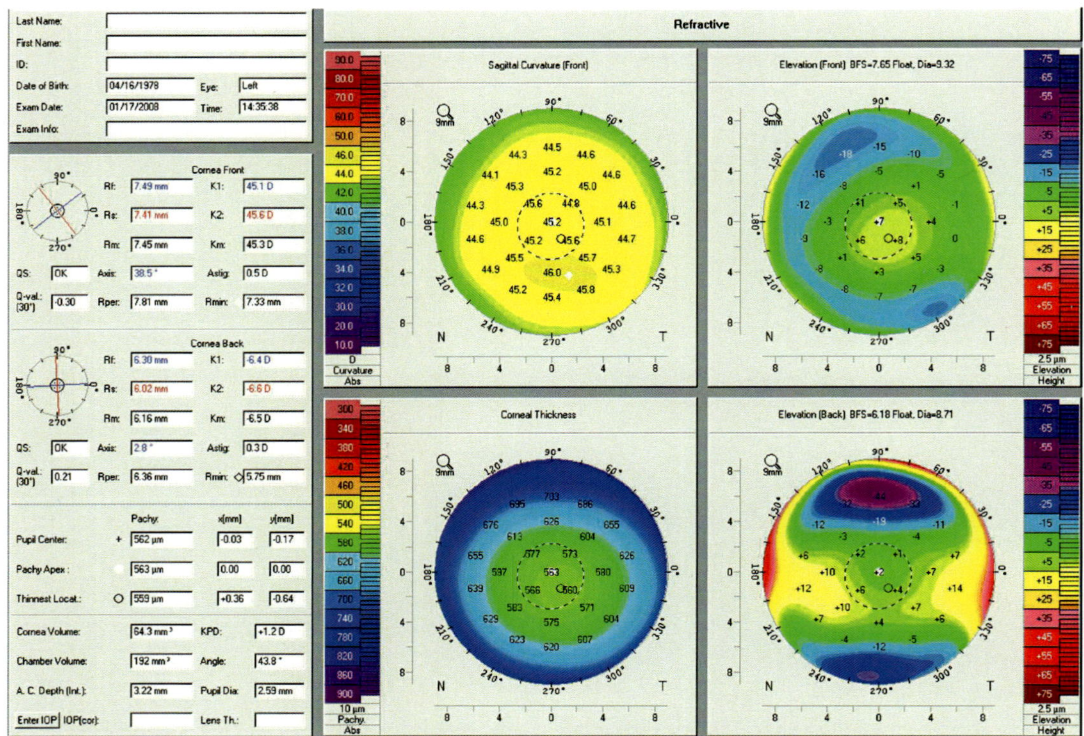

Fig. 5.11: Astigmatism manifests as a "saddle" pattern on the posterior surface

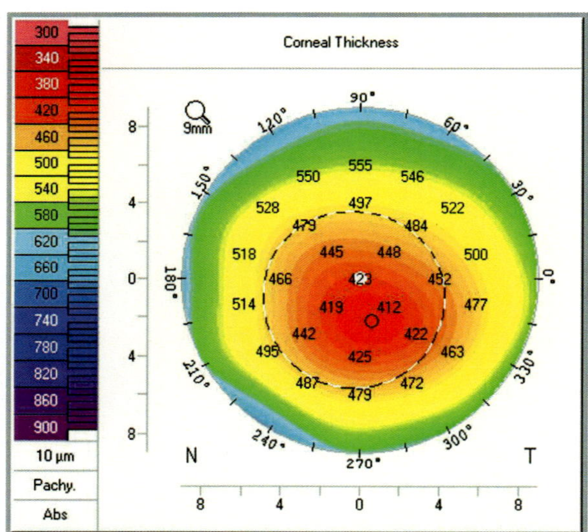

Fig. 5.12: A pachymetry map of a patient with keratoconus. Note the displacement of the thinnest point, and the overall reduction of corneal thickness

good repeatability in pachymetry measurements[16, 17] and strong correlation[18] such that authors suggested Pentacam pachymetry may be substituted for ultrasound in the post-LASIK patient.[19]

POSTERIOR SURFACE

As a tomographer, the Pentacam measures the posterior surface directly, as shown in Figure 5.13A. Calculations are based on the Gullstrand eye model. Values are negative, due to the negative refractive index of the cornea and aqueous humor. Table 5.4 lists the values suggested for clinical ectasia.

Literature reports suggest good repeatability for the posterior Best Fit Sphere (BSF),[20,21] with significant differences when compared to Orbscan (Fig. 5.13B). Hashemi et al studied LASIK patients using the Orbscan and Pentacam pre- and postoperatively. They reported that, the Orbscan II yielded larger posterior elevation values before and after surgery, and significant postoperative changes in Posterior Corneal Elevation and Posterior Maximum Elevation compared to the Pentacam.[22]

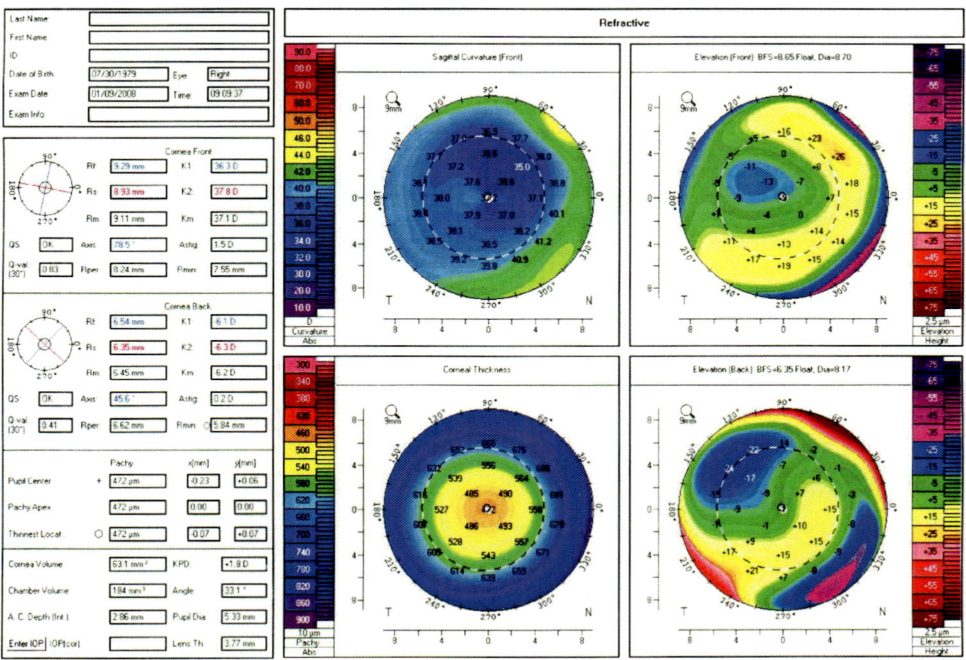

Fig. 5.13A: Posterior corneal surface in a patient with a history of LASIK using the posterior surface using the Best Fit Sphere. No significant ectasia was noted on the Pentacam, and pachymetry was similar to ultrasound value (480 microns)

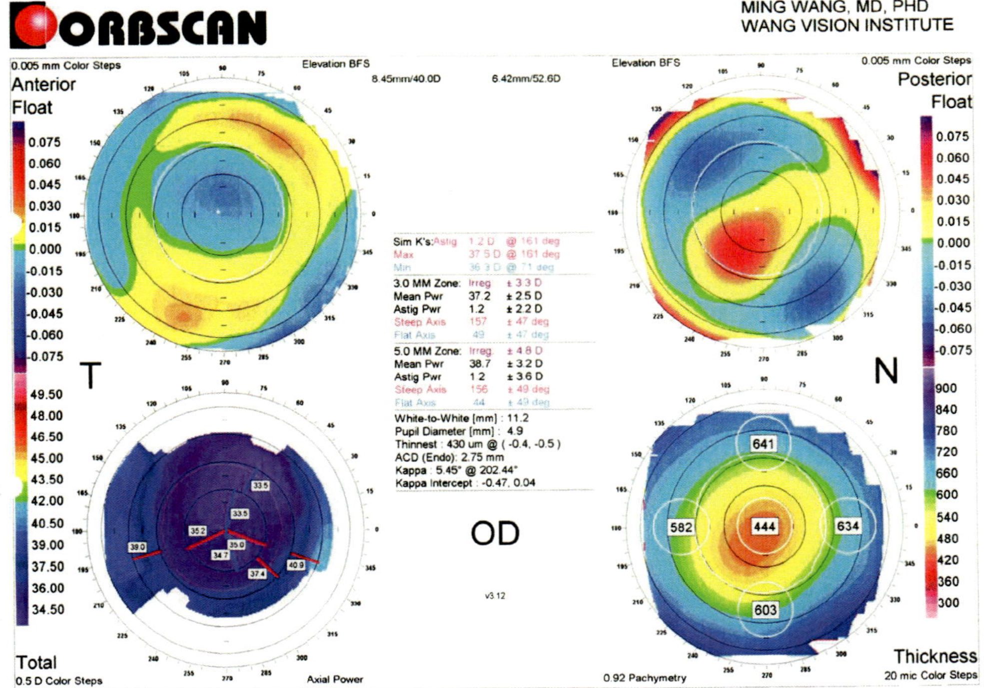

Fig. 5.13B: Orbscan quad map of the eye shown in Figure 5.13A. Note the difference in the appearance of the posterior float map, which indicates ectasia. The pachymetry was 444 microns, significantly different from 472 of Pentacam and ultrasound (480 microns)

Table 5.4: KC screening guidelines for anterior and posterior elevation

	Normal	*Suspect*	*Pathological*
Anterior	Less than 12 µm	12 to 15 µm	Greater than 15 µm
Posterior	Less than 17 µm	17 to 20 µm	Greater than 20 µm

Ciolino found no statistically significant difference in posterior corneal displacement between the LASIK and PRK patients as measured by the Pentacam and suggested ectasia may not routinely occur after LASIK.[23] Quisling et al found the Pentacam and Orbscan IIz measure similar thinnest points but differ in posterior elevations above the best-fit sphere, despite similar radii of curvature. They were not able to determine if the Pentacam underestimated posterior vault or if Orbscan overestimates the height.[24]

KERATOCONUS SCREENING

The "Keratoconus Screening" display incorporates the keratometry, pachymetry, anterior chamber information, corneal volume, and thickness assessment relative to the thinnest point. "Rings" with diameters of 1 mm, 2 mm, 3 mm, 4 mm, and 5 mm around the thinnest point are created, and mean corneal thickness and corneal thickness progression are illustrated in graphical displays, as show in Figure 5.14. Various indices, described in Table 5.1 are used to determine the level of KC risk, and suspect values appear in red, as show in Figure 5.15. Note these indices are calculated using only the anterior surface. Numerical values describing normal, suspect and pathological values for these indices are listed in Table 5.5. The KC index describes the risk of keratoconus using a 4 stage classification based on those of Amsler and Muckenhirm. Selecting "Keratoconus Level Topography" opens the table which describes classical signs of keratoconus used by the KC index. Clinical assessment must be incorporated as these should not be used for diagnosis alone.

Parameters listed on the KC display are based on studies indicating differences exist among those with KC and healthy corneas. Emre et al found that with

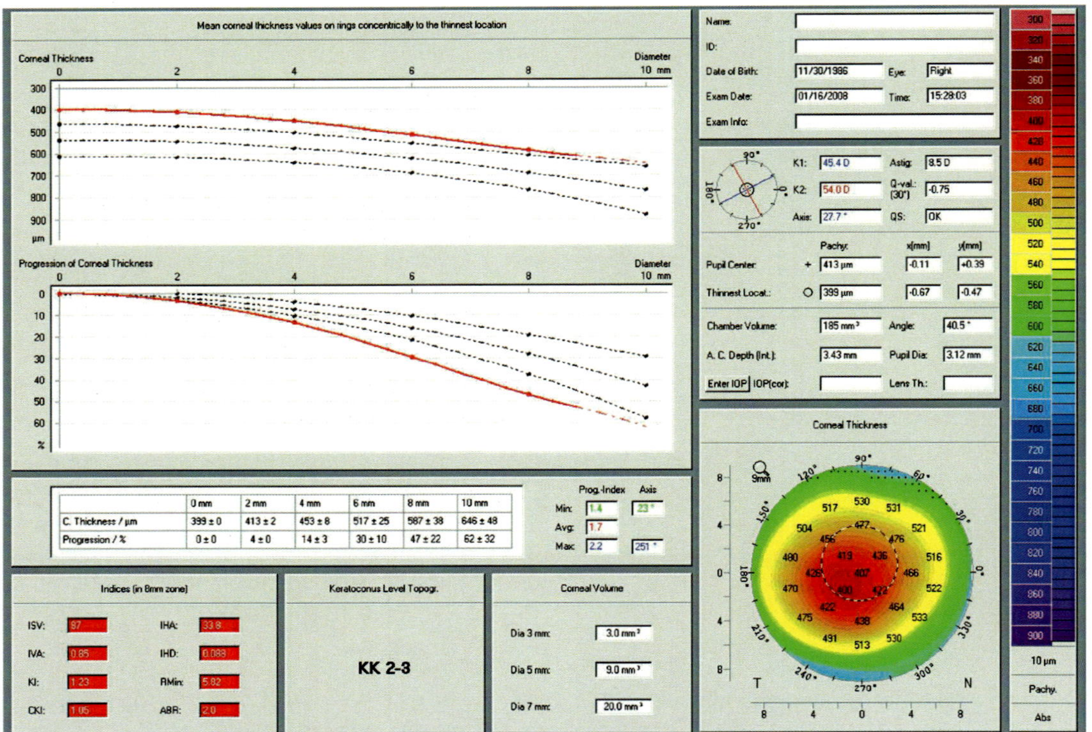

Fig. 5.14: Keratoconus display. Note suspicious indices appear yellow and red

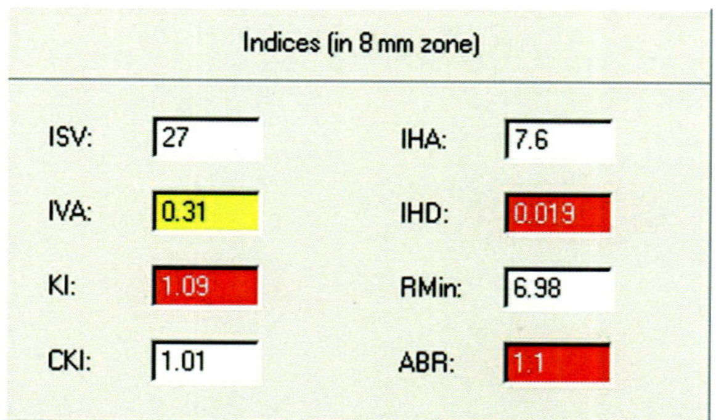

Fig. 5.15: Various indices, described in Table 5.5, are used to determine the level of KC risk, and suspect values appear in red

Table 5.5: KC index levels

Index	*Abnormal (yellow)*	*Pathological (Red)*
Index of surface variance (ISV)	≥37	≥41
Index of vertical asymmetry (IVA)	≥0.28	≥0.32
Keratoconus index (KI)	>1.07	>1.07
Center keratoconus index (CKI)	≥1.03	≥1.03
Radii minimum (Rmin)	<6.71	<6.71
Index of height asymmetry (IHA)	≥19	≥21
Index of height decentration (IHD)	≥0.014	≥0.016
Aberration coefficient (ABR)	≥1	≥1

progression of disease, total corneal thickness and anterior chamber depth were statistically different and there were statistically significant differences in anterior chamber angle and corneal volume measurements between the mild keratoconus and severe keratoconus groups.[25]

Ambrosio et al studied mild to moderate keratoconic eyes compared with normal eyes using the Pentacam. Corneal-thickness spatial profile, corneal-volume distribution, percentage increase in thickness, and percentage increase in volume were different between keratoconic corneas and normal corneas.[26]

CATARACT EVALUATION

Evaluation of cataracts can be objectively performed using Densometry, show in Figure 5.16. The tomography display (Fig. 5.17) can also be used to educate patients on the level of cataract development, and is tremendously valuable for patients presenting for elective vision correction with mild cataracts. Pentacam imaging has been reported to be helpful in the evaluation of penetrating eye injury and intralenticular foreign body,[27] as well as diagnosis and management of CBDS, posterior capsular haze,[28] and subclinical manifestations of electric cataract injuries.[29] Note that when the goal of the examination is densitometry, the 'enhanced dynamic' examination scanning mode should be selected. This lengthens the exposure time per Scheimpflug image during the scan. Progress may be monitored when the same number of images during the scans is selected upon the patient's subsequent visits.

IOL CALCULATION

The Holladay Report (Fig. 5.18) was developed to assist surgeons in calculation of IOL power in patients with a history of refractive surgery. Changes in the central topography may produce "refractive surprise", an unwanted result in this age of high patient expectation. Typical keratometry fails to estimate the true corneal power in patients with surgically altered topography. Errors result because keratometers assume the ratio of power between the anterior and posterior cornea is 82 percent, as in a virgin eye. They calculate corneal power using an index of 1.3375. Because excimer treatment alters this ratio, the calculation is inaccurate, and the lens implant power fails to properly correct the refractive error. The Pentacam calculates the front and back surface power, and produces the "Equivalent K Readings" or EKR's. The EKR's are used with IOL calculation formulas to obtain correct IOL powers for patients with surgically altered corneas.

The calculation of EKR's is related to the pupil center rather then the corneal apex as in keratometry, and utilizes the refractive power map rather than the

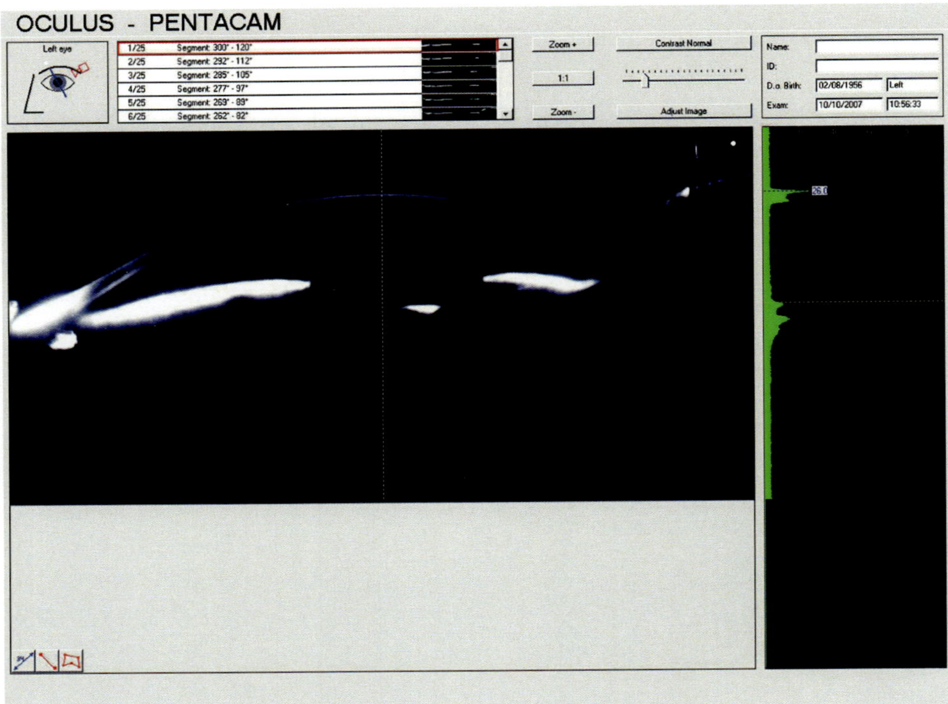

Fig. 5.16: Densitometry in a patient with an ASC. The spike in the level of opacification corresponds directly to the placement of the cursor, and allows the clinician numerical assessment of the lens to track progression of cataracts

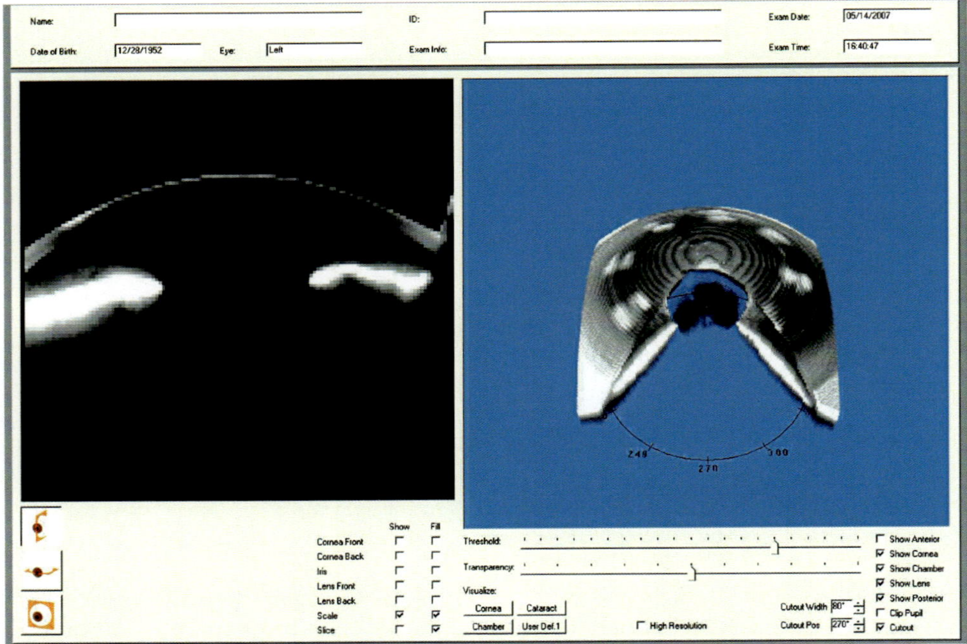

Fig. 5.17: The tomography display can also be used to educate patients on the level of cataract development, and is especially valuable for patients presenting for enhancement following keratorefractive correction with mild cataracts. This patient had a history of conductive keratoplasty and presented with complaints of decreased reading vision. Cataract surgery was recommended rather than additional refractive surgery

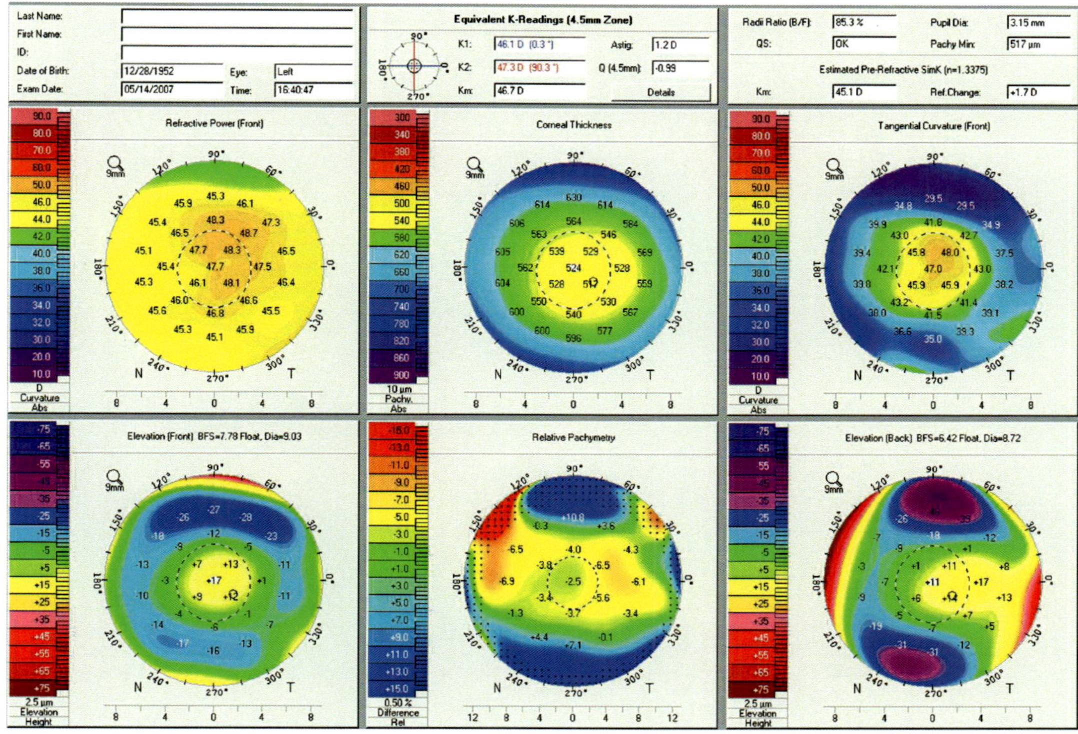

Fig. 5.18: The Holladay Report is useful when calculating intraocular lens power in patients with a history of refractive surgery

curvature map. The calculation is based on the ratio of the anterior and posterior surface radii within the 4.5 mm zone, shown to be the most pertinent for patients with a history of excimer treatment.

The detailed report (Fig. 5.19) shows the EKR's for manually selected zone measurements, and may be of value when other zones may be better options, such as in patients with a history of radial keratotomy (RK), trauma, or severe irregular astigmatism.

ANTERIOR CHAMBER EVALUATION

The Pentacam presents data regarding anterior chamber depth and volume, as well as assessment of the chamber angle. The anterior chamber display is shown in Figure 5.20. The chamber volume is calculated directly, while the distance between the cornea's posterior surface and the iris are integrated in a 12 mm diameter around the corneal apex. The angle should not be evaluated while the pupil is dilated, and may be used to evaluate patients for glaucoma risk due to narrow angle. Anterior chamber information can also be used when evaluating patients for phakic lens implants.

Nemeth et al compared the ultrasound and Pentacam Anterior Chamber Depth (ACD) measurements in phakic and pseudophakic eyes. They reported similar ACD measurements with the Pentacam and ultrasound in phakic eyes, with significantly lower measurements using the Pentacam in pseudophakes, however.[30]

Elbaz et al compared ACD measurements taken from Pentacam, ultrasound A-scan and IOLMaster (Carl Zeiss Meditach, Jena, Germany). Measurements of ACD by the Pentacam differed significantly from those of ultrasound and IOLMaster. Authors concluded measurements of ACD and corneal curvature using these machines may not be interchangeable.[31] In contrast, when comparing Pentacam and Orbscan ACD measurements, Lackner et al studied the differences of ACD values as well as inter- and

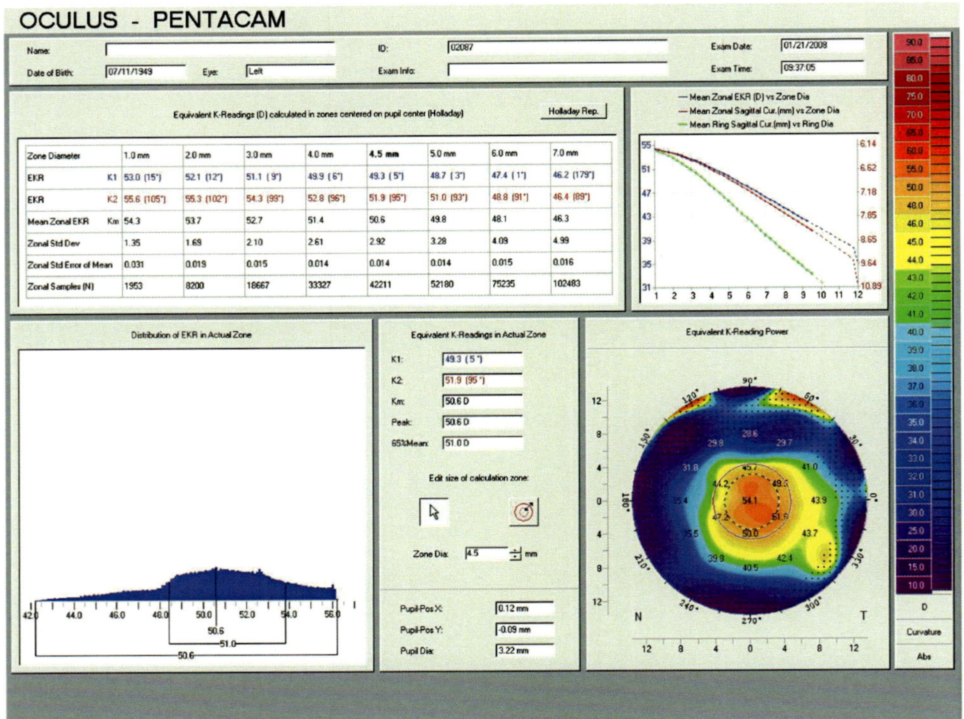

Fig. 5.19: Various optical zones may be needed for cases of severely irregular astigmatism, such as shown in the EKR detail report in a patient with a history of repeated LASIK surgeries and central corneal scarring

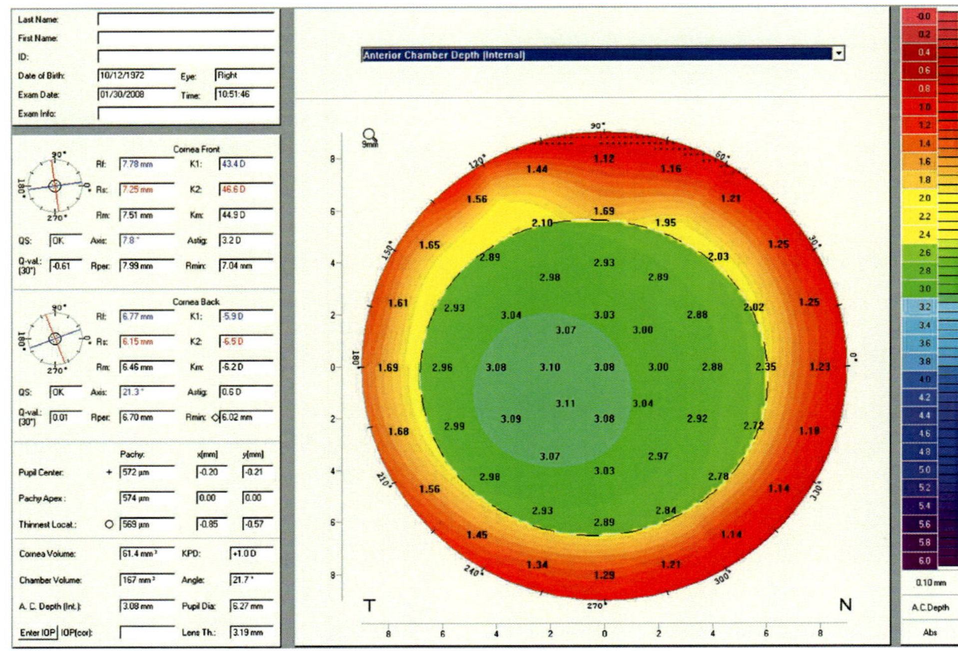

Fig. 5.20A: Anterior chamber display in a patient evaluated for increased IOP after Visian lens (Staar, Irvine, CA) implantation

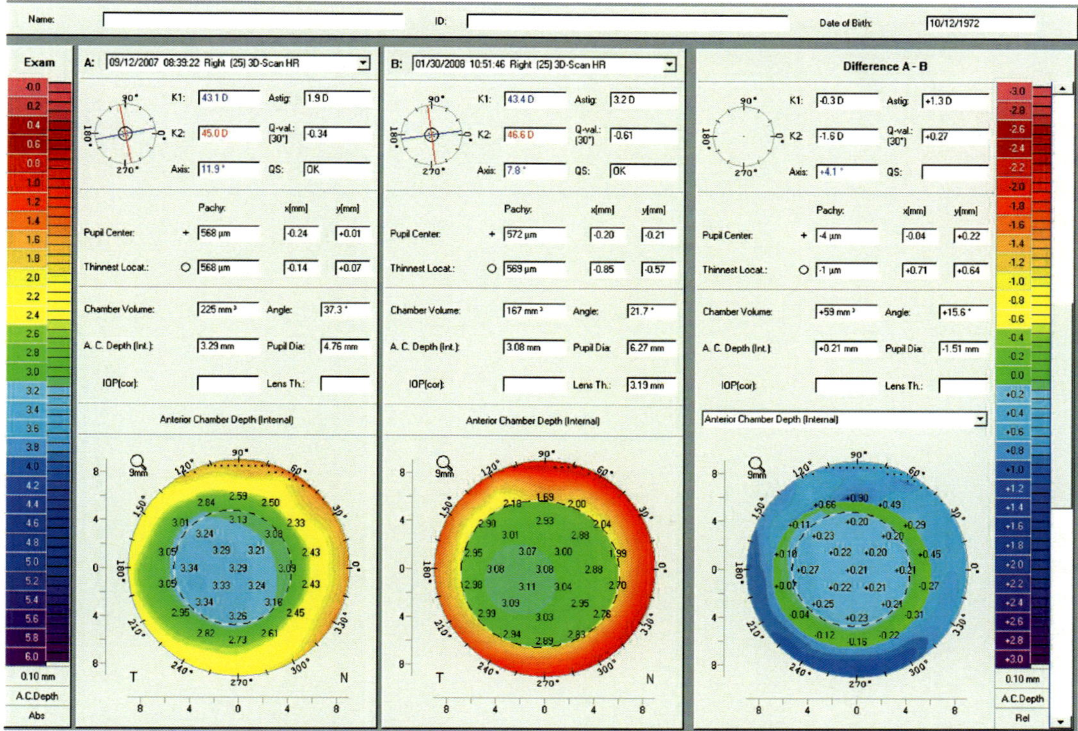

Fig. 5.20B: A difference map showing the AC information preoperatively, and after a Visian lens implantation. The plateau iris and physical bowing of the iris cause a mid-dilated pupil block, and increased pressure. The Scheimpflug image demonstrated the architecture of the iris was the cause of the pupil block. Note the decrease in the chamber angle

intraobserver variability measured with Orbscan and Pentacam were such that the two modalities can be regarded as interchangeable.[32]

Angle anatomy relative to angle-closure glaucoma may be assessed using the Pentacam as well. Rabsiber et al found the good reliability with anterior chamber assessment, and suggested the Pentacam may be used to classify the potential risk for angle-closure glaucoma.[33]

CORNEAL WAVEFRONT EVALUATION

Pentacam describes the wavefront error based on height data for the anterior and posterior surface. Note this is different from a wavefront aberrometer, which measures the whole eye wavefront error. Zernicke analysis is performed without a reference body, but rather compared to normative data (from healthy eyes). Abnormal values are highlighted for ease of detection. An Example is shown in Figure 5.21. The Zernicke coefficients are used to calculate the aberration coefficient. A value of 0 denotes no aberration. Values greater than 1.0 may be visually significant.

ANTERIOR CHAMBER PHAKIC LENS SIMULATION

The software simulation was created to assist surgeons with implantation of phakic lenses into the anterior chamber. Posterior chamber lenses cannot be imaged, as the Pentacam is not able to image structures behind the iris. Lens type and power can be chosen from the database, and software calculates the refractive lens power based on the manifest refraction entered by the clinician. Distances between the phakic lens, crystalline lens, and endothelium are displayed, and aging simulations are also available.

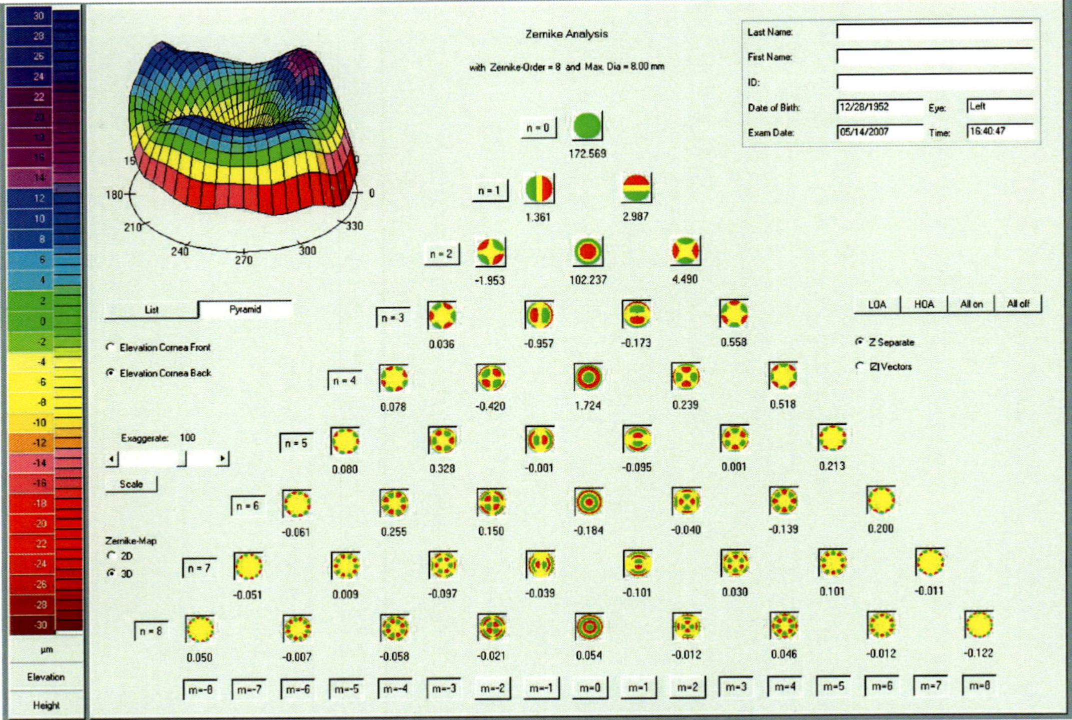

Fig. 5.21: Corneal wavefront maps for the patient in Figure 5.5 with a history of CK

The software assumes that crystalline lens grows at a rate of 18 microns per year, which over time would cause the iris to move toward the cornea with age, crowding the anterior chamber and putting the endothelium at risk.

CONCLUSION

The Pentacam serves many purposes for the refractive surgeon: elevation topography, cataract and anterior chamber evaluation, high resolution corneal imaging, corneal wavefront, pachymetry, and tomography. Applications include clinical diagnosis of ectasia, cataracts, glaucoma risk, etiology of reduced best corrected vision, and keratoconus, as well as aids for patient education. Its versatility makes it beneficial for the corneal and refractive surgeon.

REFERENCES

1. Maus M, Krober S, Swartz T, Belin M, Michaelson M, Sutphin J, et al. Pentacam. In Wang M, (Ed): Corneal Topography in the Wavefront Era, Slack, Inc; Thorofare, NJ. 2006.
2. Holladay J. Tomography and Tomography Course Handout, AAO November 5, 2007. New Orleans, LA. http://www.docholladay.com/handouts/Topography and Tomography Course Handout Color Nov07.pdf accessed January 22, 2008.
3. Lackner B, Schmidinger G, Pieh S, Funovics MA, Skorpik C. Repeatability and reproducibility of central corneal thickness measurement with Pentacam, Orbscan, and ultrasound. Optom Vis Sci 2005;82(10):892-9.
4. Barkana Y, Gerber Y, Elbaz U, Schwartz S, Ken-Dror G, Avni I, et al. Central corneal thickness measurement with the Pentacam Scheimpflug system, optical low-coherence reflectometry pachymeter, and ultrasound pachymetry. J Cataract Refract Surg 2005;31(9):1729-35.
5. O'Donnell C, Maldonado-Codina C. Agreement and repeatability of central thickness measurement in normal corneas using ultrasound pachymetry and the OCULUS Pentacam. Cornea 2005;24(8):920-4.
6. Rosa N, Lanza M, Borrelli M, Polito B, Filosa ML, De Bernardo M. Comparison of central corneal thickness measured with Orbscan and Pentacam. J Refract Surg 2007;23(9):895-9.
7. Amano S, Honda N, Amano Y, Yamagami S, Miyai T, Samejima T, et al. Comparison of central corneal thickness measurements by rotating Scheimpflug camera, ultrasonic pachymetry, and scanning-slit corneal topography. Ophthalmology 2006;113(6):937-41.

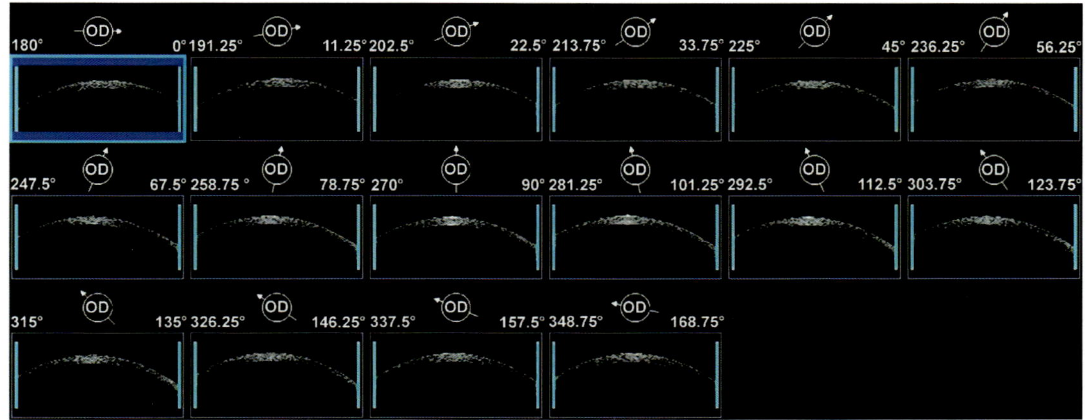

Fig. 6.3: Global pachymetric map is created from 16 modified high res images as noted in this figure

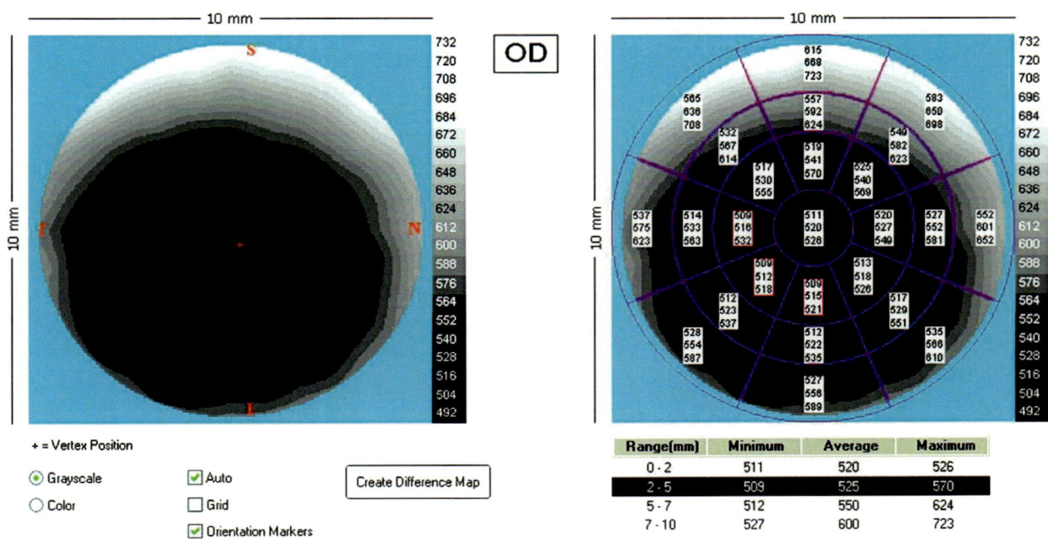

Fig. 6.4: Global pachymetric map of the right eye, shows an infero-temporal thinning of the cornea

California, USA). Slight interior steepening of the right eye prompted concerns of possible forme fruste keratoconus. A Global Pachy Map of both eye (Figs 6.3 to 6.5) revealed an infero-temporal thinning, consistent with bilateral infero-temporal steepening on the topography. Diagnosis of forme fruste keratoconus was confidently made and patient was encouraged to continue with his regular corrective methods and not consider excimer laser therapy at this time.

To counter balance the previous example, here is a case of a 13-year-old male patient with rapidly progressive keratoconus. He underwent standard penetrating keratoplasty 11 months earlier in his left eye. In the span of 11 months his keratometric measurement in his fellow right eye has progressed from mean of 48 diopters to 58 diopters. His vision has also declined from best corrected 20/20 to 20/400. In his preoperative evaluation for IntraLase Enabled Keratoplasty, the Pachy Map (Fig. 6.6)

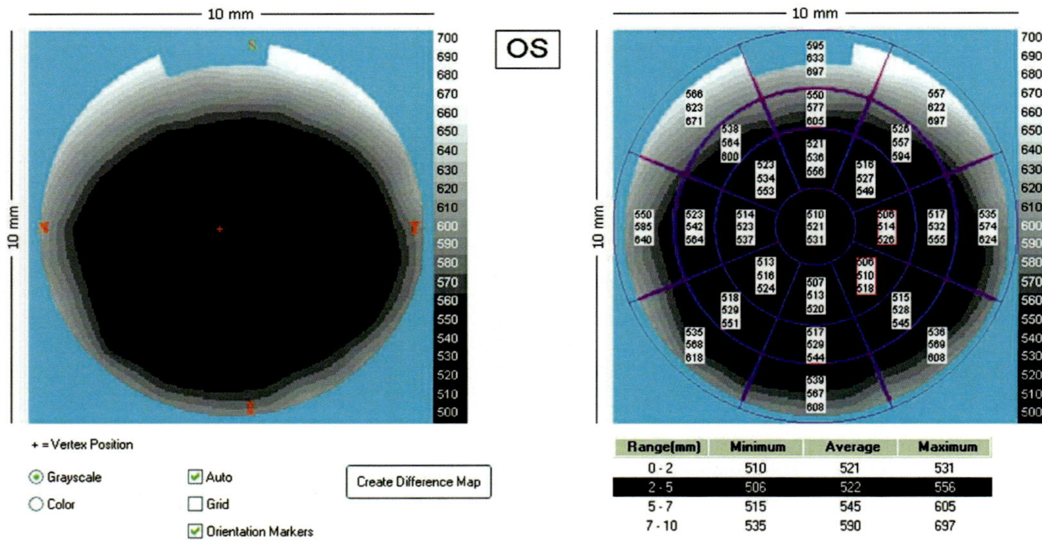

Fig. 6.5: Global pachymetric map of the left eye showing infero-temporal thinning of the cornea

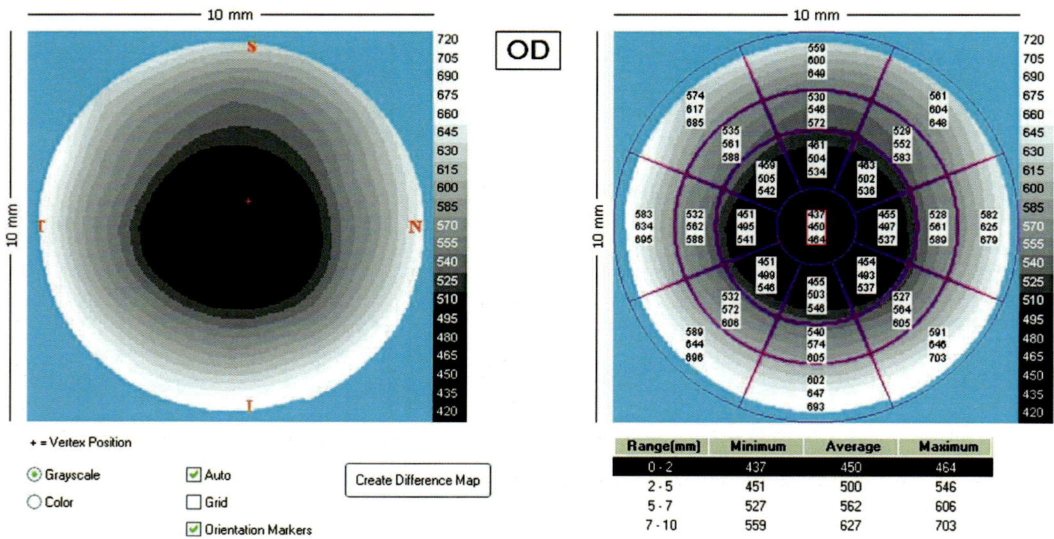

Fig. 6.6: Pre-IntraLase enabled keratoplasty Visante pachymetric mapping of patient with advanced keratoconus and central keratometric readings of 58 diopters

revealed a perfectly normal pattern of pachymetric distribution, despite the clearly pathologic cornea. This case is to demonstrate that one must consider the pachymetric mapping only as an augmentation of information in consideration of LASIK surgery and may appear normal despite such advanced pathology.

Angle Evaluation

In case of a refractive patient, one must never overlook the ophthalmic care that may be required. A fifty-five-year-old female patient with 2.00 diopters of hyperopia presented for LASIK eye surgery. Preoperative Visante evaluation, Figure 6.7, revealed narrow angles of approximately 10 degrees.

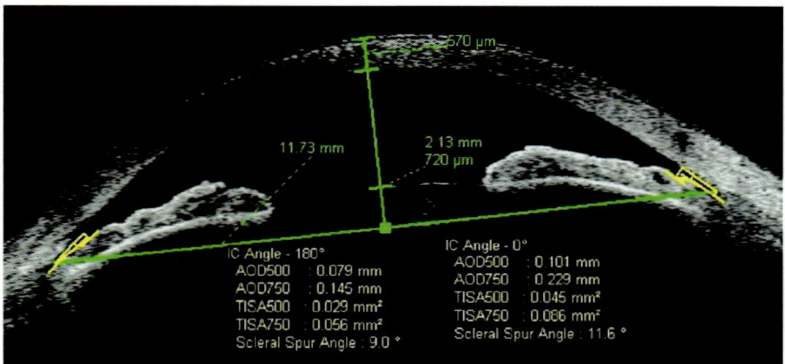

Fig. 6.7: Preoperative evaluation of the anterior segment of a patient with 2 diopters of hyperopia in consideration of LASIK

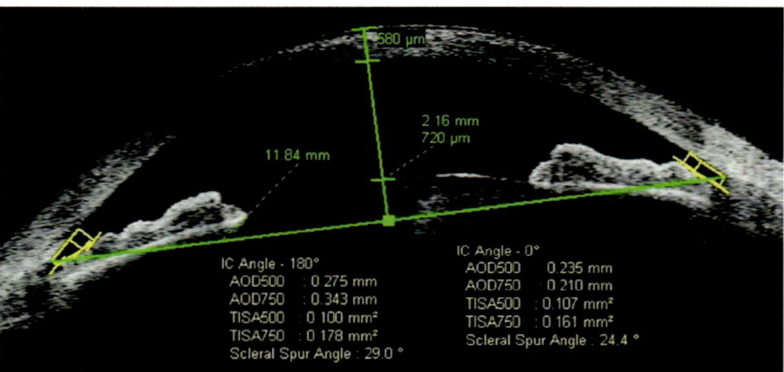

Fig. 6.8: Post-iridotomy evaluation of the same patient as Figure 6.1, showing greater opening of the angle and flatting of the posterior pigmented iris line

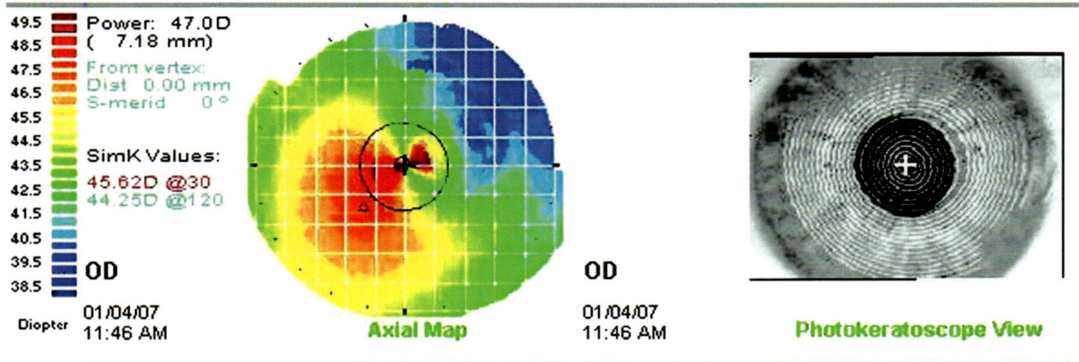

Fig. 6.9: Corneal topography prior to PRK showing area of flattening associated with corneal scar at 2 o'clock paracentral position

Moderate anterior bowing of the posterior iris pigmented line can be noted. Peripheral iridotomies were performed weeks prior to her LASIK eye surgery. After the iridotomy (Fig. 6.8), despite the fact that the pupil is larger compared to the pre-operative image, the angles are significantly more open at approximately 25 degrees with near complete flattening of the posterior pigmented iris lines. As compared with standard slit lamp gonioscopic examination of the eye, the angle is identified quantitatively with multiple methods of calculated angle area and distance measurements. Trabecular-iris space area (TISA) and angle opening distance (AOD) are both measured at 500 microns and 750 microns away from the scleral spur. The AOD is defined as the distance perpendicularly away from the trabecular meshwork/endothelial surface to the surface of the iris. The TISA is a trapezoidal area bordered by the AOD at 500 µm or 750 µm, and a line drawn perpendicularly from the scleral spur to the iris. The ability to acquire and present all this information in real-time to a patient represents a major advance in both diagnosis and patient education.

Corneal Pathology

A forty-four-year-old female contact lens user has developed a corneal ulcer in her dominant eye five years earlier with complete healing and resolution; however, best corrected visual acuity had been reduced to 20/40. The patient was seeking consultation for LASIK eye surgery. Her cornea was noted to have a paracentral scar with concordant flattening on the topographic map (Fig. 6.9). Her preoperative refraction was –4.00-1.50 × 110 leading to 20/40 vision. The Visante was used to measure the depth of tissue

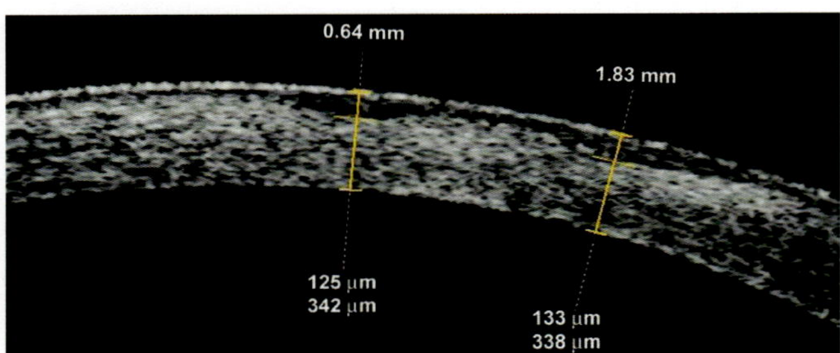

Fig. 6.10: Corneal scar of the same patient as Figure 6.9 showing loss of corneal tissue and filling with epithelium

loss, epithelial filing and the corneal scar (Fig. 6.10). A decision was made to correct this eye conservatively with stepwise approach. As such treatment of only –2.25-1.50 × 110 was delivered via photorefractive keratectomy. Six months after the PRK patient was elated with 20/25+ uncorrected visual acuity and correctable to 20/20 with plano –0.75 × 135. The corneal topography (Fig. 6.11) can also be noted to have improved mire rings. The corneal scar although not obliterated by the excimer laser was reduced in thickness and opacity intensity (Fig. 6.12). Additionally, the epithelial pooling over the depressed scar area is also noted to be significantly less. It can also be noted that the Bowman's membrane noted as a black line under the white epithelium in Figure 6.10 is obliterated and nonexistent in Figure 6.12 after PRK.

Flap Evaluation

In evaluation of post-operative LASIK patients who may be considering enhancement, the Visante can provide detailed information that would be essential to the safety of the procedure. The Visante can provide details of corneal flap shape and regularity. The LASIK flaps are created using either a mechanical microkeratome or a femtosecond laser. An example of a mechanical microkeratome flap, created using the Amadeus II (Ziemer Ophthalmic Group AG, Switzerland) (Fig. 6.13) can be noted to have a tapered edge with thicker peripheral flap and

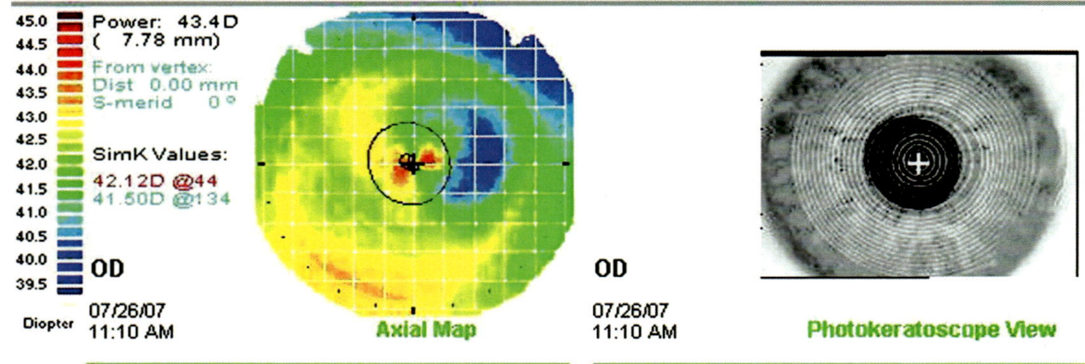

Fig. 6.11: Corneal topography of the same patient as Figure 6.9 after her PRK

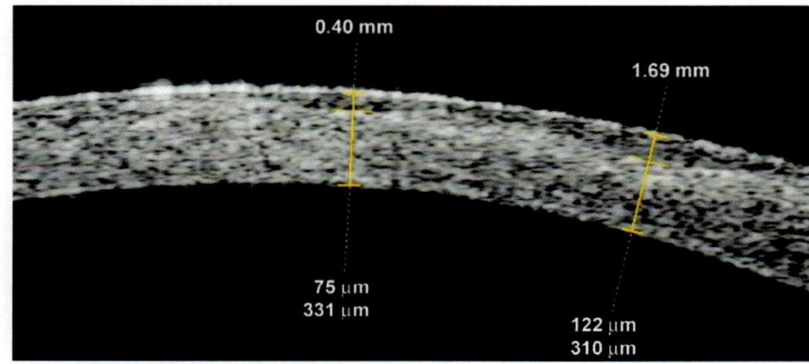

Fig. 6.12: Corneal scar of the same patient as Figure 6.9 after PRK

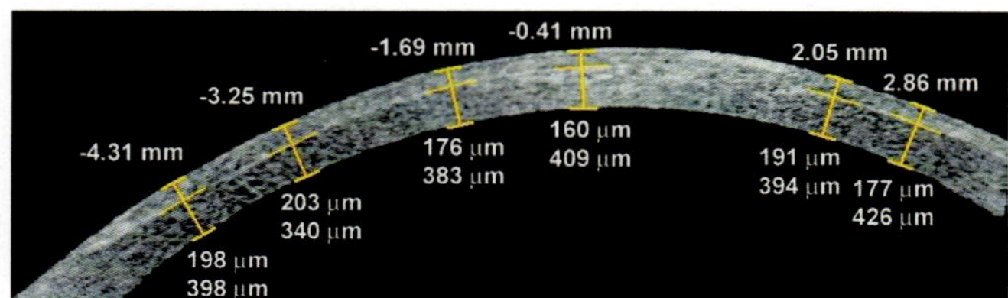

Fig. 6.13: Amadeus II microkeratome created flap showing the tapered flap edge and meniscus flap configuration

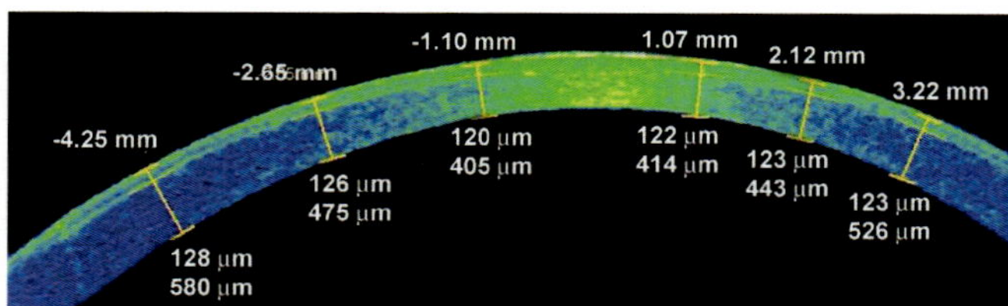

Fig. 6.14: IntraLase created LASIK flap with vertical edge and linear flap configuration

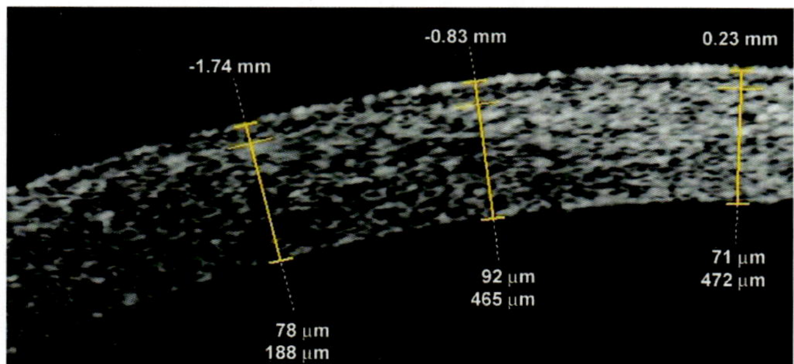

Fig. 6.15: Patient asking for enhancement 5 years after initial LASIK surgery

thinner central flap. This configuration is referred to as the meniscus flap. An example of a femtosecond laser flap created using the IntraLase (Advanced Medical Optics, Inc, Santa Ana, California, USA) shows a sharp 70 degree flap edge and an evenly thick flap throughout (Fig. 6.14). This flap configuration is referred to as the linear flap

A thirty-five-year-old male patient had LASIK eye surgery 5 years previously elsewhere and no records were available. A LASIK flap with jagged edge could be noted peripherally. The Visante was able to demonstrate presence of a very thin LASIK flap (Fig. 6.15). A decision was made to perform a surface ablation rather than to try to lift the previous LASIK flap. The patient obtained 20/15 vision postoperatively.

A thirty-five-year-old female with a refraction of –8.00-2.75 × 020 with central corneal thickness of 515 microns had CustomVue, IntraLase LASIK eye surgery with Iris Registration (iLASIK) (Advanced Medical Optics, Inc., Santa Ana, California, USA). One can note in Figure 6.16, the central residual stromal bed remaining after the initial iLASIK is only in the range of 280 microns. Postoperative refraction stable

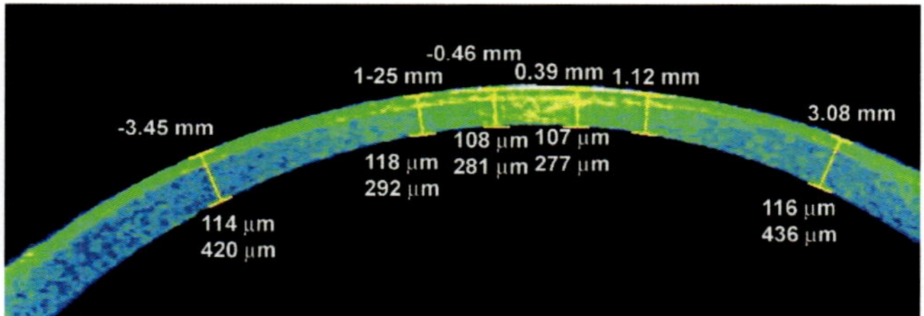

Fig. 6.16: Highly myopic patient after iLASIK in need of minor enhancement

over 6 months is –0.25-1.75 × 010. There may be as many opinions and options regarding the safety of LASIK and its enhancements in this patient as there are residual microns left, but the data provided allows the individual patient and surgeon to discuss the plan and practice the art of medicine in this case. In this iLASIK case one may note the 70 degrees flap edge on the left side of the image and the linear flap thickness created by the IntraLase femtosecond laser. Although the range of the flap thickness is measured from 107 to 118 microns, one must also note the limitation in gradation of the flap tool in the Visante software that may be stepwise and in accordance to the resolution limits of the hardware. In specific, the axial resolution of the Visante is 18 microns and has a repeatability of +/– 7 microns in measurement of the flap and +/– 11 microns in the measurement of the stromal tissue. It should also be noted that flap visibility is diminished over time. The sensitivity at 1 day is noted at 99 percent, and 95 percent at 6 months.

Complication Evaluation

A thirty-eight-year-old male, who had LASIK eye surgery 8 years previously elsewhere with no records available, presented for LASIK enhancement. The Visante was able to clearly demonstrate the flap and residual stromal bed thickness. Patient was assured that LASIK enhancement via lifting of the flap could be performed. The patient however developed epithelial ingrowth post-enhancement. The patient with uncorrected 20/15 vision after the enhancement chose not to have any intervention. The Visante is able to identify the leading edge of the epithelial ingrowth and allow for very precise monitoring overtime. The

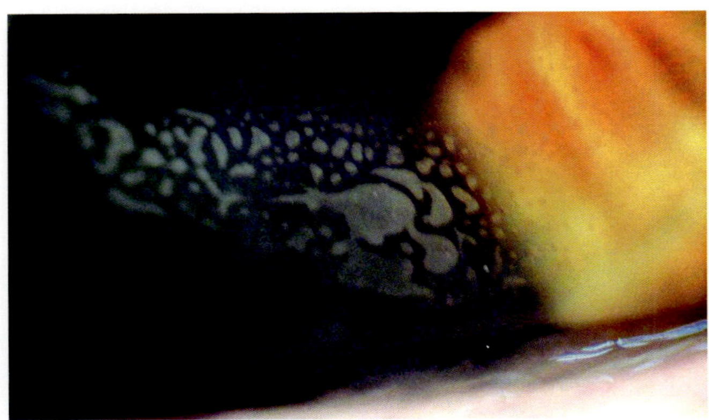

Fig. 6.17: Epithelial ingrowth after LASIK enhancement

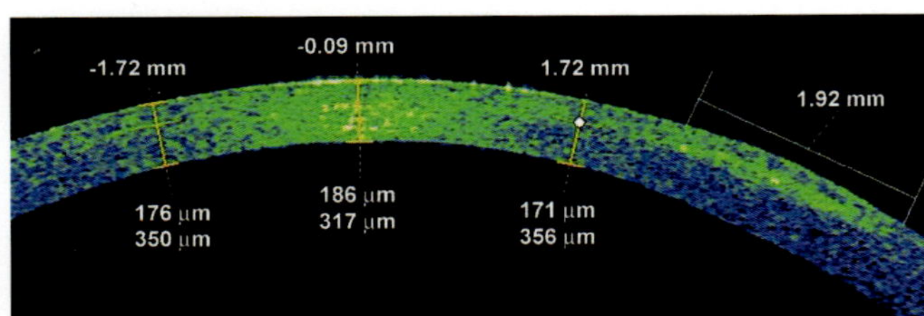

Fig. 6.18: Visante (standard High Res Mode) 2 months after LASIK enhancement

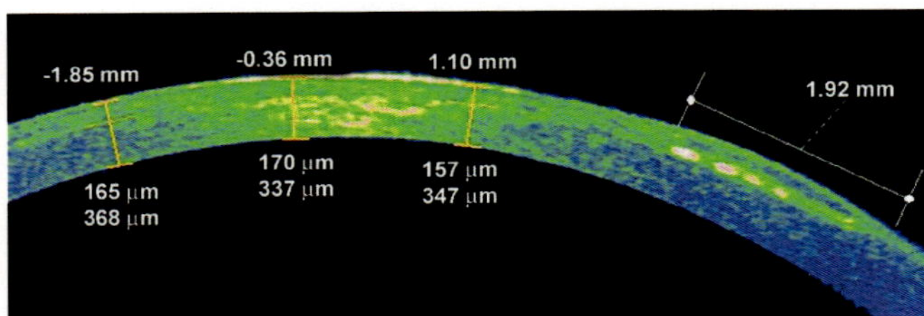

Fig. 6.19: Visante (Enhanced High Res Mode) 8 months after LASIK enhancement

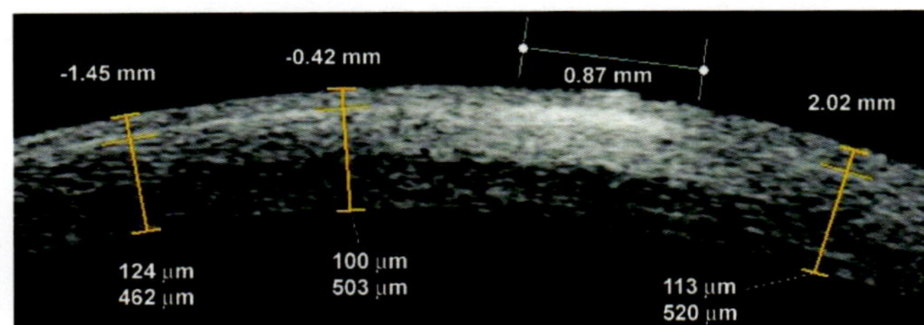

Fig. 6.20: Visante image of inter-flap space ulcer

clinical appearance of the epithelial ingrowth at 2 months can be noted in Figure 6.17. The Visante Image (Fig. 6.18), in regular High Res Mode in rainbow color scheme, performed at 2 months after the LASIK enhancement demonstrates the leading edge of the epithelial ingrowth from the flap edge. At a follow-up visit 6 months later (8 months postoperative) clinical appearance was unchanged. The Visante Image (Fig. 6.19), was however acquired in the Enhanced High Res Mode. In this Enhanced format, 4 high resolution images are composited together to provide an enhanced view with reduced graininess and increased contrast within the image. Please note that the epithelial ingrowth on the Visante has remained identical.

A sixty-three-year-old male patient, one year post-LASIK, acquired a new kitten. The kitten with her very sharp, narrow claws punctured the LASIK flap and seeded the inter-stromal space with a small infiltrate forming ulcer (Fig. 6.20). The ulcer was treated conservatively with very close evaluation intervals, without lifting of the flap, with combined aminoglycoside (tobramycin) and fluoroquinolone (moxifloxacin) for complete resolution without any loss of visual acuity.

A fifty-six-year-old male patient with history of initial refractive errors of –0.50-3.00 × 050 right eye and –0.75-2.25 × 115 left eye with pre-LASIK corneal topographies as noted in Figure 6.21 underwent LASIK eye surgery elsewhere. The patient later underwent 2 enhancement procedures for correction of residual refraction in the right eye and one enhancement procedure in the left eye. Patient presented for second opinion in regards to his progressively declining vision. The Visante (Fig. 6.22) was able to demonstrate that despite the residual stromal tissue of at least 300 microns, ectasia of the cornea was clearly notable. Patient underwent a corneal transplant surgery for the right eye and was fitted with hard contact lens in the left eye.

As demonstrated in the case presentations above, the Visante anterior segment OCT is very useful in evaluation of LASIK patients preoperatively. Evaluation of the corneal pachymetric map as an adjunct to the corneal topographic map and quantitative assessment of the angles are examples. The postoperative care is also enhanced in evaluation of patients for

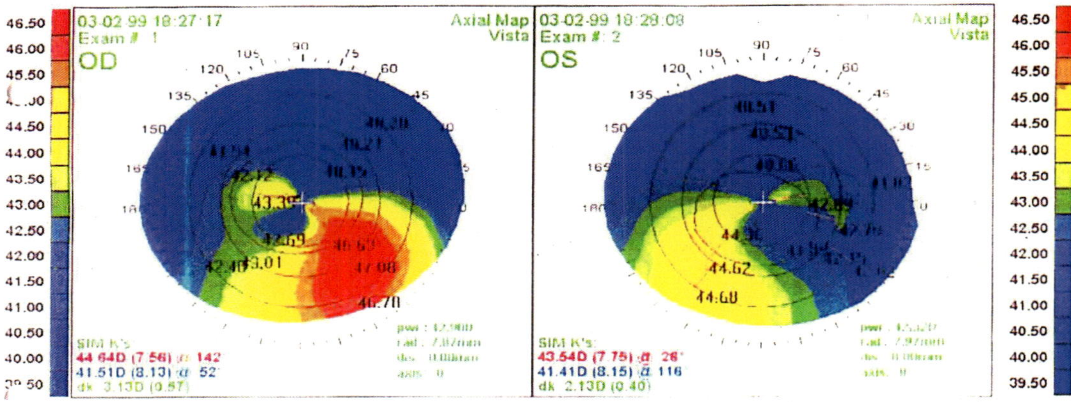

Fig. 6.21: Pre-LASIK topography of patient in Figure 6.22

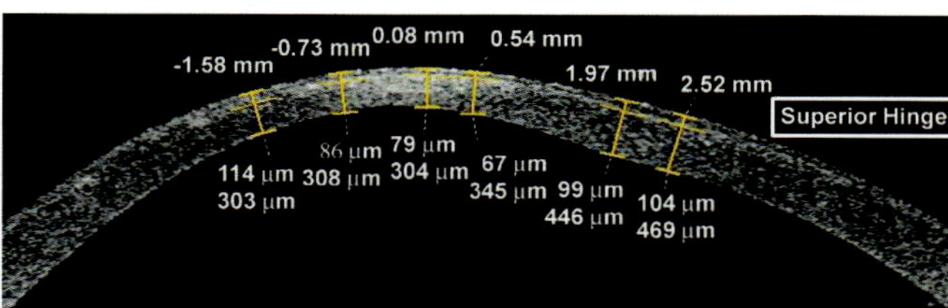

Fig. 6.22: Corneal Ectasia after LASIK

enhancement and also for management of complications.

PHAKIC INTRAOCULAR LENSES

Phakic intraocular lenses (phakic IOLs) are relatively new in the United States market. However, they have enjoyed much greater acceptance and use internationally. At the time of writing this chapter in January 2008, there are only two approved phakic IOLs that are approved by the United States Food and Drug Administration, the Verisyse (Advanced Medical Optics, Inc., Santa Ana, California, USA), and the Visian ICL (Staar Surgical, Inc., Monrovia, California, USA). Both of the phakic IOLs are only approved for correction of myopia in the USA. The Verisyse is an anterior chamber lens that is enclavated to the iris (Fig. 6.23). The Visian ICL is a posterior chamber lens that rests in the sulcus space anterior to the crystalline lens. There are many other lenses available in the international markets and also in clinical trials in the United States.

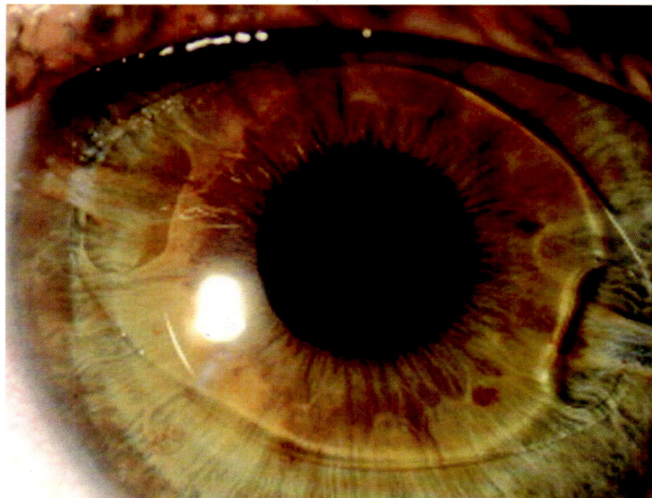

Fig. 6.23: Image of an eye implanted with Verisyse

Endothelial Clearance

The inner lining of the cornea is populated by the corneal endothelium cells. With placement of the phakic IOLs, there is always a concern of the lifetime consequences that placement of these prostheses may pose on the population of these cells. Two of the risk factors noted and emphasized by Advanced Medical Optics, Inc., are the 1.5 mm minimal clearance of the anterior aspect of the prosthesis to the corneal endothelium and the minimum anterior chamber depth of 3.2 mm. AMO has a computer software program called the VeriCalc. This program requires the patient's prescription in sphere and cylinder, along with anterior chamber depth and the corneal keratometric

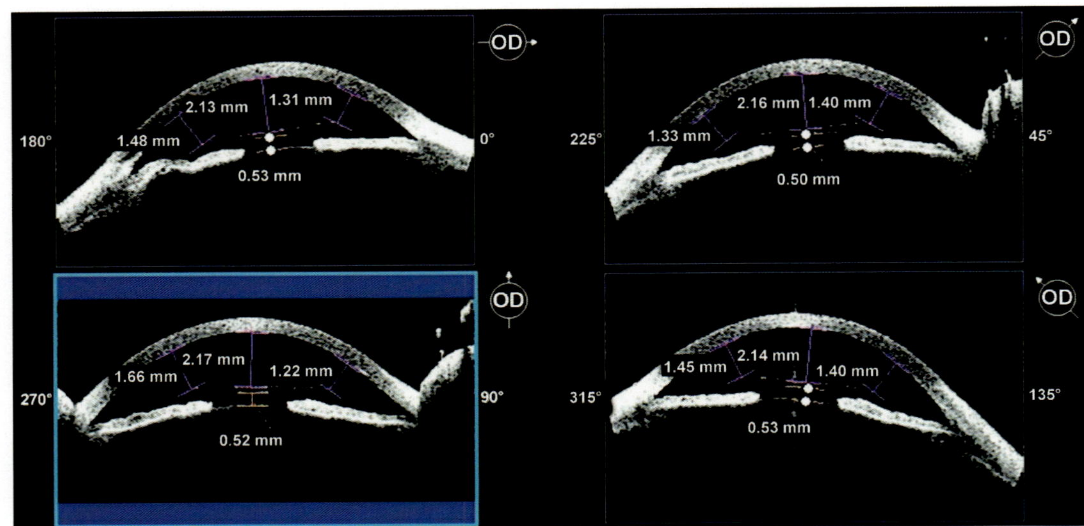

Fig. 6.24: Visante images (Quad scan) of the right eye implanted with Verisyse

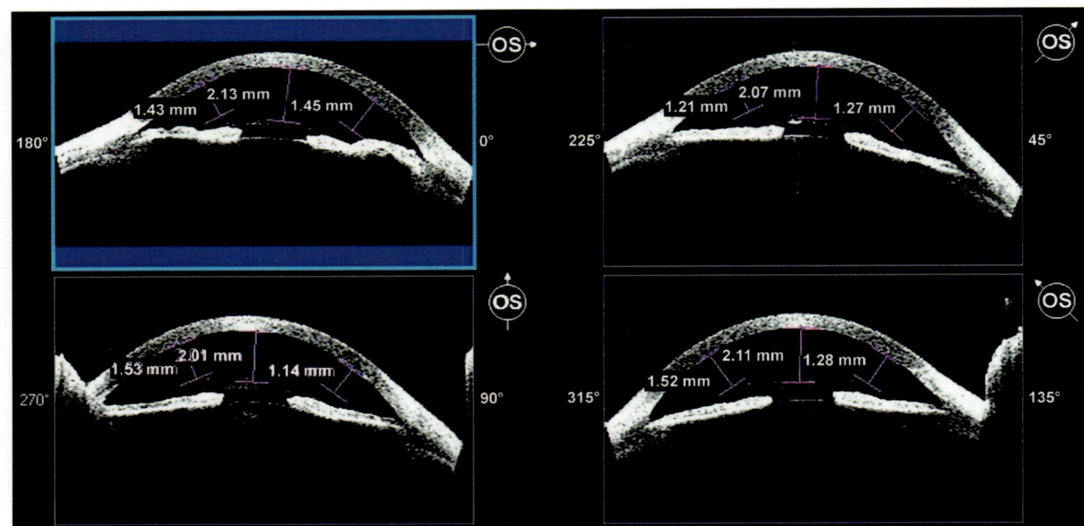

Fig. 6.25: Visante images (Quad scan) of the left eye implanted with Verisyse

measurements. Although the VeriCalc is helpful, the Visante with its new phakic IOL module may provide a much more accurate assessment of acceptable implantation requirements.

The next case is a patient that had Verisyse implantation prior to availability of the Visante and its phakic IOL module. A twenty-eight-year-old female with prescription of right eye –15.00–1.50 × 165, and the left eye –14.25-1.25 × 175, with the VeriCalc was estimated to have a postoperative minimal endothelial clearance of 1.56 and 1.65 in the right and left eye respectively. However, on post-operative evaluation, (Figs 6.24 and 6.25) the patient was noted to have significantly less endothelial - Verisyse clearance, ranging from 1.22 to 1.66 mm right eye, with average of 1.41 mm, and ranging from 1.14 to 1.53 mm left eye with average of 1.35 mm.

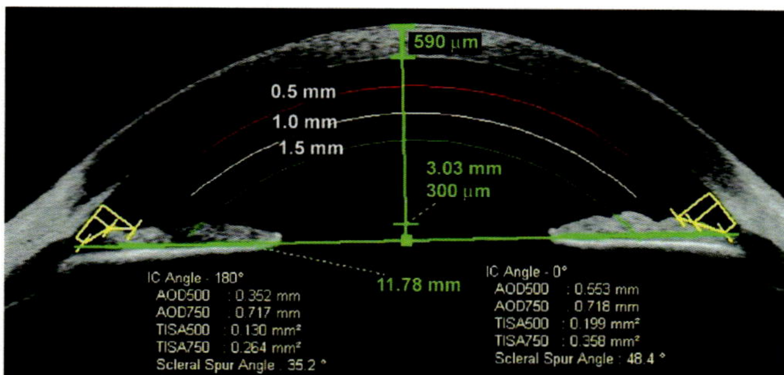

Fig. 6.26: Preoperative evaluation of eye for Verisyse. Evaluations of the angles, crystalline lens rise, anterior chamber depth, and safety endothelial distance clearance are noted

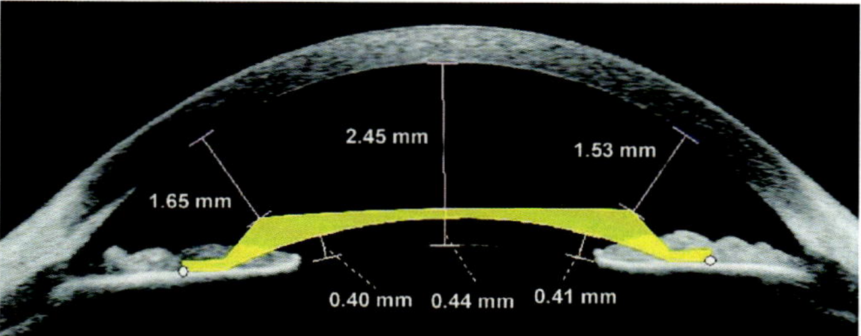

Fig. 6.27: Preoperative Verisyse model placement using the Visante. The Verisyse model and power are programmed and placed properly. The lens-endothelial clearance and the vault distances are measured preoperatively

Crystalline Lens Rise

In the following case presentation however, the patient was evaluated with the new Phakic IOL module available with the Visante 2.0 software. A twenty year-old male with right eye refraction of –14.25 -2.75 × 115 leading to 20/40 vision, with slight amblyopia, was evaluated for the Verisyse implantation. In Figure 6.26 one can evaluate the angles, anterior chamber and the gross endothelial clearance with the "rainbow" module. The anterior chamber depth (ACD) in this case equals to the anterior lens surface to endothelial distance (3.03 mm) plus the corneal thickness (590 microns = 0.59 mm). Therefore, the ACD would equal to 3.03 mm + 0.59 mm = 3.62 mm. Baikoff has described the crystalline lens rise (CLR) as measurement of lens rise above or below the horizontal line across the deepest portion of the angles. Note that although the angle measurements are done from the scleral spur, these measurements are done from the deepest angle positions. In this case the CLR is found to be 300 microns. Baikoff describes a form of pigment dispersion syndrome (PDS) in 9 patients, 8 of whom had a CLR greater than 600 microns. This form of PDS is a direct result of iris pigment liberation from traumatized iris tissue in between the phakic IOL and the crystalline lens. As an example the patient in Figure 6.7, has a CLR of 720 microns and would neither have sufficient clearance of ACD nor the CLR and would not be a Verisyse candidate.

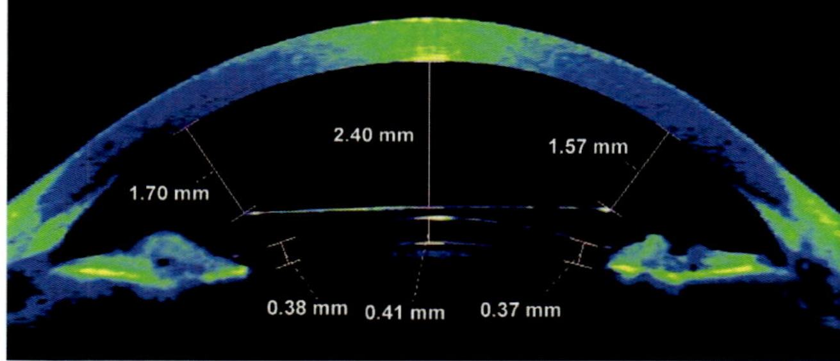

Fig. 6.28: Postoperative actual Visante scan of eye implanted with Verisyse. Endothelial clearance and vault distances are measures. The iris claw hooks are noted as black spots in the iris tissue

Preoperative Phakic IOL Model

After the initial quick evaluation (Fig. 6.27), one may proceed to a much more in depth evaluation with the Verisyse model number and power. Once the model is aligned just anterior to the posterior iris pigmented epithelium, and centered, the measurement via the safety lines and the lens vault can be placed. The safety lines are to evaluate for the anterior surface of the phakic IOL to the posterior aspect of the cornea. The vault caliper is used to evaluate the distance from posterior aspect of the phakic IOL to the anterior crystalline lens distance.

This patient did subsequently undergo Verisyse implantation and was evaluated by the Visante (Fig. 6.28). The VeriCalc had calculated the minimum endothelial clearance as 1.92 mm. The Visante model calculated an average of 1.59 mm phakic IOL to endothelium clearance, and a vault distance of 41.67 microns. The actual postoperative data revealed a 1.64 mm phakic IOL to endothelial clearance and a vault distance of 38.67 microns.

Dynamic Changes of the Anterior Chamber with Accommodation

Verisyse as currently available in the United States is a solid PMMA lens available in 6.0 mm or 5.0 mm optics, and as such must be inserted through a similar size wound. Artiflex is a foldable version of the same and may be inserted through a smaller wound. Jose Guell and colleagues published a study where they implanted Verisyse in one eye and Artiflex in the second eye. They then did an accommodative dynamic study on each eye of the 11 patients in their study. Using the optometer, accommodation was induced in the patient's eye, one diopters at a time, up to seven diopters. Their conclusion was that there were no clinical differences in how both phakic IOLs behaved relative to each other; however with accommodation, there was a total anterior movement of the iris-lens diaphragm of up to a maximal 250 microns at the center of the phakic IOL to the endothelial distance. It must be noted that the distance of the phakic IOL edge to the endothelium is much less than the center and may prove to be more significant than the measurement of the center of the lens. Additionally, a maximal 1.5 mm pupillary constriction with accommodation was noted. Accommodation did not cause significant change in the vault distance between the crystalline lens and the posterior aspect of the phakic IOL.

In another study, Kiovula and Kugelberg studied the Phakic Refractive Lens (Medennium, Inc., Irvine, California, USA), which is not currently approved by the FDA in United States. The PRL is a posterior chamber lens that floats in the posterior chamber and rests on the zonules and freely rotates. In their study, in the hyperopic group there were no contacts between the crystalline lens and the PRL at baseline, however with accommodation, contact was noted in 3 cases (27%) and a decrease in the distance noted in another 6 cases (55%). In the myopic group, with the lens model PRL 100, there was one case of contact (10%) at base line, 2 crystalline lenses had contact with the PRL with accommodation (20%), and 3 cases (30%) had decrease in the distance between the PRL and the crystalline lens. In the myopic PRL 101, 2 cases (6%) had baseline PRL-Crystalline lens contact at base line and another lens came in contact with accommodation for a total of (10%), and 21 cases (68%) exhibited decrease in the PRL-crystalline lens distance without contact. There was a mean of 84 micron reduction in the PRL-crystalline lens distance in the PRL models 101 and 200; however, there was no reduction in the PRL model 100. The authors suggest that the smaller size of this model prevents the reduction in the PRL-crystalline lens caused by pupillary constriction and the anterior lens movement. They also suggest that despite greater prosthesis – crystalline touch, the reason for fewer cataract complications of this lens compared to the sulcus fixated posterior chamber Visian ICL phakic IOL, is that the lens rotation allows for aqueous exchange.

In evaluation of the phakic IOL candidate the Visante Anterior Segment OCT plays a crucial role in safely evaluating the anterior chamber depth, the crystalline lens rise, the endothelial–phakic IOL distance, the phakic IOL–crystalline lens vault and the dynamic accommodative changes of the anterior segment.

CONCLUSION

In one of the most commonly performed refractive surgeries, namely, cataract surgery or clear lens extraction, there is also a significant role for the Visante anterior segment OCT in those cases as well. With increasing emphasis on the premium IOL, including the accommodative lenses, the Visante becomes invaluable in demonstrating the efficacy of the lenses. Visante can be used to induce accommodation using the build-in optometer as noted under the phakic IOL section. An example of CrystaLens implanted in a patient is presented, however, no measurable movement in the lens could be noted (Fig. 6.29).

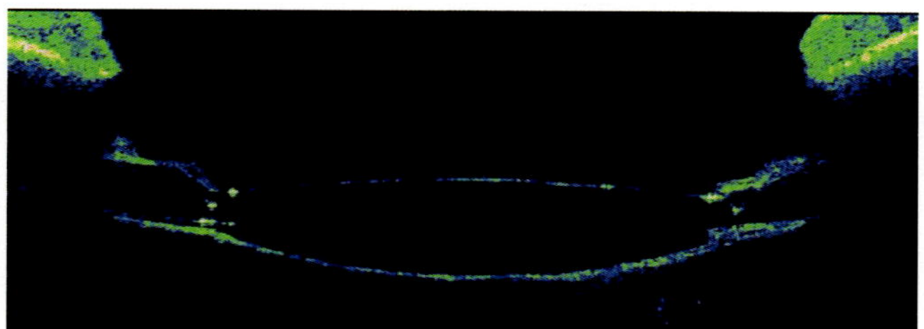

Fig. 6.29: CrytaLens implanted in the eye. The optic and the hinges are clearly noted

As demonstrated through case presentations, the Visante Anterior Segment Optical Coherence Tomography System is a powerful non-contact, real-time imaging system of the eye that shows excellent accuracy. In care of the excimer laser patients, from the preoperative stages the patients' candidacy may be enhanced with additional information such as pachymetric mapping of the cornea. The health of the eye may be assessed beyond its refraction, such as the quantitative measurement of the angle as opposed to the qualitative capabilities of the standard slit lamp gonioscope. Corneal pathologies, such as scars, infections, flap configurations, and irregularities are quantitatively noted and are only some of the examples of the usefulness of the Visante in the care of a past, present, and future refractive patient.

REFERENCE

1. Roger F Steinert, David Hwang: Anterior Segment Optical Coherence Tomography; Slack , USA, 2008.

7 Corneal Topographers and Wavefront Aberrometers: Complementary Tools

Tracy Schroeder Swartz, Ming Wang, Arun C Gulani

INTRODUCTION

The accessibility of the cornea and the non-intraocular designation of its anatomical status makes it the focus of refractive surgery. The cornea has therewith enjoyed this privilege for decades of refractive surgery. These very advantages also have us refractive surgeons constantly vying to make this delicately transparent yet inherently elastic tissue more predictable.

Thus began our search for that perfect tool which could study and analyze the cornea and also determine our consistency for cornea-based refractive surgery. Corneal topographers have been the gold standard for understanding of corneal shape which is the basis of laser refractive surgery. Recently with the advent of aberrometers, the bar has been raised. We have a new technology as well as a new language to address the cornea with and thereby translate the same into effective and accurate surgical outcomes.

This bridge from topography to wavefront technology is actually an adjunct and not about the past or future. These are complementary technologies as of now and this chapter therewith addresses the application of the two.

With the advent of complex topographic systems and wavefront aberrometers, ophthalmologists now benefit from a deeper understanding of optics of the cornea and their effect on vision.

KERATOMETERS

The first instrument to measure the surface of the cornea was the ophthalmometer. This device measured the curvature of the cornea using reflected rings. It is important to remember the following assumptions related to keratometry:[1]

- The formula used is based on spherical geometry. The cornea however is not spherical but is a prolate (flattened) ellipsoid. Thus, the central radius is slightly steeper than actually measured.
- Keratometry is based on four data points within the central 3 mm of the cornea. It provides no insight into the area inside or outside of the 3 mm ring.
- Keratometry theory assumes paraxial optics. While the approximation may be clinically acceptable for fitting contacts or estimating corneal astigmatism, it may not be when measuring peripheral curvature.
- Keratometers assume alignment of the corneal apex, line of sight and instrument axis. However, this rarely occurs during actual measurement.
- The formula used to calculate the radius (r) approximates the distance to the convex focal point, which in the case of the Reichert keratometer, may introduce up to 0.12D of error. This error may increase if the instrument is not correctly focused or the operator accommodates during measurement.

- Since the indexes may differ between manufacturers, one must be careful comparing the readings in diopters between different instruments.

CORNEAL TOPOGRAPHY

Such assumptions result in significant errors when considering the peripheral cornea, especially in eyes with irregular surfaces such as in keratoconus or S/P keratorefractive surgery. With the growth of computers came the corneal topography systems widely used today to evaluate the shape characteristics of the cornea.

Early videokeratoscopes used axial power maps to illustrate the information from captured raw data. The power at each point was calculated according to the Javal ophthalmometer convention, and suffered many of keratometry's assumptions.

The axial map is a traditional but poor descriptor of corneal refraction because it does not take into account spherical aberration.[2,3] Despite its limits, the axial map became known as "the corneal topography map". With the development of arc-step algorithms, placido systems could not only approximate axial power, but also measure corneal shape. Elevation maps became available. An example of an axial and elevation map of an eye with with-the-rule astigmatism is shown in Figure 7.1.

In the early to the mid 1990s, the explosion of excimer laser refractive surgery necessitated more accurate optical instruments to create more detailed representation of the corneal surface. At this point, the path divided as two parallel paths emerged. Some believed the answers to problems encountered in refractive surgery could be answered using elevation-based topography, while others supported wavefront aberrometry-based platforms.

ELEVATION BASED TOPOGRAPHY

Placido disk imaging systems are limited to evaluation of the anterior cornea only, and calculate rather than directly measure elevation data. Systems emerged which directly measured corneal elevation, and evaluated anatomy posterior to the anterior cornea. The PAR Corneal Topography System (PAR CTS) was the first system to directly measure anterior elevation topography, using principles of triangulation. The distortion of a grid projected on to the cornea was mathematically compared to the true grid in a reference plane. Because the geometry of the reference surface and the grid projection is known, rays can be intersected in three-dimensional space to compute the X, Y and Z coordinates of the surface.[4] This system was generally accepted to be more accurate when measuring complex bicurve and multicurve test surfaces, but poor reproducibility was reported.

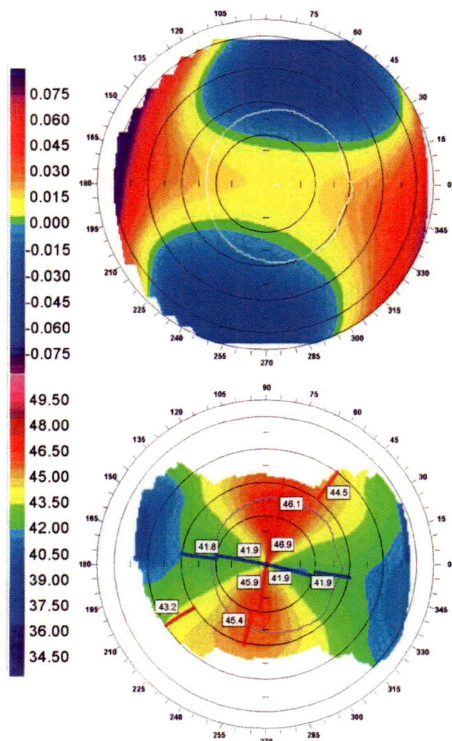

Fig. 7.1: An axial (bottom) and elevation (top) map of an eye showing with-the-rule astigmatism

Slit-scanning technology addressed both the need for direct measurement of elevation as well as evaluation of the posterior structures within the eye. The Orbscan II (Bausch and Lomb, Roschester, New York) combined a placido disk to measure curvature and slit scanning to measure both surfaces of the cornea. The most commonly used display for this system is the Quad map, shown in Figure 7.2. A

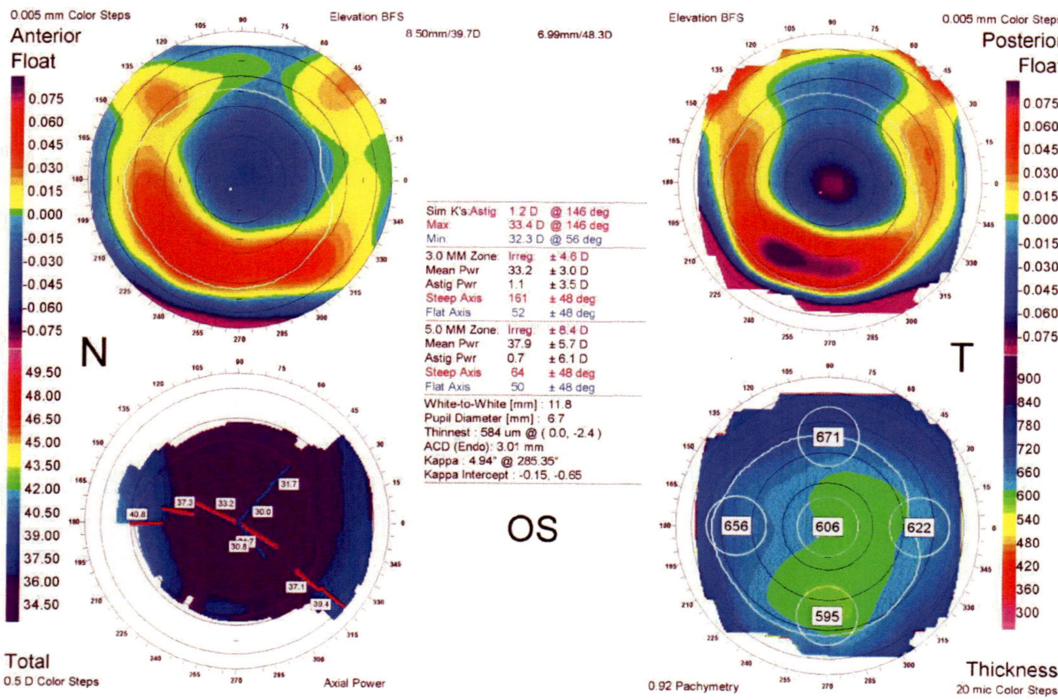

Fig. 7.2: An example of a quad map in a patient S/P myopic LASIK

placido image is captured to evaluate curvature data. Then, over 1.5 seconds, two scanning slit lamps project a total of 40 images each at 45 degrees of the video axis. A proprietary tracking system reduced eye movements. It produced pachymetry and anterior chamber depth information for the first time. This system remains the only type capable of evaluation of the posterior surface. Thus, there is no way to validate the information found in the posterior map.

Another technology was developed to address two problems associated with currently used topographic technology: assumptions inherent to power calculation and paracentral measurement of the cornea. The Pentacam (Oculus) addressed these deficiencies. It is a rotating Scheimpflug camera which provides a complete picture from the anterior surface of the cornea to the posterior surface of the lens, as shown in Figure 7.3.

As topographic systems advanced, understanding of the optics resulting from changes in shape induced by disease or refractive surgery, and the need to correct optical problems grew. Unfortunately, significantly irregular corneas, dry eyes, and scarring may cause topographic systems to fail.

Programs such as the Custom Corneal Ablation Planner (Custom CAP) utilized elevation data and computer analysis to create custom ablation profiles in an attempt to correct decentered ablations and relieve patients of visual distortion. An example is shown in Figure 7.4. Topography-driven programs fail to address the refractive error, however, and refractive changes induced by such treatments were somewhat unpredictable.

WAVEFRONT: ANOTHER VIEW OF CORNEAL OPTICS

Just as topographic analysis was facilitated by computers, so was measurement of optical aberrations. This advance in technology occurred slightly later and parallel to the growth of topography. The most common types of aberrometers are the Hartmann-Shack and the raytracing models. Hartmann-Shack

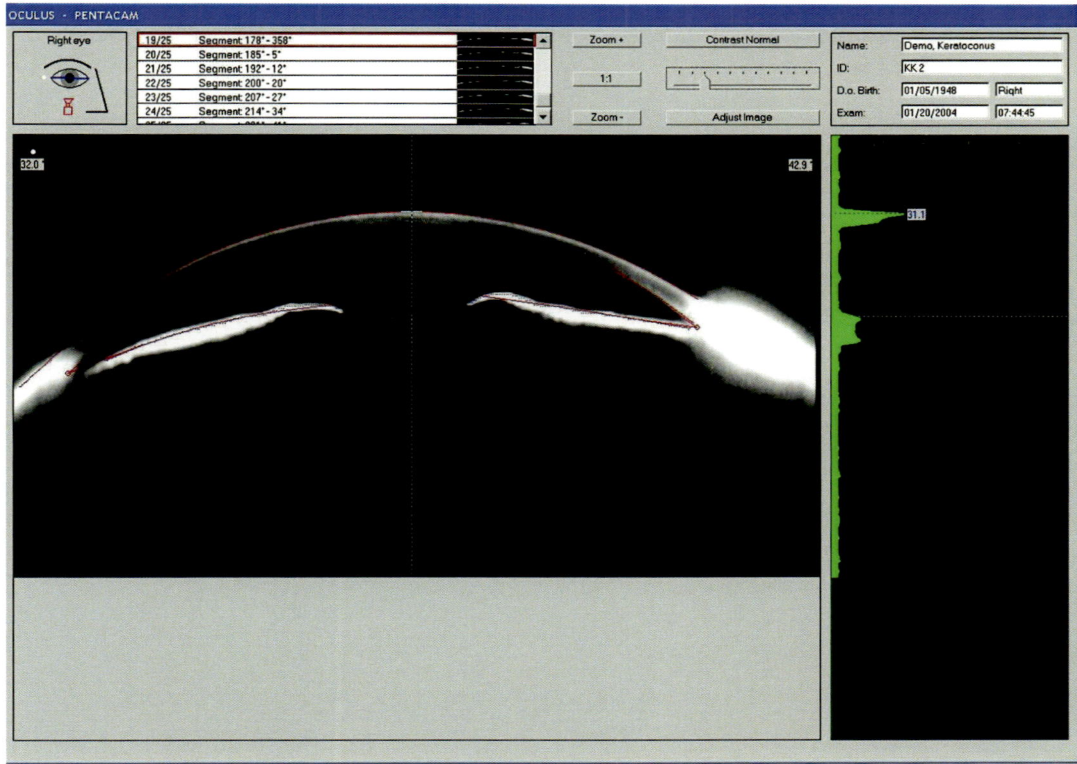

Fig. 7.3: Scheimpflug image

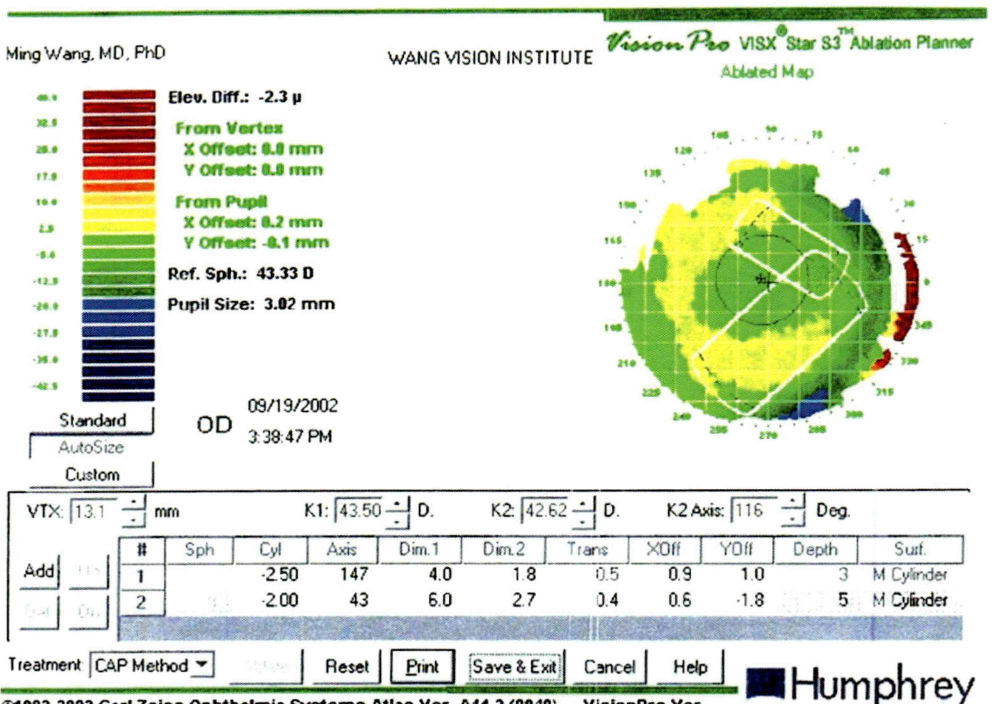

#	Sph	Cyl	Axis	Dim.1	Dim.2	Trans	XOff	YOff	Depth	Surf.
1		-2.50	147	4.0	1.8	0.5	0.9	1.0	3	M Cylinder
2		-2.00	43	6.0	2.7	0.4	0.6	-1.8	5	M Cylinder

Fig. 7.4: Custom CAP case

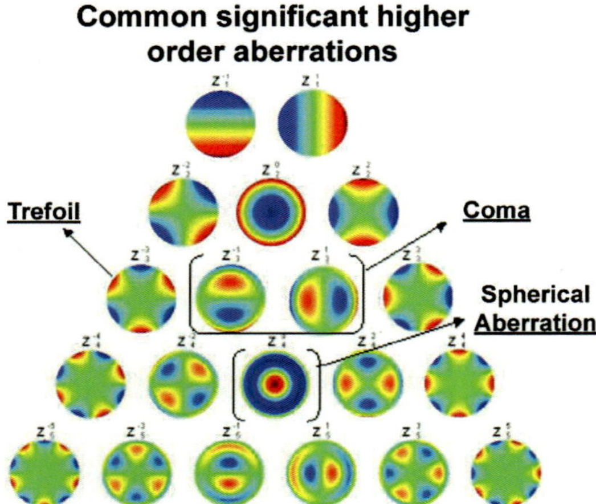

Fig. 7.5: Zernicke polynomial pyramid

models utilize several hundred lenslets to measure the wavefront. Raytracing models utililize individual rays of light to measure the wavefront. Both models measure aberrations as a deviation from the plane wave in microns, and measurements are limited by pupil size. This is problematic in eyes with smaller pupils.

The shape of the wavefront is then mathematically described, most commonly using Zernicke polynomials.[5] Figure 7.5 shows this polynomial pyramid. Zernicke polynomials are a combination of radial trigometric functions which describe the wavefront mathematically. While second order terms of defocus and astigmatism are addressed by the manifest refraction, the irregular astigmatism primarily attributed to the cornea can be described by higher order terms such as coma, spherical aberration, and trefoil.

Just as topographers exhibit difficulty capturing irregular corneal surfaces, aberrometers falter on irregular wavefronts (typically due to irregular astigmatism). This is especially true for diseased eyes and those S/P keratorefractive procedures. Smolek and Klyce studied zernicke fitting methods for corneal elevation and reported 4th order Zernicke polynomials may not be adequate in their description of corneal aberrations in significantly aberrant eyes.[6]

Because topography failed to address lower order aberrations, and aberrometry failed to address focal topography irregularities, advanced methods were needed. Several case examples later in this chapter demonstrate how using several systems to gain information about the topography and aberrometry combined is beneficial in determination of the etiology of the visual complaint. It is also beneficial in creating a management plan for surgery.

As the limitations of wavefront became apparent, interest turned to corneal wavefront measurements—the ability to measure the amount of aberration attributable to the cornea alone. Systems which subtracted the corneal wavefront from the total ocular wavefront emerged. The EyeSys system is capable of using Wavefront aberrometry and corneal topography to develop a corneal Wavefront map. Figures 7.6A and B illustrate the aberrations found in a keratoconic patient with a 4 mm pupil (A) as well as the topography (B). Figure 7.7 illustrates the cornea and internal aberrations of the same eye.

It has been suggested that surgeons consider the rule of three when considering corneal surgery: for every 3 microns of distortion from the ideal shape of the cornea, about +1 micron difference in the OPD map and -1 micron difference in the wavefront error map exists. It should be noted, however, that the precision of both excimer lasers and wavefront aberrometers far surpasses that of human healing.

CASES

As previously suggested, rather than look at the technologies as separate, it is advantageous to consider them in conjunction with each other. Using both topography and wavefront measurements to determine the etiology of a visual complaint can be advantageous in the clinical setting. This is illustrated by the following case discussions.

Case I: Double Vision Complaints S/P LASIK

Patient WR presented complaining of "terrible night vision OS after LASIK. Preoperatively, he was significantly nearsighted, and correctable to 20/20. Postoperatively, he refracted to –2.75+1.75 × 160, with a BVA of 20/30. An RGP improved his vision to

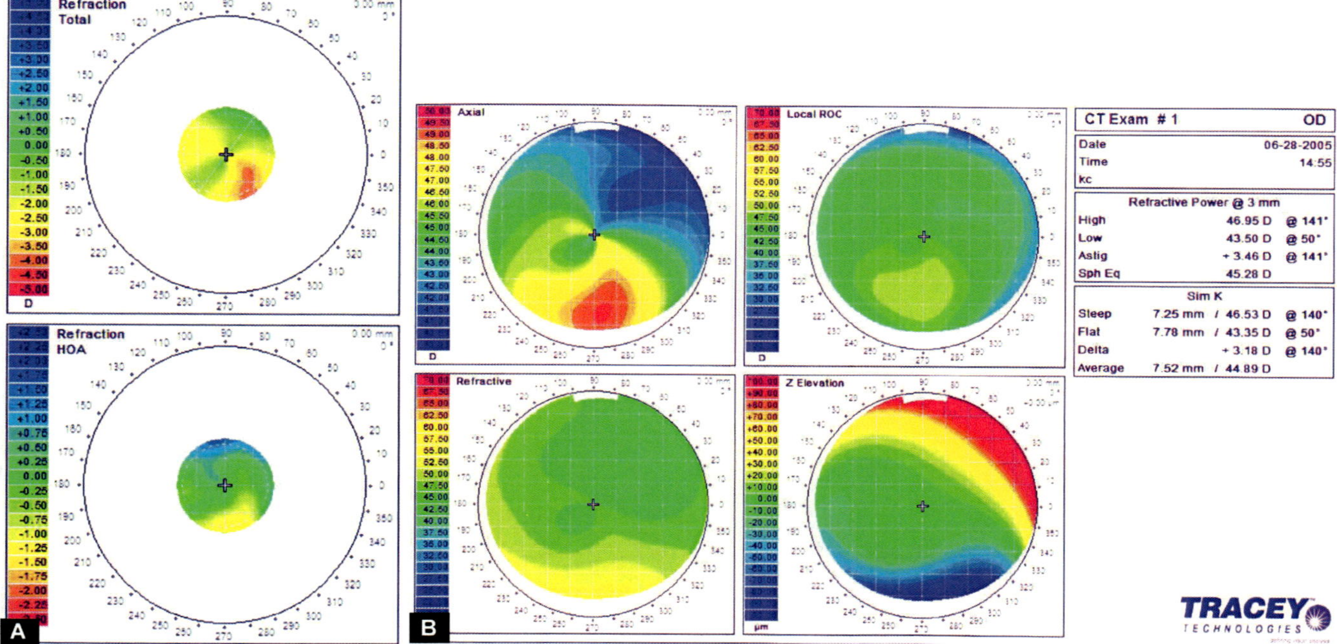

Figs 7.6A and B: The aberrations found in a keratoconic patient with a 4 mm pupil (A) and the topography (B) of the same eye

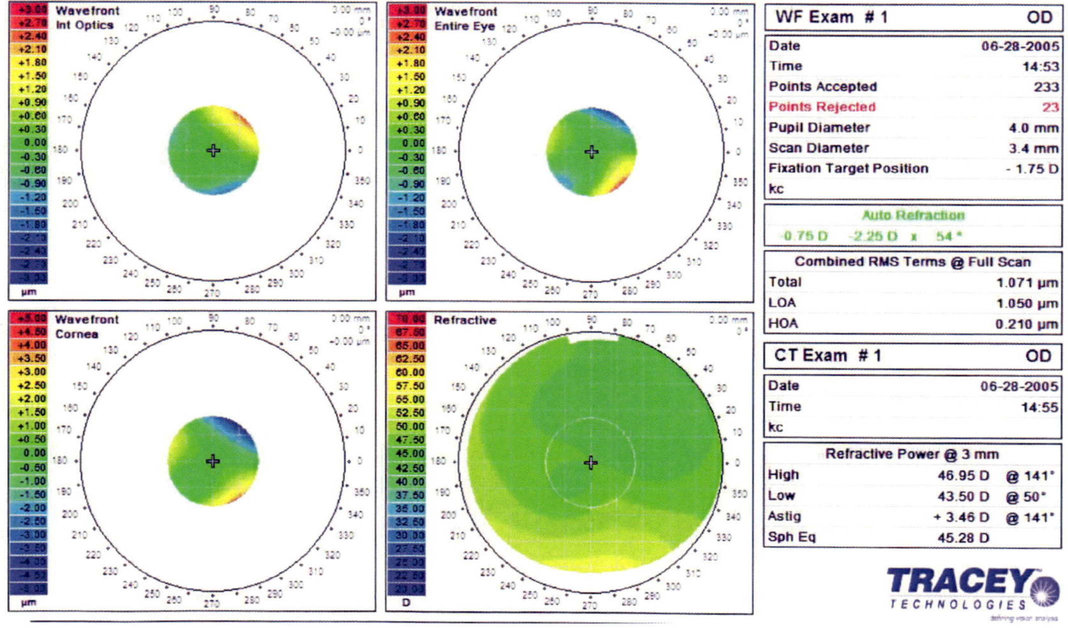

Fig. 7.7: Corneal and internal aberrations of the same eye

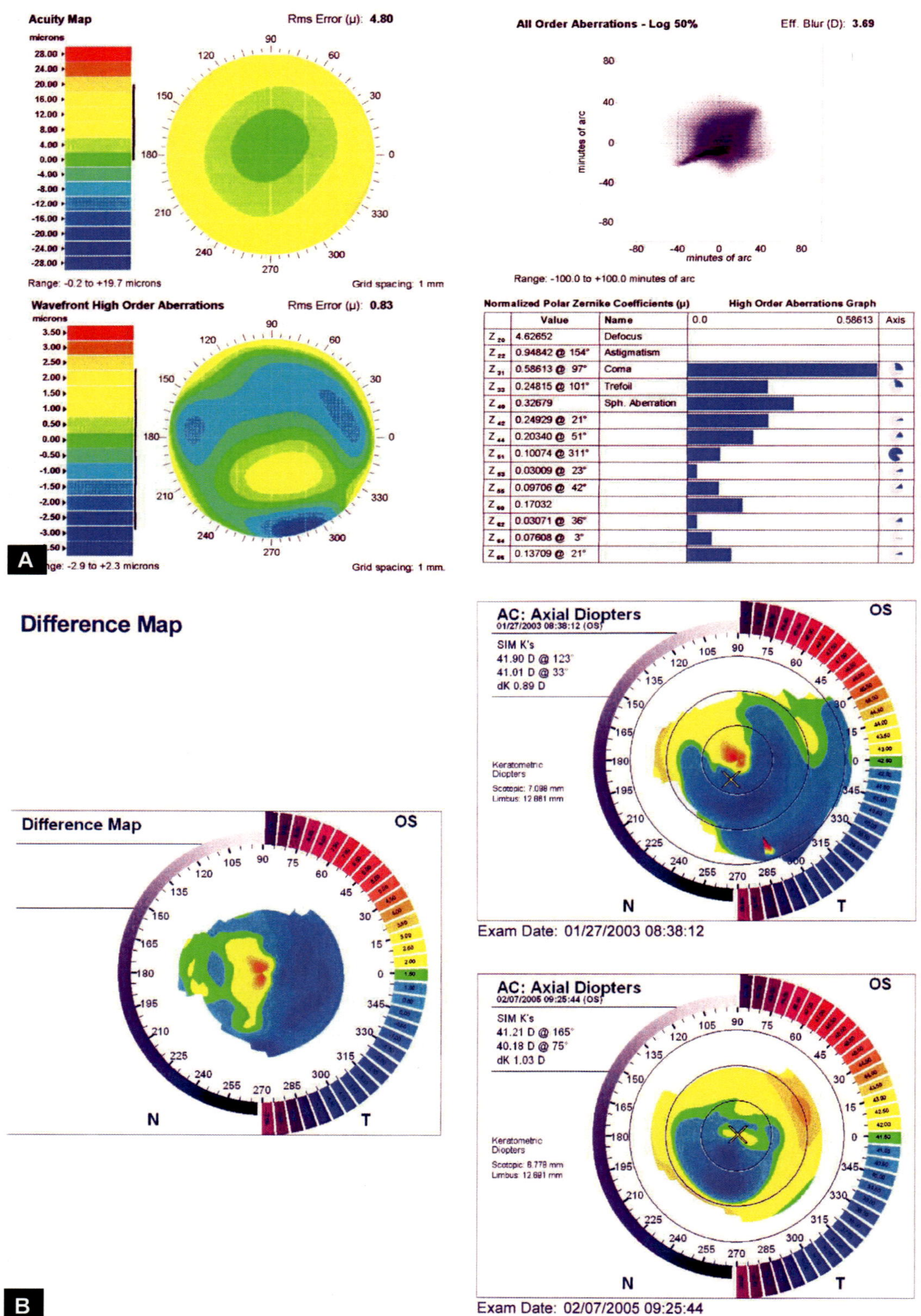

Figs 7.8A and B: Preoperative WaveScan map, and topography difference map showing the change in topography following a Custom CAP treatment

20/20 with a significant reduction in monocular diplopia. His preoperative WaveScan map is shown in Figure 7.8A, with the preoperative topography in the upper right corner of the difference map shown in Figure 7.8B. Elevation mapping revealed a decentered ablation. Significant coma is evident in the aberrometry map, as expected with decentered ablations. We performed a Custom-CAP treatment, which treats the decentered ablation directly without taking the refractive error into account, and the visual distortion improved significantly, indicated by the drop in the RMS value shown in Figure 7.9.

Case II: Night Vision Complaints S/P LASIK

Patient WR presented with complaints of "terrible night vision, starbursts and halos" after LASIK in 2000. Preoperatively, she was –2.50 DS. Postoperatively, she refracted to –1.00+0.25 × 160, with a BVA of 20/30 OD, her dominant eye. Figure 7.10A shows her topography, revealing central irregularities. WaveScan, found in Figure 7.10B, revealed coma and trefoil. We suspected the central irregularities were exaggerated by her dry eye, and treated her aggressively with punctual occlusion, Restasis BID, and Liqugel nightly. Her symptoms improved slightly, and she is waiting for more advanced custom treatment.

Case III: Complaint of Multiple Images after Hyperopic LASIK

Patient TD presented complaining of light sensitivity, ghosting, halos and starbursts at night. Preoperatively she was +4.50D OU. Postoperatively she refracted to PL, 20/25+ OD, +0.25+0.50 × 150, 20/25+ OS. Despite her unaided 20/20- Snellen acuity, she complained bitterly about her quality of vision. Topography found a smaller optical zone OS with greater steepening in the dominant left eye, as shown on the axial map in Figure 7.11A. WaveScan found significant spherical aberration (Figure 7.11B). Note the spherical aberration is negative due to the hyperopic treatment. We have prescribed Alphagan

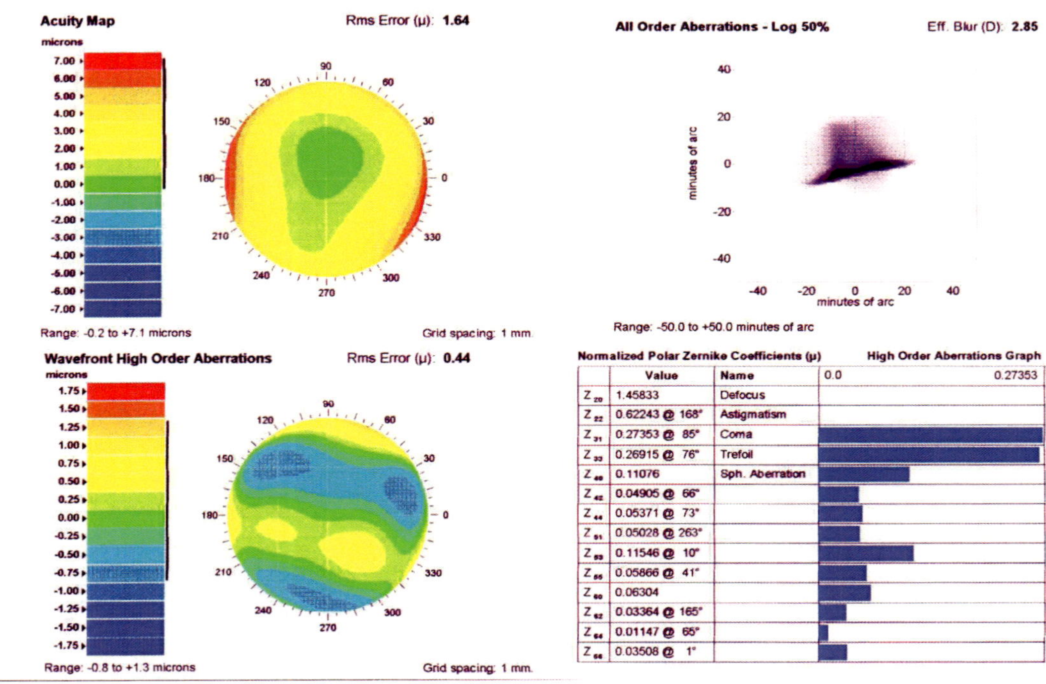

Fig. 7.9: Wavescan S/P Custom Cap treatment

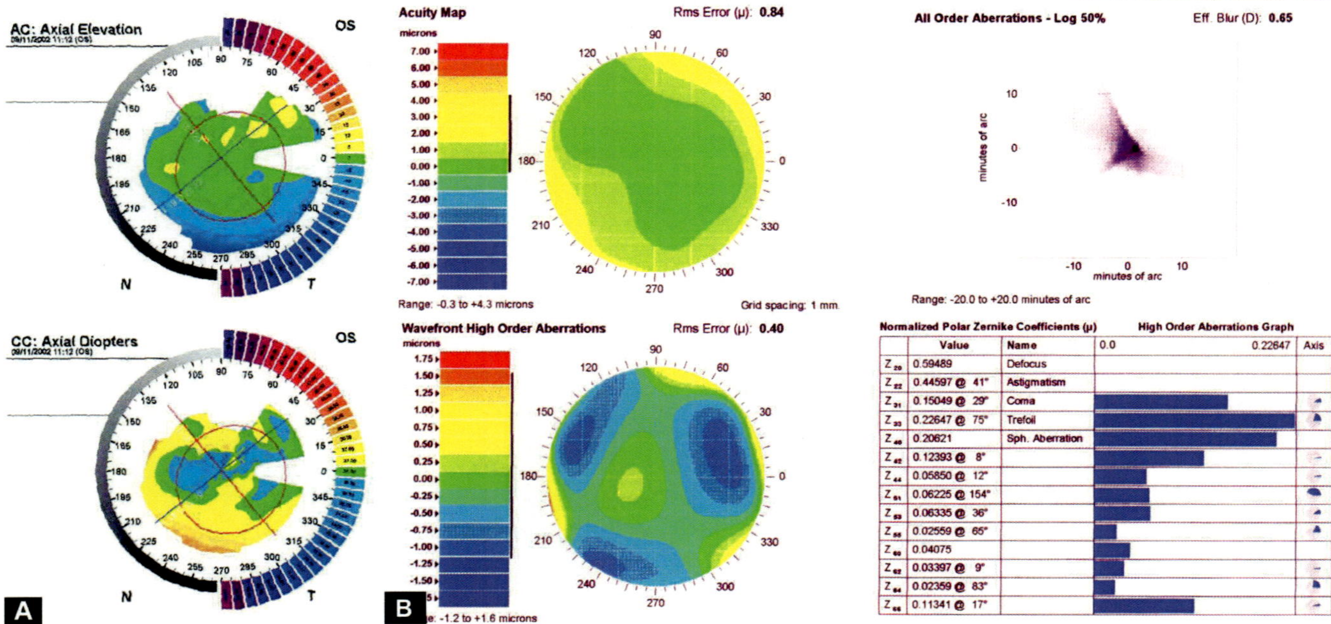

Figs 7.10A and B: Central irregularities were revealed with topography, while aberrometry found coma and trefoil. Dry eye treatment only partially resolved this patient's complaints

P in an attempt to decrease the pupil size and minimize the night vision issues, and fit the patient with gas perm lenses.

Case IV: Double Vision with Loss of Best Correction S/P LASIK

Patient RD presented for evaluation of double vision S/P LASIK, even with glasses. Preoperatively, he was –4.75+0.75 × 105, with a BVA of 20/20. After his original surgery, he underwent two enhancements and astigmatic keratotomy in the affected eye, leaving him –2.00. He was fitted with an RGP, which he reported did not resolve the diplopia, so he rarely wore the lens. Clinical notes from the fitting doctor report BCCLVA of 20/25. The topography was surprisingly regular in the pupillary zone despite the repeated corneal surgery. Wavefront analysis found significant COMA and trefoil, and can be seen in Figure 7.12. We attribute this to early lenticular changes, and elected to monitor rather than proceed with corrective ablation.

Case V: Hyperopic Keratorefractive Surgery Results in Steep Cornea

A 19-year-old female presented for LASIK evaluation. Manifest refraction was +1.75+05.0 × 25 OD (20/40) and +0.75 OS (20/25). Cycloplegic found latent hyperopia: +4.25 OD (20/50) and +1.50 (20/40) OS. Her preoperative topography was normal, and is shown in Figure 7.13A. After considerable discussion, she elected to undergo LASIK in both eyes. The latent hyperopia OD was partially addressed, and the goal was a correction of +2.75 OD, +1.00 OS. She underwent bilateral femtosecond laser assisted keratomileusis using a VISX Star 4 laser.

S/P LASIK, the patient complained of blurred vison OD, and the UCVA dropped to 20/50. Manifest refraction found +1.50+1.25 × 180 while the cycloplegic again revealed the latent hyperopia: +3.00+1.25 × 180, yielding a VA of 20/30. Her visual complaint was relieved with simple hyperopic correction, and the patient underwent an enhancement by relift of +1.50+1.25 × 180.

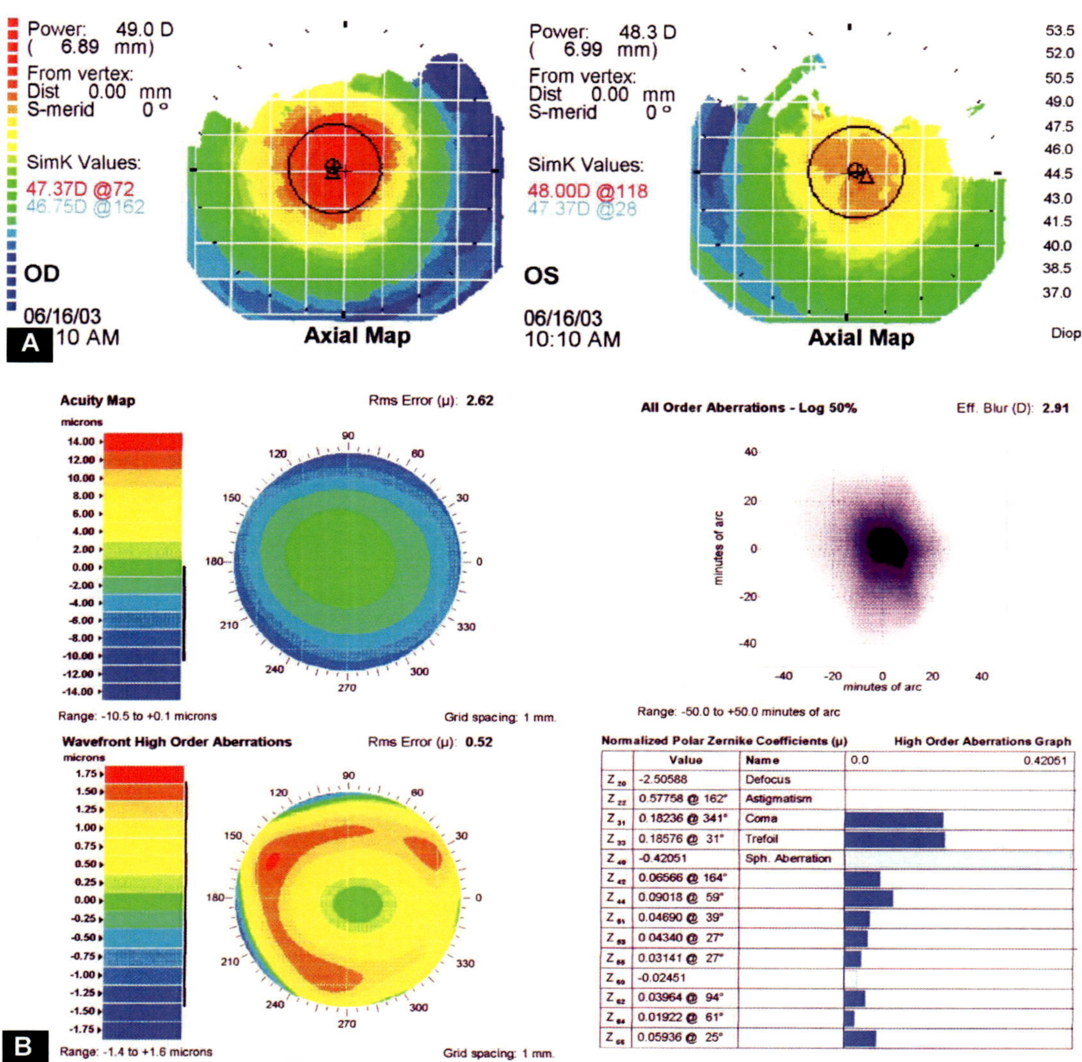

	Value	Name	0.0 — 0.42051
Z_{20}	-2.50588	Defocus	
Z_{22}	0.57758 @ 162°	Astigmatism	
Z_{31}	0.18236 @ 341°	Coma	
Z_{33}	0.18576 @ 31°	Trefoil	
Z_{40}	-0.42051	Sph. Aberration	
Z_{42}	0.06566 @ 164°		
Z_{44}	0.09018 @ 59°		
Z_{51}	0.04690 @ 39°		
Z_{53}	0.04340 @ 27°		
Z_{55}	0.03141 @ 27°		
Z_{60}	-0.02451		
Z_{62}	0.03964 @ 94°		
Z_{64}	0.01922 @ 61°		
Z_{66}	0.05936 @ 25°		

Figs 7.11A and B: This patient complained of glare and night vision disturbances secondary to the HOA caused by the small area of central steepening OS

At one month, she presented complaining of decreased vision OD, multiple images, and "an unbalanced feeling". Manifest refraction found –1.50+0.75 × 75, and corrected her to only 20/50. Her elevation maps reveal marked central steepening OD as seen on the elevation map in Figure 7.13A. Her wavefront aberrometry measurements revealed coma OD, shown in Figures 7.13B and C. Interestingly, the Wavescan and I-Trace both found hyperopic refractions. The coma suggested a decentered apex, and topography revealed a significant steepening just above the geographical center.

Neither correction of the manifest refraction with a soft lens nor Alphagan-P to change the pupil size corrected the patient's complaint. While a gas permeable lens did restore the functional vision, the patient is not able to tolerate the lens. It appears that the patient only uses the tip of the cornea for vision, resulting in the preferred myopic refraction. As time progressed and the natural smoothing of the cornea

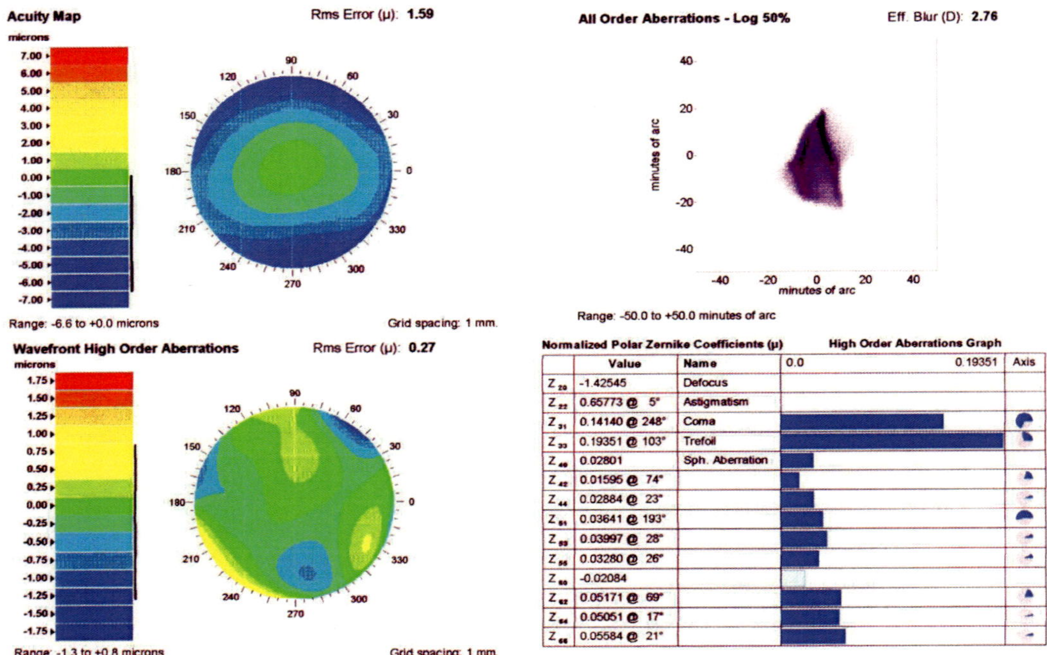

Fig. 7.12: Aberrometry revealed the cause of the patient's complaint when topography found a relatively normal shape: early cataracts

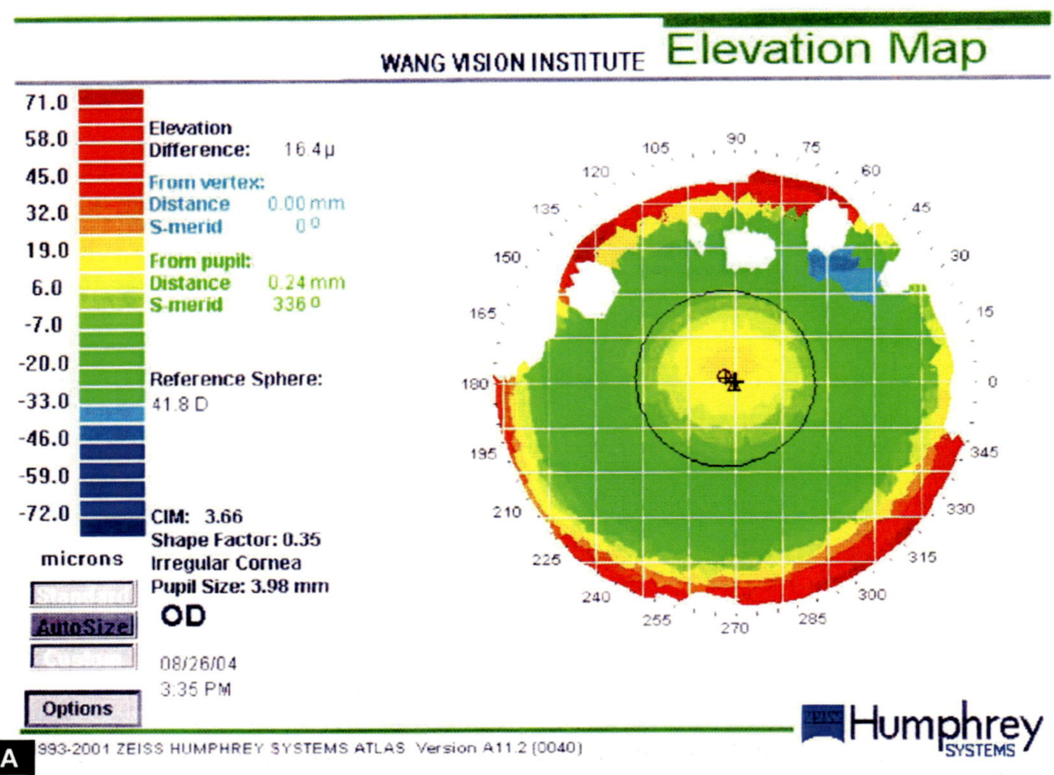

Fig. 7.13A

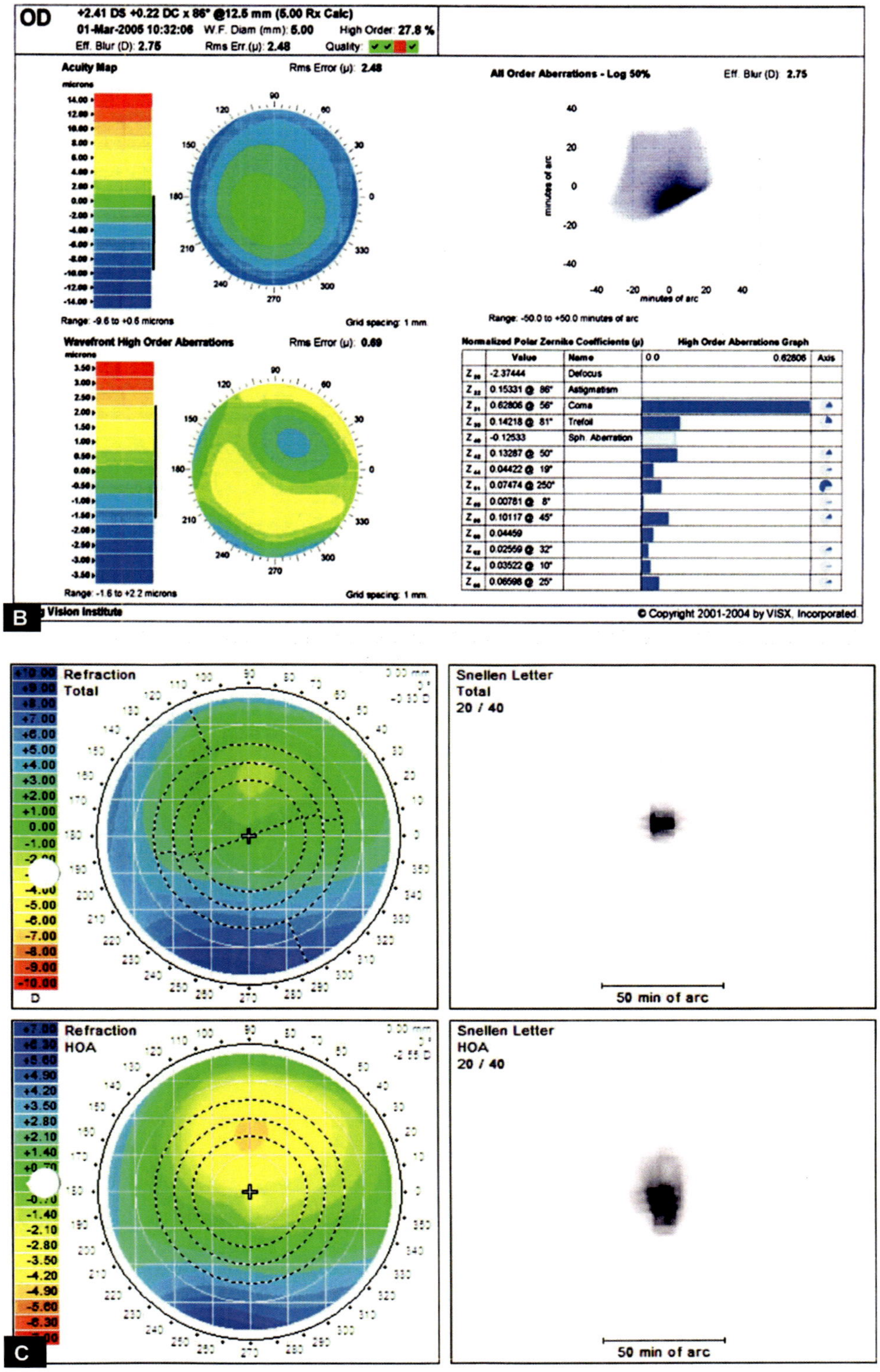

OD +2.41 DS +0.22 DC x 86° @12.5 mm (5.00 Rx Calc)
01-Mar-2005 10:32:06 W.F. Diam (mm): 5.00 High Order: 27.8 %
Eff. Blur (D): 2.75 Rms Err.(μ): 2.48 Quality:

Acuity Map — Rms Error (μ): 2.48

Range: -9.6 to +0.6 microns — Grid spacing: 1 mm

All Order Aberrations - Log 50% — Eff. Blur (D): 2.75

Range: -50.0 to +50.0 minutes of arc

Wavefront High Order Aberrations — Rms Error (μ): 0.69

Range: -1.6 to +2.2 microns — Grid spacing: 1 mm

Normalized Polar Zernike Coefficients (μ) — High Order Aberrations Graph

	Value	Name
Z	-2.37444	Defocus
Z	0.15331 @ 86°	Astigmatism
Z	0.62806 @ 56°	Coma
Z	0.14218 @ 81°	Trefoil
Z	-0.12533	Sph. Aberration
Z	0.13287 @ 50°	
Z	0.04422 @ 19°	
Z	0.07474 @ 250°	
Z	0.00781 @ 8°	
Z	0.10117 @ 45°	
Z	0.04459	
Z	0.02559 @ 32°	
Z	0.03522 @ 10°	
Z	0.06598 @ 25°	

B

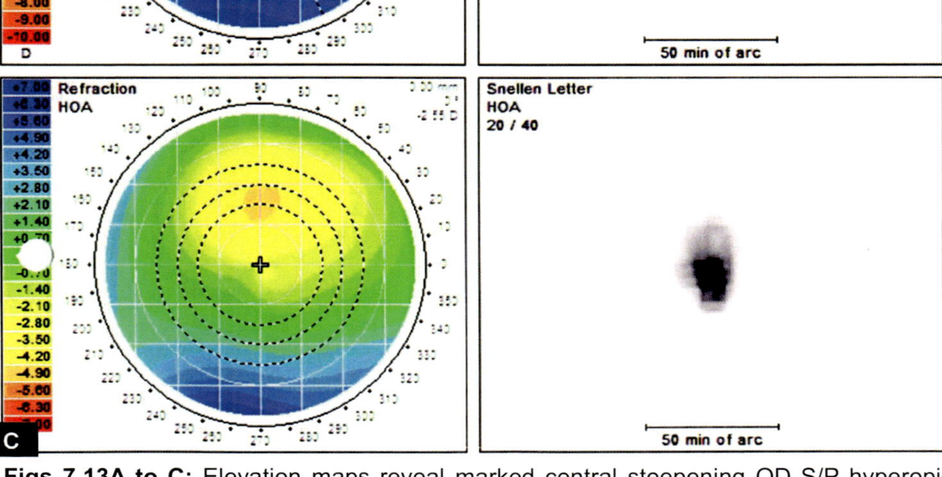

C

Figs 7.13A to C: Elevation maps reveal marked central steepening OD S/P hyperopic lasik with hyperopic enhancement, as seen on the elevation map (A). Her WaveScan map (B) and Itrace map (C) revealed coma, and reported hyperopic refractions despite a manifest of –1.50 DS occurs, her symptoms are lessening and we may perform a custom treatment in the future.

CONCLUSION

While topographers and aberrometers may work well in virgin eyes, for surgeons striving for technology to address irregular astigmatism, current systems fall short. Improved understanding of the relationship between aberrometry, topography and corneal optics must be gained with continued advancement of the current technology.

Several generalizations can be made regarding the relationship between topography and wavefront aberrometry. The loss of the prolate cornea results in an increase in spherical aberration. Irregular astigmatism may be associated with an increase in coma and trefoil. Decentered ablations have been linked to increased coma. The irregular surface associated with dry eyes has been found to be improved with punctal occlusion and accompanied by a secondary reduction in HO aberrations.[7]

For patients with visual complaints S/P keratorefractive surgery, it is advantageous to obtain information from various sources about the etiology of the visual complaint. Using wavefront aberrometry and corneal topography to investigate the source of the patient's problem, and better understand the visual system as a whole, will better enable us to manage our patient's. Systems such as the Advanced Corneal Ablation Pattern (VISX), which combine topographic and wavefront information to create computerized simulations for surgery, may enable correction of irregular surfaces as well as refractive errors.

REFERENCES

1. Horner DG, Salmon TO, Soni PS. Chapter 17, Corneal Topography. In Benjamin WJ (Ed): Borish's Clinical Refraction. WB Saunders Company: Philadelphia 1998.
2. Klein SA. A corneal topography algorithm that produces continuous curvature. Optom Vis Sci 1992;69:829-34.
3. Roberts C. The Accuracy of "Power" maps to display curvature data in corneal topography systems. Invest Ophtalmol Vis Sci 1994;35:3524-32.
4. Belin MW, Cambier JL, Nabors JR, Ratliff CD. PAR Corneal Topography System (PAR CTS): the clinical application of close-range photogrammetry. Optom Vis Sci 1995;72:828-37.
5. Campbell C. A new method for describing the aberrations of the eye using zernike polynomials. Optometry and Vision Science 2003;80(1):79-83.
6. Smolek MK, Kyce SD. Zernicke polynomial fitting fials to represent all visuall signficant corneal aberrations. Invest Ophthalmol Vis Sci 2003;44: 4676-81.
7. Pepose J, Huang B, Mirza A, Qazi M. Effect of punctal occlusion on wavefront aberrations in dry eyes after LASIK. Invest Ophthalmol Vis Sci 2003 44: E-Abstract 2628.

8 Aberrometry and Topography in the Vector Analysis of Refractive Laser Surgery

Noel A Alpins, Gemma Walsh B Optom

INTRODUCTION

Refractive laser surgery techniques such as laser in situ keratomileusis (LASIK) and photorefractive keratectomy (PRK) are effective methods of treating spherical myopic errors up to 12D and hyperopic errors up to 6D, with good visual outcomes. However, generally more than half of the people who are suitable candidates for refractive surgery have enough astigmatism to warrant its inclusion in the surgical correction. As astigmatism has both direction and magnitude, its incorporation into the treatment makes planning more complex. It has been shown that vector analysis could likely improve the visual outcome of spherocylindrical treatments by combining the topographic and refractive astigmatic components to target a reduced level of corneal astigmatism compared to using refractive parameters alone.[1-4,7]

MEASUREMENT OF ASTIGMATISM

There are three differing categories of astigmatism; naturally occurring regular astigmatism, naturally occurring irregular astigmatism and secondary irregular astigmatism associated with ocular trauma, disease, infection or previous ocular surgery.[1] There are many different ways to measure astigmatism, some assessing corneal astigmatism only, and the others measuring refractive astigmatism including the internal optics of the eye. It is important in routine clinical practice to utilize more than one method in the preoperative examination.

The manifest subjective refraction is a measure of the spherocylindrical correction required for the patient's perception of their best vision. The principal contribution to the cylindrical error is the corneal astigmatism, but also includes astigmatism from the internal optics of the eye (such as the crystalline lens) as well as the interpretation of the image by the cerebral cortex. The measured result depends on many variables such as chart illumination and contrast, test distance and room lighting. The newer technology of wavefront analysis provides a spatially oriented refractive map of the pathway of light through the eye, which provides a greater amount of information on the refractive system than the manifest refraction data alone. It too includes the internal optics of the eye, but unlike subjective responses does not include the conscious percept of the cerebral cortex, thus giving no information regarding the non-optical interpretation of astigmatism images on the retina and visual cortex. This subjective value conventionally forms part of the ablative treatment and is an important component for patient satisfaction. The application of wavefront analysis in the treatment plan is discussed further on.

Keratometry is a useful objective test to measure average corneal curvature at the paracentral region of the cornea. However, as it requires the manual alignment of optical mires to identify the steepest and flattest corneal axes, there is a potential problem with reproducing reliable results due to variability between different observers. Corneal topography, or computer assisted videokeratography (CAVK), provides a more detailed quantified view of the corneal astigmatism displayed as a map based on the measurement of refractive power of thousands of separate points over the entire cornea. Average topographical astigmatism can be represented by a simulated keratometry value, which is a mean value derived from a number of constant reference points. It is a best fit compromise, and determined in various ways by the different types of topographers.

SURGICAL PLANNING—REFRACTION, TOPOGRAPHY OR BOTH?

In an ideal world the goal of astigmatic refractive surgery is to completely eliminate astigmatism from the eye and its optical correction. However, it has been recognized that this is not possible in the majority of cases due to the inherent differences between corneal astigmatism (represented by the simulated keratometry value from topography) and refractive astigmatism (represented by lower [second] order aberrations from aberrometry) correcting the eye.[6,7] Most surgeons traditionally treat the refractive value alone based on the principle that treating what the patient perceives to give their best corrected vision will provide a superior visual outcome.

However, this is not necessarily the case. Disregarding the shape of the cornea while changing it flies in the face of the fundamental principles of corneal surgery. In fact, simple arithmetic analysis shows that an excessive amount of corneal astigmatism may be left if treatment is applied exclusively based on the parameters derived from the refractive cylinder magnitude and axis.[2,5] This occurs because failing to align the maximum ablation closer to the flattest corneal meridia results in off-axis loss of effect when reducing corneal astigmatism. Consequently, lower (second) order astigmatic aberrations and (third order) coma would not be minimized, with more remaining than otherwise necessary.[1] This may result in post-surgical symptoms such as reduced visual acuity and contrast sensitivity, creating difficulty with night driving and thus actually diminishing satisfaction in a proportion of patients.

It becomes particularly important to consider this in patients with form fruste or mild keratoconus as there is usually a large discrepancy between the refractive and corneal astigmatism in these cases. It has been shown that optimizing the PRK treatment by combining the refractive parameters with the corneal topography can improve the total astigmatic and visual outcomes for these patients.[3]

As it becomes more widely recognized that a zero overall astigmatism is mostly unattainable, effective contemporary methods target astigmatism outcomes that combine both the refractive and topographic measurements in the analytical planning process. This should ensure the distribution of the remaining astigmatism to achieve the optimal outcome. That is, choosing a maximal treatment that leaves the minimum amount of astigmatism and in the most favorable orientation. With-the-rule astigmatism is more prevalent in the younger population undergoing laser vision correction, and is thought to be more visually tolerable to refractive perception than against-the-rule astigmatism (Javals rule).[5,7,10]

VECTOR ANALYSIS BY THE ALPINS METHOD

The surgical planning and analysis process is expedited by the implementation of computer and software technology. Calculations performed for the publication of this chapter utilized the ASSORT® program developed by the first author (the Alpins Statistical System for Ophthalmic Refractive surgery Techniques). It employs the principles of vector planning and analysis[1-8] and can utilize a paradigm that favors with-the-rule astigmatism that minimizes measurable postoperative refractive astigmatism quantified as second order aberrations.

The amount and axis of astigmatic change that the surgeon intends to induce is called the target induced astigmatism vector (TIA). This is determined by using an optimal combination of refractive and topographic data, as seen in the example later on. The surgically induced astigmatism vector (SIA) is the astigmatic change actually induced by the surgery. It is possible to determine whether the treatment was on-axis or off-axis, and also whether too much or too little treatment was applied by examining the various relationships between the SIA and TIA. The Correction Index (CI) is the ratio of the SIA to TIA and ideally is 1.0. An overcorrection occurs if the CI is greater than 1.0 and less than 1.0 for an undercorrection. The Magnitude of Error (ME) is the arithmetic difference between the magnitudes of the SIA and TIA. This is positive for overcorrections and negative for undercorrections. The angle of error (AE) is the angle contained by the SIA and TIA vectors. If the achieved correction is orientated counterclockwise (CCW) to where it was intended then the AE is positive. If the achieved correction is clockwise (CW) to the intended axis then the AE is negative.

An absolute measure of success of the surgery is described by the difference vector (DV). This is the induced astigmatic change that would enable the initial surgery to achieve its initial intended target, and is ideally zero. The DV is a useful dioptric measure of uncorrected astigmatism. A relative measure of success is the Index of Success (IOS) which is calculated by dividing the DV by the intended change, the TIA. This is also preferably zero.

As previously mentioned, the corneal and refractive astigmatisms are rarely equivalent. This difference may be represented vectorially by the ocular residual astigmatism (ORA).[11] In other words, the ORA is the noncorneal component of total refractive astigmatism, and quantifies by magnitude and axis orientation the minimum intraocular second order astigmatism aberrations. It is also the amount of corneal astigmatism expected to remain after treatment guided by refractive values alone, to neutralize this intraocular astigmatism.

ABERROMETRY AND WAVEFRONT GUIDED TREATMENT

Wavefront technology offers theoretical guidance to reduce spherical aberrations by achieving the most effective prolate aspheric profile. However, wavefront-assisted Lasik does not address the amount of resultant corneal astigmatism, and therefore is similar to Lasik based on manifest refraction. In addition, as aberrometry includes the internal optics of the eye in its calculations, any changes over time to the crystalline lens may undermine any benefit gained from the wavefront ablation.[1,9]

Furthermore, if wavefront guided ablation corrects all ocular aberrations at the corneal surface, it would produce an uneven corneal treatment resulting in induced corneal irregularities. This might be an undesirable result when it is widely recognized that a regular cornea with orthogonal and symmetrical astigmatism gives a superior visual result.[1,8] Permanently changing regional corneal shape in this manner is also complicated by the fact that this form of treatment may in fact be neutralized by epithelial healing.[9] Despite these potential limitations wavefront technology does provide useful refractive information. Rather than employing wavefront data exclusively, it can be combined with the vector planning method described in this chapter to produce an optimal treatment with reduced post-surgical aberrations.

COMBINING WAVEFRONT ANALYSIS AND TOPOGRAPHY WITH VECTOR PLANNING

A typical wavefront analysis is depicted in Figure 8.1. The spherocylindrical refraction as measured by the wavefront device at the spectacle plane is +0.52/ –1.83 × 3. The two-dimensional illustration of the wavefront analysis on the left shows a moderate level of mixed astigmatism with a typical saddle appearance. The higher order spherical aberrations are quantified as root-mean-square values in the lower right hand corner of the display. The spherical component of the correction (+0.52) is shown as the defocus. The cylindrical component is displayed beneath this. Third order aberrations (coma and trefoil) are listed separately, with 4th order spherical aberrations. 'Other terms' indicates 5th order and higher order aberrations.

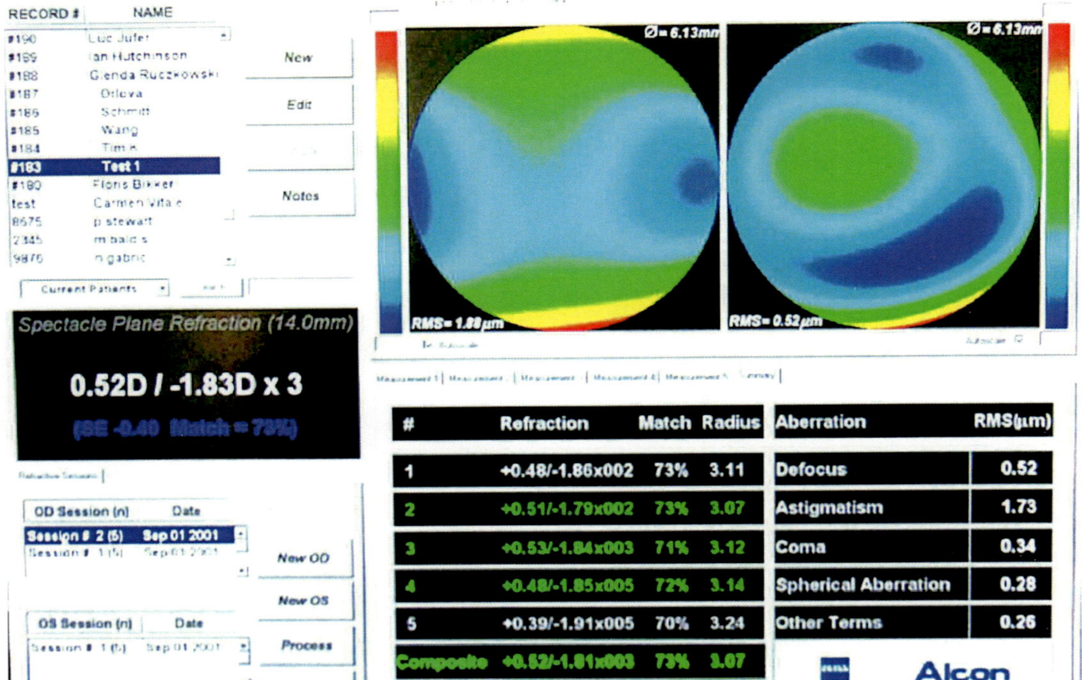

Fig. 8.1: A typical wavefront analysis display

Figure 8.2 displays a topographical map of the matching astigmatic eye. The typical bow-tie appearance of the regular corneal astigmatism is evident. In this example the astigmatism measures 2.62 D at the steepest meridian of 96 degrees as quantified by the simulated keratometry values. These parameters can then be examined together with those from the wavefront analysis spherocylindrical (second order) values to produce an optimal treatment by using the Alpins method contained in the ASSORT® program. This is shown in the treatment planning screen in Figure 8.3. In this diagram the treatment has been set to a base of 100 percent emphasis for correction of refractive astigmatism parameters.

This treatment screen in Figure 8.3 has been disassembled further for ease of understanding the various components. Figure 8.4 is the top central section on the ASSORT® treatment screen, displaying the preoperative spherocylindrical refractive values taken from the wavefront analysis and also the corneal plane conversion. The cylindrical component here is 1.81D of astigmatism at axis 3. This figure also displays the spherocylindrical target for the treatment, which in this case is zero.

The treatment vector being employed is shown in the polar diagram in Figure 8.5. Here the TIA is 1.81D at axis 3. The pre- and postoperative target astigmatism values are shown in Figure 8.6. The postoperative refractive target value is zero with the target corneal astigmatism value (obtained from Fig. 8.7 below) displayed in blue.

The simulated keratometry values from the preoperative topographical map are shown in Figure 8.7. Also displayed here are the ORA and the target for the corneal postoperative astigmatism. A vectorial calculation is used to determine the ORA, which in this case is 0.84 D. That is, there is a calculated amount of 0.84 D of intraocular astigmatism that cannot be eliminated from this eye. As the spherocylindircal refractive target has already been guided to zero, this can only leave the whole of the remaining astig-

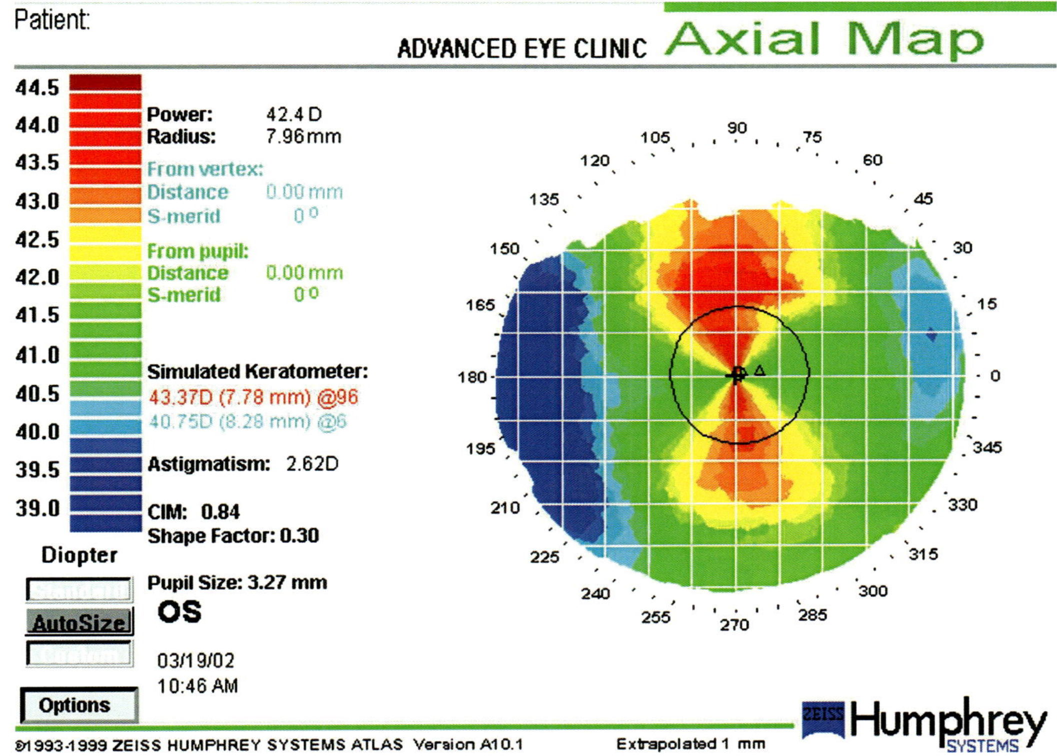

Fig. 8.2: Topographical analysis of the same eye

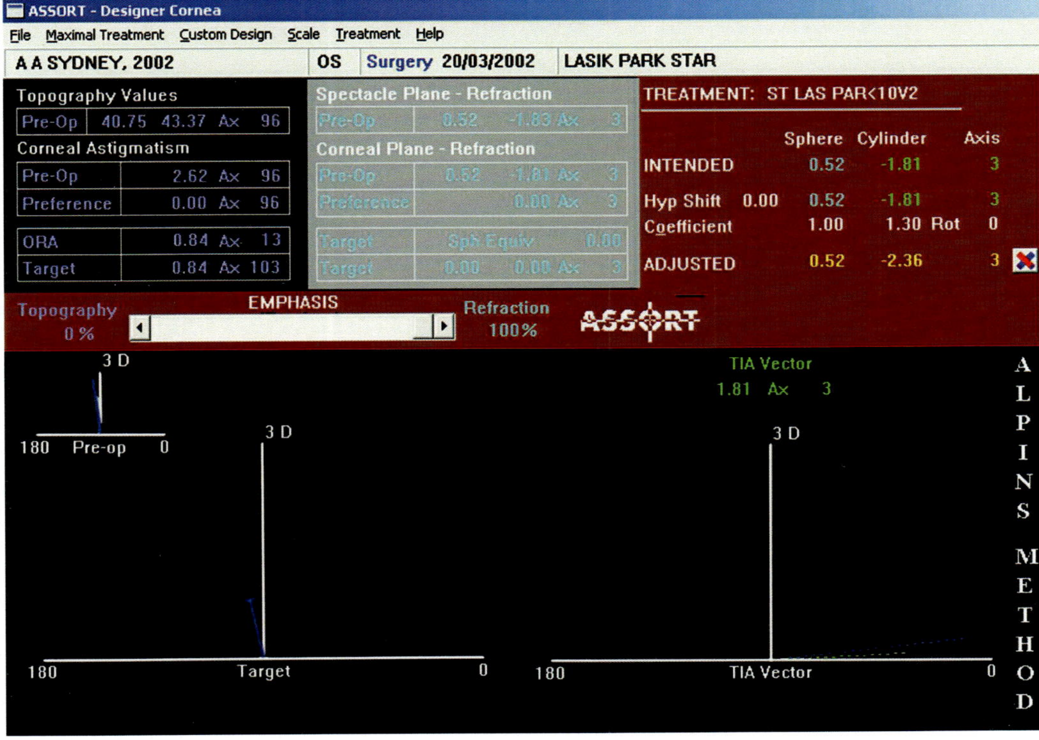

Fig. 8.3: The ASSORT surgical planning module for this eye

Spectacle Plane - Refraction

Pre-op	0.52	-1.83	Ax	3

Corneal Plane - Refraction

Pre-op	0.52	-1.81	Ax	3
Preferemce	0.52	0.00	Ax	3

Target	Sph Equiv			0.00
Target	0.00	0.00	Ax	3

Fig. 8.4: The top central section of the ASSORT screen displaying the preoperative refractive data obtained from the wavefront analysis (both spectacle and corneal plane values) and the chosen refractive spherocylindrical target

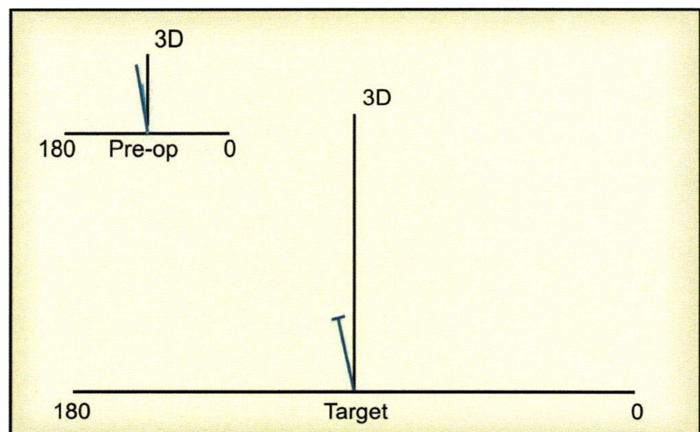

Fig. 8.6: Preoperative and postoperative target astigmatism vectors. The postoperative refractive target value is zero with the target corneal astigmatism vector displayed in green

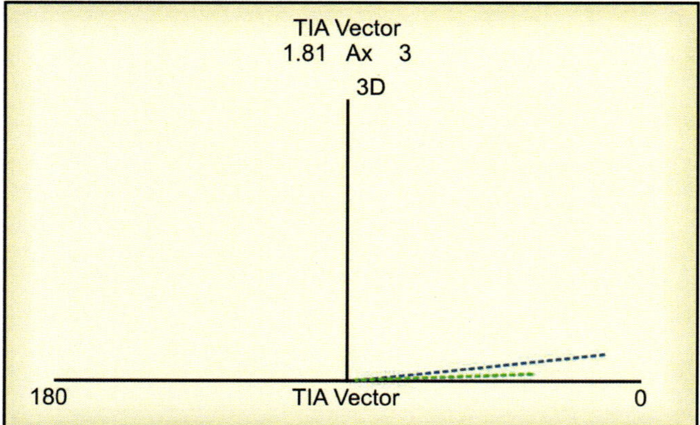

Fig. 8.5: The lower right hand graph on the ASSORT screen with a polar display of the TIA vector

Topography Values

Pre-op	40.75	43.37	Ax	96

Corneal Astigmatism

Pre-op	2.62	Ax	96
Preference	0.00	Ax	96

ORA	0.84	Ax	13
Target	0.84	Ax	103

Fig. 8.7: The top left hand box of the ASSORT screen displaying the corneal topographical preoperative values and the targeted corneal postoperative value. The minimum amount of astigmatism is displayed as the ORA, which in this case matches the magnitude target for the corneal astigmatism and is 90 degrees away

matism on the cornea at a near vertical meridian of 103 degrees to neutralize the ORA 90 degrees away, as seen in the target value of Figure 8.7.

However, as the emphasis is shifted towards the left, the treatment is more closely aligned to the principal corneal meridian. Figure 8.8 shows the optimal treatment for this eye, with the emphasis placed at 33 percent topography and 67 percent refraction. The ORA is still 0.84 D, but now it is apportioned between the refraction and the cornea. Here less corneal astigmatism is targeted and has been reduced to 0.56 D at an unchanged meridian 103 (Fig. 8.9). The remaining 0.28 D which is included in the spherocylindrical target of a spherical equivalent of zero, is not necessarily detected by the perceptive system at these levels, particularly as it is orientated favorably towards with-the-rule. Thus, with this method of vectorial planning, although the targeted spherocylindrical outcome is not zero, but 0.14/ –0.28 × 103 as displayed in Figure 8.10, the measured postoperative refractive and wavefront astigmatism is likely to be negligible.

Despite not targeting a zero spherocylindrical outcome, by directing the remaining astigmatism away from the cornea the overall astigmatism is also

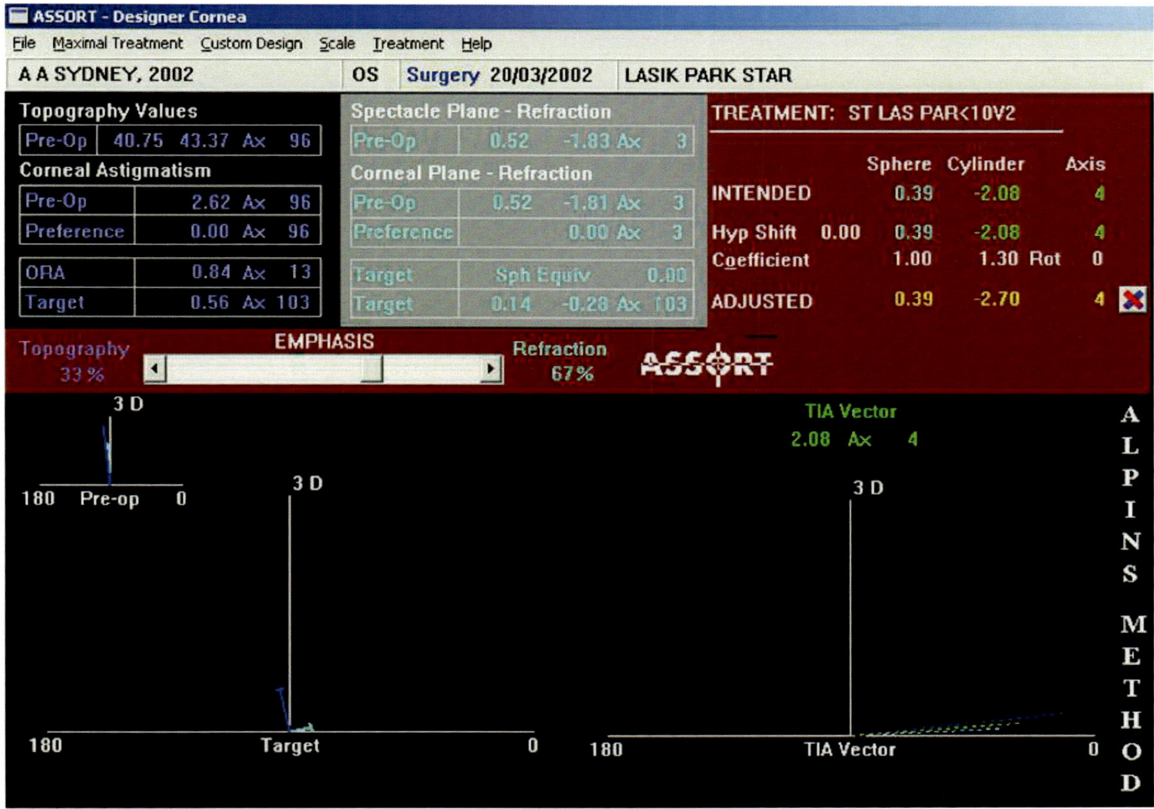

Fig. 8.8: The ASSORT treatment screen displaying the optimal treatment for the same eye. Here the emphasis bar has been shifted 33 percent towards the left so that not all of the surgical emphasis is placed on complete refractive astigmatism correction

Topography Values				
Pre-op	40.75	43.37	Ax	96
Corneal Astigmatism				
Pre-op		2.62	Ax	96
Preference		0.00	Ax	96
ORA		0.84	Ax	13
Target		0.56	Ax	103

Fig. 8.9: The optimal treatment for the same eye. Here the amount of corneal astigmatism remaining after treatment has been reduced by one third to 0.56 D, though the total ORA remains unchanged at 0.84 D

Spectacle Plane - Refraction				
Pre-op	0.52	-1.83	Ax	3
Corneal Plane - Refraction				
Pre-op	0.52	-1.81	Ax	3
Preference		0.00	Ax	3
Target	Sph Equiv			0.00
Target	0.14	-0.28	Ax	103

Fig. 8.10: The new spherocylindrical target for this eye is not zero, but 0.14/–0.28 × 103. This distributes the ORA between the postoperative refractive and corneal modes to produce a more favorable corneal shape and therefore less second order aberrations following surgery. The favorably orientated and minimal refractive target is not likely to be perceived by the patient

less, and there are fewer aberrations remaining. This treatment results in an overall higher patient satisfaction.

TREATMENT OF IRREGULAR ASTIGMATISM

Differences in the two opposite superior and inferior hemidivisions of the corneal topographical contour map are widely prevalent. This is known as irregular astigmatism and occurs if the two sides of the bow-tie representation differ in magnitude (asymmetrical) or are not aligned at 180 degrees to each other (non-orthogonal), or most commonly a combination of the two.[1,8] Irregular astigmatism may also be identified optically using wavefront devices. Unlike other methods of astigmatism analysis, the method described in this chapter may theoretically also be applied independently to each hemidivision in a cornea displaying pre-existing idiopathic irregularity. This would theoretically allow analysis and treatment of this irregular astigmatism to produce an orthogonal, symmetrical cornea.

The target refractive and corneal astigmatism values must be considered separately for each hemimeridian, with individual treatment plans required for both the superior and inferior topographic magnitudes and meridian values with the common refractive astigmatism value. From this, minimum target astigmatism values may be calculated for each part of the cornea, and their orientations are used to guide the choice for the optimal TIA for that side.[8]

The vectorial difference between the two opposite semimeridian values for magnitude and axis in each corneal part is called the topographic disparity (TD). When displayed on a 720 degrees double-angle vector diagram, the TD quantifies the irregular astigmatism of the cornea in dioptres, and the treatment required to reduce or eliminate the irregular astigmatism can be determined from this.[8]

The information gained from computerized topography regarding the corneal height (either directly such as the Z dimension on the Orbscan device, or indirectly inferred from slope measurement) may be translated into planned tissue ablation patterns using the Munnerlyn formula. This ablative pattern may then be applied at specific points on the corneal surface to reduce the irregularity.[1] There are various methods to link topographical information with tailored ablation, though a real-time preoperative link is yet to be achieved.

In this way, the corneal shape may be manipulated by asymmetrical surgical treatment to the irregular hemidivisions of the cornea, allowing the achievement of any corneal shape (thus producing regular astigmatism where selected). In cases of irregular astigmatism a rearrangement rather than a reduction of the corneal astigmatism may be of benefit, as regularizing the cornea may improve best corrected visual acuity to better approach the goal of supernormal vision.

SUMMARY

Due to natural differences in the vast majority of eyes between total astigmatism as measured by refraction and corneal astigmatism, it is impossible to completely eliminate astigmatism from the eye's optical system and its correction. It can therefore be beneficial to combine both these elements when considering the plan for refractive laser surgery to produce an optimal, individualized outcome. If the treatment plan utilizes manifest refraction data alone, it may actually increase the postoperative aberrations, thereby reducing the final visual result.

The Alpins method of vector planning utilizes information from both corneal topography and manifest refraction/wavefront data to target less postoperative corneal astigmatism and minimize postoperative aberrations. Though this often means that the postoperative refractive astigmatism target is not zero, this minor refractive error (with a spherical equivalent of zero) that remains postoperatively in a favorable orientation may not be significant enough for patient perception. In fact, overall the patient satisfaction is potentially higher due to the lesser amount of lower order aberrations.

This method of vector planning and analysis may also be used to optimize treatment for each separate hemimeridian of the cornea in cases of irregular astigmatism. This would enable the surgeon to rearrange the corneal astigmatism and regularize the cornea, thus producing a potential increase in the best corrected visual acuity. Though a real-time preoperative link to the topographical and wavefront information for this specialized ablation is yet to be formed, this integration of these diagnostic modalities utilizing vector planning may be a reality in the future.

REFERENCES

1. Goggin M, Alpins N, Schmid L. Management of irregular astigmatism. Current Opinion in Ophthalmology 2000; 11:260-6.
2. Alpins NA. Astigmatism by the Alpins Method. J Cataract Refract Surg 2001;27:31-49
3. Alpins NA, Stamatelatos G. Customized photoastigmatic refractive keratectomy using combined topographic and refractive data for myopia and astigmatism in eyes with form fruste and mild keratoconus. J Cataract Refract Surg 2007;33:591-602.
4. Alpins NA, Stamatelatos G. Clinical outcomes of Lasik using combined topography and refractive wavefront treatments for myopic astigmatism. J Cataract Refract Surg 2008; (in print).
5. Croes, KJ. The Alpins Method: A breakthrough in astigmatism analysis. Medical Electronics, 1998.
6. Alpins NA. A new method of analyzing vectors for changes in astigmatism. J Cataract Refract Surg 1993;19: 524-33.
7. Alpins NA. New method of targeting vectors to treat astigmatism. J Cataract Refract Surg 1997;23:65-75.
8. Alpins NA. Treatment of irregular astigmatism. J Cataract Refract Surg 1998;24:634-46.
9. Alpins NA. Wavefront technology: a new advance that fails to answer old questions on corneal vs refractive astigmatism correction. J of Refractive Surg 2002;737-9. *Discusses wavefront technology and the benefits of incorporating it into the refractive laser surgery plan.*
10. Javal E. Memoirs d'Ophthalmometrie. 1890, G Masson, Paris
11. Duke-Elder S, (Ed). System of Ophthalmology. Ophthalmic optics and refraction. St Louis, Mosby, 1970; 5:275-8.

9 Endothelial Evaluation Role in Refractive Surgery

Ajay V Kulkarni, Murali K Aasuri, Satish Gupta

INTRODUCTION

The corneal endothelium is the most important cellular monolayer responsible for maintenance of corneal transperancy, which is vital for normal vision. The endothelial cells spread themselves on a scafolding provided by the Descemet's membrane. The endothelial cell count at birth is approximately 350,000 cells (3000 cells/mm^2) arranged in a continuous monolayer.[1] The polygonal cells are closely apposed forming a uniform paving stone mosaic 4 to 6 μ thick. The individual cell is about 20 μ in diameter, with a surface area of 250 μ^2.[2] Each cell has 5 to 7 sides.[1] The endothelial population is uniformly distributed over the cornea and is symmetrical in both eyes of an individual. The cells become more irregular as they merge into the trabecular endothelium. With increasing age the endothelial cells die and disappear, while some cells enlarge in response to ageing and disease, while other cells remain of the same size. Since the human endothelial cells do not have the capacity to divide rapidly enough to replace the ageing or injured endothelial cells, they enlarge, reorganize and migrate to maintain an intact monolayer.

The endothelial cells are rich in mitochondria, endoplasmic reticulum, Golgi apparatus and free ribosomes which demonstrate that these cells are active in metabolism and secretions. The posterior surface of the cell membrane bulges into the anterior chamber and is thrown into microvilli and marginal folds, thereby, exposing greater cell surface area to aqueous humor. The endothelial cells are closely interdigitated with several junctional complex structures (zonula occludens, macula occludens, macula adherens), except desmosomes. In addition, gap junctions, 2 to 3 nm in size, between the adjacent endothelial cells permit penetration of small molecules and electrolytes between the endothelial cells. The interconnected endothelial cell layer provides a "leaky" barrier to aqueous humor.

The lateral plasma membrane of the endothelial cells contains Na^+-K^+ ATPase, an enzyme essential for endothelial pump function. It maintains the electro-chemical gradient for sodium and is directly involved in active transport of sodium across the endothelial cells.

The delicate balance between fluid entering the corneal stroma (barrier function) and fluid eggressing the stroma (pump function) maintains the corneal hydration at a fixed level of 78 percent. Any derangement in this delicate balance can result in corneal edema.

EVALUATION OF CORNEAL ENDOTHELIUM

Broadly, methods for endothelial evaluation are classified into *in vivo* (clinical) and *in vitro* (laboratory). There are three clinical methods for evaluating the corneal endothelial cell function: (i) pachymetry, by

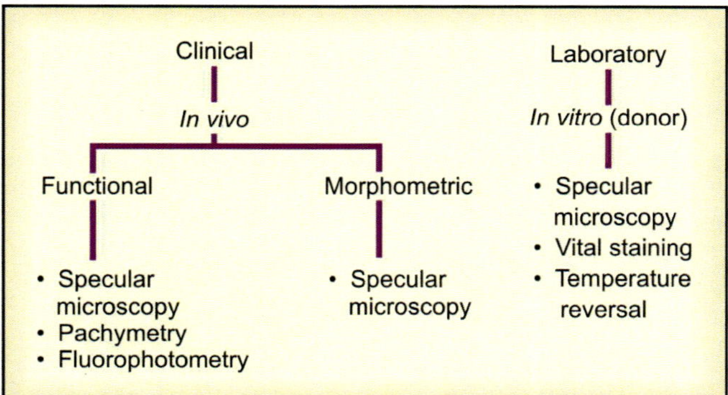

Fig. 9.1: Evaluation of corneal endothelium

optical or ultrasonic means, is an indirect measure of endothelial function that appraises corneal thickness, (ii) specular microscope studies the morphology of the endothelium, delineating cell size, density and distribution, and (iii) fluorophotometry which is a direct gauge of endothelial barrier function and acts as a barometer of fluid transport (Fig. 9.1).

SPECULAR MICROSCOPY

The first direct visualization of corneal endothelium was demonstrated by Vogt in 1918.[3] Unfortunately, factors such as continuous eye movement, limited magnification and annoying light reflexes precluded routine systematic study of endothelium for sometime thereafter. It was David Maurice[4] in 1968 who modified the metallurgical microscope and using the principle of reflective microscope obtained specular reflections from the endothelial surface through a fluid medium at high magnification. Later, Bourne and Kaufmann[5] and Laing et al[6] made further modifications which allowed routine clinical examination and photography of the endothelium. The major drawback of these models was a narrow field of view (0.04 mm^2). Current specular microscopes have multiple advantages such as wider field of view (1 mm^2) and improved optics which minimize annoying light reflections. In addition, higher resolution power, video cameras and recording systems have aided in capturing high quality pictures of the endothelium.

There are two basic types of clinical specular microscopes available today: (i) contact type, and (ii) the noncontact type. In the contact type the objective lens and the dipping cone lie directly on the corneal surface and eliminate the epithelial light reflection, whereas in the noncontact type, the observer finds the zone of specular reflection, as with the slit lamp. The ease of use, higher magnification and better resolution are the advantages of contact specular microscopes. However, the manipulation of the cornea may induce artifacts and the patients are less tolerant of the corneal contact. The noncontact type is generally difficult to use as it is more cumbersome to maintain a view in the field of specular reflection. Although the field of view is wider, the resolution is generally less.

Principle of Specular Microscopy

The specular reflection is the one in which the angle of incidence is equal to the angle of reflection. The reflected and back scattered light coming from the illumination source is collected into the objective lens of specular microscopes which is focussed on a film which shows four zones:

- A dark zone—part of aqueous humor
- Endothelial region—shows cell pattern
- Homogeneous area of stroma
- A bright zone—reflection of tear film or contact medium.

The interface between zones 3 and 4 is termed as dark boundary. This represents an area of separation of illuminated cornea from the nonilluminated more posterior structures. The interface between zone 2 and 3 is known as bright boundary. This separates the endothelium from the stroma. The normal endothelial cells are compact and regular with uniform cell size and cell area. The angulations and interjunctions are linear and regular.

Patient set-up: for noncontact specular microscopy First the procedure is explained to the patient. Once the patient is comfortably seated on a stool and the chin rests on the chin rest of the slit lamp, the head is fixed with a head band. The patient is asked to look straight ahead. Positioning of the eye is best achieved with a fixation light (Fig. 9.2).

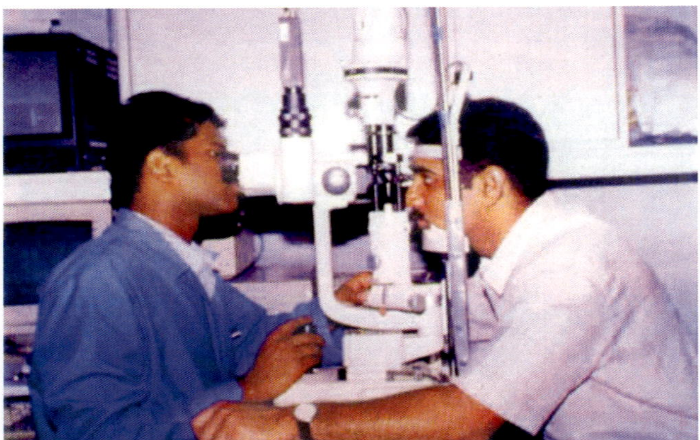

Fig. 9.2: Evaluation with noncontact specular microscope

The illumination system is turned on and is set at an angle of 40 to 60° with the observation system. The height of the beam is 2 mm and the width 0.8 mm. Then slowly the system is moved towards the eye of regard and the zone of specular reflection is located. This zone is reached when one sees the pattern of endothelial mosaic. With fine adjustment the image of the endothelium which is displayed on a monitor is focussed and multiple photographs of the endothelium are taken. This completes the procedure of recording the endothelial picture.

The analysis is done by the computer after the observer selects a particular endothelial photograph.

Clinical specular microscopy can be done using a narrow slit of light or wide slit of light which gives a larger field but a reduced contrast of the endothelial cell layer and loss of cellular definition.

Qualitative Evaluation of Endothelium

Qualitative analysis is based on morphologic appearance of the endothelial mosaic. It identifies abnormal endothelial structures and grades the endothelium either according to the number or size of the abnormal structures or on the basis of an overall assessment of endothelial appearance.

Following parameters are considered for evaluation:[7]

- Cell conformation
- Cell boundaries and their intersections

Fig. 9.3: The specular photomicrograph of normal endothelium showing a quasiregular pattern of endothelial mosaic. Note the uniformity of size and shape of individual cells

- Posterior corneal surface (configuration of the dark boundary)
- Presence of acellular structures.

Cell conformation The endothelial mosaic of the normal cornea is seen as a quasiregular pattern of contiguous cells having well-defined boundaries. The central endothelial cells are of approximately same size (100-400 μ^2 according to age) and the cell area distribution is approximately normal (gaussian). In young normal endothelium, cell side lengths are all roughly equal. Angles of intersection are approximately 60° at all ages (Fig. 9.3).

Cell boundaries and intersection Cell boundaries appear dark in the endothelial photomicrograph as the light incident on cell boundaries is scattered and does not return to the collection optic. Commonly they appear as straight narrow lines. They intersect in such a way that three angles of intersection are formed of approximately 60° each. Angles of intersection which vary considerably from 60° suggest that they are formed by abnormal cells.

The dark boundary The dark boundary represents the interface between the endothelial cell pattern and the adjacent dark zone produced by the aqueous humor. It gives information regarding posterior corneal surface. The boundary will be straight if the surface is smooth and regular. The four basic possible types of dark boundaries are smooth and straight, rough, wavy and excressed. A combination of any of the above can also be seen.

Presence of acellular structures These may be both intra- or intercellular and may be either dark or bright in appearance.

Intracellular structures

- Bright structure vary in size and are typically contained in a single endothelial cell. They can be single or multiple and are commonly seen in enlarged stressed cells.
- Bright structure spanning several endothelial cells appear white or orange in color and sparkles. They are thought to correspond to pigmented endothelial deposits.
- Two additional intracellular dark bodies have also been noted. The first type is a small, central or paracentral and well defined. Presumably, it represents the base of endothelial cilia. The second type is larger with indistinct edges and represent intracellular vacuoles or blebs.

Intercellular structures Dark structures which tend to be of uniform size with random distribution mostly lying at the endothelial cell intersection are seen in patients with anterior uveitis and are believed to represent invading inflammatory cells. Guttate are seen as intercellular dark structures which may be smaller or larger than individual endothelial cells (Fig. 9.4).

Fig. 9.4: The specular photomicrograph of endothelium showing dark areas representing guttate excrescences. Note the disruption of endothelial pattern

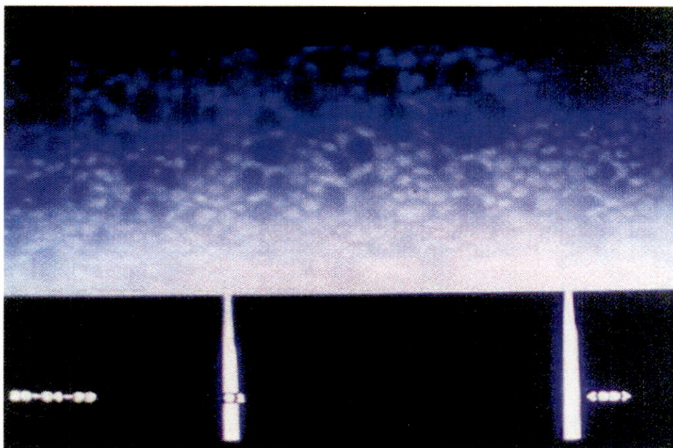

Fig. 9.5: The specular photomicrograph of endothelium showing variation in size (polymegathism) and shape (pleomorphism)

Quantitative Morphometric Analysis

Quantitative morphometric analysis is done with an aim or assigning a number or a set of numbers to the specular photomicrograph that can provide a measure of endothelial status.

The morphologic parameters which can be quantified are:

- Cell size (Fig. 9.5) (cell area and cell density)
- Polymegathism (variation of cell size such as coefficient of variation of mean cell area)
- Pleomorphism (variation of cell shape such as percentage of hexagonal cells or coefficient of variation of cell shape
- Cell perimeter
- Average cell side length
- Cell shape.

Two equivalent parameters have been used to quantify endothelial cell size:

- Mean cell area expressed in units of square microns (μ^2)
- Cell density (cell count) obtained by dividing the number of cells by the area of that frame, expressed in units of cells per square millimeters (cells/mm^2). These two quantities are related as:

$$\text{Mean cell area} = \frac{10^6}{\text{cell density (cells/mm}^2\text{)}}$$

Two different methods can be used to measure either of these two parameters of cell size: (i) fixed frame analysis, and (ii) variable frame analysis.

Fixed frame analysis In this method the number of cells within a frame of constant area are counted. All cells lying completely within the frame are counted as whole cells. The cell that lies only partly within the frame is counted as half cell. This is regardless of the fractional area of that cell within the frame.

- Cell count = sum of the number of whole and half cells within the frame
- Cell density (cells/mm^2) = $\dfrac{\text{cell count}}{\text{area of the frame}}$
- The area of the frame must be referred to the endothelium $= \dfrac{\text{Actual area of the frame}}{(\text{linear magnification of specular microscope})^2}$
- Mean cell area = $\dfrac{\text{Area}}{\text{Cell count}}$

In practice, a minimum of 35 contiguous cells (preferably 50-100 cells) should be within the counting frame otherwise one lands up with too large an error associated with counting.

Variable frame analysis Here one measures the variable area occupied by an integral number of cells by tracing around a contiguous group of cells. It eliminates the problem of counting fractional cells along the boundary and hence gives a more accurate determination of mean cell size as compared to fixed frame analysis. Each cell is marked and then the computer calculates the density by dividing the marked cells by the area of the frame. This results in a small counting error. It also gives an additional information regarding the range of cell densities or cell areas.

Individual Cell Analysis

Individual cell can be analyzed after tracing it or digitizing it during a variable frame analysis. It gives more information about endothelial cell pattern. It is probably the most accurate method of determining cell density and can be done manually, semiautomatically or fully automatically.

Computerized Morphometric Analysis[3]

A specular photograph is chosen on the basis of clarity of cell boundary and is enlarged to 400 times. Before the specular photograph is printed a calibration negative is taken with the same camera and is placed in an enlarger to ensure accurate cornea-to-print magnification. One hundred individual cells are numbered consecutively to minimize sampling and analysis error. Individual cells are digitized by marking each cell apex with a graphic tablet pen. The coordinates are entered into a digitizing tablet and analyzed by endothelial analysis software.

- Polymegathism is calculated as:
  $$\frac{\text{Standard deviation of mean cell area}}{\text{mean cell area}}$$
- Coefficient of variation (polymegathism)
  It is a dimensionless index and provides quantitative measurement of cell variation.[8] The coefficient of variation of normal cornea is 0.25.
- Cell shapes are described by the number of apices of each cell and the variation is analyzed automatically by digitizing the apex of each cell (pleomorphism). Both pleomorphism and polymegathism reflect compensatory mechanisms of the endothelium to accommodate stress and are thought to be more sensitive and reliable in giving the idea regarding the cell loss when compared to cell area and cell density measurement alone.

Little correlation has been seen between the cell density and the functional capacity of endothelial mosaic. In addition there is no direct correlation between cell density and endothelial function as indicated by corneal thickness measurement.[9]

PACHYMETRY

Corneal thickness is an important indicator of corneal endothelial function. The collagen fibers of stroma run along the plane of cornea from limbus to limbus, and any increase in corneal hydration can manifest itself only in increase in the corneal thickness[9] as the length of the collagen fibers cannot increase.

The normal central corneal thickness is 0.52 mm $\pm$ 0.02 mm, with thickening in the periphery to about

0.65 to 0.75 mm. The value of pachymetry lies in estimating the functional reserve of the endothelium in a clear cornea and is very useful when subclinical edema is suspected.

Methods of Pachymetry

Optical Doubling[10]

A special attachment to the slit lamp gives a split image of the corneal section. The corneal thickness can be read directly from a dial when the amount of doubling can be adjusted so that the anterior surface of one image lines up with the posterior surface in the other image. Measurement of the thickness must be made perpendicular to the cornea, failure to do so is a major source of error in the measurement. This error is circumvented in some pachymeters by the incorporation of two small lamps attached to the extended plate of the pachymeter with the narrow aperture for the passage of the slit beam. While measuring, the images of the two small lamps must be on the epithelial line and equidistant from the horizontal dividing line. This ensures the perpendicular alignment of the optical section.

Optical Focusing

Certain specular microscopes are calibrated so that when the endothelium is in focus, the thickness of the cornea is automatically displayed digitally. At the start of the measurement, care must be taken to establish the zero by focusing on the interface between the contact element and the epithelial layer.

Ultrasonic Pachymetry[11]

A refinement in ultrasonographic techniques has made it possible to measure corneal thickness. The techniques used are along the principles of ultrasonographic measurement of axial length of the globe. It is a rapid and accurate test, it can be used in supine or sitting positions and it readily scans the entire cornea.

The ultrasonic pachymeter averages multiple readings taken in 1 to 2 sec by the sound waves of a probe when it is held within 10 degrees of the perpendicular to the corneal surface. Although various studies suggest that the inter- and intraobserver ultrasonographic reading errors are less than 0.005 mm, the degree of accuracy depends on the measurement size. Even small movements of the probe from initial measurement location invalidate the accuracy of the values recording changes in thickness produced by measuring adjacent parts of the cornea. Some assessment errors using this method result from incorrect alignment of the ultrasonic probe, varying speeds of sound through corneal tissue, difficulty in relocating exactly the same area to measure corneal thickness sequentially. With skill and good deal of practice the reading error is about + or –2 percent. Accuracy in pachymetry readings is particularly important while determining the depth of incisions in refractive corneal surgery.

FLUOROPHOTOMETRY

The barrier function of the endothelium can be evaluated by measurement of its permeability to various substances, e.g. fluorescein.[9] Fluorescein can be injected intravenously or can be ingested (10% fluorescein sodium 5 mg/kg of body wt) or may be driven into the corneal stroma from the surface by iontophoresis, and the diffusion across the endothelium can be measured. Fluorophotometer measures the fluorescein concentration in the corneal stroma and aqueous.

In the peripheral cornea fluorescein enters the corneal stroma directly from the limbal vessels but in the center the dye is transferred exclusively from the aqueous across the endothelium.

The fluorescein concentration in aqueous and corneal stroma changes with time. In the aqueous almost 100 percent of the fluorescein is free for diffusion, while in the cornea significant amount is protein bound and only 57 percent is diffusible and is in equilibrium with aqueous fluorescein. The transfer coefficient, the index of endothelial permeability, is increased when the barrier function of the endothelium is affected. The transfer coefficient is approximately 0.4 hr^1 and the permeability of the endothelium is approximately 3.5×10^{-4} cm/min.[9]

ENDOTHELIAL CHANGES FOLLOWING REFRACTIVE SURGERY

Refractive procedures to correct myopia, hyperopia and astigmatism are generally performed on healthy eyes. These can be extraocular (corneal) or intraocular. All of them have a potential to cause endothelial damage.

Endothelial damage can be acute, short-term or prolonged leading to progressive decrease in cell density. Several mechanisms have been noted, the most common being direct and indirect mechanical trauma (direct cut, stretching, folding, shock waves and cavitation bubbles generated in the stroma). Other effects such as increase in temperature and mutagenic effects may also be responsible. Implants or their storage solutions may produce toxic effects. Long-term metabolic effects after refractive procedures such as, changes in glucose diffusion, can also alter the endothelial cell layer.[12]

INCISIONAL PROCEDURES

Radial Keratotomy (RK)

In the initial days during the evolution of RK Sato et al[13] gave incisions on the posterior cornea in addition to the anterior cornea. In most of these patients bullous keratopathy developed more than 10 years after surgery. Endothelial integrity with anterior RK (90-100% thickness) has been studied extensively.

Yamaguchi et al[14] reported endothelial cell damage and distended intracellular spaces beneath anterior radial incisions in rabbits. Posterior protrusion of Descemet's membrane was also noted. The endothelium recovered in 3 months, but the distended intracellular spaces persisted.

Studies on monkeys have demonstrated inflammatory cell infiltrate on the endothelium in the first 2 weeks associated with marked intercellular vacuolation and intracytoplasmic condensation. These changes were not detected after six months and no long-term progressive cell damage could be detected.[15]

Dunn et al[16] have reported increased polymegathism and coefficient of variation for cell area and cell perimeter for 1 month postoperatively following which the values returned to normal. Several studies in humans have reported central endothelial density losses (Table 9.1) averaging between 3 and 10 percent.

Table 1: Endothelial cell loss after RK

Authors	*Percentage of cell loss*	*Duration after RK (months)*	*No of incisions*	*No of eyes*
Rowsey et al[17]	5.6	1	8-16	99
	6.9	6	8-16	39
Hoffer et al[18]	9.0	3	16	48
	2.6	6	8	14
Chiba et al[19]	5.6	6-30	8	24
MacRae et al[20]	3.3	12	8	11

Risk factors for increased endothelial damage in RK include:

- Intraoperative microperforations
- Increased number of incisions
- Smaller optical zone diameter.

Recently MacRae et al[21] compared long-term results in 25 RK eyes with eyes of noncontact lens wearers. Up to 7 years after surgery, no significant differences in endothelial cell density, hexagonality and coefficient of variation could be detected.

LAMELLAR PROCEDURES

Keratophakia and Keratomileusis

In 1981 Aquavella et al[22] reported on 27 eyes undergoing keratomileusis and keratophakia. Central endothelial cell loss was 6.2 percent in myopic keratomileusis and 18 percent when it was combined with cataract extraction and in hyperopic keratomileusis in aphakes. Busin et al[23] reported no alteration of endothelial cell density after 2 years in 8 patients undergoing epikeratophakia using prelathed lyophilized tissue.

CORNEAL INLAYS

Hydrogel Lenses

Nonhuman primate studies have confirmed good biocompatibility of the inlays up to 8 years postoperatively and a mean endothelial cell loss of 7.5 percent at 2 years.[24,25]

Barraquer et al[26] reported no alteration in endothelial cell count in 10 eyes with intracorneal lenses at the end of a 6-year follow-up.

Intracorneal Ring Segments (ICRS)

These rings achieve indirect central flattening induced by peripheral steepening related to the ring segments. The material used is polymethylmethacrylate (PMMA).

Assil et al[27] evaluated ICRS in 10 nonfunctional human eyes. At the end of 1 year following the surgery, endothelial cell counts were unaffected by the ICRS.

Similar results were also reported by Cochener et al[28] in 47 patients with ICRS followed for 3 to 18 months. No significant changes in endothelial cells and central corneal thickness were noted.

LASER PROCEDURES

Excimer Laser

Photorefractive Keratectomy (PRK)

The effect of deep radial excision of corneal tissue by 193 nm ultraviolet (UV) light has been carefully investigated. It causes endothelial cell loss similar to that of RK with a blade. Marshall et al[29,30] have demonstrated in rabbits that radial excision with excimer laser damages the endothelium only if the cut is within 40 m of the Descemet's membrane.

Fantes et al[31] demonstrated a normal endothelium and absence of newly produced material in Descemet's membrane after –2.0 to –8.0 D PRK in monkeys. In humans both Descemet's membrane and endothelium remained normal after laser lamellar keratectomy up to 60 μ depth.[32]

Stulting et al[32] prospectively investigated 142 eyes of 142 patients who had PRK for myopia between –2.0 to –6.0 D. There was no difference in central endothelial cell density at 3 months and 1 year postoperatively. Wojoiechowska[34] reported no statistically significant difference in endothelial cell density in patients undergoing PRK between preoperative and 12 month postoperative examinations.

Perez-Santonja et al[35] based on the results of 14 PRKs postulated cell migration from the peripheral to the central cornea. They found unchanged central endothelial density and hexagonality but, significantly decreased coefficient of variation in cell size after PRK.

Laser in-situ Keratomileusis (LASIK)

Endothelial cell loss has been reported after LASIK. Pallikaris et al[36] reported an average endothelial cell loss of 2.43 percent at 2 years in 43 patients undergoing LASIK. One patient had a transient endothelial decompensation.

Perez-Santonja[37] compared endothelial cell loss in eyes with and without contact lenses with those undergoing LASIK. He reported increased central endothelial cellular density at 6 months in LASIK and contact lens group along with increased hexagonality at 3,6,12 months. The coefficient of variation was noted to be decreased in all visits.

Thermokeratoplasty

This procedure achieves steepening of the central cornea by producing peripheral corneal burns with a cautery of holmium laser. Available data on effects on endothelial cells are controversial.

Neuman et al[38] did not find any change in central and peripheral endothelial cell counts in 15 human eyes before and 6 or 12 months after the procedure.

In rabbits, Feldman et al[39] observed endothelial damage directly under the burn and extending circumferentially with a radius of 300 μ. The expected endothelial cell loss after standard thermokeratoplasty is 5 to 14 percent.

PHAKIC INTRAOCULAR LENSES

High level of myopia can be corrected with great accuracy by implanting minus power anterior or posterior chamber lenses in phakic eyes. Endothelial trauma during this intraocular surgery is one of the most serious complications of the procedure. Phakic

IOLs can be anterior chamber angle fixated or iris claw lenses or posterior chamber lenses. The more anterior the location, greater are the chances of endothelial damage. Various modifications in the lens design have occurred in last few years towards minimizing endothelial damage.

Anterior Chamber Phakic IOL (ACIOL)

In a series of 62 eyes with Worst-Fechner iris claw lens, Fechner et al[40] noted two eyes in which the mean endothelial cell count decreased from 3000 to 4000 cells/mm^2 to 1500 cells/mm^2 which was attributed to surgical trauma and at least in one case to relatively shallow anterior chamber prior to surgery. In a later study[41] the same author showed a marked endothelial cell loss in 10 of 109 eyes. Three eyes required penetrating keratoplasty. The author suggested that rubbing the myopic eye with low scleral rigidity causes transient lens-endothelial touch which is responsible for the damage. With the first generation Baikoff lenses endothelial cell loss was reported to be 10 to 15 percent one year after the surgery.

Praeger et al[42] showed 5.3 percent endothelial cell loss postoperatively but was not progressive on a 3-year follow-up examination. Mimouni et al[44] reported endothelial cell loss in central and paracentral areas in 15 patients with Baikoff AC implants. In 36.3 percent patients a loss of more than 20 percent and in 54.4 percent patients a loss of less than 10 percent was noted.

Baikoff et al[44] in a retrospective study quantitatively and topographically analyzed the corneal endothelium in 20 eyes and found that most of the endothelial cell loss occurred in the second postoperative year with a wide standard deviation and the cell loss was seen to be higher in higher power implants.

Perez-Santonja et al[44] reported on long-term endothelial cell loss after implantation of Worst-Fechner and Baikoff ZB5M ACIOLs. Preoperative and serial postoperative microscopy was performed. The results are summarized in Table 9.2. Baikoff suggests that ACIOL should be removed if endothelial cell count is less than 50 percent of normal count.

Table 9.2: Endothelial cell loss after phakic anterior chamber intraocular lens (IOL)

Lens type	No of eyes	Cell loss	
		One year (Percentage)	Two years (Percentage)
Worst Fechner	30	13	17.60
Baikoff	28	12.33	12.30

Posterior Chamber Phakic IOL (PCIOL)

Theoretically these lenses are expected to be safer as compared to ACIOL as far as endothelial cell damage is concerned. Fyodorov et al[46] have reported mean decreases in the endothelial cell density of 5 percent with silicone posterior chamber phakic IOL and Assetto et al[47] found mean losses of 4 percent in 15 eyes that received the Staar collamer IOL.

SUMMARY

All the available refractive procedures do result in variable degrees of endothelial injury. Preoperative status of endothelium, intraoperative complications and postoperative management play a critical role. It is absolutely essential for the surgeon to have an understanding of the nature of the surgical procedure and its impact on the health of the endothelium before undertaking the procedure. This will help in proper patient selection, avoidance of postoperative surprises and legal litigations.

REFERENCES

1. Edelhauser HF, Van Horn DL, Records RE. Cornea and sclera. In Duane TD, Jaeger EA (Eds): Biomedical Foundations of Ophthalmology Harper and Row: Hagerstown 1982;2(4).
2. Sturrock GD, Sherrad ES, Rice MSC. Specular microscopy of the corneal endothelium. Br J Ophthalmol 1978;62:809.
3. Yee RY. Widefield clinical specular microscopy and computerized morphometric analysis. In Podos SM, Yanoff M (Eds): Textbook of Ophthalmology: External Diseases, London, Mosby: St Louis 1994;8(7):10-2.
4. Dickstein S, Maurice DM. The metabolic basis of the fluid pump in the cornea. J Physiol 1972;221:29-41.
5. Bourne WM, Kaufman HE. Specular microscopy of human corneal endothelium. Am J Ophthalmol 1976; 81:319-23.

6. Laing RA, Sandstrom MM, Leibowitz HM, et al. In vivo photomicrography of the corneal endothelium. Arch Ophthalmol 1975;93:143-5.
7. Laing RA, Sandstrom MM, Leibowitz HM, et al. Clinical specular microscopy II—qualitative evaluation of corneal endothelial photomicrographs. Arch Ophthalmol 1979; 97:1720.
8. Rao GN, Waldron W, Aquavella J. Morphology of graft endothelium and donor age. Br J Ophthalmol 1980;64: 523-7.
9. Mishima S. Clinical investigations on the corneal endothelium. Ophthalmology 1982;89:525-30.
10. Mishima S. Corneal thickness. Surv Ophthalmol 1968; 13:57.
11. Ytteborg J, Dohlman CH. Corneal edema and intraocular pressure II—clinical results. Arch Ophthalmol 1965;74: 477.
12. Fruch BE, Bohnke M. Endothelial changes following refractive surgery. J Cataract Refract Surg 1996;22(4):490-6.
13. Sato T, Shibata H, Akiyama K. Surgery of myopia, incision of corneal posterior surface. Acta Soc Ophthalmol Jpn 1952;56:1137-9.
14. Yamaguchi T, Polack FM, Velenti J, et al. Endothelial damage after anterior radial keratotomy—an electron microscopic study of rabbit cornea. Arch Ophthalmol 1981;92: 153-71.
15. Jester JV, Steel D, Salz J, et al. Radial keratotomy in nonhuman primate eyes. Am J Ophthalmol 1981;92:153-71.
16. Dunn S, Jester JV, Arthur J, et al. Endothelial cell loss following radial keratotomy in a primate model. Arch Ophthalmol 1984;102:1666-70.
17. Rowsey JJ, Balyeat HD. Preliminary results and complications of radial keratotomy. Am J Ophthalmol 1982;93:437-55.
18. Hoffer KJ, Darin JJ, Pettit TH, et al. Three-year experience with radial keratotomy—the UCLA study. Ophthalmology 1983;90:627-36.
19. Chiba K, Tsubota K, Oak SS, et al. Morphometric analysis of corneal endothelium following radial keratotomy. J Cataract Refract Surg 1987;13:263-7.
20. MacRae SM, Matsuda M, Rich LF. The effect of radial keratotomy on the corneal endothelium. Am J Ophthalmol 1985;100:538-42.
21. MacRae SM, Rich LF. Morphometric analysis of the long-term effects of RK on the corneal endothelium—ARVO abstract 1785. Invest Ophthalmol Vis Sci 1994;35:1637.
22. Aquavella JV, Barraquer F, Rao GN, et al. Morphological variations in corneal endothelium following keratophakia and keratomileusis. Ophthalmology 1981;88:721-3.
23. Busin M, Spitznas M, Hockwin O. Evaluation of functional and morphologic parameter of the cornea after epikeratophakia using prelathed, lyophilized tissue. Ophthalmology 1990;97(3):330-3.
24. Werblin TP, Peiffer RL, Binder PS, et al. Eight years experience with permalens intracorneal lenses in nonhuman primates. Refract Corneal Surg 1992;8:12-22.
25. McDonald MB, McCarey BE, Storie B, et al. Assessment of the long-term corneal response to hydrogel intrastromal lenses implanted in monkey eyes for upto 5 years. J Cataract Refract Surg 1993;19:212-22.
26. Barraquer MJI, Gomez ML. Permalens hydrogel intracorneal lenses for spherical ametropia. J Cataract Refract Surg 1997;13(4):342-8.
27. Assil KK, Barrett AM, Fouraker BD, et al. One year results of intrastromal corneal ring in nonfunctional human eyes—intrastromal corneal ring study group. Arch Ophthalmol 1995;113(2):159-67.
28. Cochener B, Le Floch G, Colin J. Intracorneal rings for the correction of weak myopias. J Fr Ophthalmol 1998; 21(3): 191-208.
29. Marshall J, Trokel S, Rothery S, et al. An ultrastructural study of corneal incisions induced by an excimer laser at 193 nm. Ophthalmology 1985;92:749-58.
30. Marshall J, Trokel S, Rothery S, et al. A comparative study of corneal incisions induced by diamond and steel knives and two ultraviolet radiation from an excimer laser. Br J Ophthalmol 1986;70:482-501.
31. Fantes FE, Hanna KD, Waring GO III, et al. Wound healing after excimer laser keratomileusis (photorefractive keratectomy) in monkeys. Arch Ophthalmol 1990; 108:665-75.
32. Taylor DM, L'Esperance FA Jr, Del Pero RA, et al. Human excimer laser lamellar keratectomy—a clinical study. Ophthalmology 1989;96:654-64.
33. Stulting RD,Thompson KP, Reddik DE, et al. The effect of 193 nm excimer laser photorefractive keratectomy (PRK) on the human corneal endothelium—ARVO abstract 1843. Invest Ophthalmol Vis Sci 1994;35:1650.
34. Wojoiechowska R, Borek S, Gierek-Ciaciura S, et al. Corneal endothelium after photorefractive keratectomy procedures. Klin Ozna 1996;98(3):361-3.
35. Perez-Santonja JJ, Meza J, Moreno E, et al. Short-term corneal endothelial changes after photorefractive keratectomy. J Refract Corneal Surg 1994;10:5194-8.
36. Pallikaris IG, Siganos D. Laser in-situ keratomileusis to treat myopia—early experience. J Cataract Refract Surg 1997;23:39-49.
37. Perez Santonja JJ, Sakla HF, Gobbi F, et al. Corneal endothelial changes after laser in-situ keratomileusis. J Cataract Refract Surg 1997;23:177-83.
38. Neumann AC, Sanders D, Raanan M, et al. Hyperopic thermokeratoplasty—clinical evaluation. J Cataract Refract Surg 1991;17:830-8.
39. Feldman ST, Ellis W, Frucht-Pery J, et al. Experimental radial thermokeratoplasty in rabbits. Arch Ophthalmol 1990;108:997-1000.
40. Fechner PU, Van der Heijde GL, Worst JGF. The correction of myopia by lens implantation into phakic eyes. Am J Ophthalmol 1989;107:659-63.

41. Fechner PU, Strobel J, Wichmann W. Correction of myopia by implantation of a concave worst-iris claw lens into phakic eyes. Refract Corneal Surg 1991;7:286-98.
42. Praeger DL, Mamose A, Muroff LL. Thirty-six month follow up of a contemporary phakic intraocular lens for the surgical correction of myopia. Ann Ophthalmol 1991;23: 6-10.
43. Baikoff G. The refractive IOL in a phakic eye. Ophthalmic Pract 1991;9:58-61.
44. Mimouni F, Colin J, Koffi V, et al. Damage to the corneal endothelium from anterior chamber intraocular lenses in phakic myopic eyes. Refract Corneal Surg 1991;7:277-81.
45. Perez-Santonja JJ, Iradier MT, Sanz-Iglesiaz L, et al. Endothelial changes in phakic eyes with anterior chamber intraocular lenses to correct high myopia. J Cataract Refract Surg 1996;22:1017-22.
46. Fyodorov SN, Zuyev VK, Tumanyan MR, et al. Clinical and functional follow up of minus IOL implantation in high grade myopia. Ophthal Surg 1993;2:12-7.
47. Assetto V, Benedetti S, Pesando P. Collamer intraocular contact lens to correct high myopia. J Cataract Refract Surg 1996;22:551-6.

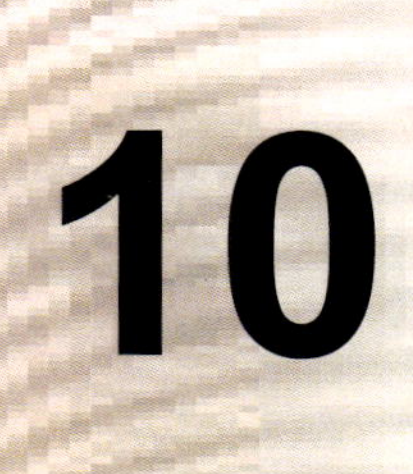

10 The Importance of a Preoperative Examination in LASIK and PRK

Dimitrios S Siganos

INTRODUCTION

The importance of carrying out a preoperative examination and evaluation cannot be stressed too strongly; and this examination must be of the most thorough and meticulous type.

Every patient is not suited to laser surgery and many may be excluded because of an ocular or systemic disease, by history or by other external factors.

CONTRAINDICATIONS

Ocular

- Active ocular contraindications could include, but not be limited to, Sjögren's disease
- Residual ocular contraindications could include herpes simplex virus
- Recurrent ocular contraindications could include corneal scarring.

The refractive result is unpredictable in eyes with scarring because the excimer laser ablation rate will be different over the scar tissue and the elasticity of the cornea is not uniform. Any refractive procedure performed on scarred eyes may well result in irregular astigmatism which, in turn, requires a second operation and/or hard contact lenses in order to achieve the preoperative best corrected visual acuity (BCVA). This should be clearly explained both verbally and on the consent form to be signed before any procedure takes place.

Systemic

In systemic, the contraindications include pregnancy, lactation or women who may be pregnant—laser-induced teratogenesis is potentially dangerous, as are the possible contraindications of drugs that may be required in the postoperative period. Contraceptive pills have also been reported to induce temporary myopia and the patient should be encouraged to bring any and all medication which they are currently taking to the ophthalmologist in order to ascertain that there will be no contraindications and that the assessment of the degree of refractive error will be accurate.

Collagen vascular diseases, rheumatoid arthritis, systemic lupus erythematosus (SLE) and Sjögren's disease are also examples of when the ophthalmologist should be wary of performing a laser procedure. Diabetes, too, is a major stumbling block as epithelial healing can be vastly reduced. Refraction is not usually stable and diabetics develop cataracts earlier than nondiabetics (as supported by the PRK Summit initial FDA data). Diabetics also have a much higher susceptibility to infection.

Contact lens wearers should be advised that they should stop wearing their soft lenses at least three weeks before evaluation and surgery or their hard lenses for at least three months prior to evaluation and surgery, in order for the cornea to regain its "normal" shape and to avoid misdiagnosing corneal warpage syndrome.

THE EXAMINATION

Basically, the examination and subsequent evaluation will have two parts: (i) invasive and (ii) noninvasive tests.

The patient's unaided visual acuity (UVA) must be measured under optimum conditions, as well as the near UVA and BCVA manifest refraction. Signs of subclinical keratoconus, corneal warpage syndrome and/or irregular astigmatism are all potential exclusion factors.

BCVA manifest refraction is of paramount importance and could even be termed the single most important factor to evaluate. Postoperative UVA is a useful aid in measuring efficacy, but safety of a procedure is BCVA. Moderate and high myopes should be evaluated by the use of a soft contact lens for preference or by a hard if necessary, and that having a spherical equivalent as close as possible to the patient's refraction. All powers of contact lenses should ideally be available in order for the patient's refraction to be properly determined. At this stage, one should point out that overrefraction should never be more than $\pm$ 2.5 diopters. Contact lens determination of BCVA in myopia over 6.5 diopters and in hyperopia over 4 diopters is a good rule to follow.

In myopias with astigmatism, the surgeon should be prepared to deal with a discrepancy in manifest and cycloplegic axis. In high myopias, a large amount of tissue is removed, the possibility of potentially induced astigmatism is high, and the patient should be informed of the probability of a second "enhancement" procedure being performed for the correction of the remaining astigmatism and/or myopia.

We move on now to stability of refraction and among the questions to be posed of the patient are the following:

- Is the patient at least 18 years old?
- What is the patient's earlier refractive status?
- What is the patient's frequency of changing glasses or contact lenses?
- What is the discrepancy between manifest and cycloplegic refraction?
- What are the results of checking the clarity or condition of the topical media?
- Is there a suspicion of keratoconus or cataract in progression, or corneal warpage syndrome?

Corneal Topography

Corneal topography must be performed and forms an essential part of the preoperative evaluation. In no circumstances should it be overlooked. Subclinical keratoconus can only be diagnosed by corneal topography and may well be missed in a slit lamp or keratometer examination.

Contrast Sensitivity

Contrast sensitivity testing is the most vital measurement of procedure safety and should be performed carefully and thoroughly, as should all the preoperative tests. LASIK and PRK treat the stroma of the cornea so there is healing in the interface; because of this healing, potential reduction of clarity and, in turn, contrast sensitivity may be induced. In very high myopes, it is sometimes difficult with the available tests to measure contrast sensitivity and every attempt should be made to record a measurement, which is always done with the patient having his best contact lens correction.

There is a slight possibility, seen in approximately 4 percent of patients, of ptosis following LASIK or PRK and, although some patients believe their eyelids never recovered from this, almost all cases are temporary. This is usually due to steroids although the actual reasoning behind this is not currently understood. It might be an idea, although it is not yet a legal requirement, to take "before and after" photographs for medicolegal reasons and to avoid any retribution after the event.

Ocular Motility

Preoperative latent or undocumented ductions, versions, tropias and phorias may become manifest following refractive surgery. This is why the patient should be properly diagnosed and informed accordingly. High anisometropics may also develop binocular diplopia.

Slit Lamp Examination

Slit lamp examination is another mandatory preoperative test, used in order to rule out various conditions and/or diseases before surgery is performed. Lids should be checked for blepharitis or other indications that all is not well and treatment should be completed before the refractive procedure is carried out.

Corneal Thickness

The cornea should be examined for clarity, scars, the presence of dystrophies and degenerations, especially keratoconus, although it is not an absolute contra-indication for LASIK. A preoperative corneal thickness of at least 480 μ and refractive stability are absolute prerequisites for moderate to high myopes in LASIK. The refraction may have suboptimal results, the condition may deteriorate and a corneal transplant may even become necessary. The refractive surgeon should also be vigilant about neovascularization as a result of contact lens wear as, in LASIK, the suction produced by the microkeratome often ruptures these vessels, resulting in conjunctival hemorrhage. Although not a major complication, visibility during surgery may be decreased and the patient may become anxious.

The anterior chamber should be checked for active iritis and the crystalline lens examined under full mydriasis. **A 50-year-old patient, for example, with –11 diopters and nuclear sclerosis or other peripheral lens opacity would benefit more from a clear lens extraction than from LASIK.**

Schirmer's Test

The Schirmer's test is performed in order to avoid operating on a patient with xerophthalmia, something which often delays the healing process. This is more important in photorefractive keratectomy than in laser-in-situ keratomileusis (LASIK). Symptoms of xerophthalmia may be exacerbated due to the preservatives contained in the drugs used following surgery or by the surgery itself.

Pupil Size

The pupil size should be measured in dim light and this is important to avoid postoperative glare problems. The thickness of the corneal tissue to be removed is proportional to the ablation zone diameter and, since LASIK is usually used to correct moderate and high degrees of myopia where large corrections are attempted, small zones are utilized to avoid getting too deep in the cornea. Prismatic effects of the reshaped corneal optics are liable to induce glare and halo phenomena more commonly than PRK if a transition zone or multipass technique is not used. As a general rule of thumb, such effects are to be expected, and are more pronounced the greater the correction if the dim light pupil diameter is less than 5 mm.

Endothelioscopy

Noncontact endothelioscopy should be performed in older patients who may later require an intraocular procedure, e.g. cataract operation, or in patients in whom a secondary, refinement procedure is expected, i.e. patients with very high myopic spherical equivalent, or high astigmatism in whom predictability is expected to be suboptimal. Although LASIK and PRK do not appear significantly to influence the endothelial cell population, owing to the very deep ablations that may be required in relatively thin corneas, it is an examination that should be done on the above patient.

Cycloplegic Refraction

To determine cycloplegic refraction, one drop of phenylephrine 5 percent and one drop of cyclopentolate 1 percent (the latter is repeated five minutes later) should be instilled and refraction taken about 30 to 40 minutes later. For reasons mentioned earlier, contact lenses should be used in moderate and high myopes and, more noticeably, in hyperopes. It should be noted here that, although hyperopes present high spasms of accommodation, cases have been seen in myopes with differences of more than 2 diopters between manifest and cycloplegic refraction. The patient should be rechecked at a later date when the cycloplegic refraction is lower than the manifest as this spasm may be caused by a simple overcorrection of spectacles or contact lenses. If there is still an obvious difference after rechecking, then cycloplegic refraction corrected to the corneal plane is used as the attempted correction.

Pachymetry

Taking pachymetry readings also form an obligatory and integral part of preoperative evaluation. If the corneal thickness is less than 480 microns, LASIK is not recommended.

IOP and Glaucoma

Commonly used tonometers are the applanation ones. Flattening the cornea means that the cornea is already applanated and we may get falsely low IOP readings.

IOP after PRK: 1.6 – [0.4 × (SEq)]

SEq = Preoperative spherical equivalent.

The preoperative IOP should be recorded, as should the amount of intended correction.

We should be cautious, as glaucoma is a vision-threatening disease, and medicolegal implications as well as liability claims to both refractive surgeons and ophthalmologists who have not recognized the disease are pending ... For all the above reasons, PRK or LASIK candidates with ocular hypertension are better avoided. Having stated that, glaucoma is not an absolute contraindication for LASIK.

Some of the major concerns are:

- the period for which steroids are prescribed may totally destabilize the patient's IOP
- the corneal epithelium may be found to be suffering from antiglaucomatous drug-related epitheliopathy
- the condition of ocular vessels in glaucomatous eyes is suboptimal and the sudden rise of pressure produced by most microkeratomes during the LASIK procedure may provoke intraocular hemorrhage.

Fundus Examination

Another vital examination, which must be performed under full mydriasis, is that of the fundus. Numerous peripheral retinal degenerations, holes, tears and breaks have been encountered in high myopic eyes. These could be treated with argon laser prior to LASIK. Photodocumentation and fluorescein angiography is performed, when needed, to determine macular pathology.

It is extremely important that the patient understands that correction of the refractive error is optical and not anatomical and that, as a myope, there is a strong liability to retinal detachment than the natural emmetrope.

UNILATERAL OR BILATERAL TREATMENT

Having undergone all the above examinations and having been declared a successful candidate for LASIK or PRK, the decision has to be made as to which eye should be operated first and indeed, whether both eyes should be operated simultaneously. Unless requested by the patient, the nondominant eye is selected—the nondominant eye being defined as the one having the lower BCVA and the higher astigmatism and refractive error. Patients generally ask for planorefraction, however, myopes with impending presbyopia may benefit from an intended undercorrection as it will enable them to read without glasses at least for some time. Many have never recognized that they have a reading problem and others may remove their glasses or use a deliberately undercorrected prescription in order to avoid having bi- or multifocal glasses.

Among the advantages of simultaneous treatment are: (i) the patient recovers from the bilateral error of refraction at the same time and that there are fewer postoperative visits, and (ii) the patient will not experience anisokonia or monocular vision if contact lens intolerant. Disadvantages include being unable to check for postoperative complications (such as a bilaterally decentered ablation zone) and any residual error in one eye would not be taken into account in the fellow eye.

INFORMED CONSENT

Finally, the patient should sign an informed consent form. This should be written in clear and simple language and the patient encouraged to ask any questions before signing. The surgeon should include alternative methods of overcoming the refractive error, the nature of the procedure, the expected benefits, healing time, postoperative treatment and possible complications. These may include over- or undercorrection, decrease of BCVA, glare and halos, potential driving problems, as well as rarer complications such as scarring, epithelial islands and, therefore, the possibility of a corneal transplant. All should be stated clearly and comprehensibly.

Women should further sign that they are neither pregnant, nor believe that they may be, and that they are not lactating. In any event, the consent form should never be signed with the patient under cycloplegia.

SECTION TWO

Surface Ablations

11 Excimer Laser: Fundamental Concepts

Amar Agarwal

INTRODUCTION

To understand what an excimer laser is, one should understand the fundamental concepts of the excimer.[1,2] The word LASER stands for Light Amplification by Stimulated Emission of Radiation. The word EXCIMER stands for excited dimer. If we understand these two words, then only we can understand what an excimer laser is?

ATOM

Let us first of all understand what an atom is. In an atom (Fig. 11.1) we have a nucleus. This nucleus contains protons and neutrons. The protons are positively charged and the neutrons are neutral. Around the nucleus we have electrons which are negatively charged. These electrons move around in orbits. These orbits are named K, L, M, N, etc. The first orbit K has 2 electrons. This is calculated from the formula $2n^2$, n stands for the number in the orbit. For example, in the first orbit the number of electrons present will be-

$$K = 2n^2$$

$$K = 2 \times 1^2 = 2$$

This means that in the first orbit K there can be a maximum of 2 electrons. Let us now look at the second orbit L.

$$L = 2n^2$$

$$L = 2 \times 2^2 = 8$$

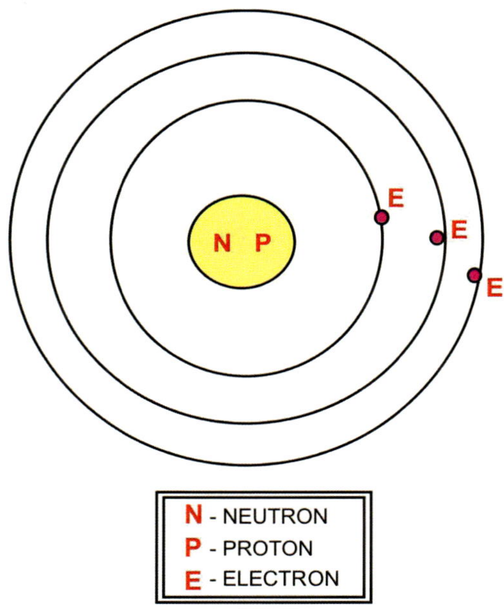

Fig. 11.1: Atom

Thus, in the second orbit L there can be a maximum of 8 electrons.

EMISSION

There are two words, which we have to understand. They are spontaneous emission and stimulated emission. Whenever an electron from a lower orbit say K moves to a higher orbit say M it cannot stay there for a long time. It has to come back to its original place. When that happens it gives off a photon of

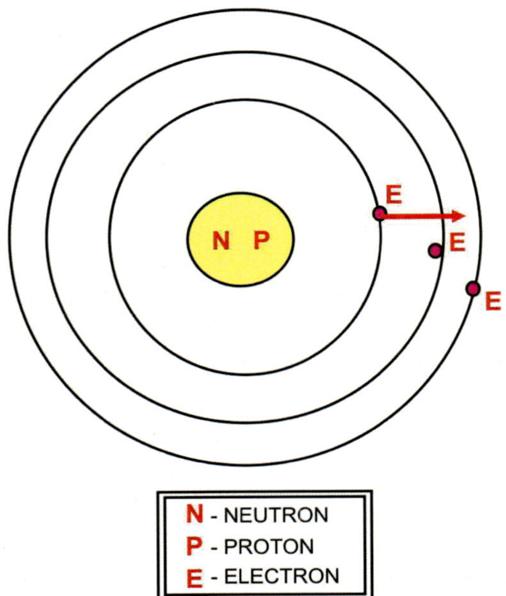

Fig. 11.2: Spontaneous emission

light. In spontaneous emission (Fig. 11.2) the electron at a lower orbit is energized spontaneously to a higher orbit. But it cannot stay there, so it decays back to the lower energy orbit level. At this time, it gives off a photon of light (Fig. 11.3). The wavelength of this light is inversely proportional to the energy lost by the

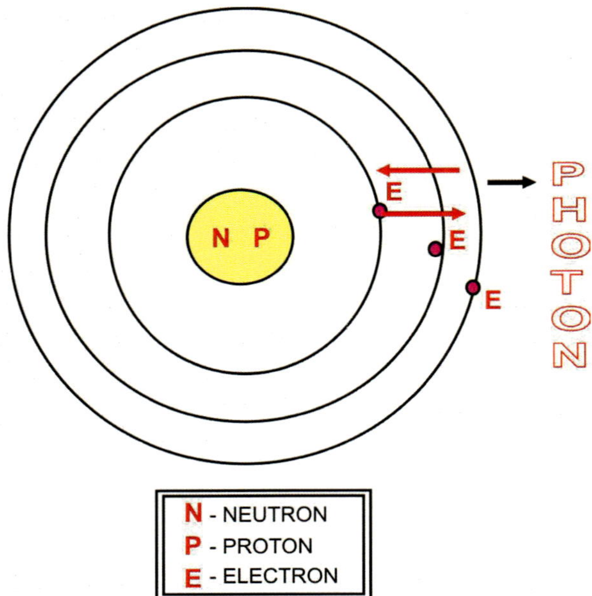

Fig. 11.3: Spontaneous emission—note the release of photon

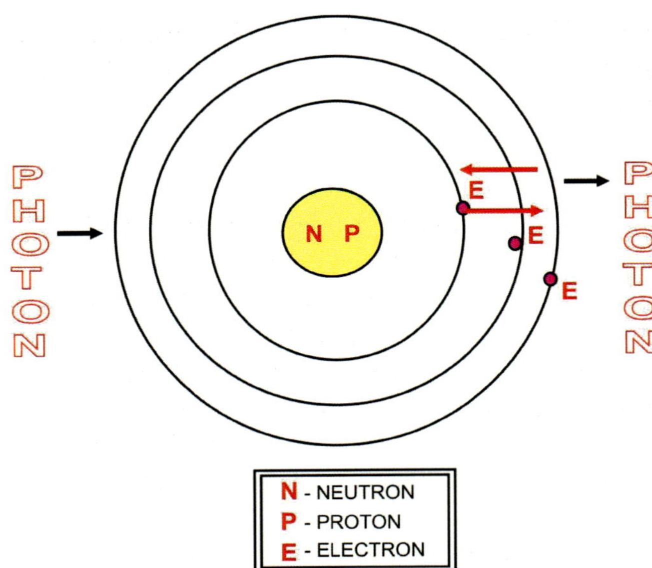

Fig. 11.4: Stimulated emission

electron, which, in turn, is dependent upon the type of atom.

If the electron is energized and sent to a higher orbit by another photon that has an identical wavelength to that which the atom will produce, then we call it as stimulated emission (Fig. 11.4). The photon stimulates the electrons, which goes from the lower orbit to a higher orbit. Once again it cannot stay there for a long time and so falls back to its original orbit level and in the process gives off another photon of light.

When this process continues it leads to an amplification process (Fig. 11.5). One photon hits an atom producing the electron from that atom going to a higher orbit. When the electron falls back to its

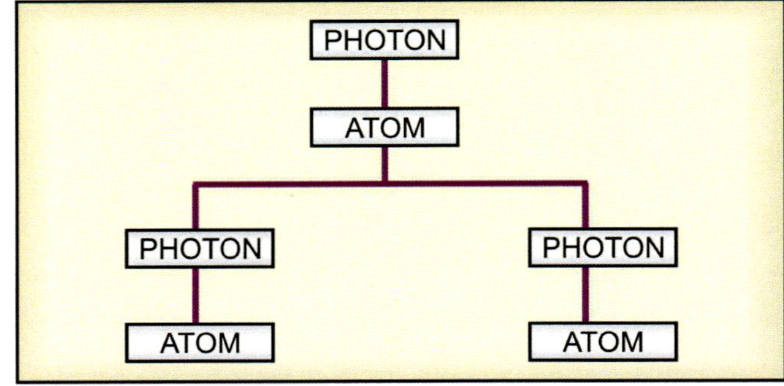

Fig. 11.5: Amplification process

original level it, in turn, releases, photons. These then hit other atoms, thus, leading to an amplification process.

LASER MEDIA AND PUMPS

Now that we have understood what an amplification process is we should understand what the laser media and laser pumps are. The laser media contains the atoms that do the lasing. The laser media can be a gas medium, which is what happens in the excimer or the argon laser. It can be a liquid medium as in the dye laser or it can be a solid medium as in the neodymium: yttrium-aluminum-garnet (Nd:YAG) or diode lasers.

From what we have read it is obvious that we need some energy to hit the atoms. The laser pump is a source of energy that is needed to energize the electrons. This can be in the form of electrical discharge or current. Alternatively it could be light energy produced by either flash lamps or another lamp.

If lasing has to occur population inversion must be present. In other words, the pumped medium must be in a state of population inversion for lasing to occur. **Population inversion is when more than half of the atoms in the medium are energized to an excited state.** An atom that is capable of being excited and then stimulated to emit a photon of light will also resonantly absorb a photon of the same wavelength when not excited. So, more atoms should be in the excited state than the nonexcited state. If there are more atoms in the nonexcited state than the excited state, the atoms will have the absorption process going rather than the stimulated emission process, and the amplification process will not occur. As one wants the amplification process to occur more atoms should be in the excited state than the nonexcited state. This is called "population inversion".

EXCITED DIMER

The word excimer is a contraction of the term excited dimer. Let us first understand what the word dimer means. **Molecules made up of two identical atoms are called dimers (Fig. 11.6).** In excimer laser, we use

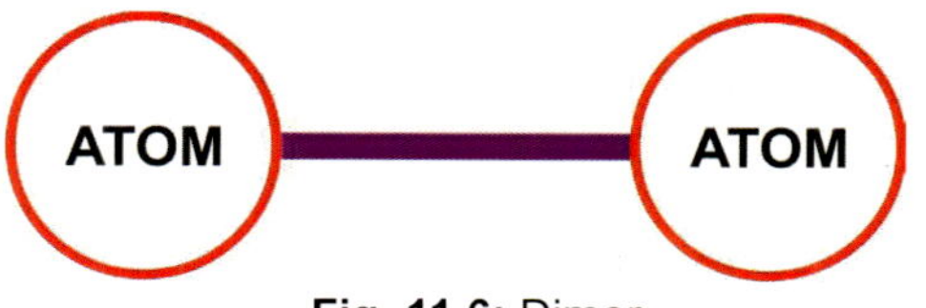

Fig. 11.6: Dimer

two atoms—an inert gas and a halide, specifically argon and fluoride. These two elements are in very small concentrations in a helium mixture known as premix. Thus, in excimer laser we do not use an actual dimer, as the two atoms are not exactly identical. This is why it is said that the word dimer is a misnomer as it applies to two of the same elements.

If two systems (atoms or molecules) do not form a strong chemical bond when they are in their ground states, but form a strong chemical bond when one of them is in an excited state, then the bound excited state is called an excimer. The excimer dissociates in the ground state and this helps maintain population inversion necessary for lasing to occur. When the excited dimer (argon and fluoride) dissociates it releases ultraviolet energy.

EXCIMER LASER

Thus an excimer laser is an excited dimer which produces a laser beam of ultraviolet energy. The excimer lasers can produce ultraviolet light energy at various wavelengths depending upon the gas elements utilized. If the ultraviolet energy released is of 248 nm, it results in potentially mutagenic behavior as evidenced by unscheduled DNA synthesis. If the ultraviolet energy is of 308 nm it can lead to cataract formation. Thus, it was found that the ideal ultraviolet energy should be 193 nm. This is really suitable for corneal ablation. The excimer laser at this wavelength has submicron precision with submicron collateral damage and minimal thermal energy effect. The excimer laser removes 0.25 microns per pulse and damages an additional 0.25 microns of adjacent corneal tissue.

LASER VS LIGHT

The laser beam is a coherent light compared to a light beam. The differences between laser and light are shown in Table 11.1.

Table 11.1: Difference between laser and light

Laser	*Light*
Monochromatic	Polychromatic
Coherent	Incoherent
Laser beam is less divergent	Light beam is more divergent
Laser is a narrow beam with small spot size	Light beam is a broad beam with large spot size

EXCIMER MACHINE

Excimer lasers usually consist of a large elongated aluminum box. This box is filled with the appropriate gas mixture. Running the full lengths of this box are two metal electrodes spaced about 2 to 3 cm apart. At one end of the box, aligned with the gap between the electrodes, a mirror is mounted and, at the other end, a window. The window is usually an uncoated optic. Outside the box, there is usually a large bank of capacitors, and these are charged using a high voltage power supply to several tons of kilovolts. A special switch called a thyraton is used to dump the energy stored in these capacitors across the electrodes inside the box. The electrical discharge through the gas between the electrodes ionizes the gas and allows the excimer molecules to form. Lasing action usually occurs within nanoseconds. The laser beam goes through a power monitoring system and is then directed by mirrors onto the patient's eye (Fig. 11.7).

FLUENCY

Once the concept of an excimer laser is understood, we have to then understand what the word fluence means. **Fluence means the amount of energy applied to the ablative area.** In other words,

Fluence = Energy/Area = millijoules/sqcm

Fluence is defined as energy applied to a given area and is expressed in units of millijoules per square centimeter and varies depending upon the laser. Fluence is the primary determinant of the amount of tissue ablated with each pulse. Different excimer machines have different fluency values. For example, the fluence of:

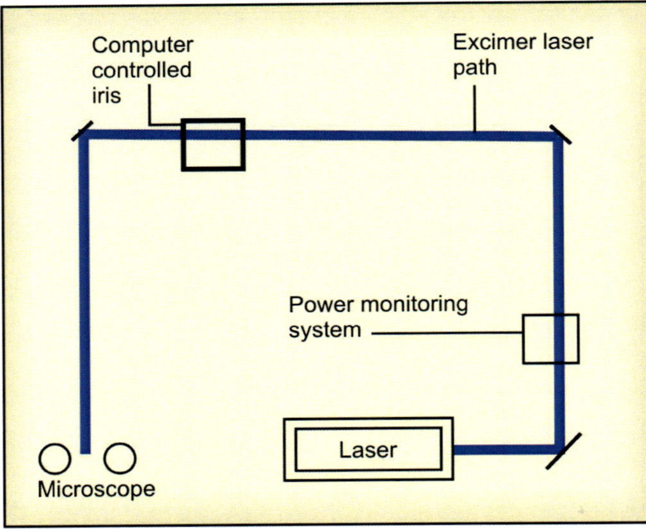

Fig. 11.7: Excimer laser machine

Summit excimer—160 mJ/cm^2
Chiron—130 mJ/cm^2
Nidek—130 mJ/cm^2

This means that when we are testing the fluence plates before starting lasik or photorefractive keratectomy (PRK), we first keep the fluence plates and convert the white plates to red in the Chiron machine. We check in the Chiron machine that once the area has become fully red, the figure in the computer shows 65 shots. If that happens then only we proceed with the case. This shows that the fluence is now 130 mJ/cm^2.

HOMOGENEITY

Homogeneity indicates the pattern of energy distribution within the exposed area. This can be shown as microhomogeneity or macrohomogeneity. Microhomogeneity shows localized variability in the energy beam density, i.e. hot and cold areas within the beam. The hot areas represent highest energy density areas and the cold areas represent lowest energy density areas. Rather than defining localized energy patterns, macrohomogeneity tends to refer to the overall energy beam profile of the laser. Macrohomogeneity can be gaussian, homogeneous or reverse gaussian. In gaussian, the greatest energy density is centrally.

In homogeneous, the energy distribution is equal throughout the beam and in reverse gaussian, the energy density is lowest centrally.

DELIVERY SYSTEMS

We have to remember with all this there has to be a delivery system, which delivers the laser beam onto the eye. The delivery systems can be broad beam or a scanning beam system. The broad beam system is similar in concept to a projection system for a 35 mm slide system. The broad beam delivery system projects the entire beam on the stromal surface. Then utilizing an iris diaphragm or variable aperture system, the broad beam is controlled to create the ablation pattern required. The scanning systems utilize a slit beam or small spot to scan the surface of the cornea. The advantages are the versatility for creating various topographical patterns—hyperopia, asymmetrical astigmatism, etc. In Figure 11.8, one can see the slit beam scanning system. The slit beam scans the corneal surface. In the flying spot system, instead of the slit beam, one has a flying spot, which delivers the excimer laser energy. In the scanning systems, one incorporates an eyetracking system, as these systems are less forgiving for even small decentrations. The advantage of the scanning beam is that as the beam is smaller, it allows for a more easily created homogeneous beam, requiring less optics and a less powerful laser head.

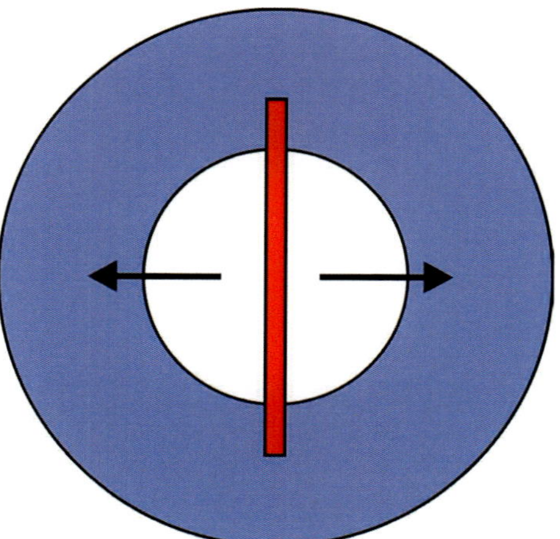

Fig. 11.8: Slit-beam scanning laser system

SUMMARY

An excimer laser has changed the management of refractive errors. It is nothing but an excited dimer, which creates a 193 nm wavelength of ultraviolet light. The excimer laser machine is a very sophisticated machine, and one should remember fluence, homogeneity and delivery systems when understanding this machine.

REFERENCES

1. Mcghee CNJ, Taylor HR, Garty DS, et al. Excimer Lasers in Ophthalmology: Principles and Practice. Martin Duntz: London, 1997.
2. Machat JJ. Excimer Laser Refractive Surgery, Slack Inc: Thorofare, 1996.

12 Painless Photorefractive Keratectomy (PRK)

F Hampton Roy, Donald G Johnson

INTRODUCTION

Many of the Lasik surgeons explain their reason for not doing PRK as being due to the pain associated with PRK. There have been many advancements in pain management after PRK.

CORNEAL EPITHELIAL REMOVAL IN PREPARATION FOR PRK

Photorefractive keratectomy (PRK) is based on surface removal of the epithelial layer. This is apparently a simple maneuver, but it can account for considerable differences between surgeons. The types of methods by which the epithelium can be removed are shown in Table 12.1.

Manual Removal of the Corneal Epithelium

Manual removal is completed after topical anesthesia and a lid speculum is placed. A blunt spatula is used to remove the epithelium starting from the periphery to the center. An optical zone marker is placed to indicate the size of treatment. In PRKs for myopia and myopic astigmatism it is 6 mm and for hyperopia and hyperopic astigmatism treatment it is generally 9 mm. One disadvantage of this method is that the removal of the epithelium is irregular at the peripheral portion. There may also be irregularity of the corneal surface as it is relatively easy to indent the cornea and to alter the local curvature and moisture content of the cornea. This may be transferred with PRK into an irregular ablation contour.

Table 12.1: Methods of epithelial removal in PRK

1. Manual removal
2. Alcohol removal
3. Amoils or pallikaris brush technique
4. Laser techniques
   a. Laser scrape
   b. No touch technique
      i. PTK mode
      ii. PRK/PTK mode

Alcohol Removal of the Corneal Epithelium

Alcohol removal of the corneal epithelium can be completed quite easily. The size of the marker that you want of the epithelium removed is put down firmly on the cornea. A solution that is two-third balance-salt solution (BSS) and one-third absolute alcohol is placed on the eye enough to cover the epithelium and left on for 30 seconds (timed) with the optical zone marker left in place. At the end of 30 seconds, the optical zone marker is removed and chilled BSS is used to rinse the cornea and rinse off the residual alcohol. A weck cell is used to remove the epithelium from that central area. The cornea is dried with a weck cell and the surgeon can proceed with the laser correction.

Amoils or Pallikaris Brush Technique

The Amoils or Pallikaris brush technique can be used to remove the epithelium. This is a rotating brush, which allows rapid debridement of the corneal epithelium and is now available commercially. It may cause a slightly larger than intended epithelium removal area but does leave a smooth surface. It is often used as the initial debridement and then a general wipe with a blunt spatula is used to remove any other residual islands of epithelium. This type of brush is frequently used for hyperopic PRK where the area of corneal epithelium removal is 9 mm and scrapping can be very prolonged and fraught with more difficulty. Transepithelial ablation of the epithelium has gone through several evolutionary steps and there are some physicians that are using each of the steps.

Laser Techniques

"Laser scrape" is a partial laser ablation over the ablation zone with PTK and then the remainder of the epithelium removed with a spatula or weck cell. "No touch" excimer laser transepithelial ablation is a technique in which topical anesthesia and then lid speculum are used. The laser is activated to remove all of the epithelium. This technique can be either a PTK mode technique or a PRK/PTK mode technique.

With a PTK mode technique a fixed depth of 43 microns of tissue is removed and then to correct for the hyperopic amount produced, –0.75 is added back to the amount treated. This technique is not as exact as the next technique described because a set of epithelial thickness is assumed, and it may not be as exact. Also, hyperopic shift is approximately –0.75 and this part may vary somewhat from surgery to surgery.

With the PRK/PTK mode technique total laser removal of the epithelium is completed. A central PRK ablation is used to "flatten" laser-wise the epithelium. Then, with the PTK mode all the epithelium is removed at the same time uniformly. As the epithelium is removed, the epithelial autofluorescence ceases for a definite end point.

With the laser procedures there is a definite edge removed of the epithelium. This can be used as a marker for central fixation for the doctor. Sometimes as the fixation target blurs, the patient may loose fixation. The ring markers in the Visx star laser head can be used to help with this centration. Secondly, the patient gets accustomed to the PRK process with the laser pulse noise and sensation. With the PTK mode, there is a much larger sensation and more noise, which may initially startle the patient.

There is recent scientific evidence to support total laser epithelium removal, as there is an improved healing response in contrast to the other methods. Dr Steve Wilson has studied corneal healing in rabbit corneas. Apoptosis is an involutional form of cell death. Electron microscopic studies reveal a connection between the epithelium and apoptosis of keratocytes. Laser "scraped" corneas had considerable apoptosis present. Epithelial cells release enzymes called "casposes" which leads to apoptosis. Therefore, laser-only removal elicits a different healing response, which leads to an improved healing time.

EXCIMER LASER ABLATION

Once the epithelium has been removed, the next step is to start the PRK treatment. Before one starts the PRK treatment one should calibrate the excimer laser machine correctly. One should enter the appropriate refractive power and cylindrical power one has to correct. When the ablation is complete, wash the cornea well with the BSS fluid.

CONTACT LENSES POST-PRK

With the improvements of lasers the ablations are smoother and heal faster, thus, there is much less discomfort. As a general rule with myopic PRK, the contact lenses are left on approximately for three days and with hyperopic PRK they are left on for an average of four days.

Pain Discomfort Level

In the early healing period the pain discomfort level from one practice was:

- 45 percent require no pain medication
- 45 percent reported mild discomfort
- 8 percent reported moderate discomfort
- 2 percent reported severe discomfort.

POST-PRK CARE

The exact modalities that are used are as follows:
- Therapeutic (bandage) soft contact lenses
- Topical non-steroidal antiinflammatory drugs (NSAIDs)
- Non-preserved topical dilute anesthetics
- Chilled artificial tears
- Systemic analgesia, narcotics, and sedation.

A therapeutic soft bandage contact lens should fit the eye comfortably. Some practitioners knowing that the initial refraction if being treated for myopic PRK will be hyperopic, put + 0.50 D lens on the eye. The author feels that it does not matter at this stage of treatment. The contact lens is cooled on ice and applied following the procedure.

Topical applications of NSAIDs have dramatically reduced and in some cases eliminated the perception of pain after PRK. Two topical NSAIDs have been approved in the United States for treatment of ocular pain: Acular (Ketorolac tromethamine—Allergan Inc.) and Voltaren (diclofenac sodium—Ciba Vision Ophthalmics).

The use of nonpreserved topical dilute anesthetic for the first 24 hours has markedly reduced the pain. Our method is to use a 3 cc sample bottle of Refresh tears with the addition of 1 cc of topical anesthetic (AK-Taine, Alcaine or Ophthetic). The patient may use this anytime from 15 to 30 minutes following surgery and for the first 24 hours and then discontinue using the drop. Anesthetics are known to prolong the healing time and we insist the drops be stopped after the first 24 hours.

Chilled artificial tears may be beneficial in reducing some of the discomfort. We are chilling the drops on ice that are used on the eye both pre- and postoperatively. This helps to cool the eye and hopefully reduces some of the haze that may occur related to a build-up of heat during the procedure (Fig. 12.1).

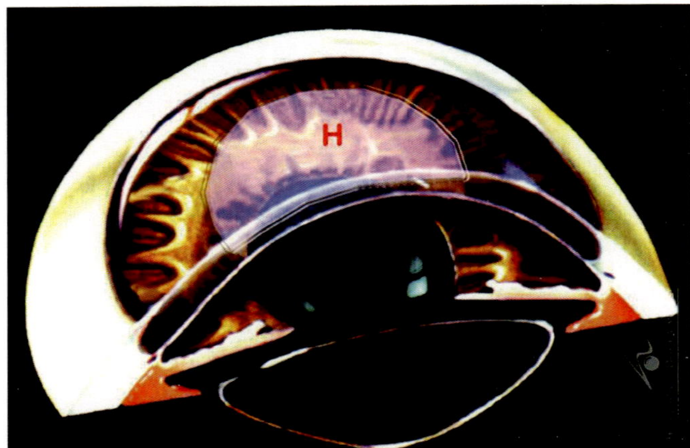

Fig. 12.1: PRK: Stromal haze formation: Some patients develop a diffuse subepithelial haze between 3 and 4 weeks following PRK. The amount of haze is not usually related to the degree of ametropia treated. It may even appear in eyes with low degrees of refractive errors. In this illustration a grade 3 haze (H) is presented, which may significantly affect the patient's visual acuity. In most cases, the haze greatly diminishes or even disappears after one year. This is a major disadvantage of PRK (*Courtesy* Highlights of Ophthalmology)

Drops used include an antibiotic such as Ocuflox, FML, Acular and anesthetic drops. Corneal infiltrates may be related to using NSAIDs and thus the use of FML (fluorometholone) following PRK is useful to help eliminating that possibility. Once the contact lenses are removed the only drop that is continued is the FML ophthalmic steroid drop, this is gradually tapered depending on the refraction. If the refraction is hyperopic at two weeks, the FML is gradually tapered at 3 days intervals. If the refraction is myopic at two weeks, the FML is continued at four times a day or the type steroid increased to Pred Forte.

Systemic analgesia, narcotics and sedation are useful to reduce pain. The author's general regime is to prescribe Demerol 50 mg (10) and Phenergan 25 mg (10), one of each every two hours as needed for pain.

BIBLIOGRAPHY

1. Johnson DG, George S. Photorefractive keratectomy retreatment—a comparison of two methods of excimer laser epithelial removal. Refractive Surgery 1998, American Academy of Ophthalmology, November 6, 1998.
2. Pallikarris IG, Karoutis AD, Lydataki SE, et al. Rotating brush for fast removal of corneal epithelium. J Refract Corneal Surgery 1994;10:439.
3. Pop M, Aras M. Photorefractive keratectomy retreatments for regression—one year follow-up. Ophthalmology 1996;103(11):1979-84.
4. Price FW Jr. Painless PRK—is it possible? Refractive Surgery 1998, American Academy of Ophthalmology, 1998;54-6.
5. Rooks WH, Maloney PJ, Shott LD, et al. The analgesic anti-inflammatory profile of kenorolac and its tromethamine salt. Drugs Exp Clin Res 1986;8:479-92.

13 From LASEK to Epi-LASEK

Massimo Camellin, Daniel Wyler

INTRODUCTION

With over nine years of follow-up, LASEK surgery has had ample time to demonstrate its many advantages, particularly in patients with high myopia.[1] LASEK can be used for all refractive defects, and unlike PRK, there have been no occurrences of epithelialization delay, or grave haze. The same advantages, which make LASEK a successful alternative to LASIK, are present in the Epi-LASEK procedure—a safe and effective improvement.

When we analyze haze level, we observe the opacity due to abnormal collagen and increased number of keratocytes.[2] This opacity however, is only the final, and most severe result of a series of lesser complications. We must also take into account the regression that leads to irregular topographical patterns, reduction of optical zones, and deterioration of visual acuity. Regression following PRK is quite common, and is taken into account by increasing the laser setting, if not already done so by the manufacturer. This regression following PRK is most likely a preliminary step of haze, where there is an activation of keratocytes, which transform into myofibroblasts. In short, after surface ablation, it is normal to have a reaction involving keratocytes, which can lead to regression, or in the worst case haze.

Postoperative haze becomes transparent with time, however, the interface between the epithelium and stroma will remain rough. This feature is clearly demonstrable in re-operations, where after removing the epithelium before surgery, we observe a completely uneven surface. This uneven interface impairs visual acuity since the refractive index of the epithelium is slightly different from that of the stroma[3]—it increases scattering and higher order aberrations. With our experience, we have observed that re-operating on a PRK eye almost always results in a broken epithelial flap in the center, which does not occur on LASEK re-operations. Following LASEK, there is a reduced stromal reaction and epithelium can re-grow with lesser adherence to the stroma. A stromal surface protected by epithelium will react less,[4] which can lead to a quieter healing process.[5-7] MMC can reduce keratocyte activation by inducing apoptosis,[8] however, long-term side effects are relatively unknown. Our personal experience is that MMC generates some variations in refraction, and may result in a rougher epithelial surface during the first few months.[9]

We have not had any problems with over 2,000 LASEK operations performed between –0.5D and –18D of myopia. Other authors who have followed our procedure have obtained the same excellent results.[10,11]

When LASEK or Epi-Lasik results are compared to PRK for low myopia, the advantages regarding haze are less evident, however, the results may be better in cases with high myopia. Therefore, we recommend critically reading all studies which state that there is no difference between LASEK or Epi-Lasik and PRK. Often, these analyses were performed on a few number of cases[12,13] or on cases with a low degree of myopia.[14-17]

LASEK VERSUS EPI-LASIK

When Epi-Lasik was developed, several studies that compared this technique to LASEK gave clear evidence to show that there are no differences with regards to haze or pain.[18] Furthermore, studies have proved the efficacy of Epi-Lasik over PRK.[19] Even if the epithelial flap in Epi-Lasik is more viable than in LASEK, the epithelium is completely renewed within one week, and the postoperative courses are likely equivalent. Some criticisms of LASEK were that the alcohol increased postoperative haze and/or pain. To investigate this, we performed a prospective study involving 63 patients. We performed the procedures bilaterally, on each patient. This type of study reduces the patient-to-patient variations since each patient receives both treatments, and all of the biological responses belong to the same patient. Therefore, comparisons between the two treatments are more easily made.

MATERIALS AND METHODS

Sixty-three patients were enrolled. Myopic (n = 51) spheroequivalent was –5.4D (SD = 2.8) and hyperopic (n = 12) spheroequivalent was +3.2D (SD1.6). Myopic astigmatism was 1D (SD = 1.1) while hyperopic astigmatism was 1.5D (SD 1.3).

Each patient was operated on bilaterally, one eye with LASEK and the other with Epi-Lasik (Centurion Epikeratome (Norwood Abbey Eye Care – Victoria, Australia)). A Schwind Esiris excimer laser (Schwind eye tech solutions -Kleinostheim, Germany) was used in each treatment (7 mm optical zone, 8 mm transition in myopia and 7 mm optical zone, 9 mm trasition in hyperopia).

Three patients were excluded for having lost the lens during the first postoperative hours. All refractive data were recorded, including corneal aberrations and topographic index of regularity (BFTI)[20] by using a topographer (Keratron Optikon 2000 s.p.a. Roma, Italy). Follow-up data were recorded for a minimum of one-year.

RESULTS EPI-LASIK VS LASEK

Pain: No significant differences were observed even though there is a trend of higher discomfort with Epi-Lasik (Fig. 13.1).

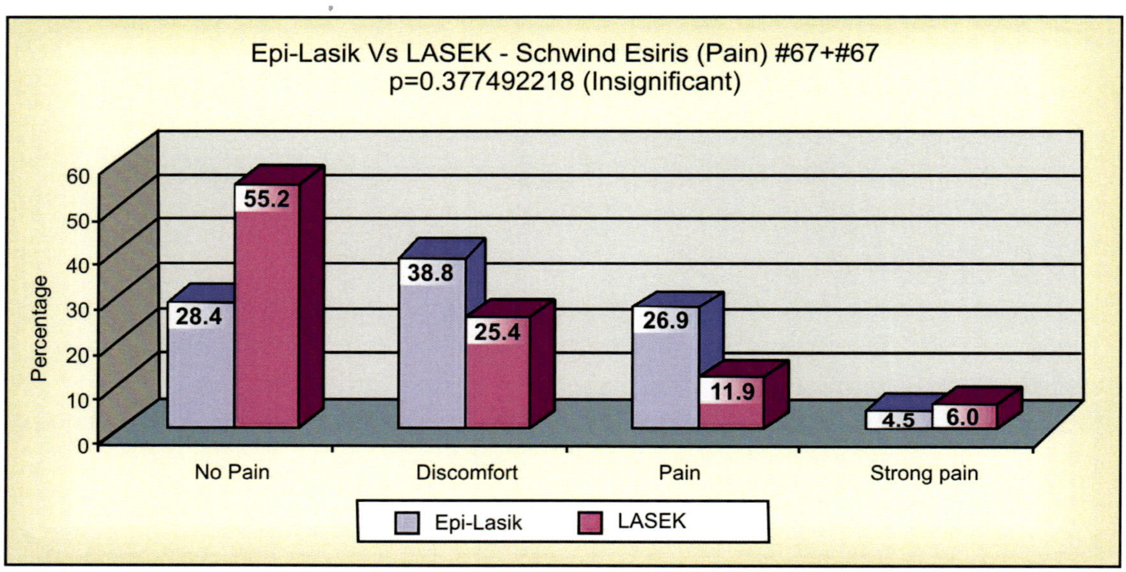

Fig. 13.1: There are no significant differences in pain, however there is a slight trend for increased discomfort with Epi-Lasik

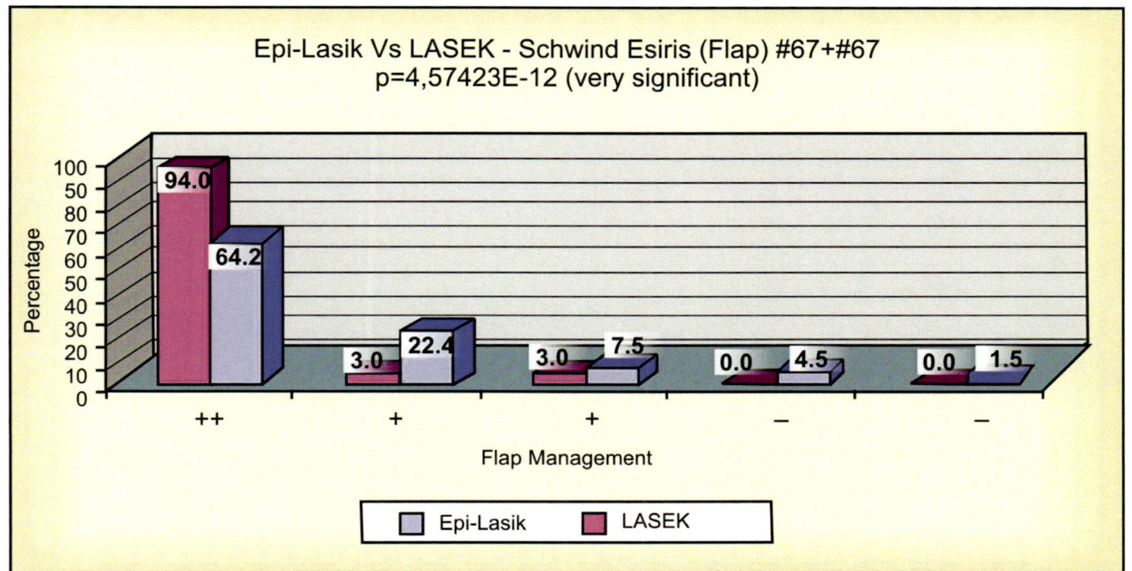

Fig. 13.2: The flap with the Epi-Lasik treatment is significantly better than with LASEK

Flap quality: Here there is a significant difference. With Epi-Lasik, the flap is almost always excellent (flap ++) while with LASEK there can be some difficult cases with broken flaps (flap^{--}). It is evident that with Epi-Lasik we were able to obtain a good flap in almost all cases (Fig. 13.2).

Hinge: Here we have divided the analysis between myopia and hyperopia because of the wider optical zone used in hyperopia (9 mm) compared to the smaller zones in myopia (8 mm). This difference leads to a more peripheral hinge in hyperopia, which can lead to an increased risk of tearing. An intact hinge is important in maintaining a stable flap during the first postoperative hours. We can see in Figures 13.3 and 13.4 that there is a difference in the quality of the hinge. In cases of myopia, the hinge quality is

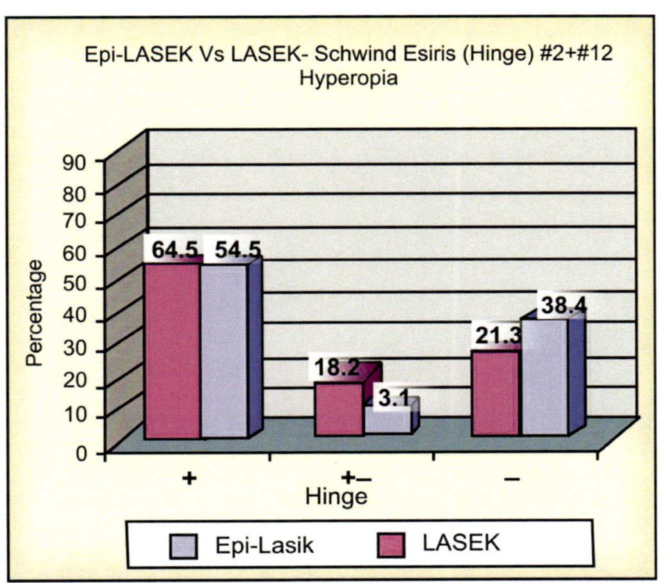

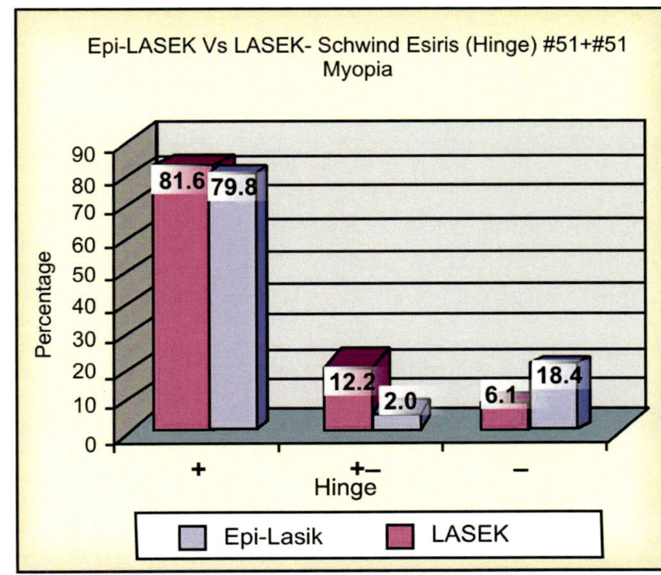

Figs 13.3 and 13.4: Hinge quality is better with the Epi-Lasik treatment in both myopic and hyperopic cases

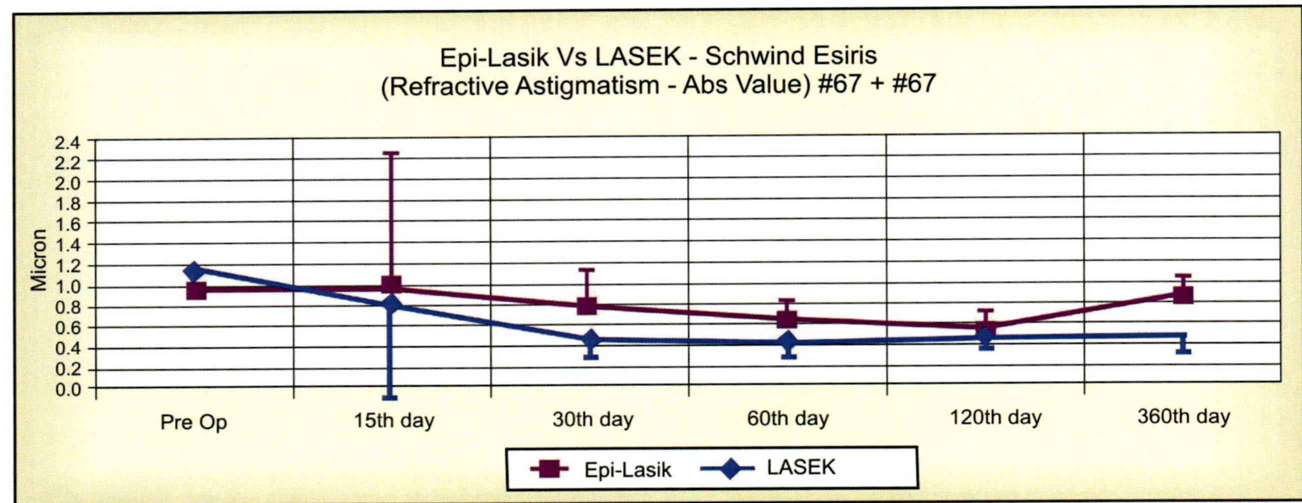

Fig. 13.5: Astigmatism is higher in the Epi-Lasik group during the first two months

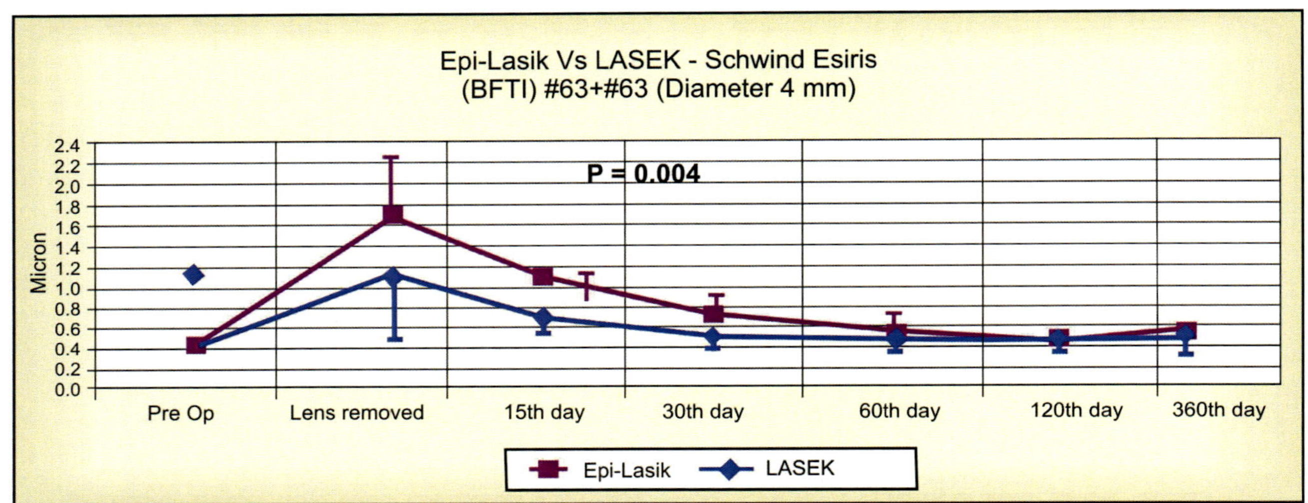

Fig. 13.6: Corneal regularity index is lower in LASEK compared to Epi-Lasik. This means there is a smoother surface with the LASEK treatment during the first two months

generally better than in hyperopia. In both groups, the Epi-Lasik treatment shows better outcomes than LASEK, and these results are significant.

Astigmatism: we noticed an increased amount of astigmatism with the Epi-Lasik treatment group, particularly during the first two months (Fig. 13.5). Topographically, this astigmatism was central and disappeared with time. Because this astigmatism was slightly irregular, it can lead to a temporarily reduced BCVA.

Corneal regularity coefficient (BFTI): This is a Maloney index present in the Keratron Scout Topographer (Optikon 2000) which takes into account the 4 mm around the pupil center. There is a difference between the Epi-Lasik (worse) and the LASEK treatment groups (better) that disappears within two months (Fig. 13.6).

Haze (Fantes scale[21]*):* It is almost always seen as traces in both groups, and disappears within three months. In hyperopia, its value is slightly higher, however, it

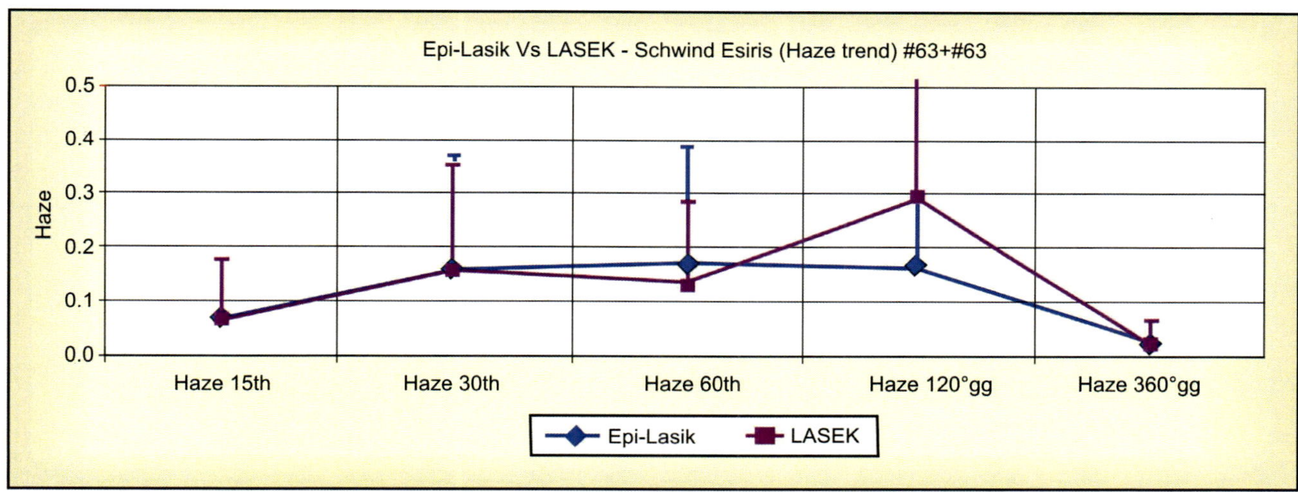

Fig. 13.7: Haze is low in both groups with a slight peak in LASEK during the fourth month

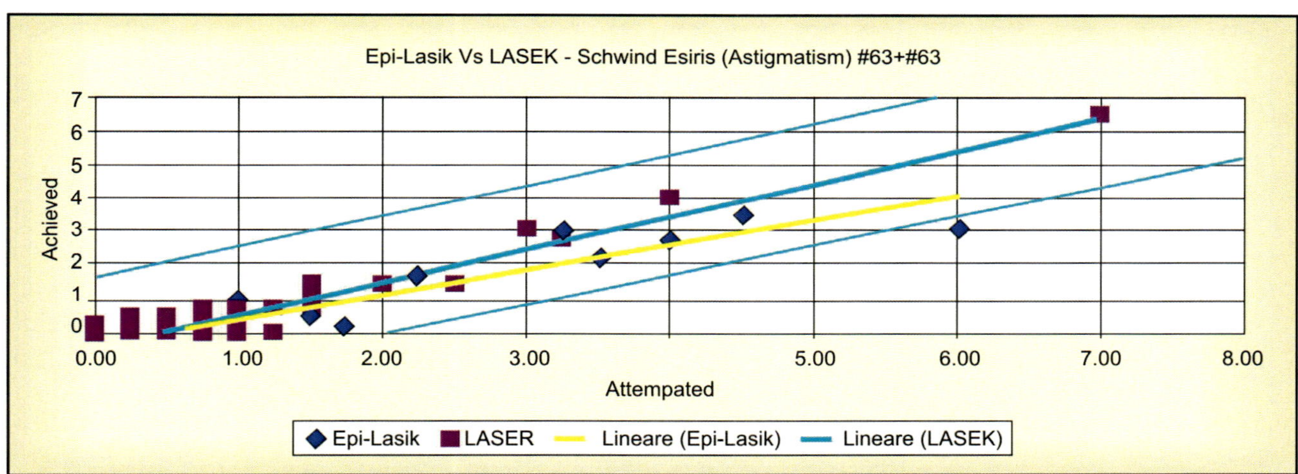

Fig. 13.8: Astigmatism is a slightly higher with the Epi-Lasik treatment

is peripheral and does not reduce the visual acuity. The only difference in haze between the two groups is a peak in the LASEK treatment during the fourth month, with an average value of 0.3 (Fig. 13.7).

Spheroequivalent predictability: Quite similar in both groups.

Astigmatism predictability: The results with LASEK are better for the on the rule astigmatism present during the first two months with the Epi-Lasik group. The computation was performed using the absolute value, so there may be a slight fault with the analysis (Fig. 13.8).

Efficacy and safety: The efficacy (UCVA post/BCVA pre) is better with LASEK (0.91) compared to Epi-Lasik (0.83) while safety (BCVA post/BCVA pre) is high in both treatments (0.99).

These results allow us to draw the conclusion that alcohol does not increase pain or haze. Epi-Lasik creates a more complete flap and hinge, however, we have observed some problems in the nasal region where the angle of attack of the blade is too acute. In these areas in some patients, the separation is not perfect and can be intra-epithelial (Fig. 13.9) or intra-basal membrane (Fig. 13.10).

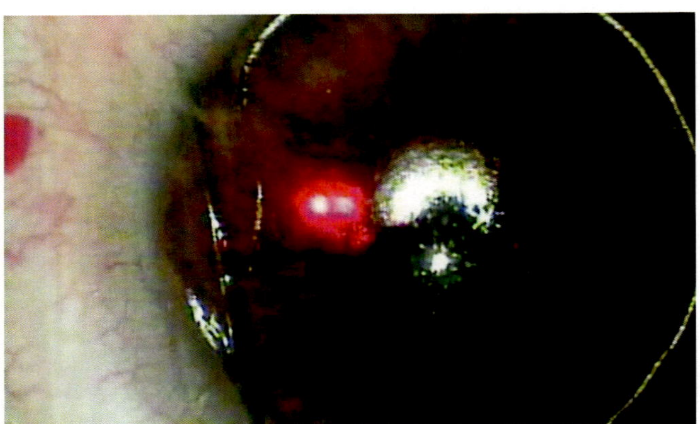

Fig. 13.9: Intraepithelial dissection following Epi-Lasik. The presence of epithelium close to the hinge is clear

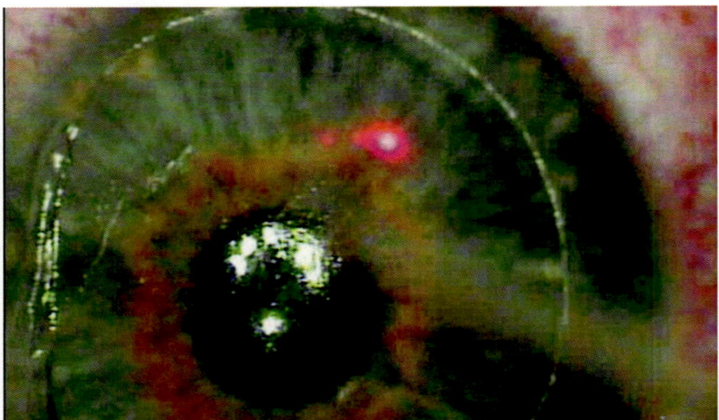

Fig. 13.10: Intrabasal membrane dissection following Epi-Lasik. We can observe a step (due to the presence of a residual basal membrane) close to the hinge that is difficult to remove

It is obvious that if we ignore these defects, the photoablation will be performed over stroma and part of the epithelium, which may cause irregularities. In fact, less stromal tissue is removed from the area where the epithelium remains. Moreover, we have seen that in the course of scraping this residual epithelial tissue, the hinge may be damaged.

Our data show that mechanical separation is not always uniform, particularly in the nasal region, and that the mechanical separation over Bowman's layer results in a rougher surface. Alcohol splits the basal membrane in two layers,[22] lamina lucida and lamina densa, and therefore photoablation is performed over the lamina densa, which is smoother than Bowman's layer. Alcohol eases the separation of the epithelium and does not increase pain or haze.

What happens when we add alcohol solution to the Epi-Lasik procedure? Alcohol helps create a new cleavage plain (between lamina lucida and lamina densa) which is easily identified by the epi-keratome; this results in a smoother treatment surface (lamina densa), and a thicker epithelial flap (for distilled water solution use) which is more elastic and manageable. The flap hinge is also wider and more complete.

EPI-LASIK VERSUS EPI-LASEK

A new prospective study was recently published[23] which has demonstrated all of the advantages of the epi-LASEK procedure (LASEK with epi-keratome). Fourty-five patients were operated on bilaterally with the Epi-Lasik treatment in one eye, and Epi-Lasik plus alcohol (which we call Epi-LASEK) in the other. Alcohol (20% with distilled water) was used for 20 seconds before making the flap in the Epi-LASEK treatment group.

Epi-LASIK Treatment

Myopic (n = 40) mean spheroequivalent was –5.6D (SD = 3.3) and hyperopic (n = 5) mean spheroequivalent was +2.9D (SD = 1.8). Myopic mean astigmatism was 1.4D (SD = 1.2), while hyperopic mean astigmatism was 0.6D (SD = 0.6).

Epi-LASEK Treatment

Myopic (n = 40) mean spheroequivalent was –5.9D (SD = 3.5) and hyperopic (n = 5) mean spheroequivalent was +3D (SD = 1.9). Myopic mean astigmatism was 1.6D (SD = 1.3), while hyperopic mean astigmatism was 0.6D (SD = 0.9).

$P > 0.05$ for all checked fields so there were no differences among groups.

We have named this new technique Epi-LASEK, which means the use of an epi-keratome with the LASEK procedure.

EPI-LASEK TECHNIQUE

Topical anesthesia is applied for a few minutes before starting the procedure and some more drops are applied to the speculum. The Shahinian well (E.

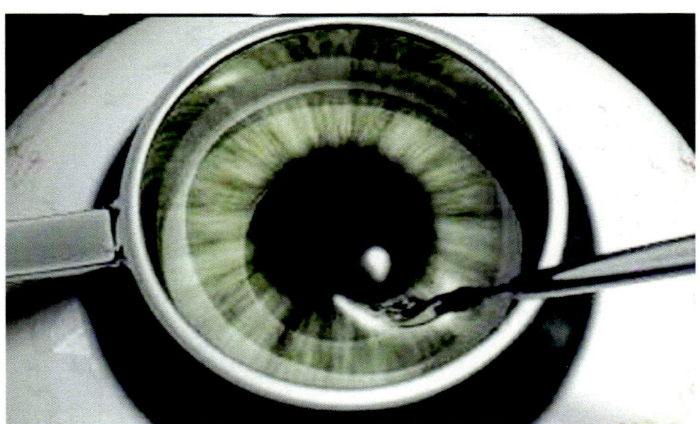

Fig. 13.11: Shahinian well containing 20 percent alcohol solution in distilled water for 20 seconds before applying the epi-keratome

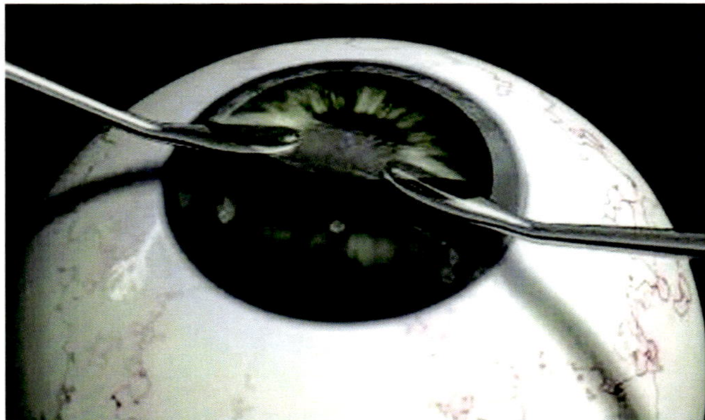

Fig. 13.13: The epithelial flap is rolled back after moistening the stromal surface with BSS

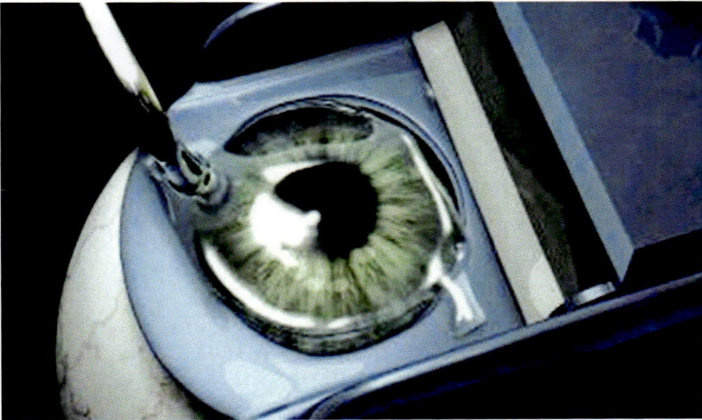

Fig. 13.12: Nordwood instrument applied slightly de-centered nasally to avoid creating the hinge in the photoablation area where it can be damaged by the laser

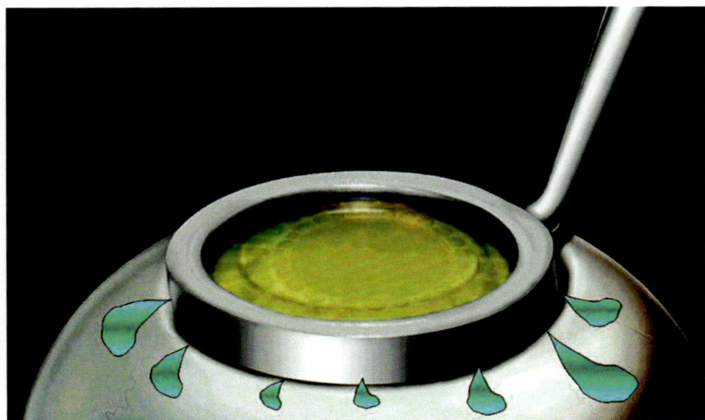

Fig. 13.14: The applanator is used to squeeze all fluid from under the flap, helping to fix the flap position

Janach - Como, Italy) is applied and filled with alcohol solution (20% in distilled water) previously warmed to 32° (Celsius).

After 20 seconds, the content is dried with a cotton sponge and rinsed with diclofenac sodium (preservative free). The surface is now rinsed with BSS (balanced salt solution) and the epi-keratome applied (we used a Nordwood Centurion) (Fig. 13.12). The parameters of the instrument were 600 (vacuum), 50 (speed), and 100 (frequency). We usually move the instrument nasally to avoid creating the hinge in the photoablation area.

If the diameter of the flap is checked with a caliper, and is determined to be too small, it is possible to enlarge it by scraping the periphery with a Hokey spatula (Janach). At this point the photoablation is performed, after which we apply some drops of BSS and roll back the flap (Fig. 13.13).

It is important to remove excess liquid from under the flap, leaving only the amount of fluid necessary to allow the flap to slide over the surface. This reduces flap mobility. Flap mobility is often a cause of post-operative pain due to the stimulation of nerves from the flap itself during lid movements. The surface can now be dried for 30 seconds to increase stability. A soft lens is fitted and an applanator is used to squeeze all fluid from under the flap (Fig. 13.14). The surface should now show a clear aspect.

At this point we apply these drugs: Netildex (Dexametazone 0.1% + Netilmicin 0.3% - S.i.f.i. Spa -

Aci S. Antonio (CT)- Italy), Voltaren Ofta (Diclofenac 0.1% - Novartis – Origgio (VA) Italy), Visumidriatic 0.5% (Tropicamide 0.5% - Visufarma – Roma - Italy) and Tetramil (Feniramine 0.3% + Tetrizoline 0.05% - Farmigea – Pisa (PI) - Italy).

Postoperative care includes Netilmicin 0.3% four times a day for 10 days, Diclofenac 0.1 percent only if necessary to reduce discomfort during the first few days, and Visucloben (Clobetazone – Visufarma Spa– Roma) (twice a day for one month) after removing the lens. Some patients may feel pain during the first day, and we suggest applying crushed ice in a small bag for 30 minutes at a time. Less than 20 percent of patients reported feeling pain (and never strong pain), with no differences between the Epi-LASIK and Epi-LASEK treatments. In a previous LASEK analysis,[24] 1 percent (myopia) to 6 percent (hyperopia) of patients reported feeling strong pain. The use of an epi-keratome seems to improve this number.

The most interesting outcome of this research was the improved hinge quality and flap integrity with the Epi-LASEK group.

86.7 percent perfect hinge in Epi-LASEK while 66.7 percent in Epi-Lasik.

97.8 percent perfect flap in Epi-LASEK while 93.3 percent in Epi-Lasik.

$P<0.05$

No differences in pain and haze were observed between the two techniques. A trend towards less astigmatism and corneal regularity came out in epi-LASEK group. A better UCVA in Epi-LASEK group was noted at the time the contact lens was just removed ($P<0.05$), and no significant differences in sphero-equivalent predictability, long-term safety and efficacy were found.

CONCLUSION

The importance of leaving an epithelial flap over the treated stroma may be debated, however there is evidence to show that there are advantages in cases of high myopia and hyperopia. If we are to accept the studies which site an advantage of leaving an epithelial flap,[25,26] we must find the most effective techniques that create the most stable flap possible, with a wide and complete hinge. The Epi-LASEK procedure combines two mechanisms, chemical and mechanical, which increase our ability to create a more stable flap and hinge.[27] This reduces the risk of creating a free-floating cap, which almost always means performing a PRK procedure. Studies that compare the Epi-Lasik and LASEK procedures show that there are few, if any, drawbacks of using an alcohol solution to help separate the epithelium. When adding the use of an epi-keratome to the LASEK procedure (epi-LASEK), patients who had hinge problems in the eye with the Epi-Lasik treatment did not have any problems in their other Epi-LASEK treated eye.

The Epi-LASEK procedure that we have developed does not change the parameters of the LASEK alcohol percentage or exposure time, nor does it change the suggested settings of the epi-keratome for speed, frequency, and vacuum. We are aware that it may be possible to reduce the alcohol percentage and time of exposure, and probably the vacuum value as well, increasing the speed of the instrument. These changes could improve safety while leaving the enhanced flap quality unaffected. A good flap is important because the basal membrane of epithelium plays a role in counteracting the negative chain of events that can lead to haze or regression, which prevents the drawbacks of a PRK treatment where Bowman's layer is removed. One day, we will hopefully have a chemical that could overcome these problems, but until then, we suggest using the safe and effective Epi-LASEK procedure.

REFERENCES

1. Camellin M. Laser epithelial keratomileusis for myopia. J Refract Surg 2003;19(6):666-70.
2. Moller-Pedersen T, Cavanagh HD, Petroll WM, Jester JV. Stromal wound healing explains refractive instability and haze development after photorefractive keratectomy. Ophthalmology 2000;107:1235-45.
3. Patel S, Marsshall J, Fitzke FW. Refractive index of the human corneal epithelium and stroma. J Refract Surg 11:100-5.
4. Hayashida Y, Nishida K, Yamato M, Yang J, Sugiyama H, Watanabe K, et al. Transplantation of tissue-engineered epithelial cell sheets after excimer laser photoablation reduces postoperative corneal haze.

Investigative Ophthalmology and Visual Science 2006;47:552-7.

5. Choi YS, Kim JY, Wee WR, Lee JH. Effect of the application of human amniotic membrane on rabbit corneal wound healing after excimer laser photorefractive keratectomy. Cornea 1998;17(4):389-95.
6. Wang MX, Gray TB, Park WC, et al. Reduction in corneal haze and apoptosis by amniotic membrane matrix in excimer laser photoablation in rabbits. J Cataract Refract Surg 2001;27(2):310-9.
7. Woo HM, Kim MS, Kweon OK, Kim DY, Nam TC, Kim JH. Effects of amniotic membrane on epithelial wound healing and stromal remodelling after excimer laser keratectomy in rabbit cornea. Br J Ophthalmol 2001;85 (3):345-9.
8. Netto MV, Mohan RR, Sinha S, Sharma A, Gupta PC, Wilson SE. Effect of prophylactic and therapeutic Mitomycin C on corneal apoptosis, cellular proliferation, haze, and long-term keratocyte density in rabbits. J Refract Surg 2006;22:562-74.
9. Camellin M. Laser epithelial keratomileusis with mitomycin C: indications and limits. J Refract Surg 2004; 20:S693-8.
10. Claringbold TV 2nd. Laser-assisted subepithelial keratectomy for the correction of myopia. J Cataract Refract Surg 2002;28:18-22.
11. Shahinian L Jr. Laser-assisted subepithelial keratectomy for low to high myopia and astigmatism. J Cataract Refract Surg 2002;28:1334-42.
12. Torres LF, Sancho C, Tan B, Padilla K, Schanzlin DJ, Chayet AS. Early postoperative pain following epi-lasik and photorefractive keratectomy: a prospective, comparative, bilateral study. J Refract Surg 2007;23:126-32.
13. Chalita MR, Tekwani NH, Krueger RR. Laser epithelial keratomileusis: outcome of initial cases performed by an experienced surgeon. J Refract Surg 2003;19:412-5.
14. Litwak S, Zadok D, Garcia-de Quevedo V, Robledo N, Chayet AS. Laser-assisted subepithelial keratectomy versus photorefractive keratectomy for the correction of myopia. A prospective comparative study. J Cataract Refract Surg 2002;28:1330-3.
15. Teus MA, De Benito-Llopis L, Sànchez-Pina JM. Learning curve of laser-assisted subepithelial keratectomy. Influence on visual and refractive results. J Cataract Refract Surg 2007;33:1381-5.
16. Hassan Hashemi, Akbar Fotouhi, Hamid Foudazi, Navid Sadeghi, Saeed Payvar. Prospective, randomized, paired comparison of laser epithelial keratomileusis and photorefractive keratectomy for myopia less than –6.50 Diopters. Journal of Refractive Surgery 2004;20(3).
17. Pirouzian A, Thornton J, Ngo S. One-year outcomes of a bilateral randomized prospective clinical trial comparing laser subepithelial keratomileusis and photorefractive keratectomy. J Refract Surg 2006;22:575-9.
18. Zhou XT, Chu RY, Wang XY, Zhou H, Yu ZQ, Wu LC et al. The clinical study of the epithelial flap of painless LASEK and Epi-Lasik 2005;41(Issue 11):977-80.
19. Gamaly TO, El Danasoury A, El Maghraby A. A prospective, randomized, contralateral eye comparison of epithelial laser in situ keratomileusis and photo-refractive keratectomy in eyes prone to haze. J Refract Surg 2007;23:S1015-20.
20 Maloney RK, Bogan SJ, Waring GO. Determination of corneal image-forming properties from corneal topography. Am J Ophthalm 1993;115:31-41.
21. Fantes FE, Hanna KD, Waring GO, Pouliquen Y, Thompson KP, Savoldelli M. Wound healing after excimer laser keratomileusis (photorefractive keratectomy) in monkeys. Arch Ophthalmol 1990;108:665-75.
22. Browning AC, Shah S, Dua HS, Maharajan SV, Gray T and Bragheeth MA. Alcohol debridement of the corneal epithelium in PRK and LASEK: an electron microscopic study. Invest Ophthalmol Vis Sci 2003;44:510-3.
23. Camellin M, Wyler D, Epi-Lasik Versus Epi-LASEK. J Refract Surg 2008;?
24. Camellin M. LASEK and As a History Technique Long-term Results. Fabiano Editore, Canelli 2006;327.
25. Long Q, Chu R, Zhou X, Dai J, Chen C, Rao SK, Lam D. Correlation between TGF-B1 in tears and corneal haze following LASEK and Epi-Lasik. J Refract Surg 2006;22:708-12.
26. Esquenazi S, He J, Bazan N, Bazan H. Comparison of corneal wound-healing response in photorefractive keratectomy and laser-assisted subepithelial keratectomy. J Cataract Refract Surg 2005;31:1632-9.
27. O'Doherty M, Kirwan C, O'Keeffe M, O'Doherty J. Postoperative pain following epi-Lasik, LASEK, and PRK for myopia. J Refract Surg 2007;23(Issue 2):133-8.

14 Advanced Surface Ablation in Thin Corneas

Miguel A Teus, Laura de Benito-Llopis, Jorge L Alió

INTRODUCTION

Excimer laser surface ablation and laser in situ keratomileusis (LASIK) have shown to be safe, effective and predictable procedures to correct different degrees of myopia.[1-7] Despite the disadvantages of surface ablation, i.e. slower visual recovery and higher postoperative discomfort, compared to LASIK, this procedure has become the technique of choice in patients with thin central corneal thickness (CCT), those at risk for trauma, and those with corneal surface problems such as dry eye, recurrent erosion syndrome or basement membrane disease.[2,8] Another potential advantage of advanced surface ablation techniques is the lower induction of higher order aberrations related to the lack of flap creation when compared to LASIK.[9,10]

RISK FACTORS ASSOCIATED WITH THE DEVELOPMENT OF ECTASIA AFTER EXCIMER LASER REFRACTIVE SURGERY

One of the most dreaded complications after excimer laser refractive surgery is secondary ectasia (Fig. 14.1). Although post-LASIK ectasia has been usually associated with a thin residual stromal bed,[11,12] deep ablations[11-13] or preoperative irregular topography,[12,14-16] this complication has also been reported after LASIK with shallower ablations[14,17-19] and in patients with no apparent preoperative risk factors,[19-21] suggesting that other factors, still undetermined and probably specific for each eye, play a role in the development of postoperative ectasia.[22] A review by Randleman et al of the published cases of ectasia after corneal refractive surgery showed that the main factor associated with the development of postoperative ectasia was a preoperative abnormal corneal topography, followed by the residual stromal bed thickness and the patient's age.[21]

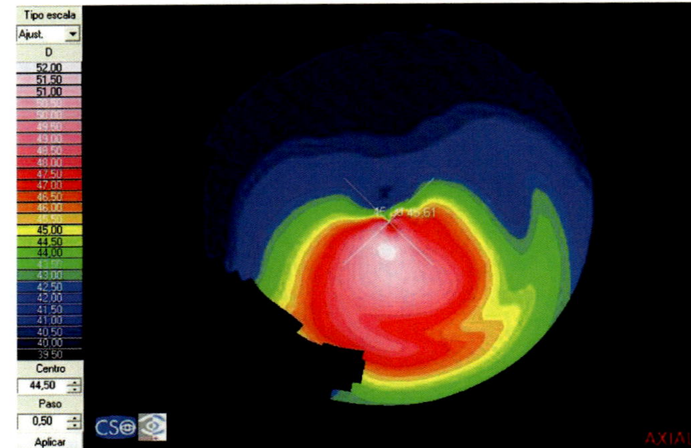

Fig. 14.1: Corneal ectasia after laser in situ keratomileusis

There have been very few reports of post-surface ablation ectasia and most of them either had preoperatively signs of primary ectasia[23-27] or did not have a complete preoperative examination to rule out the possibility of primary ectasia.[26-31] To the best of our knowledge, just one case[25] shows a thorough preoperative examination which showed an apparently normal cornea. Nevertheless, the patient had a moderately high cylindrical defect and a CCT of 509/508 μm, one patient's sibling had had penetrating keratoplasty due to an unknown cause, and the patient admitted to rub his eyes frequently, which has been associated to the development of primary ectasia.[32-34] Considering the high number of surface ablation procedures performed since the introduction of the technique, it seems that the risk of ectasia after surface ablation in eyes with no predisposing risk factors is extremely rare.

Interestingly, among the reported cases of ectasia after PRK, we found a much stronger relationship between the development of postoperative ectasia and preoperative corneal topographical abnormalities rather than preoperative CCT: in the review by Leccisotti[23] of 6453 eyes that had undergone PRK, only 5 eyes developed ectasia and all of them had preoperative topographical abnormalities or had keratoconus in the fellow eye. Among those 5 eyes, only two of them had preoperative CCT less than 500 μm. In the case of ectasia after PRK reported by Kim et al,[28] no preoperative topography was available, but the preoperative CCT was 536 μm. The case reported by Randleman et al [25] had a preoperative CCT of 509/508 μm. The unusual case of ectasia after PTK in an eye with band keratopathy reported by Miyata et al[31] had a preoperative cornea of 540 μm.

CONVENTIONAL LIMITS OF CORNEAL THICKNESS IN EXCIMER LASER REFRACTIVE SURGERY

Although no definite residual stromal bed thickness has been established as safe to avoid post-LASIK ectasia,[35] it is suggested that a residual stromal bed thinner than 250 μm or a postoperative total CCT thinner than 400 μm should be avoided.[13,15,36] In the usual clinical practice, corneas with less than 490-500 μm are generally considered a relative contraindication to undergo LASIK.[2,8,37,38]

Excimer laser surface ablation, including photorefractive keratectomy (PRK), laser-assisted subepithelial keratectomy (LASEK) and epipolis LASIK (epi-LASIK), theoretically minimizes the risk of having postoperative ectasia as it allows to leave a thicker residual stroma than LASIK,[8,39] while obtaining similar refractive and visual results.[3-7] Nevertheless, no minimal thickness in thin corneas with otherwise normal appearance (normal topography) has been established as safe to perform surface ablation.

From a statistical point of view, a cornea may be considered "normal" when its thickness falls within two standard deviations of the mean thickness described for its race.[40-45] Therefore, caution is recommended when dealing with thinner corneas, and corneal refractive surgery has usually been avoided in these cases. However, the clinical practice has shown that the preoperative corneal thickness is not in itself a risk factor for developing post-LASIK ectasia.[21,46] This observation leaves a "gray zone" between normal and abnormal corneal thickness that makes it difficult to establish a definite limit to perform excimer laser refractive surgery.

REPORTS OF EXCIMER LASER REFRACTIVE SURGERY IN THIN CORNEAS

There have been very few reports on LASIK performed in thin corneas, with good results and no development of post-LASIK ectasia[47-49] (Table 14.1). However, LASIK in this type of corneas encounters two major limitations:[47] the necessity to reduce the optical zone in order to avoid postoperative stromal bed thickness thinner than 250 μm (with the subsequent risk of night vision disturbance) and the incidence of refractive regression, which is usually higher in the group with higher preoperative myopia, whose enhancement would be obviously limited by the residual stromal bed thickness. Surface ablation seems to obtain as good results as LASIK,[3-7,50,51] while reducing those two limitations.

There are also very few reports of surface ablation performed in thin corneas. Table 14.2 briefly compares those specifically designed to study the outcomes of surface ablation in corneas with a CCT less than 500 μm. All those three studies[49,52,53] obtained initially good visual and refractive results and no case deve-

Table 14.1: Published series of laser in situ keratomileusis (LASIK) performed in corneas thinner than 500 µm

	Eyes	*Intended flap thickness*	*Min preop CCT*	*Estimated RSB thickness*	*Max myopia treated (D)*	*Min follow-up (m)*
Kremer et al[47]	98	160	456	>250	–10.00	36
Kymionis et al[49]	56	90	470	276-385	–6.50	12
He et al[48]	39	"ultra thin"	450	na	–9.50	12

CCT: central corneal thickness (in microns); RSB: residual stromal bed; na: not available; D: diopters; m: months

Table 14.2: Published series of laser surface ablation performed in corneas thinner than 500 µm

	Eyes	*MMC*	*Min preop CCT*	*Min CCT 3 m postop*	*Max preop K*	*Max myopia (diopters)*	*Min follow-up (months)*
Hashemi et al[52]	48	No	455	372	n.a.	–8.75	1
Kymionis et al[49]	68	No	453	358	<47	–6.75	12
De Benito-Llopis et al[51]	136	Yes	440	339	48	–11.00	15

MMC: mitomycin-C; CCT: central corneal thickness (in microns); K: keratometry; na: not available

loped postoperative ectasia. The study by Hashemi et al is mainly limited by its short follow-up (3 months[52]). In the study by Kymionis et al,[49] patients with preoperative keratometry of 47.00 D or greater were excluded, and they treated only low to moderate myopia (up to –6.75 D of spherical equivalent), which limits the applicability of their results to the clinical practice. In the study by De Benito-Llopis et al[51] no limit in preoperative keratometry was established and myopia up to –11.00 D was treated. Visual and refractive outcomes did not show any significant difference between the 3rd month and 15-month postoperative examinations, suggesting that thin corneas operated with laser surface ablation were stable at least one year after the surgery. Obviously, the short follow-up of these studies (15 months maximum[51]) may have prevented them to detect later regression or ectasia. Nevertheless, approximately 50 percent of the cases of post-LASIK ectasia seem to present within the first 12 months after surgery.[15,21] It is clear that it may still be possible to detect progression to ectasia in this type of corneas with longer follow-up or more cases.

Other studies support the results of those series. Lee et al[54] compared different techniques for epithelial removal in surface ablation and included patients with a preoperative thin cornea (range from 421 µm to 602 µm). They do not focus on the outcomes of the thinnest corneas, but they do not report any postoperative ectasia. Vinciguerra et al[55] reported on the results of phototherapeutic keratectomy (PTK) performed in 48 very thin corneas (range 290 to 444 µm) due to complications of previous PRK. Postoperative CCT ranged from 264 to 414 µm and did not show signs of progressive thinning during the follow-up (one year follow-up: 100% of eyes; five-year follow-up: 64.5% of eyes). They did not detect any change in the residual refractive error that would suggest progressive ectasia.

COULD THE DIFFERENCES BETWEEN LASIK AND SURFACE ABLATION JUSTIFY DIFFERENT LIMITS IN PREOPERATIVE CENTRAL CORNEAL THICKNESS?

The risk of ectasia after LASIK seems, although low, higher in comparison to surface ablation, with an estimated incidence of 0.04 to 0.6 percent depending on the series, although many cases have probably not been reported in the literature and the incidence could be higher.[15,21] In fact, there have been reports of corneal ectasia occurring after LASIK in one eye and

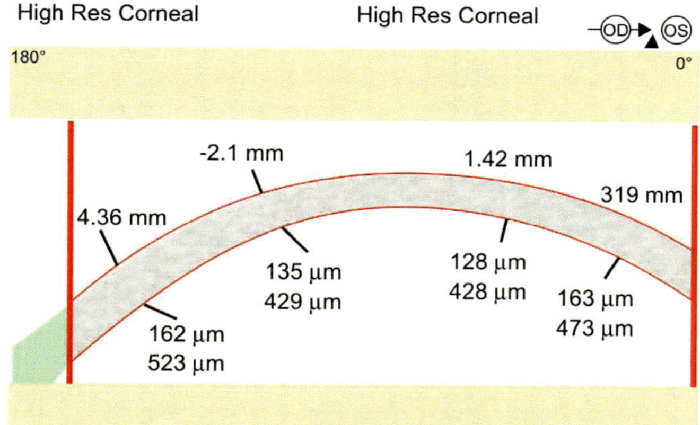

Fig. 14.2: Flap and stromal bed thicknesses after laser in situ keratomileusis measured with optical coherence tomography

not after PRK in the contralateral eye of the same patient.[56,57] Surface ablation is thought to lead to a lower risk of postoperative ectasia due to the lack of stromal flap, which may be one of the most important causes of corneal destabilization. Due to the anatomic distribution of the corneal lamellae in the cornea, with a marked anteroposterior lamellar interweave in the anterior cornea that is not seen in the most posterior part of it,[58-60] the anterior corneal layers are believed to have more biomechanical strength than the posterior ones, and are considered the ones responsible for maintaining the normal corneal curvature, specially the most anterior 100-120 µm.[58-60]

In contrast with surface ablation, LASIK first produces a disruption of the anterior corneal layers when performing the stromal flap (Fig. 14.2) that, once healed, does not re-establish the preoperative strength of the virgin stroma.[61] LASIK causes further disruption of the central corneal lamellae by the excimer laser ablation. This double aggression to the cornea makes LASIK theoretically more threatening to the corneal biomechanical stability than surface ablation.[55,56,58] Moreover, topographical suspicion of keratoconus is a contraindication of LASIK[15,21,34] and the reports of this procedure performed in clinical keratoconus[62] and in keratoconus fruste[16] have shown worsening of the primary ectasia, whereas surface ablation has been performed in several series in patients with topographic inferior steepening or keratoconus fruste[63-69] with stable results. When performing surface ablation in clinical keratoconus, authors have very rarely seen progression of the primary ectasia.[70-74] Surface ablation has even been proposed as a therapeutic procedure to avoid progression of the keratoconus in the initial phases.[73]

It is usually accepted that LASIK should not be performed in corneas with a preoperative CCT thinner than 500 µm[2,8] (490 µm for some authors[38,75]) to avoid altering the biomechanical strength of these high-risk corneas.[37] Due to the differences between LASIK and surface ablation regarding the aggression they inflict to the cornea, the limits in CCT assumed in LASIK surgery may not be applicable in surface ablation surgery.[34] The limit of 490-500 µm of preoperative CCT usually accepted in LASIK may be too restrictive in surface ablation.[76]

Compared to the agreement achieved in the necessity of leaving a minimal stromal bed of 250-300 µm after LASIK,[13,15,36] there is no consensus on the limit needed to be left after surface ablation.[34] Some authors consider it is necessary to leave a minimum of 380-400 µm.[26] Most of the series of cases with preoperative keratoconus fruste treated with PRK had as an exclusion criterion a calculated residual stromal thickness less than 350 µm[63] or even 450 µm.[64] However, this limit on preoperatively healthy corneas may also be too restrictive. In the cases treated by Vinciguerra et al[55] with PTK to treat complicated PRK cases, they left a residual CCT of 264 µm up to 414 µm and found stable results and no progressive thinning. In our series,[53] the postoperative CCT 3 months after surgery ranged from 339 to 473 µm. In fact, even the limit of 250-300 µm established in LASIK may not be definitive.[21] Condon et al[38] published a series of 107 eyes whose high myopia (> –10 D) was treated with LASIK. The calculated residual stromal bed thickness was thinner than 250 µm in 15 eyes, and only one developed ectasia. Moreover, this was the only eye with a preoperative CCT <490 µm.

CONCLUSION

In conclusion, excimer laser surface ablation seems to be safe and effective to correct myopia and myopic astigmatism in thin corneas (CCT <500 μm) with normal topography. Due to the biomechanical differences between LASIK and surface ablation, the limits of 500 μm of preoperative CCT and of 250-300 μm of residual stromal thickness established for LASIK may be too restrictive when applied to surface ablation. There is published evidence suggesting that thin corneas treated with surface ablation to correct myopia, with or without the concomitant use of MMC, are stable at least 15 months after the surgery.[51] More studies with longer follow-up are needed to further elucidate the safety of the procedure in this type of corneas.

REFERENCES

1. Sugar A, Rapuano CJ, Culbertson WW, Huang D, Varley GA, Agapitos PJ, et al. Laser in situ keratomileusis for myopia and astigmatism: safety and efficacy. A report by the American Academy of Ophthalmology. Ophthalmology 2002;109:175-87.
2. Taneri S, Zieske JD, Azar DT. Evolution, techniques, clinical outcomes and pathophysiology of LASEK: review of the literature. Surv Ophthalmol 2004; 49(6):576-602.
3. Scerrati E. Laser in situ keratomileusis versus laser epithelial keratomileusis (LASIK vs. LASEK). J Refract Surg 2001;17:S219-21.
4. Kaya V, Oncel B, Sivrikaya H, Yilmaz OF. Prospective, paired comparison of laser in situ keratomileusis and laser epithelial keratomileusis for myopia less than -6.00 diopters. J Refract Surg 2004;20:223-8.
5. De Benito-Llopis L, Teus MA, Sánchez-Pina JM, Hernández-Verdejo JL. Comparison between LASEK and LASIK for the correction of low myopia. J Refract Surg 2007;23:139-45.
6. Tobaigy FM, Ghanem RC, Sayegh RR, Hallak JA, Azar DT. A control-matched comparison of laser epithelial keratomileusis and laser in situ keratomileusis for low to moderate myopia. Am J Ophthalmol 2006;142:901-8.
7. Teus MA, de Benito-Llopis L, Sánchez-Pina JM. LASEK versus LASIK for the correction of moderate myopia. Optom Vis Sci 2007;84:605-10.
8. Netto MV, Wilson SE. Indications for excimer laser surface ablation. J Refract Surg 2005;21:734-41.
9. Yamane N, Miyata K, Samejima T, Hiraoka T, Kiuchi T, Okamoto F, et al. Ocular higher-order aberrations and contrast sensitivity after conventional laser in situ keratomileusis. Invest Ophthalmol Vis Sci 2004;45:3986-90.
10. Waheed S, Chalita MR, Xu M, Krueger RR. Flap-induced and laser-induced ocular aberrations in a two-step LASIK procedure. J Refract Surg 2005;21:346-52.
11. Pallikaris IG, Kymionis GD, Astyrakakis NI. Corneal ectasia induced by laser in situ keratomileusis. J Cataract Refract Surg 2001;27:1796-802.
12. Rad AS, Jabbarvand M, Saifi N. Progressive keratectasia after laser in situ keratomileusis. J Refract Surg 2004;20:S718-22.
13. Seiler T, Koufala K, Richter G. Iatrogenic keratectasia after laser in situ keratomileusis. J Refract Surg 1998;14:312-7.
14. Amoils SP, Deist MB, Gous P, Amoils PM. Iatrogenic keratectasia after laser in situ keratomileusis for less than –4 to –7 diopters of myopia. J Cataract Refract Surg 2000; 26:967-77.
15. Randleman JB. Post-laser in situ keratomileusis ectasia: current understanding and future directions. Curr Opin Ophthalmol 2006;17(4):406-12.
16. Seiler T, Quurke AW. Iatrogenic keratectasia after LASIK in a case of forme fruste keratoconus. J Cataract Refract Surg 1998;24:1007-9.
17. Lifshitz T, Levy J, Klemperer I, Levinger S. Late bilateral keratectasia after LASIK in a low myopic patient. J Refract Surg 2005;21:494-6.
18. Argento C, Cosentino MJ, Tytiun A, Rapetti G, Zarate J. Corneal ectasia after laser in situ keratomileusis. J Cataract Refract Surg 2001;27:1440-8.
19. Kymionis GD, Tsiklis N, Karp CL, Kalyvianaki M, Pallikaris AI. Unilateral corneal ectasia after laser in situ keratomileusis in a patient with uncomplicated photorefractive keratectomy in the fellow eye. J Cataract Refract Surg 2007;33:859-61.
20. Klein SR, Epstein RJ, Randleman JB, Stulting RD. Corneal ectasia after laser in situ keratomileusis in patients without apparent preoperative risk factors. Cornea 2006;25:388-403.
21. Randleman JB, Woodward M, Lynn MJ, Stulting RD. Risk assessment for ectasia after corneal refractive surgery. Ophthalmology 2008;115:37-50.
22. Binder PS. Ectasia after laser in situ keratomileusis. J Cataract Refract Surg 2003;29:2419-29.
23. Leccisotti A. Corneal ectasia after photorefractive keratectomy. Graefe's Arch Clin Exp Ophthalmol 2007;245:869-75.
24. Malecaze F, coullet J, Calvas P, Fournié P, Arné J-L, Brodaty C. Corneal ectasia after photorefractive keratectomy for low myopia. Ophthalmology 2006;113:742-6.
25. Randleman JB, Caster AI, Banning C, Stulting RD. Corneal ectasia after photorefractive keratectomy. J Cataract Refract Surg 2006;32:1395-8.
26. Lovisolo CF, Fleming JF. Intracorneal ring segments for iatrogenic keratectasia after laser in situ keratomileusis or photorefractive keratectomy. J Refract Surg 2002;18: 535-41.
27. Holland SP, Srivannaboon S, Reinstein DZ. Avoiding serious corneal complications of laser assisted in situ

keratomileusis and photorefractive keratectomy. Ophthalmology 2000;107:640-52.
28. Kim H, Coi J-S, Joo C-K. Corneal ectasia after PRK. Clinicopathologic case report. Cornea 2006;25:845-8.
29. Parmar D, Claoué C. Keratectasia following excimer laser photorefractive keratectomy. Acta Ophthalmol Scand 2004;82:102-5.
30. Chiou A G-Y, Bovet J, de Courten C. Management of corneal ectasia and cataract following photorefractive keratectomy. J Cataract Refract Surg 2006;32:679-80.
31. Miyata K, Takahashi T, Tomidokoro A, Oshira KOT. Iatrogenic keratectasia after phototherapeutic keratectomy. Br J Ophthalmol 2001;85:247-8.
32. Karseras AG, Ruben M. Aetiology of keratoconus. Br J Ophthalmol 1976;60:522-5.
33. Krachmer JH. Eye rubbing can cause keratoconus. Cornea 2004;23:539-40.
34. Binder PS, Lindstrom RL, Stulting RD, Donnenfeld E, Wu H, McDonnell P, et al. Keratoconus and corneal ectasia after LASIK. J Cataract Refract Surg 2005;31:2035-8.
35. Reinstein DZ, Srivannaboon S, Archer TJ, Silverman RH, Sutton H, Coleman DJ. Probability model of the inaccuracy of residual stromal thickness prediction to reduce the risk of ectasia after LASIK part II: quantifying population risk. J Refract Surg 2006;22(9):861-70.
36. Tabbara KF, Kotb AA. Risk factors for corneal ectasia after LASIK. Ophthalmology 2006;113:1618-22.
37. Guirao A. Theoretical elastic response of the cornea to refractive surgery: risk factors for keratectasia. J Refract Surg 2005;21:176-85.
38. Condon PI, O'Keefe M, Binder PS. Long-term results of laser in situ keratomileusis for high myopia: risk for ectasia. J Cataract Refract Surg 2007;33:583-90.
39. Camellin M. Laser epithelial keratomileusis for myopia. J Refract Surg 2003;19:666-70.
40. La Rosa FA, Gross RL, Orengo-Nania S. Central corneal thickness of Caucasians and African Americans in glaucomatous and nonglaucomatous populations. Arch Ophthalmol 2001;119:23-7.
41. Doughty MJ, Zaman ML. Human corneal thickness and its impact on intraocular pressure measures: a review and meta-analysis approach. Surv Ophthalmol 2000;44:367-408.
42. Chakrabarti HS, Craig JP, Brahma A, Malik TY, McGhee CNJ. Comparison of corneal thickness measurements using ultrasound and Orbscan slit-scanning topography in normal and post-LASIK eyes. J Cataract Refract Surg 2001;27:1823-8.
43. Shimmyo M, Ross AJ, Moy A, Mostafavi R. Intraocular pressure, Goldmann applanation tension, corneal thickness, and corneal curvature in Caucasians, Asians, Hispanics, and African Americans. Am J Ophthalmol 2003;136:603-13.
44. Aghaian E, Choe JE, Lin S, Stamper RL. Central corneal thickness of Caucasians, Chinese, Hispanics, Filipinos, African Americans, and Japanese in a glaucoma clinic. Ophthalmology 2004;111:2211-9.
45. Yo C, Ariyasu RG. Racial differences in central corneal thickness and refraction among refractive surgery candidates. J Refract Surg 2005;21:194-7.
46. Binder PS. Analysis of ectasia after laser in situ keratomileusis: risk factors. J Cataract Refract Surg 2007;33:1530-8
47. Kremer I, Bahar I, Hirsh A, Levinger S. Clinical outcome of wavefront-guided laser in situ keratomileusis in eyes with moderate to high myopia with thin corneas. J Cataract Refract Surg 2005;31:1366-71.
48. He TG, Shi WR. Clinical study of ultrathin flap LASIK and LASEK for the treatment of high myopia with thin cornea. Zhonghua Yan Ke Za Zhi 2006;42:517-21.
49. Kymionis GD, Bouzoukis D, Diakonis V, Tsiklis N, Gkenos E, Pallikaris AI, et al. Long-term results of thin corneas after refractive laser surgery. Am J Ophthalmol 2007;144:181-5.
50. Kim JK, Kim SS, Lee HK, et al. Laser in situ keratomileusis versus laser-assisted subepithelial keratectomy for the correction of high myopia. J Cataract Refract Surg 2004; 30:1405-11.
51. De Benito-Llopis L, Teus MA, Sánchez-Pina JM. Comparison between LASEK with MMC and LASIK for the correction of high myopia (-7.00 to -13.75 D). J Refract Surg (In Press).
52. Hashemi H, Fotouhi A, Sadeghi N, Payvar S, Foudazi H. Laser epithelial keratomileusis (LASEK) for myopia in patients with a thin cornea. J Refract Surg 2004;20:90-1.
53. De Benito-Llopis L, Teus MA, Sánchez-Pina JM, Fuentes I. Stability of LASEK with and without mitomycin-C performed to correct myopia in thin corneas. A 15-month follow-up. Am J Ophthalmol 2008 (In Press).
54. Lee HK, Lee KS, Kim JK, Kim HC, Seo KR, Kim EK. Epithelial healing and clinical outcomes in excimer laser photorefractive surgery following three epithelial removal techniques: mechanical, alcohol, and excimer laser. Am J Ophthalmol 2005;139:56-63.
55. Vinciguerra P, Torres-Munoz MI, Camesasca FI, Grizzi F, Roberts C. Long-term follow-up of ultrathin corneas after surface retreatment with phototherapeutic keratectomy. J Cataract Refract Surg 2005;31:82-7.
56. Javadi MA, Mohammadpour M, Rabei HM. Keratect-ectasia after LASIK but not after PRK in one patient. J Refract Surg 2006;22:817-20.
57. Rao SK, Srinivasan B, Sitalakshmi G, Padmanabhan P. Photorefractive keratectomy versus laser in situ kerato-mileusis to prevent keratectasia after corneal ablation. J Cataract Refract Surg 2004;30:2623-8.
58. Dupps WJ, Wilson SE. Biomechanics and wound healing in the cornea. Exp Eye Res 2006;83:709-20.
59. Müller LJ, Tels E, Vrensen GFJM. The specific architecture of the anterior stroma accounts for maintenance of corneal curvature. Br J Ophthalmol 2001;85:437-43.
60. Bron AJ. The architecture of the corneal stroma. Br J Ophthalmol 2001;85:379-83.
61. Dawson DG, Edelhauser HF, Grossniklaus HE. Long-term histopathologic findings in human corneal wounds

after refractive surgical procedures. Am J Ophthalmol 2005;139:168-78.
62. Buzard KA, Tuengler A, Febbraro JL. Treatment of mild to moderate keratoconus with laser in situ keratomileusis. J Cataract Refract Surg 1999;25:1600-9.
63. Bahar I, Levinger S, Kremer I. Wavefrong-supported photorefractive keratectomy with the Bausch and Lomb Zyoptix in patients with myopic astigmatism and suspected keratoconus. J Refract Surg 2006;22:533-8.
64. Koller T, Iseli HP, Donitzky C, Papadopoulos N, Seiler T. Topography-guided surface ablation for forme fruste keratoconus. Ophthalmology 2006;113:2198-202.
65. Alpins N, Stamatelatos G. Customized photoastigmatic refractive keratectomy using combined topographic and refractive data for myopia and astigmatism in eyes with forme fruste and mild keratoconus. J Cataract Refract Surg 2007;33:591-602.
66. Sun R, Gimbel HV, Kaye GB. Photorefractive keratectomy in keratoconus suspects. J Cataract Refract Surg 1999;25: 1461-6.
67. Doyle SJ, Hynes E, Naroo S, Shah S. PRK in patients with a keratoconic topography picture. The concept of a physiological "displaced apex syndrome". Br J Ophthalmol 1996;80:25-8.
68. Bilgihan K, Ozdek SC, Konuk O, Akata F, Hasanreisoglu B. Results of photorefractive keratectomy in keratoconus suspects at 4 years. J Refract Surg 2000;16:438-43.
69. Colin J, Cochener B, Bobo C, Malet F, Gallinaro C, Le Floch G. Myopic photorefractive keratectomy in eyes with atypical inferior corneal steepening. J Cataract Refract Surg 1996;22:1423-6.
70. Mortensen J, Carlsson K, Ohrstrom A. Excimer laser surgery for keratoconus. J Cataract Refract Surg 1998; 24:893-8.
71. Dausch d, Schroder E, Dausch S. Topography-controlled excimer laser photorefractive keratectomy. J Refract Surg 2000;16:13-22.
72. Kremer I, Shochot Y, Kaplan A, Blumenthal M. Three year results of photoastigmatic refractive keratectomy for mild and atypical keratoconus. J Cataract Refract Surg 1998;24:1581-8.
73. Kasparova EA, Kasparov AA. Six-year experience with excimer laser surgery for primary keratoconus in Russia. J Refract Surg 2003;19:S250-4.
74. Cennamo G, Intravaja A, Boccuzzi D, Marotta G, Cennamo G. Treatment of keratoconus by topography-guided customized photorefractive keratectomy: two-year follow-up study. J Refract Surg 2008;24:145-9.
75. Randleman JB, Russell B, Ward MA, Thompson KP, Stulting RD. Risk factors and prognosis for corneal ectasia after LASIK. Ophthalmology 2003;110:267-75.
76. Salz JJ, Binder PS. Is there a "magic number" to reduce the risk of ectasia after laser in situ keratomileusis and photorefractive keratectomy? Am J Ophthalmol 2007;144:284-5.

15 Phototherapeutic Keratectomy (PTK)

Jes Mortenson

INTRODUCTION

In 1983, Professor Stephen Trokel suggested the use of the excimer laser in ophthalmic surgery. Since then, millions of patients have been treated successfully, mostly in the refractive area. The exact edging capability of the excimer laser has been found useful in treating superficial corneal opacities, corneal scars, dystrophies and irregularities. This part of the excimer laser use is commonly referred to as PTK or phototherapeutic keratectomy.[1-3]

PTK

PTK aims to change the corneal surface: to correct irregularities of the corneal surface or to change the refraction of the cornea, to make the epithelium adhere better to the basal membrane in recurrent erosions and in some superficial corneal dystrophies. Different techniques have been used to remove the epithelium: scraping with a knife and later a brush. Since 2000 we prefer to loosen the epithelium by exposure to 30 percent alcohol for 20 seconds in a ring. After the treatment the epithelium is rolled back and covered by a silicon lens. We have found that this procedure reduces the postoperative pain the patient has to endure. In refractive cases such as anisometropia after previous ocular surgery, LASIK is the preferred technique. Removing the epithelium gives a better situation to accurately measure the degree of the irregularity of the corneal surface, as the epithelium always conceals the minor irregularities.

WOUND HEALING OF THE CORNEA AFTER EXCIMER LASER ABLATION

The model of wound healing in the body almost always follows the same pattern: (i) Inflammation, early polymorphonuclear leukocyte invasion, late, monocyte invasion; (ii) granular tissue formation and re-epithelialization; (iii) new matrix formation and remodelling of the matrix; (iv) wound contraction; (v) collagen accumulation and normalization of the number of cells in the scar. These steps are all seen in the corneal wound healing but are modulated and down regulated resulting in a regeneration of the corneal tissue as the end product rather than scar tissue that could severely injure the function of the eye as a visual organ.

The first reaction taking place in the cornea as a reaction to a trauma (e.g. scraping of the epithelium, scalpel incision PRK, Lasik and even a viral infection in the epithelium) is a cell death of the anterior keratocytes by apoptosis thinning the stroma according to the magnitude of the injury. This was first described by Dohlman et al 1968. The understanding of apoptosis had of course not developed at that time. The apoptosis starts after one hour with a peak after approximately 4 hours. An interesting hypothesis on the selective advantage of apoptosis in the keratocytes is that it can be a way to prevent a virus infection in the epithelium from spreading to the stroma. Within a few hours after the trauma, polymorph nuclear leucocytes invade the wound followed later by mononuclear cells. These cells help to remove dead cells and stromal remnants and fight bacterial intruders. The process of repair starts with activation of the keratocytes around the acellullar zone that arises after the cell death of the keratocytes. The keratocytes develop in to fibroblasts. The fibroblasts excrete fibronectin in the wound area, which may allow the fibroblasts to migrate on the fibronectin. The altered composition of the ECM probably explains the opacity of the repair tissue. The fibroblasts also up regulate the synthesis of enzymes capable of degrading the new ECM; among these are Matrix Metalloproteinase. A gradual interleaving between the stromal collagen lamellae and the collagen lamellae at the wound edge emerges. The remodeling of the stroma to a more mature state contributes to restoration of the transparency of the cornea. A new cell type appears at the contraction phase one to two weeks after the trauma to the cornea: the myofibroblasts which are characterized by the intracellular appearance of α-smooth muscle actin. The myofibroblasts are believed to differentiate from the fibroblasts; (some studies have questioned the hypothesis showing that they are derived from the bone-marrow). Restoration of the epithelial basement membrane is crucial for the delicate balance between stromal regeneration and developing fibrotic scar tissue. Myofibroblasts often disappear after the following weeks, but if a defective basement membrane arises the wound healing would be reparative rather than regenerative with a fibrotic response due to the myofibroblasts (causing haze in photorefractive keratectomy?). Can Bowman's layer reform after removal? A study of corneas undergoing radial keratotomy 5 to 10 years earlier showed that a layer similar to Bowman's layer develops around the ectopic epithelium in the cuts. A homeostatic interaction between the epithelial cells and the keratocytes in the stroma is suggested to maintain the normal structure of the cornea. These observations suggest that the epithelium actively participates in the formation and maintenance of Bowman's layer. Re-epithelization after an abrasion as such as in PRK typically takes 48 to 72 hours. Epithelial healing is complete after six weeks when permanent anchoring is restored to the basal membrane. The epithelial restoration is crucial to restore a barrier against bacteria but also in the modulation leading to a regenerative response instead of a fibrotic repair with scar tissue. The cornea undergoes a homeostatic remodeling like the skin and other tissue with collagen matrix but with a much slower turn over. The answer to the question why the cornea often undergoes regenerative wound healing is that the cornea, as is the whole eye, is an immune-privileged site, meaning that it is relatively protected against an immune response to foreign or self antigens. The historical definition of an immune privileged site is an anatomical site where a transplanted allograft survives for an extended period of time in an immune competent host. Today the immune privilege is considered a dynamic rather than passive process. In a grafted cornea the anatomic features work together with immune-regulation to prevent rejection; this process will never stop - rejection can take place in spite of decades of silence.That would give an explanation to the permanence of the changes made by the excimer laser ablation to the corneal surface.

RECURRENT EROSION

This was first described by Hansen in 1872 and it causes episodes of acute pain, lacrimation and photophobia on waking. There may be a history of previous ocular trauma, or it may occur spontaneously – Map-dot-Fingerprint dystrophy, often the cause, is not always correctly diagnosed.

Treatment Protocol

In the beginning the PTK is performed transepthelially if the patient does not have any epithelium defect. 45 to 50 microns is treated followed by 5 microns.

If the cornea had an erosion or we found the epithelium to be very loose we scraped the epithelium off from the affected area and treated 5-8 microns through the Bowman's membrane.

Today LASEK is used: in a ring with a diameter of 8 to 9 mm, 30 percent alcohol is placed for

20 seconds. The epithelium is carefully rolled off, and after ablation of 5 to 8 microns, rolled back and a contact lens is placed for 4 to 5 days.

A thing you should be very careful about is not to treat too deeply especially if you have a emmetropic or hyperopic patient, or you might end up with unintended hyperopia and not a very satisfied patient. Videokeratography can often help you if you are not able to localise the erosion, as it will often show irregularity of the afflicted area. If the erosions are near the visual axis the treatment should always be properly centred to omit any irregularity of the surface that could disturb the visual acuity or visual quality of the eye. Post-operatively the patients were given oral painkillers and antibiotic eyedrops as recommended treatment.

CORNEAL DYSTROPHIES

Corneal dystrophies can be classified into pre-Bowman's layer, Bowman's layer, anterior stromal and stromal. The dystrophies are congenital and will recur, so the PTK treatment cannot be considered as a cure for the future problems caused by the dystrophies. This means that the procedure should offer the anatomy as little as possible, to allow for repeated treatment later. Generally, the problems most often seen with dystrophies are recurrent erosion and irregularity of the surface. Cloudiness of the stroma is a rarer cause for reduction of the visual acuity. Putting a hard contact lens on the cornea can give a good idea of what can be accomplished by the polishing of the irregular corneal surface, especially if some cloudiness is also a part of the picture.

Most eyes were treated transepithelially followed by 15 to 100 μm in the stroma; LaserVis®, methyl-cellulose or BSS were used as masking. Today LASEK is used followed by polishing by LaserVis® (Figs 15.1 and 15.2). PTK treatment of various corneal dystrophies often gives very good results, especially if the problem is due to recurrent erosion or moderate irregularity of the corneal surface.

CORNEAL SCARS, BAND KERATOPATHY, PTERYGIUM AND HIGH MYOPIA

Before treating, you have to decide the aim of the treatment: Reducing pain, increasing visual acuity, cosmetic reasons or help the eye to tolerate a contact lens. Do not treat denervated corneas or severe dry eyes. Be conservative do not promise the patient anything, severe surface irregularity is difficult to treat with the excimer laser, but sometimes nature will help you.

Figures 15.3 and 15.4 show a case of severe ischemia of the cornea after contact lens wearing. The cornea was cloudy and had severe edema. The epithelium healed with severe scarring and

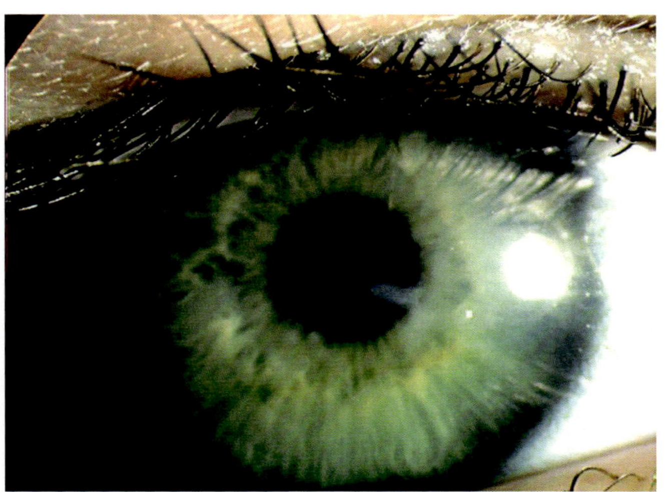

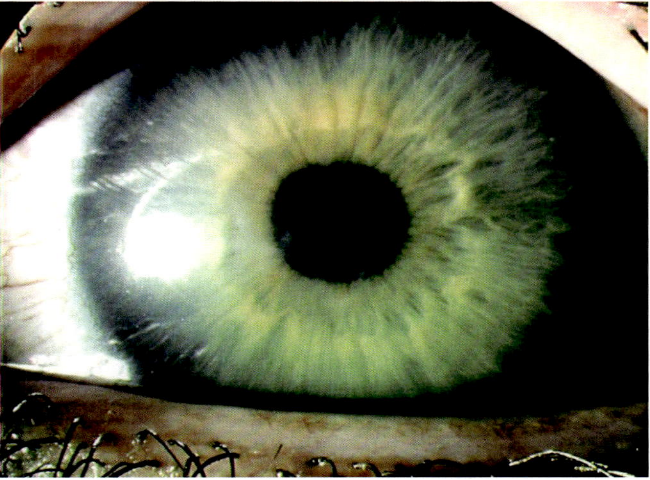

Figs 15.1 and 15.2: Cornea with Groenow´s dystrophy pre- and postoperative after PTK

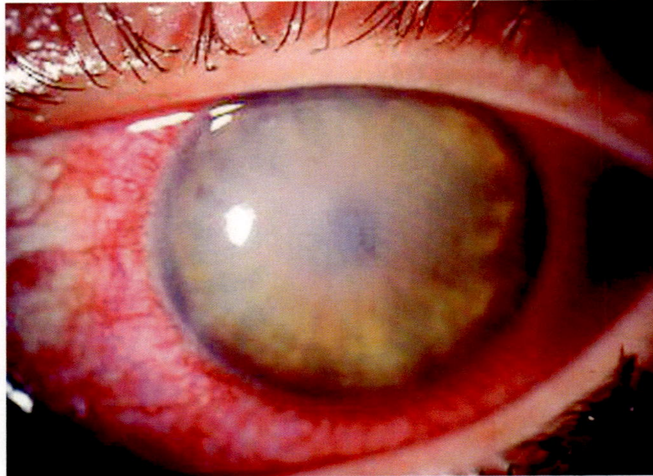

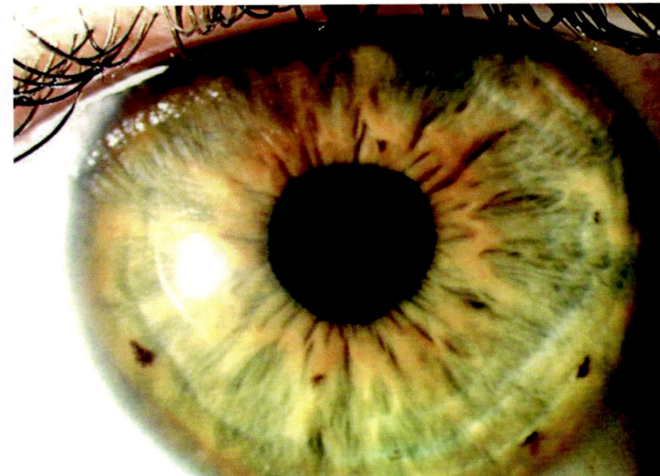

Figs 15.3 and 15.4: Cornea with severe ischemia and at follow-up 7 years later. The cornea had totally regenerated

irregularity but after three weeks increasing transparency of the cornea. Visual acuity improved from CF to 20/100. After one year 20/40 with contact lens after polishing the surface by PTK. The patient was seen after 7 years. The cornea had totally regenerated and visual acuity was 1.0 with glasses.

By treating **pterygium** we hoped to stop or reduce the recurrence of the pterygium. The pterygium was surgically excised and after that the denuded area was polished, often under masking of methylcellulose, by the excimer laser. We did not see any indication that polishing after surgical removal reduce the recurrence of the pterygium compared with only surgical excision.

SUMMARY

PTK has become an important therapeutic instrument in ophthalmology. The refractive changes are persistent even in corneas with dystrophies affected the anterior surface of the cornea.

REFERENCES

1. Agarwal A. Refractive Surgery Nightmares; Slack Inc, USA 2006; In press.
2. Agarwal S, Agarwal AT, Agarwal A. Textbook on Corneal Topography. Jaypee, India, 2005.
3. Agarwal A. Handbook of Ophthalmology. Slack Inc, USA; 2005.

SECTION THREE

ABERROPIA

16 Aberropia: A New Refractive Entity

Amar Agarwal, Athiya Agarwal

INTRODUCTION

The next evolution to come on to the visual science scene in refractive ocular imaging is the aberrometer, the Orbscan and wave front analysis. This technology is based on astrophysical principles, which astronomers use to perfect the images impinging on their telescopes. Dr. Bille, the Director of the Institute of Applied Physics at the University of Heidelberg first began work in this field while developing this specific technology for astronomy applications in the mid-1970's. For perfect imaging, astrophysicists have to be able to measure and correct the imperfect higher-order aberrations or wavefront distortions that enter their telescopic lens system from the galaxy. To achieve this purpose, adaptive optics are used wherein deformable mirrors reform the distorted wavefront to allow clear visualization of celestial objects. Extrapolating these same principles to the human eye, it was thought that removal of the wavefront aberrations of the eye might finally yield the long awaited and much desired ultimate goal of "super vision".

So far, the only parameters that could be modified to obtain the optical correction for a given patients refractive error were the sphere, cylinder and axis even though this does not give the ideal optical correction many a times. This is because the current modes for correcting the optical aberrations of the eye do not reduce the higher order aberrations. The ideal optical system should be able to correct the optical aberrations in such a way that the spatial resolving ability of the eye is limited only by the limits imposed by the neural retina, i.e. receptor diameter and receptor packing.

Thus, there may be a large group of patients whose best corrected visual acuity (BCVA) may actually improve significantly on removal of the optical aberrations. These optical aberrations are contributed to by the eye's entire optical system, i.e. the cornea, the lens, the vitreous and the retina. This study was conducted to determine the existence of a hitherto unidentified entity which we label as "**aberropia**" wherein patients with best corrected visual acuity of $\leq$ 6/9 (0.63), corneal topography not accounting for the lack of improvement in BCVA and with no other known cause for decreased vision improved by $\geq$ 2 Snellen lines after refractive correction of their wavefront aberration.

MATERIALS AND METHODS

16 eyes of 10 patients were included in this retrospective study carried out at the Dr. Agarwal's Eye Institute, India between May to December 2002. Only patients who had visual acuity less than 6/9 (0.63) prior to the procedure and whose visual acuity improved by more than or equal to two lines after the procedure were included in the study. None of these patients had any other known cause for

decreased vision and their corneal topography did not account for the lack of improvement in BCVA. The routine patient evaluation including uncorrected (UCVA) and best corrected visual acuity (BCVA), slit lamp examination, applanation tonometry, manifest and cycloplegic refractions, Orbscan, aberrometry, corneal pachymetry, corneal diameter, Schirmer's test and indirect ophthalmoscopy had been performed for all the patients. Patients wearing contact lenses had been asked to discontinue soft lenses for a minimum of 1 week and rigid gas permeable lenses for a minimum of 2 weeks before the preoperative examination and surgery. Informed consent was obtained form all patients after a thorough explanation of the procedure and its potential benefits and risks.

The Zyoptix procedure was then performed using the Bausch and Lomb Technolas 217 Z machine. The parameters used were: wavelength 193 nm, fluence 130 mJ/cm^2 and ablation zone diameters between 4.8 mm and 6 mm. The Hansatome (Bausch and Lomb) was used in all the eyes. Either the 180 µm or the 160 µm plate was used in all the eyes. The aberrometer and the Orbscan, which checks the corneal topography, are linked and a zylink created. An appropriate software file is created which is then used to generate the laser treatment file.

Postoperatively, the patients underwent complete examination including UCVA, BCVA, slit lamp examination, Orbscan and aberrometry. The mean follow-up was 37.5 days.

For statistical analysis, the Snellen acuity was converted to the decimal notation. Continuous variables were described with mean, standard deviation, minimum and maximum values.

RESULTS

16 eyes of 10 patients satisfied the inclusion criteria. The mean age of the patients was 29.43 years (range 22 to 35 years). 6 patients were females and 4 were males. The mean preoperative pupil diameter measured on aberrometer was 4.69 mm and mean postoperative pupil diameter measured on aberrometer was 4.53 mm.

The mean preoperative spherical equivalent was – 4.94 D (range –12.50 to –1.5 D). The mean spherical equivalent at 1 month postoperative period was –0.16 ± 0.68 D (range –1.0 to 1.5) . Mean preoperative sphere was –4.95 D (range-12.50 to –0.75 D) and the mean postoperative sphere was –0.13 ± 0.68 D (range-1 to 1.5) at 1 month. The mean preoperative cylinder was –1.34 D (range 0 to –3.50). The mean postoperative cylinder was –0.08 ± 0.24 D (range 0 to –0.75 D) at one month. Postoperatively, at the end of first month, 70% of the patients were within ± 0.5D and 90% were within ± 1D of emmetropia (Fig. 16.1). Preoperatively mean RMS (Root Mean square) values (Fig. 16.2) were: Z 200 Defocus –9.22, Z 221 Astigmatism 0.12, Z 220 Astigmatism 1.02, Z 311 Coma –0.041, Z 310 Coma –0.04, Z 331 Trefoil 0.23, Z 330 Trefoil 0.016, Z 400 Spherical aberration –0.054, Z 420 Secondary astigmatism 0.103, Z 421 Secondary astigmatism 0.029, Z 440 Quadrafoil –0.103, Z 441 Quadrafoil –0.021, Z 510 Secondary coma 0.025, Z 511 Secondary coma –0.015, Z 530 Secondary trefoil 0.0049, Z 531 Secondary trefoil -0.00219, Z 550 Pentafoil 0.023, Z 551 Pentafoil 0.046. Postoperative mean RMS values were: Z 200 Defocus –0.429, Z 221 Astigmatism 0.07, Z 220 Astigmatism –0.07, Z 311 Coma 0.149, Z 310 Coma –0.079, Z 331 Trefoil –0.102, Z 330 Trefoil –0.004, Z 400 Spherical aberration -0.179, Z 420 Secondary astigmatism 0.015, Z 421 Secondary astigmatism 0.031, Z 440 Quadrafoil 0.019, Z 441 Quadrafoil –0.069, Z 510 Secondary coma –0.008, Z 511 Secondary coma 0.008, Z 530 Secondary Trefoil -0.002, Z 531 Secondary Trefoil –0.014, Z 550 Pentafoil 0.006, Z 551 Pentafoil 0.026.

RMS pre- and post-laser showed a reduction in the higher order aberrations (Tables 16.1 and 16.2). 6.25 percent patients achieved 6/9, 31.25 percent patients achieved ≥ 6/6 (1.00) , 37.50 percent achieved a BCVA of 6/5 (1.25) and 25 percent achieved a BCVA of 6/4 (1.6) (Fig. 16.3). Figure 16.4 shows the pre-op Orbscan picture of a patient showing no abnormality. Figures 16.5 and 16.6 show the aberrometer maps of the right eye and left eye of a patient in which we can see the aberrations reduced post laser.

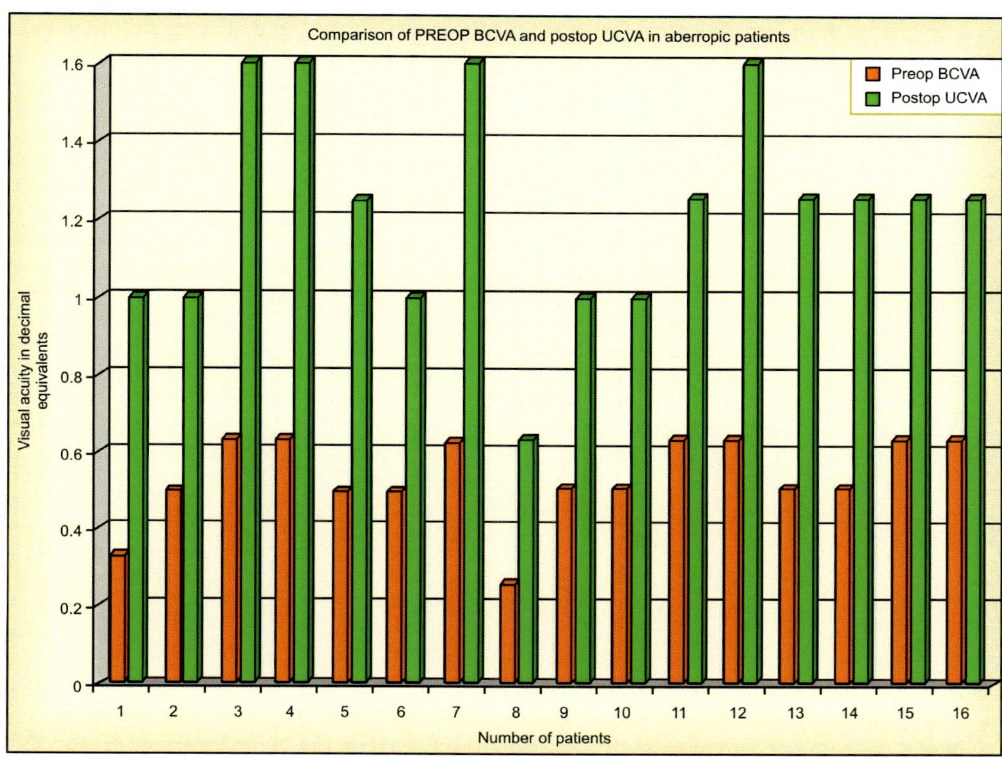

Fig. 16.1: Preoperative BCVA versus postoperative UCVA

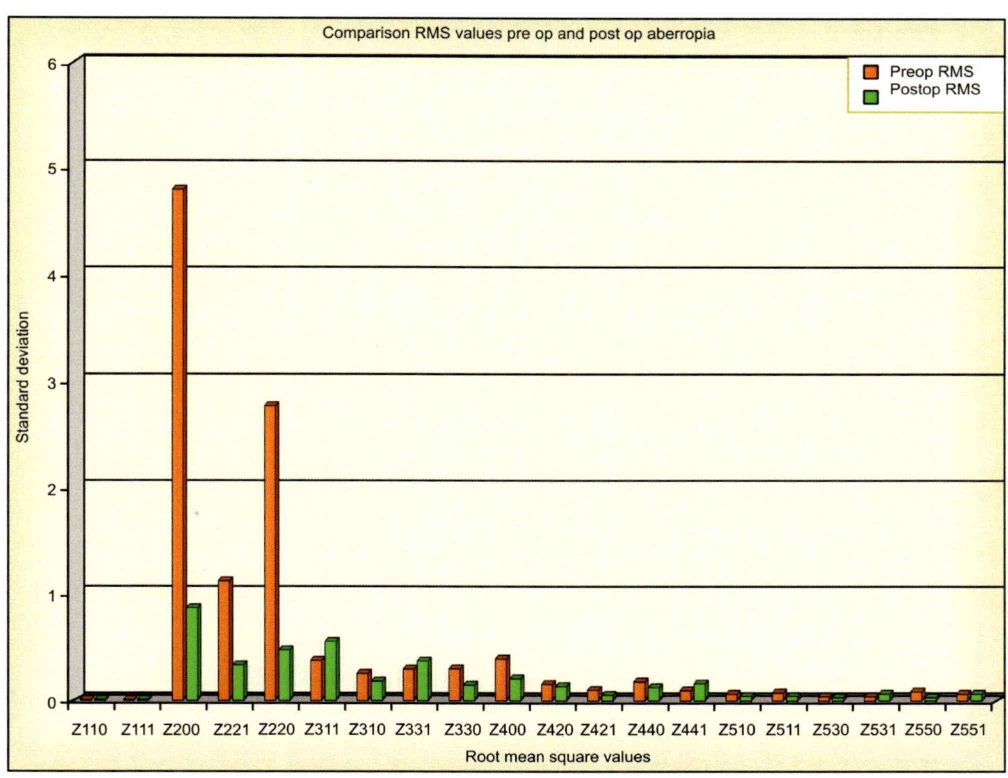

Fig. 16.2: RMS values preoperative and postoperative

Table 16.1: RMS preoperative of 16 eyes

Patient No	Z 110	Z 111	Z 200	Z 221	Z 220	Z 311	Z 310	Z 331	Z 330	Z 400	Z 420	Z 421	Z 440	Z 441	Z 510	Z 511	Z 530	Z 531	Z 550	Z 551	Z 6
1	0	0	–5.77	4.055.	-6.131	0.299	–0.113	0.725	–0.44	0.009	–0.03	0.102	–0.233	0.109	0.131	0.027	–0.048	–0.041	0.052	0.039	-9999
2	0	0	–4.323	–1.719	6.005	–0.273	0.022	–0.353	0.275	0.092	0.092	–0.145	0.199	–0.013	–0.006	0.011	0.034	–0.039	0.042	0.042	-9999
3	0	0	–11.8	–0.088	0.116	0.435	–0.658	–0.444	–0.567	–0.779	–0.089	0.043	–0.202	–0.053	–0.052	–0.057	–0.04	–0.001	0.13	0.111	-9999
4	0	0	–12.46	0.514	–0.155	0.29	–0.006	0.016	0.529	–0.91	0.124	0.124	–0.431	–0.222	0.074	–0.04	0.001	–0.063	–0.141	0.119	-9999
5	0	0	–6.535	–0.123	–0.886	0.156	–0.09	0.094	–0.128	–0.084	–0.072	0.035	–0.009	–0.044	0.001	–0.031	0.01	–0.005	0.001	–0.041	-9999
6	0	0	–7.867	0.185	1.704	–0.02	0.414	0.441	0.197	0.365	0.197	0.107	–0.155	–0.002	0.123	0.026	–0.001	0.049	0.048	0.032	-9999
7	0	0	–4.28	0.167	2.571	0.007	–0.089	0.356	0.125	0.585	0.101	–0.002	–0.17	–0.062	–0.077	0.198	0.001	–0.104	–0.022	0.029	-9999
8	0	0	–10.4	0.502	–0.587	–0.007	–0.331	0.165	–0.126	–0.054	–0.071	0.036	–0.118	–0.128	0.009	0.017	–0.007	–0.026	0.063	–0.052	-9999
9	0	0	–17.15	–0.414	–1.217	0.093	–0.106	0.343	–0.18	–0.254	0.009	0.002	0.001	–0.025	0.007	–0.022	–0.007	–0.042	0.037	0.04	-9999
10	0	0	–16.78	–0.162	–0.637	0.122	–0.159	0.279	0.2	–0.181	0.115	0.007	–0.002	0.042	–0.034	–0.028	0.021	–0.043	–0.006	–0.017	-9999
11	0	0	–4.513	2.916	4.661	–0.634	–0.205	0.477	0.44	0.094	0.377	0.058	–0.201	0.101	0.133	–0.147	0.009	0.011	–0.055	0.118	-9999
12	0	0	–5.736	–1.501	5.195	–1.126	0.32	0.665	–0.254	0.218	0.479	0.122	–0.253	–0.045	0.099	–0.025	0.012	–0.006	–0.05	0.11	-9999
13	0	0	–15.46	1.605	2.754	0.378	0.443	0.208	0.458	0.643	–0.083	0.09	0.407	–0.006	–0.021	0.09	0.033	0.032	0.239	0.149	-9999
14	0	0	–15.26	–0.557	2.865	–0.26	–0.059	0.107	0.122	0.168	0.025	–0.256	–0.003	0.257	0.007	0.051	0.136	–0.061	–0.114	0.124	-9999
15	0	0	–4.955	0.735	0.383	–0.401	0.003	0.62	–0.494	–0.676	0.391	0.163	–0.421	–0.264	0.039	–0.261	–0.079	0.241	0.103	–0.067	-9999
16	0	0	–4.367	–0.195	–0.238	0.28	–0.04	0.021	0.11	–0.112	0.084	–0.022	–0.061	0.013	–0.018	–0.063	0.004	0.063	0.044	0	-9999

Table 16.2: RMS postoperative of 16 eyes

Patient No	Z 110	Z 111	Z 200	Z 221	Z 220	Z 311	Z 310	Z 331	Z 330	Z 400	Z 420	Z 421	Z 440	Z 441	Z 510	Z 511	Z 530	Z 531	Z 550	Z 551	Z 6
1	0	0	–0.022	0.74	–1.294	0.117	–0.067	0.141	0.052	–0.063	–0.076	0.1	0.054	–0.037	–0.028	0.001	0.008	0.007	0.013	0.006	-9999
2	0	0	–0.508	0.12	0.194	–0.085	0.039	–0.12	–0.018	-9999	-9999	-9999	-9999	-9999	-9999	-9999	-9999	-9999	-9999	-9999	-9999
3	0	0	–1.398	–0.606	0.697	–0.558	–0.351	0.841	0.345	–0.39	0.392	0.038	–0.303	–0.038	–0.001	0.103	–0.066	–0.105	–0.021	0.137	-9999
4	0	0	–2.05	–0.499	–0.375	–0.027	–0.269	–0.534	–0.289	–0.58	0.114	0.058	0.236	–0.161	0.034	–0.083	0.004	0.039	0.01	–0.077	-9999
5	0	0	0.229	0.1	–0.123	-9999	-9999	-9999	-9999	-9999	-9999	-9999	-9999	-9999	-9999	-9999	-9999	-9999	-9999	-9999	-9999
6	0	0	–0.036	–0.17	0.425	–0.002	0.069	–0.045	–0.042	–0.342	–0.032	0.094	0.075	–0.05	0.068	0.03	0.064	–0.014	0.012	0.002	-9999
7	0	0	0.687	0.128	–0.028	–0.117	–0.043	0.062	0.088	–0.178	0.179	0.024	–0.045	0.055	0.013	0.016	–0.034	–0.013	–0.013	0.059	-9999
8	0	0	–2.164	0.279	–0.696	–0.25	–0.398	–0.147	–0.128	–0.581	–0.238	0.02	0.032	–0.088	–0.129	0.028	–0.029	0.007	0.089	0.059	-9999
9	0	0	–0.298	0.002	–0.311	0.158	–0.206	0.129	–0.116	–0.105	–0.045	–0.043	–0.1	–0.1	-9999	-9999	-9999	-9999	-9999	-9999	-9999
10	0	0	0.109	0.241	–0.503	0.233	–0.119	–0.16	–0.204	-9999	-9999	-9999	-9999	-9999	-9999	-9999	-9999	-9999	-9999	-9999	-9999
11	0	0	0.034	–0.092	0.076	0.013	–0.03	–0.067	0.003	-9999	-9999	-9999	-9999	-9999	-9999	-9999	-9999	-9999	-9999	-9999	-9999
12	0	0	0.187	0.061	0.004	–0.097	0.015	0.067	0.035	-9999	-9999	-9999	-9999	-9999	-9999	-9999	-9999	-9999	-9999	-9999	-9999
13	0	0	–0.701	0.291	0.598	2.161	0.349	–1.062	–0.201	–0.428	–0.013	0.204	0.258	–0.636	–0.082	0.113	0.069	–0.239	0.062	-9999	-9999
14	0	0	–0.638	0.094	0.391	0.517	–0.328	–0.336	0.188	–0.118	–0.077	0.003	0.157	0.034	–0.006	–0.025	0.004	0.018	–0.066	-9999	-9999
15	0	0	–0.148	0.493	0.017	0.261	0.017	–0.354	0.302	–0.111	0.053	0.07	–0.019	–0.084	–0.007	–0.051	–0.052	0.063	0.011	-9999	-9999
16	0	0	–0.161	–0.038	–0.331	0.072	0.049	–0.05	–0.086	0.025	–0.008	–0.059	–0.028	-9999	-9999	-9999	-9999	-9999	-9999	-9999	-9999

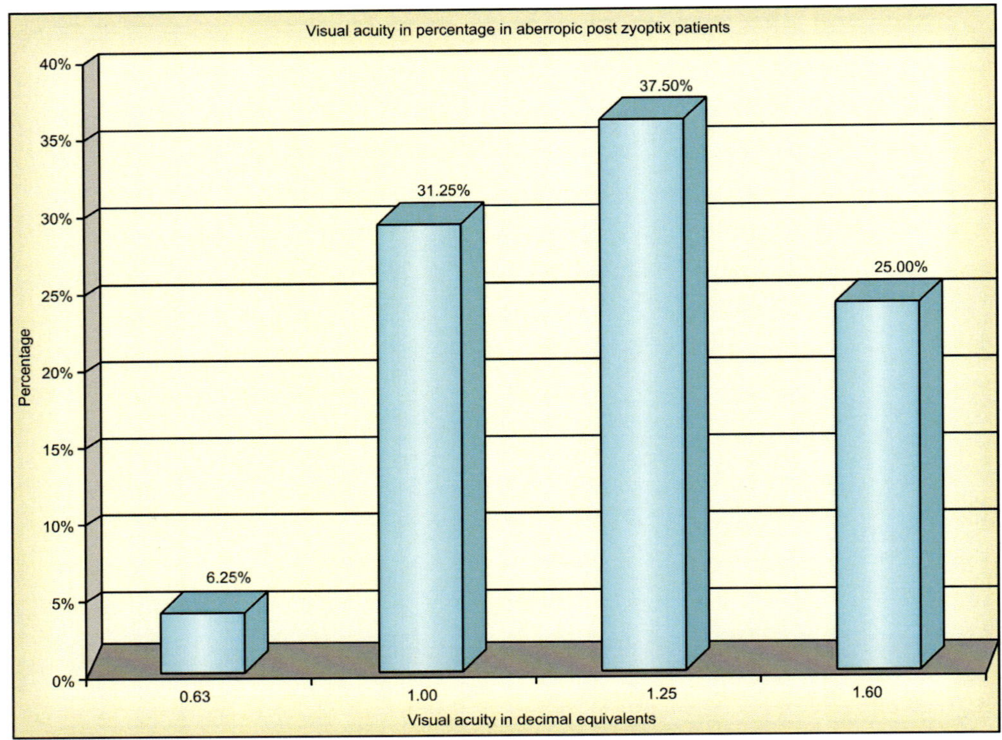

Fig. 16.3: Percentage values of visual acuity

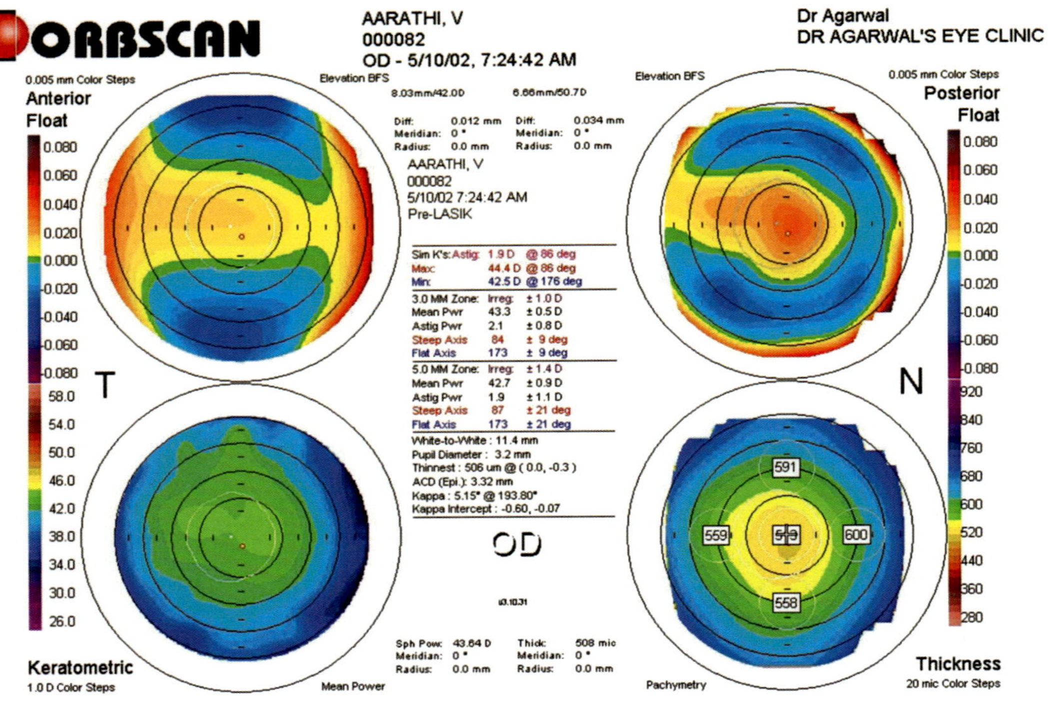

Fig. 16.4: Preoperative orbscan

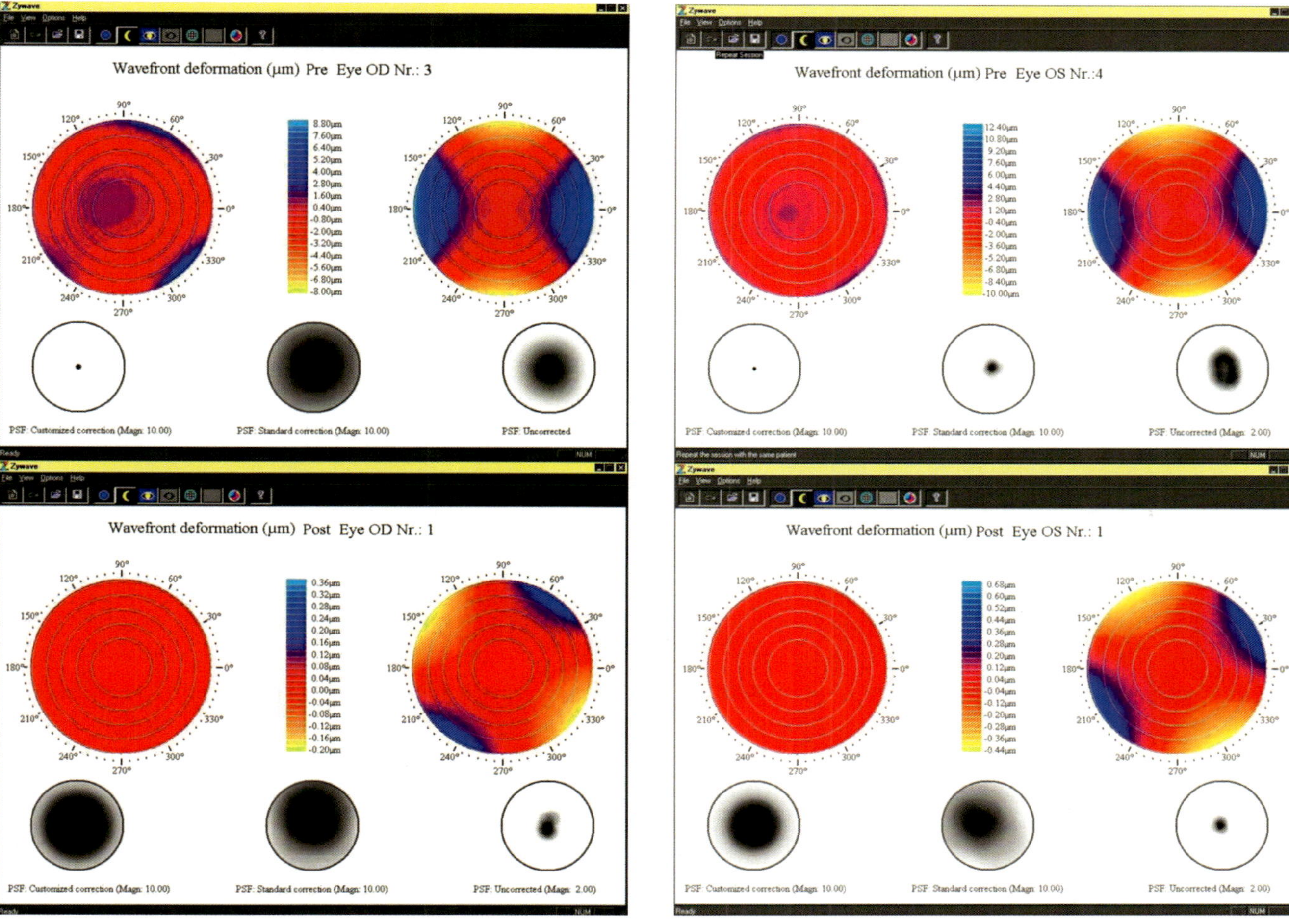

Figs 16.5 and 16.6: Pre and postoperative aberrometry of the right and left eye of the same patient showing removal of higher order aberrations

DISCUSSION

Zyoptix is the new generation of excimer laser used for the treatment of refractive disorders. Until recently, refractive disorders were treated with standard techniques, which took into consideration only the subjective refraction. Zyoptix technique on the other hand, takes into account the patient's subjective refraction, ocular optical aberrations and corneal topography, with the latter not only for the diagnosis, but also for the therapeutic treatment, in order to design a personalized treatment based on the total structure of the eye. The wavefront technology in Zyoptix uses the Hartmann Shack aberrometer based on the Hartmann-Shack principle[1] demonstrated by Liang et al[2] to measure the eye's wave aberration. This wavefront sensor has been improved by increasing the density of samples taken of the wave-front slope in the pupil.[3] All Hartmann-Shack devices are outgoing testing devices in that they evaluate the light being bounced back out through the optical system. A narrow laser beam is focused onto the retina to generate a point source. The out coming light rays which experience all the aberrations of the eye pass through an array of lenses which detects their deviation. The wavefront deformation is calculated by analyzing the direction of the light rays using this lenslet array. Parallel light beams indicate a good wavefront and non-parallel light beams indicate a wavefront with aberrations, which does not give equidistant focal points. This image is then captured onto a CCD camera and the wavefront is reconstructed. The data are explained mathematically in three-dimensions with polynomial functions. Most investigators have chosen the Zernike method for this analysis although Taylor series can also be used for the same purpose.[4] Data from the wavefront map are presented as a sum of Zernike polynomials each describing a certain deformation. At any point in the pupil, the wavefront aberration is the optical path difference between the actual image wavefront and the ideal spherical wavefront centered at the image point.[5]

Any refractive error which cannot be corrected by spherocylindrical lens combinations is referred to by physicists as higher order aberrations, i.e. comma, spherical aberration, chromatic aberration. The Zernike polynomials, which describe ray points, are used to obtain a best fit toric to correct for the refractive error of the eye. The points are described in the x and y coordinates and the third dimension, height, is described in the z-axis. The local refractive correction of each area of the entrance pupil can be determined by calculating from the wavefront polynomial the corresponding local radii of curvature and hence the required spherocylindrical correction[6]. Thus each small region of the entrance pupil has its own three parameters that characterize the local refractive correction: sphere, cylinder and axis.[6] The global aberrations of the entire optical system including the cornea, lens, vitreous and the retina are thus measured. The great advantage of wavefront analysis is that it can describe these other aberrations.

The first order polynomial describes the spherical error or power of the eye. The second order polynomial describes the regular astigmatic component and its orientation or axis. Third order aberrations are considered to be coma and fourth order aberrations are considered to be spherical aberration. Zernike polynomial descriptions for wavefront analysis typically go up to the tenth order of expression. The first and second orders describe the morphology of a normal straight curve. More local maximum and minimum points require higher orders of the polynomial series to describe the surface. Normal eyes exhibit spherical[7,8] and coma[9,10] aberrations in addition to exhibiting defocus and astigmatism.

Ideally, the difference in the magnitude of the local refractive correction of each area of the entrance pupil should not exceed 0.25 D. Lower spherocylindrical corrections are generally associated with lower wavefront aberrations.[6] These observations regarding variation in local ocular refraction along different meridians are also confirmed by Ivanoff[11] and Jenkins.[12] Van den Brink[13] also commented on the change in refraction across the pupil. Clinically significant changes of at least 0.25 D in one or both components of the spherocylindrical correction might normally be expected for decentrations of about 1 mm. Rayleigh's quarter wavelength rule states that if the wavefront aberration exceeds a quarter of a wavelength, the quality of the retinal image will be impaired significantly.[14] Thus the aberration in eyes starts to become significant when the pupil diameter exceeds 1-2 mm.[6] Thus it is not possible to correct the entire wavefront aberration with a single spherocylindrical lens. As conventional refractive procedures such as Lasik also reduce only the second order aberrations, the visual acuity will still be limited by aberrations of third and higher order aberrations. These patients are likely to undergo tremendous improvement in their BCVA after correction of their aberrations by Zyoptix.

In the Zyoptix system, the aberrometer and the Orbscan, which checks the corneal topography, are linked and a zylink created. An appropriate software file is created which is then used to generate the laser treatment file. The truncated gaussian beam shape used in Zyoptix combines the advantages of the common beam shapes, i.e. flat top beam and the gaussian beam, creating a maximized smoothness and minimized thermal effect. Thus Zyoptix gives a smoother corneal surface, reducing glare and increasing visual acuity. The larger optical zones reduce haloes. Zyoptix also causes a reduction of the ablation depth by 15-20 percent and a reduced enhancement rate

In a patient with higher order aberrations, lasik does not remove the higher order aberrations and the point-spread function is a large blur. Zyoptix on the other hand, performs customized ablation and removes the higher order aberrations thus minimizing the wavefront deformation. The point-spread function is therefore a small spot of light.

In our study, the mean preoperative spherical equivalent improved from –4.78 D to –0.16 D ± 0.68 and the mean preoperative cylinder improved from –1.34 D to –0.08 D ± 0.24. The aberrations were reduced drastically in all the eyes and the BCVA improved in all cases by ≥ 2 lines. Reduction of the aberrations of the eye can thus result in an improved BCVA postoperatively.

Improving the optics of the eye by removing aberrations increases the contrast and spatial detail of the retinal image. Reduction of higher order aberrations may not improve high contrast acuity much more in eyes where spherocylindrical lenses alone improve the BCVA to 6/3 (2.00) or better. In contrast, in otherwise normal eyes where the BCVA is limited to 6/9 (0.50) or 6/6 (1.00) due to optical aberrations, reduction of higher order aberrations should improve visual acuity.

Realization of the best possible unaided visual acuity may be limited at the cortical, retinal and the spectacle, corneal, or implant level. All maculae may not be able to support 6/3 (2.00) vision. Insufficient cone density or sub-optimal orientation of cone receptors or a sub-optimal Stiles-Crawford profile of the macula may make 6/3 (2.00) vision impossible. Clinical or sub clinical amblyopia may make achievement of super vision impossible. But, in spite of this, there may be a certain patient population who have the potential for an improved BCVA on removal of their wavefront aberrations. The corneal topography does not account for the decreased preoperative visual acuity in these patients, neither do they have any other identifiable cause for the decrease in acuity except for an abnormal wavefront. It is important that this subgroup of patients are identified and their optical aberrations neutralized so that they are not deprived of the opportunity to gain in their BCVA.

Wavefront sensing technology, at present, does not in most cases define the exact locale of the pathology causing the aberration. Hence, clinical examination and other refractive tools, such as corneal topographic mapping, along with sound clinical judgment is required for proper understanding of the eye and its individual refractive status. Also, wavefront aberrations may not remain static. Numerous authors,[15-18], have shown that ocular optical aberrations probably remain constant between 20 and 40 years of age but increase after that. Aberrations also change during accommodation[19,20] and may be affected by mydriatics.[21] Thus, the patient should be informed about these possibilities while taking the consent for the procedure. Long term studies are required to determine the stability of the postoperative refraction, residual aberrations and changes in BCVA if any.

The question of magnification factor improving visual acuity does not arise as these patients preoperatively did not improve with contact lenses. Further the refractive error in some of these patients was not very large.

CONCLUSION

In conclusion, removal of the wavefront aberration may extend the benefit of an improved BCVA to patients with an abnormal wavefront. The subgroup of patients with higher order aberrations, normal corneal topography and no other known cause for decreased vision may thus benefit immensely with wavefront guided refractive surgery. Customized refractive surgery tailor-made for these individual patients, aimed at neutralizing the wavefront aberrations of the eye is safer, more predictable, provides better visual acuities and reduces the incidence of unsatisfactory outcomes. Further studies are required to assess the long-term outcomes.

Till now, when we discuss refractive errors we discuss about spherical and a cylindrical correction. But in todays world we have to think of a third parameter which is the aberrations present in the eye which can be anywhere in the optical media. These can be corrected in the corneal level by the laser treatment.

REFERENCES

1. Platt B, Shack RV. Lenticular Hartmann screen. Opt Sci Center News (University of Arizona) 1971;5:15-6.
2. Liang J, Grimm B, Goelz S, Bille J. Objective measurement of the wave aberrations of the human eye with the use of a Hartmann-Shack wavefront sensor. J Opt Soc Am 1994;11:1949-57.
3. Liang J, Williams DR, et al. Aberrations and retinal image quality of the normal human eye. J Opt Soc Am A 1997; 14(11):2873-83.
4. Oshika T, Klyce SD, Applegate RA, et al. Comparison of corneal wavefront aberrations after photorefractive keratectomy and laser in situ keratomileusis. Am J Ophthalmol 1999;127:1-7.
5. Fincham WHA, Freeman MH. Optics (9th ed). London: Butterworths, 1980.
6. WN Charman, G Walsh. Variations in the local refractive correction of the eye across its entrance pupil. Optometry and Vision Science 1989;66(1):34-40.
7. Rosenblum WM, Christensen JL. Objective and subjective spherical aberration measurement of the human eye. In Wolf E (Ed): Progress in Optics, (North-Holland, Amsterdam, 1976;13:69-91.
8. Campbell MC, Harrison EM, Simonet P. Psychophysical measurement of the blur on the retina due to optical aberrations of the eye. Vision Res 1990;30:1587-1602.
9. Howland HC, Howland B. A subjective method for the measurement of monochromatic aberrations of the eye. J Opt Soc Am 1977;67:1508-18.
10. Walsh G, Charman WN, Howland HC. Objective technique for the determination of monochromatic aberrations of the human eye. J Opt Soc Am A1 1984;987-92.
11. Ivanoff A. About the spherical aberration of the eye. J Opt Soc Am 1956;46:901-3.
12. Jenkins TCA. Aberrations of the eye and their effects on vision. Part 1. Br J Physiol Opt 1963;20:59-91.
13. Van den Brink G. Measurements of the geometric aberrations of the eye. Vision Res 1962;2:233-44.
14. Born M, Wolf E. Principles of Optics (2nd ed). New York: Macmillan, 1964:203-32.
15. Kaemmerer M, Mrochen M, Mierdel p, et al. Optical aberrations of the human eye. Nature Medicine (in press).
16. Oshika T, Klyce SD, Applegate RA, et al. Changes in corneal wavefront aberration with aging. Invest Ophthalmol Vis Sci 1999;40:1351-5.
17. Calver RI, Cox MJ, Elliot DB. Effect of aging on the monochromatic aberrations of the human eye. J Opt Soc Am A 1999;16:2069-78.
18. Guirao A, Gonzalez C, Redondo M, et al. Average optical performance of the human eye as a function of age in a normal population. Invest Ophthalmol Vis Sci 1999;40: 203-13.
19. Krueger R, Kaemerrer M, Mrochen M, et al. Understanding refraction and accommodation through "ingoing optics" aberrometry: a case report. Ophthalmology (in press).
20. He JC, Burns SA, Marcos S. Monochromatic aberrations in the accommodated human eye. Vis Res 2000;40:41-8.
21. Fankhauser F, Kaemerrer M, Mrochen M, et al. The effect of accommodation, mydriasis, and cycloplegia on aberrometry. ARVO abstract 2248. Invest Ophthalmol Vis Sci 2000;41:S461.

17 Differences between Various Aberrometer Systems

Ronald R Krueger

INTRODUCTION

Custom ablation is a very broad term. It can refer to treatment of the cornea that does not depend on recent technological advances: surgeon-oriented customization occurs, for instance, if the surgeon decides to treat a small zone for a central island that has developed following laser vision correction.

The implied meaning of custom ablation today does involve recent advances. Custom ablation can be guided by topography, and more recently by wavefront mapping. Wavefront guided customization will be the most successful method of corneal ablation in the future. Most companies in the ophthalmic vision correction industry are focusing their resources on this technology because it promises to yield all the information needed for doing customized laser treatment.

MAPPING A PROFILE OF THE WHOLE EYE

The wavefront sensing device provides a new and objective way of mapping the profile of refraction and of higher order defects in the eye such as coma and spherical aberrations. Whereas corneal topography allows us to map a profile of the corneal surface, wavefront mapping makes it possible to map a profile of the whole eye.

Wavefront analysis is a more sophisticated method of defining aberrations that the surgeon is trying to correct through refractive surgery. Until the present time the basis for diagnosis has essentially been corneal topography.

DIFFERENT METHODS AVAILABLE

Wavefront technology originated from two main sources more than 100 years ago. A physicist named Hartmann developed principles of subjectively measuring optical aberrations in a reproducible way. This system was later developed into what is called the Hartmann-Shack wavefront analyzing device, which is used by most manufacturers today (Fig. 17.1). Tscherning, an ophthalmologist working in the late 1800's, devised another method of doing wavefront mapping. Tscherning's method was further developed by Howland and Howland in the 1970's and more recently, Theo Seiler modified this method for clinical use, as adopted by two German manufacturers. The Tscherning's principle is also utilized in a retinal tracing method applied with the Tracey technology.

A third method is used by the group at Emory University in Atlanta, Georgia. Their method involves a spatially resolved refractometer which evaluates the wavefront profile by soliciting the patient's subjective response to a series of light rays entering the eye. Still another method of wavefront analysis, which Nidek is using, operates more by retinoscopic principles.

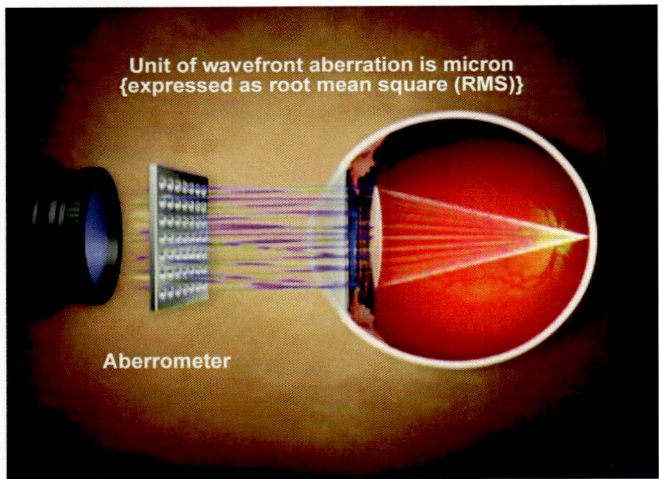

Fig. 17.1: Hartmann Shack aberrometer
(*Courtesy* Dr Agarwal's Eye Hospital, India)

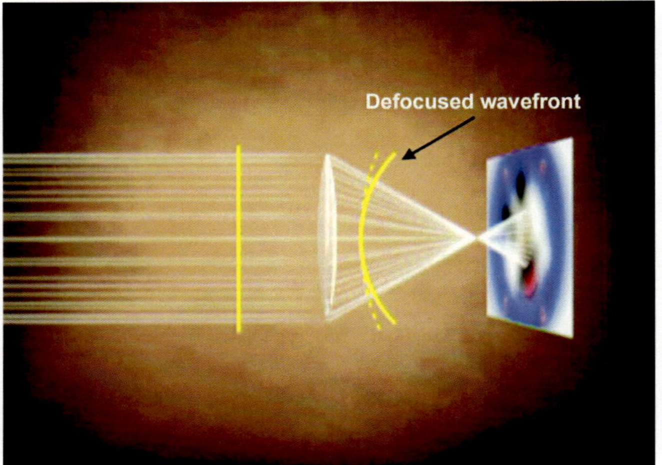

Fig. 17.2: Defocussed wavefront
(*Courtesy* Dr Agarwal's Eye Hospital, India)

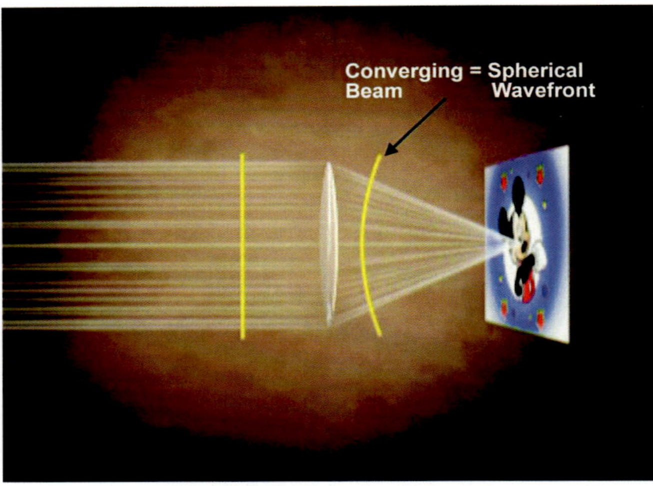

Fig. 17.3: Spherical wavefront
(*Courtesy* Dr Agarwal's Eye Hospital, India)

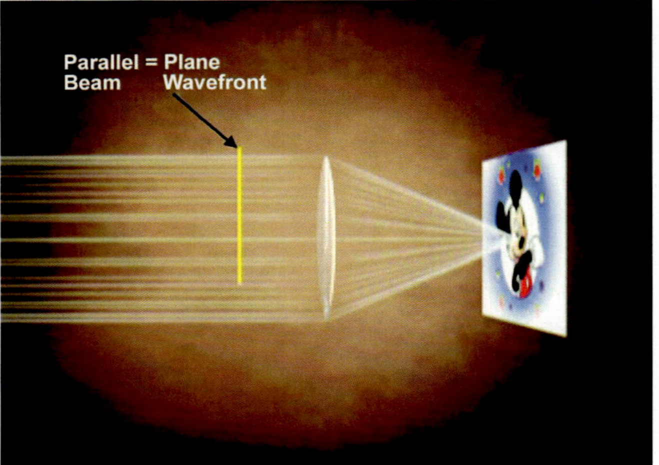

Fig. 17.4: Plane wavefront
(*Courtesy* Dr Agarwal's Eye Hospital, India)

THE MECHANISMS OF WAVEFRONT DEVICES

Light passing in and out of the eye has to go through multiple structures like the vitreous, lens and the back and front surfaces of the cornea. Aberrations inside the eye can affect the passage of the light (Figs 17.2 to 17.5). Ultimately, seeing where the light is emitted from the eye in relation to the cornea allows the ophthalmologist to predict the change in corneal shape needed to give the patient perfect focus.

Wavefront devices can be categorized into four groups. With "outgoing" wavefront analysis, the wavefront is defined by the foveally reflected laser

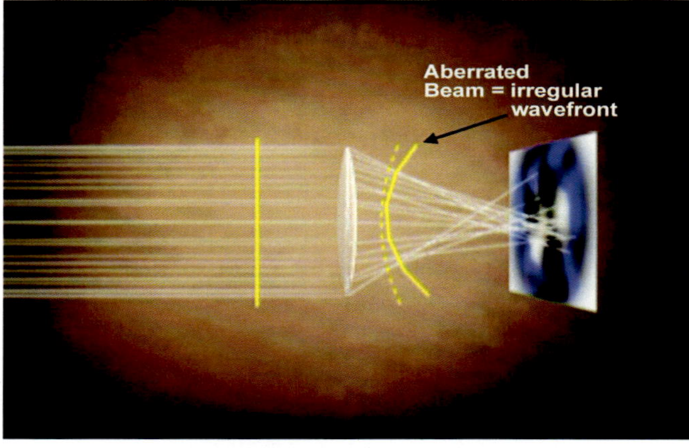

Fig. 17.5: Irregular wavefront
(*Courtesy* Dr Agarwal's Eye Hospital, India)

light going out of the eye. The Hartmann-Shack devices represented by Alcon, Visx, Bausch and Lomb, Meditec and Topcon are all based on this form of wavefront analysis. The Tscherning device, named after a prominent ophthalmologist from the late 1800's, is based on "retinal imaging" wavefront analysis. The Tscherning device involves a grid of laser energy shone into the eye. The way the grid deviates as it enters the eye and is imagined on the retina defines the wavefront pattern. This device uses the retina to obtain the wavefront pattern. It has been popularized through the efforts of Dr Theo Seiler, who introduced the technology to two German companies, Wavelight, and Schwind. The Tracey retinal ray tracing method sequentially delivers one ray at a time which is imaged on the retina in a rapid (<10 mSec) fashion. The third method is an ingoing adjustable way of determining the wavefront pattern. It measures the light rays coming in, being manually adjusted by the patient to a central retinal focus. The Spatially Resolved Refractometer use this mechanism. The final method uses a double pass (in and out) method of analyzing the wavefront by slit Skioloscopy, using retinoscopic principles. The Nidek OPD scan uses this mechanism.

BENEFITS OF WAVEFRONT ANALYSIS

Probably the best analogy to the development of wavefront technology relates to the early days of radial keratotomy in refractive surgery. At that point, before the age of corneal topography, all the surgeon needed to know was the keratometry value and certain other numbers about the shape of the cornea. The advent of corneal topography allowed us to map a whole profile of the shape of the cornea, giving us much more information for diagnosis.

Approaching patients with spherocylindrical refraction, we base the laser treatment on the refractive error with sphere, cylinder and axis. But those are only three numbers, just as keratometry is defined with only a few numbers. Our goal is to get the whole profile of refraction, with an equivalent value at every point within the pupillary aperture. Once this information is obtained, the ophthalmologist can use the laser to create the perfect optical surface.

LINKING DIAGNOSTIC INFORMATION FROM WAVEFRONT MAPPING TO LASER TREATMENT

It is already possible to link diagnostic information obtained from wavefront analysis to the excimer laser treatment. Several companies are actively doing this form of customized treatment in studies performed in non-US countries. Alcon is using the technology as part of clinical trials in cooperation with the US Food and Drug Administration (FDA). Autonomous Technologies Corp., which had a very effective scanning spot laser, was purchased by Summit Technologies, which owns many patents in the US. Now Summit has been acquired by Alcon. Alcon is now refining their LADARVision excimer laser to be used with the custom cornea wavefront device. The specific aberrations can be used to obtain diagnostic information. Then, with the laser, that diagnostic information can be directly applied to the treatment. This custom cornea platform of Alcon was recently approved in the US for the correction of myopia.

All the companies that have excimer lasers are developing their own unique wavefront devices. Alcon has the LADARWave Wavefront Device. Visx has the WaveScan device, Bausch and Lomb has the Zywave device and Zeiss-Meditec has the Wavefront Sciences Device as part of their WASCA program. Each of these modified Hartmann-Shack devices uses "outgoing optics" to define the wavefront pattern. WaveLight and Schwind have their own wavefront devices based on Tscherning's design of "retinal imaging" optics. Nidek has the OPD Scan, which is a special device based on slit Skioloscopy, using a modification of retinoscopic principles.

Because there is variation among all these types, it would not be wise to obtain a device from Alcon and a laser from Nidek, because the two may not correspond to allow for custom ablation. At this point in the development of the technology no one really knows which is the best device, and comparative studies are yet to be done. The best approach is to examine the technology, consider the manufacturers behind the various devices, and try to predict which are likely to be successful.

WAVEFRONT ANALYSIS IN CONJUNCTION WITH CORNEAL TOPOGRAPHY

Ophthalmologists have learned to depend on corneal topography devices to help screen for disease before surgery and to monitor patients after surgery. More and more we will use the wavefront device for diagnostic testing before and after surgery. Wavefront mapping in conjunction with corneal topography will provide the most complete picture. Although it is uncertain whether corneal topography will continue to be used a decade from now as technology continues to advance, there is definitely a place for it now. Meanwhile, the wavefront device provides even more detailed information about what the patient is likely to see because it measures the light passage into the eye focusing on the retina. Whereas the shape of the cornea is important, it is more important to ensure that the focus on the retina is perfectly sharp.

PERSONALIZED LASIK NOMOGRAMS

At present there is considerable interest in developing a commercial database system for nomograms. A number of researchers and companies are working on programs tailor-made for collecting data and determining individual nomograms. There may be several ways to achieve this goal. You can obtain your own Excel file. Using this file you can compare the attempted correction to what is achieved, and then assess the difference. Through regression analysis according to different variables, a nomogram can be derived.

In the future wavefront mapping may be used to refine some of these measures. However, at present with custom cornea wavefront guided treatment, a nomogram is not necessary, but rather simply an offset feature which can be adjusted according to a particular surgeon, climate and environment.

18 Corneal Wavefront-guided Excimer Laser Surgery

Jorge L Alio, David P Pinero, Mohamad Rosman

INTRODUCTION

Higher-order corneal aberrations (HOAs) can result in significant visual symptoms and visual impairment, especially in some patients who have undergone corneal refractive surgery. Advancements in excimer laser refractive surgery have led to the introduction of wavefront-guided excimer laser refractive surgery. Wavefront-guided excimer laser refractive surgery, based on correcting global (or total) aberrations of the eye, has been shown to reduce the induction of higher-order aberrations during PRK and LASIK of normal eyes and has also been shown to reduce the amount of higher-order aberrations in highly aberrated eyes. However, as 80 percent of the refractive power of the eye is attributed to the first corneal surface, higher-order aberrations from the corneal surface will have a greater impact on visual quality. Hence, the correction of corneal higher-order aberrations, as opposed to the correction of total higher-order aberrations, may have a greater impact to visual quality in the long-term. This chapter will illustrate the rationale and clinical results of corneal wavefront-guided excimer laser surgery for the correction of eye aberrations.

IMPACT OF HIGHER-ORDER ABERRATIONS

Higher-order aberrations in significant amount may cause symptomatic visual impairment, especially among patients who have undergone corneal refractive surgery. Symptoms of glare, haloes and starburst are associated with spherical, coma and other types of aberrations.[1,2] Coma-like aberration of the eye has been shown to significantly affect contrast sensitivity function,[3] cause haloes[2] and may also cause monocular diplopia.[1,4] While the effect of these higher-order aberrations may not be significant when the pupil is small (3 mm), they play a substantial role in degrading visual performance when the pupil is large, i.e. in scotopic light conditions.[5,6] Hence, resulting in significant night vision symptoms.

The normal cornea has a positive 4th order spherical aberration that changes with age, with mirror symmetry between the right and left eyes.[7,8] The amount of higher-order aberrations measured in normal eyes vary among subjects and increases with age.[7-9] Wang et al reported that there is a wide range of individual variability among normal individuals in aberrations with ranges of individual Zernike terms from –0.579 to +0.572 µm. The mean coefficient of the 4th order spherical aberration (SA) (Z_4^0) was 0.280 +/– 0.086 µm and was positive in all corneas. The mean root-mean-square (RMS) values were 0.479 +/– 0.124 µm for HOA, 0.281 +/– 0.086 µm for SA (Z_4^0) and (Z_6^0), and 0.248 +/– 0.135 µm for coma (Z_3^{-1}), (Z_3^1), (Z_5^{-1}), and (Z_5^1).[7] Changes on the cornea due to surgery and disease can result in changes in higher-order aberrations which may be visually significant. Laser refractive surgery, in particular, is well-known to induce higher-order aberrations.[6]

Myopic laser refractive surgery induces a positive spherical aberration while hyperopic corrections induce a negative spherical aberration.[10-12] These induced aberrations are increased when higher corrections are attempted. PRK and LASIK have also been noted to increase ocular higher-order aberrations differently. The difference between the two types of surgery may be correlated with the change of the corneal shape, the conversion of biodynamics, the healing of the corneal cut, and re-structured corneal epithelium and/or the stroma.[13] Studies have also shown that significant higher-order aberrations are induced in eyes which have undergone LASIK with a microkeratome-created flap compared to eyes which have undergone LASIK with an intralase-created flap.[14-16] The induction of higher-order aberrations is further exaggerated in eyes with complications during laser refractive surgery.[17] On average, eyes with central islands had the most vertical coma while eyes with central islands and decentered ablations had elevated amounts of spherical aberration compared with successful postoperative LASIK eyes.[18]

Of all the aberrometric components, the primary spherical aberration and coma aberration are the most symptomatic and the most frequent after refractive surgery. As mentioned, the most frequent aberration after an uncomplicated refractive surgery is spherical aberration. The primary spherical aberration is a higher order aberration corresponding to the fourth order of the Zernike decomposition. Basically this error is due to the difference of refractive power between the central and the peripheral area of the optical ocular system (between the ablated and the non-ablated area). As a result, all the light rays passing through the system do not focus at the same point. Several light rays will be focused in front of the retinal plane, whereas others will be focused behind it. This phenomenon generates a concentric circle of blurred light around the focused point or halo. The higher the aperture of the system (the pupil diameter), the halo generated is more significant, because the aberrated peripheral area has a greater impact on the retinal image. Thus, this optical situation induces significant disturbances and discomfort in the patient under scotopic conditions (Figs 18.1 and 18.2).

To a certain extent, newer aspheric ablation profiles may reduce the induction of spherical aberrations in uncomplicated laser refractive surgery,[19] while more advanced eye-tracking systems have reduced the risk of decentered ablations and thereby reduced the risk of coma aberrations. However, the risk of visually significant higher-order aberration after laser refractive surgery and other causes, like corneal surgery or diseases, still persists. The challenge to all refractive surgeons is how to treat such patients and to reduce the amount of higher-order aberrations which are present.

WAVEFRONT-GUIDED REFRACTIVE SURGERY

The concept of wavefront-guided ablations in excimer laser refractive surgery was introduced in 2000.[20,21] The aim of wavefront-guided excimer laser refractive surgery was to correct pre-existing individual optical aberrations while correcting the refractive error during excimer laser refractive surgery. Thus, it has the potential advantage of reducing post-LASIK night-vision problems and may even result in improved post-LASIK vision.

The basic concept of wavefront-guided LASIK involves the measurement of the wavefront aberrations with a wavefront analyser such as the Hartmann-Shack aberrometer and to transfer the aberrations into an appropriate ablation pattern to be performed by a scanning-spot excimer laser. However, the results of wavefront-guided LASIK are influenced by other variables in the LASIK procedure, which includes accurate centration of the laser spot, creation and replacement of the corneal flap and wound healing. Cyclotorsion in the supine position may also influence the spot position as related to the aberrometer data.

Studies have shown wavefront-guided LASIK to be as safe and efficacious as conventional LASIK.[22-25] Wavefront-guided LASIK has also been shown to reduce the amount of induced higher-order aberrations compared to conventional LASIK.[26] But other studies have shown that wavefront-guided LASIK only reduced higher-order aberrations in less than 50 percent of eyes.[27] Furthermore, the clinical benefits of performing wavefront-guided LASIK compared to conventional LASIK in a normal eye may not be apparent.[28]

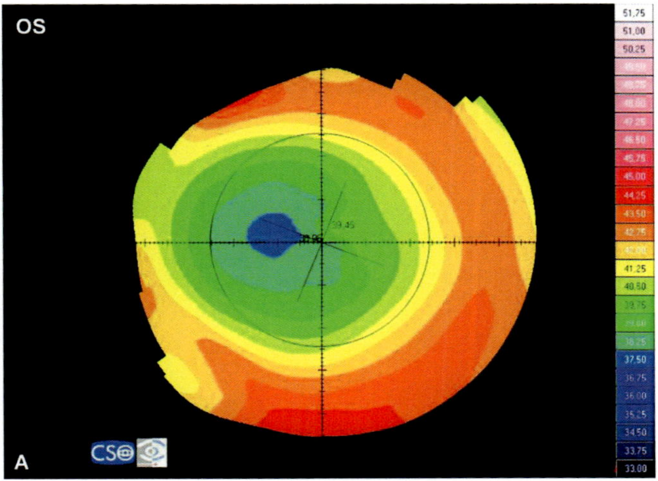

Perhaps the value of wavefront-guided excimer laser treatment lies in correcting aberrated eyes with significant visual symptoms and the retreatment of LASIK for residual refractive errors. Wavefront-guided LASIK appears to be superior to conventional LASIK when used to correct residual refractive errors after excimer laser refractive surgery as it induces less high-order aberrations and is less likely to cause a reduction in contrast sensitivity.[29,30]

Patients who are more likely to benefit from wavefront-guided excimer laser treatment include those with significant aberrations after uneventful conventional refractive surgery, patients with complications during refractive surgeries and patients with aberrated corneas due to corneal surgery or diseases. In general, the treatment of aberrated cornea with wavefront-guided LASIK results in significant reduction in higher-order aberrations. Patients also noticed a reduction in their pre-existing visual symptoms and reported improvement in quality of

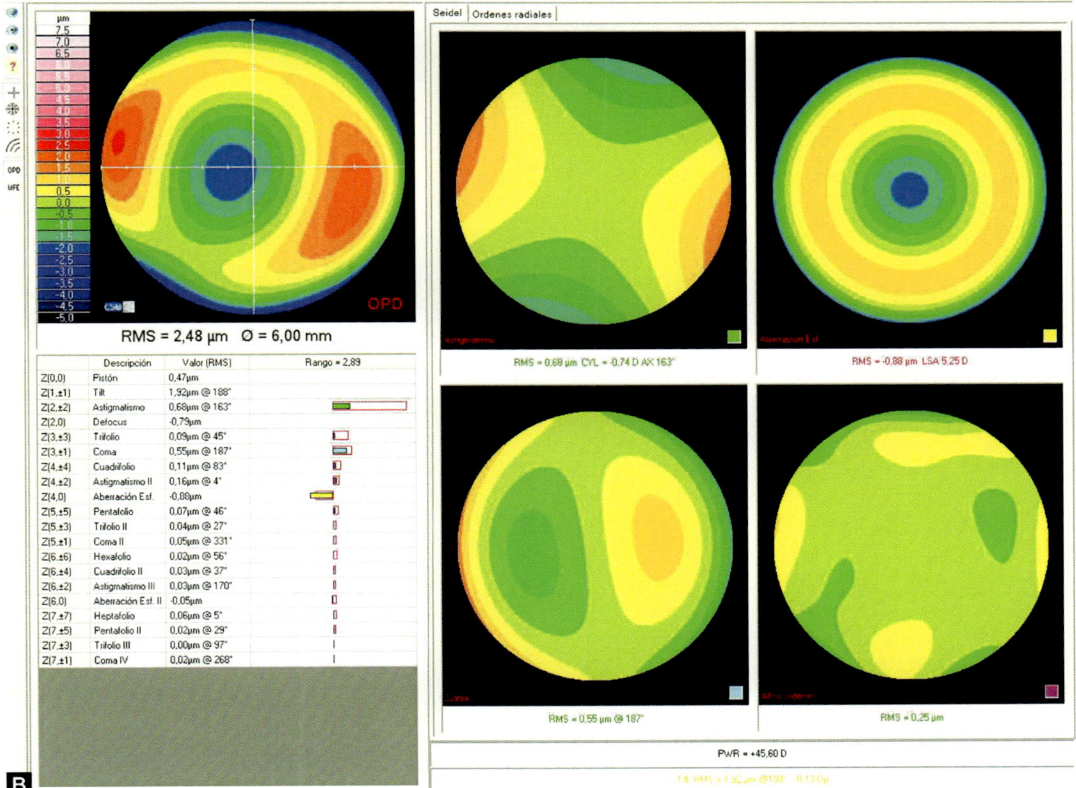

Figs 18.1A and B: Corneal topography showing increased spherical aberration after LASIK

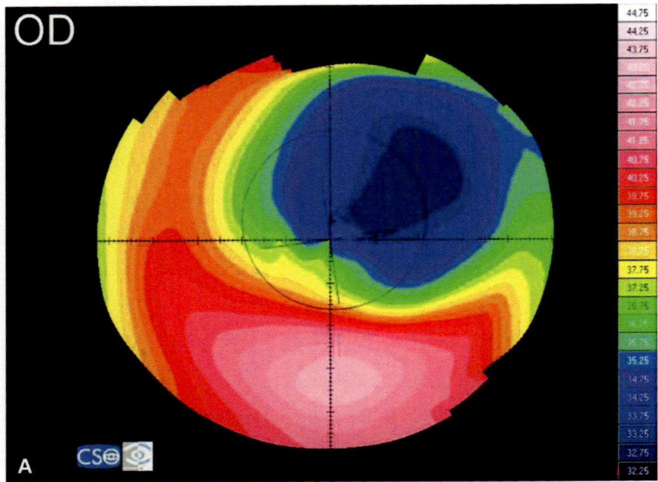

Fig. 18.2A: Coma aberrations are commonly associated with decentered treatments which results in asymmetry in the cornea. This produces an enlargement of the image light distribution along an axis, generating a comet-like image of a point source light object

vision.[31-37] Wavefront-guided PRK has also been reported to be effective in treating a patient with visual symptoms secondary to coma and a loss of best corrected visual acuity due to a LASIK flap button hole.[38]

CORNEAL WAVEFRONT-GUIDED REFRACTIVE SURGERY

Having established the efficacy of wavefront-guided excimer laser treatment for cases of retreatment and the treatment of aberrated corneas, the debate now lies between the efficacy of wavefront-guided (total wavefront) treatments versus corneal wavefront-guided treatments. Current technology enables the measurement of both corneal and total ocular aberrations. Global (or total) aberrations are analysed by wavefront sensors such as the Hartmann-Shack

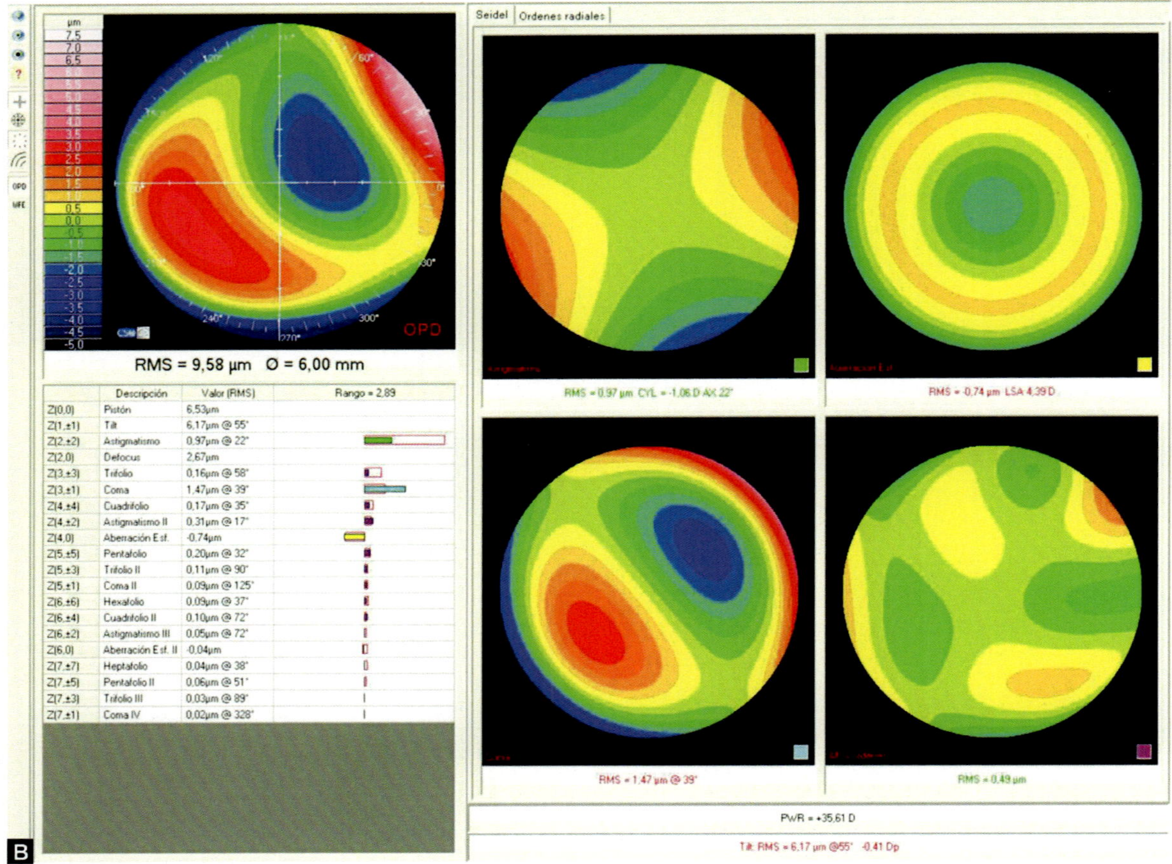

Fig. 18.2B: Corneal topography showing increased coma aberrations due to decentered ablation

aberrometer, while corneal aberrations are obtained by a mathematical transformation from corneal topography.

In the normal eye, 90 percent of the total aberrations are caused by the corneal optics; this proportion is largely the majority of the global aberration pattern of the eye when the cornea shows some degree of irregularity. Thus, targeting the corneal aberrations instead of the global aberration may be more efficacious in the treatment of highly aberrated corneas.

Global wavefront sensors available today only analyse up to 1452 points.[39] It is usually ineffective to register data of highly irregular corneas, and its information is limited to the pupil size area and by accomodation. The data is also affected by intraocular optics. With topographical systems, more than 6000 points can be studied and an exhaustive analysis performed. About 90 percent of the corneal surface can be analysed with a higher resolution of 1 μm (compared to 210 μm for global wavefront aberrometry). Thus, corneal aberrometry, as mathematically transformed from corneal topography, offers data from nearly the whole cornea, providing a larger quantity and more specific information about the optical performance of the anterior corneal surface. Moreover, this measurement is not influenced by intraocular optics and accommodation.

The terms *topography guided* and *corneal wavefront-guided* can be confusing. Systems that try to reduce corneal irregularity by changing the corneal shape without considering corneal wavefront analysis are called topography guided. These systems are less accurate and thus were improved by the introduction of corneal wavefront data derived from corneal elevation data in the calculation of the ablation profile.

In summary, the justifications for the use of corneal wavefront-guided treatment for the treatment of highly aberrated corneas are:

1. The first refractive interface corresponding to air-cornea is the most important contributor to the total power of the eye because the greatest difference in refractive indices between mediums in the eye is found at that point.
2. In highly aberrated corneas with previous keratorefractive procedures, the contribution of the aberrations in the cornea generated by the surgery will be the most significant source of optical errors.
3. The sampling provided by most ocular wavefront sensors or aberrometers is more limited than that obtained with corneal topographers.
4. Ocular wavefront sensors or aberrometers have limitations in the analysis of highly aberrated eyes. These include the crowding or superimposition of the light spots or the assumption of a flat slope for each analyzed portion of the wavefront (Hartmann-Shack devices).

Computerized Corneal Topography and Corneal Wavefront Analysis

In our centre, corneal aberrations were derived from the CSO corneal topography system (CSO, Florence Italy). The CSO topography system is a corneal topographer that is capable of evaluating the optical function of the anterior corneal surface, in addition to the topography. The CSO topography system measures 6144 points on the anterior corneal surface enclosed in a circular annulus defined by an inner radius of 0.33 mm and an outer radius of 10 mm respective to the cornea vertex. This is performed by projecting 24 placido rings into the cornea and then capturing the images of these rings using a high-resolution camera. The software of the CSO, Eye Top/ Eye Image V.6.4, analyzes the perceived placido rings and then constructs different topographic maps, which also provide the wavefront error or corneal aberration demonstrated in a wavefront map.

The CSO corneal topographer/aberrometer makes the conversion of the corneal elevation profile into corneal wavefront data using the Zernike polynomials, taking into account that deviations in the topography are directly proportional to wavefront deviations of the anterior surface of the cornea. Higher order aberrations values are expressed as root-mean-square (RMS) values in micrometers. Eye alignment and the tear film stability are of extreme importance during topography acquisition. Pupil position and its size in low mesopic conditions also are provided.

Ablation Design

Data obtained from the CSO topographer are then transferred to the Optimized Refractive Keratectomy software (ORK-W or ORK-CAM; Schwind, Kleinostheim, Germany), which transforms the wavefront data into a three-dimensional ablation profile. These softwares allow the surgeon to modify and select the corneal aberrations to be treated by the laser, and modify the size of the optical and transition zones in the treatment profile. The ORK-CAM software is an upgraded version of the ORK-W software and is currently in use at our centre. Data from ORK-W or ORK-CAM Schwind softwares are then transferred and used by the ESIRIS/Schwind Laser platform (Schwind Eye-Tech Solutions) to ablate the cornea.

Surgical Technique and Ablation Profile

The ESIRIS/Schwind excimer laser (Schwind Eye-Tech Solutions) has a flying-spot technology with a repetition rate of 200 Hz and a para-Gaussian profile spot diameter of 0.8 mm. The ESIRIS eye-tracker has 330 Hz and 6 to 8 milliseconds mean response time.

The ablation profile used was generated by the ORK-W or the ORK-CAM software based on the data obtained from the CSO topographer. In general, the main intention of the customized corneal wavefront-guided ablation was to reduce higher-order aberrations which were considered significant, in particular spherical-like and coma-like aberrations.

In most cases of previous LASIK, the original flaps were re-lifted where possible. However, PRK was performed in eyes with previous PRK or with inadequate residual stromal bed.

RESULTS OF CORNEAL WAVEFRONT GUIDED REFRACTIVE SURGERY

Several studies have reported the results of corneal wavefront-guided technology in highly aberrated corneas,[40-46] such as after complicated refractive surgery, keratoplasty, or corneal penetrating injuries. The results confirm the applicability of these excimer laser profiles.

We will now highlight our experience in the treatment of highly aberrated corneas with corneal wavefront-guided excimer laser surgery.

Corneal Wavefront-guided Retreatments for Significant Night Vision Symptoms after Myopic Laser Refractive Surgery[47]

We evaluated the safety and efficacy of corneal wavefront-guided retreatments with aspheric profiles for patients with significant night vision disturbances and high positive corneal spherical aberrations (SA) induced by conventional myopic laser refractive surgery. Previous studies of conventional and wavefront-guided laser refractive surgery found a factor of between 2.2 and 9.4 for SA induction after myopic ablation.[11,24,27,48,49] Clinically, patients with night vision symptoms (glare, haloes and starbursts) after myopic laser refractive surgery had significantly higher SA than asymptomatic patients.[18,50] Although determination of a cut-off level is not always possible, it was postulated that SA (Z_4^0) higher than 0.5 µm can lead to significant night vision symptoms.[51] Based on these facts, we treated eyes with significant night vision disturbances and more than 0.5 µm of positive corneal SA (Z_4^0) induced by previous myopic ablation.

METHODS

We performed corneal wavefront-guided retreatments for 28 eyes (16 men, 12 women) (14 right and 14 left) of 20 patients with significant postoperative night vision symptoms that did not improve after a trial of corrective lenses for at least for three months. Mean patient age was 41.0 +/- 14.6 years (range, 24 to 63 years).

Inclusion criteria were:

1. Availability of preoperative and six-month postoperative visual symptom evaluation.
2. Topography maps with no missing data points within the central 7.0 mm zone.

3. No intraoperative or postoperative complications.
4. SA (Z_4^0) higher than 0.5 µm.
5. No contact lens wear for two weeks before the baseline retreatment examination.
6. Stable refractive error for at least two months before surgery.
7. Stable refraction achieved at least three months after the procedure.

Exclusion criteria were:

1. Ectasia.
2. Keratoconus suspect.
3. Decentration as evidenced by corneal topography.
4. Active ocular or systemic disease likely to affect corneal wound healing.
5. Pregnant or nursing.
6. Inability to comply with postoperative follow-up regimen.

The main outcome measures were visual symptoms, change in corneal SA (Z_4^0), and corneal asphericity (Q-value).

Evaluation of Subjective Symptoms

Before and after the retreatment, patients underwent a grading of night vision symptoms that was recorded using a subjective scale (Table 18.1). All patients underwent a full ophthalmologic examination including manifest and cycloplegic refraction, determination of uncorrected visual acuity (UCVA), best-corrected visual acuity, computerized videokeratography with the CSO topographer (CSO, Firenze, Italy), slit-lamp biomicroscopy, Goldmann applanation tonometry, binocular indirect ophthalmoscopy, and ultrasonic pachymetry before and after retreatment. Before surgery, pupil diameter was measured using the Procyon P2000D pupillometer (Procyon Instruments, Ltd, London, United Kingdom) under low mesopic condition (3 cd/m^2). Postoperative assessments were performed routinely at one day, one month, three months, and six months after surgery. An independent survey was made regarding the night vision symptoms of the patients recorded from different examinations.

Table 18.1: Grading of the night vision symptoms[47]

Grade	*Symptoms*
0 (None)	No symptoms
1 (Mild)	Halos, starburst, or acuity distortion noted to affect light sources at night but not interfering with functions
2 (Moderate)	Halos or starburst noted to affect usual activities; especially while driving or looking at light sources at night
3 (Disturbing)	Halos or starburst forcing the patient to refrain from certain activities at night, such as driving or looking at light sources
4 (Incapacitating)	Patients cannot drive at night at all

Analysis of Corneal Aberrations

Corneal aberrations were derived from the CSO corneal topography system. The software of this topography system, the EyeTop 2005 (CSO, Firenze, Italy), performed the conversion of the corneal elevation profile into corneal wavefront data. Taking into account specific coefficients of the Zernike decomposition of the corneal wavefront, different root mean square (RMS) values were calculated. Specifically, the RMS for total wavefront aberration (TWA), coma-like aberration ($Z_3^{+/-1}$, $Z_5^{+/-1}$), spherical-like aberration (Z_4^0, Z_6^0), spherical Seidel aberration (Z_4^0), coma Seidel aberration ($Z_3^{+/-1}$),and Strehl ratio were compared before and after surgery. In all cases, the aberrometric study was performed for a 7 mm zone.

Ablation Algorithm

Enhancement surgery was planned to remove residual refractive error and corneal SA (Z_4^0) in all (n = 28) eyes. Using custom ablation manager software (ORK-CAM; Schwind Eye-Tech Solutions, Kleinostham, Germany) and data derived from the CSO corneal topographer, specific ablation profiles for treating corneal aberrations were created. The main intention of customized ablation was to reduce SA (Z_4^0), but accompanying high coma and other HOAs also were treated when they were significant considering the physiologic level of each kind of Zernike error. Customized ablation for the correction of SA (Z_4^0) and coma ($Z_3^{+/-1}$) was performed in 18 of 28 eyes, for the correction of only SA (Z_4^0) in five eyes, all HOA in three eyes, and all third- and fourth-order aberration in two eyes. The age of the patient, subjective spherocylindrical refraction, central corneal thickness, and flap thickness also must be introduced for the calculation of the ablations with this software. Using all these data, an ablation profile was generated and modified until the more appropriate profile (regarding the corneal asphericity) was obtained for the specific case. The software automatically calculates the optical and transition zones, taking into account the low mesopic pupil diameter, corneal thickness, and specific targeted Zernike terms.

The designed algorithms of the ORK-CAM software had an adjustment of the sphere correction depending on the level of SA corrected. This adjustment factor depended on the features of each specific case. The potential change in corneal aberrations was always calculated according to the ORK-CAM eye model, always having, as an objective a postoperative asphericity, –0.25 μm (approximately the mean value of the corneal asphericity in the normal population).

Primary Refractive Surgery

All eyes had myopia or compound myopic astigmatism before primary refractive surgery. All eyes underwent refractive surgery for myopia using the Planoscan algorithm with the Technolas 217-Z (Bausch and Lomb, Rochester, New York, USA). Twenty-three (82%) of 28 eyes underwent LASIK and five (18%) of 28 eyes underwent PRK as primary surgery. Of the 23 eyes that underwent LASIK as primary surgery, a flap was created using a femtosecond laser (Intralase, Inc, Irvine, California, USA) in 14 eyes and using a mechanical microkeratome in nine eyes (Moria M2 [Moria, Antony, France], eight eyes; Hansatome [Bausch and Lomb], one eye).

Surgical Technique

The enhancement procedure was performed after a minimum follow-up of six months after the initial surgery. Retreatments were performed under topical anesthesia. The original LASIK flap was relifted in 21 (75%) of 28 eyes, whereas the remaining seven (25%) eyes underwent PRK because of previous PRK (five eyes) or inadequate residual stromal bed (two eyes). Patients underwent corneal wavefront-guided laser refractive surgery retreatment with the ESIRIS/SCHWIND excimer laser system (Schwind Eye-Tech Solutions). The ablation was centered on the pupil center in all eyes. The mean optical zone was 6.50 +/– 0.27 mm (range, 6.00 to 7.00 mm), and the treatment zone was 7.54 +/– 0.34 mm (range, 6.88 to 8.39 mm). No intraoperative complications occurred. All eyes had one retreatment, and no additional retreatment was performed in any eye.

RESULTS

Night Vision Symptoms

Before surgery, all patients reported symptoms of significant night vision disability (moderate [grade 2] or disturbing [grade 3]). After surgery, night time glare and halo symptoms subjectively improved to none or mild (grade 1) in all patients at the six-month follow-up. The mean preoperative pupil diameter under low mesopic condition was 6.68 +/– 0.62 mm (range, 5.69 to 7.68 mm). Eight (28.5%) of 28 eyes had pupil diameters of more than 7 mm under low mesopic conditions.

Aberrations

The mean preoperative corneal TWA significantly decreased from 3.03 +/- 1.33 μm to 2.44 +/–1.55 μm after surgery (P = 0.002). Of the 28 eyes treated, 22 (79%) had a decrease in corneal TWA, 24 (86%) had a decrease in spherical-like aberrations, 19 (68%) had a decrease in coma-like aberrations, 25 (89%) had a decrease in SA (Z_4^0), and 22 (79%) had a decrease in coma ($Z_3^{+/-1}$) after enhancement.

We observed an increase in SA (Z_4^0) in three (11%) of 28 eyes after the retreatment, but the average magnitude of increase was low (mean, 0.09 μm; range, 0.002 to 0.16 μm). These three eyes had a mean myopic correction of –1.71 diopters.

Asphericity

The mean asphericity (Q-value) under the 4.5 mm zone decreased significantly after enhancement, whereas it did not change significantly under the 8.0 mm zone.

DISCUSSION

Treatment of eyes with significant night vision disturbances and more than 0.5 µm of positive corneal SA (Z_4^0) induced by previous myopic ablation using a topographic corneal WF-guided customization with aspheric profile resulted in a significant improvement in night vision symptoms and a decrease in corneal SA. Although we targeted SA in all eyes, treatment of corneal aberrations other than SA might have contributed to the improvement in the night vision in our patients.

Corneal Wavefront-guided LASIK Retreatments for Correction of Highly Aberrated Corneas following Refractive Surgery[52]

We evaluated the use of customized anterior surface corneal wavefront-guided excimer laser surgery in improving visual quality, best spectacle-corrected visual acuity (BSCVA), and refractive outcome in symptomatic patients with elevated higher order aberrations following LASIK.

METHODS

Seventy-five consecutive eyes of 59 patients (27 men and 32 women) were included in this prospective consecutive, observational non-randomized, non-comparative study. The eyes had previously undergone LASIK procedures for myopia or hyperopia (dioptric range: –8.00 to +4.00) between 2001 and 2004 and were referred with significant visual symptoms. Mean patient age was 31.5+/–4.8 years.

The eyes included in this study were divided into two groups for analysis of results. The night symptoms group included 37 (49.3%) eyes that suffered from significant night vision disability in the form of halos and glare under low illumination in the presence of uneventful primary LASIK surgery. The corneal complications group included 38 (50.7%) eyes that had corneal complications following the primary surgery; these complications included flap complications, decentration, and an irregular ablation profile evidenced by topography in the form of micro- and macro-irregularities.

Inclusion criteria were patients with:

1. No other eye disease or corneal problem that could be related to the visual symptoms.
2. Significant symptoms affecting visual performance in at least one activity of daily living, associated with a decrease in at least one line of BSCVA.
3. An interval of at least 6 months following the LASIK procedure.
4. Presence of an abnormal increase in the normal limits of global (if measurable) and corneal higher-order aberrations following the first surgery.

In addition, eyes were required to have at least a total higher-order aberration > 0.50 µm for the night symptoms group and 0.80 µm for the corneal complications group. No eye was excluded because of an excessive corneal irregularity.

Exclusion criteria were:

1. Moderate or severe dry eye syndrome.
2. Detectable slit-lamp changes in crystalline lens.
3. Cornea thickness <400 µm at any location in the cornea.

All patients underwent a complete ophthalmologic examination that included manifest and cycloplegic refraction, pre-dilatation computerized corneal topography (CSO, Florence, Italy), and post-dilatation corneal wavefront measurement using the 7.5 mm central corneal area (CSO). For all eyes, data concerning corneal point spread function (PSF) was measured as obtained from the corneal topography at each visit. The examinations were performed preoperatively and at 1, 3, and 6 months postoperatively. Patients were also asked about the presence of visual symptoms (e.g. halos, glare, and double vision) for each eye, whether the symptoms were significant enough to limit their normal day or night activities, and whether these symptoms were eliminated by the surgery.

Analysis of Corneal Aberrations and Surgical Technique

Corneal wavefront measurements were performed using the CSO topography system. Data from the CSO topographer were then transferred to the Optimized Refractive Keratectomy software (ORK-W, Schwind Eye-Tech Solutions) which transforms the wavefront data into a three-dimensional ablation profile. In this study, a large optical zone of 6 to 6.5 mm with a standard transition zone of 1 to 1.5 mm was used in all cases. Data from the ORK-W Schwind software were then transferred and used by the ESIRIS/Schwind Laser platform to ablate the cornea.

The surgical technique performed in this study was similar in all the eyes. Flap elevation was performed followed by laser ablation on the corneal stroma.

RESULTS

Visual Outcome

Uncorrected visual acuity: In the night symptoms group, mean preoperative UCVA was 20/32 (0.6+/–0.2 decimal value) and 6 months postoperative UCVA was 20/25 (0.8+/–0.2 decimal value). In the corneal complications group, mean preoperative UCVA was 20/40 (0.5+/–0.2 decimal value) and 6 months postoperative UCVA was 20/30 (0.7+/–0.2 decimal value). The difference between preoperative and postoperative UCVA was statistically significant in both groups ($P < 0.001$).

Best spectacle-corrected visual acuity: In both groups, mean preoperative and 6-month postoperative BSCVA were 20/25 (0.8+/–0.2 decimal value). The difference between preoperative and postoperative BSCVA in both groups was not statistically significant ($P = 0.219$ for the night symptoms and $P = 0.149$ for the corneal complications group).

Safety and efficacy indices: The safety index was 1.1 in both groups, and the efficacy index was 0.93 in the night symptoms group and 0.92 in the corneal complications group.

Refractive Outcome

Sphere: In the night symptoms group, mean sphere was –0.20+/–0.90 D preoperatively and –0.20+/–0.40 D at 6 months postoperatively; this difference was statistically significant ($P = 0.005$). In the corneal complications group, mean sphere was 0.80+/–1.60 D preoperatively and 0.30+/–0.70 D at 6 months postoperatively; this difference was not statistically significant ($P = 0.100$).

Cylinder: In the night symptoms group, mean cylinder was –0.70+/–0.40 D preoperatively and –0.50+/–0.50 D at 6 months postoperatively; this difference was not statistically significant ($P = 0.122$). In the corneal complications group, mean cylinder was –1.20+/–0.80 D preoperatively and –0.70+/–0.70 D at 6 months postoperatively; this difference was statistically significant ($P < 0.001$).

Spherical equivalent refraction: In the night symptoms group, mean spherical equivalent refraction was –0.50+/–0.80 D preoperatively and –0.01+/–0.50 D at 6 months postoperatively; this difference was not statistically significant ($P = 0.006$). In the corneal complications group, mean spherical equivalent refraction was 0.12+/–1.60 D preoperatively and -0.04+/-0.70 D at 6 months postoperatively; this difference was not statistically significant ($P = 0.639$).

Corneal Aberrations

Total higher-order aberrations: In the night symptoms group, mean total higher-order aberrations decreased from 1.25+/–0.39 µm preoperatively to 0.92+/–0.31 µm at 6 months postoperatively. In the corneal complications group, mean total higher-order aberrations decreased from 1.64+/–0.55 µm preoperatively to 1.25+/–0.43 µm at 6 months postoperatively.

Tilt: In the night symptoms group, mean tilt decreased from 1.38 +/– 0.88 µm preoperatively to 1.03 +/– 0.52 µm at 6 months postoperatively. In the corneal complications group, mean tilt decreased from 2.38 +/– 1.35 µm preoperatively to 1.65 +/– 0.95 µm at 6 months postoperatively.

Spherical aberrations: In the night symptoms group, mean spherical aberrations decreased from 0.89 +/– 0.35 µm preoperatively to 0.69 +/–0.29 µm at 6 months postoperatively. In the corneal complications group, mean spherical aberrations decreased from 1.03 +/–0.55 µm preoperatively to 0.86 +/–0.46 µm at 6 months postoperatively.

Coma: In the night symptoms group, mean coma decreased from 0.76 +/–0.32 µm preoperatively to 0.58 +/–0.21 µm at 6 months postoperatively. In the corneal complications group, mean coma decreased from 1.18 +/–0.47 µm preoperatively to 0.87 +/–0.36 µm at 6 months postoperatively. The differences between the preoperative and postoperative values for corneal aberrations were statistically significant in both groups.

Point Spread Function (PSF)

The PSF percentage represents the relation in percentage between the light intensity peak obtained in our cases and that corresponding to the theoretical perfect eye (only diffraction-limited eye). In the night symptoms group, mean PSF percentage increased from 11.60 +/–7.17 preoperatively to 19.22 +/–10.90 at 6 months postoperatively. In the corneal complications group, mean PSF percentage increased from 7.66 +/–5.33 preoperatively to 10.75 +/–6.786 at 6 months postoperatively. The differences between preoperative and postoperative PSF were statistically significant in both groups.

DISCUSSION

In this study, the corneal aberrations were measured and used as a base for the treatment performed by the excimer laser. Approximately, 50 percent of patients in the night symptoms group did not complain of decreased visual acuity but had significant complaints regarding night vision disability such as halos and glare. Eyes in the corneal complications group were more complicated cases because of previous corneal refractive surgery. Marked improvement occurred in both groups with regard to total aberrations, tilt, and improvement of spherical aberrations and coma, as well as in PSF, UCVA, and BSCVA.

The eyes in both groups had a mean improvement in UCVA of 2 lines. In the night symptoms group, 30 (81.1%) of the eyes retained their BSCVA or gained at least 1 line of BSCVA compared with 34 (89.5%) eyes in the corneal complications group. All patients experienced improvement of their visual acuity, double vision problem, and night vision capabilities, which could be explained by the improvement in their PSF values.

The stability of the spherical equivalent refraction was another factor that added to the success of the surgery. The difference between mean preoperative and postoperative spherical equivalent refraction was +0.50 +/–0.99 D in the night symptoms group and –0.12 +/–1.50 D in the corneal complications group. This means the ablation performed by the laser during customized retreatment caused a shift within +/-0.50 D from the original refraction. This result means the software used in the ablation profile (ORK-W ablation for ESIRIS excimer laser) played an important role in compensating the ablation performed by the laser maintaining the curvature of the cornea within the pretreatment range.

The treatment of LASIK-induced symptoms associated with significant higher-order aberrations using corneal wavefront-guided technology is safe and effective in this select group of patients whose corneas were of adequate thickness and who had no additional lenticular or corneal pathology.

Corneal Wavefront-guided Retreatments for Corneas with High Levels of Corneal Coma Aberration after LASIK[53]

We evaluated the improvement in visual and optical performance after corneal wavefront-guided LASIK enhancement with the ORK-CAM system (Schwind Eye-Tech Solutions) in patients with high levels of corneal coma aberration and complaints about their quality of vision resulting from decentered primary LASIK procedures.

METHODS

We studied 34 consecutive symptomatic eyes of 29 patients with a hyperopic or myopic spherical equivalent (SE) who had unsuccessful primary LASIK.

Inclusion criteria were previous LASIK surgery with residual symptomatic myopia, hyperopia, or astigmatism and a significant level of primary corneal coma aberration. Thus, corneas with relevant asymmetry after surgery caused by improper centration were selected. The level of corneal coma was considered significant when the associated root mean square (RMS) for the corneal primary coma (measured over a pupil of 6.0 mm) was higher than 0.5 µm.[7,51] This criterion was chosen based on previously reported physiologic levels of corneal HOAs. The 0.5 µm cutoff point was selected because the associated probability of it being a normal value was less than 1 percent.[7,51]

Exclusion criteria were:

1. Corneas with flap-related problems at the time of surgery
2. Postoperative inflammation at the interface
3. Epithelial ingrowth under the flap
4. Corneal opacity
5. A formal contraindication to LASIK

In all cases, primary LASIK had been performed at least 6 months before the evaluation for enhancement. No treatment was performed if the refraction was not stable at 2 consecutive examinations performed at least 3 weeks apart. The target postoperative refraction was emmetropia in all cases. The postoperative follow-up was 6 months.

Preoperative Examination

The preoperative examination included uncorrected decimal visual acuity (UCVA); best spectacle-corrected decimal visual acuity (BSCVA); manifest and cycloplegic refractions; slitlamp biomicroscopy; applanation tonometry; ultrasonic pachymetry (DHG500 US pachymeter, DHG Technology, Inc.); scotopic, low, and high mesopic pupillometry (Procyon Pupillometer P2000SA, Procyon Instruments Ltd.); corneal topography (CSO system, Costruzione Strumenti Oftalmici); and fundus evaluation. Corneal aberrations were derived from corneal topography following the protocol described below in Corneal Aberrations. In addition, patients were asked to evaluate the levels of halos and glare they perceived at night using the following qualitative scale: none, low, moderate, high, or severe.

Corneal Aberrations and Ablation Profile

Corneal aberrations were derived from the data of the anterior surface of the cornea obtained with the CSO topography system. The corneal elevation profiles were converted into corneal wavefront data with the system's software (EyeTop 2005).

The corneal wavefront–guided customized ablation was designed and calculated using commercially available ORK-CAM software. The main goal of the designed ablation in all cases was to minimize the primary coma ($Z_3^{+/-1}$). The spherical aberration (Z_4^0) was treated if it was significant (55.9% of cases). The aim was to create a corneal surface with an elevation profile that would generate a minimally distorted wavefront. In addition, all treatments were designed to leave an expected residual stromal bed thicker than 250 mm in the central cornea.

Surgical Technique

All LASIK procedures were performed by the same surgeon (JLA) at Vissum Instituto Oftalmologico de Alicante using the Esiris excimer laser (Schwind Eye-Tech Solutions).

The optical zone of the treatment was selected according to the preoperative scotopic pupil size. Depending on the pachymetry, optical zones with a diameter at least as large as the scotopic pupil were targeted to prevent unwanted optical phenomena.

RESULTS

The mean age of the 29 patients was 40.82 +/− 9.79 years (range 26 to 64 years). The mean preoperative SE was +0.47 +/− 1.16 diopters (D) (range −1.75 to +3.00 D).

		Mean ± SD (Range)		
		Postoperative		
Parameter	*Preoperative*	*1 month*	*3 months*	*6 months*
UCVA (decimal)	0.63 ± 0.19 (0.20 to 1.00)	0.62 ± 0.25 (0.20 to 1.00)	0.72 ± 0.20 (0.30 to 1.00)	0.75 ± 0.20(0.20 to 1.00)
Spherical (D)	+ 1.13 ± 1.30 (–1.00 to + 5.00)	+ 0.35 ± 0.52 (–0.75 to + 1.50)	+ 0.41 ± 0.50 (–0.50 to + 1.50)	+ 0.31 ± 0.66 (–0.75 to + 1.50)
Cylinder (D)	–1.32 ± 0.74 (–4.50 to –0.50)	–0.84 ± 0.65 (–2.50 to 0.00)	–0.83 ± 0.70 (–3.00 to 0.00)	–0.76 ± 0.61 (–2.25 to 0.000)
SE (D)	+ 0.47 ± 1.16 (–1.75 to + 3.00)	–0.06 ± 0.57 (–1.50 to +1.25)	–0.01 ± 0.50 (–1.00 to + 0.88)	–0.02 ± 0.58 (–1.25 to 0.88)
BSCVA (decimal)	0.85 ± 0.18 (0.30 to 1.20)	0.76 ± 0.23 (0.30 to 1.00)	0.86 ± 0.15 (0.50 to 1.00)	0.86 ± 0.18 (0.35 to 1.20)
Efficacy	—	0.73 ± 0.23 (0.20 to 1.00)	0.83 ± 0.16 (0.43 to 1.19)	0.88 ± 0.12 (0.67 to1.06)
Safety	—	0.91 ± 0.22 (0.44 to 1.42)	1.00 ± 0.13 (0.83 to 1.50)	1.03 ± 0.16 (0.78 to 1.50)

BSCVA = Best spectacle-corrected visual acuity;SE = Spherical equivalent; UCVA = Uncorrected visual acuity

Thirteen eyes (38.2%) had a myopic SE and 21 eyes (61.8%), a hyperopic SE. The mean preoperative scotopic pupil size was 6.43 +/– 0.76 mm and the mean optical zone, 6.56 +/– 0.28 mm (range 6.00 to 7.00 mm). The mean total ablation zone designed with ORK-CAM software was 7.71 +/– 0.40 mm (range 6.88 to 8.50 mm).

Refractive Outcomes

Statistically significant reductions were observed in sphere and cylinder at 1 month (both $P < 0.01$). At 6 months, the mean efficacy index was 0.88 +/–0.12 (range 0.67 to 1.06) and the mean safety index was 1.03 +/–0.16 (range 0.78 to 1.50). The improvement in both parameters at 1 month was statistically significant ($P = 0.01$ for efficacy and $P < 0.01$ for safety). After that, there were no statistically significant changes.

Six months postoperatively, the UCVA was statistically significant better ($P = 0.01$). The loss of 2 lines in 1 eye (2.94%) was due to the proliferation of a superior epithelial ingrowth, which was responsible for an unpredictable irregularity. In addition, in 2 eyes with a loss of 1 line of BSCVA, corneal alterations (significant punctuate keratitis in 1 eye and proliferation of epithelial ingrowth in the other) were found at the 6-month examinations.

Corneal Aberrations

At 1 month, there was a statistically significant reduction in total RMS ($P = 0.01$), astigmatic RMS ($P = 0.01$), and primary coma RMS ($P < 0.01$). The (Z_4^0) coefficient changed significantly to negative values ($P < 0.01$). There were no significant changes in these aberrometric parameters at 3 months and 6 months.

Subjective Symptoms

Complications

The existing flaps were lifted without complications in all cases, and all procedures were centered at the pupillary center. No eye required retreatment during the postoperative follow-up.

DISCUSSION

Corneal wavefront–guided LASIK enhancement using the ORK-CAM software was useful in treating cases of high levels of primary coma caused by a previous decentered refractive surgery procedure. It provided excellent safety and efficacy for correction of 2nd-order components. In addition, primary coma was significantly reduced and night-vision symptoms were decreased. Spherical aberration can also be corrected using this technique.

The improvement observed in corneal aberrations after the corneal wavefront–guided enhancement was related to a reduction in the bothersome symptoms perceived by patients preoperatively. Specifically, the presence of night halos and glare was studied because patients with highly aberrated corneas often report these symptoms and they are easy to describe and understand. An increase in HOAs increases the incidence of night-vision complaints, especially after refractive surgery. These optical errors significantly increase image distortion, especially when the pupil dilates because the most aberrated part of the ocular optical system takes part in the generation of the retinal image. We did not report other symptoms associated with aberrated vision, such as double vision or ghost images.

LIMITATIONS OF CORNEAL WAVEFRONT-GUIDED REFRACTIVE SURGERY

Currently, one limitation of customized refractive surgery is the size of the laser spot. The ideal spot for complete correction of HOAs is 0.5 mm or smaller.[54] This will allow a smoother and more precise ablation profile. The Esiris laser has a spot size of 0.8 mm, which could be responsible for the partial correction of some HOAs. However, with the advent of newer excimer lasers with laser spot size of 0.5 mm or smaller, for example, the Amaris excimer laser (Schwind Eye-Tech Solutions); the results of customized laser ablations are likely to improve.

Another limitation of customized refractive surgery is the wound-healing response of the cornea. The cornea is made of complex structural composite material that undergoes biomechanical changes and healing responses after damage or injury.[55] The ablation of tissue with the excimer laser could generate subtle unexpected modifications that could limit the effect of a customized ablation.[56] Therefore, although the ablation profile was planned to achieve a more regular corneal surface, biomechanical changes and wound-healing responses could reduce the effectiveness of the customized ablation.

CONCLUSION

Higher-order aberrations are correlated with bothersome visual symptoms and night-vision disturbances. These aberrations are usually seen in post-refractive surgery patients, especially in eyes with complications. Corneal wavefront-guided excimer laser retreatments in such eyes have been shown to reduce the amount of higher-order aberrations with resulting improvement in visual quality and reduction in visual symptoms.

REFERENCES

1. Chalita MR, Xu M, Krueger RR. Correlation of aberrations with visual symptoms using wavefront analysis in eyes after laser in situ keratomileusis. J Refract Surg 2003;19:S682-6.
2. Villa C, Gutierrez R, Jimenez JR, Gonzalez-Meijome JM. Night vision disturbances after successful LASIK surgery. Br J Ophthalmol 2007;91:1031-7.
3. Oshika T, Okamoto C, Samejima T, et al. Contrast sensitivity function and ocular higher-order wavefront aberrations in normal human eyes. Ophthalmology 2006;113:1807-12.
4. Melamud A, Chalita MR, Krueger RR, Lee MS. Comatic aberration as a cause of monocular diplopia. J Cataract Refract Surg 2006;32:529-32.
5. Liang J, Williams DR. Aberrations and retinal image quality of the normal human eye. J Opt Soc Am A Opt Image Sci Vis 1997;14:2873-83.
6. Joslin CE, Wu SM, McMahon TT, Shahidi M. Higher-order wavefront aberrations in corneal refractive therapy. Optom Vis Sci 2003;80:805-11.
7. Wang L, Dai E, Koch DD, Nathoo A. Optical aberrations of the human anterior cornea. J Cataract Refract Surg 2003;29:1514-21.
8. Wang L, Koch DD. Ocular higher-order aberrations in individuals screened for refractive surgery. J Cataract Refract Surg 2003;29:1896-903.
9. Netto MV, Ambrosio R Jr, Shen TT, Wilson SE. Wavefront analysis in normal refractive surgery candidates. J Refract Surg 2005;21:332-8.
10. Yoon G, MacRae S, Williams DR, Cox IG. Causes of spherical aberration induced by laser refractive surgery. J Cataract Refract Surg 2005;31:127-35.
11. Wang L, Koch DD. Anterior corneal optical aberrations induced by laser *in situ* keratomileusis for hyperopia. J Cataract Refract Surg 2003;29:1702-8.
12. Kohnen T, Mahmoud K, Buhren J. Comparison of corneal higher-order aberrations induced by myopic and hyperopic LASIK. Ophthalmology 2005;112:1692.

13. Wang Y, Zhao KX, He JC, et al. Ocular higher-order aberrations features analysis after corneal refractive surgery. Chin Med J (Engl) 2007;120:269-73.
14. Tran DB, Sarayba MA, Bor Z, et al. Randomized prospective clinical study comparing induced aberrations with IntraLase and Hansatome flap creation in fellow eyes: potential impact on wavefront-guided laser *in situ* keratomileusis. J Cataract Refract Surg 2005;31:97-105.
15. Medeiros FW, Stapleton WM, Hammel J, et al. Wavefront analysis comparison of LASIK outcomes with the femtosecond laser and mechanical microkeratomes. J Refract Surg 2007;23:880-7.
16. Lim T, Yang S, Kim M, Tchah H. Comparison of the IntraLase femtosecond laser and mechanical microkeratome for laser *in situ* keratomileusis. Am J Ophthalmol 2006;141:833-9.
17. Tanabe T, Miyata K, Samejima T, et al. Influence of wavefront aberration and corneal subepithelial haze on low-contrast visual acuity after photorefractive keratectomy. Am J Ophthalmol 2004;138:620-4.
18. McCormick GJ, Porter J, Cox IG, MacRae S. Higher-order aberrations in eyes with irregular corneas after laser refractive surgery. Ophthalmology 2005;112:1699-709.
19. Zhou C, Chai X, Yuan L, et al. Corneal higher-order aberrations after customized aspheric ablation and conventional ablation for myopic correction. Curr Eye Res 2007;32:431-8.
20. Mrochen M, Kaemmerer M, Seiler T. Wavefront-guided laser *in situ* keratomileusis: early results in three eyes. J Refract Surg 2000;16:116-21.
21. Mrochen M, Kaemmerer M, Seiler T. Clinical results of wavefront-guided laser *in situ* keratomileusis 3 months after surgery. J Cataract Refract Surg 2001;27:201-7.
22. Caster AI, Hoff JL, Ruiz R. Conventional vs wavefront-guided LASIK using the LADARVision4000 excimer laser. J Refract Surg 2005;21:S786-91.
23. Bahar I, Levinger S, Kremer I. Wavefront-guided LASIK for myopia with the Technolas 217z: results at 3 years. J Refract Surg 2007;23:586-90, discussion.
24. Aizawa D, Shimizu K, Komatsu M, et al. Clinical outcomes of wavefront-guided laser *in situ* keratomileusis: 6-month follow-up. J Cataract Refract Surg 2003;29:1507-13.
25. Nuijts RM, Nabar VA, Hament WJ, Eggink FA. Wavefront-guided versus standard laser *in situ* keratomileusis to correct low to moderate myopia. J Cataract Refract Surg 2002;28:1907-13.
26. He R, Qu M, Yu S. Comparison of NIDEK CATz wavefront-guided LASIK to traditional LASIK with the NIDEK CXII excimer laser in myopia. J Refract Surg 2005;21:S646-9.
27. Kohnen T, Buhren J, Kuhne C, Mirshahi A. Wavefront-guided LASIK with the Zyoptix 3.1 system for the correction of myopia and compound myopic astigmatism with 1-year follow-up: clinical outcome and change in higher order aberrations. Ophthalmology 2004;111:2175-85.
28. Phusitphoykai N, Tungsiripat T, Siriboonkoom J, Vongthongsri A. Comparison of conventional versus wavefront-guided laser *in situ* keratomileusis in the same patient. J Refract Surg 2003;19:S217-20.
29. Schwartz GS, Park DH, Lane SS. CustomCornea wavefront retreatment after conventional laser *in situ* keratomileusis. J Cataract Refract Surg 2005;31:1502-5.
30. Alio JL, Montes-Mico R. Wavefront-guided versus standard LASIK enhancement for residual refractive errors. Ophthalmology 2006;113:191-7.
31. Kanellopoulos AJ, Pe LH. Wavefront-guided enhancements using the wavelight excimer laser in symptomatic eyes previously treated with LASIK. J Refract Surg 2006;22:345-9.
32. Hiatt JA, Grant CN, Wachler BS. Complex wavefront-guided retreatments with the Alcon CustomCornea platform after prior LASIK. J Refract Surg 2006;22:48-53.
33. Durrie DS, Stahl JE, Schwendeman F. Alcon LADARWave CustomCornea retreatments. J Refract Surg 2005;21:S804-7.
34. Carones F, Vigo L, Scandola E. Wavefront-guided treatment of abnormal eyes using the LADARVision platform. J Refract Surg 2003;19:S703-8.
35. Montague AA, Manche EE. CustomVue laser *in situ* keratomileusis treatment after previous keratorefractive surgery. J Cataract Refract Surg 2006;32:795-8.
36. Mrochen M, Krueger RR, Bueeler M, Seiler T. Aberration-sensing and wavefront-guided laser *in situ* keratomileusis: management of decentered ablation. J Refract Surg 2002;18:418-29.
37. Salz JJ. Wavefront-guided treatment for previous laser *in situ* keratomileusis and photorefractive keratectomy: case reports. J Refract Surg 2003;19:S697-S702.
38. Chalita MR, Roth AS, Krueger RR. Wavefront-guided surface ablation with prophylactic use of mitomycin C after a buttonhole laser *in situ* keratomileusis flap. J Refract Surg 2004;20:176-81.
39. Rozema JJ, Van Dyck DE, Tassignon MJ. Clinical comparison of 6 aberrometers. Part 1: Technical specifications. J Cataract Refract Surg 2005;31:1114-27.
40. Alio JL, Belda JI, Osman AA, Shalaby AM. Topography-guided laser *in situ* keratomileusis (TOPOLINK) to correct irregular astigmatism after previous refractive surgery. J Refract Surg 2003;19:516-27.
41. Cosar CB, Acar S. Topography-guided LASIK with the wavelight laser after penetrating keratoplasty. J Refract Surg 2006;22:716-9.
42. Kanellopoulos AJ. Topography-guided custom retreatments in 27 symptomatic eyes. J Refract Surg 2005;21: S513-8.
43. Koller T, Iseli HP, Donitzky C, et al. Topography-guided surface ablation for forme fruste keratoconus. Ophthalmology 2006;113:2198-202.
44. Lee DH, Seo SJ, Shin SC. Topography-guided excimer laser ablation of irregular cornea resulting from penetrating injury. J Cataract Refract Surg 2002;28:186-8.

45. Rajan MS, O'Brart DP, Patel P, et al. Topography-guided customized laser-assisted subepithelial keratectomy for the treatment of postkeratoplasty astigmatism. J Cataract Refract Surg 2006;32:949-57.
46. Toda I, Yamamoto T, Ito M, et al. Topography-guided ablation for treatment of patients with irregular astigmatism. J Refract Surg 2007;23:118-25.
47. Alio JL, Pinero D, Muftuoglu O. Corneal wavefront-guided retreatments for significant night vision symptoms after myopic laser refractive surgery. Am J Ophthalmol 2008;145:65-74.
48. Erdem U, Muftuoglu O. Optical factors in increased best spectacle-corrected visual acuity after LASIK. J Refract Surg 2006;22:S1056-68.
49. Kim TI, Yang SJ, Tchah H. Bilateral comparison of wavefront-guided versus conventional laser *in situ* keratomileusis with Bausch and Lomb Zyoptix. J Refract Surg 2004;20:432-8.
50. Chalita MR, Chavala S, Xu M, Krueger RR. Wavefront analysis in post-LASIK eyes and its correlation with visual symptoms, refraction, and topography. Ophthalmology 2004;111:447-53.
51. Vinciguerra P, Camesasca FI, Calossi A. Statistical analysis of physiological aberrations of the cornea. J Refract Surg 2003;19:S265-9.
52. Alio J, Galal A, Montalban R, Pinero D. Corneal wavefront-guided LASIK retreatments for correction of highly aberrated corneas following refractive surgery. J Refract Surg 2007;23:760-73.
53. Alio JL, Pinero DP, Plaza Puche AB. Corneal wavefront-guided enhancement for high levels of corneal coma aberration after laser *in situ* keratomileusis. J Cataract Refract Surg 2008;34:222-31.
54. Krueger RR. Technological requirements for customized corneal ablation. In: McRae SM, Krueger RR, Applegate RA, (Eds). Customized Corneal Ablation; the Quest for SuperVision. Thorofare, NJ: Slack; 2001;133-48.
55. Dupps WJ Jr, Wilson SE. Biomechanics and wound healing in the cornea. Exp Eye Res 2006;83:709-20.
56. Roberts C. Biomechanics of the cornea and wavefront-guided laser refractive surgery. J Refract Surg 2002;18: S589-92.

19 Ocular Higher-order Aberration Induced Decrease in Vision: Aberropia

Amar Agarwal, Soosan Jacob, Dhivya A Kumar, Rahul Tiwari, Athiya Agarwal

ABERROPIA

We describe two patients who had been diagnosed to have amblyopia and underwent wavefront guided refractive surgery (Zyoptix) for correction of co-existing myopia. Both patients had a significant increase in their best corrected high contrast visual acuity (HCVA) and low contrast visual acuity (LCVA) over preoperative levels. An analysis of their pre- and postoperative higher-order aberrations (HOA) lead to the conclusion that this increase in HCVA and LCVA must have been due to an alteration in their HOA.

We propose and classify a new refractive error – aberropia which we define as a refractive error which results in a decrease in the visual acuity or quality due to HOA and which is not correctable by standard sphero-cylindrical correction. This is due to a net detrimental HOA, post-interaction between different types of aberrations so that there is deterioration in the visual performance of the patients. We also propose that selected cases of so-called "amblyopia" may actually be aberropia and these patients have the potential to gain significantly in their visual acuity on correction of aberropia.

INTRODUCTION

Astrophysicists have to be able to measure and correct the imperfect higher-order aberrations (HOA) or wavefront distortions that enter their telescopic lens system from the galaxy for perfect imaging. To achieve this purpose, adaptive optics are used wherein deformable mirrors reform the distorted wavefront to allow clear visualization of celestial objects. Extrapolating these same principles to the human eye raises the question of whether removal or alteration of the wavefront aberrations of the eye might result in a significant improvement in the preoperative best corrected visual acuity.

Prior to the advent of wavefront guided LASIK, the only parameters that could be modified to obtain optical correction for a given patient's refractive error were the sphere and cylinder. This would often not give the ideal optical correction, many a times resulting in poor visual quality in an otherwise 20/20 post-refractive surgery patient and in some patients, even resulting in a decrease in best spectacle corrected visual acuity (BSCVA). This situation is usually because of either the persistence or induction of significant amounts of higher order aberrations after LASIK.

There may therefore be a large group of patients, either with virgin eyes or post-refractive surgery, whose best corrected visual acuity (BCVA) or visual quality may actually improve significantly over preoperative levels on altering their optical aberrations. These optical aberrations are contributed to by the eye's entire optical system, i.e. the cornea, lens, vitreous and the retina.

We report two patients with subnormal visual acuity throughout their lives in the eye that underwent wavefront guided LASIK, both of whom had a significant improvement in their best corrected visual acuity to better than normal levels post-wavefront guided refractive surgery. They had both been diagnosed as being amblyopic preoperatively.

CASE REPORT

Both patients underwent routine preoperative patient evaluation including uncorrected and best corrected high and low contrast visual acuity, slit-lamp examination, applanation tonometry, manifest and cycloplegic refractions, Orbscan, aberrometry, corneal pachymetry, corneal diameter, Schirmer's test and indirect ophthalmoscopy. Patients wearing contact lenses had been asked to discontinue soft lenses for a minimum of 1 week and rigid gas permeable lenses for a minimum of 2 weeks before the preoperative examination and surgery.

The Zywave machine has a real time pupillometer setting, which can be used for measuring exact pupil size. We examined the visual acuity and aberrometry at the same mesopic pupil size. The Matlab 7.1 version software was used to generate wavefront maps (Figs 19.1A and B), the modulation transfer function (MTF) (Figs 19.2A and B), phase transfer function (PTF) (Fig. 19.2B), point spread function (PSF) (Figs 19.3A and B), and the individual polynomial RMS from the preoperative and postoperative file of zernicke coefficients (Zerfiles) at mesopic pupil size and at 6 mm pupil. Zernicke polynomial ordering was

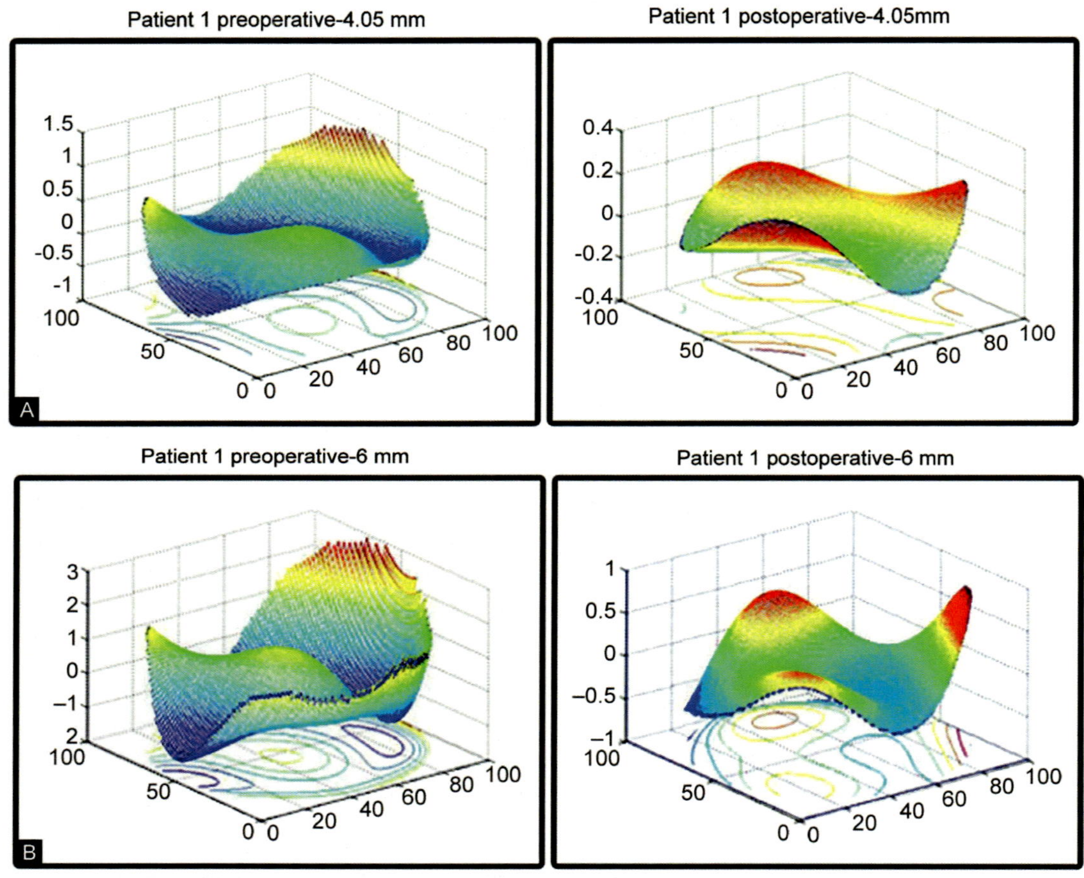

Figs 19.1A and B: Pre- and postoperative 3D wavefront maps for patient 1 for mesopic (4.05 mm) and 6 mm pupils

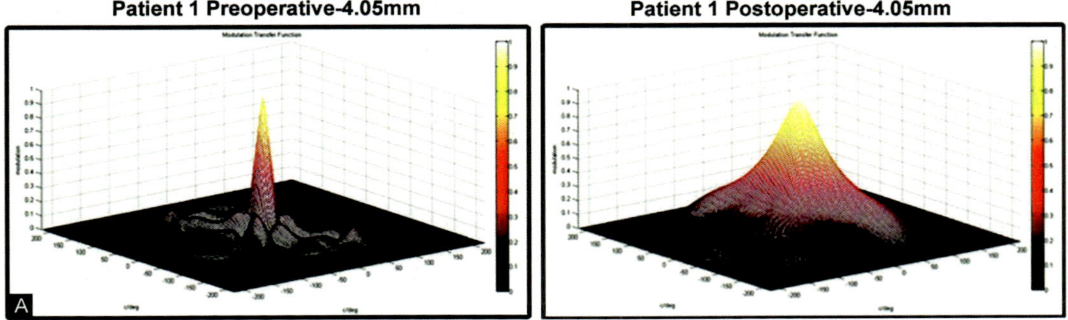

Fig. 19.2A: Pre- and postoperative modular transfer function with mesopic pupil for patient 1 showing improvement

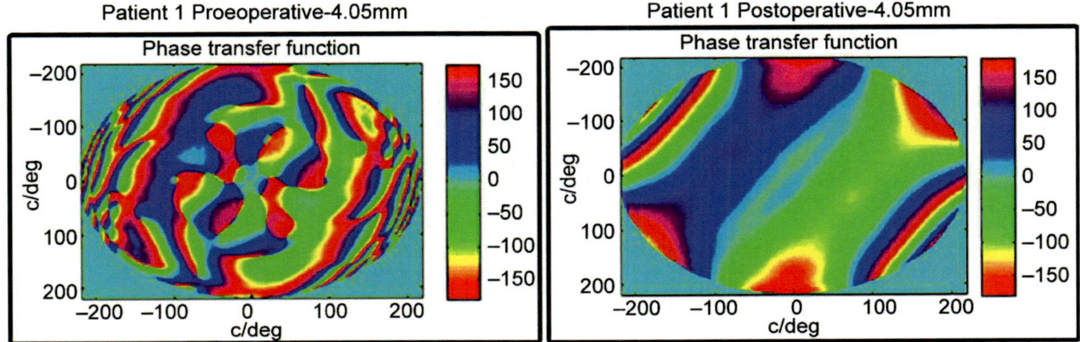

Fig. 19.2B: Pre- and postoperative phase transfer function with mesopic pupil for patient 1 showing improvement

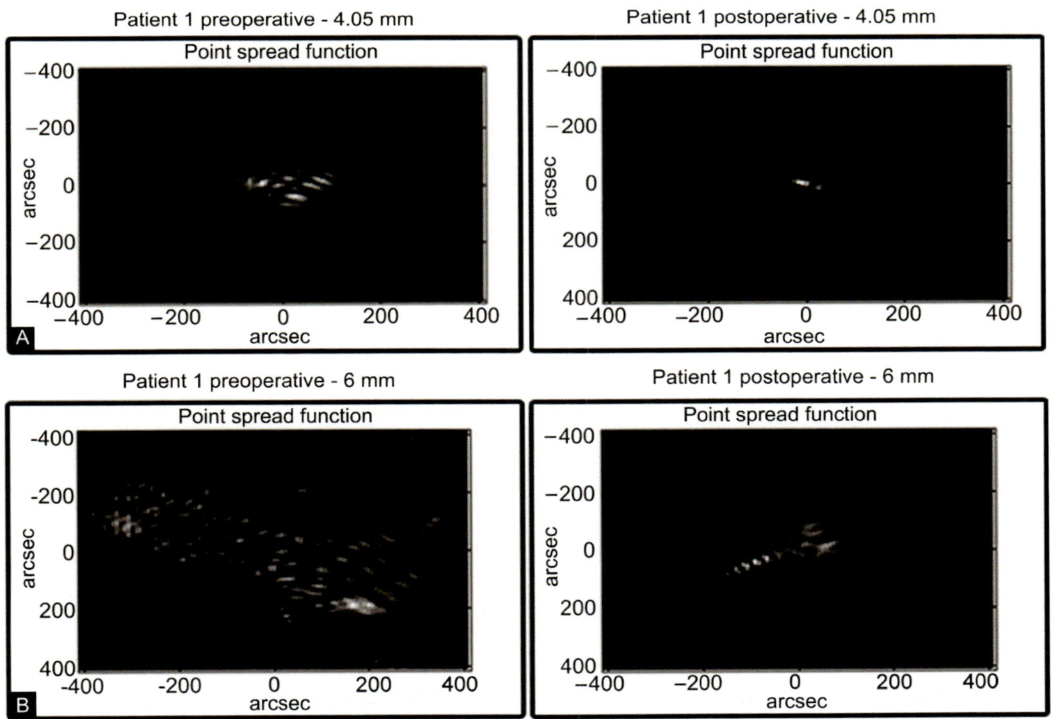

Figs 19.3A and B: Pre- and postoperative point spread function for patient 1 for mesopic (4.05 mm) and 6 mm pupils showing decrease in size

done based on OSA/VSIA standards. Strehls ratio was also calculated for preoperative and postoperative higher-order aberrations. Equivalent defocus was calculated for both mesopic pupil size and 6 mm.

Patient 1

The first patient was a 23 years old female patient with history of decreased vision in left eye (OS) never having improved to more than present levels and with history of wearing glasses since childhood. Cycloplegic refraction was –5DS/–2.5DC at 132 degrees. The uncorrected HCVA was 20/800, best corrected HCVA was 20/30 and the best corrected LCVA was 20/50, none improving further with pin hole and/or contact lens. Preoperative slit-lamp examination showed a normal anterior segment. Extraocular movements were normal and fundus evaluation showed temporal crescent and a tessellated appearance. Macula was normal.

Orbscan showed astigmatism of 1.7D at 50 degrees with irregularity coefficient ± 1.3D and ± 2D at 3 mm and 5 mm zones respectively. Central corneal thickness measured was 569 microns. Anterior segment OCT was within normal limits.

The mesopic pupil size of the patient was 4.05 mm and aberrometry was taken at this pupil size. Preoperative total RMS was 1.77 micrometers, HORMS was 0.05 micrometers, third order RMS was 0.08 and fourth order RMS was 0.04 micrometers for 4.05 mm pupil. We then dilated the pupil to 6 mm with topical phenylephrine 1 percent and again performed aberrometry.

The patient underwent wavefront guided LASIK with Zyoptix work station which includes Zywave (Hartmann Shack aberrometer with Orbscan) and Technolas 217 laser system. Postoperative uncorrected HCVA was 20/10 while the LCVA was 20/20. Orbscan showed astigmatism of 0.6 D at 70 degrees with irregularity coefficient ±1.7 D and ± 2.7D at 3 mm and 5 mm zone respectively. Central corneal thickness measured was 424 microns postoperatively. Post-operative total RMS was 0.47 micrometers, HORMS was 0.020, third order RMS was 0.038 and fourth order RMS was 0.008 microns respectively

Table 19.1: RMS, equivalent defocus and Strehl's ratio for patient 2

Patient 1 pupil diameter 4.05 mm	*Root mean square (RMS) micrometers*		*Equivalent Defocus Diopters*	
	Preoperative	*Postoperative*	*Preoperative*	*Post-operative*
Total RMS	1.77	0.470	2.988	0.795
Horms	0.05	0.020	0.091	0.034
3rd order	0.08	0.038	0.145	0.064
4th order	0.04	0.008	0.075	0.064
5th order	0.009	0.002	0.016	0.037
Strehl ratio	0.66	1.2		

(Table 19.1). At the three months postoperative follow-up examination, the patient maintained the same distance uncorrected HCVA of 20/10.

Patient 2

The second patient was a 19 years old male with history of wearing glasses since early childhood. He also gave history of visual acuity in OS never improving beyond present levels with either glasses or contact lenses since early childhood. His distance uncorrected high contrast visual acuity (HCVA) in OS measured by Snellen visual acuity chart was 20/2000 which improved to 20/40 with spectacle correction. His best spectacle corrected low contrast visual acuity (LCVA) detected by CSO digital contrast sensitivity projector was 20/60. There was no further improvement over these levels with either contact lens and/or pinhole. The cycloplegic refraction in OS was found to be –7.5DS. Anterior segment by slit-lamp evaluation was normal. Corneal topography obtained by Orbscan showed 1.6D astigmatism at 99 degrees with irregularity coefficient ±0.8D and ±1.4D at 3 mm and 5 mm zone respectively. Central corneal thickness measured was 513 microns. Anterior segment OCT was within normal limits. Fundus evaluation was within normal limits.

The mesopic pupil size of the patient was 4.18 mm. Preoperatively, total RMS was 2.34 micrometers, HORMS was 0.019 micrometers, third order RMS was

Table 19.2: RMS, equivalent defocus and Strehl's ratio for patient 1

Patient 2 pupil diameter 4.18 mm	*Root mean square (RMS) micrometers*		*Equivalent defocus Diopters*	
	Pre-operative	*Post-operative*	*Pre-operative*	*Post-operative*
Total RMS	2.343	0.47	3.716	0.744
Horms	0.019	0.017	0.0311	0.0275
3rd order	0.038	0.022	0.059	0.035
4th order	0.005	0.022	0.007	0.035
5th order	0.001	0.002	0.002	0.003
Strehl ratio	1.2	1.22		

0.038 and fourth order RMS was 0.005 micrometers before surgery.

The patient underwent wavefront guided LASIK in OS with the Zyoptix work station. On the first postoperative day, the patient's uncorrected HCVA and LCVA was 20/15 which improved to 20/10 with –0.5DS. After 2 months follow up, the patient still has best corrected HCVA of 20/10. Post operatively, the total RMS was 0.47 and HORMS was 0.017. Third order RMS and fourth order RMS were 0.022 and 0.022 microns respectively (Table 19.2). Postoperatively, his Z_0^4 showed a change from positive spherical aberration (+ 0.010) to negative spherical aberration (–0.048). Orbscan showed 0.9D at 87 degrees with irregularity coefficient ±1.1D and ± 2.8D at 3 mm and 5 mm zone respectively. Central corneal thickness measured was 402 microns.

DISCUSSION

Wave front guided LASIK is a relatively new technology which takes the patient's subjective refraction, ocular optical aberrations and corneal topography into consideration not only for diagnosis, but also for therapeutic treatment, in order to design a personalized treatment based on the total structure of the eye. The wavefront technology in Zyoptix uses the Hartmann-Shack aberrometer based on the Hartmann-Shack principle[1] demonstrated by Liang et al[2,3] to measure the ocular aberrations. The Bausch and Lomb Technolas 217 Z laser into which the topography and aberrometry data is fed provides individualized treatments set to correct lower and higher order aberrations. The treatment is mainly aberrometry based, though it also takes certain parameters such as pachymetry from the Orbscan data into account. Zernike polynomials are used to describe ocular aberrations.[4-6]

Considering our two patients, both had subnormal visual acuity but after refractive surgery, they were able to read up to 20/10. These patients had been diagnosed preoperatively as being amblyopic and therefore, it was surprising to see this improvement in their BCVA as refractive surgery in adulthood should not correct amblyopia since amblyopia functions at the cortical and not the optical level. So, was it the alteration brought about in their higher order aberrations that made possible a visual acuity that was never before experienced by the patients by any means?

We hypothesize that amongst the large sub-group of so called "amblyopia" patients, there will be a subset of patients who are not actually amblyopic but only aberropic but since ordinary testing methods do not reveal HOA and hence aberropia, the patient would have all along been mistakenly labelled as having amblyopia.

The role of higher order aberrations (HOA) in defining visual acuity has not yet been fully understood. There have been studies which state that as aberrations increase, the visual performance decreases but this study included patients with gross abnormalities such as keratoconus, penetrating keratoplasty, corneal trauma, etc.[7] and this inverse correlation between aberrations and acuity was found to much lesser in eyes over a lower aberration range.[8,9] Recently, Applegate and associates[10] found that for low levels of aberration, the root-mean-square (RMS) wavefront error is not a good predictor of visual acuity. Levy Y et al[11] also stated that the amount of ocular HOAs in eyes with natural supernormal vision (UCVA) ≥ 20/15) is not negligible, and is comparable to the reported amount of HOAs in myopic eyes.

It is important to know the effectiveness of correcting HOA in improving the visual acuity over this lower aberration range that compose the majority of normal and refractive surgery patients. Two important points should be kept in mind while considering this.[12] One is that because the magnitude of the Zernicke coefficient reflects its relative contribution to the total wavefront RMS error, it does not indicate that the largest Zernike coefficient will affect vision the most. This is because different Zernicke modes affect vision to different extents. Secondly, we also need to consider the effect of aberrations when they interact with each other. Combinations of Zernike polynomials have been known to improve or worsen visual performance.[12] Thus, some beneficial aberrations overcome the detrimental effects of other aberrations and help in reducing the point spread function from a large blur to a smaller spot of light. This interaction for the better or worse occurs independently of the increase or decrease in the total wavefront error, i.e. they may interact for the better, leading to better visual performance, despite an overall increase in the wavefront error. Analysis of the first patient's wavefront map showed an overall flattening in the central area overlying both 4 and 6 mm pupil as compared to the preoperative map which might have been responsible for the improvement in vision (Fig. 19.1). Previous studies[10] have contended that the greater the area in the center of the pupil over which the wavefront error is reasonably flat, the better the visual acuity. Patient 1 had an overall decrease in HORMS, 3rd, 4th and 5th order RMS postoperatively (Fig. 19.4).

Analysis of Patient 2 showed that though the HO-RMS and 3rd order RMS decreased slightly postoperatively, the 4th and 5th order RMS increased (Fig. 19.5). These changes in the HOA along with interaction must have been responsible for his increase in vision, both HCVA and LCVA. This interaction can especially be beautifully demonstrated by the fact that his BCVA further improved from 20/15 to 20/10 on addition of –0.5 DS. Analysis of his

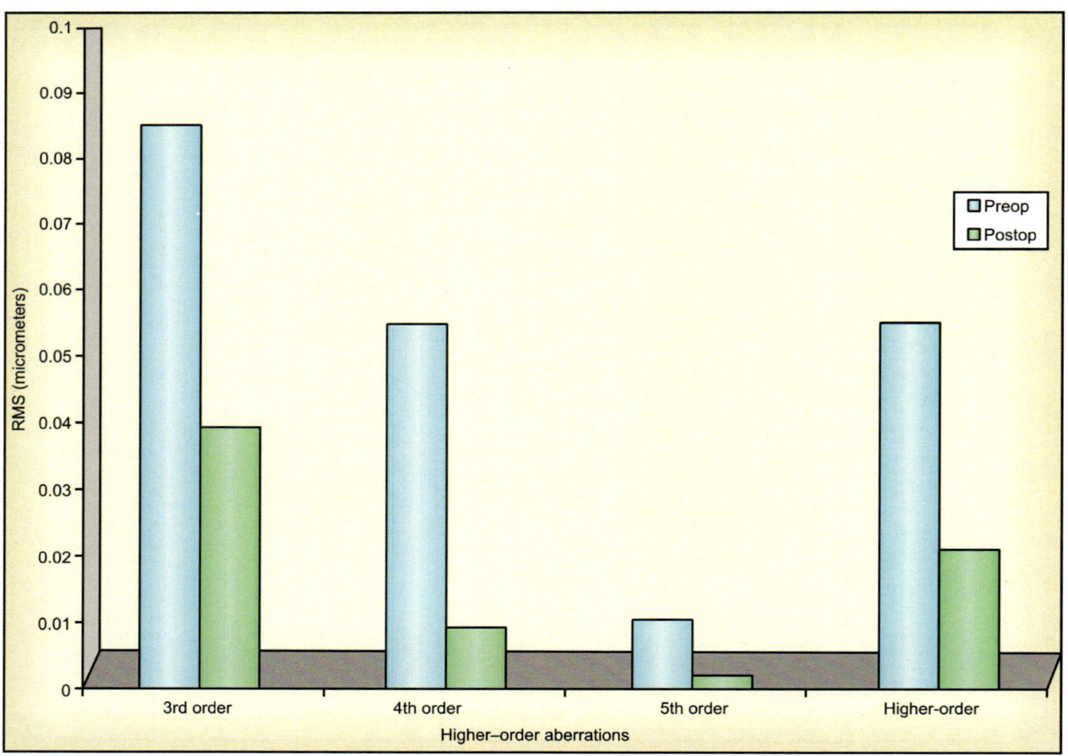

Fig. 19.4: Comparison of pre- and postoperative HOA for patient 1

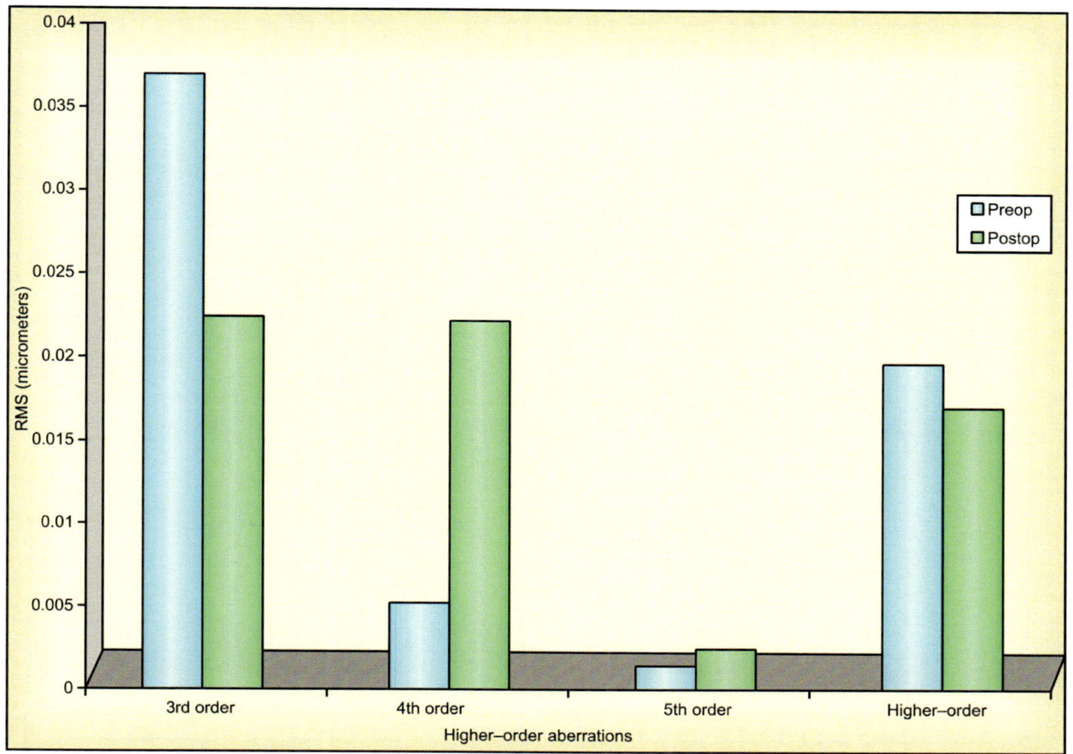

Fig. 19.5: Comparison of pre- and postoperative HOA for patient 2

postoperative wavefront map (Figs 19.6A and B) shows a predominant negative spherical aberration at both 4.18 and 6 mm pupils. Applegate et al have stated that Zernike modes with like signed coefficients 2 radial orders apart (e.g. radial orders 2 and 4) and having the same angular frequency (e.g. angular frequencies 0, –2, or 2) can interact positively[12] and this is seen well in our case.

Logically, in the perfect scenario, a zero higher order aberration would provide the best visual performance. A zero higher order aberration system is a pure diffraction limited system. In a pure diffraction limited system, Fraunhofer diffraction produces an Airy disc, the diameter of which varies inversely with the diameter of the pupil, hence the best possible vision would be obtained with a larger pupil size. Considering a similar scenario, with a zero order aberration system in the eye extending over the entire scotopic pupil size, i.e. in an aberration free, diffraction limited system, an increase in the size of the pupil would result in better visual acuity. Pupil size smaller than 3 mm would of course lead to deteriorating vision (in a pure diffraction limited aberration free system) due to Fraunhofer diffraction which leads to a larger Airy disc diameter with a smaller pupil size.

In the less than perfect but more common situation, it is an advantage to have positively interacting wavefront aberrations to cancel or neutralize the wavefront aberrations that deteriorate visual quality. In our case report, the patients had an improvement in their BCVA to never before experienced levels which could not be explained by any other reason. The patients did not postoperatively have an aberration free optics and therefore, the improved visual acuity in these patients must have been due to obtaining a set of aberrations which interacted positively to improve visual performance. The question of magnification factor improving visual acuity does not arise as these patients preoperatively did not improve with contact lenses. Further the

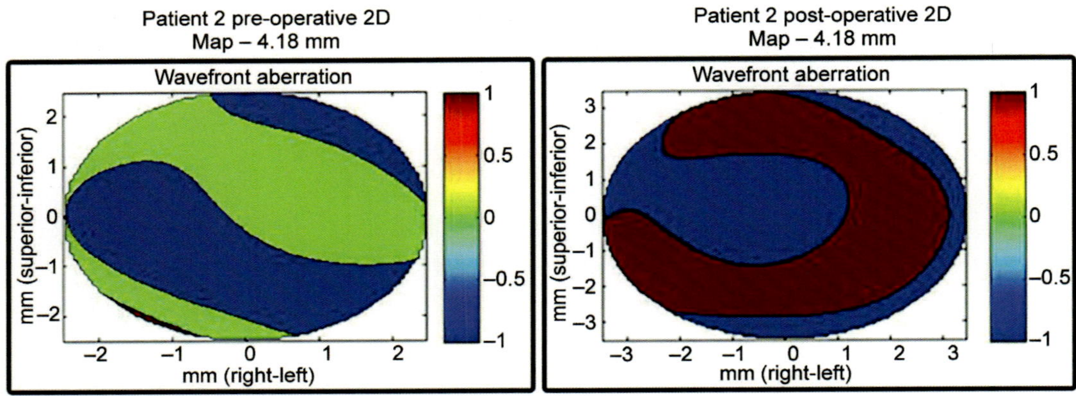

Fig. 19.6A: Comparison of pre- and postoperative 2D map at 4.18 mm (mesopic pupil)

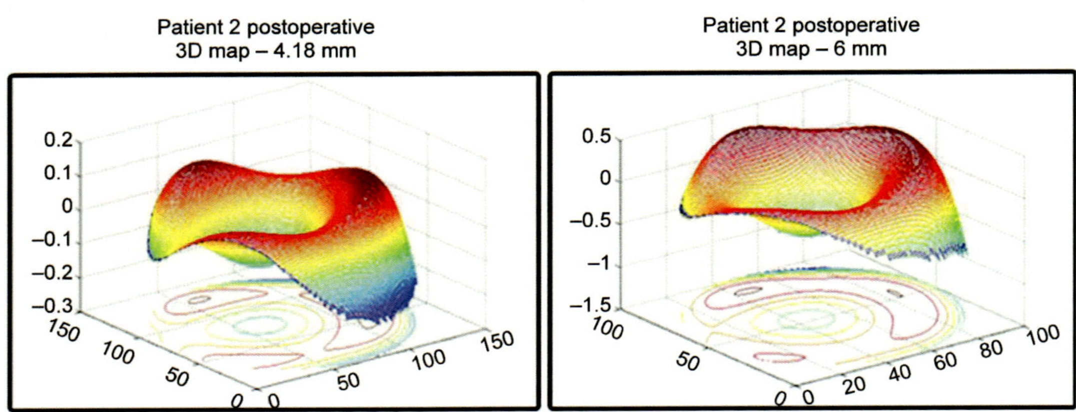

Fig. 19.6B: Postoperative 3D wavefront map at mesopic and 6 mm pupil size showing negative spherical aberration

refractive error in these patients was not very large.

Our case report included two patients with an improvement in best corrected HCVA and LCVA postrefractive surgery. Aberropia need not be limited to this but would refer to any significant improvement in the visual acuity or quality which is brought about by altering/removing the wavefront error.

Considering the reverse of these two cases, there would also be post LASIK patients who have a decrease in their best corrected visual acuity or visual quality which is not correctable by spherocylindrical combinations and which cannot be explained as being due to media opacities, such as epithelial ingrowth, etc. These could be due to decentered aberrations, central islands, etc. which are conditions that operate in the higher ranges of aberrations. There is also a group of post LASIK patients whose total wavefront error is not too large but who still do not improve with spherocylinders. These patients despite being in the lower aberration range may be having net detrimental aberrations. It might at least theoretically, be possible to treat them either by inducing aberrations which interact positively with these detrimental aberrations or more ideally, by bringing the total wavefront error to zero, i.e. making it an aberration free optics.

In healthy eyes with pupil_size more than 3.0 mm and having clear media, the wavefront error is the main contributor to image degradation. These aberrations present in the eye can be anywhere in the optical media and can be corrected at the corneal plane. Thus, correction of any significant wavefront error in patients with unexplained decreased visual performance might give them the benefit of improved visual acuity or quality. Identification of this subgroup of patients, possibly with preoperative testing with customized wavefront glasses, adaptive optics or some other such modality might allow one to perform customized wavefront guided LASIK and if the treatment is applied over at least the scotopic pupil size, it should neutralize their optical aberrations and allow them improved visual performance. It would be necessary to develop ways of testing these patients in the clinical set-up.

Of course, it is true that getting the best possible optical system and consecutively the best possible retinal image is only the first step in the entire process of visual perception. Limitations are still imposed by the neural transfer function and the sensory system which exists right from the photoreceptors to the cortical level. Also, it has been proposed that each person is adapted to his/her own aberrations (neuroadaptation) and so, the visual acuity with the person's original, less than perfect wavefront may still be better than the visual acuity obtained with a changed but better wavefront.[13]

But would this mean that presenting a better optical sytem would degrade visual quality in every patient? In our two patients, neuroadaptation as well as limits imposed by the neural transfer function would have been expected to bring about an increase in vision to preoperative best corrected visual acuity and not any better than that. The fact that these patients gained significantly in their lines of vision to levels never before experienced by the patient shows that this must have been due to the alteration brought about in their wavefront.

In the present day scenario, with the current limitations in wavefront guided treatment platforms as well as techniques, one may not be totally successful in trying to correct or alter the higher-order aberrations during refractive surgery. But in the future, with greater technological advances, if one can precisely determine preoperatively using either adaptive optics or any other newer modalities which may become available in the future as to what type of correction if applied would lead to an improved or enhanced visual outcome and if the technology for extremely precise application of this wavefront correction to the patients cornea can be developed, then it would definitely be worthwhile to try and do a wavefront "correcting" refractive surgery for every patient. Further research is required to make this kind of wavefront correction a reality and this would be possible only by further improvements in diagnostic modalities as well as refinements in the present wavefront guided LASIK systems available.

We have proposed two systems of classification for this newly defined refractive error based on the etiology and also on the magnitude of aberropia. These are shown in Tables 19.3 and 19.4.

Keeping all these facts in mind, we venture forwards to propose a new refractive error –

Table 19.3: Classification of aberropia based on etiology

I. Congenital aberropia

Here, the person is born with these aberrations. If unilateral and large enough to interfere with normal binocular interaction between the two eyes, these could possibly lead to amblyopia in that eye.[16,17]

II. Acquired aberropia

- A. Post-surgical
  - a. Corneal:
    - i. Post-penetrating keratoplasty
    - ii. Post-refractive surgery
  - b. Lenticular:
    - i. IOL induced aberrations: either inherent in the IOL or due to malpositioned IOL
    - ii. Aberrations due to capsular abnormalities
- B. Others
  - a. Corneal:
    - i. Keratoconus and other ectatic disorders
    - ii. Corneal trauma, scars, etc.
    - iii. Other causes of irregular astigmatism
  - b. Lenticular:
    - i. Incipient cataract
    - ii. Lenticonus
    - iii. Subluxated lens, coloboma lens
  - c. Vitreous: Vitreous opacities and floaters
  - d. Retinal:
    - i. Thickened posterior hyaloid
    - ii. Very fine ERMs not causing traction on the retina

Table 19.4: Classification of aberropia based on magnitude

Higher range aberropia: Keratoconus, post-penetrating keratoplasty, corneal trauma, lenticonus, etc. Here the visual performance has a good correlation with the amount of higher order aberrations.

Lower range aberropia: Majority of normal and refractive surgery patients, where the correlation between the range of aberrations and the visual performance is no longer present. This loss of correlation is due also to interaction between the different aberrations besides other factors such as neural transfer function, etc.

aberropia which was first published by us in 2002.[14-17] We define this as a refractive error which results in a decrease in the visual quality that can be attributable to higher order aberrations.[18] This is either due to the helpful aberrations being inadequate in overcoming the detrimental aberrations or due to a situation where there are only detrimental aberrations present in the eye. Thus, we have coined this term for a refractive error which is due to a net detrimental HOA, post-interaction between different types of aberrations. Correction of this refractive error could be by changing the different aberrations so that they interact differently, thus having a net effect of clear visual performance despite the fact that the total wavefront error is not zero. Correction could also be achieved by bringing down the total wavefront error to zero. Both these situations would yield improved visual performance. Extremely asymmetric HOA between the two eyes during the period of plasticity of the visual system could similarly lead to aberropia induced amblyopia[18-20] (Table 19.3).

All this does cause one to think what happens when a person with aberropia who is treated presents with age related changes in his wavefront aberrations, either due to loss of accommodation or due to lens changes or any other causes. This would be similar to the present day problem of calculating IOL power for post LASIK patients. One may have to treat the patient further for his/her wavefronts or use customized wavefront glasses, contact lenses or even IOLs. There may also develop in the future, some newer modality of optical correction utilizing adaptive optics as done in astrophysics at present.

CONCLUSION

We know that not all wavefront aberrations may be bad for the eye and that these aberrations may sometimes interact positively or negatively to increase or decrease visual performance. We propose a new refractive entity – aberropia, where there is a net negative interaction between the higher order aberrations so that there is deterioration in the visual performance of the patients. We hypothesize that selected cases of unexplained poor vision and so called "amblyopia" maybe actually be due to aberropia and that these are treatable and these patients can obtain an improvement in the BCVA/ visual quality. Thus, similar to the conventional "hyperopia", "myopia" and "astigmatism" which are corrected with spherocylinders, it is only logical that this HOA induced loss of vision would be a new refractive entity – aberropia, which could be correctable by removing or altering these aberrations.

This new field definitely needs a lot of research before attaining its full potential but as research has always been stimulated by what has not been fully understood, and as identification is the first step towards understanding, it is essential that we first recognize and identify aberropia as a new refractive error and try to understand it fully so that all venues are opened for obtaining, not supervision in terms of 20/10 or better, but the best possible vision that is optically possible for a particular person. It will be interesting to see what the future holds.

REFERENCES

1. Platt B, Shack RV. Lenticular Hartmann screen. Opt Sci Center News (University of Arizona) 1971;5:15-6.
2. Liang J, Grimm B, Goelz S, Bille J. Objective measurement of the wave aberrations of the human eye with the use of a Hartmann-Shack wavefront sensor. J Opt Soc Am 1994;11:1949-57.
3. Liang J, Williams DR, et al. Aberrations and retinal image quality of the normal human eye. J Opt Soc Am A 1997; 14(11):2873-83.

4. Thibos LN, Applegate RA, Schwiegerling JT, Webb R. Standards for reporting the optical aberrations of eyes; VSIA Standards Taskforce Members. OSA Trends in Optics Photonics 2000;35:232-44.
5. MacRae SM, Krueger RR, Applegate RA. Customized Corneal Ablation: the Quest for Supervision. Thorofare, NJ, Slack, 2001; appendix 1:347-61.
6. Thibos LN, Applegate RA, Schwiegerling JT, Webb R. Standards for reporting the optical aberrations of eyes. J Refract Surg 2002;18:S652-61.
7. Applegate RA, Hilmantel G, Howland HC, et al. Corneal first surface optical aberrations and visual performance. J Refract Surg 2000;16:507-14.
8. Hong X, Thibos LN, Bradley A, et al. Impact of monochromatic aberrations on polychromatic image quality and vision. Invest Ophthalmol Vis Sci 2001;42(suppl): S162.
9. Cheng X, Bradley A, Hong X, Thibos LN. Relationship between refractive error and monochromatic aberrations of the eye. Optom Vis Sci 2003;80:43-9.
10. Applegate RA, Marsack JD, Ramos R, Sarver EJ. Interaction between aberrations to improve or reduce visual performance. J Cataract Refract Surg 2003;29:1487-95.
11. Levy Y, Segal O, Avni I. Ocular higher order aberrations in eyes with supernormal vision. AJO 2005;139:225-8.
12. Applegate RA, Sarver EJ, Khemsara V. Are all aberrations equal? J Refract Surg 2002;18:S556-62.
13. Artal P, Chen Li, Fernandez EJ, et al. Neural compensation for the eye's optical aberrations. Journal of Vision 2004;4:281-7.
14. Agarwal A, Jacob S, Agarwal A, et al. Aberropia: a new refractive entity. Ocular Surgery News, US Edition, 2002; 20(19):14-9.
15. Agarwal A, Jacob S, Kanjani N, et al. Aberropia: A New Refractive Entity. In: Boyd BF, Agarwal A (Eds). Wavefront Analysis, Aberrometers and Corneal Topography. Panama, Republic of Panama: Highlights of Ophthalmology International; 2003;333-42.
16. Aberropia: A new Refractive Entity. Highlights of Ophthalmology. Indian Edition 2003;1:29-35.
17. Chalita MR, Krueger RR. Refractive Surgery In: Agarwal A (Ed). Handbook of Ophthalmology. Thorofare, NJ: Slack Incorporated 2006;630-2.
18. Agarwal A, Jacob S, Agarwal A. Aberropia: A new refractive entity. JCRS (In Press).
19. Prakash G, Sharma N, Chowdhary V, et al. Association between amblyopia and higher-order aberrations. J Cataract Refract Surg 2007;33:901-04.
20. de Faber. Higher-order aberrations: Explanation of idiopathic amblyopia? J Cataract Refract Surg 2007; 33:753.

SECTION FOUR

LASIK, Customised LASIK and Femtosecond Laser

20 Predictive Formulas for LASIK

Louis E Probst, Jonathan Woolfson, Michiel Kritzinger

INTRODUCTION

The predictive formulas for laser-in-situ keratomileusis (LASIK) have two components: (i) *the excimer laser ablation nomogram*, and (ii) the *adjustment factors*. The excimer laser ablation nomogram controls the relative distribution of the refraction correction into one or more zones. In some of the newer excimer lasers such as the Visx Star, the excimer ablation nomogram is controlled by the laser's computer, while in other excimer lasers such as the Chiron Technolas 116, the ablation nomogram is fully programmable by the surgeon. The adjustment factors allow surgeons to refine the treatment protocol to reflect their particular refractive situation. For these formulas to be predictive, a high level of consistency must be achieved in the application of both the ablation nomograms and adjustment factors. Other extraneous variables such as the methods of preoperative refraction, the room temperature and humidity, and room air quality and flow, surgical technique and time, and the postoperative medications must be tightly controlled to avoid deviations from the intended correction.

It is crucial to remember that the predictive formulas including both the excimer laser ablation nomogram and the adjustment factors must be individualized for each surgeon. Direct extrapolations from the experience of one surgeon or one center will likely lead to an unexpected deviation of the surgical results from emmetropia. Since it is impossible to control every aspect of surgery, each surgeon must develop his or her own predictive formula once his or her technique has become standardized and his or her postoperative result can be analyzed. For the novice LASIK surgeon, conservative corrections are preferable as enhancements are easy to perform while overcorrections can be much more challenging.

Once the excimer ablation nomogram and the adjustment factors have been standardized and individualized for each excimer laser surgeon, the final uncontrolled variable with LASIK is the healing pattern of the cornea. While there is a clear tendency for greater amounts of regression after LASIK for higher levels of myopia, often the degree of regression after LASIK is unpredictable. Younger patients (< 25 years) often demonstrate significant regression while older patients (> 50 years) may not regress at all. **We have often observed regression of 1.0 to 2.0 D in one eye and no regression in the other eye after bilateral simultaneous LASIK in which the excimer nomogram, the adjustment factors, surgical technique, and extraneous variables were all exactly the same for the correction of both eyes. This unpredictable healing pattern of the cornea represents the limitation of corneal refractive surgery.** In order to avoid LASIK overcorrections, it is best to plan for a 10 to 20 percent enhancement rate for lower myopes and even higher rates with high myopes, which will allow retreatment for those patients that have regressed.

EXCIMER LASER ABLATION NOMOGRAMS FOR PHOTOREFRACTIVE KERATECTOMY

The excimer laser nomograms for LASIK have been developed from the excimer LASIK experience with photorefractive keratectomy (PRK). The concepts of laser pretreatment to prevent central islands and multizone ablations to decrease ablation depth and smooth the laser contour evolved as the worldwide PRK experience as well as the technological capabilities of the excimer lasers increased.

Pretreatment Protocols

Pretreatment protocols have been added to the ablation profiles of the broad beam excimer lasers such as the Visx Star, Summit Omnimed, and Chiron Technolas Keracor 116 to reduce the incidence of postoperative central islands.[1] The Visx Star pretreatment is automatically calculated by the central island factor (CIF) 4.01 software and incorporated into the excimer ablation protocol. Approximately 1 micron per diopter of spherical correction plus an additional 2 microns is added to each ablation protocol and is performed at 2.5 mm. The Chiron Technolas Keracor 116 pretreatment is surgeon programmable. Generally, 1 micron per diopter plus 2 to 4 microns is added to each ablation protocol and is performed at 3.0 mm.[2] The Summit Omnimed excimer laser has a gaussian beam distribution for which a relatively greater amount of laser energy is produced in the center of the ablation circle, so less pretreatment is required. A pretreatment of 1 to 2 microns per diopter is generally performed using the patient training "A" mode with optical zone of 2.6 to 2.8 mm. The newer scanning excimer laser systems such as the Chiron Technolas 217 excimer laser do not need pretreatment protocols as this phenomena of undertreatment of the central cornea is avoided with these scanning laser systems

Single and Multizone Ablation Protocols

All excimer laser refractive procedures modify the refracting power of the cornea by altering the anterior corneal curvature by the process of photoablation. The correction of myopia involves the relative flattening of the central cornea compared to the peripheral cornea, which reduces the anterior corneal curvature, hence, reduces the refractive power of the treated area. Because the maximal corneal stromal tissue will be photoablated from the central cornea, the thickness of the central cornea becomes important when LASIK is performed for high refractive errors with large ablation depths.

Many excimer ablation techniques have evolved. The initial single zone techniques increased from 4.0 to 6.0 mm,[3,4] to improve the quality of the postoperative vision and reduce the incidence of halos and regression. The multipass multizone technique was developed by Mihai Pop, for the Visx excimer laser[5,6] and the multi-multizone technique was developed by Jeffery J Machat, for the Chiron Technolas excimer laser.[1] **These multizone techniques divide the myopic treatment into multiple zones, which decreases the ablation depth and creates a smoother ablation surface.** This blending and smoothing effect of the mutlizone protocols has helped to reduce the incidence of post-PRK regression and haze particularly for the treatment of high myopia.[6]

Recently, Alpins *et al*[7] from the Melbourne Excimer Laser Group have compared the algorithms and results of three different multizones (Tables 20.1 to 20.3) PRK ablation programs designed for the Visx 20/20 excimer laser. While each algorithm had a maximum ablation zone of 6.0 mm, they differed in the number of zones employed, the proportion of treatment assigned to each zone, and the treatment of astigmatism. The Melbourne multizone equally divided the treatment into a maximum of three zones at 4.5, 5.0, and 6.0 mm. The Pop multizone technique utilized a pretreatment with treatment bias for the smaller zones to a maximum of six zones at 3.5, 4.0, 4.5, 5.0, 5.5, and 6.0 mm. The Alpins multizone technique also utilized a pretreatment and equally divided the treatment up to a maximum of six zones at 3.5, 4.0, 4.5, 5.0, 5.5, and 6.0 mm. Although all the algorithms were effective in the reduction of myopia, statistical analysis indicated that the Alpins multizone

Table 20.1: Melbourne excimer laser group multizone PRK treatment algorithm

	Diopters at corneal plane															
Ablation zone (mm)	−3	−4	−5	−6	−7	−8	−9	−10	−11	−12	−13	−14	−15	−16	−17	−18
4.5	–	–	–	–	–	–	–	–	−3.67	−4	−4.33	−4.67	−5	−5.33	−5.67	−6
5.0	–	–	–	−3	−3.5	−4	−4.5	−5	−3.67	−4	−4.33	−4.67	−5	−5.33	−5.67	−6
6.0	−3	−4	−5	−3	−3.5	−4	−4.5	−5	−3.67	−4	−4.33	−4.67	−5	−5.33	−5.67	−6

Table 20.2: Pop multizone PRK treatment algorithm

	Diopters at corneal plane															
Ablation zone (mm)	*−3*	*−4*	*−5*	*−6*	*−7*	*−8*	*−9*	*−10*	*−11*	*−12*	*−13*	*−14*	*−15*	*−16*	*−17*	*−18*
2.5 (pre-treatment)	−1.5	−1.5	−1.5	−1.5	−1.5	−1.5	−1.5	−1	−1	−1	−1	−1	−1	−1	−1	−1
3.5	–	–	–	–	–	–	–	–	–	–	–	–	–	–	−4	−4
4	–	–	–	–	–	–	–	–	−4	−4	−4	−4	−4	−4	−4	−4
4.5	–	–	–	−3	−4	−4	−4	−4	−2	−2	−3	−4	−3	−4	−2	−2
5	–	−2	−3	−1	−1	−2	−2	−2	−2	−2	−2	−2	−2	−2	−2	−2
5.5	−2	−1	−1	−1	−1	−1	−2	−2	−2	−2	−2	−2	−2	−2	−2	−2
6	−1	−1	−1	−1	−1	−1	−1	−2	−1	−1	−1	−2	−2	−2	−2	−2

Table 20.3: Alpins multizone PRK treatment algorithm

	Diopters at corneal plane															
Ablation zone (mm)	−3	−4	−5	−6	−7	−8	−9	−10	−11	−12	−13	−14	−15	−16	−17	−18
2.5 (pre-treatment)	−1.5	−1.5	−1.5	−1.5	−1.5	−1.5	−1.5	−1	−1	−1	−1	−1	−1	−1	−1	−1
3.5	–	–	–	–	–	–	–	–	–	–	–	–	–	−2.67	−2.83	−3
4	–	–	–	–	–	–	–	–	–	–	−2.6	−2.8	−3	−2.67	−2.83	−3
4.5	–	–	–	–	–	–	–	−2.5	−2.75	−3	−2.6	−2.8	−3	−2.67	−2.83	−3
5	–	–	–	–	−2.33	−2.67	−3	−2.5	−2.75	−3	−2.6	−2.8	−3	−2.67	−2.83	−3
5.5	–	−2	−2.5	−3	−2.33	−2.67	−3	−2.5	−2.75	−3	−2.6	−2.8	−3	−2.67	−2.83	−3
6	−3	−2	−2.5	−3	−2.33	−2.67	−3	−2.5	−2.75	−3	−2.6	−2.8	−3	−2.67	−2.83	−3

algorithm achieved better visual acuity and refractive results.

EXCIMER LASER ABLATION NOMOGRAMS FOR LASIK

The creation of the corneal flap and the routine correction of higher levels of myopia with LASIK introduced new considerations into the excimer nomograms. The depth of the ablation and the size of the ablation zones have become recognized as crucial consideration to achieve a good quality and quantity of correction while maintaining the safety of the procedure and the stability of the cornea. If all of these factors are considered, LASIK has correction limits of 10 to 15 D of myopia depending on which ablation nomogram is used.

Basic Tenets of LASIK

There are four critical values or dimensions that must be considered when performing LASIK which are: (i) the flap thickness, (ii) the amount of residual corneal stroma, (iii) the diameter of the excimer ablation, and (iv) the depth of the excimer ablation. These values determine the key concepts of LASIK which are the safety and stability of the procedure, and the quality and quantity of the laser correction (Doane JF, Nordan LT, Baker RN *et al:* Basic tenets of lamellar refractive surgery. Unpublished course material).

The *flap thickness* must be sufficient to prevent irregular astigmatism while not so excessive to remove stroma potentially available for ablation. We generally use a 160 mm flap for thin corneas or large refractive corrections (> 10.0 D), a 180 mm flap for average corneas and moderate corrections (> 6.0 D), and a 200 mm flap for thick corneas and small corrections (≤ 6.0 D). Sufficient *residual posterior stroma* must be left after the LASIK procedure to avoid a decrease of the corneal integrity and the subsequent development of corneal ectasia. Since iatrogenic keratoconus has been observed after automated lamellar keratoplasty (ALK) with 200 mm of remaining posterior stromal tissue, we generally elect to leave at least 250 mm of posterior stromal tissue. The *diameter* of the excimer ablation should be at least 6.0 mm to create a functional postoperative optical zone of at least 4.0 mm which will allow for sufficient *quality* of vision. Finally, the *depth* of the excimer ablation determines the *quantity* of myopia that can be safely treated while preserving adequate residual corneal stroma.

Ablation Depth Per Diopter

Each excimer laser ablates a different amount of stromal tissue per diopter of refractive correction because of the differences in the ablation zone diameters, amount of pretreatment, and the ablation protocols. **The Munnerlyn formula[8] (depth of ablation = diopters of correction × ablation diameter^2 ÷ 3) indicates that each spherical equivalent (SE) diopter of myopic correction performed at a 6.0 mm *single zone* will ablate 12 microns of tissue.** Pretreatment protocols added to the ablation profile of broad beam excimer lasers such as the Visx Star and the Chiron Technolas Keracor 116 will increase the depth per SE diopter to 17 to 20 microns for low corrections (1-2 diopters) and 15 to 17 microns for higher corrections (3 or more diopters). The Summit Omnimed will ablate 13.0 to 14.0 microns per SE diopter for all levels of myopia with pretreatment.

The *multipass multizone* ablation technique used with Visx Star "international cards" has an average stromal ablation of 12.5 microns per SE diopter. The *full multi-multizone* ablation technique with the ablation pattern distributed between 3.6 and 6.2 mm reduces the average stromal ablation to approximately 10 microns per SE diopter.[1] While the *full multi-multizone* protocol significantly reduces ablation depth, it should only be used for LASIK when necessitated by a thin cornea associated with high myopia because of the compromised quality of postoperative night vision.

Correction Limits for Primary LASIK

The average central corneal thickness is approximately 550 ± 100 mm.[9] Since the flap thickness during the LASIK procedure is generally 160 mm, the average cornea will have 390 mm of posterior stromal bed left after the flap creation. Therefore, the maximal myopic correction that should be performed on a patient with a 550 mm cornea using a *full multi-multizone* technique is generally less than 14 D while leaving a residual posterior stromal bed of 250 microns. A partial multizone ablation as performed with the Chiron Technolas 116 and the Visx Star would allow a maximal correction of approximately 12.0 D, and a single zone ablation would allow a maximal myopic correction of 10.0 D.[10]

VISX STAR: PREDICTIVE FORMULAS FOR LASIK

The Visx Star utilizes a propriety multizone nomogram developed from the PRK multizone experience with the Visx 20/20 excimer laser. A pretreatment is combined with a multizone ablation that is not surgeon programmable. While this limits the flexibility of the laser for adjusting ablation zone size, which would be beneficial for patients with large pupils, it does reduce the variation in the techniques of surgeons and therefore allows for good comparisons between centers.

Early in the LASIK experience with the Visx Star excimer laser, it became clear that this laser would tend to overcorrect if the unmodified PRK correction was utilized for LASIK. Surgeons developed "adjustment factors" that were used to modify the refractive correction before it was programmed into the excimer laser in order to avoid overcorrections. These values usually involved reduction in the value of the spherical component of the refraction by 10 to 30 percent.

Any number of factors may contribute to the increased effectiveness of the Visx Star excimer laser when used for LASIK. The vacuum nozzle of this machine may decrease stromal hydration, increasing the effect of the excimer ablation. The slower pulse frequency may allow the cornea to dehydrate. Surgeon factors such as the time taken to perform the procedure and the methods of drying the cornea have also been considered.

Once several centers gained more experience with the Visx Star laser patterns, a pattern began to emerge regarding the "adjustment factors". The nomograms for 15 surgeons that have performed more than 500 LASIK procedures each on the Visx Star laser were compared (Table 20.4). The range of the myopia treated and the enhancement rates were recorded to ensure that most surgeons were achieving a similar level of predictability with their procedures. The temperature room and the humidity range of the procedure rooms did not correlate with the adjustment factors used at each center. Most surgeons did not use drying techniques.

The altitude emerged however as a consistent factor that seemed to be related to the adjustment factor. When the two factors were correlated it was found that there was a statistically significant correlation between the altitude of the refractive center and the surgeon spherical adjustment factor ($r = 0.75$, $n = 15$, $p = 0.002$, slope 0.0032). This allows us to calculate that a city with an altitude at sea level such as New York should be using an adjustment factor of 12.8 percent, while Denver at an altitude of 5280 feet should have an adjustment factor of 29.7 percent ($12.8 + 0.0032 \times 5280$).

This variation in the effectiveness of the excimer laser at different altitudes is probably a function of the changes in air density. The Ideal Gas Law solved for density is $D=P/(T \times R)$ where D is the air density, P is the station pressure at the altitude of the refractive center, T is the temperature in Kelvin, and R is the gas constant. Increased humidity will actually decrease the air density, however, its effect on the air density is minimal and most refractive centers have humidity control systems installed. Temperature is usually well controlled so it is unlikely that this would introduce significant variation in results. The station pressure is the direct barometer reading. Two variables affect the barometer reading, the air pressure of the weather systems and the altitude of the center, which will decrease the air pressure significantly at higher altitudes. While we currently adjust the spherical component of the Visx Star ablation by a constant value that seems to be related to altitude, perhaps our adjustments in the future will be based on the daily barometric reading and the corresponding calculations of air density.

VISX S2 SMOOTHSCAN: PREDICTIVE FORMULAS FOR LASIK

The adjustment factors utilized for the Visx S2 Smoothscan excimer laser upgrade are very similar to those used for the Visx Star laser. Most surgeons have made only minor adjustments to their Visx Star reduction factor. Increasing the frequency of the excimer pulse to 10 Hz reduces the laser time by almost 50 percent but does not affect the degree of refractive correction. The spherical reduction factor that we currently utilize at TLC, Chicago is outlined (Table 20.5).

Table 20.4: Nomogram comparison table

Location	*ENH Rate (Percentage)*	*Preop MR Range (–)*	*Altitude*	*Temp Range*	*Humidity Range*	*Drying*	*Age Adjust*	*Sphere Adjust (–) (Percentage)*	*Cylinder Adjust (–)*
Tulsa, OK	21	1.00 to 16	711	60 to 65	30 to 40	None	No	10	No
Oklahoma city, OK	10	1.00 to 17	1208	65 to 70	40 to 60	None	No	20	No
Garden city, NY	15	1.00 to 16	0	65 to 76	30 to 60	Subjective	Yes	Sliding: 14-18	10%
Seattle, WA	5	1.00 to 15	260	60 to 65	30 to 40	None	No	7.70	No
Brea, CA	8	0.75 to 13.75	650	65 to 70	45 to 50	Periodic	No	8	No
Indianapolis, IN	8	1.00 to 15	770	60 to 65	35 to 40	Periodic	Yes	20	No
Denver, CO	25	1.00 to 20	5280	60 to 65	35 to 45	None	No	30	No
Rockville, MD	15	0.75 to 16	0	60 to 65	35 to 40	None	Yes	Sliding: 15-20	No
Fairfax, VA	15	0.75 to 16	0	60 to 65	35 to 40	None	Yes	Sliding: 15-20	No
New york, NY	10	0.50 to 22	15	65 to 68	30 to 35	None	Yes	Sliding: 10-20	No
Charlotte, NC	15	1.00 to 16	765	65 to 70	35 to 40	None	No	15	No
Rockville, MD	7	1.00 to 16	0	60 to 65	35 to 40	None	Yes	15	10
Fairfax, VA	7	1.00 to 16	0	60 to 65	35 to 40	None	Yes	15	10
Greenville, SC	10	1.00 to 16	950	65 to 70	35 to 50	Subjective	No	10	No
Johnson city, TN	10	1.00 to 16	1700	65 to 70	30 to 45	Subjective	No	20	No

Table 20.5: Probst Nomogram for Visx S2 SmoothScan

	< 25 years	*25–45 years*	*> 45 years*
< 2.0 D myopia	100%	100%	100%
> 2.0 D myopia	90%	86%	84%

For hyperopic corrections, we utilize the 5.0 mm optical zone with a 9.0 mm blendzone for hyperopic LASIK with the Hansatome. For hyperopes, we add between 10 and 20 percent to the spherical refractive error to account for the greater amount of regression that occurs with the treatment of hyperopia.

CHIRON TECHNOLAS 116: PREDICTIVE FORMULAS FOR LASIK

With the Chiron Technolas 116, the ideal zone depth for each step of the multizone LASIK ablation was initially felt to be 15 to 20 mm to create the smoothest blended multizone ablation[2] (Table 20.6). This algorithm was similar to those used for PRK and provided a smooth blend of the myopic ablation with zones that extended from 3.6 mm to 6.2 mm for maximum seven zones. This full multizone ablation allowed the treatment of high levels of myopia as the total ablation depth was minimized with the smaller zone size. Unfortunately, the smaller zone sizes resulted in a significant reduction in the effective optical zone observed on corneal topography following LASIK. High myopes treated with the full multizone algorithm demonstrated effectively an optical zone that was often less than 4.0 mm. Clinically, this resulted in complaints of visual distortion and halos at night in the same manner in which the early small zone PRK ablations were associated with these difficulties. Decentrations are poorly tolerated with the small zone ablations as the refracted light for the edge of the ablation could be in close proximity to the visual axis.

Machat has found that the size of the ablation zones should be increased so that most of the treatment is performed at a 5.5 mm or larger ablation zone.[11] This increases the depth of ablation to 30 to 40 mm per zone in the *partial multi-multizone* protocol which accounts for the hydration effects of the deeper stroma

Table 20.6. Previous Machat Chiron 116: LASIK nomogram for high myopia

Important points

- No vertex distance correction.
- Pretreatment 1 micron per diopter plus 2 to 4 microns total
- Depth at 3 mm for Chiron Technolas Keracor 116 to compensate for central island formation.
- All treatment zones of equal depth (not including pretreatment step)
- All zones ideally between 15 and 20 microns
- Goal is to achieve at least 6–mm effective optical zone
- Compressed air is used intraoperatively to control hydration.

LASIK nomogram for –13 D attempted correction

Optical zone	*Dioptric distribution*	*Percentage of treatment*	*Micron depth*
3 mm	–5.4 D	Pretreatment (1 μm/D + 3)	16
3.6 mm	–3.63 D	27.9	17
4.2 mm	–.258 D	18.9	17
4.8 mm	–1.90 D	14.6	17
5.4 mm	–1.46 D	11.2	17
5.8 mm	–1.23 D	9.5	17
6 mm	–1.14 D	8.8	17
6.2 mm	–1.06 D	8.15	17

Eight zones of equal micron depth. Each zone 0.6 mm larger than the previous zone, with two additional zones within 0.2 mm of 6-mm optical zone to ensure adequate peripheral blend for reduced spherical aberration and night visual disturbances.

and the masking effect of the corneal flap. By increasing the size and depth of ablation of each zone to 30 to 40 mm and decreasing the number of zones, the effective postoperative optical zone on videokeratography can be increased, and night vision difficulties minimized (Table 20.7). This *partial multi-multizone* ablation that we now use for LASIK ablations removes 12.5 microns of stroma per SE diopter. While the quality of the night vision is improved with these new algorithms, the depth of ablation per diopter must be increased with the corresponding increase in zone size. This limits the quantity of myopia that can be safely corrected to approximately 15.0 D in an eye with an average corneal thickness.

Table 20.7: TLC the laser center: Chiron 116 nomogram

Correction	*Pretreatment*	*Percentage*	*Zone diameter*	*Zone depth*	*Total depth*
0–3.5		100	6.5		
–3.50		54.5	6.1		
		45.5	6.6		
–5.75	3.1@3	60	5.5	41.25	
		40	6.6	42	91
–6	–3.15@ 3	60	5.5	43.25	
		40	6.6	43.75	97
–6.5	–3.35@ 3	60	5.5	46.75	
		40	6.6	47.25	104.25
7	–3.5@3	41	5.5	34.5	
		32	6.1	34	
		27	6.6	34.5	114
–7.5	–3.65@3	41	5.5	37	
		32	6.1	36.5	
		27	6.6	36.75	121.75
8	–3.85@3	41	5.5	39.25	
		32	6.1	38.75	
		27	6.6	39.5	129.5
–8.5	–4@3	41	5.5	41.75	
		32	6.1	41.25	
		27	6.6	41.75	137.25
		45	5	37	
		30	6.1	38.25	
		25	6.6	38.75	127
		48	4.5	31.25	
		31	5.5	31.5	
		21	6.5	31.25	106.5
–9	–4.15@3	41	5.5	44.25	
		32	6.1	43.75	
		27	6.6	44.25	145.25
		45	5	39.25	
		30	6.1	41	
		25	6.6	41	134.25
		48	4.5	33.25	
		31	5.5	33.5	
		21	6.5	33.25	113
–9.5	4.25@3	41	5.5	46.75	
		32	6.1	46	
		27	6.6	46.75	153
		45	5	41.75	
		30	6.1	43.25	
		25	6.6	43.25	141.5
		48	4.5	35	
		31	5.5	35.25	
		21	6.5	35.25	119
–10	–4.45@3	45	5	43.5	
		30	6.1	45.5	
		25	6.6	45.5	148.5
		48	4.5	36.75	
		31	5.5	37.25	
		21	6.5	37	125
–10.5	–4.6@3	48	4.5	38.75	
		31	5.5	39	
		21	6.5	38.75	131
		40	4	25	
		25	5	25.5	
		19	6.1	30.5	
		16	6.6	30.75	126.25
–11	–4.75@3	48	4.5	40.5	
		31	5.5	41	
		21	6.5	40.75	137.25
		40	4	26	
		25	5	26.75	
		19	6.1	31.75	
		16	6.6	32	131.5
11.5	–4.9@3	48	4.5	42.25	
		31	5.5	42.75	
		21	6.5	42.5	143
		40	4	27.25	
		25	5	28	
		19	6.1	33.25	
		16	6.6	33.5	137.5
–12	–4.75@3	48	4.5	44.25	
		31	5.5	44.5	
		21	6.5	44.25	148
		40	4	28.5	
		25	5	29	
		19	6.1	34.75	
		16	6.6	35	142.25
–13	–5.1@3	48	4.5	47.75	
		31	5.5	48.25	
		21	6.5	48	160
		40	4	30.75	
		25	5	31.5	
		19	6.1	27.5	
		16	6.6	38	153.75

Early in our LASIK experience with the Chiron Technolas 116, we experienced undercorrections. For PRK we used the vertex corrected refraction, however, for LASIK we found that the nonvertex corrected refraction produced more accurate results. The surgical technique was modified to allow treatment of the central corneal hydration. Filtered compressed air is applied to the central stroma during the pretreatment and for the first three seconds of each zone. An additional three seconds are applied during the middle of the last zone. By adhering to the partial multizone ablation nomogram and applying these techniques consistently, we have achieved very predictable results.

KRITZINGER NOMOGRAM FOR TECHNOLAS 217 EXCIMER LASER

The success of excellent postoperative visual results does not only depend on the nomogram, but other factors come into play are

- Environmental factors in the operating room; temperature, humidity and drafts in the air
- Surgical technique of the surgeon
- Preoperative refraction of the patient
- Postoperative medication to the patient
- Type and make of the laser in use, broad beam/ scanning

General Rules

- Room temperature: 16°-18°C
- Room humidity: 45–50 percent
- Exact superimposition of red and green HeNe beam critical—or undercorrections will occur
- Use 6 × magnification—not larger, because you can loose your orientation to the visual axis
- Correctly align patient prior to lifting the flap, to limit exposure time of stroma before the treatment starts—thus, it will give you more accurate and consistent visual results
- The Kritzinger 217 nomogram differs moderately from the Probst 217 nomogram (Table 20.8)
- Lift flap with a Colibri—do not use BSS cannula as this may introduce moisture to the bed. Do not use a spatula, since foreign material, e.g. epithelium may be introduced into the interface
- Begin laser treatment, and let the assistant press the "enter" key to give continuous treatment without breaks, so that you make the treatment time and the stromal exposure time as short as possible
- Avoid contact with the stromal bed—do not wipe whilst lasering the stroma—*this is totally contraindicated*, because it will give overcorrections with the 217 laser
- Minimum residual cornea after ablation 250 micron (excluding flap thickness)
- Ideal treatment zone 4-6 mm
- It is advisable not to use a smaller zone diameter than 4.0 mm (night vision glare) and a maximum zone diameter of 6 mm (unnecessary vertex ablation and overcorrections will result).

Kritzinger Nomograms

Myopia

- For treatment of –1.0 to –13.0 spherical equivalent diopters
- Use *subjective* spectacle correction for minus spheres
- Add 10 percent to sphere and cylinder
- Subtract or add the calculated cylindrical correction from or to the calculated spherical correction, because:
  i. 20 percent *hyperopic* coupling shift with *negative* cylinders, on the spherical diopters, and
  ii. 10 percent *myopic* coupling shift with *plus* cylinders, on the spherical diopters.

Table 20.8: Probst nomogram for Chiron Technolas 217 planoscan version 2.422

		Zone	*Sphere*	*Cylinder*	*Comment*
Myopia	Kritzinger	5.5	add 10%	add 10%	add 20% –cyl to –sph
(minus cyl)	Probst	6.0	add 10%	no change	
Hyperopia	Argento	4.2–5.5	add 50–75%	add 25%	add +sph >40 yrs
(plus cyl)	Kritzinger	5.5	add 15%	add 10%	subtract 10% of cyl from sph
	Probst	6.0	add 20%	no change	
Mixed	Kritzinger	5.5	add 10%	add 10%	add 1/3 +cyl to –sph
(plus cyl)	Probst	6.0	no change	no change	add 1/3 +cyl to –sph

Hyperopia

- For treatment of + 1.0 to + 3.0, (rarely up to +4.0 D) spherical equivalent diopters
- Selection of treatment program, of the (217) laser (hyperopia/myopia) is dependent on the sphere, and not the cylinder
- Use *subjective* spectacle correction
- Add 15 percent to sphere and 10 percent to the cylinder
- Subtract or add the calculated cylindrical correction from or to the calculated spherical correction, because:
  i. 20 percent *hyperopic* coupling shift with *negative* cylinders, on the spherical diopters, and
  ii. 10 percent *myopic* coupling shift with *plus* cylinders, on the spherical diopters.

Information

- Hyperopic treatment regresses more than myopic treatments
- **If one has a high plus sphere and any strength minus cylinder, one should do a *transposition* to a plus cylinder (less tissue ablation, shorter treatment time, less gas consumption)**
- Most plus spheres are treated in the plus cylinder prescription—therefore, a transposition is often required.

Table 20.9: The Casebeer LASIK personal calibration nomogram (based on Arizona's dry climate)

The Visx Star excimer laser was used on patients with myopia and
astigmatism. Pretreatment was per the laser program, ablation took place on a dry stromal bed, and there was no intraoperative wiping.

Refraction	*20 to 25*	*26 to 30*	*31 to 35*	*36 to 40*	*>40*
–1	–1	–.98	–.95	– .9	–.85
–1.5	–1.5	–1.46	–1.43	–1.35	–1.28
–2	–2	–1.95	–1.9	–1.8	–1.7
–2.0	–2.5	–2.44	–2.38	–2.25	–2.13
–3	–3	–2.93	–2.85	– 2.7	–2.55
–3.5	–3.33	–3.24	–3.15	–2.98	–2.8
–4	–3.8	–3.7	–3.6	–3.4	–3.2
–4.5	–4.28	–4.16	–4.05	–3.83	–3.6
–5	–4.75	–4.63	–4.5	–4.25	–4
–5.5	–5.23	–5.09	–4.95	–4.68	–4.4
–6	–5.7	–5.55	–5.4	–5.1	–4.8
–6.5	–5.85	–5.69	–5.53	–5.2	–4.88
–7	–6.3	–6.13	–5.95	–5.6	–5.25
–7.5	–6.75	–6.56	–6.38	–6.4	–6
–8.5	–7.65	–7.44	–7.23	–6.8	–6.38
–9	–8.1	–7.88	–7.65	–7.2	–6.75
–9.5	–8.08	–7.84	–7.6	–7.13	–6.65
–10	–8.5	–8.25	–8	–7.5	–7
–10.5	–8.93	–8.66	–8.4	–7.88	–7.35
–11	–9.35	–9.08	–8.8	–8.25	–7.7
–11.5	–9.78	–9.49	–9.2	–8.63	–8.05
–12	–10.2	–9.9	–9.6	–9	–8.4
–12.5	–10.63	–10.31	–10	–9.38	–8.75
–13	–11.05	–10.73	–10.4	–9.75	–9.1
–13.5	–11.48	–11.14	–10.8	–10.13	–9.45
–14	–11.9	–11.55	–11.2	–10.5	–9.8
–14.5	–12.33	–11.96	–11.6	–10.88	–10.15

ADJUSTMENT FACTORS FOR THE REFRACTIVE CORRECTION OF LASIK

Aside from the altitude of the refractive center, patient age is the other commonly considered adjustment factor. Patient age has been used in the past predominantly for the radial keratotomy and astigmatic keratotomy nomograms.[12] Age adjustments have been less consistently applied for LASIK. Since a refractive stability is achieved with LASIK by 3 to 6 months postoperatively, the hyperopic drift that occurred with RK is not a concern with LASIK. Slight overcorrection of 0.5D is preferable in patients under the age of 25 years, as the vision will be excellent and small buffer is created against a future regression of effect. Middle-aged patients between 25 and 50 years are best treated with the full refractive correction, unless monovision is planned in the nondominant eye. Older patients (<50 years) are usually best undercorrected by 0.5 D as they tend to have a greater response to the excimer ablation and are less tolerant to overcorrections. Casebeer has described his nomogram for LASIK based on the dry climate of Arizona[13] (Table 20.9). The nomogram used at the TLC Chicago center makes similar adjustments on a simpler scale (Table 20.5).

SUMMARY

LASIK is a procedure in evolution. While LASIK surgeons originally performed corrections over 20.0 D,[14] we now limit our corrections to much lower levels of myopia to preserve the integrity of the cornea and the quality of postoperative vision. As the worldwide LASIK experience increases, the variables affecting our results are being controlled and minimized. However, each year new excimer lasers are becoming available that have different ablation nomograms and therefore will have some variation in their predictive formulas. A slow conservative initial approach to these innovations will lead to the best results for our patients.

REFERENCES

1. Machat JJ. PRK complications and their management. In Machat JJ (Ed): Excimer Laser Refractive Surgery. Slack Inc: Thorofare, 1996.
2. Machat JJ. LASIK Procedure. In Machat JJ (Ed): Excimer Laser Refractive Surgery. Slack Inc: Thorofare, 1996.
3. Gartry DS, Kerr Muir MG, Marshall J. Photorefractive keratectomy with an argon fluoride excimer laser—a clinical study. Refract Corneal Surg 1991;7:420-35.
4. Talley AR, Hardten DR, Sher NA, et al. Results one year after using the 193-nm excimer laser for photorefractive keratectomy in mild to moderate myopia. Am J Ophthalmol 1994;118:304-11.
5. Pop M, Aras M. Multizone/multipass photorefractive keratectomy—six-month results. J Cataract Refract Surg 1995;21:633-43.
6. Pop M. The Multipass/Multizone PRK technique to correct myopia and astigmatism. In Machat JJ (Ed): Excimer Laser Refractive Surgery. Slack Inc: Thorofare, 1996.
7. Alpins NA, Taylor HR, Kent DG, et al. Three Multizone photorefractive keratectomy algorithms for myopia. J Refract Surg 1997;13:535-44.
8. Munnerlyn CR, Koons SJ, Marshall J. Photorefractive keratectomy—a technique for laser refractive surgery. J Refract Surg 1988;14:46-52.
9. Emara B, Probst LE, Tingey D, et al. Correlation of intraocular pressure and corneal thickness in normal myopic eyes and following LASIK. J Cataract Refract Surg 1997.
10. Probst LE, Machat JJ. The Mathematics of LASIK for high myopia. J Cataract Refract Surg 1997.
11. Probst LE, Machat JJ. LASIK enhancements techniques and results. In Buratto L (Ed): LASIK: Principles and Techniques, Slack IncL Thorofare, 1997;325-38.
12. Committee on Ophthalmic Procedures Assessment, American Academy of Ophthalmology: Radial keratotomy for myopia. Ophthalmology 1993;100(7):1103-15.
13. Casebeer JC. A systemized approach to LASIK. In Buratto L (Ed): LASIK: Principles and Techniques Slack Inc: Thorofare, 1997;225-8.
14. Salah T, Waring GO III, Maghraby AE, et al. Excimer laser in situ keratomileusis under the flap for myopia of 2 to 20 diopters. Am J Ophthalmol 1996;121:143-55.

21 Microkeratomes for LASIK

Rasik B Vajpayee, Tanuj Dada

INTRODUCTION

The microkeratome is the basic instrument required to make a corneal flap to facilitate intrastromal excimer laser ablation during laser-in-situ-keratomileusis (LASIK). The purpose of the microkeratome is to create a uniform and homogenous corneal flap of precisely calculated diameter and thickness by cutting across the corneal lamellae. The cutting action of the microkeratome is derived from a blade which is powered by an electromechanical system (or turbine system). The microkeratome motor is powered through a cable and activated by a foot pedal control.The following components are included in an assembled microkeratome:

Head—contains the thickness plate, blade holder and blade

Handle—contains the motor

Footplate—to stabilize and pressurize the eye

Console—for power control.

An ideal microkeratome should be simple to assemble and operate, cheap to use , easy to clean and reassemble or readily disposable, allow visibility of the cornea during creation of the flap and demonstrate dependability, durability and repeatability in several consecutive cases.

A number of different microkeratomes have been developed by various scientists around the world and are available for clinical use. There are several more microkeratomes referred to in the literature, that are still under development and not in commercial use.This chapter gives a brief description of the various microkeratomes used for LASIK.

BARRAQUER'S MICROKERATOME

Jose Ignacio Barraquer designed the original microkeratome (Fig. 21.1) that served as the basis for the development of all subsequent microkeratomes. Barraquer's original microkeratome consisted of a head with a steel blade that was passed manually over the cornea.The system had the following components.

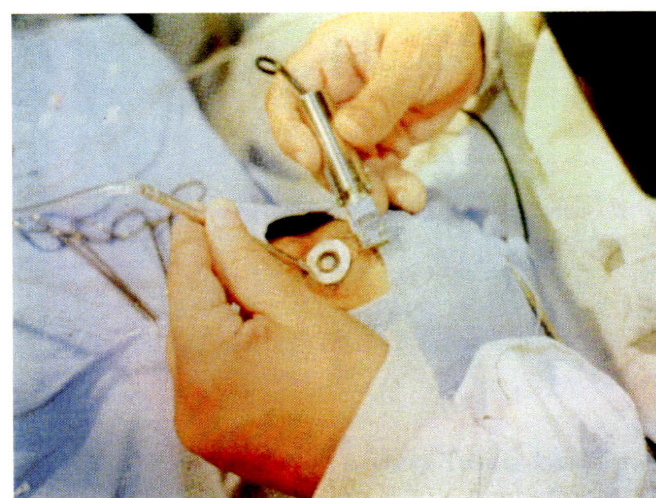

Fig. 21.1: Barraquer's microkeratome. This was used for keratomileusis and keratophakia (*Courtesy:* Dr. Agarwal's Eye Hospital)

Blade

It is a precision surgical blade with a dot marked on its surface to indicate the correct orientation since it can be mounted only in one way onto the blade holder. The rear of the blade contains a groove that must face posteriorly to engage the eccentric pin of the motor providing oscillatory movement with a lateral excursion of approximately 2.5 mm of the blade holder and blade.

Plate

The thickness plate is made of plastic or stainless steel. It allows the surgeon to set the depth of the lamellar cut. These plates come in multiple thicknesses and can be changed to give flaps of the required thickness. The thickness plate is fitted in a specific groove situated in the anterior portion of the microkeratome head. With traditional microkeratomes, the absence of the plate or its incorrect insertion into the head of the microkeratome, could cause a full-thickness cut through the cornea. This could lead to damage of the iris and the lens and even vitreous loss. Although every step in the assembly of the microkeratome is important, the proper fitting of the thickness plate is of vital importance.

Suction Ring

A suction ring is an integral part of the microkeratome. Besides helping in fixing the eyeball and raising the intraocular pressure (IOP) to facilitate creation of the corneal flap, it contains a track which engages the microkeratome and allows the surgeon to regulate the accurate movement of the microkeratome. The suction plate is made up of steel and the original microkeratome had 10 different sized rings for different diameter corneal cuts. The newer microkeratomes utilize a single suction ring and differing diameters of corneal tissue are cut by adjusting the height of the ring. The suction ring has a hollow handle to which a silicone tube is attached to transmit suction from the suction pump in the console. To achieve an ideal cut, the suction should increase the IOP to 60 to 65 mm Hg. This needs to be carefully checked with an applanation tonometer before using the microkeratome. Inadequate suction will result in a small or incomplete flap.

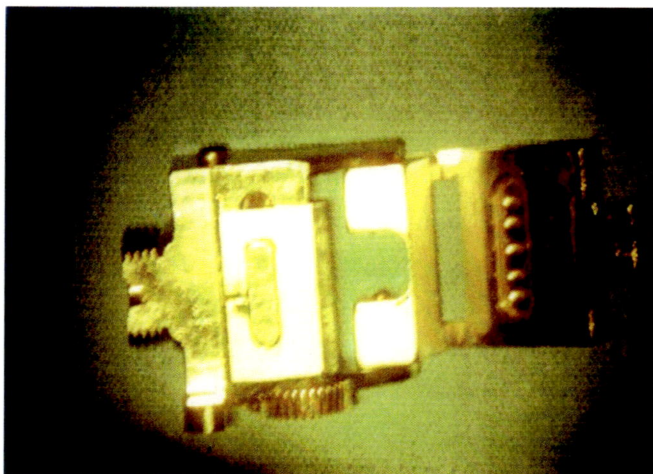

Fig. 21.2: Automated corneal shaper, before installation (*Courtesy:* Dr. Agarwal's Eye Hospital)

AUTOMATED CORNEAL SHAPER

The automated corneal shaper (ACS) (read chapter 22) has been designed by Luis Ruiz and is produced by Hansa of Miami, Florida. Although it is fundamentally similar to the Barraquer's microkeratome, the key difference is that it has an automated advancement mechanism that acts through a gear system to advance the blade in a uniform and regular way. It is available in two forms: (i) combined ALK/LASIK unit, and (ii) dedicated LASIK unit. The ACS (Fig. 21.2) has the following parts.

Shaper Head

The keratome head houses the blade which is driven by an electric motor at a rate of 8000 rpm. The side of the shaper head has three gears that constitute the core of the instrument's automated movement system. These gears are driven by the electric motor in the handle that also operates the oscillating blade. The first gear transmits a rotatory impulse to the other two gears and engages a gear track on the suction ring, thereby, driving the microkeratome across the cornea. A stop mechanism has been incorporated in the shaper head to limit the complete run of the microkeratome along the track. This leaves an incomplete hinged flap rather than a free flap. The depth of the corneal cut is controlled by a thickness plate that is fitted in the designated groove on the anterior portion of the shaper head. These plates are numbered progressively and the thickness of the plate used determines, the thickness of the corneal flap. If a thin plate is used the space between plate and the blade would be larger allowing a greater exposure of the corneal tissue to the microkeratome, and this will create a thicker flap. For LASIK, a plate which allows creation of a 160 mm thick corneal flap is employed.

Motor

The motor of the microkeratome is a 12 volt micromotor that is housed in a cylindrical handle. This handle connects to the posterior aspect of the shaper head and drives both the oscillating blade and the gears. The motor is connected through a cable to the control box. The motor is activated by a two-mode foot pedal that can be pressed for changing the direction of the direct current, for forward and backward movements of the microkeratome.

Pneumatic Fixation Ring

The suction ring serves primarily to stabilize the globe. Other uses of the ring include guiding the microkeratome to move on its gear track and facilitating smooth passage of the cutting blade, increasing the IOP prior to the cutting of the cornea and determining the position of the flap. The ring is made up of steel and has a rectangular chamber on its underside. This chamber is connected to a suction pump in the control unit through the tubing attached to the handle of the suction ring. The suction pump creates a vacuum within the chamber. The optimal vacuum for LASIK is in the range of 22 to 27 mm Hg.

Control Unit

The control unit contains the suction pump for the pneumatic suction ring and provides the power to both the suction pump and motor of the microkeratome. On the front panel of the control unit, there are 2 meters to show the levels of vacuum created in the suction ring and amplitude of power delivered to the motor of the microkeratome. The voltage meter indicates the power delivered for the advancement and reversal of the microkeratome (optimal requirement is 12 volts).

Foot Pedal

Two separate foot pedals are supplied with the control unit—suction pedal and power pedal. To initiate and maintain the suction, the suction pump is activated by simply depressing and releasing the suction pedal. After the completion of the LASIK procedure, the suction is disengaged and the pneumatic ring released by pressing and releasing the suction pedal for a second time. The power pedal has two parts: one to activate and advance the microkeratome across the cornea to create the corneal flap, and the other to reverse the microkeratome after the completion of the corneal cut.

SCHWIND MICROKERATOME

Schwind microkeratome is produced by Herbert Schwind and has been designed and developed by Hoffmann and Seiler. This microkeratome is different from traditional microkeratomes such as the Automated Corneal Shaper and has the following design characteristics.

- The device comes as a single unit with accompanying power pack and foot controls
- The microkeratome blade is reusable and is made up of sapphire. Each blade can be used approximately for 400 cuts. The angle of contact of blade with cornea is 0 degree as compared to 26 degree angle of other microkeratomes, which allows for a low oscillation speed (1600-1800 rpm) during the cut
- The blade is electrically propelled and its progression is automated. Its movement is straight and harmonic. The progression speed of the blade is 1.33 mm/sec for a total of 6 seconds. The thickness plate is fixed and only allows corneal cuts of 150 μm depth. Both anterior and posterior parts

of the plate are transparent, and the surgeon can directly view the action of the blade on the corneal tissue during the entire procedure
- The vacuum system of the unit contains two suction rings. The rings are fixed and nonadjustable. One ring fixes the eyeball in the peripheral cornea and the other stabilizes the corneal flap during the incision
- The electrical motor system of the device is situated in the instrument's console and two metal drive cables transmit the advancing and oscillatory movements of the blade
- This microkeratome cuts a 150 μm thick flap of 9 mm diameter with 0.5 mm hinge.

The disadvantages of this keratome are: (i) the marked vibration of the instrument, (ii) the low oscillation speed of the blade, and (iii) the use of metal cables to transmit power.

TURBOKERATOME (SCMD MICROKERATOME)

Under the aegis of SCMD Ltd, this turbine microkeratome has been developed by John Livecchi of the University of Philadelphia. It has the following characteristics:
- The keratome head is fixed and does not have a thickness plate. The keratome produces a fixed 150 μm flap thickness
- There is a bifaceted blade made up of metal. The angle of attack on the cornea is 20 degrees and its oscillating cycles range from 10,000 to 24,000 rpm although the recommended oscillation speed of operation is 13,800 rpm. The direction of blade movement is sidewise.
- The microkeratome is independent of electrical power and the oscillations of the blade are powered by a turbine with nitrogen protoxide propulsion.
- The microkeratome does not have an automated progression system and is advanced manually by the surgeon.
- A digital micrometer with adjustment screws between the handle and the head of the microkeratome permits the surgeon to set the stop point and therefore determine the length of the cut.
- The unit has multiple suction rings and can create flaps of varying diameter, and there are four stop rings that give varying hinge dimensions.
- The device does not enable the surgeon to directly visualize the operative field during the creation of the corneal flap.

UNIVERSAL KERATOME

The Universal keratome has been developed by Phoenix Keratek Inc. of Scottsdale under the guidance of Perry S Binder. The keratome has the following innovative features:
- Keratome comes as a single unit and has a suction ring incorporated in it. There are no separate handled suction rings.
- The thickness plate and suction ring are fixed and provide only a hinged flap of preset thickness and diameter.
- The metal blade is unifaceted and its attack angle on to the cornea is 0 degree.
- The blade is powered by a piezoelectric motor and blade oscillations have a speed of 14,000 rpm. The blade has a straight pendular movement.
- The device is automatically advanced using an electrical motor drive.
- The device has a unique computer-controlled console to regulate the resistance and the cutting speed on the cornea.
- The system is unique in that it has a series of polymethylmethacrylate (PMMA) disks that can be used for refractive resections for the correction of myopia and hyperopia.
- The surgeon has a direct view of the corneal cutting during the procedure and can observe whether the cut has been performed correctly.

MASTEL-BUZARD MICROKERATOME

Mastel-Buzard microkeratome has been designed and developed by Mastel Precision Surgical Instruments Inc under the guidance of David Mastel and Kurt Buzard. The microkeratome has the following specific features:
- The device is built as a single piece with integrated vacuum as a part of it.

- The unit has a diamond blade that is advanced manually by the surgeon.
- The microkeratome creates a hinged flap of a fixed diameter of 8.5 mm with the hinge being parallel to the eyebrow.
- The incision is created by advancing the diamond blade with the surgeon's thumb after engaging the cornea, and then pushing the thumb piece to the stop, which completes the cut.

AUTOMATED DISPOSABLE KERATOME

Automated disposable keratome has been designed by Luis Antonio Ruiz and has been developed by Laser Sight Technologies Inc. The automated disposable keratome has the following features.

- It comes as a single, preassembled, individually sterile, packaged, single-use, moulded plastic device.
- The microkeratome has a vacuum safety ridge that can establish dual vacuum chambers to decrease the likelihood of vacuum port occlusion and false suction.
- The components of the device are of transparent plastic allowing the surgeon a direct view of the operative surface.
- The thickness plates are an integral part of the head and cannot be removed. Two types of the devices are available for creation of flaps of either 130 µm or 160 µm.
- The gears of the device are covered to minimize the chances of entrapment of lids or lashes, or injury.
- The unit has a tandem track drive that can eliminate the torque seen in single track units.
- The metal blade has a speed of 10,000 rpm and is advanced automatically.
- The device can create both horizontal and vertical flaps.

INNOVATOME

Innovatome has been developed by Innovative Optics Inc. Its distinctive design features are as follows:

- It is a lightweight, moulded plastic microkeratome, weighing only 37 gm on the eye.
- The microkeratome has an automated advancement system and is driven by a single flexible cable. There are no gears or mechanical assemblies.
- The unit has a disposable steel blade that is 100 micron thick and 1 mm wide. The blade is electrically driven and has a oscillation speed of 12,000 rpm.
- The microkeratome allows the creation of either horizontal or vertical flaps. The flap diameter can range from 8.5 to 10 mm.
- The device has a clear sapphire applanator that allows the surgeon to directly view the operative field. The applanator is marked to enable the surgeon to predict the location of hinge.
- The pneumatic fixation ring is integrated in the device and is mechanically grooved to provide infinite points of suction.

MICROPRECISION'S MICROLAMELLAR KERATOME

Microprecision's microlamellar keratome system is distributed by Eye Technology Inc. The device has the following design characteristics:

- The unit has a metal blade that is bifaceted and angulated at 9 degrees. The blade drive has a sideways movement with 20,000 oscillations per minute.
- The blade drive is powered by a pneumatic turbine and has six times the torque of electric motors.
- The microkeratome is manually advanced by the surgeon
- The device has an adjustable thickness plate which allows creation of a range of corneal flaps from 0 to 466 µm in 1 µm increments. The calibration of thickness plate is verified with a micrometer.
- The unit comes with multiple suction rings that allow for flaps of varying diameters.
- The suction rings and microkeratome head have dual dove-tail rail systems to create the hinge which decreases the risk of jumping and causes fewer chatter marks in the stroma leading to a smoother keratectomy bed.

- The device has a "stop-pin" system to create a hinged flap but does not allow the surgeon to directly visualize the operative field.

FLAPMAKER DISPOSABLE MICROKERATOME

Flapmaker disposable microkeratome is being manufactured and distributed by Refractive Technologies Inc, Cleveland, Ohio. The device has the following design features.

- **The device comes as a preassembled, single-use, moulded plastic unit and is completely disposable.**
- The unit does not have any gears and is driven by flexible shafts that provide a uniform motion of the microkeratome.
- The device has a metal blade made from surgical stainless steel which has an oscillation speed of 12,500 cycles per minute. It is driven across the cornea at 6.8 mm per second and only oscillates in the forward motion.
- The resection depth is prefixed at 130 μm or 160 μm and the flap produced has a fixed diameter of 10.5 mm.
- The unit is made of clear acrylic and allows the surgeon to directly visualize the operative field.

CLEAR CORNEAL MOLDER

Dr Ricardo Guimaraes of Brazil has developed this microkeratome for use in LASIK. The microkeratome has the following distinctive features:

- The device comes as a single piece integrated instrument unit that includes the head with a dual axis motor, the handle, the suction ring and the plate.
- The device has a diamond or steel blade which is powered by an electrical motor and has an oscillation rate of 12,000 per minute with a 0 degree angle of attack on the cornea.
- The diameter and the thickness of the corneal flap cut by the device can be varied.
- The device has only one pneumatic fixation ring whose height is adjustable in relation to the blade.
- The device has a transparent surface and allows the surgeon to directly visualize the operative field during the surgery.

The blade movement can be stopped at a preset point with a lever on the handle of the microkeratome which allows both free caps or hinged flaps to be obtained.

DRAEGER LAMELLATING ROTOKERATOME

Draeger lamellating rotokeratome was the first automated microkeratome and is now no longer in use. It was designed in conjunction with Draeger and was distributed by Storz Inc. The device has the following design characteristics:

- The device comes as a single unit that contains a circular cutting blade, a dual axis motor, a single thickness plate and a suction ring.
- The device has a metal blade and is powered by an electric motor. It is mechanically advanced and the angle of its attack on cornea is 0 degree. The blade has a rotary motion with a speed of 500 revolutions per minute.
- The device has a single suction ring that has a central opening of 12 mm. It is fitted with a silicon ring with 12 openings that act as a vacuum chamber.
- The device allows the surgeon to directly view the surgical field intraoperatively.

LAMELLAR KERATOPLASTY SYSTEM (PLANCON INSTRUMENTS MICROKERATOME)

Lamellar keratoplasty system is manufactured by Plancon Instruments of Anatony, France and is distributed by Moria of France. It has the following features:

- It is a nonautomated microkeratome in which the head is advanced manually.
- The device has a bifaceted metal blade that oscillates 15,000 cycles per minute. The blade oscillations are powered by a turbine which is driven by nitrogen gas, and the blade attack angle is 21.5 degrees.

- The microkeratome has four thickness plates allowing cut thickness of 120, 140, 160 and 180 μm.
- The unit comes with multiple suction rings depending on the diameter of the flap desired and the suction rings are less bulky as compared to other rings available which is helpful to create an adequate exposure in eyes with a narrow palpebral fissure.
- There are four metal stop rings which enables the surgeon to create a corneal hinge of diameters ranging between 1.5 and 2.5 mm.

EYE-TECH MICROKERATOME

Eye-tech microkeratome is a modified version of the BKS 1000 system developed by Swinger and Krumeich in 1983.The salient features are as follows:

- The blade enters the cornea at an angle of 26 degree and oscillates at a frequency of 8,000 to 14,000 cycles per minute.
- A Teflon coating is provided on the sliding surfaces of the microkeratome which minimizes the friction between the two steel surfaces.
- An adjustable micrometer is located at the junction of the head and the handle which limits the excursion of the keratome to the exact point as set by the surgeon.

STORZ MICROKERATOME

Storz microkeratome can be used for lamellar keratoplasty as well as LASIK and is produced and marketed by the Storz Inc. It is a one piece instrument with the following components and features.

- The instrument has two motors which provide a rotatory and advancing movement of the blade which cuts in only one direction unlike the back and forth cut of the oscillating blade.
- A flat rotating blade is used to create the flap and lamellar cuts can be performed without transferring vibrations or irregularities to the underlying tissue, a feature which is a major advantage over the oscillating blade.
- The thickness plate is adjustable with a micrometer which varies the height of the plate with respect to the corneal plane exposed to the suction ring, and thus, allows for modifications in the thickness of the cut.
- A plexiglass pressure plate is provided which allows the surgeon to evaluate precisely the diameter of the cut by studying the applanation image of the corneal tissue in relation to the reticule.

HANSATOME

Hansatome (read chapter 25) has been developed by Chiron Vision Corp. It is a device that further refines the ability of the automated corneal shaper (ACS) devised by Ruiz. The microkeratome has the following design characteristics.

- The microkeratome head has a fixed depth plate and a permanent nonadjustable stop device.
- The device utilizes a disposable metal blade and comes with an integrated plastic holder.
- The unit has a single suction ring that has an elevated, curved gear rack that aligns with the single gear of the hansatome (Fig. 21.3).
- The hansatome creates a superiorly placed hinge at 12 o'clock position which can be protected by the upper lid and the average diameter of the flap is 9.5 mm (Fig. 21.4).

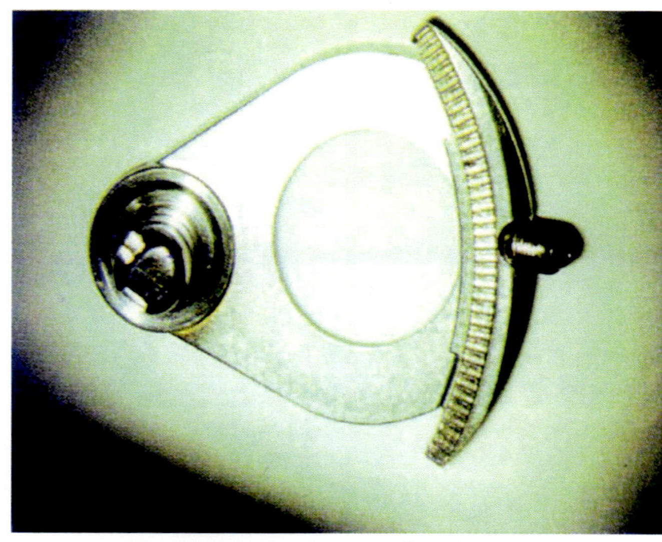

Fig. 21.3: Hansatome suction ring seen (*Courtesy:* Dr. Agarwal's Eye Hospital)

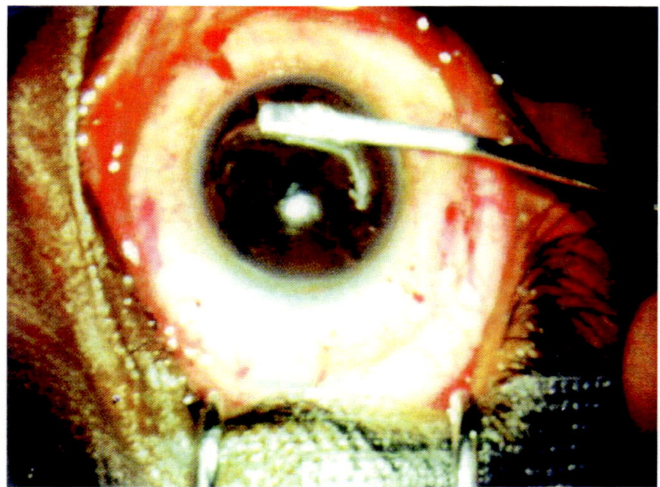

Fig. 21.4: Superior flap being lifted. The hinge is superiorly placed (*Courtesy:* Dr. Agarwal's Eye Hospital)

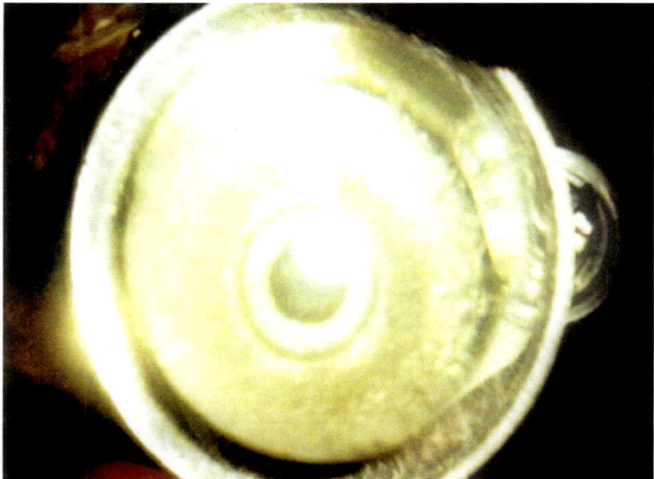

Fig. 21.5: Intraocular pressure (IOP) checked with Barraquer's tonometer (*Courtesy:* Dr. Agarwal's Eye Hospital)

- Two heads with fixed thickness plates are provided which cut flaps of preset thickness:160 µm and 180 µm.
- There is a left or right eye adapter that fits over the microkeratome head and the motor is positioned vertically,which enables the microkeratome head to pass over the suction ring on an elevated rack away from the speculum and the eyelids.
- The cutting action of the microkeratome cannot be started until the appropriate vacuum level is reached and the cutting stops if the vacuum falls below a certain level (Fig. 21.5).

VISIJET HYDROKERATOME

Visijet hydrokeratome uses a *waterjet* technology to create a *cleavage* in between the corneal lamellae.This is accomplished by fatiguing and breaking the collagen bonds between the corneal lamellae while preserving the integrity of the lamellae and the keratocytes. Since the cornea is a highly sectile tissue, cleavage rather than cutting is the best mechanism for tissue separation with minimal tissue damage. Therefore, this procedure is less traumatic and much safer as compared to the mechanical microkeratomes which cut across the corneal tissues.The anticipated advantages of the hydrokeratome are: (i) a decrease in epithelial ingrowth, (ii) irregular astigmatism, (iii) haze, (iv) regression, and (v) flap or suction-related complications.

The Visijet hydrokeratome uses a continuous beam of ultrahigh pressure saline that is only 36 microns in diameter to cut a flap across the cornea. The key to the hydrokeratome's success is the extreme high pressure (over 15,000 psi.) combined with a tightly collimated waterjet beam. Under these "ultrafluidic conditions" the water molecules leave the orifice of the instrument at a speed in excess of 800 mph and take on almost metallic properties. The device has the following design features.

- The device uses a high pressure waterjet beam to cleave the cornea.
- The surgeon controlled foot switch activates the suction ring vacuum, the waterjet aspiration and the high pressure waterjet beam.
- A handpiece translates the waterjet across the cornea. The angle of attack of the water beam on the cornea is 0 degree.
- The end point of water jet operation is preprogrammed by the surgeon depending on the selected hinge length and flap diameter.
- The water pressure and waterjet beam position are continuously monitored by an image tracking technology.

- The flap thickness can be varied from 100 to 200 microns, depending on the thickness plate used. The flap diameter ranges from 8 to 11 mm.
- The applanating surface is made up of lexan, a special plastic and has a diameter of 12 mm. The surface is transparent and the surgeon has full visualization of the visual axis at all times.

Since this keratome is easy to use, has a low cost and an increased safety, this is expected to gain wide acceptance among LASIK surgeons in the coming years.

PICOSECOND LASER MICROKERATOME

Picosecond laser microkeratome is the microkeratome of the future, still under development.The laser microkeratome is used as an intrastromal cutting tool based on picosecond intrastromal photodisruption. It causes separation and removal of a small amount of stromal collagen from within the cornea by focusing highly transmissive infrared laser light through the cornea. The main advantages of this technique are the precision and reproducibility of the laser in producing flaps of uniform thickness and the smoothness of the flap interphase. Suction rings and the cutting blades are also not required in this procedure. Currently, the limitations of this laser technology are: (i) the small flap diameter, (ii) poor centration, (iii) increased intraoperative time, and (iv) difficulty in dissection. Research is on to develop a solid state ultraviolet laser which can be used both for cutting the flap and intrastromal ablation.

22 Automatic Corneal Shaper

Amar Agarwal, T Agarwal, J Agarwal

INTRODUCTION

Automatic corneal shaper (ACS) is an excellent microkeratome manufactured by Chiron Vision (Bausch and Lomb). It allows for cutting of a precise corneal disk of preselected thickness and diameter. When LASIK (laser-in-situ keratomileusis) was started it was not that successful. Later on three important techniques improved and changed the success of LASIK. These were: (i) an automated microkeratome, (ii) the development of a hinged flap technique, and (iii) the development of the sutureless technique. For all three, the ACS was excellent and the results of LASIK improved drastically with this microkeratome.

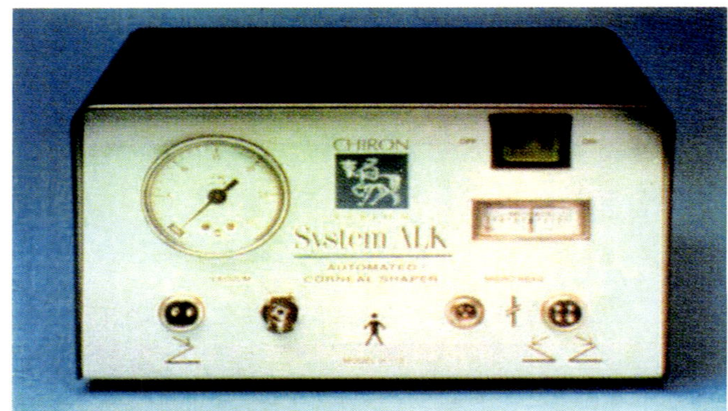

Fig. 22.1: Power pack for the automatic corneal shaper (ACS)

PRESURGICAL SET-UP

The ACS consists of three basic units:

- Power pack
- Suction ring
- Microkeratome.

All three have to be set up for the machine to work smoothly and comfortably.

Power Pack

The Power pack (Fig. 22.1) provides electric current for the suction pump and microkeratome. On the front panel you have sockets as seen in Figure 22.1 to which the cords of the suction ring and microkeratome are connected (Fig. 22.2). In the rear panel there is a receptacle for the main power cord. One should place the ACS power pack on a firm, level surface. In the Chiron 217 excimer laser (LASIK laser) there is no need of a separate power pack. The power pack is inbuilt in the excimer laser itself (Fig. 22.3). Note in Figure 22.3, the Chiron 217 and the tubings of the suction ring and the cords for the microkeratome are protruding out of the machine.

Suction Ring

The suction pump is connected to the suction ring handle (Fig. 22.4) by a disposable tubing. This comes in a sterile package (Fig. 22.5). On opening this package, we will find not only the tubing but also a disposable blade for the microkeratome (Fig. 22.6).

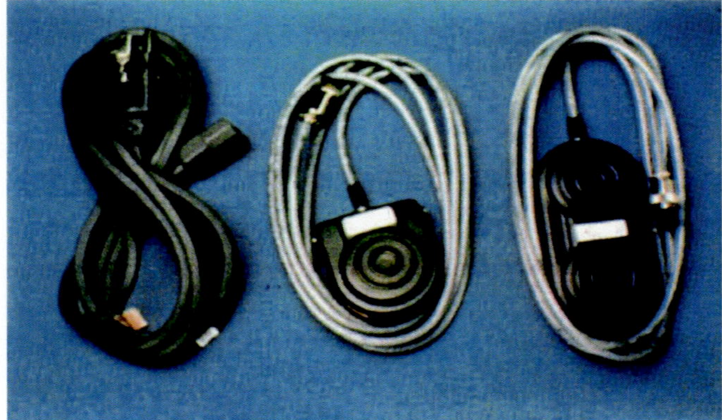

Fig. 22.2: Cords for the power pack, suction ring and microkeratome

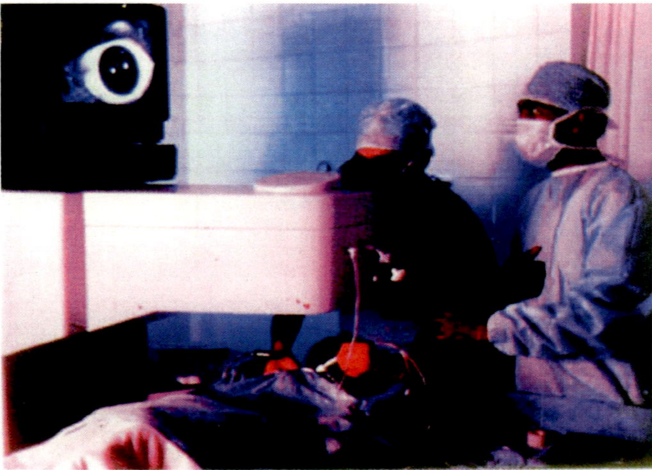

Fig. 22.3: Chiron 217 Excimer (LASIK) Laser

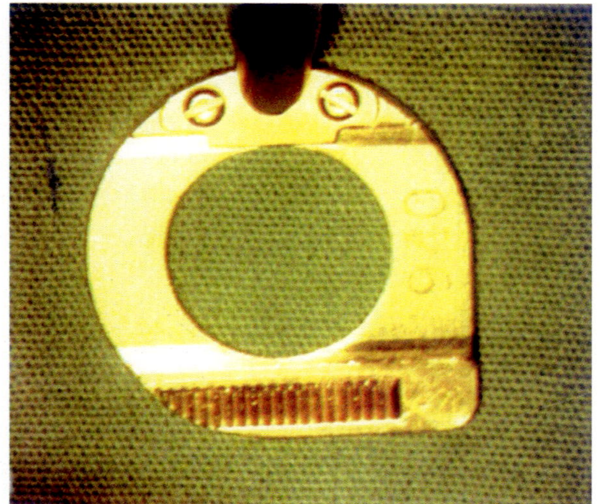

Fig. 22.4: Suction ring handle. Note the track for the gears in the suction ring

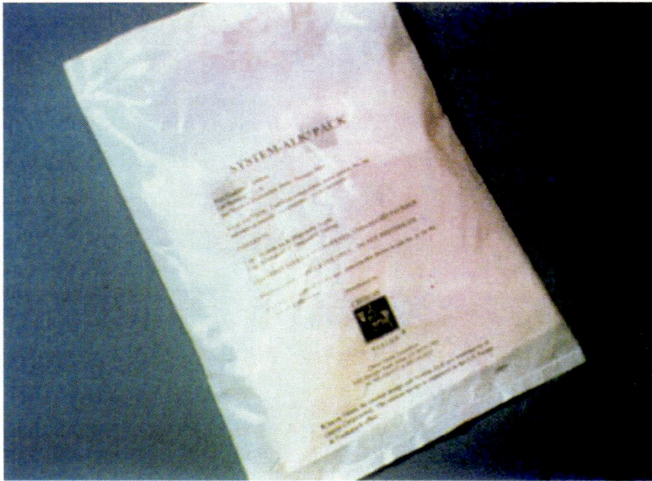

Fig. 22.5: Disposable tubing pack

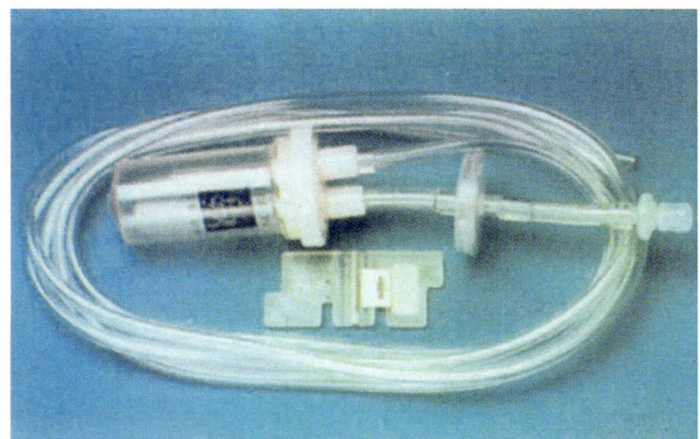

Fig. 22.6: Disposable tubing with a disposable microkeratome blade

The suction ring consists of the suction handle, the ring and the track on which the gears of the microkeratome move (See Fig. 22.4). The suction handle screws onto the suction ring. The handle is hollow and is in turn connected to the power pack via the disposable suction tubing. The handle is hollow so that the suction can be applied once the foot switch of the suction pump is switched on. Once the suction ring is placed on the eye to encircle the cornea and the foot switch of the suction pump pressed, the intraocular pressure (IOP) should be raised to 65 mm of Hg. This is necessary so that the microkeratome can create a nice pass and resect the cornea. The advantages of the suction ring are: (i) to fixate the eye,

(ii) to increase the IOP, and (iii) to have the track for the microkeratome to move.

Microkeratome

Take the corneal shaper head (Fig. 22.7) from the instrument tray. Check the gears (which are seen in Fig. 22.7) by your thumb and see that there is resistance-free movement. If this does not occur then repeat the cleaning process. Place the corneal shaper head with the serial number facing up (Fig. 22.8). Remove the locking ring on the rear of the corneal shaper head. Holding the shaper so that the serial number is facing up, open the hinged cover to expose the blade holder. The blade holder should be completely dry. If the blade holder does not move smoothly, clean the blade holder and cavity of the shaper head again. Remember that the slot should face the rear of the shaper head and the blade shoulder should face up. Take out the blade from the disposable tubing package. Open the blade carrier to expose the blade.

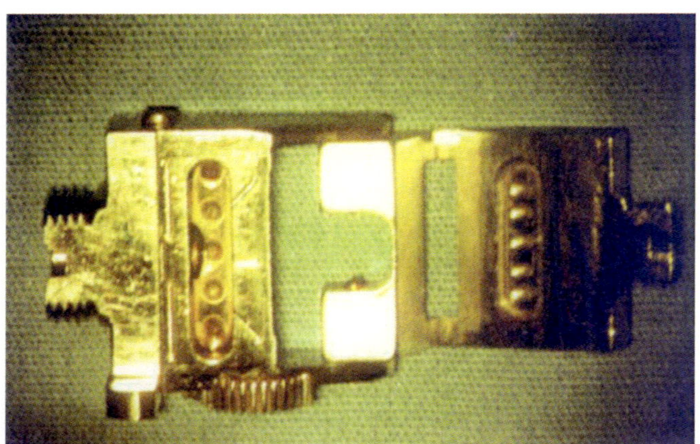

Fig. 22.7: Corneal shaper head

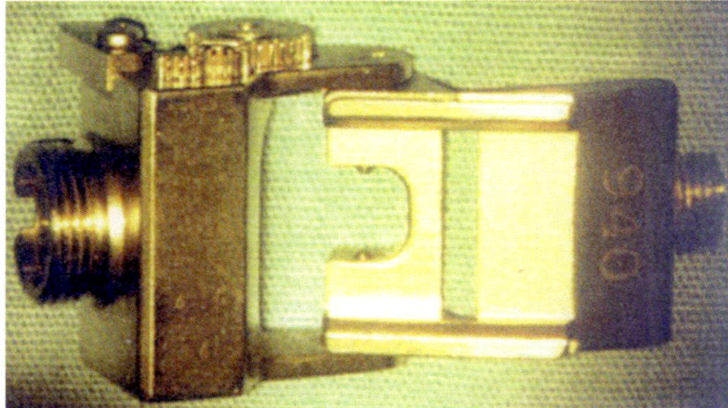

Fig. 22.8: Corneal shaper head (other side of corneal shaper head with serial number facing up)

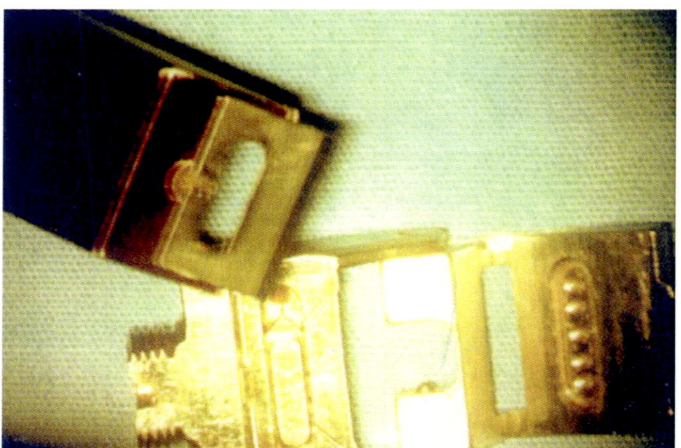

Fig. 22.9: Corneal shaper head exposing the blade holder. The blade is adjacent to it. Note the magnet holding the blade so that one does not damage the sharp edge of the blade

The blade is packaged in the carrier with the square edge of the slot on the left and the round edge on the right to correspond with the correct placement of the blade in the shaper head. Pin the unsharpened, back edge of the blade down with your left forefinger so that it will not jump up to the magnet of the blade insertion tool. With the blade insertion tool in your dominant hand, carefully position the tool over the sharp edge of the blade and allow the magnet to grasp the blade. Lift the blade straight up and off the carrier (Fig. 22.9). Position the blade slot over the raised shoulder of the blade holder and press the blade down firmly with the tool. Pin the blade down in the shaper head with your nondominant hand's fore-finger and lift the tool off and away. Invert the blade tool and use one or both of the front tines to press down on the blade in several places to assure it is properly seated. Be careful not to contact the sharp edge of the blade. Gently close the shaper head and replace the locking nut with the knurled portion facing out. The head should close flush without force. Test the movement of the blade by placing the test shaft into the rear of the shaper head. Rotate the test shaft to feel the oscillation of the blade, which should

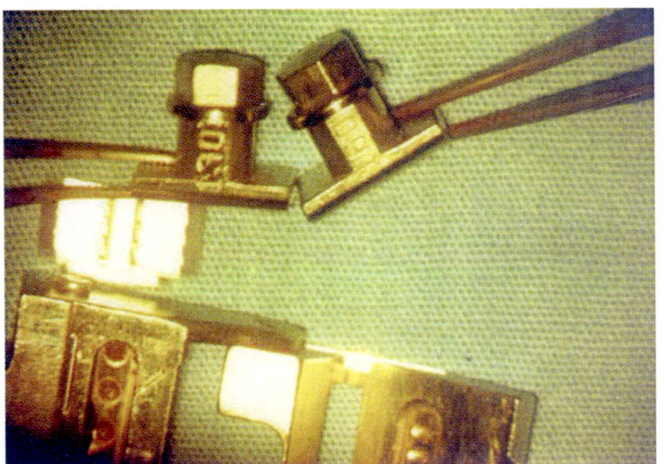

Fig. 22.10: Thickness plates of 130 microns and 160 microns. Note the number on the thickness plates

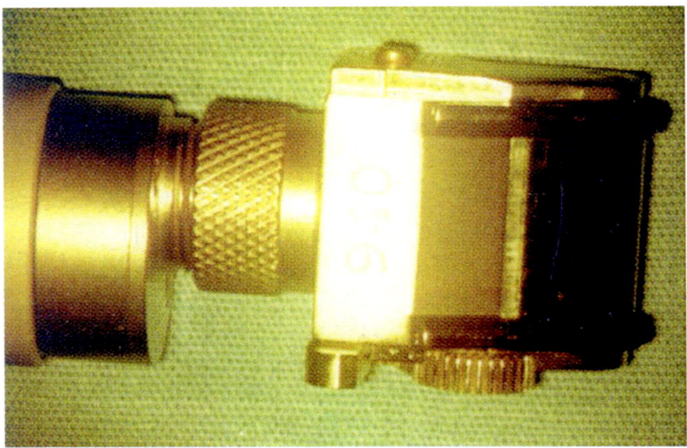

Fig. 22.11: Assembled microkeratome

be absolutely smooth and free of resistance. While rotating the test shaft, visually confirm that the blade is moving side to side to verify that the blade holder has been installed properly. If the blade movement is restricted, carefully remove the blade and confirm that all surfaces of the shaper head and blade holder are clean and perfectly dry. Replace the blade and check again. If resistance is still detected, install another blade and repeat the testing process until you feel absolutely no resistance. *Do not proceed with a blade with restricted movement, as this could cause the unit to jam or create a less than optimal cut.*

Remove the desired thickness plate (Fig. 22.10) from the tray by placing the locking wrench onto the hex nut of the plate and tilting back. Place your forefinger on the plate to keep it from falling off the wrench and lift out of the tray. The thickness plates can be of 130 microns or 160 microns. This means if we use the 130-micron thickness plate the flap will be of 130 microns. If we use the 160-micron thickness plate the flap created will be of 160-micron thickness. *Always confirm the engraved number on the plate with your surgical plan.* **If the corneal pachymetry is not much or the refractive error to correct is a lot, one might use the 130-micron thickness plate so that we get an extra 30 microns to ablate. But by and large in our hospital, we prefer to use the 160-micron thickness plate, as the flap created by this is better. By using the 130-micron thickness plate we found the flap a bit thin and so we shifted to the 160-micron thickness plate in all cases.**

The plate has a nut and washer, which must be slightly loosened to allow the plate to be installed into the shaper head. Stabilize the plate with your forefinger on the front and slide the plate completely into the notch on the front of the shaper head. You should feel and hear the plate snap into place so that it is perfectly flush to the front of the shaper head. Secure the plate by rotating the nut clockwise with the wrench. The plate must be perfectly flush to the shaper head and locked firmly in place so that it will not come loose during a surgical procedure. *If the thickness plate is not fixed properly or if we forget to fix the thickness plate we will create a perforation in the anterior chamber.*

Once the microkeratome is fully installed (Fig. 22.11) it has to be fixed to the motor cord which in turn is fixed to the power pack (Fig. 22.12). Insert the motor cord into the keyed receptacle at the back of the motor. A click indicates that a positive lock has been achieved. With the motor foot switch, run the motor in each direction and listen for any irregular sounds from the operation of the motor. Place the shaper head on the motor shaft and carefully rotate the shaper head until it is firmly attached.

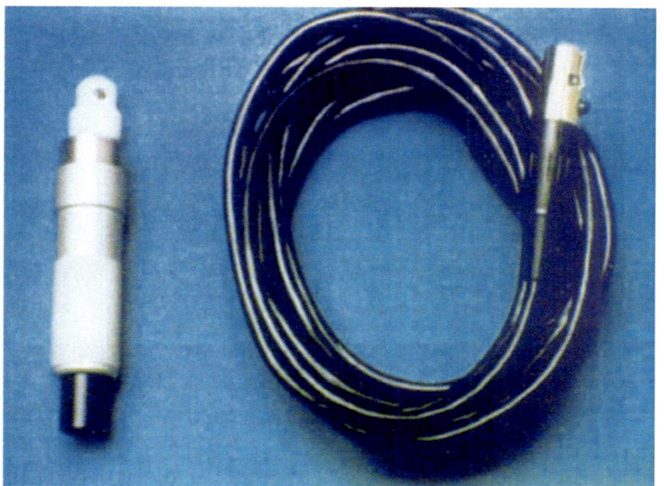

Fig. 22.12: Motor cord to connect the microkeratome to the power pack

CHECK

Before starting the procedure on the patient, check if everything is working. Check the gears, check the movement of the blades, etc. Most important, install the microkeratome (shaper head) onto the suction ring (Fig. 22.13). Engage the dovetail side first then rotate the shaper flat against the ring. The dovetail of the head should be kept parallel to the track. Gently advance the shaper until the gears are engaged. Press the forward switch of the motor with your foot.

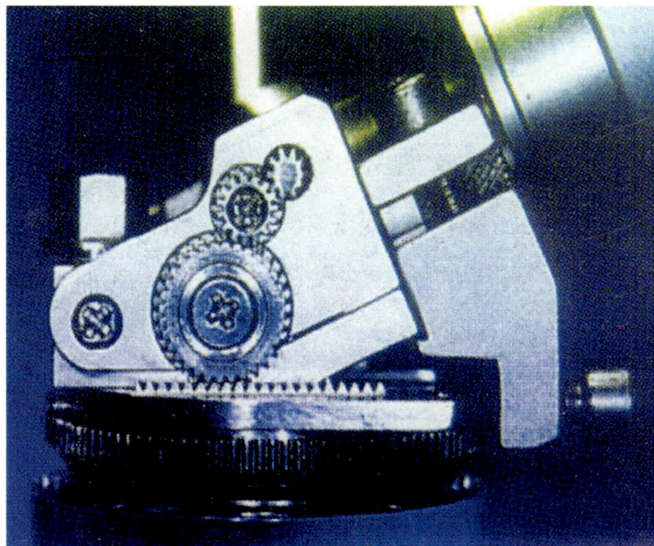

Fig. 22.13: Automatic corneal shaper (ACS) head with permanent stopper for use with fixed suction ring

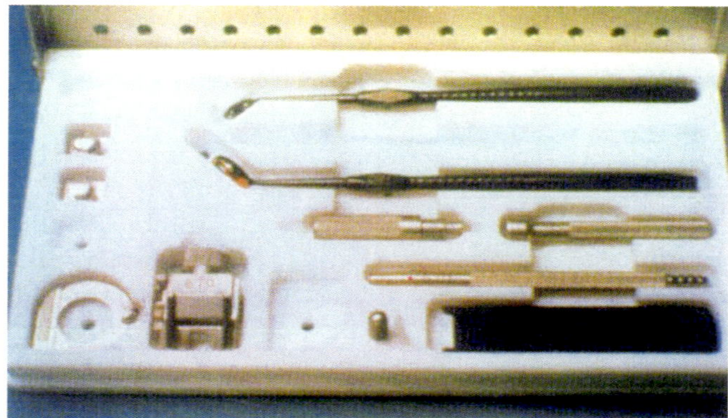

Fig. 22.14: Instruments in the set of ACS

Promptly release the foot switch when the permanent stopper abuts the suction ring and stops the forward progress of the shaper. Press the reverse foot switch to retract the shaper head and remove it from the suction ring. The forward and reverse travel of the shaper head across the suction ring must be completely smooth. If binding or resistance is encountered, do not attempt the surgical procedure. Repeat the cleaning process and once again the functional test. If everything has been checked and found alright, the ACS is ready for use in a surgical procedure.

SURGICAL TECHNIQUE

The ACS consists of state-of-the-art instrumentation designed for performing lamellar corneal resections. Figures 22.14 and 22.15 show the instruments of the

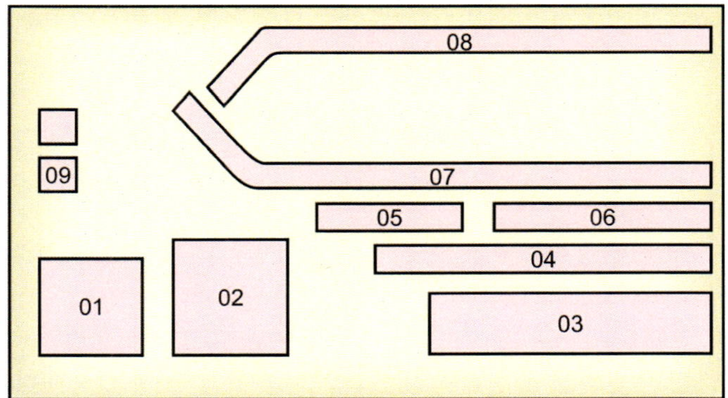

Fig. 22.15: Diagrammatic representation of instruments for ACS as seen in Figure 22.14: 01—suction ring, 02—shaper head, 03—blade tool, 04—suction handle, 05—test shaft, 06—locking wrench, 07—reference marker, 08—spatula, 09—thickness plates

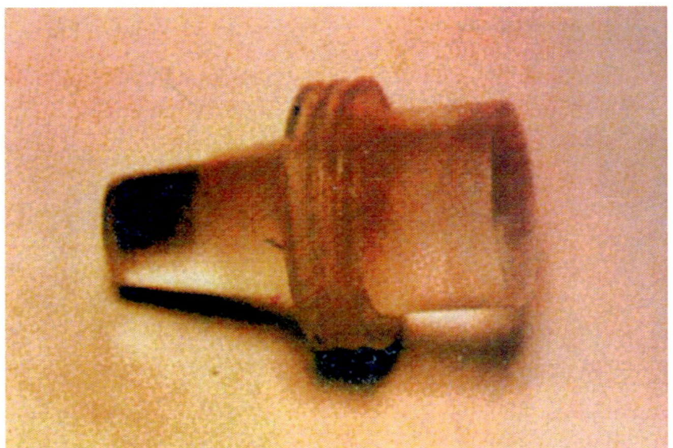

Fig. 22.16: Presurgical tonometer

ACS. Once the ACS is ready for use, one can start the LASIK procedure. The excimer laser is set up for the required refractive power correction and calibration done (the authors have a Chiron 217 Excimer in their Chennai hospital and a PDI—Photon Data Incorporated Excimer in their Bangalore hospital in India).

Once the surgical drape is applied, care being taken that the lashes do not come in the surgical field, the procedure is started. A reference mark is made and the suction ring fixed onto the eye. The presurgical tonometer (Fig. 22.16) is used to check if the IOP is sufficient. Then the microkeratome (corneal shaper head) is adjusted onto the suction ring till the gears are in place. Then the forward footswitch is pressed and the microkeratome moves forward. It stops at the permanent stopper to prevent a free cap from occurring. Then the reverse footswitch is pressed and the microkeratome moves back. The corneal shaper head is removed. *The authors do not remove the suction ring as yet. This helps to stabilize the eye and move it so that the excimer beam is perpendicular to the ablation zone.* **Dr (Mrs) T Agarwal started this technique and the authors noticed that even with the IOP high for the duration of ablation no complications occurred. On the other hand, it solved problems of patients being uncooperative and getting decentered ablations.**

Once the cornea is flapped and the ablations completed, the stroma and the flap are cleaned with the balanced salt solution (BSS) fluid. Then a wet Merocel sponge is taken and the flap cleaned with both sides of the Merocel sponge. This helps to prevent epithelial ingrowths. Then the cannula attached to a syringe with BSS fluid is taken and placed under the flap. It is moved to the junction of the flap and the cornea and gradually the flap lifted with it so that the flap falls back into its original position over the cornea. *This method appears to be an excellent method to reposit back the corneal flap.* When the flap is in position one should check if the corneal reference markers are in apposition. Check if any foreign body is present in the interface. Wait for a couple of minutes and check if the flap has stuck or not. Then carefully take out the speculum.

Both eyes are done simultaneously by the authors. The patient is then seen on the slit lamp after about half an hour and sent home without any pad or shield. The patient is put on topical steroids and artificial tears for 2 to 3 weeks. The patient is seen the next day. On the first postoperative visit, one should generally see only subconjunctival hemorrhages due to the suction ring and nothing on the cornea. **The cornea should look like a normal cornea on the slit lamp.** Check the vision, which should generally be normal without glasses. The authors call the patient next after a month. This is advantageous so that if regression has occurred then the flap is again lifted and reablation done. It is quite easy to lift the flap within a month of the laser. The patient if alright is called after 6 months. Figure 22.17 shows a postopera-

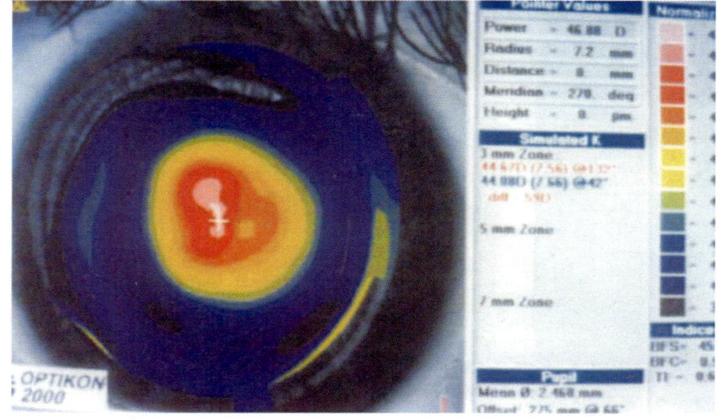

Fig. 22.17: Postoperative topograph of a hyperopic lasik. Note the flatenning in the periphery as seen in blue color

tive topograph of a hyperopic LASIK in which one can see the excellent result with the flattening of the periphery as seen by the blue color.

PROBLEMS DURING SURGERY

Certain problems can occur while performing the keratectomy. **Most important is to remember to put the thickness plates on the corneal shaper head otherwise there will be a perforation into the anterior chamber.** Check the IOP carefully because if the pressure is not high enough the flap will be very thin. Before starting the keratectomy apply a little bit of fluid on the cornea to make it wet so that the keratectomy is smooth. Do not apply too much of fluid for otherwise the gears can get stuck with too much of fluid. Check that the lids will not get stuck in the movement of the microkeratome. Sometimes, temporally the lid gets stuck in the microkeratome and this stops the microkeratome in the middle of the procedure. **Always ablate in the pupillary area so that you do not get a decentered ablation. The ablation should always be perpendicular to the cornea and not oblique.** When the flap is being cleaned and reposited one should be careful that the flap does not tear. Wait for a couple of minutes before taking off the speculum otherwise the flap might shift. If after half an hour the flap has moved as seen on the slit lamp then take the patient back to the theater and correct the flap displacement.

TROUBLE SHOOTING

Corneal Shaper Head/blade Holder

Rough Gear Movement

If the gears of the shaper head are completely bound up or moving roughly as you run your thumb over them, it is most likely due to a residue of cleaning solution or BSS left inside the gear cavity. First, try immersing the shaper head in sterile water and running your thumb over the gears to purge the residue. If this does not help loosen up the gears, repeat the cleaning process with the toothbrush and cleaning solution, rinse completely with distilled water and dry before sterilizing again.

Blade Holder Not Moving Freely

The blade holder may be restricted within the cavity of the shaper head because of a residue of cleaning solution, BSS or Cidex. Remove the blade holder and thoroughly clean it and the cavity of the shaper head with a toothbrush in the cleaning solution. Make sure to completely rinse the components with distilled water and dry them before sterilizing again.

Restricted Blade Movement with Shaft

If the blade holder moved freely when tested by itself, but feels restricted with a blade installed and the shaper head closed, remove the thickness plate and open the shaper head to confirm that the blade is properly seated on the blade holder and that all surfaces are perfectly clean and dry. One may use a fiber-free surgical sponge to absorb any moisture in the cavity. Close the shaper head and test the blade again. If the movement still feels restricted, the blade may have been crimpled in the installation process. Replace the blade with another and check with the test shaft again. Proceed only if the blade movement is absolutely smooth and resistance-free.

No Blade Movement with Shaft or Motor

If the blade does not move at all, remove the test shaft or motor from the shaper head. Look into the back of the shaper head to see if the blade holder is inserted properly. If you do not see the groove, open the shaper head and remove the blade. Take the blade holder out and insert properly, then replace the blade, close the shaper head and retest.

Thickness Plate not Fitting into the Shaper Head

When you have difficulty in inserting or seating a plate, it is probably because the hex nut of the plate is fully tightened. By rotating the locking wrench counterclockwise between your fingers, you will back the hex nut off enough to allow the plate to be installed. If the plate still does not fit flush into the head, check for debris or blockage in the recess of the head or on the post of the thickness plate and clean as necessary.

Suction Ring

Shaper Head Feeling Rough When Passed Through Ring

If the manual movement of the shaper head through the guide ring feels less than perfectly smooth, inspect the dovetail and gear track of the guide ring as well as the dovetail tracks on the shaper head for residue or debris. Clean both the shaper head and guide ring as necessary. Rinse the components in distilled water only. Tap water may leave deposits.

Suction not Enough

If the suction is not enough, check the tubing. The tubing might be cracked. So change the tubing. There could also be some blockage in the suction system.

Corneal Shape Motor

Motor Shaft not Rotating When not attached to the Shaper Head

If the motor shaft does not rotate when the foot switch is depressed, check to see that the unit is turned on. Also confirm that the foot switch and power cord are properly connected.

Motor not Attaching to the Shaper Head

If the motor does not attach to the shaper head, check to see that the locking nut is installed with the knurled portion out and the smooth portion in. Correct as necessary. Also, confirm that the blade holder is properly installed with the notch facing out towards the back of the shaper head. If not, disassemble the shaper head and remove the blade so that the blade holder may be removed and properly installed.

Table 22.1: Sterilization of automatic corneal shaper (ACS) and its components

ACS component	*Autoclave*	*ETO*	*Cidex*	*Alcohol*
Instrument tray and contents	Yes	Yes	No	No
Applanation lens	No	Yes	Yes	No
Tonometer	No	Yes	Yes	No
ACS motor	No	No	No	Wipe only
Motor cable	No	Yes	No	Wipe only

CARE AND HANDLING

Problems can be avoided by keeping the ACS as clean as possible. Oscillation of the blade and the passage of the shaper head must be absolutely smooth and resistance-free. The ACS device must be cleaned thoroughly after each use. One should clean with a cleaning solution consisting of 2 parts green Palmolive dishwashing liquid to 100 parts warm water. The type of soap present in Palmolive helps provide lubrication for the device. All parts must be thoroughly rinsed with distilled water after cleaning with the solution. It is best not to perform any cleaning steps in or over a sink, as many of the components are small and could be lost in the drain. Use small plastic bowls or basins instead.

STERILIZATION

Sterilization of the ACS is extremely important. In Table 22.1 the various sterilization techniques are shown.

23 Care and Handling of Microkeratomes

Nicholas C Caro, Paul Graczyk, Carmelita Coronel

METICULOUS CARE AND HANDLING OF MICROKERATOMES

The microkeratome is a very precise and intricate part of the LASIK (laser in situ keratomileusis) procedure. Although there are many different microkeratomes in the market today, they all have one thing in common, i.e. all microkeratomes need to be maintained and kept in excellent working condition. Having a support staff that realizes the importance of this highly important piece of equipment will provide a physician with his or her most important piece of mind, preventing and eliminating any unnecessary outcomes during surgery.

The authors hope this chapter will give some guidance towards the proper handling and care of the many microkeratomes in the market today. These guidelines are here to help in becoming familiar with the different processes and the rationales why they are practiced. You may want to read and follow your manufacturer's suggestions, so as not to deviate from the suggested guidelines for your specific microkeratome, but the basic cleaning procedures should remain universal.

CAUTION

- Microkeratomes are high precision delicate instruments, and one should read all owner's manual instructions for assembly, operations, cleaning and storing of the equipment safely.
- Do not test or use on any other material other than ocular tissue. Use on or contact with any other material may seriously damage the microkeratome equipment.
- The microkeratome heads are solid nonsterile and must be sterilized prior to each use.
- Before inspecting, cleaning, or sterilizing this instrument you must first be trained in the proper handling techniques of the equipment.
- Do not wipe down the keratome head or component parts with anything other than lint-free materials, i.e. (lint free) PVA (polyvinyl alcohol) surgical instrument wipes, (PVA) eye spears and soft bristled toothbrushes.
- Polyvinyl alcohol or acetal (PVA) materials contain no fibers and will not shed debris into the operative site and is an ideal material to use in the cleaning of your microkeratomes.
- Cellulose (hydrocellular) materials can leave thread-like fibers (debris) on the surface as well as in the recessed areas of the microkeratomes during cleaning. This material can damage the inner workings of the microkeratome and in certain cases be deposited directly into the stromal interface through the microkeratome head during LASIK procedures. Cellulose materials should be avoided in all situations during LASIK procedures and in the cleaning of your equipment.
- Do not clean equipment with anything other than surgically approved instrument cleaners and solutions.

- Do not sterilize any piece of the equipment that appears to have a surface deposit such as cellular debris and/or a protein build-up. Clean and reinspect the equipment prior to sterilization and use.

PREPARATION METHODS: INSPECTION OF EQUIPMENT

All new microkeratome component parts should be inspected under a minimum of 10 × magnification or higher for defects such as blade defects, misalignment of the blade, scratches or burrs on the head assembly, plates (if applicable) tracks, bearing (if applicable), dovetails, suction rings and drive assembly to ensure that they will operate properly. If any part is found to be defective it should be sent back to the manufacturer for immediate service.

PREPARATION STEPS: ASSEMBLY OF THE EQUIPMENT

The individual microkeratome manufacturer's instructions should be followed for proper assembly of the equipment. Extra care needs to be taken while each component part of the microkeratome is put together and assembled to ensure that it will function properly during surgery.

Each component part must go together easily (without stress or forcing the parts together), visually inspect each part to make sure it is free of any debris, burrs or scratches and (if applicable) the bearings and tracks of the microkeratome head assembly are moving freely.

Once you have visually inspected the new equipment to make sure it is operating properly, disassemble the component parts and prepare them for cleaning and sterilization.

- Prior to actual surgical use the assembled microkeratome handpieces (head and suction ring) are handed to the physician, the pedal is pressed to activate the keratome head to ensure that it is operating properly.
- If any part of the microkeratome head assembly is not operating properly *do not use the microkeratome.*

The following steps and procedures will apply to new and in use surgical keratomes.

RECOMMENDED CLEANING SUPPLIES: SET-UP

Prepare three cleaning bowls: the first with an approved surgical instrument cleaning solution and lubricant and a new soft toothbrush, the second bowl is filled with distilled water, the third bowl is also filled with distilled water and a new soft toothbrush.

CLEANING SOLUTIONS

Cleaning solutions with a neutral pH level of 7.0 to 8.5 pH is used for general surgical instruments, however, with surgical specialty instruments, i.e. eye, ENT, neuro, etc. a 7.0 to 10.5 pH dilution ratio is recommended. An extremely alkaline detergent (higher than 10.5) may stain and might cause breaks, and extremely low acid detergent (lower than 6.0) may cause an instrument to pit.

- Keep on hand a lint-free disposable towel, canned air, dry soft toothbrush, PVA surgical instrument wipes and PVA surgical spears. Several Brush-Pix's™ or plastic toothpicks can be kept in the cleaning area for use in those very hard to reach recessed areas in the microkeratome head and dovetails. This will aid in dislodging and removing baked on cellular debris, protein build-up or baked on lubricating gels.

MANUAL CLEANING: HAND WASHING OF INSTRUMENTS

Automated or Manual Microkeratome Head Cleaning Procedures (with Plates)

- Break down the microkeratome head. The keratome blade is removed from the head assembly, then using the toothbrush begin scrubbing the head using the surgical instrument cleaning solution. Be sure to concentrate on the gears and the underside of the head to remove all tissues and debris. Special attention should be paid to the dovetail of the rings and the head.
- In the second bowl of distilled water thoroughly rinse the microkeratome head, rings and all

component parts used during the procedure. Visually inspect all component parts carefully. "Pay special attention to all recessed areas of the microkeratome head, blade holder areas, tracks, gears and dovetails for any debris or burrs".

- In the third bowl of distilled water once again using a clean soft toothbrush clean the microkeratome head concentrating on all recessed areas, tracks, gears, dovetails and the underside of the head to remove any debris. Visually inspect all component parts carefully. If any cellular debris or burrs are found, repeat step one and step two in the cleaning process.
- Set the microkeratome head on a lint-free towel while you repeat the process with the suction ring and any other additional component parts.
- After manual cleaning you will dry the microkeratome head, suction ring and all component parts. Go to the "drying instruments" section for additional procedures to follow.

ULTRASONIC CLEANING: MACHINE WASHING OF INSTRUMENTS

"Certain microkeratome manufacturers do not recommend the use of an ultrasonic cleaner with their units". If you have any questions regarding this issue please refer to your owner's operating manual.

Ultrasonic Cleaners

"Ultrasonic cleaners work by transforming sonic energy into mechanical energy, thus, creating tiny bubbles on all of the instrument surfaces. These tiny bubbles implode and the minivacuum removes all foreign matter from the instrument, particularly in the hard-to-reach areas, like the box locks, scissors locks and other crevice-like areas. Ultrasonic cleaners also remove all lubrication from instruments, therefore, all clean instruments should be bathed in a water-soluble instrument milk (if a multipurpose cleaner and lubricant is not used) after ultrasonic cleaning". Ultrasonic cleaning is 16 times more effective than hand washing of surgical instruments.

Although ultrasonic cleaners remove over 90 percent of the soil and contaminants deposited on your surgical instruments, it does not preempt the need for sterilization.

Caution

Microsurgical instruments must not come in contact with one another during ultrasonic cleaning. The unit's vibrations may cause premature wear of instruments' precision tips, use ultrasonic cleaners with frequencies set at 43 to 60 Hz. Also,

- When using an ultrasonic cleaner you should always change or discard the cleaning solution after every use to avoid bacterial growth. Bacterial growth can occur in these solutions after the instruments have been cleaned and the solution is left in the ultrasonic cleaner for any period of time.
- After the instruments have been ultrasonically cleaned: (i) discard the used cleaning solution, (ii) rinse the inside of the tank with clean distilled water, (iii) wipe it dry with a soft lint free towel, (iv) then, wipe down the inside and outside surfaces of the ultrasonic unit with a disposable alcohol wipe to disinfect the unit.
- The ultrasonic cleaner is now ready for storage or it can be refilled with a new batch of cleaning solution to process additional instruments.

Automated or Manual Microkeratome Head Ultrasonic Cleaning Procedures (without Plates)

- Prepare two (optional 3) cleaning bowls: the first with an approved surgical instrument cleaning solution and lubricant and a new soft toothbrush, the second bowl is filled with distilled water and a new soft toothbrush, and the third (optional) bowl is filled with distilled water and a new soft toothbrush.
- Break down the microkeratome head, the keratome blade is removed from the head assembly, then using the toothbrush begin scrubbing the head using an approved surgical instrument cleaning solution and lubricant. Be sure to concentrate on the gears and the underside

of the head to remove all tissues and debris. Special attention should be paid to the dovetail of the rings and the head.

- The microkeratome head, suction ring and all component parts are then cleaned in an ultrasonic bath using an approved surgical instrument cleaner and lubricant for 5 to 7 minutes.
  Caution—All microkeratome manufacturers do not recommend the use of ultrasonic cleaners with their units. Please refer to your owner's manual for recommended procedures.
- Remove the microkeratome head, suction ring and all component parts and rinse them completely in the second bowl of distilled water. Visually inspect all component parts carefully. "Pay special attention to all recessed areas of the microkeratome head, blade holder areas, tracks, gears and dovetails for any debris or burrs". If any debris is found repeat the previous three steps. If any damage to the microkeratome head or component parts is observed that should be returned to the manufacturer for immediate service. Discard the used cleaning solution.

SOAKING INSTRUMENTS

If after several repeated tries the cellular debris, protein build-up or lubricant gel has not become loosened up and removed during normal cleaning steps, some additional steps may become necessary. Using an approved concentrated surgical instrument cleaner, place the microkeratome head and the component parts into a small tray. Use enough concentrated surgical instrument cleaner to cover the instruments in the tray and allow the instruments to soak for several hours. Visually inspect each component and where it is necessary use the BrushPix's™ or plastic toothpick (like a dentist pick) to gently loosen and remove the debris from the recessed areas. Several attempts may be necessary to completely clean these areas. Once this is done repeat your normal cleaning procedures. Then, visually inspect all components again to make sure they are clean and working properly.

- Set the microkeratome head, the suction ring and all component parts on a lint-free towel.

DRYING INSTRUMENTS

After cleaning, the instruments should be dried quickly to prevent water spots and mineral stains from forming on the microkeratome head and component parts. Mineral deposits on the surface of the delicate microkeratome head, tracks, dovetails and bearing assembly will prevent the smooth operation of the microkeratome.

- Pat down the microkeratome head and all component parts with the lint-free towel or PVA surgical instrument wipe to remove all excess water.
- Dry the microkeratome head with the canned air and use the PVA surgical eye spears and PVA instrument wipes to dry any hard to reach areas. Remember while drying, concentrate on the gears being certain that they spin with no resistance. Visually inspect all component parts carefully.
- Buff the microkeratome head with a soft dry toothbrush. Insert the blade holder into the microkeratome head and rock it back and forth. Be sure the blade holder is moving freely with no resistance. If the blade holder is not moving freely, repeat drying process.
- Lubricating the microkeratome head, suction ring and any additional component parts should be done in water-soluble instrument milk (bath) for a period of approximately 30 seconds. This will apply a light surface lubricant to the instrument ensuring that it will operate smoothly following sterilization. Visually inspect all component parts carefully.

LUBRICATION OF INSTRUMENTS

It is recommended that the instruments be lubricated after every cleaning process to guard against mineral deposits and other water system impurities, which may lead to stains, rust and corrosion. Also, prior vigorous cleaning removes all lubricants, which may result in "frozen" areas of the microkeratome equipment. To impede the growth of bacteria in the lubricant bath, only water-soluble lubricants are recommended and discarded after every use.

- Set the microkeratome head, suction ring and any additional component parts into its sterilization case. Then place the case into the autoclave for the full cycle.
- When finished, the case is now ready for storage. Then discard the used instrument cleaning solution and instrument milk (bath).

STERILIZATION OF INSTRUMENTS

Steam Sterilization

The most common and practical form of sterilizing instruments is steam sterilization. The autoclave has to be in good working order and operate perfectly in both steam and drying cycles. Instruments loaded into the autoclave chamber should not be too cold, as they can cause steam condensation, water spotting and staining. In some instances, it may be advisable to preheat the load (using the drying cycle) to warm up the instruments before sterilization. Try this first whenever you encounter water stains after sterilization. Also, it is very important not to open the chamber immediately after sterilization, but rather, to crack the door for a few minutes (7-10 minutes, as per the manufacturer's recommendations), while the drying cycle is on. In any case, the instruments should come out bone dry, without any condensation moisture anywhere on the instruments or in the instrument packs. To minimize steam staining, use water in the autoclave, which is distilled deionized. Also, all autoclaves should be flushed according to manufacturer's time schedules and recommendations.

Cold Sterilization (Germicidal Solution Bath)

Contrary to popular opinion, cold sterilization is not better than steam sterilization for instruments. Remember, most professional offices leave the instrument in germicide for hours and days at a time. Even though the germicides are slightly corrosive, it is the extra long time of immersion, which takes its toll on the instrument surface. A short (20 to 30 minute) steam exposure is much less corrosive and also less dulling to sharp edges of scissors and knives, than long exposure to cold sterilization. Also, some of the solutions are highly alkaline (high pH—more than 7), or highly caustic (very low pH—less than 7), and can cause staining and corrosion when autoclaved after a germicidal bath. Make sure to rinse very thoroughly after taking the instruments out of the germicidal bath.

SAMPLE (ONLY) OVERVIEW: CLEANING, STERILIZATION AND DISINFECTING THE MICROKERATOME COMPONENT PARTS

Please refer to your owner's manual for exact processing steps. Table 23.1 is used only as an example.

MICROKERATOME CONSOLE

The exterior of the microkeratome console should be cleaned with a soft cloth dampened in a mild soap and water solution, any stainless steel components on the face of the console may be polished with a commercial metal polish if desired.

Also, the microkeratome console may be cleaned and disinfected by wiping down the exterior surfaces of the unit with sterile disposable alcohol wipe.

STORAGE OF INSTRUMENTS

The main problem in this respect is moisture. Always store instruments (after drying them thoroughly) in a moisture-free area. Sterile packs can be stored the same way for any period of time, as recommended by the manufacturer of the sterilizer. If instruments are kept in drawers, make sure that they do not touch each other. Keep the tips and edges of all instruments protected to avoid damage with, i.e. silicone tubing, cork or other specially designed materials for your equipment.

Well-defined storage procedures reduce the chance of bent, broken and dulled instruments.

Do not bounce, or weight down instruments. Treat them gently, handle them individually or in small quantities. Masses of entangled instruments cause

Table 23.1: Cleaning, sterilization and disinfecting the microkeratome component parts

Microkeratome components	*Steam sterilization temperature: 135°C/275°F duration time: 20 minutes*	*Surface "alcohol" wipe*	*Disinfecting soak*
Applanator lenses	No	No	No
Operating room	Yes *270° for three minutes	No	No
Tonometer	Yes	Yes	No
Turbine motor	Yes	Yes	Yes
Microkeratome head	Yes	Yes	Yes
Vacuum suction ring	Yes	Yes	Yes
Vacuum fixation handle	Yes	Yes	Yes
Stop rings	Yes	Yes	Yes
Instrument tray	No	Yes	No
Turbine hose	No	Yes	No
Suction tubing			

damage. Do not cram a large instrument kit into a small tray. Place heavier instruments in the tray bottom with the lighter weight instruments on the top.

Instruments should be arranged accordingly

- Place instruments in a holder to keep them in an open position to prevent damage from occurring
- Instruments with pointed or curved components should be all point in the same direction
- For purposes of instrument protection, the edges should not come in contact with other instruments.

SUMMARY

A few pointers for persons using surgical instruments:

- All instruments are designed for a special purpose, and should be used only for the purpose intended. All instruments should be cleaned after every use as soon as possible, and kept in a clean and moisture-free environment.
- Instruments with metal to metal contact areas should be lubricated with recommended lubricants.
- Any instrument found not to be in perfect working order should either be repaired or replaced as soon as possible. "Damaged instruments should not be used under any circumstances".
- All instruments should be given routine maintenance by qualified instrument manufacturers or repair facilities.

Because repairs can be costly, a specifically scheduled preventive maintenance program based on usage is the best alternative.

Particular steps include:

- Inspection and evaluation
- Repassivation
- Clean and lubricate
- Replacement of worn and missing parts
- Restoration of finish (i.e. grind out scratches and gouges and repolish)
- Final adjustment to insure an instrument works easily and is properly aligned.

Implementing the above program restores your instruments to surgical grade quality before major repairs and/or possible replacement becomes necessary. Although your instrument repair costs may rise, your new instrument costs will decline over the long run, an important factor to consider in the present economy.

24 LASIK: The Technique

Howard V Gimbel, Ellen E Anderson Penno

BACKGROUND

Laser in situ keratomileusis (LASIK) was developed from the previously well-established techniques of lamellar keratoplasty and photorefractive keratectomy (PRK).[1-5] The basic history and development of the LASIK techniques are discussed in depth in a number of excellent texts.[6-10] However, as is occurring with all refractive surgery techniques, the instrumentation and techniques of LASIK are continually being refined. In order to serve the patient well and continue to improve outcomes, refractive surgeons need to be aware of both the fundamental principles of LASIK as well any new developments in techniques and technology.

LASIK FUNDAMENTALS

There are three basic steps that should be taken to optimize the results of LASIK surgery: (i) proper assessment of the patients preoperative motivations and expectations, (ii) thorough preoperative testing with selection of the appropriate refractive surgical technique, and (iii) good intraoperative and postoperative techniques including an understanding of how to manage complications.

As in all surgical procedures, good outcomes begin with proper patient selection (Table 24.1). Many patients requesting refractive surgery are well informed about various refractive surgery techniques and may have friends or relatives that have undergone surgery already. In spite of this, the surgeon must be careful to thoroughly explain the surgical techniques and what the patient can expect as an outcome. It is important to ask all patients directly about their motivations for surgery. For example, a presbyope with mild myopia whose occupation involves near work might simply state their motivation is to be free from corrective lenses, it is imperative that the surgeon must educate the patients with regard to the need for reading glasses postoperatively and inform the patients that while they may be free from glasses for driving and some sports they have to wear corrective lenses for their work. For some patients a trial of monovision in contact lenses might be appropriate. Similarly, a patient with amblyopia will need to understand that refractive surgery is not likely (except in rare circumstances) to improve their best-corrected visual acuity (BCVA). There are many circumstances in which the preoperative discussion can be used to correct misconceptions and provide additional information, and these discussions must be tailored to each individual patient. Understanding the patient's visual requirements in terms of work and hobbies as well as motivations for surgery are essential in preoperative counseling. Appropriate expectations lead to more satisfied postoperative patients.

The preoperative work-up for LASIK patients should include a careful medical and ophthalmic

Table 24.1: Preoperative factors indicating increased risk*	
Patient history	• Inappropriate motivations or expectations • Contact lens use (verify when last used—should be discontinued 48 hours prior to testing for soft lenses, and 2 weeks for hard lenses) • Previous ocular surgery or corneal injuries predisposing to poor exposure or suction failure • History of steroid-induced ocular hypertension or medication allergies • Collagen vascular diseases (risk for corneal melt) • Hormonal status or diabetes (refractive instability) • Systemic medications such as steroids (refractive instability or mydriasis)
Age	• Presbyopes or near presbyopes should be counseled carefully (consider monovision) • Verify a stable refraction in all patients especially if less than 30 years of age
Refraction	• Refraction stable for 1 year prior to surgery • Consider cycloplegic refraction in all patients
Pachymetry	• Inadequate pachymetry risk for postoperative ectasia
Manual keratometry	• Overly steep or flat corneas may be prone to flap complications
Pupil size	• Large pupils (risk of night vision difficulties especially important in high corrections). Corneal surgery may not be advisable
Slit-lamp examination	• Lid abnormalities (poor exposure risk for flap dislocation) • Blepharitis (increased risk for infections or infiltrates) • Corneal dystrophies (risk for epithelial problems, may need PTK)

*These are examples of factors which may indicate an increased risk for unsatisfactory outcomes or complications from LASIK surgery. All patients should have dilated indirect ophthalmoscopic examination, higher myopes and patients with prior history of retinal problems should have retinal drawings. Any pathology should be noted and referred for treatment if needed. *The surgeon must be vigilant when assessing patients preoperatively and carefully consider all factors which may increase the risk of complications so that the patient can be counseled accordingly*

history, uncorrected visual acuity (UCVA) and BCVA measurements, assessment of refractive stability based on their current lenses or previous records, pupil measurements in bright and dim light, assessment of ocular motility, tonometry, slit-lamp examination, dilated funduscopic examination with retinal drawings, pachymetry, manual keratometry, and corneal mapping. Any lid or orbital abnormalities should also be noted as this may affect the ability to place the suction ring or microkeratome during the LASIK procedure. It is helpful if the examiner also notes any extreme nervousness when attempting tonometry or placing drops, as these patients may need additional counseling in oder to ensure that they can cooperate with the surgeon during the LASIK surgery.

Once the preoperative testing is complete and assessment can be made as to the patient's appropriateness for refractive surgery and with regard to which technique or techniques would be most appropriate, we currently offer LASIK to all myopes including moderately high myopes if pachymetry is adequate. Generally a residual stromal bed of 250 microns is desirable and the Munnerlyn formula ($T = [Dh^2]/3$, T = thickness in microns, D = power in diopters, h = diameter of optical zone in millimeters) can be used in the clinic to assess the theoretical ablation depth. Pupil size in high hyperopes and in myopes must be carefully assessed due to the risk of night vision effects if a small optical zone is used in an effort to conserve corneal tissue. High myopes with marginal pachymetry are asked to consider phakic intraocular lenses (phakic IOLs) implants or refractive lensectomy (for presbyopes) as alternatives. For patients with low to moderate myopia, the options of intrastromal corneal rings (ISCR) and PRK are discussed in addition to LASIK. Hyperopes can undergo LASIK up to about + 4 D. Patients have undergone LASIK for higher degrees of hyperopia with good results. However, above that range consideration should be given to refractive lensectomy for presbyopes and phakic IOL (if the anterior chamber depth is adequate). It is helpful for each surgeon to assess LASIK outcomes on an ongoing basis in order to counsel patients as accurately as possible with regard to complication rates and enhancement rates.

After the patient has been counseled with regard to the surgical options for the correction of their individual refractive error, and decided upon LASIK, it is wise to ask the patient if they have any additional questions. In some cases, an ophthalmologist or optometrist other than the surgeon may have done the initial preoperative work-up and in these cases the surgeon should always have a discussion prior to surgery emphasizing particularly important factors such as presbyopia and the potential need for reading glasses postoperatively or the potential for night vision disturbances for patients with large pupils. The surgeon must also review the testing results and double check that the pachymetry is adequate for high corrections.

The patient is asked to sign the informed consent and is then ready to undergo LASIK surgery. The fundamental principles of good intraoperative LASIK techniques are attention to detail, good exposure, careful fluid management, and a feather-light touch. This is discussed in detail.

INTRAOPERATIVE LASIK TECHNIQUE

Each procedure begins with a series of careful checks. The microkeratome and suction ring are checked under the microscope for correct assembly and for any dried salt crystals, lint, or other debris that might interfere with proper functioning. The microkeratome is then put through a dry run before each case. It is essential that the surgeon and surgical staff be familiar with the specifics of the microkeratome system in use to ensure that the appropriate checks are made and that any irregularities in functioning can be detected during the preoperative inspection (Fig. 24.1).

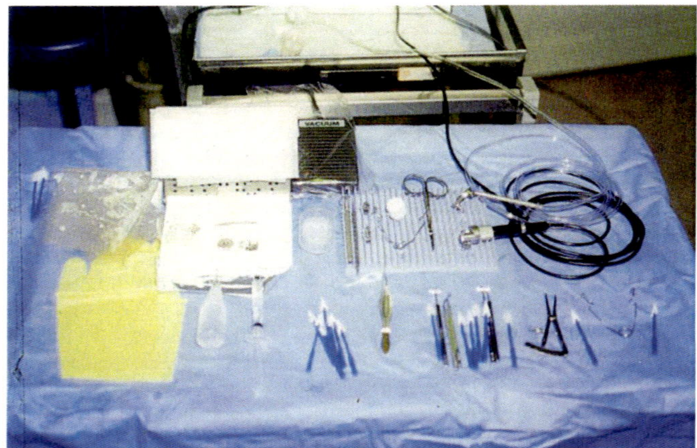

Fig. 24.1: Example of set-up for LASIK surgery. The surgeon and staff should be familiar with the specifics of the microkeratome system in use and ensure that all the appropriate preoperative checks are made before each case

The surgeon must also be thoroughly familiar with the laser system in place so as to position the patient correctly and give appropriate instructions with regard to fixation lights and system noise. A well-informed patient will have better fixation and is less likely to startle when beginning the excimer ablation, thus, optimizing results. The surgeon should also check the laser input against the patient record to ensure that all parameters have been entered correctly.

Positioning of the patient is similar to that required in cataract surgery (Fig. 24.2). As with all ophthalmic surgeries done under topical anesthesia, the patient is instructed not to move his or her arms or legs and to warn the surgeon if he or she need to shift position or cough. The patient is also told to keep both eyes open but to continue to blink normally, and to avoid squeezing the eyes as this can result in a Bell's phenomenon in the operative eye. Optimizing exposure is an essential component to complication-free surgery; the patient's chin should be slightly elevated such that the cornea is well centered such that the lids and drapes will not interfere with the microkeratome pass. To aid in exposure, the drape should be applied carefully without creation of a pseudopalpebral fissure (Fig. 24.3) which may result from edges of the drape adhering to each other. The scrub assistant can

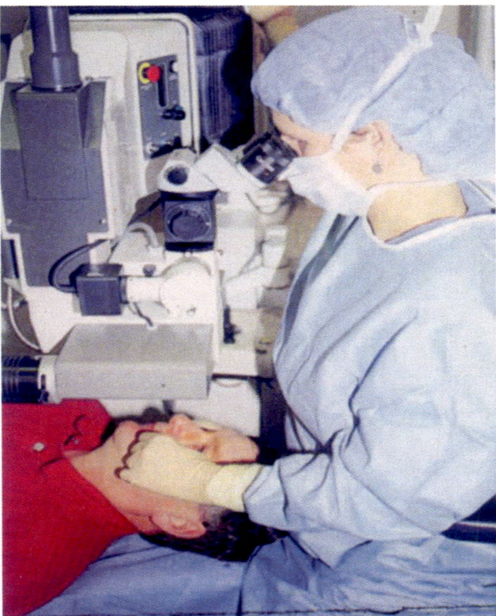

Fig. 24.2: The position of the patient should be similar to that required in cataract surgery. Often it is helpful to have a slight chin-up position such that the brow does not interfere with exposure. As the patient is positioned, instructions are given with regard to fixation lights and system noise to aid in his or her ability to cooperate with laser ablation

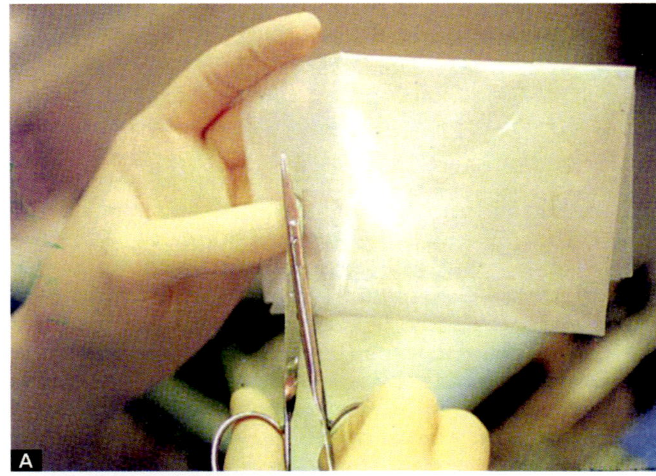

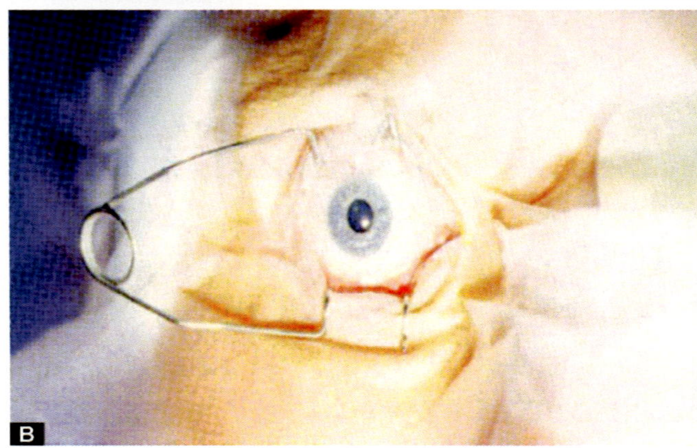

Figs 24.3A and B: (A) Optimal exposure is essential for complication-free surgery. Special attention should be paid to avoid creation of a pseudopalpebral fissure medially or laterally. To avoid this we routinely cut our drapes preoperatively, and (B) avoid any overlap in the drape at the medial or lateral canthus. The patient is also instructed to avoid squeezing the eyes and to concentrate on keeping the fellow eye open to aid in avoiding a Bell's phenomenon in the operative eye

place gentle pressure downward and outward on the lid speculum to aid in exposure during the microkeratome pass and avoid obstruction of the microkeratome by lids or drapes.

In addition to optimization of exposure another key to obtaining the best results with LASIK surgery is careful fluid management. Preoperative topical anesthetic drops should be minimized. The fornix is gently cleared of excess fluid prior to marking the cornea. Three asymmetric marks are made to assist in correct flap replacement. The surgeon should have the footpedal ready prior to placing the suction ring to avoid any delays between placing the ring and starting the microkeratome pass (Fig. 24.4). After placement of the suction ring the cornea is wiped with a sponge soaked in proparacaine. During this maneuver it is helpful to reassure the patient that it is normal to feel sensation on the lids and that the surface of the eye is numbed. Proparacaine is used instead of balanced salt solution (BSS) to avoid salt crystals forming in the microkeratome gears which may cause jamming of the gear mechanism (Fig. 24.5). The patient is warned that the vision will dim out temporarily and that he or she will feel pressure on the lids and in the eye as suction is placed. It may be helpful to use downward pressure in the suction ring during the microkeratome pass (after the lower lid is cleared when using down-up cutting instruments) to decrease the risk of a buttonhole. Once the pass is complete it alleviates patient anxiety to tell the patient that the flap is intact. After the microkeratome pass the laser should be centered, the laser armed, and the patient instructed to concentrate on the fixation light prior to lifting the flap to minimize the time between

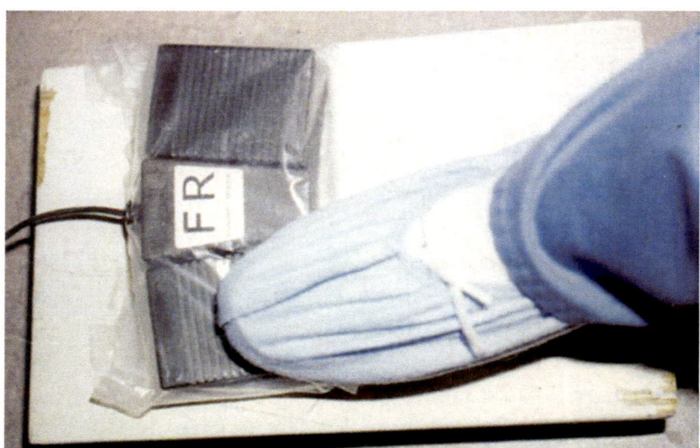

Fig. 24.4: The surgeon should have the footpedal ready prior to placing the suction ring to avoid any delays between placing the suction ring and starting the microkeratome pass

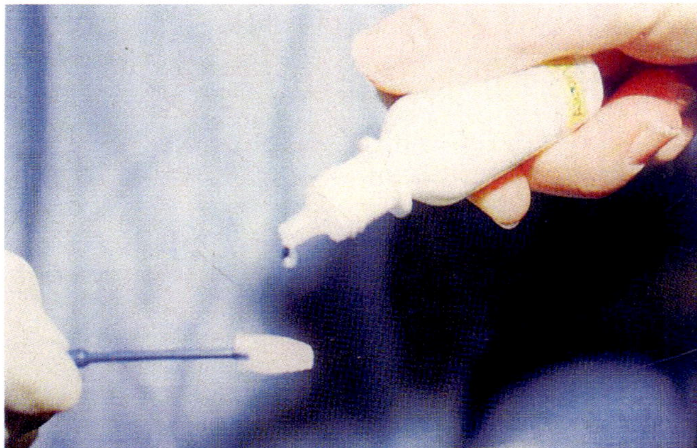

Fig. 24.5: After placing of the suction ring and just prior to placing the microkeratome the cornea should be moistened slightly using topical anesthetic drops. Balanced salt solution (BSS) is avoided due to the possibility of salt crystals forming in the microkeratome gears which may lead to jamming of the gear mechanisms and a partial pass

flap lifting and laser ablation and avoid excessive dehydration of the stromal bed. The flap is carefully laid onto a moistened Chayet or Gimbel-Chayet sponge maintaining its cup-like shape. This technique prevents drying or wrinkling of the flap during the laser application. After laser ablation is completed minimal fluid should be used when refloating the flap. Excessive fluid may result in stromal or epithelial edema and may also cause debris to float up from the cul-de-sac. A moistened sponge is used with a feather-light touch to express fluid from the interface, to wick fluid out from the flap edges, and to help to settle the flap into place. All movements at this stage should start at the hinge and movements should be away from the hinge.

Throughout the LASIK procedure attention should be given in maintaining the epithelial integrity. In some cases there can be loose epithelium superiorly. If any loose or torn epithelium is encountered after the microkeratome pass, it should be carefully smoothed into place prior to turning the flap. Small areas of loose or torn epithelium do not require placement of a bandage contact lens, however, larger areas may necessitate a contact lens for comfort. Patching should be avoided due to the risk of flap dislocation. In most cases epithelium can be replaced and need not be removed. Often epithelium may stretch and replacement may require the use of a dry sponge to coax epithelial fragments into place. It is important that no epithelium remain under the flap as this is a risk for epithelial ingrowth, this is of particular importance when performing enhancement surgery. If a tag of epithelium is seen at the edge of the stromal bed during either primary or enhancement surgery, it should be reflected back until the flap is replaced and then repositioned. When using large transition zones such as when treating hyperopia, care should be taken to shield the hinge area if necessary since ablation that spills over onto the epithelium may also pose an increased risk of epithelial ingrowth. **Minimization of topical anesthetic drops preoperatively also aids in preventing epithelial complications.** While typically a transient problem, epithelial tears and abrasions can lead to increased discomfort and blurred vision in the immediate postoperative period.

After the flap is repositioned an inspection is made to check on the position (using the marks made prior to the microkeratome pass) and to check for interface debris. The illumination systems will vary depending on the laser system being used, and the surgeon should be familiar with the variety of settings available. The Nidek laser used at our center has a slit beam capability which is quite helpful during this inspection. We also advise turning the room lights

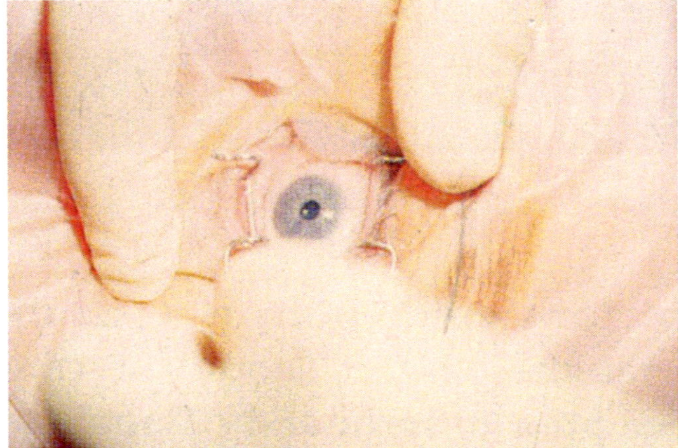

Fig. 24.6: As the speculum is removed the patient is cautioned not to squeeze the lids, and to continue looking straight ahead. The lids are stabilized with the thumb and forefinger as the speculum is removed to avoid the possibility of flap dislocation at this stage

down during this step as this enhances visibility of the interface. The beam and magnification will need to be varied to allow a thorough inspection and in particular when viewing small air-bubbles which can sometimes be difficult to distinguish from debris. If debris are identified near the edge, it may be irrigated out using a cannula and BSS without having to refloat the entire flap. If debris are noted in the center or if a flap appears shifted or wrinkled it is advisable to refloat the entire flap. Once the interface has been determined to be clean and the flap is in good position, some surgeons will wait up to 4 minutes prior to removing the drape and speculum to ensure flap adherence. This interval will be determined by each surgeon and may vary depending on the hinge location, surgeon experience, and technique.

Finally, the procedure is not complete until the lid speculum is removed and the blink test performed. When removing the speculum the patient must be cautioned not to squeeze the lids and to look straight ahead to avoid flap dislocation at this step (Fig. 24.6). As the drapes are removed the lids should be stabilized with the thumb and forefinger and again the patient should be instructed not to squeeze the lids (Figs 24.7 and B). Once the speculum and drapes are removed the patient is instructed to close the eyes gently while excess fluid is removed from the lids with a dry sponge (Fig. 24.8). The patient is then told to blink normally and a final inspection of the flap is made. Depending on the microkeratome being used and the location of the hinge, consideration should be given as to whether a postoperative check should be made within 30 to 45 minutes following LASIK surgery. We no longer routinely do this immediate postoperative check when using the Hansatome which creates a superior hinge.

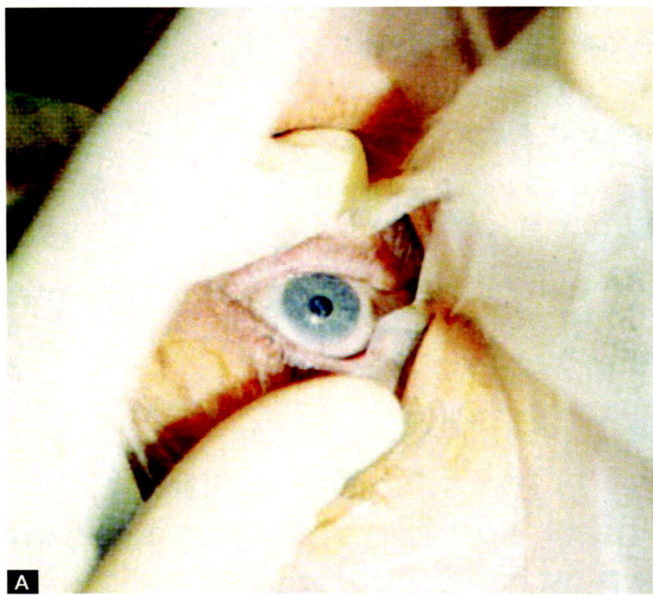

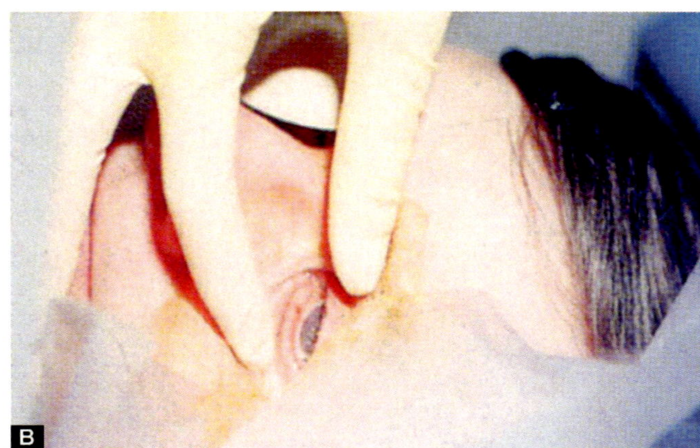

Figs 24.7A and B: (A) The thumb and forefinger are again used as the drape is removed, this may often require switching hands at the midpoint when the drape is removed, and (B) the patient is again instructed not to squeeze and to continue looking straight ahead to avoid any possibility of the flap becoming dislodged during this maneuver

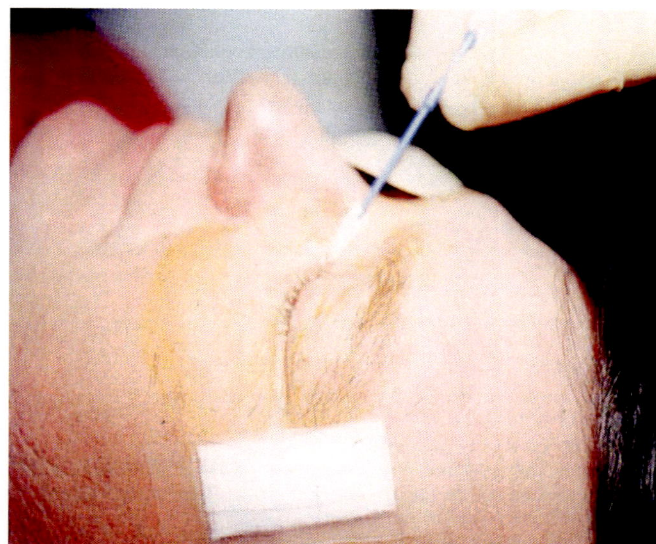

Fig. 24.8: Excess fluid is removed from the lids with a dry sponge. Also visible in this picture is the sponge used to catch any excess fluid at the temple. These maneuvers are important in maintaining patient comfort and ensuring good patient cooperation during the procedure

POSTOPERATIVE CARE OF LASIK PATIENTS

It is helpful to counsel the patients as to what to expect in terms of discomfort and vision. We generally tell patients that the amount of discomfort will be minimal, that there may be a foreign body sensation, and that these symptoms should clear within several hours to one day. They are told that the vision will be somewhat blurry for the first 6 to 24 hours and that for some patients it can take up to 48 hours to clear. Patients are also advised that the amount of discomfort and blurred vision can vary slightly between the two eyes.

The use of moisture chambers following surgery is recommended to decrease the likelihood of flap dislocation in the early postoperative period. Patients are also urged to avoid rubbing or squeezing the eyes and not to swim for at least two weeks. The postoperative medications will vary slightly from surgeon to surgeon but should include a broad-spectrum antibiotic and usually a mild steroid for approximately one week postoperatively.

Postoperative checks should continue until the epithelium is healed and then at 3 to 5 weeks and at 3 months. Patients are instructed that enhancement surgery will not be performed prior to 1 month for simple undercorrections and that it may be necessary to wait up to 3 months or longer depending upon the type of residual refractive error.

LASIK COMPLICATIONS

There are myriad of intraoperative and postoperative complications that may occur when performing LASIK surgery. These are outlined in Tables 24.2 and 24.3. The management of intraoperative and postoperative complications is touched on briefly in the tables mentioned above.

Following careful protocols of preoperative testing will identify patients with anatomic features such as steep corneas (risk for buttonhole) which may put patients at an increased risk for complications. Adhering to the principles of appropriate patient instruction, meticulous preoperative checking of the microkeratome assembly and laser input, adequate exposure, appropriate fluid management, a feather-light touch, and proper management of epithelium will help to minimize the risk of intraoperative complications. Finally, proper postoperative care including prophylactic topical antibiotics and the use of moisture chambers will help to decrease the incidence of postoperative complications.

Because many complications are rare it is imperative that the novice surgeon work with a more experienced surgeon for a period of time, it is also helpful to review the literature including the several texts that are available on the subject of LASIK.[4,6,8-14] When managing complications the same fundamental principles as outlined above (including fluid management, adequate exposure, and a feather-light touch) apply.

CONCLUSION

While LASIK is a quick procedure and may seem simple, the theory and reality of proper technique is more complex. It is important for the novice surgeon to be well trained and in addition to the short courses that are offered to learn this technique, observation

Table 24.2: Intraoperative complications	
Inadequate exposure	
Possible cause	Orbital anatomy (deep-set eyes, small palpebral fissure, prior trauma, or surgery), poor draping technique, poor lid speculum
Results	Difficulty placing suction ring, inadequate suction, incomplete pass
Avoidance	Careful draping, strong spring or locking speculum, good head positioning, assistant to put downward pressure on lid speculum during pass
Management	Lateral canthotomy or consider PRK if appropriate
Inadequate suction	
Possible cause	• Inadequate exposure • Small corneal diameter resulting in conjunctival tenting and blockage of the suction port • Manipulations of suction ring, drape or speculum leading to loss of suction
Results	Thin flap, or buttonhole
Avoidance	• Attention to techniques which optimize exposure • Hold suction ring firmly against globe when turning suction on, avoid manipulations of the suction ring, drapes, or speculum
Management	Measure IOP with Barraquer tonometer, do not rely on the suction gauge, remeasure IOP if any manipulations made
Thin flaps and buttonholes	
Possible cause	Inadequate suction, corneal anatomy (excessively steep, irregular), poor blade quality
Results	Inability to perform laser ablation, risk of epithelial ingrowth, risk of irregular astigmatism
Avoidance	Do not make the microkeratome pass if adequate IOP not verified, consider deeper depth plate on steep corneas, check microkeratome and blade prior to each use, use a new blade for each patient
Management	Replace the thin flap or buttonholed flap carefully managing the epithelial edges, inspect the flap meticulously and verify adherence, laser ablation may not be done in the case of a thin flap with ridges on the bed or with only a very thin cut of stroma, recut the flap with a thicker depth plate at a later date (2 to 3 months later)
Free cap	
Possible cause	Failure to advance the stopper sufficiently on the corneal shaper, corneal anatomy large and flat (< 41.00 mean keratometry)
Results	Free cap, ablation can proceed
Avoidance	Carefully check the entire microkeratome assembly including the stopper prior to each case, corneal marks should be asymmetric to aid in proper cap replacement
Management	Place the free cap in an antidesiccation chamber or keep covered in the microkeratome while the ablation is done, carefully replace the cap stromal side down with attention to orientation as aided by preoperative corneal marks, assure adherence by waiting 3 to 5 minutes after cap replacement, sutures are not necessary in most cases
Incomplete pass	
Possible cause	Poor exposure obstruction by drapes, lid, or speculum, debris or conjunctiva on suction ring tracks, improper assembly or cleaning of the microkeratome
Results	Inability to proceed with the ablation if the pass stops within the central 6 to 7 mm zone
Avoidance	Proper techniques to ensure adequate exposure including lateral canthotomy in rare cases, careful assembly, cleaning and inspection of microkeratome and suction ring prior to each use. Do a complete forward and reverse cycle with the microkeratome prior to each eye to ensure proper functioning, avoid excess fluid prior to microkeratome use (BSS) crystals may lead to motor head dysfunction in subsequent cases)
Managment	If proceeding with laser ablation, shield the hinge with a sponge, if unable to perform ablation (if the pass stops within the central 5 mm) replace the flap and recut at a later date with the same depth plate

Contd...

Table contd...

Corneal perforation	
Possible cause	Failure to place the depth plate into the microkeratome assembly, improperly seating the depth plate
Avoidance	Meticulous assembly and inspection of the microkeratome prior to each use
Management	Dependent on the depth of the cut, corneal transplantation and IOL implantation may be needed in severe cases
Shifted flap intraoperatively	
Possible cause	Movement of the eye when doing the striae test, patient squeezing eyes as drapes and speculum are being removed
Results	Flap dislocation or wrinkling
Avoidance	Have patient concentrate on the light when doing the striae test, ask the patient to avoid squeezing and to look straight ahead as drapes and speculum are being removed, hold the lids open with thumb and forefinger as the drapes and speculum are being removed
Management	Immediately refloat the flap into position
Wrinkled flap intraoperatively	
Possible cause	Improper flap positioning during the ablation, excessive drying of the flap, rough handling of the flap leading to stretching and microwrinkles when repositioning
Results	Wrinkles can lead to irregular astigmatism and visual disturbances
Avoidance	Carefully lay the flap in a cupped position on a damp sponge during the ablation, use a delicate touch with a wet sponge and begin smoothing at the hinge with subsequent motions away from the flap center, do not leave any fluid under the flap
Management	Refloat into position with only a gentle manipulation, epithelial wrinkles will often disappear without additional repositioning in a short time
Interface debris	
Possible cause	Poor fluid management drawing debris from cul-de-sac, lint from sponge, particles from microkeratome, debris from the cannulas, syringe or bottle
Results	Flap needs to be irrigated or possibly refloated if noted only postoperatively
Avoidance	Irrigate and wipe cul-de-sac to remove mucous preoperatively, avoid excess fluid on the surgical field, carefully inspect microkeratome prior to each use, carefully clean and rinse with clean water all reusable cannulas, use disposable syringes
Management	Inspect the interface and flap carefully prior to removing drapes and speculum, edge irrigation may be used for peripheral debris, lift flap and reposition after irrigation for centrally located debris
Flap edema	
Possible cause	Prolonged flap manipulation, excessive irrigation
Results	Flap edge retraction
Avoidance	Minimize handling of flap, minimize irrigation under the flap
Management	Attempt to gently stretch flap into place with a dry sponge as it begins to adhere, sutures may be necessary in some cases.
Flap shrinkage	
Possible cause	Excess drying due to delays in surgical technique
Results	Necessitates stretching and/or sutures
Avoidance	Plan carefully such that the patient is centered at the laser and in good position prior to turning flap
Management	Attempt to gently stretch flap into position, if necessary sutures may be placed
Flap stretching	
Possible cause	Prolonged manipulation, excessive force during smoothing or positioning maneuvers
Results	Difficulty in positioning flap and/or epithelium, visually significant striae
Avoidance	Minimize flap manipulations, use a light touch with a soaking wet sponge when smoothing or positioning the flap
Management	Gently reposition, trim redundant epithelium, place a contact lens as necessary

Contd...

Table contd...

Epithelial complications	
Possible cause	Excessive preoperative drops, improper draping, rough corneal marking, patient squeezing when placing/removing microkeratome, failure of the blade to move, basement membrane dystrophy, forceps damage
Results	Abrasions, loose epithelium, loss of gentian violet marks
Avoidance	Limit properative drops, instruct patients not to squeeze and to look straight ahead while inserting and removing drapes and speculum, a gentle touch when marking or handling the flap, warn patients with basement membrane dystrophy that they are at higher risk for epithelial complications
Management	Carefully smooth the epithelium into position, remove excess tags. A contact lens may be placed in select cases with severe epithelial disruption, moisture chambers should be used in all patients
Intraoperative bleeding	
Possible cause	Superficial corneal pannus, larger flap size (hansatome)
Results	Delays in ablation due to the need to remove blood from the stromal bed, additional steps may be needed to remove interface blood
Avoidance	A Chayet or Gimbel-Chayet sponge may be positioned to wick blood away from the hinge area
Management	Pause the ablation, wick excess blood away from the bed, irrigate the bed and gently wipe away any excess blood at edges after ablation, irrigate any blood remaining in the interface and milk it from the flap edge using a damp sponge or if necessary the shaft of a cannula

Table 24.3: Postoperative complications

Postoperative keratitis	
Possible cause	Infections (rare), toxic (Sands of the Sahara)
Results	Pain, blurred vision
Avoidance	Careful cleaning of all cannulas and syringes using fresh sterile distilled water for ultrasound cleaning, washing and rinsing, careful clearing and inspections of microkeratome assembly and blade, treatment of blepharitis preoperatively, sterile technique, avoid excess irrigation intraoperatively, prophylactic postoperative topical antibiotic/steroid solution, recommend no swimming or hot tubs for 2 weeks postoperatively
Management	Patent steroid drops q 1-2 hours, topical NSAID drops, topical antibiotics, close observation.
Shifted flap postoperatively	
Possible cause	Squeezing lids, eye rubbing, poor blink, lid or orbital abnormalities resulting in poor wetting, lateral canthotomy, loose epithelium leading to poor flap adherence, poor adherence, postoperative trauma
Results	Necessity for repositioning, risk of epithelial edema, abrasions, epithelial ingrowth, possibly will need sutures
Avoidance	Careful attention to any lid or orbit abnormalities preoperatively, check adherence with the striae test at the end of the case, moisture chambers in all patients, counsel patient to avoid squeezing lids and to wear moisture chambers for 24 hours and then every night for one week postoperatively
Management	Tips of dry sponges may be used to stretch flap after it adheres to stromal bed (if the epithelium is intact), suture flap edges in cases with persistent wrinkles and/or loose epithelium, clear off epithelium from flap edges if shifted flap $\geq$ 24 hours postoperatively, verify correct position by examining the gutter width circumferentially
Epithelial ingrowth	
Possible cause	Poor flap edge adhesion, epithelial abrasions at the flap edge, flap misalignment, buttonholes, spillover of ablation at the bed margins, irregularities or epithelial tags at the bed margins on enhancements

Contd...

Table contd...

Results	Decreased visual acuity, irregular astigmatism, discomfort (relating to surface irregularities), risk of stromal melt
Avoidance	Meticulous attention to epithelium on primary and enhancement surgeries, approximate carefully all torn epithelium at edges of flap, clear any epithelium, tags or debris from stromal bed prior to flap repositioning, avoid large transition zones on small beds and shield hinge area as necessary
Management	Very small area at flap edge with vision changes can be monitored carefully, visually significant ingrowth or an area of epithelial ingrowth of less than 1 to 2 mm requires treatment, lift the flap after clearing edges of epithelial tags or debris with the Paton spatula, debride the stromal surface and undersurface of flap edges using a clean sponge for each pass.
Irregular astigmatism	
Possible cause	Wrinkles or folds in flap, epithelial ingrowth, interface debris, decentration
Results	Loss of BCVA, symptoms such as glare, blurring, or ghosting
Avoidance	Meticulous technique
Management	Directed towards underlying cause
Undercorrection overcorrection	
Possible cause	Improper data entry, poor calibration of laser, discrepancy between manifest and cycloplegic refraction
Results	Need for enhancement
Avoidance	Careful preoperative work-up with cycloplegic refraction, ongoing outcomes analysis with algorithm adjustments as necessary, meticulous cross-checking of data entry
Management	Enhancement by lifting flap when refraction is stable, spectacles or contacts if needed in the interim

of a more experienced surgeon with mentoring if possible is advised.

The experienced surgeon can also benefit from the experience of colleagues and the wealth of information that is available in the literature, in texts, and at meetings. Refractive surgery including LASIK will continue to advance as techniques change and technology advances, and an attitude of continuous improvement and lifetime learning will always be an important part of excellent surgical outcomes.

REFERENCES

1. Waring III GO. Development and classification of refractive surgical procedures. In Waring III GO (Ed): Refractive Keratotomy for Myopia and Astigmatism Mosby Year Book: St Louis 1992;145-66.
2. Trokel SL, Srinivasan R, Braren B. Excimer laser surgery of the cornea. Am J Ophthalmol 1983;96:710-15.
3. Pureskin NP. Weakening ocular refraction by means of partial stromectomy of cornea under experimental conditions. Vestnik Oftalmologii 1967;80(1):19-24.
4. Buratto L, Ferrari M, Rama P. Excimer laser instrastromal keratomileusis. Am J Ophthalmol 1992;113:291-5.
5. Pallikaris I. Development of LASIK. In Machatt JJ (Ed): Excimer Laser Refractive Surgery: Practice and Principles SLACK Inc: Thorofare 1986;268-88.
6. Wu HK, Thompson VM, Steinert RF, et al. Refractive Surgery Thieme: New York 1999;1-492.
7. Pallikaris IG, Siganos DS. LASIK. SLACK Inc: Thorofare 1998;384.
8. Serdarevic ON. Refractive Surgery: Current Techniques and Management Igaku-Shoin: New York 1997;1-350.
9. Waring III GO. Refractive Keratotomy for Myopia and Astigmatism Mosby Year Book: St Louis 1992;1-1326.
10. Machatt JJ. Excimer Laser Refractive Surgery: Practice and Principles SLACK Inc: Thorofare 1986;1-456.
11. Gimbel HV, Penno EEA, van Westenbrugge JA, et al. Incidence and management of intra and early post-operative complications in 1000 consecutive LASIK cases. Ophthalmology 1998;105(10):1839-48.
12. Handzel A. How to shorten the learning curve. In Pallikaris IG, Siganos DS (Eds): LASIK SLACK Inc: Thorofare 1998;153-63.
13. Gimbel HV, Basti S, Kaye GB, et al. Experience during the learning curve of laser in situ keratomileusis. J Cataract Refract Surg 1996;22:542-50.
14. Gimbel HV, Anderson Penno EE. LASIK Complications: Prevention and Management SLACK Inc: Thorofare 1999;1-223.

25 Down-up LASIK

T Agarwal, Athiya Agarwal

INTRODUCTION

The Hansatome[1,2] is the latest microkeratome from Chiron Vision (Bausch and Lomb) which performs the Down-up Lasik technique. Instead of creating a nasal hinge this creates a superior hinge. The basic advantage of the hinge being superiorly is that the eyelid as it moves downward presses on the flap in that direction, thus, creating less chances of displacement of the flap.

SETTING UP OF THE HANSATOME

Power Supply Unit

The Hansatome has a power supply unit, a suction ring and a motor head. First of all place the power supply unit on a firm surface. The authors place the Hansatome power supply on the Chiron 217 excimer laser machine (Fig. 25.1). This is also called sometimes as the LASIK Laser. Attach the power cords to the power supply unit. Also attach the footswitch cords to the unit.

Suction Ring

Take the suction tubing and connect it to the appropriate receptacle in the front panel of the power supply unit. Insert the tubing connector until a positive latch is obtained. If the tubing connector is not fully latched, the vacuum panel connector will remain occluded, and no suction will be available through the tubing to the patient. Take the suction ring and the suction handle (Fig. 25.2) from the instrument tray. Screw the handle onto the suction port of the suction ring until it is snug, and place the suction tubing firmly over the end of the suction handle. The tracks on the suction ring are on the side so that one can have a down-up LASIK done. **There is an arch-shaped protrusion which blocks the microkeratome's cutting action. This is called the stop.**

Microkeratome Head

The most important step is to assemble the microkeratome head. The first step is to take the blade. Chiron supplies the blade known as the AccuGlide single-use blade. This comes in a sterile package (Fig. 25.3). It is made of steel and is mounted on a blade-holder. The blade holder is made in such a way that it can be inserted in one position only. This will prevent any assembly errors. The blade is first fixed onto the supporting instrument (Figs 25.4 and 25.5). Once that is done the blade cover is opened (Fig. 25.6) and the blade inserted in the groove in the head of the microkeratome (Figs 25.7 and 25.8). Once the blade has been successfully inserted into the Hansatome head. One should ensure that it is centered within the cavity.

The next step is to take the left/right eye adapter. Place the left/right eye adapter over the motor port

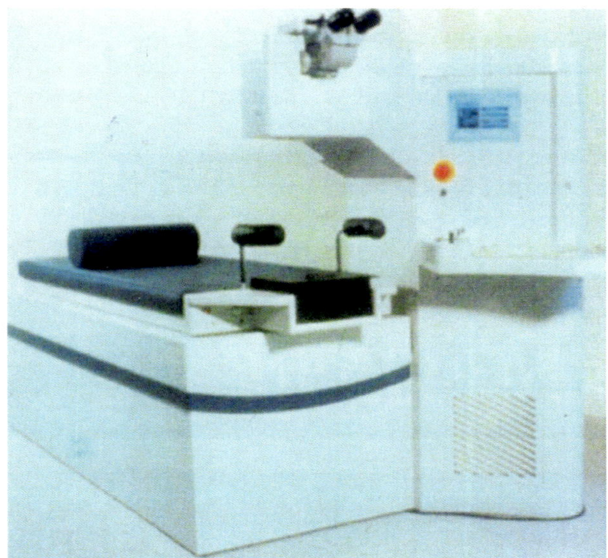

Fig. 25.1: Chiron 217 excimer laser machine

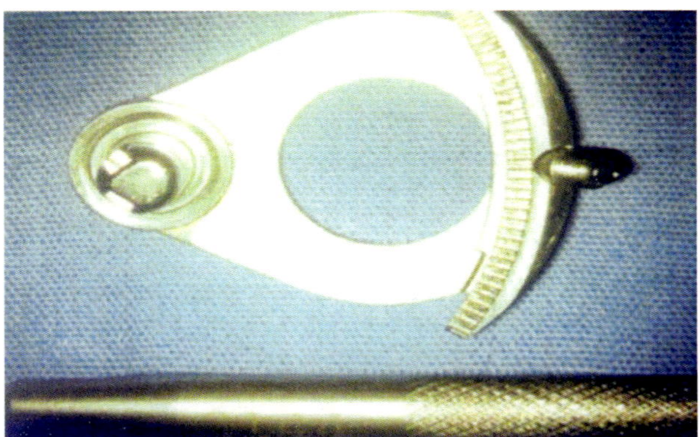

Fig. 25.2: Suction ring and handle

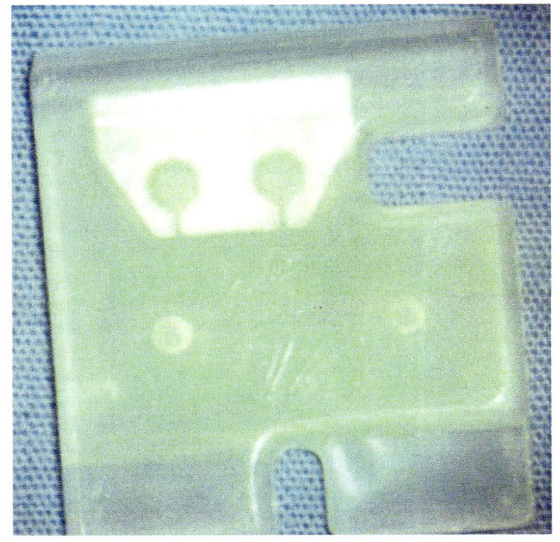

Fig. 25.3: AccuGlide single-use blade in a sterile package

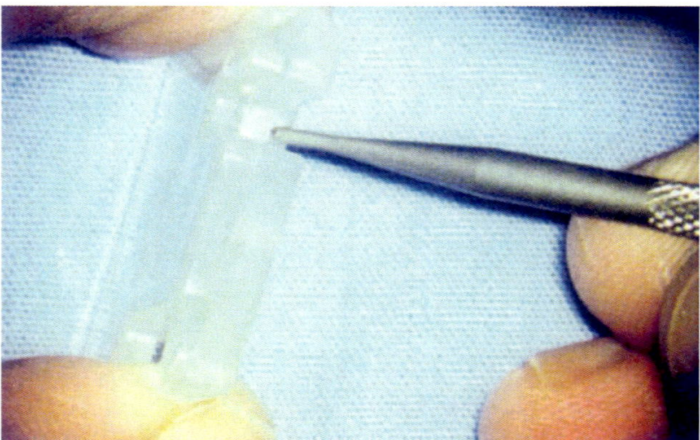

Fig. 25.4: Support for the blade being used

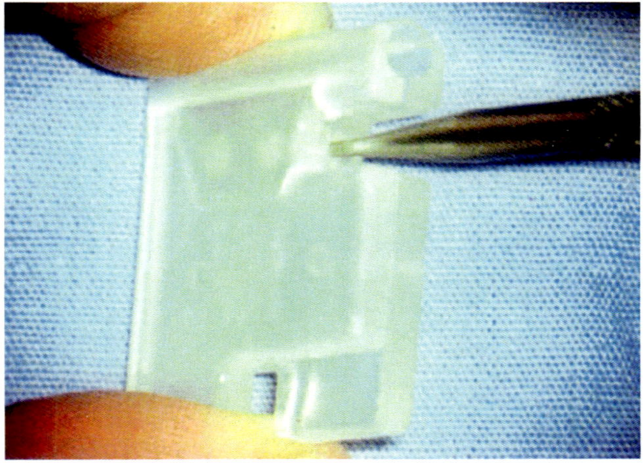

Fig. 25.5: Support for the blade fixed onto the blade

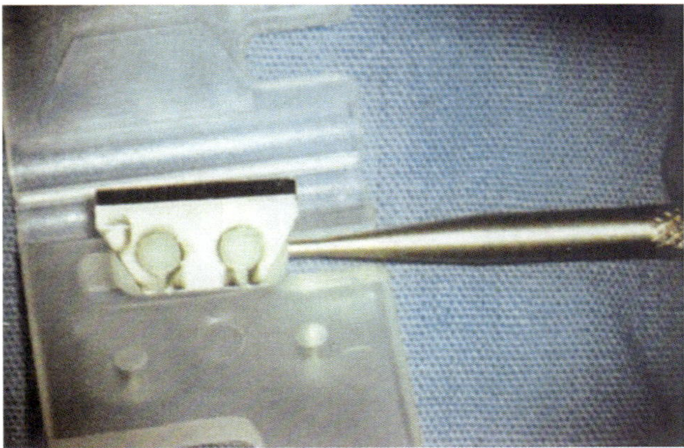

Fig. 25.6: Blade cover opened. This way one does not damage the blade

on top of the head to correspond with the eye that is to be operated on. When preparing the device for a right eye surgery, the eye adapter will effectively cover the "L" for left that is stamped on the head,

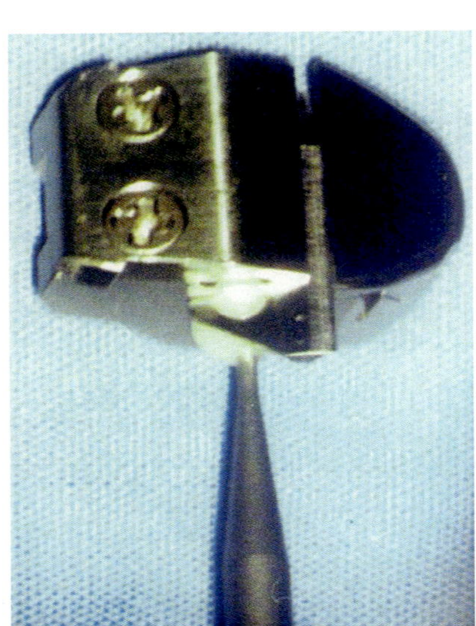

Fig. 25.7: Blade being inserted into the groove of the microkeratome's head

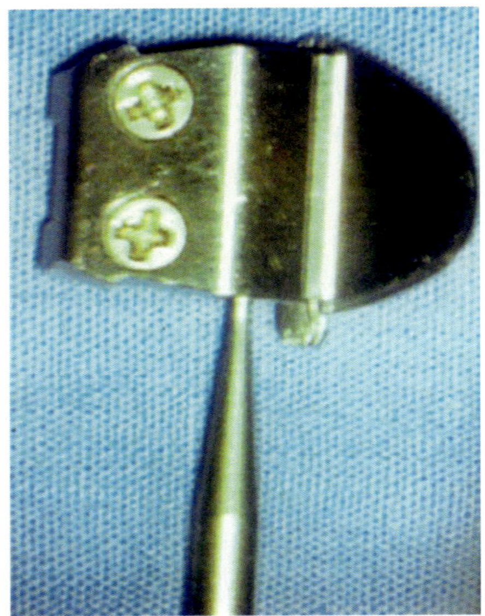

Fig. 25.8: Blade inserted into the Hansatome head

leaving the "R" for right in full view and indicating that the device is configured for a right eye surgery (Fig. 25.9). When preparing the device for a left eye surgery, the eye adapter will effectively cover the "R" for right that is stamped on the head, leaving the "L" for left in full view and indicating that the device is configured for a left eye surgery. The head

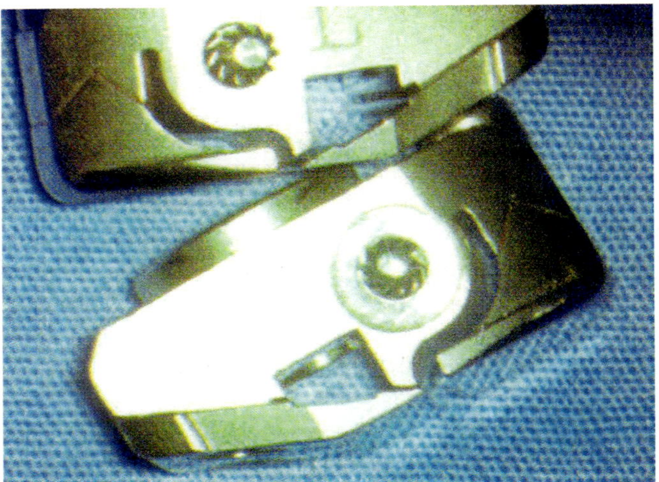

Fig. 25.9: Hansatome head showing for left and right eye

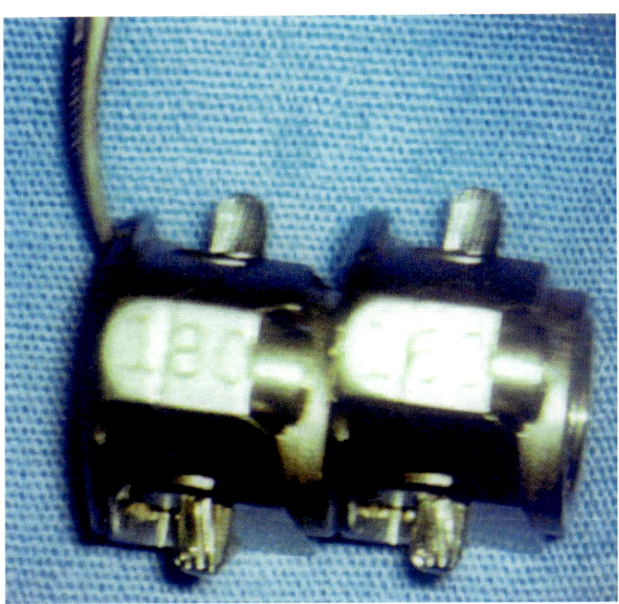

Fig. 25.10: Hansatome head showing the 180 and 160 microns thickness marks

can be 180 or 160 microns (Fig. 25.10). This means that if we use the 180 microns head the microkeratome will create a flap of 180 microns and if we use the 160 microns head the flap thickness will be 160 microns.

Once the head and the adapter are fixed (Figs 25.11 and 25.12) the motor of the keratome is taken and screwed onto the head of the microkeratome (Figs 25.13 and 25.14). The cord (Fig. 25.15) is

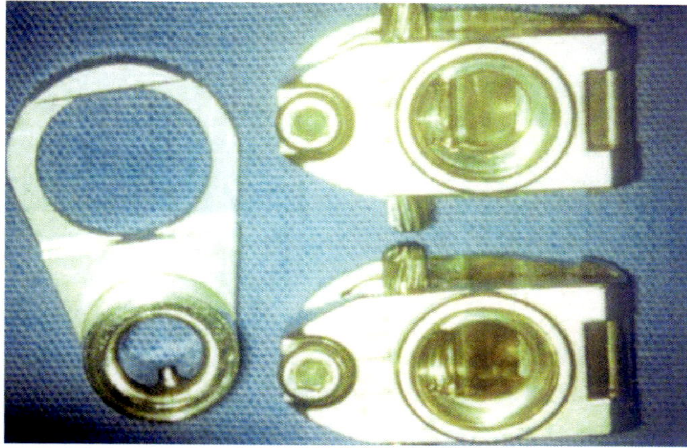

Fig. 25.11: Left/right eye adapter with head

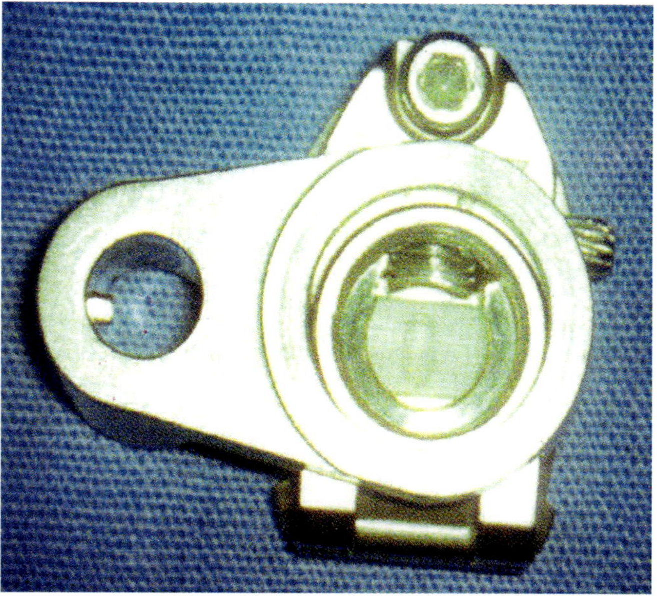

Fig. 25.12: Head fixed on the adapter

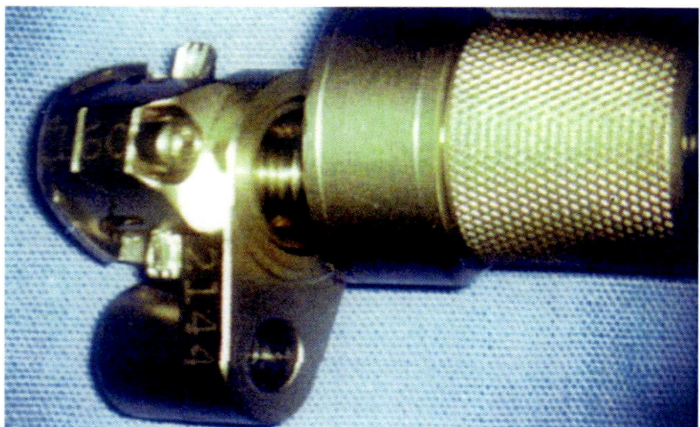

Fig. 25.13: Motor of the microkeratome being screwed onto the head

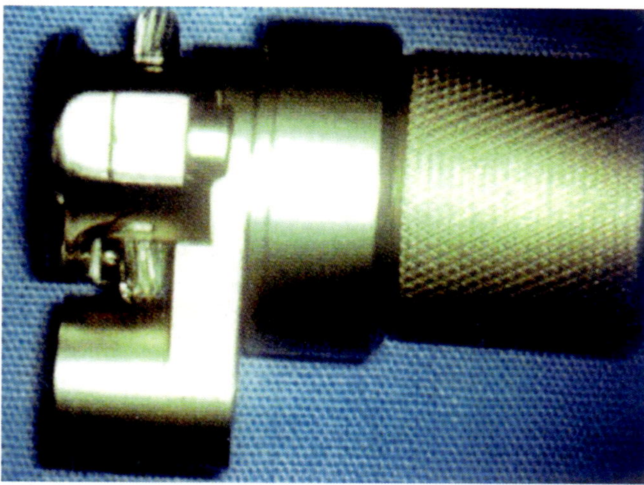

Fig. 25.14: Motor fixed onto the head of the microkeratome. Note the 160 microns head is used

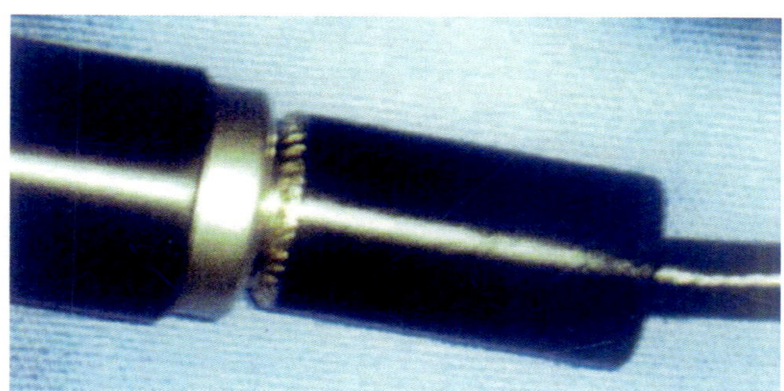

Fig. 25.15: The motor connected to the cable which in turn is connected to the power supply

connected to the motor, which in turn is connected to the power supply. Once the motor has been screwed into place, the blade will swing from right to left with a slow regular movement. This indicates that the instrument has been assembled correctly.

Test the Microkeratome

Place the assembled Hansatome head onto the suction ring (Fig. 25.16) by guiding the left/right eye adapter over the pivot pin of the suction ring. Align the head over the approximate starting position appropriate to the selected eye, left or right. This will allow the head/adapter assembly to drop down all the way on the pivot pin. Move the rolling gear

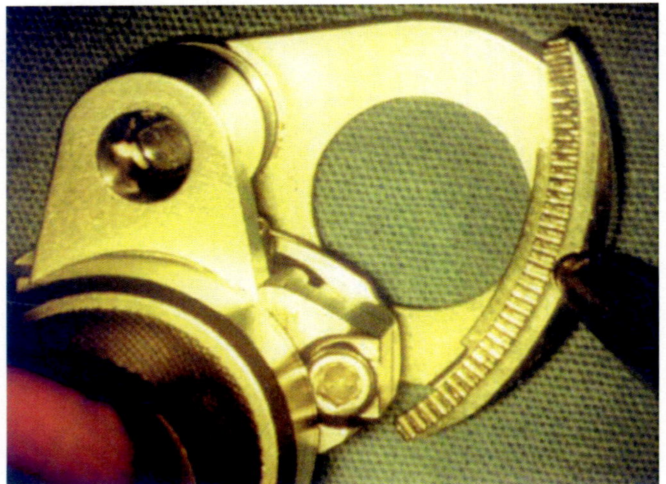

Fig. 25.16: Head placed on the pin of the suction ring

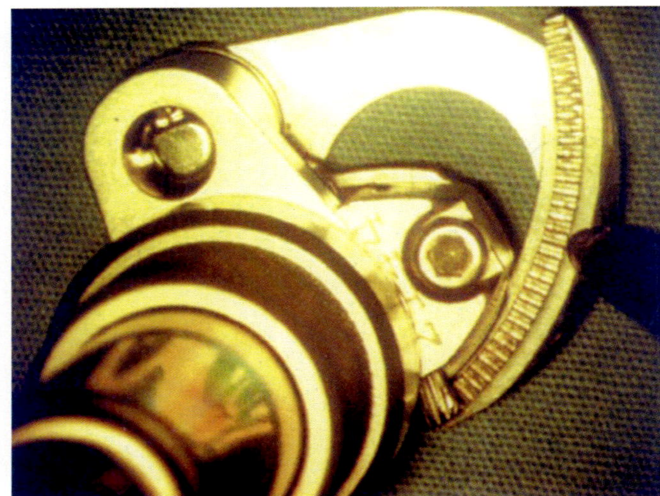

Fig. 25.17: Head moving on the tracks of the suction ring

up to the first gear tooth of the rack. While lightly supporting the motor, press the forward pedal (labeled F) of the motor footswitch to start the head across the ring (Fig. 25.17). In normal operation, the head will automatically stop, with two audible beeps. This will happen when the head reaches the mechanical stop and the motor current will drop to zero. Once this happens, depress the reverse pedal (labeled R) of the motor footswitch to reverse the head back off the ring. If everything is alright then only should one proceed with using the Hansatome on the patient.

CARE AND MAINTENANCE

The mechanical components of the Hansatome should be cleaned immediately and thoroughly after each use. Delayed cleaning can leave residual debris such as stromal cells, epithelial cells and strands from surgical sponges. If the components are autoclaved, this debris may become firmly baked onto the components. To remove debris allow the components to soak in very hot distilled water for a minimum of 15 minutes, then employ the cleaning regimen outlined below and repeat until all debris has been removed. Debris allowed to build up on the Hansatome microkeratome components may affect the performance of the device and result in malfunction of the device and possible patient injury.

Chiron Vision recommends use of a cleaning solution consisting of 2 parts green Palmolive dishwashing liquid (unconcentrated product) to 100 parts warm tap water. Do not substitute. The cleaning solution used must not leave any residue. All the components must be thoroughly rinsed with distilled or sterile water after cleaning in the solution. Once this is done one should dry with a lint-free surgical wipe or blow dry with micro-filtered forced air. Since most of the components are small and could possibly be lost in a sink or drain, it is best to perform the cleaning procedure by using small bowls or basins. The bowls or basins should be made of plastic and not metal to avoid potential damage to the Chiron Vision Hansatome microkeratome mechanical components.

For cleaning the Hansatome motor, wipe the outside of the motor housing with a cloth dampened with isopropyl alcohol and clean the motor shaft with a dry toothbrush. Do not immerse it in any fluid. Do not use ethylene oxide sterilization for the motor as this can congeal the internal grease and cause potential malfunctions.

For cleaning the cord, one should wipe it with a cloth dampened with isopropyl alcohol. Do not immerse it in any fluid or autoclave it. Autoclaving will cause convolution of the initially round cable and will cause cumulative damage to the cable and electrical connectors, eventually leading to possible malfunction.

STERILIZATION

The various methods of sterilization for the Hansatome parts are shown in Table 25.1.

TROUBLESHOOTING

Head not Advancing across the Suction Ring

The head may be jammed on the first tooth of the gear track. Press the reverse pedal of the motor footswitch to release, then place the head in position and try again.

Head not Fitting Properly onto the Suction Ring

Confirm that the left/right eye adapter has been oriented correctly onto the head for the eye to be operated on. Confirm that the head has been oriented near the correct starting point for the cut, at which point the adapter should drop down onto the pivot pin. Check for any obstructions or debris that may be impeding the loading of the head onto the suction ring. Clean the head, adapter and suction ring and try again.

No Suction Occurring

Check if the tubing is all right or if the attachment of the tubing to the power supply is correctly done.

SURGICAL TECHNIQUE

The surgical technique of down up LASIK starts from draping of the patient (Fig. 25.18). When one drapes the patient one should be careful that the eyelashes do not come into the microkeratome. The authors use cellotape to tape the eyelashes so that they are away from the field of the microkeratome. Then the eyelid speculum is inserted. The eyelid speculum should be a good one, which retracts the eyelids well.

Once the eyelid speculum is inserted, one should check the working of the microkeratome. The microkeratome head should be fixed on the suction

Table 25.1: Sterilization of the Hansatome

	Autoclave sterilization[5]			*EO sterilization*	*Alcohol sanitization*
Components	*250° F/121°C for 30 minutes*	*Flash cycle at 250°F/ 121°C for 10 minutes*	*Prevacuum cycle at 250°F/121°C for 3 minutes*	*12/88/EO cycle of 100 minutes at 125°F/52°C at EO conc. of 600 mg/L level*	*N/A*
Instruments tray and contents Hansatome head Left/right eye Adapter Suction ring Suction handle Reference marker Blade handling pin	Yes	Yes	Yes	Yes	No
Applanation tonometer	No	No	No	Yes	No
Hansatome motor[4] Motor power cord	No	No	No	No	Yes

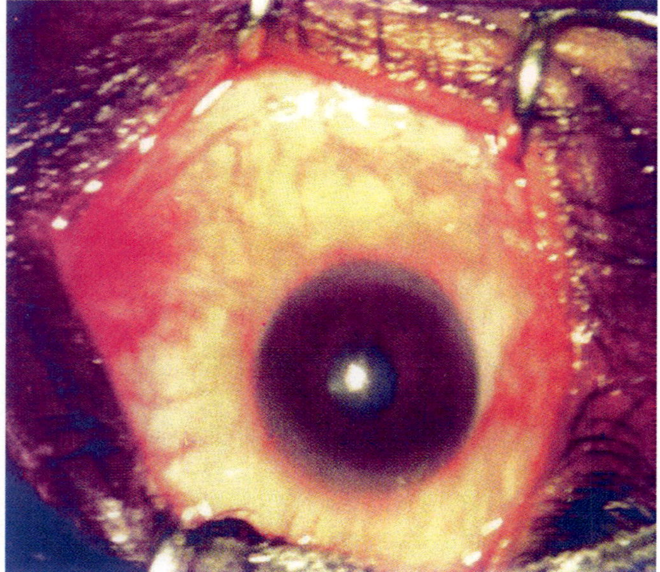

Fig. 25.18: Eye draped and speculum inserted

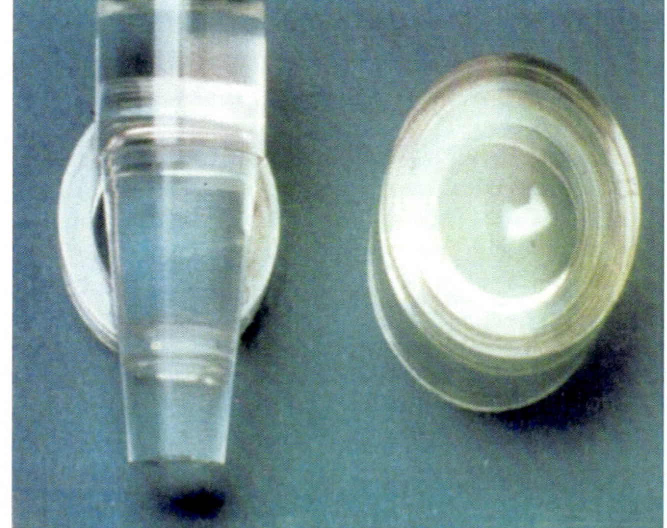

Fig. 25.20: Barraquer's presurgical tonometer

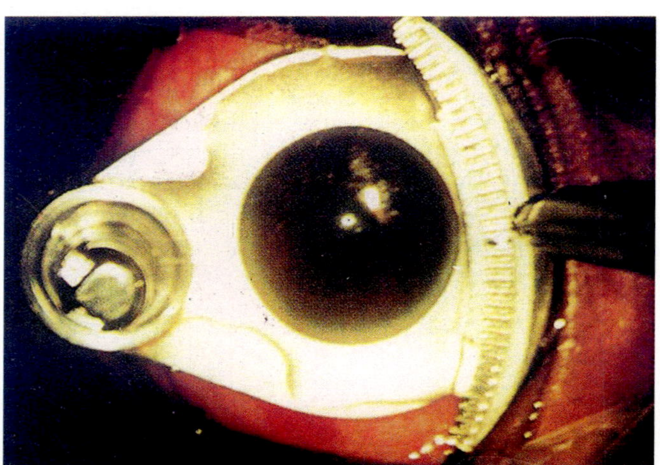

Fig. 25.19: Suction ring of the Hansatome fixed

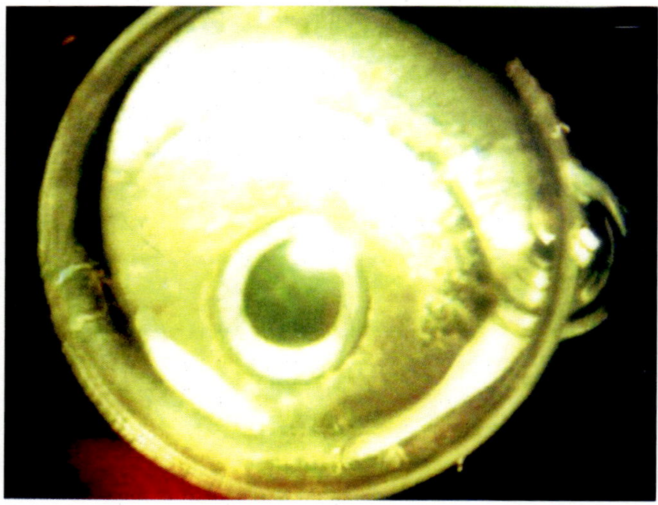

Fig. 25.21: Barraquer's tonometer on the cornea. Note the black ring in the center is smaller than the white ring just beyong it

ring and the movement of the microkeratome checked. One should check that the microkeratome moves smoothly on the tracks of the suction ring.

Using the reference marker a mark is made on the cornea. Then the suction ring is taken and placed properly on the eye (Fig. 25.19). Once the suction ring is fixed in the proper position, the footswitch of the vacuum is pressed so that the suction comes on. The tracks of the suction ring should be placed nasally. Once the suction is on one should check the intraocular pressure (IOP) of the eye using the Barraquer's presurgical tonometer (Fig. 25.20). This creates a black ring in the center. The black ring should be smaller than the white ring seen in the Barraquer's tonometer (Fig. 25.21). If this happens, then the IOP is greater than 65 mm of Hg and the case can be proceeded with. If it is larger than the white ring then something is wrong with the suction.

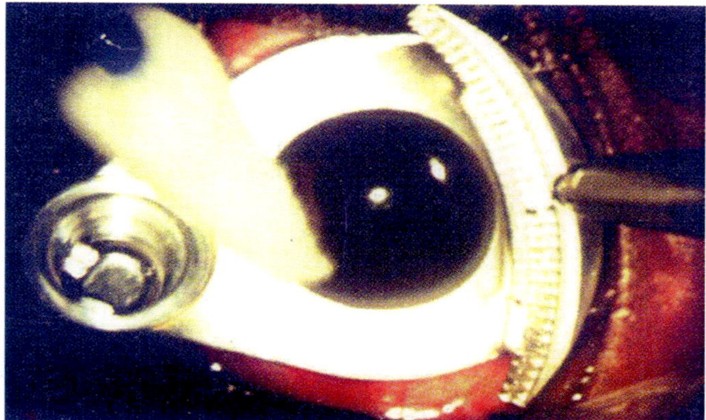

Fig. 25.22: Excess fluid wiped with the merocel sponge. This is done to prevent the fluid from jamming the microkeratome movement

So, release the suction and start the process once again. Once everything is alright swab the area so that excess fluid is not present (Fig. 25.22).

When the suction ring is fixed in position, the microkeratome head is now fixed onto the pin of the suction ring. There are notches on the pin of the suction ring, which coincide with the head so that the head gets properly fixed (Fig. 25.23). Then the forward footswitch is depressed and the microkeratome moves on the tracks of the suction ring. This will automatically stop when the head hits the stop mechanism (Fig. 25.24). When this happens two beeps will be heard. Then press the reverse footswitch and the head will move in the reverse direction. Once it has come back fully, release the suction and take off both the suction ring and the microkeratome head (Fig. 25.25).

Use a fine spatula or repositor and lift the flap from the inferior area. Lift the flap so that the hinge is superior and the flap lies superiorly (Fig. 25.26). Before the whole LASIK procedure was started, one should have calibrated the excimer laser machine and the required refractive power entered. The authors use a Chiron 217 excimer laser machine and overcorrect by 10 percent. The ablation is then started. One can use an eye tracking system or alternatively fixate the eye with a forceps and start the ablation. One should be careful that a decentered ablation does not occur. **See to it that the excimer laser hits perpendicular to the cornea and not obliquely. The laser should hit the pupillary area. In cases of astigmatism, one should be careful that the eye is not rotated otherwise the axis of the astigmatism will become different.**

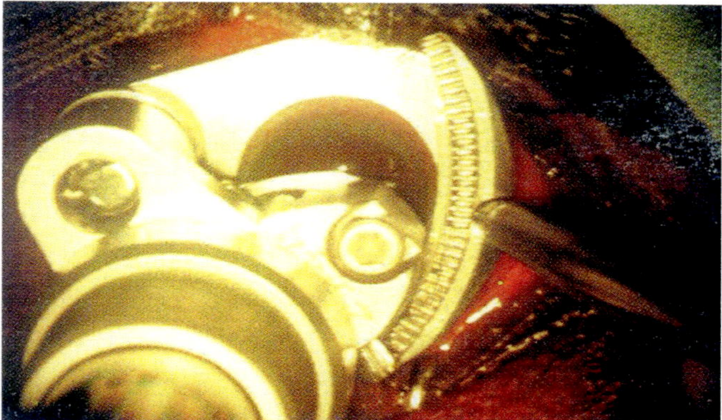

Fig. 25.23: Microkeratome head fixed on the suction ring

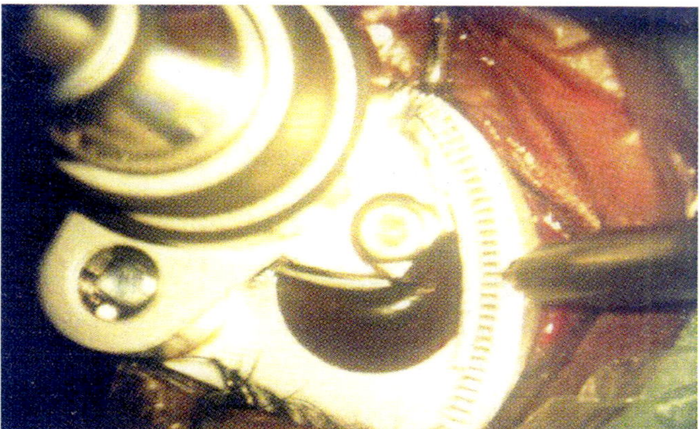

Fig. 25.24: Microkeratome head hits the stop mechanism. Now the reverse footswitch should be depressed

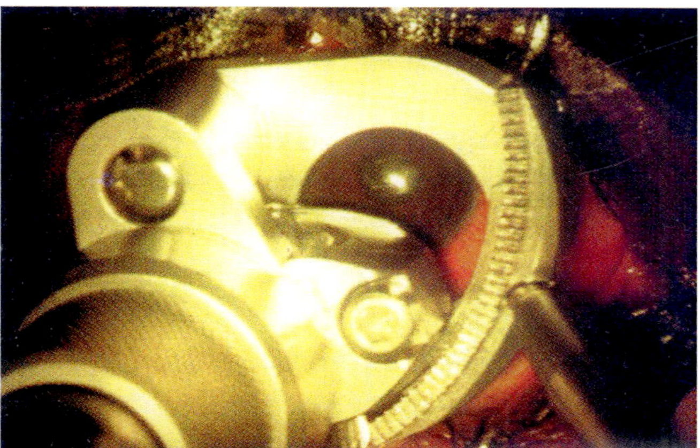

Fig. 25.25: Keratectomy done. Suction ring and microkeratome head released from the eye

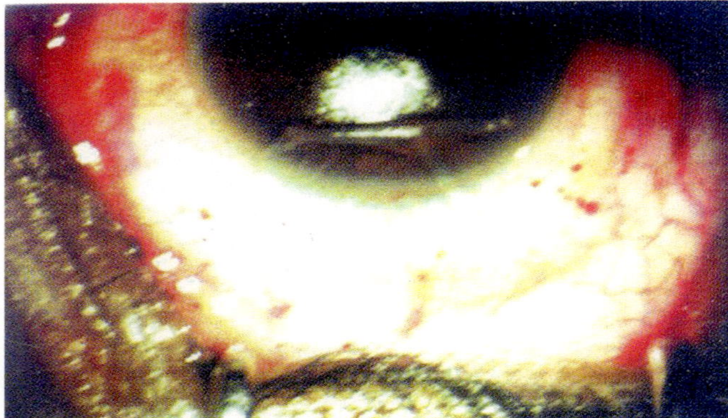

Fig. 25.26: Superior flap made. Excimer ablations started

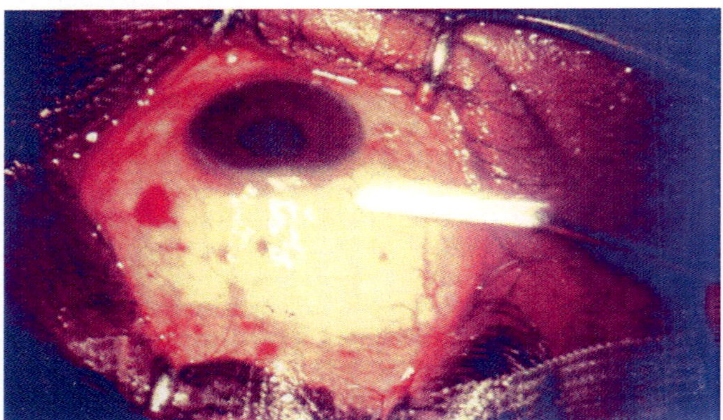

Fig. 25.27: Superior flap reposited with a spatula. One can use an irrigating cannula to do the same thing

When the ablation of the excimer is completed, one should wash the stroma with the irrigating fluid (balanced salt solutions—BSS). Wash the flap well. See to it that there is no foreign body lying on the stroma. Take a wet Merocel sponge and clean the flap with both ends of the sponge. This will prevent epithelial ingrowths. Then take the syringe with BSS and pass the cannula under the flap. While irrigating lift the flap and the flap will fall back into its original position onto the stroma. One can use a spatula also to reposit the flap (Fig. 25.27). Once the flap has been repositioned check that the reference marks coincide. Then wait for a couple of minutes so that the flap is stuck (Fig. 25.28). Carefully take out the speculum without disturbing the flap.

The authors see the patient on the slit lamp after half an hour and if everything is all right the patient goes home without a patch. Both eyes are done simultaneously. The patient is put on artificial tears, antibiotic and steroid drops for 2 to 3 weeks only. The patient is seen again the next day. When seen on the slit lamp it should be as if no treatment was done, except for slight subconjunctival hemorrhages due to the suction ring being present. The patient is seen again after a month and if necessary relasik is done by lifting the flap. This is done if regression has occurred. In such cases one need not again make the cut, but lift the same flap back.

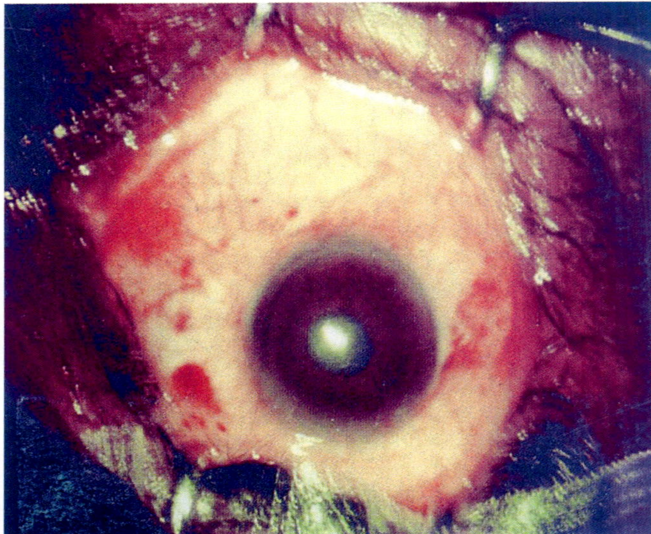

Fig. 25.28: Flap back in position. Note the cut edges of the flap. The hinge is superior

FACTORS RESPONSIBLE FOR SECURING THE FLAP

There are basically four factors[3] responsible for securing the flap in position.

- The natural capillary attraction of the tissues and mucoproteins. This occurs rapidly within seconds to minutes
- The endothelial pump action. This occurs within minutes to hours.
- Epithelial covering along the margin starts from 12 to 24 hours
- Scarring along the cut edge of Bowman's layer occurs weeks to months later.

ADVANTAGES

The main advantage of the down-up LASIK technique is that as the eyelid moves downwards it presses on the flap which has a superior hinge and thus does not displace the flap. The same does not apply to a flap, which has a hinge nasally. Gravitational forces also help in positioning the flap properly. The compression effect of the eyelid also helps to smoothen the flap. Another advantage of the down up LASIK technique is that it creates a large flap. The ablation pattern of the excimer requires a large flap preferably in cases of hyperopia treatment. Further chances of the flap getting shot with the excimer do not occur with the down up LASIK.

DISADVANTAGES

There are disadvantages of the down up LASIK technique also. One problem is the large flap. If the patient is wearing contact lenses, they can have peripheral vascularization of the cornea. On cutting the cornea, as the flap is large these blood vessels bleed and it takes some time for the bleeding to stop. Another problem with the Hansatome is that the palpebral fissure should be large. If the fissure is small then the suction ring of the Hansatome does not fit in the eye, and one would have to resort to a canthotomy. In such cases, the authors prefer to use the automatic corneal shaper (ACS). Yet another problem with the Hansatome is that when the cut has been completed the suction ring and the keratome head are removed so that when the laser is being applied there is nothing to stabilize the eye. One can use the eye tracking system to get accurate ablation. **The advantage of the ACS in contrast is that once the keratome cuts the cornea the suction ring is not removed and this can stabilize the eye well. The suction is not stopped till the entire ablation is completed. One can move the eye in such a way as the suction is still on so that the excimer lasers are perpendicular to the cornea, thus, preventing decentered ablations. This is not possible with the Hansatome.**

REFERENCES

1. Chiron Vision Hansatome Microkeratome operator's manual.
2. Buratto L. Down Up Lasik with the New Chiron Microkeratome Milano, Italy, 1997
3. Machat JJ. Excimer Laser Refractive Surgery Slack Inc: Thorofare 1996.

26 Pediatric LASIK

Athiya Agarwal

INTRODUCTION

Spectacle correction and contact lenses are the commonly availed options to correct myopia. Contact lenses have the advantages of a bigger field and better quality of vision especially in higher refractive errors. The visual performances of high myopic patients are better with contact lenses than spectacles as analyzed by contrast sensitivity testing.[1] In cases of uniocular high refractive errors with difference of more than 3 D, it has been shown that the eyes are prone to anisometropic amblyopia and retard the development of binocular single vision if left uncorrected. Diagnosis of anisometropic amblyopia at the age of four seems to be efficacious for cure of most cases though it has been shown by some that response is better if treated at two years of age.[2]

The critical factors predicting a successful outcome are the amount of anisometropia, visual acuity at the start of treatment, and compliance of the patient[3] which are usually poor in children. They usually develop diplopia and intolerance if corrected with glasses, and contact lenses are presently the preferred mode of correction in such cases. Contact lenses are used for therapeutic treatment of aphakia, anisometropia, myopia, hyperopia, some types of esotropia, irregular astigmatism and nystagmus in children.[4] But contact lenses are difficult to maintain by children.

Radial keratotomy (RK) reduces the refractive power for high myopic patients.[5] But the safety of RK in children has not been proven. Photorefractive keratectomy (PRK) has been showing promising results in such selective patients. Studies have shown that the results of PRK for myopia in pediatric eyes with anisometropic amblyopia are encouraging.[6,7] We did laser in situ keratomileusis (LASIK) laser in such selective patients at our center and present a retrospective study of 16 consecutive eyes of children below the age of 11 years that underwent the procedure to correct myopia.

PEDIATRIC LASIK

A total of 16 eyes that underwent LASIK laser correction for uniocular high myopia was retrospectively analyzed (Tables 26.1 and 26.2). The patients were subjected to LASIK laser correction for myopia only if there was a refractive error difference of more than 4 D between the eyes, and who failed in conventional amblyopia therapy based on varying combinations of spectacles, contact lenses and occlusion therapy. LASIK was advised only in these eyes as we felt the eye will go in for irreversible amblyopia because of our inability to aid in binocular vision. A fully informed consent was obtained from the parents before the procedure. Previous intraocular surgery, any other associated posterior segment pathology, active inflammations, and infections, corneal scarring, pachymetry values less than 450 μ, keratoconus, intraocular pressure (IOP) more than 19 mm Hg, patients with a narrow palpebral fissure, any associated astigmatism, and a Schirmer's test of less than 5 mm were the exclusion criteria.

Table 26.1: Demographics

Patients characteristics	*Demographics*
No of eyes	16
Mean age (Yrs)	8.4 ± 1.83
Male: female	7:9
OD:OS	7:9
Follow-up period	12 months
Mean preoperative spherical eq	–14.88 ± 3.69
Mean postoperative spherical eq	–1.44 ± 1.14
Mean preoperative BCVA	0.53 ± 0.28
Mean postoperative BCVA	0.54 ± 0.27

Routine preoperative best-corrected visual acuity (BCVA), cycloplegic refraction, estimation of the palpebral aperture, anterior segment evaluation, measurement of the corneal diameter, Schirmer's test, corneal topography, pachymetry, IOP evaluation by noncontact tonometry (IOP), and a detailed fundus evaluation by indirect ophthalmoscopy were done.

Chiron Technolas Keracor 217 was used for the excimer laser. Laser fluence was checked before every procedure by verifying the homogeneity and symmetry of the pulses according to optimal values of 65 ± 1 shots. Automatic corneal shaper (ACS) microkeratome was used for creating the lamellar corneal flap. Careful attention was paid to avoid excess air-borne debris in the operating room by ultrafiltration of air, and ultraviolet exposure of the laser device was done 24 hours before the day of surgery. The patients were sedated using intravenous Ketamine® (2 mg/kg as a bolus dose followed by 0.5 mg/kg intermittently as required) under a qualified anesthetist's supervision and were carefully monitored. The eye to be treated was confirmed and data entered in the computer and programmed. A speculum kept the palpebral fissure open. The pupillary center was marked with a gentian violet tip marker. The ACS microkeratome was assembled by the surgeon to create a 160 μ lamellar corneal flap and was test run on the base plate before each individual procedure. The suction ring was centered on the corneal marking and was activated. Intraocular pressure was confirmed to be more than 60 mm Hg.

Table 26.2: Pediatric LASIK results

S no.	*Age*	*Sex*	*Eye*	*BCVA (preop)*	*BCVA (12 mon)*	*UCVA-post (12 mon)*	*Sph Eq (preop)*	*Sph Eq (12 mon)*	*Follow-up (months)*	*Remarks*
1	9	M	LE	0.66	0.50	0.25	–9.00	0	12	free cap + persistent Gr. 2 haze
2	8	F	LE	1.00	1.00	0.66	–12.75	–0.5	12	—
3	9	F	RE	1.00	1.00	0.25	–14.50	–2.5	12	—
4	8	F	LE	1.00	1.00	0.17	–14.50	–2	12	—
5	10	F	RE	0.50	0.50	0.25	–15.00	–1.5	12	—
6	10	F	LE	0.50	0.50	0.33	–13.75	–1	12	—
7	11	M	RE	0.17	0.17	0.17	–13.25	–0.5	12	—
8	10	M	RE	0.33	0.33	0.10	–21.00	–3	12	Gr. 2 haze (resolved)
9	11	M	LE	0.33	0.25	0.05	–23.00	–4	12	Persistent Gr. 2 haze
10	6	F	LE	0.66	0.66	0.66	–14.50	0	12	—
11	5	F	RE	0.50	0.66	0.17	–14.50	–2	12	—
12	6	M	RE	0.33	0.33	0.17	–13.00	–1.5	12	—
13	6	M	LE	0.66	0.66	0.66	–11.50	0	12	free cap
14	7	M	LE	0.33	0.50	0.33	–11.00	–1	12	—
15	9	F	RE	0.33	0.33	0.10	–17.25	–1.5	12	—
16	9	F	LE	0.33	0.33	0.17	–19.50	–2	12	

The microkeratome then fashioned a lamellar corneal flap with a nasal hinge. The flap was carefully lifted with a blunt instrument and reflected on its hinge. The laser procedure was then performed taking care for accurate centration of the laser. The flap was shielded from the laser using a cellulose strip. After the procedure was performed, the flap was repositioned and the interface thoroughly washed, to clear it of any particulate and cellular debris. Care was taken to ensure there were no striae in the flap during repositioning. The suction ring was gently removed. A minimal interval of 3 minutes was allowed for the flap to settle down before padding the patients for 6 hours. The eyes were padded up as we felt children might not cooperate in keeping the flap in place and as we also felt the flap could get disturbed in the recovery phase after anesthesia.

Two patients had a free cap during the procedure which was duly replaced based on the alignment marks and sutured using four interrupted 10-0 mersiline sutures which were removed when they reported for the follow-up in the sixth month. The patients were advised postoperative tobramycin 0.3 percent with dexamethasone 0.1 percent eyedrops to be applied 4 times a day for one month. The patients were reviewed on the first postoperative day, on the first week, after one month, sixth month and after one year. When they reported for their follow-up visits, Uncorrected visual acuity (UCVA), best-corrected visual acuity (BCVA), refraction (noting induced astigmatism, if any), detailed anterior segment evaluation, grading of haze based on a 5 point scale (with 0 as no haze, +1 trace, +2 mild haze, +3 moderate haze, +4 severe haze), IOP corneal topography, and a detailed fundus evaluation was done.

RESULTS

The demographic data are shown in Tables 26.1 and and Figure 26.1. All the 16 eyes could be followed up for 12 months (Table 26.2) and the charts were analyzed at the end of the twelfth month. Students *t*-test was used for statistical analysis. The mean

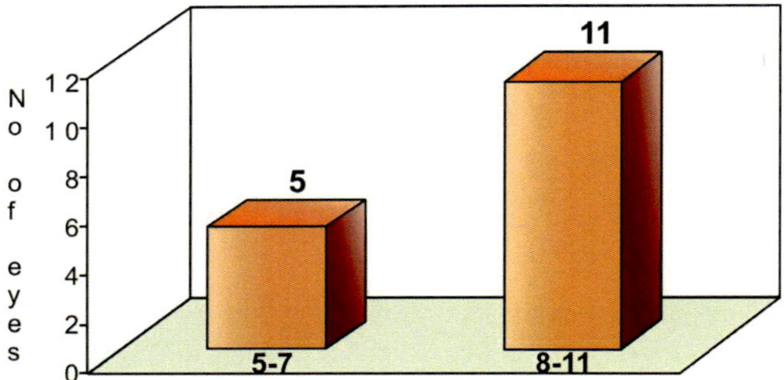

Fig. 26.1: Age ratio

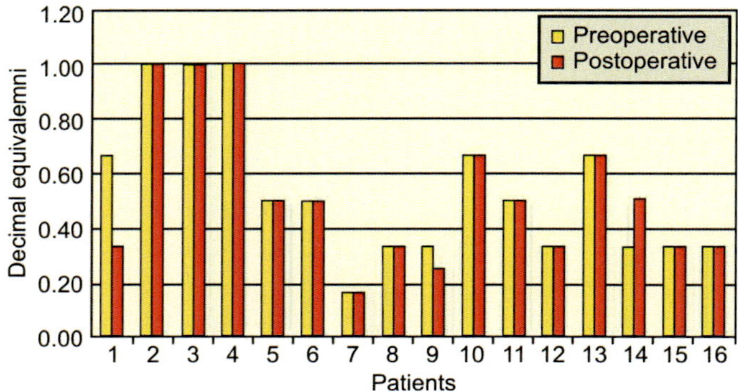

Fig. 26.2: Best-corrected visual acuity (BCVA)

preoperative BCVA in decimal equivalent was 0.53 $\pm$ 0.28 SD (range 0.17 to 1) and the mean postoperative BCVA decimal equivalent at the twelfth month was 0.54 $\pm$ 0.27 SD (range 0.17 to 1) [p value 0.77] (Fig. 26.2). The mean UCVA at the twelfth month was 0.28 $\pm$ 0.2 SD (range 0.10-0.66). The *safety index* (Mean postoperative BCVA/mean preoperative BCVA) was 1.01 and the *efficacy index* (mean postoperative UCVA/mean preoperative BCVA) was 0.53.

Two patients had a free flap during the procedure of which one had a drop in its BCVA by one line due to persistent grade 2 haze. Two eyes which had a preoperative spherical equivalent of more than –18 D and one eye which had a free cap developed grade 2 haze, one of which (–21.00 D) spontaneously resolved by the visit at the sixth month. The other two had persistent haze even up to the twelfth month follow-up and subsequently had a drop in their BCVA by one line. None of the patients developed a corneal haze more than grade 2, 12 eyes regained their BCVA after the procedure and two eyes improved by one line BCVA. None of the eyes developed rise in IOP or any retinal complication.

The mean preoperative spherical equivalent was –14.88 ± 3.69 SD (range –9 D to –23 D). The mean postoperative spherical equivalent was –1.44 ± 1.14 SD (range 0 D to –2.5 D) [p value < 0.05] (Fig. 26.3). None of the eyes had an induced astigmatism of more than 0.5 D. Only two patients had an induced astigmatism of 0.5 D evident on corneal topography but were not significantly contributing in refractive correction. Twelve months postoperatively, 3 eyes were emmetropic, 2 eyes had –0.5 D, 2 eyes had –1.0 D, 3 eyes had –1.5 D, 3 eyes had –2.0 D, 1 eye had –2.5 D, 1 eye –3.0 D and 1 eye had a residual power of –4.0 D (Fig. 26.4).

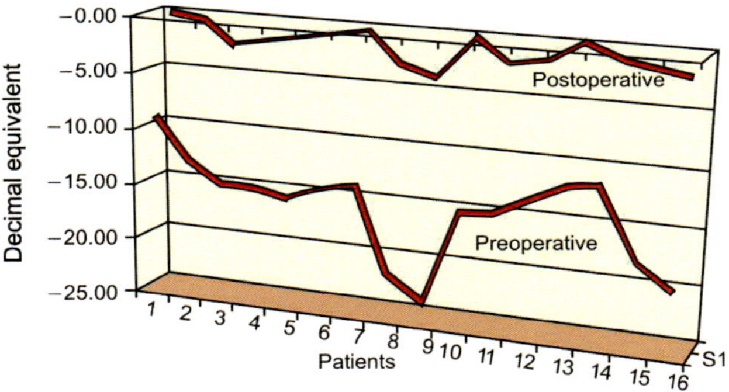

Fig. 26.3: Shift in decimal equivalent

DISCUSSION

Myopia is a common refractive error in children. Spectacle correction and contact lenses have been popular modes of correction. In uniocular high myopia, it has been found that if the refractive error was more than 3 D, there was a high incidence of intolerance due to dissimilar image size and optical aberrations. They subsequently go in for anisometropic amblyopia if left uncorrected. Children are not always compliant to conventional amblyopia therapy. Contact lenses do not minify images, do not have any optical aberration and do not have any problem of anisometropia. But some children develop intolerance to contact lenses and have problems in maintaining them. As PRK has been shown to offer promising results in such selective group of patients having uniocular high refractive errors,[6,7] and as the safety of RK in children is not fully established, we attempted LASIK laser correction of uniocular high myopia in such selective patients. LASIK is a viable method for correction of high myopia with fewer complications and has advantages over keratomileusis and PRK as it combines the best features of both methods (preserves Bowman's layer and has the excimer laser precision).[8] LASIK is effective and predictable in the correction of high myopia but is more accurate for myopia up to 12 D.[9,10] A stable refraction and a predictable outcome occur much earlier with LASIK

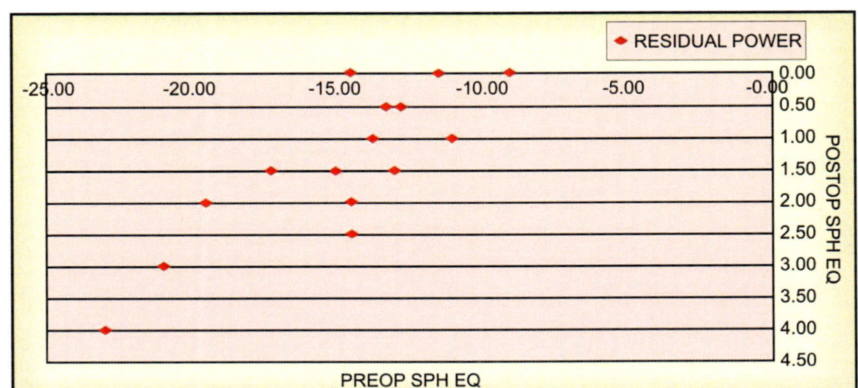

Fig. 26.4: Power residue

than with PRK.[11] We are not aware of any study which showed LASIK laser correction in pediatric eyes and present our results after a one year follow-up.

Studies show LASIK laser correction in adults is accurate and predictable.[11] LASIK laser is usually not done in children because myopia is not stable till early adulthood. But, treatment-resistant anisometropic amblyopia forms a strong medical indication for treating with LASIK laser. It was our goal to equalize the refractive power and thereby retard or, if possible, reverse amblyopia.

The children were sedated for obvious reasons. But as the children could not fixate the light the footplate of the ACS was used to aid fixation. The eyes were padded up so that the flap is not disturbed in its immediate postoperative period. Two patients had a free cap, which was duly sutured, in place aided by the gentian violet marking. Retrospectively, they were found to have a keratometry value of 39 D. Of the two, one lost one line in its BCVA because of flap striae and persistent grade 2 haze. Two eyes improved in their BCVA probably because of reversal of amblyopia or due to better quality of vision after the refractive correction.

Our results show encouraging results showing LASIK as a safe alternative to correct pediatric cases during the one year follow-up. However, long-term follow-up of these patients and a bigger study is essential to prove the long-term safety and efficacy of the procedure.

REFERENCES

1. Collins JW, Carney LG. Visual performance in high myopia. Curr Eye Res. 1990;9(3):217-23.
2. Lithander J, Sjostrand J. Anisometropia and strabismic amblyopia in the age group 2 years and above—a prospective study of the results of treatment. Br J Ophthalmol. 1991;75(2):111-6.
3. Beardsell R, Clarke S, Hill M. Outcome of occlusion treatment for amblyopia. J Pediatric Ophthalmol Strabismus 1999;36(1):19-24.
4. Jurkus JM. Contact lenses for children. Optom Clin 1996;5(2):91-104.
5. Pak KH, Kim JH. Radial keratotomy for the purpose of reducing glasses power in high myopia. Korean J Ophthalmol 1992;6(2):83-90.
6. Nano HD (Jr), Muzzin S, Irigaray LF. Excimer laser photorefractive keratectomy in pediatric patients. J Cataract Refract Surg 1997;23:736-39.
7. Alio JL, Artola A, Claramonte P, et al. Photorefractive keratectomy for pediatric myopic anisometropia. J Cataract Refract Surg 1998;24:327-30.
8. Marinho A, Pinto MC, Pinto R, et al. Lasik for high myopia—one year experience. Ophthalmic Surg Lasers 1996;27(5)(Suppl):517-20.
9. Perez Santonja JJ, Bellot J, Claramonte P, et al. Laser in situ keratomileusis to correct high myopia. J Cataract Refract Surg 1997;23(3):372-85.
10. Guell JL, Muller A. Laser in situ keratomileusis for myopia from –7 to –18 diopters. J Refract Surg 1996;12(2):222-8.
11. Condon PI, Mulhern M, Fulcher T, et al. Laser intrastromal keratomileusis for high myopia and myopic astigmatism. Br J Ophthalmol.

27 Femtosecond Lasers

Takeshi Ide, Terrence O'Brien

OVERVIEW

Although current automated mechanical microkeratomes have improved in design and safety to attain a high level of efficient clinical experience, outcome viability and patient anxiety remain concerns. In fact, flap creation with an automated mechanical microkeratome is responsible for considerable morbidity in LASIK, with intraoperative and postoperative complications occurring in a significant percents of cases.[1-3]

The complications most commonly involve mechanical abrasions of the epithelium, buttonhole flap, incomplete flap, free cap, unintentional thin/thick flap, flap dislocation, diffuse lamellar keratitis (DLK), ectasia, macro- and microstriae, and epithelial ingrowth. Even with normal function, the accuracy and precision of a mechanical microkeratome contrasts significantly with that of the submicron precision of the subsequent excimer laser ablation of the corneal stroma. Surgeon control of an automated microkeratome is limited, with little flexibility to accommodate individual surgical requirements imposed by corneal thickness, pupil location, or refractive state.

Development of a laser-based keratome was intended to address the shortcomings of traditional mechanical microkeratome technology, thereby improving the efficacy and safety of LASIK procedures. Femtosecond laser technology was chosen for this application because it has the capability to be delivered inside the corneal stroma with micron-level precision. Femtosecond solid-state lasers are gaining more popularity in many fields of medicine. With lamellar-based laser vision correction procedures, there is an evolving trend from automated mechanical to laser-assisted corneal flap creation (Fig. 27.1).

WHAT IS FEMTOSECOND?

Increasing familiarity with the concept of a "femtosecond laser" reinforces the notion that a femtosecond operates at very short time duration. Femtosecond lasers are mainly used for creation of the flap in LASIK surgery, even though there are

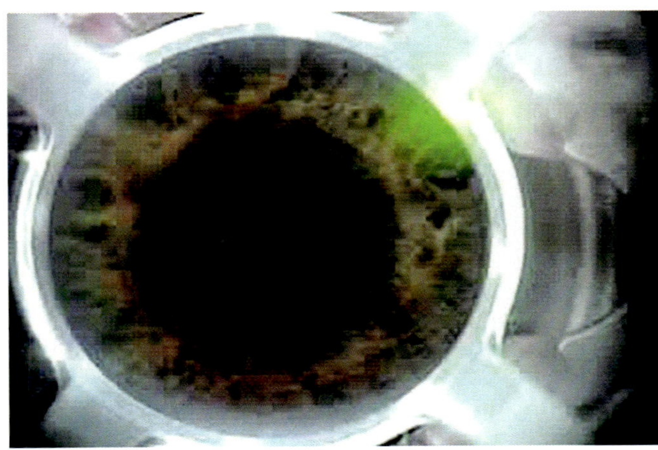

Fig. 27.1: Femtosecond laser flap creation

numerous other evolving applications of the technology in ophthalmology.

Metric prefixes are often applied as factors of ten such as "kilometer (km)", "megabyte (MB)", "gigabyte (GB)", "millisecond (ms)", or "microgram (μg)", allowing a greater appreciation for what these metrics mean, but a "femtosecond" is not a familiar metric in daily life.

Atoms and molecules have an enormously complex 'sociology'. Ever since their discovery, scientists have been concerned with their behavior in matter. However, the entire time span of the journey during any transformation is billion trillion times shorter than the human lifespan. That is why for twenty-four centuries, since its conception, the atom's motion in real-time was invisible. For atoms and molecules, the scale of time involved is awesome—its unit is the femtosecond; the prefix femto meaning 10^{-15} is from femton, the Scandinavian word for 'fifteen'. Put in comparative terms, a femtosecond is to a second as a second is to 32 million years. In one second, light travels about 186,000 miles (300,000 kilometers), almost from here to the moon and light could travel the distance around the earth about 7 1/2 times in one second; in one femtosecond, light travels 300 nanometers (0.000 000 3 meter), the dimension of virus. With femtosecond timing, the atom's motion becomes visible. Flashing a molecule with a femtosecond laser pulse can be compared to the effect of a stroboscope flash or the opening of a camera shutter.

WHAT IS FEMTOSECOND TECHNOLOGY?

Though difficult to comprehend as a basic level, the use of ultrashort pulses has a variety of potential advantages.[4,5] In short, they include three principal advantages in time, space, and wavelength.

Time

Due to the ultrashort pulsation (pulse duration), it is possible to obtain a high-frequency pulse, high signal/noise(S/N) ratio, optical nonlinearity and high peak intensity. For example, this can be utilized in ultrahigh-speed optical transmission and signal processing.

Space

An ultrashort optical pulse occupies an extremely short distance in space and propagates at the velocity of light, and this means a possibility to precisely control the delay time in a small dimension and thus the overall optical device and circuit can be very compact.

Wavelength

Ultrashort pulse has a large spectral width due to the pulse shape-spectrum interdependence deduced directly from Fourier transform relationship, and this merits the use of various photonic functions in wavelength division, such as the extraction of multichannel wavelengths from an ultrashort pulse, and also the wavelength conversion and pulse waveform shaping by applying this property. The extraction of 200 wavelength channels has been shown using a femtosecond pulse.[6]

LASER-TISSUE INTERACTION AND PHOTODISRUPTION

Laser-tissue interaction can be classified into at least five categories: thermal effects (photocoagulation; typically achieved with argon lasers), photochemical effects (photoablation; excimer laser), mechanical effects (photodisruption), evaporation effects (CO_2 laser) and photochemistry(photodynamic therapy—PDT).

The physics of the femtosecond laser-tissue interaction are based on photodisruption, the same mechanism as Nd:YAG laser commonly used for posterior capsulotomy and iridotomy. Unlike excimer laser ablation, photodisruption does not depend on the inherent absorption of the laser wavelength by corneal tissue.

Semi-transparent materials such as biological tissues do not strongly absorb light in the visible range. However, the intensity of a tightly-focused femtosecond laser pulse can be high enough to cause nonlinear absorption of laser energy by the tissue leading to permanent material change.[7] In fact, it is the ability to focus the femtosecond laser pulse through the superficial cornea to a specific location in the stroma that makes its use as a laser keratome practical.

Photodisruption begins with process called laser-induced optical break down (LIOB). LIOB occurs when a strongly focused, short duration laser pulse generates a high intensity electric field, leading to the formation of a mixture of free electrons and ions known as a plasma.[8] The free electron then generates other free electrons by collision, in a process known as avalanche ionization. The free electrons are extremely energetic.

The hot plasma expands with supersonic velocity, displacing surrounding tissue.[9-12] As the plasma expansion slows, the supersonic displacement front propagates through the tissue as a shock wave. The shock wave loses energy and velocity as it propagates, relaxing to an ordinary acoustic wave that dissipates harmlessly.[13] The cooling plasma vaporizes a small volume of tissue, eventually forming a cavitation bubble. The volume of cavitation bubble is small and very precise. In the cornea, the cavitation bubble consists mainly of CO_2, N_2 and H_2O, which can diffuse out from the tissue.[14] The specific process of photodisruption depends largely on the pulse duration, energy intensity and focusing geometry of a particular laser system. The shorter the pulse, the lower is the fluence threshold necessary to vaporize the target tissue. This reduces the required pulse energy and also the size of the cavitation bubble.

On the other hand, longer pulse duration systems, such as the widely used Nd:YAG laser, require relatively large energies to initiate LIOB. These large energies translate into large shock waves and cavitation bubbles, producing significant collateral tissue effects. For this reason, use of the Nd:YAG laser is limited to procedures such as capsulotomy and iridotomy, which are relatively far from sensitive structures.[15]

That is also why the ultrashort-pulse femtosecond laser is selected for application to the sensitive corneal tissue, not the longer duration nanosecond(10^{-9}) or picoseconds(10^{-12}) laser. (Currently the attosecond (10^{-18}) laser is unavailable in clinical ophthalmology). As just described, reducing the pulse duration of the laser decreases the threshold energy for LIOB.

The small amount of energy deposited in tissue and the rapid plasma expansion prevent significant heat transfer to surrounding tissue. Narrow collateral tissue damage zones have been demonstrated in tissue experiments with femtosecond photodisruption.[9-13,16]

In addition, the larger the numerical aperture (NA), the smaller the focal spot volume, and the smaller the energy threshold for LIOB.[9-13] To Increase the NA, we can increase the lens diameter and decrease focal length. For these reasons, in clinical practice the applanator is large, space-occupying and cumbersome for its high price. Surgeons very often experience difficulty in manipulating the applanator and have to create sufficient clearance between the patient's nose and the laser by tilting the head for proper docking.

The clinical experience with development of laser technology for corneal flap creation reflects the above relationship of pulse duration and threshold energy fluence. Initially proposed in 1995, the first laser keratome utilized the state of the art picosecond laser technology. While able to create corneal flaps clinically,[17] the relatively large damage range and cavitation bubble size of the picosecond laser, as well as the limited repetition rates of available systems, restricted clinical and commercial practicality of this approach. Practical pulse durations for surgical photodisruptive lasers appear to fall in several hundred femtosecond range.[18-20] The threshold for photodisruption decreases as the pulse duration falls dramatically from nanoseconds to a few hundred femtoseconds, but much more slowly as pulse duration reduced further. Consequently, the use of pulses shorter than a few hundred femtoseconds does not greatly reduce the photodisruption threshold. In contrast, other properties of ultrashort pulses (large optical bandwidth and high intensities) make generation and amplification of pulses shorter than a few hundred femtoseconds difficult and prone to undesirable nonlinear phenomenon (self-phase modulation, self-focusing, etc) at the required surgical energies. (Actually, 4 commercially available femtosecond laser systems employ this range of pulse duration).

LASER REFRACTIVE SURGERY

The femtosecond laser is a device initially designed to entirely carry out an intrastromal refractive procedure without having to cut a stromal flap. Early clinical trials accomplishing refractive error correction with current state femtosecond technology have not surpassed the results obtained with excimer laser technology. Therefore, the use of an excimer laser is obligatory to achieve the desired refractive correction at this point. In short, the femtosecond laser is the ideal instrument to carry out stromal tissue cuttings, whereas the excimer laser remains the ideal tool to sculpt the corneal stroma. [The clinical research for femtosecond lenticular extraction (FLEx) is now ongoing with VisuMax system (Carl Zeiss Meditec AG, Jena, Germany). This procedure is conducted by femtosecond laser alone, though requires creation and elevation of the flap.]

FLAP CREATION (PRIMARY APPLICATION)

The first commercially available FDA-approved femtosecond laser applied in ophthalmology, the IntraLase(AMO, Santa Clara, CA,USA) has a considerable clinical experience with flap creation for LASIK. We here demonstrated the straightforward IntraLase flap making technique. (We don't show setting parameters. This is because other machines and even the IntraLase (15, 30, 60kHz) have different parameters depending on the laser profiles. Please ask manufacturers or experienced surgeons).

Docking

A typical case begins with docking of the suction ring on the patient's eye under the excimer laser microscope. Some doctors advocate marking the center of the pupil with the surgical marking pen under the microscope as a centering guide. The suction ring and the cone on the laser port are applanated to give a fixed distance to facilitate application of the laser energy to a specific distance within the cornea.

Bed Change

We then swing the patient's bed from beneath the excimer laser to the IntraLase laser. (If swing bed is not available, patients move to IntraLase bed.)

Adjustment

By squeezing the suction ring, we expand it a little bit to "grab" the docking cone and adjoin the laser to the cornea. When everything is aligned and the peripheral air meniscus part is gone after joystick steering, flap centration can be adjusted by the computer mouse to center the corneal cap on the pupil. Excessive mouse centration movement will reduce the corneal flap diameter. This is automatic reduction, though the caution appears on the screen. Therefore, surgeons have to take care, especially when the treatment requires a large flap diameter (i.e. hyperopic treatment, high astigmatism treatment).

Laser

After achieving proper centration, the surgeon steps on the foot pedal to start the bed cut. The first pulses are delivered along the hinge. A pocket is first created for the gas generated during treatment to go into. Then, the raster pattern is used for bed making. This raster pattern was reported to be superior to spiral pattern with IntraLase.[21] The laser puts down a layer of bubbles in a single predetermined plane at whatever flap depth has been set. The edge of the flap are prepared last with a variable

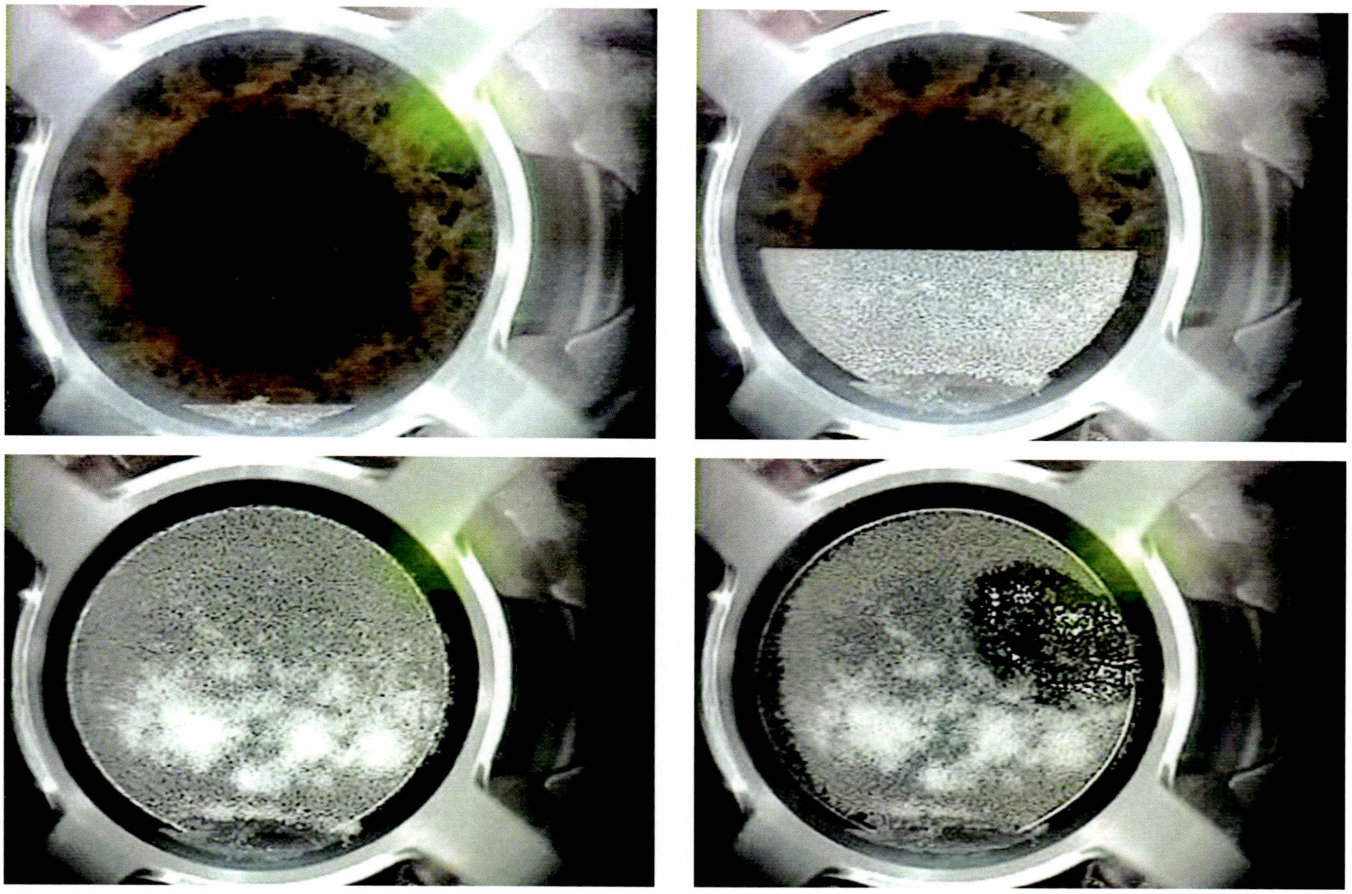

Figs 27.2 to 27.5: IntraLase flap creation

angle chosen by the operator. Following IntraLase, the suction ring is released off (Figs 27.2 to 27.5)

Second Bed Change

We again swing the patient bed to the excimer laser.

Lift the Flap and Excimer Laser

The flap is lifted with a blunt spatula, starting next to the hinge and cutting bridging residual tissue. After lifting the flap, the excimer procedure is conducted (Fig. 27.6).

FEMTOSECOND LASER-ASSISTED PENETRATING KERATOPLASTY (PKP)

There are several goals of using laser trephination instead of a conventional blade punch trephine during corneal transplantation. The first is to obtain better quality of vision, with less total astigmatism and fewer aberrations. Second, recovery of useful functional vision should be faster. The third goal is to obtain stronger wound healing, which is safer for

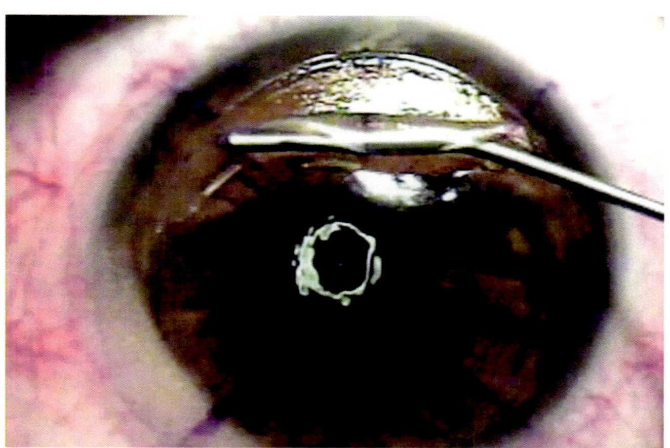

Fig. 27.6: Flap lift and excimer ablation

the patient and gives the surgeon the option of earlier suture removal.[22]

Sources of astigmatism and other aberrations derive from the alignment of the donor and host as well as the impact of the suture and uneven wound healing. Ideally, alignment of the donor to host anterior surface is a precise Bowman layer-to-Bowman layer apposition, which must be uniform over 360°. The only way to ensure this is to have some form of lamellar cut in both donor and host that is able to withstand the impact of variables including intraocular pressure. The other source of misalignment is rotational. Sutures play a role, either through excessive or uneven tension. Uneven postoperative wound healing may lead to distortion in a transplant during the postoperative period, even if the surgery is performed well. The studies explored the advantages of a shaped edge in improving resistance to wound leakage.[23,24]

The commercially released software in some laser now includes radial alignment marks that are precisely placed on the donor and the host, improving the surgeon's accuracy in precise placement of the corneal graft.

FEMTOSECOND LASER-ASSISTED SUTURELESS ANTERIOR LAMELLAR KERATOPLASTY (FALK)

Anterior lamellar keratoplasty (ALK) is a partial-thickness corneal transplantation used in eyes with pathology limited to the anterior layers. ALK provides several advantages over conventional PKP. Avoiding a full-thickness trephination minimizes potential intraoperative complications and allows for faster visual and refractive recovery. Maintaining the recipient endothelial layer decreases the rate of graft rejection. Furthermore, with the advancements in Descemet's stripping endothelial keratoplasty, ALK, and ultimately, cultured corneal cell transplantation, we can perform multiple corneal transplantations from one donor's cornea.[25-27]

The major limitations with ALK are the technical challenges of performing manual dissections and the resulting stromal interface irregularities between the donor and recipient interface that could result in stromal interface haze, induced irregular astigmatism, and loss of best-corrected visual acuity (BCVA). The improvements in automated micro-keratomes and artificial anterior chambers (ACs) minimize these difficulties.[28-32]

Recently femtosecond laser technology provides a new surgical modality in corneal surgery. Surgeon can better customize the shape and corneal dimensions of the donor and recipient, improving the resulting fit and leading to less induced irregular astigmatism and interface haze. These features may result in faster and better wound healing, without the need for sutures, though we still have several problems in adjustment of thickness and energy settings (Fig. 27.7 to 27.10). FALK in patients with anterior corneal scarring seems to be an alternative to conventional anterior LK and PK without significant short-term complications. The femto-second laser, with its ability to perform precise preprogrammed corneal dissections at a variety of depths and orientations, is a powerful tool for anterior LK, especially when combined with anterior segment OCT findings.[33]

INTRACORNEAL RING SEGMENT

Intracorneal ring segment (ICRS) [Intacs (Addition Technologies, Fremont, CA), Ferrara ring (Ferrara Ophthalmics, Belo Horizonte, Brazil), implantation is a refractive procedure that has been used for the correction of mild-to-moderate myopia, surgical management of keratoconus, pellucid corneal marginal degeneration, and iatrogenic postoperative corneal ectasia. There are two methods for creating intrastromal corneal tunnels for ICRS insertion. The first method is a mechanical approach, where a side cut is made by inserting a blade into the desired corneal depth. A specialized blunt dissecting instrument is then aided through the cornea, with the use of a suction centering device guide. The second method utilizes a femtosecond laser, creating a channel in the desired depth and location in the cornea.

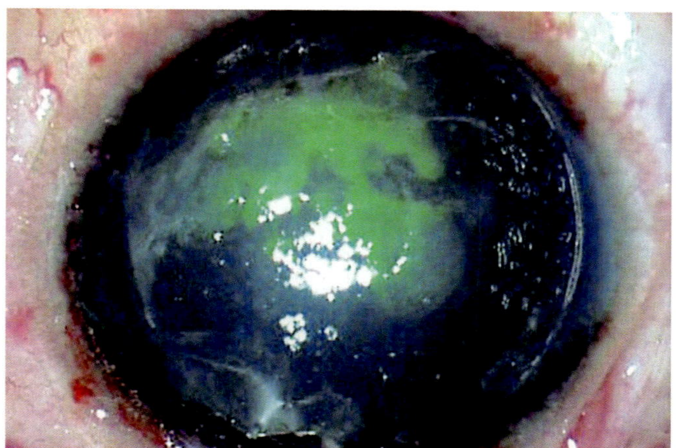

Fig. 27.7: Preoperative clinical picture of the patient showing anterior stromal opacities with lattice lines and diffuse stromal haze. Fluorescein staining shows loss of epithelium

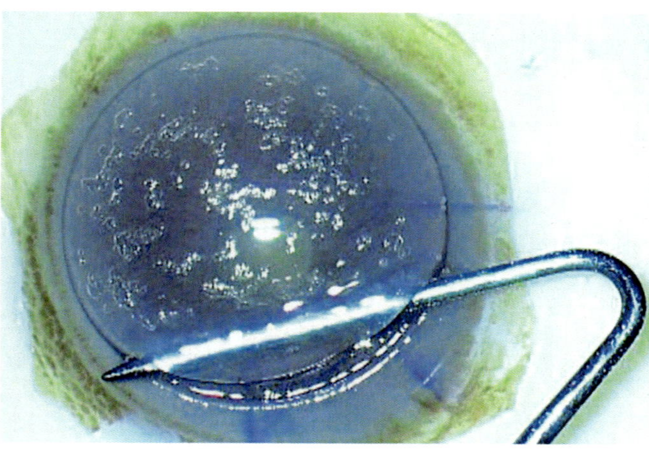

Fig. 27.8: Donor corneal tissue dissected femtosecond assisted lamellar keratoplasty (FALK) with IntraLase FMTM laser at 350 microns depth and 8.5 mm diameter

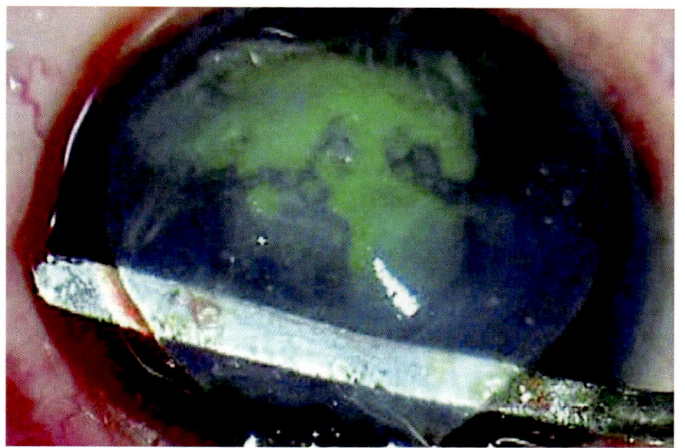

Fig. 27.9: Recipient corneal tissue excised with IntraLase FMTM laser at 350 microns depth and 8.5 mm diameter

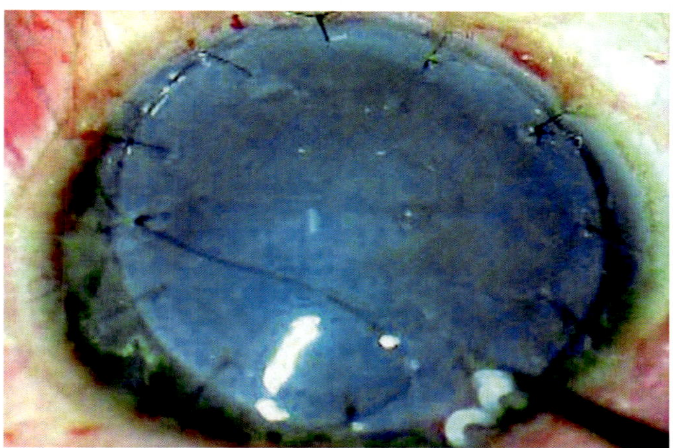

Fig. 27.10: Donor tissue placed over recipient bed and sutured with interrupted sutures

Fig. 27.7 to 27.10: Femtosecond laser-assisted anterior lamellar keratoplasty (FALK) (*Courtesy:* Dr. Agarwal's Eye Hospital)

It was reported that the femtosecond laser, compared with mechanical channel dissection, boasted greater refractive improvement.[34-36]

There are, however, some drawbacks to femtosecond laser-assisted ICRS insertion. Generally, segments are intended for insertion at a corneal depth of 70%. With the femtosecond laser, however, the maximal depth is fixed. Another disadvantage is that inadequate separation of corneal stroma may be seen in some eyes that require blunt dissection of the stroma. Also, in case of high energy levels, postoperative fibrosis is possible at the incision site. There is another risk of decentered placement of the tunnel in relation to the pupil.

In conclusion, the femtosecond laser for ICRS implantation offers significant safety and advantages including less corneal trauma, sterilization issues, and reproducibility of the channel over the mechanical technique, though there are, some limitations that must be improved.

CORNEAL INLAY

Though corneal inlay[AcuFocus (Bausch and Lomb, Rochester, NY), ReVision (formerly IntraLens) (ReVision Optics Inc, Lake Forest, CA), InVue (Biovision AG, Brüggs, Switzerland)] treatment is still experimental as of 2008, but clinical studies are progressing and seem encouraging. This method treats presbyopia by inserting a very tiny lens into the central cornea. This method of treatment is less invasive than lens-based surgery including cataract removal and clear lens insertion. In addition it is reversible because we can remove the inlay relatively easily. For the pocket/flap creation for corneal inlay, femtosecond laser can be used instead of the microkeratome or pocket maker.

ASTIGMATIC KERATOTOMY (AK)

Correcting high astigmatism with the excimer laser is problematic, and manual astigmatic keratotomy for such eyes is unreliable and unpredictable. Hammonds et al reported the results of AK using a femtosecond laser both in natural occurring and post-PKP eyes.[37] In the procedure, laser pulses are stacked on each other to create an angled cleavage plane that is then opened manually in an instrument-assisted procedure. He concluded that it can be an effective method of reducing corneal astigmatism and improving uncorrected visual acuity. With this new flexibility, it may be possible in the future to use the laser to fine-tune even lesser degrees of astigmatism. It is important to note, however, that each laser system has maximum depth of cut. For example, IntraLase was approved to go only 400 microns deep and it did one cut per procedure. New parameters are now available through the keratoplasty software which allows two incisions to be created simultaneously at different depths and deeper (1200 microns).

ASTIGMATIC KERATECTOMY

For the high astigmatism which may not be correctable with spectacles or contact lenses, existing surgical methods used to treat astigmatism include excimer laser treatment, relaxing incisions, compression sutures, and corneal wedge resections. Ghanem and Azar report using the femtosecond laser to perform a controlled arcuate wedge resection. A standardized technique was developed to use the femtosecond laser to create corneal incisions in a peripheral wedge-shaped orientation. The corneal tissue was removed and the area of wedge resection was closed with interrupted 10-0 nylon sutures, resulting in significant improvement of the astigmatism.[38]

POSTERIOR LAMELLAR KERATOPLASTY

Complications of full-thickness keratoplasty include high or irregular astigmatism, slow visual recovery, traumatic wound dehiscence, and suture-related problems. In cases of isolated posterior corneal pathology, these problems may be significantly reduced by transplanting only the diseased posterior cornea and leaving the remaining normal anterior layers intact. Despite the distinct advantages of anterior lamellar keratoplasty (ALK) surgery, penetrating keratoplasty (PK) remains the most common procedure largely because lamellar surgery is more technically demanding and time consuming, and interface irregularity arising from manual lamellar dissection often results in suboptimal visual outcomes. Recent improvements of surgical technique and advances in instrumentation such as microkeratome-assisted lamellar transplantation have contributed to improved visual quality with lamellar keratoplasty (LK) surgery. But, at the same time, we have to admit microkeratomes have some limitations in geometry predictability and customization of the tissue. To overcome this, femtosecond laser-assisted posterior lamellar keratoplasty (DSAEK, DLEK) with the femtosecond laser has been advocated and performed. Risk of endothelial cell loss and decreased visual acuity after host/donor preparation with the femtosecond laser has not been evaluated in a large study, but femtosecond-laser-assisted posterior lamellar keratoplasty seems promising.[39-45]

FEMTOSECOND LENTICULAR EXTRACTION (FLEX)

This new innovation in corneal surgery uses a femtosecond laser alone (VisuMax, Carl Zeiss Meditec AG, Jena, Germany), compared with other procedures that use an excimer plus femtosecond laser. FLEx is not LASIK; the healing responses of the two procedures are quite different. The cornea is not ablated during FLEx. Therefore, energy is not lost at the periphery of the ablation, and prolate refractive zones are similar to wavefront-optimized excimer laser ablation results. Preliminary results with FLEx, which is a single-step procedure were good.[46] During FLEx, the femtosecond laser creates a refractive and a nonrefractive cut in a single step. After the flap is lifted, a piece of stromal corneal tissue (i.e. refractive lenticule) is removed. Next, the flap is repositioned in the usual fashion. This new procedure has a potential, though we don't have enough data yet.

FEMTOSECOND LASERS IN THE MARKET

Due to increased application, adoption, interest and reduced risk of femtosecond laser, the market for this technology is growing. Currently, four US Food and Drug Administration (FDA) approved laser systems are available in the market: Femtec (20/10 Perfect Vision, Heidelberg, Germany), Femto LDV(formerly known as the Da Vinci) (Ziemer Ophthalmic Systems, Port, Switzerland), IntraLase FS laser (IntraLase Corp.,Irvine, California), and VisuMax (Carl Zeiss Meditec AG, Jena, Germany).

FLAP THICKNESS

It is almost intuitively claimed that standard deviation for mean femtosecond laser flap thickness was smaller than that for mechanical microkeratome, although newer microkeratomes may do similarly well.[47-54] The flap thickness by microkeratome is decided by a variety of biological variables, blade integrity and assembly, but femtosecond-assisted flap is unlikely to be affected by such factors. The possible reason for flap thickness variability with femtosecond laser is that there are still some mechanical interfaces needed that link the patient's eye to the femtosecond laser. These disposable docking cones or plates have considerable manufacturing tolerance and the compressing pressure changes the corneal thickness, thus limiting the predictability of flap thickness.

The ability to make reliable thin flap by femtosecond laser provides both surgeons and patients with greater biomechanical stability, reducing potential iatrogenic corneal ectasia, though large and thin flaps may increase the risk of flap striae, and slippage in these corrections where the stroma underlying the flap undergo important geometrical modifications.

DRY AND WET PROCEDURE

Keratectomy by mechanical microkeratome is wet procedure and we need lubrication for the keratome. After making flap, stromal bed must be dried prior to excimer laser ablation. This step can induce debris and epithelial cells on stromal bed and unequal hydration can cause unequal ablation. On the other hand, femtosecond laser ablation has much less risk for those issues, because this is basically dry procedure.

DRY EYE AND STEEPER FLAP EDGE CONFIGURATION

With a microkeratome, the edge configuration is about 25° to 35°. We need to enter at that angle to make a flap without risking extremely deep penetration or anterior perforation. With the femtosecond laser (except Femto LDV), the side-cut angle can be usually bigger than microkeratome one. An increased angle can allow the flap to seat more easily and, more importantly, create an entry that's a powerful barrier to epithelial cells. In addition, this steeper angle can spare corneal nerves. This can lessen the severity of long-term dry eye symptom. Femto-LDV does not perform separate bed and rim cuts. Femto-LDV steers the beam in a zig-zag pattern and relies on the natural downward slope of the cornea as it curves away from the applanation plate as a means of providing a rim cut.

THE FLAP SHAPE AND THE HINGE

The microkeratome creates a D-shaped stromal bed, leaving less room for the flap diameter we need. Therefore, we need larger flap diameter to accommodate ablation diameter. With femtosecond laser, we can decide how big the hinge is. If we are well centered on the pupil, we will have the full flap diameter we want. In addition, thanks to steeper edge configuration, we can utilize the entire stromal bed for ablation.

BED SMOOTHNESS

We often hear it said that stromal bed cut with microkeratome is superior/comparable to that with femtosecond laser because after femtosecond laser spots, theoretically a blunt spatula must mechanically dissects the bridging tissue between the microbubbles to separate the flap from the stromal bed, resulting in a less perfect surface. It is partly true, but at the same time, we have to remember that many surgeons usually use the single blade for bilateral surgeries, though in experimental study they use the blade only once. In addition, as mentioned in the comparison of 4 lasers, each system must have different bed surface depending on the laser profiles.

COST EFFECTIVENESS

One may argue that femtosecond lasers could attract more patients. Once this laser has lost its novelty, however, potential patients may be discouraged by the additional expenses that they pay for out-of-pocket. Therefore, the cost associated with the femtosecond flap-cut procedure must be taken into account in the business model of the eye center. The increased cost for femtosecond device and the use of disposable components must be compensated for and the patient's workflow rate must increase. The alternative is to cut down the profit margin per procedure.

TIME CONSUMPTION

Current femtosecond flap-cut technology does not reduce surgical time. Even the fastest femtosecond machines deliver flap cuts in approximately 20 seconds, whereas a mechanical microkeratome flap cuts last less than 15 seconds. Moreover, patients must be transferred from the femtosecond bed to the excimer laser bed or we have to rotate the laser bed from femtosecond laser to excimer laser, and some opaque bubble layer (OBL) requires extra time for gas bubbles to clear up, because the excimer laser's eye tracker would not find the pupil, and because the OBL could affect the laser efficiency. Both cause additional time when compared with conventional mechanical LASIK.

ABERRATION, CONTRAST SENSITIVITY, PREDICTABILITY OF TARGET REFRACTION

Regarding the difference in these issues after refractive surgery between mechanical microkeratome and femtosecond laser, there is still controversy and have been reports only on IntraLase as of January 2008. In addition, as mentioned before, each femtosecond laser system uses different energy, repetition rate, spot separation and so on, we cannot simply say that which is better than which. But they report the trend that femtosecond laser is better than mechanical microkeratome, though further study with a larger patient population is warranted to determine whether these differences are statistically significant and if the same can be true to all the laser systems.[55--58]

WOUND HEALING AND DIFFUSE LAMELLAR KERATITIS (DLK)

Femtosecond technology does not eliminate interface complications after LASIK, as an interface within the corneal stroma is still created. The comparison study in wound healing showed that stromal cell necrosis associated with femtosecond laser flap formation likely contributes to greater inflammation after LASIK performed with the femtosecond laser than with mechanical microkeratome. The incidence of diffuse lamellar keratitis (DLK) was significantly greater in the femtosecond laser group than in the mechanical group despite more intense postoperative steroid treatment. Confocal microscopy revealed a higher wound healing opacity index in the femtosecond laser group. The femtosecond laser produced stronger flap adhesion postoperatively, especially at the flap edge.[59-62] This stronger wound healing is not always bad, because this can work for more resistance to trauma/ectasia. Also in this issue, however, only IntraLase has been studied in the literature and we have to compare other lasers in the future.

DILEMMA

The ease of flap lift after femtosecond laser is related to the energy setting, proximity and number of laser pulses; few pulses, further apart = harder lift, more pulses, closer together = easier lift, more pulses = more treatment time. More energy = easier lift.

Even if it is easy for lifting flap, more pulses and more energy can take time and cause DLK/inflammation. To deal with this dilemma, new-concept LASIK flap lifter is also available.[63]

NEED NOMOGRAM MODIFICATION BETWEEN MICROKERATOME AND FEMTOSECOND LASER?

The microkeratome makes meniscus flap and the femtosecond laser makes planar flap. The former is wet, the latter is dry procedure and femtosecond laser tend to cause stronger wound healing.

In addition, the exact amount of tissue consumed during plasma generation may vary with the level of energy required to achieve the tissue cleavage. In a patient who had femtosecond flap cuts in both eyes, without subsequent excimer photoablation (i.e. bioptic procedure), a slight decrease in the corneal pachymetry is reported,[64] though it is hard to prove that this reduction would be consecutive to tissue plasmatization or stromal remodeling. OBL can reduce the excimer laser efficiency.

Considering these factors, we may have to adjust the nomogram depending on the technique used; microkeratome or femtosecond laser.

MICROKERATOME AND FEMTOSECOND LASER

The automated mechanical microkeratome is an excellent device in the hands of an experienced surgeon, but we have to admit that even the best surgeons experience inconsistent and unpredictable problems out of their control due to biological/ mechanical variation blade integrity/assembly and microkeratome precision. Thin/thick flap, small/ large flap, wide/narrow hinge, free flap, inconsistent bed hydration, epithelial defects, epithelial ingrowth, incomplete flap, buttonhole flap, striae, difficulty with small palpebral fissures, water, debris, bacteria swept into bed.

On the other hand, femtosecond laser flap creation is not sensitive to corneal geometric factor, such as preoperative keratometry, intraocular pressure, or corneal diameter,[65] nor is it affected by mechanical factors, such as vacuum level, variance in blade manufacture, and blade translation velocity.[65,66]

What femtosecond laser has brought us are safety, predictability, reproducibility, uniformity, maximal surgeon control, minimal complications and high patient/surgeon satisfaction and relaxed surgery in spite of a little longer time and higher cost, more early foreign body sensation and photophobia, giving the surgeon the best of both PRK and LASIK. Moreover, the versatility of femtosecond systems allows the surgeon to precisely plan the hinge position, flap diameter, thickness, and centering over the cornea. It permits different flap thicknesses-thinner than mechanical ones-saving more tissue for the ablation. Therefore, higher refractive errors may be treated, even in thinner corneas.

But at the same time, head-to-head studies comparing mechanical microkeratomes with the femtosecond laser have conflicting results[67-71] and the other studies have shown no significant difference.[72,73]

In conclusion, we apparently see more advantages of the femtosecond laser than automated mechanical microkeratome, but it does not always mean that we have to move to the femtosecond laser. Depending on practice type and experience, preference of doctors, each surgeon must carefully address the costs and benefits of switching from razor (mechanical microkeratome) to laser (femtosecond technology).

FUTURE DEVELOPMENT

The currently available femtosecond laser systems are already well-established and continuously software-updated. However, we would like to describe what we want in the future femtosecond laser system based on our clinical experiences.

CENTRATION

The femtosecond laser has brought doctors new level of precision in corneal surgeries. The femtosecond laser likely has several advantages over the microkeratome, including a more predictable flap dimensions.[74,75] Aside from unavoidable/inherent drawbacks described above, however, we often experience another major problem in making flap.

The flap position often tends to be off-centered unwantedly, though we always center the superimposed image of the incision on the screen over the patient's pupil/cornea after apparent ideal centered applanation.

The location of the pupil is an important factor in determining effective optics.[76,77] It is now generally accepted that the line from the fovea through the center of the pupil should be used in calculating the aberrations of the eye.[78,79]

We may think the decentration is a trifle in laser vision correction, because current excimer laser machines are equipped with pupil trackers. However, this must be a big problem especially in hyperopic or astigmatic treatment which require larger optical zone and intracorneal ring segment insertion which needs strict centration.

The pupillary center shift under different illumination, pharmacological, and psychological, intraocular pressure conditions, tilted applanation, surgeons' wrong handling of applanator, and large angle kappa seems to be among the reasons for centroid shift.[80-83]

To avoid this decentration, marking the pupillary center on the natural corneal position before the applanation seems to be the only available method now. Installing pupil tracker which is already used in excimer laser system can be a probable future development in femtosecond laser system.

CALIBRATION

Because each femtosecond laser unit has different characteristics even within the same line of product, it is critical that one takes the time at the outset to refine and optimize the machine's parameter settings as we do for excimer laser. We totally agree with this but, even after the optimizing, we actually observe the fluctuation in the easiness for lifting the flap. This is just our personal impression, but we think that this is not due to patient-to-patient difference, but day-to-day one.

Each femtosecond laser system has internal calibration system and it calibrate itself at the daily start up. Prior to surgery, the software automatically performs multiple pre-procedure system checks to verify the readiness of the laser and multiple calibration checks are also available to the surgeon. But this calibration system does not look like the one equipped with the excimer laser calibration system. Therefore, we would like to have more fine-tuning calibration system, after which we can obtain a consistent flap making, and intended accurate incision.

CUSTOM-DESIGNED FLAP

Though it is still controversial, sub-Bowman's keratomileusis (SBK) will become the next trend in laser refractive surgery, and will offer patients the better compromise between the early visual rehabilitation and comfort offered by LASIK and the safety and long-term stability of PRK and other surface ablation procedures. The early study results showed superior/parallel to PRK in UCVA, BCVA, ocular response analyzer (ORA), higher order aberration (HOA), and contrast acuity but at the same time authors warn that too thin flaps are more prone to complications like buttonholes, microstriae, possible haze with treatment given very thin flap and proximity to the epithelium, flap tear, especially with attempted lift and retreatment.[84-86]

In SBK, a femtosecond laser is used to create a corneal flap just below the level of Bowman's membrane (in most cases, 80 to 100 microns). Epithelial layer is meniscus shaped (thinner centrally and thicker peripherally) and therefore the thinnest flap parameter should be decided depending on the thickest epithelial layer within the flap diameter, but the thickness changes under several conditions like dryness and applanation pressure, so we can only guess the target flap thickness.

We always lose epithelium in PRK. We are not sure of the effect of alcohol in LASEK. EpiLASIK keratome sometimes injure stroma.[87] In EpiLASIK we are not sure of being able to have intended optical zone. In LASIK, postoperative corneal stability decreases.

Considering these possible complications in various laser vision corrections, we think that the best and ultimate way in making flap is femtosecond laser assisted intra-Bowman's keratomileusis (FIBK) or femtosecond laser assisted EpiLASIK (F-EpiLASIK). In these procedure, femtosecond laser should target just within (FIBK)/above(F-EpiLASIK) the Bowman's layer. By developing laser system, this must be done without epithelial breakthrough which is sometimes seen during femtosecond flap creation.[88] However, in the worst case scenario that we have flap complications, we can scrape the epithelium and perform PRK, because the flap does not have corneal stroma in FIBK and F-EpiLASIK. To be able to do this procedure, we have to combine ultrafast 3D imaging modality which can detect each corneal layer, ultrafast feedback system which can control precision femtosecond laser ablation in different depth (Z-axis) depending on the place in X-Y plane and ultrafast depth-variable femtosecond laser. This will be the final concept of flap-based refractive surgery, though we may have alternative technologies instead of femtosecond laser.

Next, with the current femtosecond laser system, we can make anterior planar flap, because the focus of laser is fixed for the surface of applanator. Considering that the shape of the cornea is meniscus shaped, we have meniscus-shaped posterior corneal tissue after removing anterior flap. Descemet's stripping automated endothelial keratoplasty (DSAEK) is becoming popular and the preparation of donor tissue with femtosecond laser has been reported.[89,90] The shape of the DSAEK donor tissue varies depending on the ratio of anterior and posterior curvature, which can be among the reasons which cause unpredictable refractive outcome after DSAEK.[91,92] To decrease the refractive surprise as much as possible, planar DSAEK donor tissue is desirable. Also for this purpose, above-mentioned ultrafast devices (3D imaging, feedback system and depth-variable femtosecond laser) are wanted.

OTHER OPHTHALMIC APPLICATIONS

When the price of the femtosecond laser goes down, and the probe for slit lamp and surgical microscope or the handy probe are available, we can use this laser for surgeries such as, sclerectomy, iridotomy, and fistulizing trabecular meshwork,[93-95] because the energy and shockwave, collateral damage is very small. And this low energy profile may enable us to perform precision capsulorhexis for cataract surgery, capsulotomy for posterior capsule opacification (PCO) or rhexis of Descemet's membrane for Descemet's stripping automated endothelial keratoplasty (DSAEK). In addition, many other possible ophthalmic procedures with femtosecond laser must be under development all over the world.

REFERENCES

1. Pallikaris IG, Saiganos DS. Excimer laser in situ keratomileusis and photorefractive keratectomy for correction of high myopia. J refractive Refract Surg 1994;10:498-510.
2. Azar DT, Farah SG. Laser in situ keratomileusis versus photorefractive keratectomy: an update on indications and safety. Ophthalmology 1998;105:1357-8.
3. Carr ID, Stulting RD, Thompson KP, et al. Laser in situ. keratomileusis. Refract Surg 1997;10:533-42.
4. Diels JC, Rudolph W. Ultrashort laser pulse phenomena: fundamentals, techniques, and applications on a femtosecond time scale. Academic Press, San Diego, CA, 1996.
5. Kamiya T. Femtosecond Technology - From Basic Research to Application Prospects. Kamiya T, Saito F, Yajima H, Wada O (Ed): (Berlin: Springer) Ch I-1, 1-11.
6. Nuss MC, Knox WH, Koren U. Scaleable 32 channel chirped-pulse WDM source. Electron Lett 1996;32:1311-2.
7. Stuart BC, Feit MD, Herman S, et al. Nanosecond-to-femtosecond laser-induced breakdown in dielectrics. Phys Rev B Condens Matter 1996;53:1749-61.
8. Bloembergen N. Laser-Induced electric breakdown in solids. IEEE JQE 1974;10:375-86.
9. Fujimoto JG, Lin WZ, Ippen EP, et al. Time-resolved studies of Nd:YAG laser-induced breakdown. Plasma formation, acoustic wave generation, and cavitation. Invest Ophthalmol Vis Sci 1985; 26:1771-7.
10. Zysset B, Fujimoto JG, Puliafito CA, et al. Picosecond optical breakdown: tissue effects and. reduction of collateral damage. Lasers Surg Med 1989;9:193-204.
11. Vogel A, Hentschel W, Holzfuss J, et al. Cavitation bubble dynamics and acoustic transient generation in ocular surgery with pulsed Neodymium:YAG lasers. Ophthalmology 1986;93:1259-69.
12. Glezer EN, Schaffer CB, Nishimura N, et al. Minimally disruptive laser-induced breakdown in water. Opt Lett 1997; 22:1817-9.
13. Vogel A, Schweiger P, Frieser A, et al. Intraocular Nd:YAG laser surgery: light-tissue interaction, damage range, and reduction of collateral effects. IEEE JQE 1990;26:2240-59.
14. Habib MS, Speaker MG, Schatter W. Mass spectometry analysis of the by-products of intrastromal photorefractive keratectomy with the Nd:YLF picosecond laser. Ophthalmic Surgery and Lasers 1995;26:481-3.
15. Steinert RF, Puliafito CA. The Nd:YAG Laser in ophthalmology. Philadelphia, Pa: WB Saunders; 1985.
16. Lubatschowski H, Maatz G, Heisterkamp A, et al. Applications of ultrashort laser pulses for intrastromal refractive surgery. Graefe's Arch Clin Exp Ophthalmol 2000;238:33-9.
17. Krueger RR, Marchi V, Gualano A, et al. Clinical analysis of the neodymium:YLF picosecond laser as a microkeratome for laser in situ keratomileusis. Partially Sighted Eye Study. J Cataract Refract Surg 1998;24:1434-40.
18. Loesel FH, Niemz MH, Bille JF, et al. Laser-induced optical breakdown on hard and soft tissues and its dependence on the pulse duration: experiment and model. IEEE J. Quantum Electron 1996;32:1717-22.
19. Kurtz RM, Liu X, Elner VM, et al. Plasma-mediated ablation in human cornea as a function of pulse width. J Refr Surg 1997;13:653-8.
20. Loesel FH, Tien AC, Backus S, et al. Effect of reduction of laser pulse width from 100 ps to 20 fs on the plasma-mediated ablation of hard and soft tissue. Proc SPIE 1998;3565:1325-8.
21. Sarayba MA, Maguen E, Salz J, et al. Femtosecond laser keratome creation of partial thickness donor corneal buttons for lamellar keratoplasty. J Refract Surg 2007; 23:58-65.
22. Steinert RF, Ignacio TS, Sarayba MS. Top hat shaped penetrating keratoplasty using the femtosecond laser. Am J Ophthalmol 2007;143:689-91.
23. Meltendorf C, Schroeter J, Bug R, et al. Corneal trephination with the femtosecond laser. Cornea 2006;25:1090-2.
24. Seitz B, Brünner H, Viestenz A, et al. Inverse mushroom-shaped nonmechanical penetrating keratoplasty using a femtosecond laser. Am J Ophthalmol 2005;139:941-4.
25. Ide T, Nishida K, Yamato M, et al. Structural characterization of bioengineered human corneal endothelial cell sheets fabricated on temperature-responsive culture dishes. Biomaterials 2006;27:607-14.
26. Nishida K, Yamato M, Hayashida Y,. Corneal reconstruction with tissue-engineered cell sheets composed of autologous oral mucosal epithelium. N Engl J Med 2004;351:1187-96.
27. Vajpayee RB, Sharma N, Jhanji V, et al. One donor cornea for 3 recipients: a new concept for cornel transplantation surgery. Arch Ophthalmol 2007;125:552-4.
28. Elkins BS, Casebeer JC, Kezirian GM. Sutureless homoplastic lamellar keratoplasty. J Refract Surg 1997;13:185-7.
29. Hafezi F, Mrochen M, Fankhauser F II, et al. Anterior lamellar keratoplasty with a microkeratome: a method for managing complications after refractive surgery. J Refract Surg 2003;19:52-7.
30. Jiménez-Alfaro I, Pérez-Santonja JJ, Gómez Tellería G, et al.Therapeutic lamellar keratoplasty with an automated microkeratome. J Cataract Refract Surg 2001;27:1161-5.
31. Vajpayee RB, Vasudendra N, Titiyal JS, et al. Automated lamellar therapeutic keratoplasty (ALTK) in the treatment of anterior to mid-stromal corneal pathologies. Acta Ophthalmol Scand 2006;84:771-3.
32. Li L, Behrens A, Sweet PM, et al. Corneal lenticule harvest using a microkeratome and an artificial anterior chamber system at high intrachamber pressure. J Cataract Refract Surg 2002;28:860-5.
33. Yoo SH, Kymionis GD, Koreishi A, et al. Femtosecond Laser-Assisted Sutureless Anterior Lamellar Keratoplasty. Ophthalmology. in press
34. Ratkay-Traub I, Ferincz IE, Juhasz T, Kurtz RM, Krueger RR et al. First clinical results with the femtosecond

neodynium-glass laser in refractive surgery. J Refract Surg 2003;19:94-103.
35. Ertan A, Kamburo?glu G, Bahadir M. Intacs insertion with the femtosecond laser for the management of keratoconus- One year results. J Cataract Refract Surg 2006;32:2039-42.
36. Ertan A. Intacs for keratoconus: comparison of mechanical versus femtolaser channeldissection. [Presented at: American Avademy of Ophthalmology AnnualMeeting; October 10-14, 2007; Las Vegas]
37. Meeting Reporter is reported live from AAO 2006, Las Vegas Accessed Apr 4 2008. http://www.eyeworld.org/article.php?sid=3516andstrict=andmorphologic=andquery
38. Ghanem RC, Azar DT. Femtosecond-laser arcuate wedge-shaped resection to correct high residual astigmatism after penetrating keratoplasty. J Cataract Refract Surg 2006; 32:1415-9.
39. Soong HK, Mian S, Abbasi O, et al. Femtosecond laser-assisted posterior lamellar keratoplasty: initial studies of surgical technique in eye bank eyes.Ophthalmology 2005; 112:44-9.
40. Mian SI, Soong HK, Patel SV, et al. In vivo femtosecond laser-assisted posterior lamellar keratoplasty in rabbits. Cornea 2006; 25:1205-9.
41. Goldman D, Koreishi A, Yoo S, et al. Sutureless anterior lamellar keratoplasty (SALK) performed with a femtosecond laser [abstract]. In: Federated Societies Scientific Session 2006; 10th November 2006; Las Vegas. Washington, DC: Eye Bank Association of America and the Cornea Society; 2006; p. 15.
42. Cheng YY, Pels E, Cleutjens JP, et al. Corneal endothelial viability after femtosecond laser preparation of posterior lamellar discs for Descemet-stripping endothelial keratoplasty. Cornea 2007;26:1118-22.
43. Cheng YY, Pels E, Nuijts RM. Femtosecond-laser-assisted Descemet's stripping endothelial keratoplasty. J Cataract Refract Surg. 2007 Jan;33:152-5.
44. Suwan-Apichon O, Reyes JM, Griffin NB, et al. Microkeratome versus femtosecond laser predissection of corneal grafts for anterior and posterior lamellar keratoplasty. Cornea. 2006;25:966-8.
45. Terry MA, Ousley PJ, Will B. A practical femtosecond laser procedure for DLEK endothelial transplantation: cadaver eye histology and topography. Cornea 2005;24:453-9.
46. Sekundo W. Femtosecond Lenticular Extraction. Cataract and Refractive Surgery Today Europe 2007 Apr: 72-73.[Accessed Apr 4 2008. http://ww.crstodayeurope.com/Issues/0407/0407_f5_sekundo.pdf]
47. Binder PS. Flap dimensions created with the IntraLase FS laser. J Cataract Refract Surg 2004;30:26-32.
48. Gimbel HV, Penno EA, van Westenbrugge JA, et al. Incidence and management of intraoperative and early postoperative complications in 1000 consecutive LASIK cases. Ophthalmology 1998;105:1839-47.
49. Hofmann RF, Bechara SJ. An independent evaluation of second generation suction microkeratomes. Refract Corneal Surg 1992;8:348-54.
50. Lin RT, Maloney RK. Flap complications associated with lamellar refractive surgery. Am J Ophthalmology 1999;127:129-36.
51. Wilhelm FW, Giessmann T, Hanschke R, et al. Cut edges and surface characteristics produced by different microkeratomes. J Refract Surg 2000;16:690-700.
52. Spadea L, Cerrone L, Necozione S, et al. Flap measurements with the Hansatome microkeratome. J Refract Surg 2002;18:149-54.
53. Binder PS, Moore M, Lambert RW, et al. Comparison of two microkeratome systems. J Refract Surg 1997;13:142-53.
54. Shemesh G, Dotan G, Lipshitz I. Predictability of corneal flap thickness in laser in situ keratomileusis using three different microkeratomes. J Refract Surg 2002;18:S347-S351.
55. Medeiros FW, Stapleton WM, Hammel J, et al. Wavefront analysis comparison of LASIK outcomes with the femtosecond laser and mechanical microkeratomes. J Refract Surg. 2007;23:880-7.
56. Tran DB, Sarayba MA, Bor Z, et al. Randomized prospective clinical study comparing induced aberrations with IntraLase and Hansatome flap creation in fellow eyes: potential impact on wavefront-guided laser in situ keratomileusis. J Cataract Refract Surg 2005;31:97-105.
57. Lim T, Yang S, Kim M,et al. Comparison of the IntraLase femtosecond laser and mechanical microkeratome for laser in situ keratomileusis. Am J Ophthalmol. 2006;141: 833-9.
58. Krueger RR, Dupps WJ Jr.Biomechanical effects of femtosecond and microkeratome-based flap creation: prospective contralateral examination of two patients. J Refract Surg. 2007;23:800-7.
59. Gil-Cazorla R, Teus MA, de Benito-Llopis L, et al.Incidence of diffuse lamellar keratitis after laser in situ keratomileusis associated with the IntraLase 15 kHz femtosecond laser and Moria M2 microkeratome. J Cataract Refract Surg 2008;34:28-31.
60. Netto MV, Mohan RR, Medeiros FW, et al. Femtosecond laser and microkeratome corneal flaps: comparison of stromal wound healing and inflammation. J Refract Surg 2007;23:667-76.
61. Javaloy J, Vidal MT, Abdelrahman AM, et al. Confocal microscopy comparison of IntraLase femtosecond laser and Moria M2 microkeratome in LASIK. J Refract Surg 2007;23:178-87.
62. Kim JY, Kim MJ, Kim TI,et al. A femtosecond laser creates a stronger flap than a mechanical microkeratome. Invest Ophthalmol Vis Sci 2006;47:599-604.
63. Ide T, Yoo SH, O'Brien TP. New LASIK flap lifter. Cataract and Refractive Surgery Today 2007 Nov/Dec:41-43.[Accessed Apr 4 2008. http://www.crstoday.com/PDF%20Articles/1107/CRST1107_06.pdf]

64. Gatinel M. The femtosecond laser: is it the gold standard yet? Cataract and Refractive Surgery Today Europe 2007 Apr: 51-52.[Accessed Apr 4 2008. http://www.crstodayeurope.com/Issues/0407/0407_f1_gatinel.pdf]
65. Nordan LT, Slade SG, Baker RN, et al. Femtosecond laser flap creation: Six month follow-up of initial US clinical series. J Refract Surg 2003;19:8-14.
66. Leung AT, Rao SK, Cheng AC, et al. Pathogenesis and management of laser in situ keratomileusis flap buttonhole. J Cataract Refract Surg 2000;26:358-62.
67. Kim JY, Kim MJ, Kim TI, et al. A femtosecond laser creates a stronger flap than a mechanical microkeratome. Invest Ophthalmol Vis Sci 2006;47:599-604.
68. Touboul D, Salin F, Mortemousque B, et al. Advantages and disadvantages of the femtosecond laser microkeratome. J Fr Ophthalmol 2005;28:535-46.
69. Durrie DS, Kezirian GM. Fentosecond laser versus mechanical keratome flaps in wavefront-guided laser in situ keratomileusis: prospective contralateral eye study. J Cataract Refract Surg 2005;31:120-6.
70. Alió JL, Piñero DP. Very high-frequency digital ultrasound measurement of the LASIK flap thickness profile using the IntraLase femtosecond laser and M2 and Carriazo-Pendular microkeratomes. J Refract Surg 2008;24:12-23.
71. Kezirian GM, Stonecipher KG. Comparison of the IntraLase femtosecond laser and mechanical keratomes for laser in situ keratomileusis. J Cataract Refract Surg 2004;30:804-11.
72. Tran DB, Sarayba MA, Bor Z, et al. IntraLase and Hansatome flap creation in fellow eyes: potential impact on wavefront-guided laser in situ keratomileusis. J Cataract Refract Surg 2005;31:97-105.
73. Montés-Micó R, Rodríguez-Galietero A, Alió JL, et al. Contrast sensitivity after LASIK flap creation with a femtosecond laser and a mechanical microkeratome. J Refract Surg 2007;23:188-92.
74. Durrie DS, Kezirian GM. Femtosecond laser versus mechanical keratome flaps in wavefront-guided laser in situ keratomileusis: prospective contralateral eye study. J Cataract Refract Surg 2005;31:120-6.
75. Kezirian GM, Stonecipher KG. Comparison of the IntraLase femtosecond laser and mechanical keratomes for laser in situ keratomileusis. J Cataract Refract Surg 2004;30:804-11.
76. Bara S, Mancebo T, Moreno-Barriuso E. Positioning tolerances for phase plates compensating aberrations of the human eye. Appl Opt 2000;39:3413-20.
77. Guirao A, Williams DR, Cox IG. Effect of rotation and translation on the expected benefit of an ideal method to correct the eye's higher-order aberrations. J Opt Soc Am A Opt Image Sci Vis 2001;18:1003-15.
78. Thibos LN, Applegate RA, Schwiegerling JT, et al. Report from the VSIA taskforce on standards for reporting optical aberrations of the eye; VSIA Standards Taskforce Members. J Refract Surg 2000;16:S654-S655.
79. Mrochen M, Eldine MS, Kaemmerer M, et al. Improvement in photorefractive corneal laser surgery results using an active eye-tracking system. J Cataract Refract Surg 2001;27:1000-6.
80. Walsh G. The effect of mydriasis on the pupillary centration of the human eye. Ophthalmic Physiol Opt 1988;8:178-82.
81. Wyatt HJ. The form of the human pupil. Vision Res 1995;35:2021-36.
82. Wilson MA, Campbell MCW, Simonet P. Change of pupil centration with change of illumination and pupil size; the Julius F. Neumueller Award in Optics. Optom Vis Sci 1992;69:129-36.
83. Ertan A, Kamburo?glu G. Analysis of centration of Intacs segments implanted with a femtosecond laser. J Cataract Refract Surg. 2007;33:484-7.
84. Durrie DS. SBK outcomes encouraging in prospective, contralateral eye-controlled study.[Accessed Apr 4 2008.http://www.escrs.org/PUBLICATIONS/EUROTIMES/07sept/SBKoutcomesencouraging.pdf]
85. Advanced surface ablation, sub-Bowman's keratomileusis equally safe, effective 6 months postop. Ophthalmology Times. Nov 9, 2007.[Accessed Apr 4 2008. http://www.ophthalmologytimes.com/ophthalmologytimes/2007+AAO+News/Advanced-surface-ablation-sub-Bowmans-keratomileus/ArticleStandard/Article/detail/471796?contextCategoryId=42078]
86. O'Brien TP. Handicapping the Future:PRK versus EpiLASIK? [Accessed Apr 4 2008. http://asacongress.com/presentations/Obrien_ASAfuture.pdf]
87. Trattler WB, Claringboldd T II,Krueger RR. Stromal divot. Cataract and Refractive Surgery Today 2007 Nov/Dec:45-47.[Accessed Apr 4 2008. http://www.crstoday.com /PDF%20Articles/1107/CRST1107_07.pdf]
88. Seider MI, Ide T, Kymionis GD, et al. Epithelial breakthrough: a complication during IntraLase flap creation for laser in situ keratomileusis. J Cataract Refract Surg (in press).
89. Mian SI, Shtein RM. Femtosecond laser-assisted corneal surgery. Curr Opin Ophthalmol 2007;18:295-9.
90. Cheng YY, Pels E, Nuijts RM. Femtosecond-laser-assisted Descemet's stripping endothelial keratoplasty.J Cataract Refract Surg 2007;33:152-5.
91. Koenig SB, Covert DJ.Early results of small-incision Descemet's stripping and automated endothelial keratoplasty.Ophthalmology 2007;114:221-6.
92. Price MO, Price FW Jr.Descemet's stripping with endothelial keratoplasty: comparative outcomes with microkeratome-dissected and manually dissected donor tissue. Ophthalmology 2006;113:1936-42.
93. Bahar I, Kaiserman I, Trope GE, et al. Non-penetrating deep sclerectomy for glaucoma surgery using the femtosecond laser: a laboratory model. Br J Ophthalmol 2007;91:1713-4.
94. Ngoi BK, Hou DX, Koh LH, et al. Femtosecond laser for glaucoma treatment: a study on ablation energy in pig iris. Lasers Med Sci 2005;19:218-22.
95. Toyran S, Liu Y, Singha S, et al. Femtosecond laser photodisruption of human trabecular meshwork: an in vitro study. Exp Eye Res 200;81:298-305.

28 Ziemer FEMTO LDV™ Femtosecond Laser

Gregg Feinerman, Richard Foulkes,
Timothy Peters, Kim Nguyen, Tammo Ripken

INTRODUCTION

The desire to offer patients an "All-laser LASIK" option has stimulated demand for femtosecond lasers. They offer the potential of extreme precision in the cutting of corneal tissue with extremely short laser pulses and minimizing the production of heat. For years, surgeons have reported favorable outcomes and patient satisfaction with femtosecond technology. However, the sheer bulk and inflexibility of most available femtosecond lasers, coupled with their complex operation and maintenance, have been obstacles to their widespread acceptance. For the first time, surgeons now have a choice of two different femtosecond laser platforms.

Ziemer's FEMTO LDV™ (Port, Switzerland) is the newest femtosecond laser for creating the corneal flap and it has several unique features, which we will discuss in detail (Fig. 28.1). The FEMTO LDV™ laser is a compact and mobile femtosecond surgical laser. It provides a powerful and versatile platform for a wide spectrum of applications in corneal surgery. The FEMTO LDV™ laser incorporates all the developments in femtosecond technology over the past decade. Of particular significance, the physics of this system are fundamentally different from other femtosecond lasers being produced.[1]

All femtosecond lasers use ultra short laser pulses to dissect corneal tissue. The interaction process for cutting is based on photodisruption. However, the femtosecond laser platforms accomplish photodisruption in significantly different ways. This chapter will give a brief overview of the main differences between current femtosecond technologies.

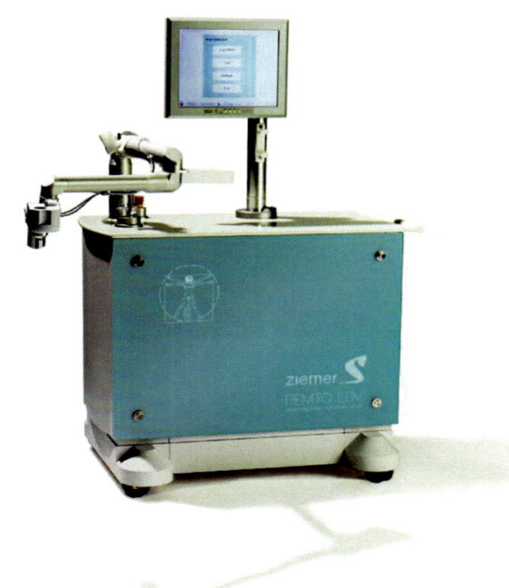

Fig. 28.1: Ziemer FEMTO LDV™

FEMTOSECOND LASER PHYSICS

Laser-Tissue Interaction

All femtosecond lasers accomplish the corneal lamellar dissection due to nonlinear absorption and consecutive disruption of the tissue followed by a cavitation bubble and a residual gas bubble. Nonlinear absorption means the tissue is transparent to the infrared laser radiation at moderate intensities and no absorption occurs.

Only at very high intensities, which can be achieved by compressing the laser pulse in time (ultra short) and in space (strong focussing), some photons can be absorbed co-instantaneously by the tissue. The narrowness of the region of photodisruption depends on the degree to which the beam is strongly focused and is never, in practice, a single point in z-axial space. However, nonlinear interaction gives the surgeon three-dimensional tissue processing. The absorption process is not limited to the surface anymore.[2-5]

While photodisruption scales with pulse intensity (W/cm^2), the unwanted side effects like thermal heating, stress and shockwaves, and large residual gas bubbles scale with pulse energy (J). Thus, it is better to minimize pulse energy while keeping the pulse intensity over the photodisruption threshold level (Fig. 28.2). Consequently, two important principles in creating the most precise lamellar cut are strong focussing and pulse shortening.

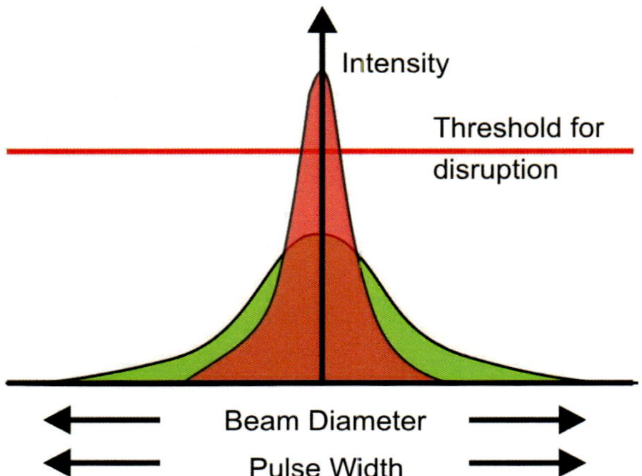

Fig. 28.2: *Threshold* for disruption scales with pulse *intensity* many, many photons on the same place, at the same time. *Unwanted* side effects (bubbles, collateral damage) scales with pulse *energy.* Photon energy is converted into heat, kinetics, and chemistry

Maximizing Cutting Precision: Achieved by Minimizing Energy

Shortening the pulse duration is related to the spectral bandwidth of the laser medium. The pulse duration of typical femtosecond laser systems is around 200 to 800 fs (1 fs = 10^{-15} sec). In this range the energy threshold for optical breakdown increases almost linearly with pulse duration. Thus, the shorter pulse duration of Ziemer's Femto LDV™ (approx. 250 fs) is related to a lower pulse energy threshold than the AMO's IntraLase® (approx. 600 fs).

Another way to decrease the energy is to decrease the focal volume of the laser spot. The focal volume of a Gaussian laser beam depends on the axial extension, the so-called Rayleigh range ($z = pw_0^2/l$) and the beam waist $w_0 = fl/pw_L$, where f is the focal length of the focusing lens, l the laser wavelength and w_L the radius of the beam at the focusing lens. **In other words, the focal volume varies inversely with the fourth power of the numerical aperture NA** = w_L/f of the focusing optics. **The larger NA the smaller is the focal spot and finally, the less pulse energy is needed to cause photodisruption** (Fig. 28.3).

There are two ways to increase the NA. The first is to increase the lens diameter (w); however, this requires large and expensive optical components. Another means of increasing the NA is to decrease

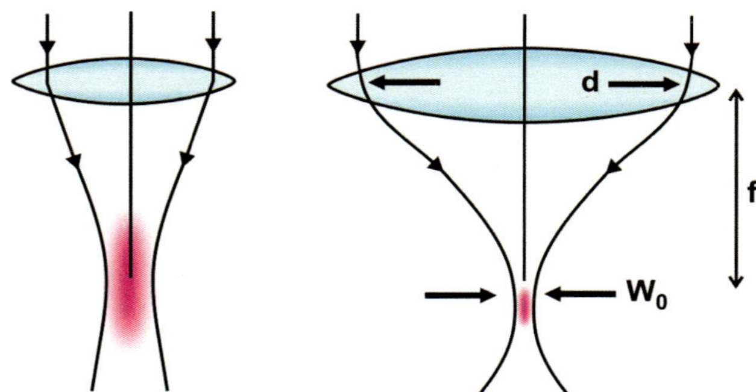

Fig. 28.3: The volume of the femtosecond laser spot scales with the numerical aperture **NA** = w_L/f of the focusing lens. The larger the NA, the smaller the focal spot. Two ways to increase the NA are increasing the lens diameter (IntraLase®, etc.) or decreasing the focal length (FEMTO LDV™)

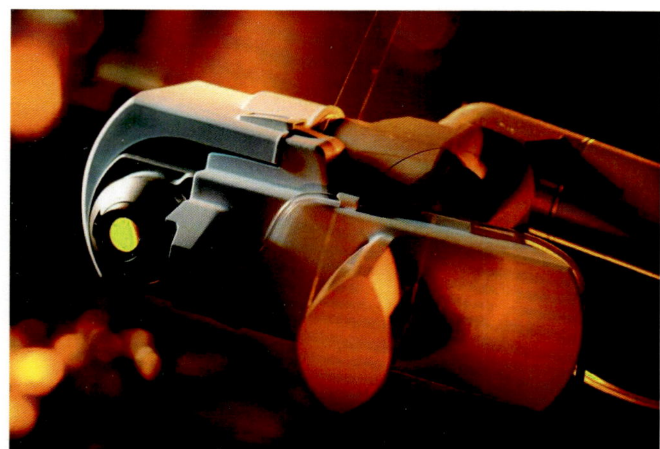

Fig. 28.4: The FEMTO LDV™ Handpiece brings the laser optics within 2 mm of the cornea. This significantly increases the numerical aperture

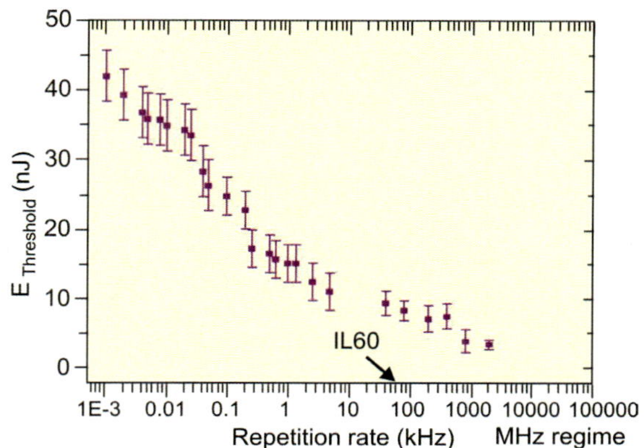

Fig. 28.5: The energy threshold in water decreases with increasing femtosecond laser frequency. The energy threshold for MHz lasers is about half of kHz lasers

the focal length of the focusing objective (f), which reduces the working distance of the laser system. The Ziemer's FEMTO LDV™ laser optics are located only 2 millimeters away from the corneal stroma. This focal length is much shorter than that of other lasers, leading to a tighter focal spot and less pulse energy. The shorter focal length results in a large **numerical aperture** and more accurately focused laser power (Fig. 28.4).

Additionally, the laser's laser frequency (repetition rate) has an important influence on the pulse energy threshold. The higher the laser frequency the less pulse energy is needed for cutting. Ziemer's Femto LDV™ uses a high repetition rate (MHz vs. kHz in other femtosecond laser platforms).

The Femto LDV repetition rate is on the order of magnitude faster than all other femtosecond platforms, which leads to the Femto LDV™ needing significantly lower pulse energy. Thus, it causes less thermal heating and less side effects (Fig. 28.5).

Groups of Femtosecond Lasers

Femtosecond surgical lasers can be classified into two groups:

1. High pulse energy with low pulse frequency
   - Amplified femtosecond laser systems, which are used to deliver pulse energies in the range of 1 μJ to the cornea.
   - The typical repetition rate is about some kHz (AMO IntraLase®, 20/10 Perfect Vision).
2. Low pulse energy with high pulse frequency
   - Consists *only* of the Ziemer FEMTO LDV™, which delivers lower (nJ) pulse energies to the eye.
   - FEMTO LDV™ uses faster (MHz) repetition rates.

Both of these differences are on the order of magnitude in size.

The cutting method is different for each group. Cutting is driven by mechanical forces in the "high pulse energy" laser group, which are applied by expanding bubbles that disrupt the tissue. The radius of the disrupted tissue is larger than the laser spot, which makes the cutting process very efficient. Thus, the spot separation of the scanned laser pulses can be larger than the spot diameter (Fig. 28.6A). However, the "high pulse energy – low pulse frequency" lasers have less focusing accuracy. The larger gas bubbles produced can lead to opaque bubble layer (OBL), rougher corneal stromal bed surfaces, transient light sensitivity (TLS) and occasional anterior chamber bubbles. OBL can cause delays in surgery while the surgeon waits for it to resolve, because the OBL blocks the excimer laser's eye tracking system.

Using low pulse energy, the cutting process is more accurately confined by the focal spot size of the

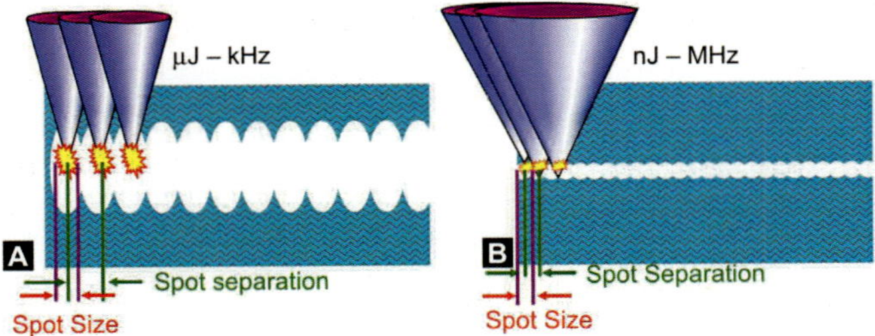

Figs 28.6A and B: Two different concepts in photodisruption process. For higher pulse energy / lower laser frequency lasers the cutting effect is driven predominantly by mechanical forces of the expanding cavitation bubble (A). Conversely, MHz laser frequencies (high frequency) can offer many more pulses that are needed for cutting using lower pulse energies and larger numerical aperture (B). Consequently, the size of the cut is defined solely by the focal spot size, not the expanding bubble

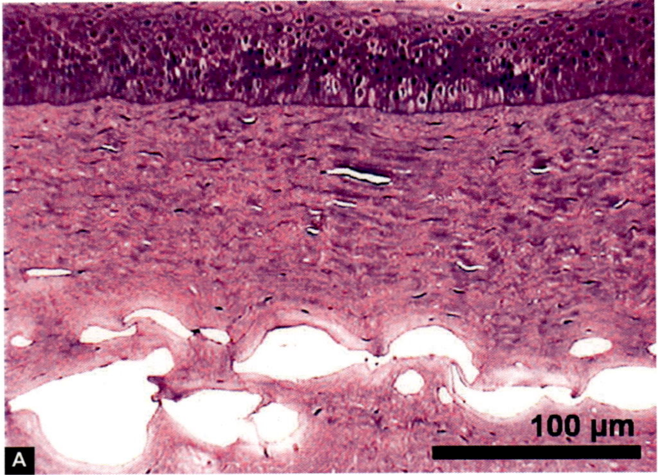

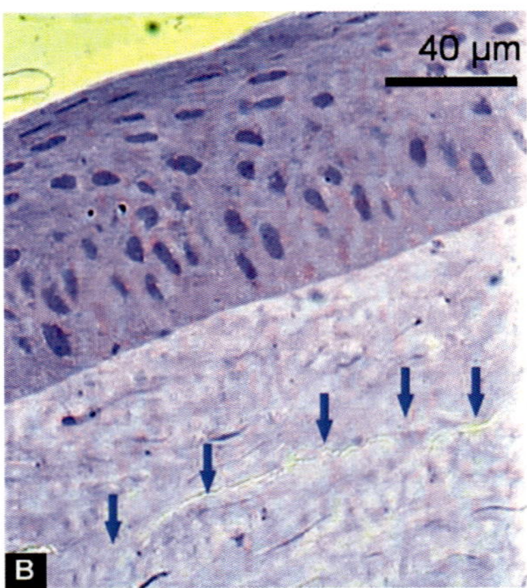

Figs 28.7A and B: Histological sections of porcine cornea cut with High Energy/Low Frequency (2 µJ pulse energy, 930 fs pulse width) (A) vs. Low Energy/Rapid Frequency (30 nJ, 250 fs) (B)

laser pulse. As a consequence, more pulses are needed to cut the same area. Higher repetition rates are used to keep the operation time at a reasonable level (Fig. 28.6B). Since the Ziemer FEMTO LDV™ uses a pure femtosecond laser oscillator (which can travel at the speed of sound), it delivers numerous pulses and is very stable and robust against environmental influences compared to amplified femtosecond lasers.

The clinical benefits of "low pulse energy – high frequency" are the absence of TLS, no OBL, and they never produce anterior chamber bubbles. Due to the very small amount of gas located precisely in the cutting plane, no gas pocket is needed and no waiting time has to be considered.

Figures 28.7A and B demonstrates the histological differences in both femtosecond laser groups. The histological photos demonstrate lamellar corneal dissections of porcine cornea. The corneas were cut with either a 2 µJ or 30 nJ pulse energy. These pictures illustrate the effect of high pulse energy with large disruptive bubbles compared to the low pulse energy laser with smaller spot sizes and smaller bubbles.

Consequently, the best method of femtosecond laser induced optical breakdown to cut corneal stromal tissue is with "low pulse energy – high frequency" laser (Ziemer's FEMTO LDV™). Additionally, the femtosecond laser oscillator makes the FEMTO LDV™ compact and robust because it delivers low pulse energy at high frequencies. The FEMTO LDV™ has unparalleled preciseness due to the high focussing optics located only 2 mm from the treated corneal stroma, giving it the highest numerical aperture. The low energy pulses reduce bubble formation during the cutting process.[6] The smaller the bubbles, the more precise the cut can be positioned. This makes the FEMTO LDV™ the best laser for sub-Bowman Keratomileusis (SBK).

Short pulse duration, fast repetition rate and more accurately focused power are key attributes that allow Ziemer's FEMTO LDV™ to achieve tissue disruption at an energy level in the low ***nanojoule*** range, a level far lower than other currently available femtosecond lasers that operate in the ***microjoule*** range, such as the IntraLase® FS, Ziess or 20/10 lasers. Lasers such as IntraLase® work by amplifying infrared light to achieve the desired tissue disruption effect. Instead, Ziemer's FEMTO LDV™ delivers tightly spaced, smaller spots of shorter duration at a much faster rate. The spots are less than 2 µm; pulse duration is 200-300 femtoseconds; and the repetition rate is faster than 1 megahertz (Table 28.1).

Ziemer's FEMTO LDV™ unique technological characteristics allow surgeons to create large, cleanly dissected, easily lifted flaps with a smooth treatment surface. Additionally, the laser's small footprint and portability make it space and cost efficient. It is possible for the laser to be placed in a relatively small laser operating room alongside the excimer laser. Thus, patients can have their All-laser LASIK procedure performed on the same operating bed. The Ziemer laser can easily be shared among multiple laser centers. Ziemer made the FEMTO LDV™ portable and smaller by eliminating the complex and sensitive laser amplification seen on other femtosecond lasers. All of these characteristics translate into benefits for our patients.

CLINICAL BENEFITS OF THE ZIEMER FEMTO LDV™

No Tissue Disorganization

Lower pulse energy and more precise focusing of the laser power mean a high percentage of the applied

Table 28.1: Comparison of femtosecond lasers

	THE NEW SHAPE OF VISION INTRALASE CORP	ziemer	FEMTEC®	ZEISS VisuMax
Type of FS	Amplified	Non-Amplified	Amplified	Amplified
Pulse width	> 600 femtosec	250 femtosec	> 500 femtosec	400 femtosec
Spot size	> 1 µm	< 1 µm	> 1 µm	1 µm
Repetition rate	60 kHz	> 1 MHz	40 kHz	120 kHz
Pulse energy	1 µJ	nJ	> 1 µJ	< 1 µJ
Laser time (9.5 mm flap)	30 sec	30 sec	1 min	< 40 sec
Surface quality	Good	Excellent	Good	Good
Centration after suction	Yes; but smaller diameter flap if re-center	No	No	Yes
Hinge position	N,S,T,I	N,S,T,I	?	?
Numerical aperture	0.2	> 0.4	0.2	0.5
Focus predictability	Fair	Excellent	Fair	Good
Interface bubbles	++++++	+	++++++	?
Bubbles in anterior chamber	Occasionally	No	Occasionally	?
Suction press (mm Hg)	> 70	< 50	> 70	< 40
Mobility	No	Yes	No	No

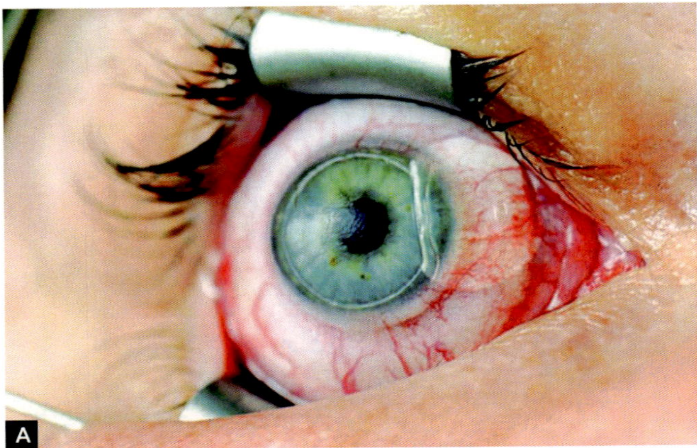

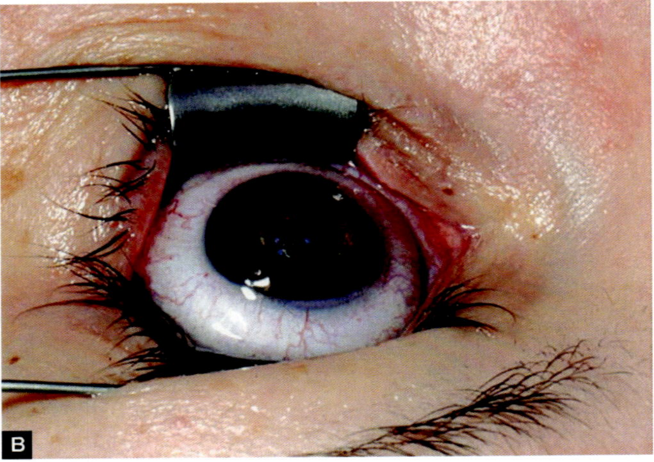

Figs 28.8A and B: Smooth stromal bed created with FEMTO LDV™ complete dissection of the stromal bed leads to easy lift of flap with forceps

energy goes into tissue disruption. Thermal side effects in neighboring tissue are minimized. Thermal zones that could prompt inflammation do not form in the corneal tissue.

No "Tissue Bridges"

Since the laser spots overlap, they result in complete dissection of the stromal bed. The resulting corneal stromal bed is smoother and the flap can be easily lifted with forceps alone (Figs 28.8A and B). In contrast, IntraLase® and other microjoule femtosecond lasers generate larger spots in the corneal tissue. The spots are separated and not overlapping in order to avoid unacceptably high energy levels. A large cavitation bubble must complete the dissection and no tissue disruption occurs in areas between spots. These areas manifest as tissue bridges that can make lifting the flap very difficult due to adherence. This is made more difficult when the cavitation bubbles make their way down from the dissection plane.

No Opaque Bubble Layer (OBL)

OBL can block the excimer laser system's eye tracker and also make's lifting the flap a challenge. It can be thought of as inflation of the corneal stroma. The lower energy produced by the Ziemer FEMTO LDV™ (nanojoule) eliminates the OBL created by high-energy (microjoule) femtosecond lasers. Ziemer's FEMTO LDV™ generates some microscopic bubbles, but they occur only in the interface liquid and not in the tissue. They dissipate immediately upon lifting the flap, or within a couple of minutes if the flap is not lifted. Consequently, if the surgeon wants to make another lamellar flap (deeper, thinner or at the same depth), it can be done within a minute or two after the first Ziemer femtosecond flap is made. A second pass can be done immediately, because there is no cavitation pressure seen in the high-energy approach.

The high-energy (microjoule) laser cavitation unavoidably and randomly produces zones of gas bubbles above and below the ablation plane, sometimes reaching into the anterior chamber. This can obscure the patient's pupil and interfere with the excimer laser's eye tracker. Furthermore, corneal tissue inflated with gas does not ablate at the same rate as corneal tissue without gas (unpublished data). The result is less accurate transfer of the excimer ablation pattern. Because part of the mechanism of dissection for microjoule femtosecond lasers assumes inflation of the lamellar plane in areas of OBL the lift can be very difficult, putting stress on the flap and epithelium above the area. Type II microstriae (Bowman's cracks) and epithelial slide can frequently occur. Visual recovery is delayed when this occurs within the optical axis.

Ziemer FEMTO LDV™: Improved Accuracy and Smoother Stromal Bed

In contrast to microjoule cavitation events, which can be thought of as explosive (like the YAG laser), Ziemer's FEMTO LDV™ produces a uniform rising wave of energy. To handle its extremely fast pulse rate (several MHz), the Ziemer FEMTO LDV™ laser beam is scanned across the cornea in a two-step process. A fast scan rapidly sweeps the beam left and right, creating a trace of spots that is a few tenths of a millimeter wide. This swept beam is then moved in a perpendicular direction across the intended diameter of the flap. This pattern combined with the laser's low energy level results in a less traumatic flap-making procedure, yet extremely effective in creating total dissection without inciting the inflammation or TLS (transient light sensitivity) reportedly seen in 11.7% of patients treated with IntraLase®.[7]

Ziemer's FEMTO LDV™ dissects the stroma more precisely and accurately than any other femtosecond laser in its class. This translates into better post-LASIK vision for our patients because it provides a planar treatment surface for the excimer laser, without OBL or tissue bridges. The glassy-smooth and uniform treatment surface allows for a more accurate excimer ablation[8] (Fig. 28.9).

Since Ziemer's FEMTO LDV™ is different than other femtosecond lasers, and using it to create the flap for LASIK followed by excimer laser ablation has been given its own name: "Z-LASIK". Z-LASIK connotes the improved micronal accuracy in the z-axis that is delivered by the excimer laser onto this improved treatment surface.

Z-LASIK also allows the surgeon to maintain a dry treatment surface, which further increases its uniformity. Because the flap is so easily lifted, tear film is not pulled up onto the eye. When a mechanical microkeratome is used, water often comes around the back of the blade where it is immediately absorbed into the corneal stroma. When water is absorbed into the stroma, it slows the ablation. With microjoule femtosecond lasers the manipulation sometimes required to lift the flap often leads to water contamination as well as flap trauma.

The safety and predictability of LASIK is also somewhat dependent on the predictability of flap thickness. Large variability in thickness can lead to variable uptake of the excimer and loss of accuracy. The flap thickness is precisely controlled by the FEMTO LDV™ InterShield spacers, which are assembled on the laser's handpiece along with a suction ring. The spacers are accurate within one

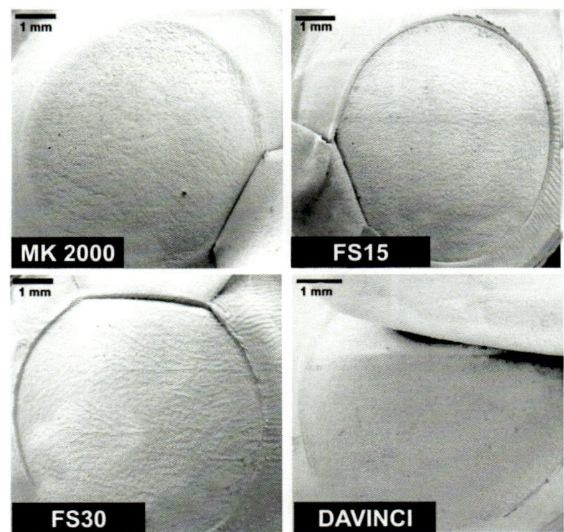

Surface roughness of the stromal bed was measured with a confocal microscope on ten eyes, each in several selected positions. In the table, the mean (± SD) of all measurements for each device is listed (left columns). In the rightmost column, the mean of the smoothest individual area found for each eye is provided.

Surface Roughness	All surface areas	Smoothest surface area per eye
Nidek MK2000	2.8 ± 1.5 μm	1.1 ± 1.1 μm
IntraLase FS15	3.1 ± 0.7 μm	2.1 ± 0.6 μm
IntraLase FS30	2.8 ± 0.6 μm	1.9 ± 0.4 μm
DAVINCI	3.0 ± 0.3 μm	2.0 ± 0.4 μm

Comparison of various femtosecond lasers and conventional microkeratomes for corneal lamellar cuts. *(Ripken T, Bernau W, Oberheide U, Schumacher S, Knorz M, Kermani O, Lubatschowski. Poster presented at the 19th Congress of German Ophthalmic Surgeons (DOC) Nuremberg, Germany, May 25-28, 2006)*

Fig. 28.9: Analysis of surface roughness.

micron. The Ziemer laser's unshielded focal distance is calibrated to 250 μm. Spacers allow surgeons to accurately adjust intended flap thickness by bringing femtosecond laser's focal plane up toward the surface. Thus, a 140 μm thick spacer is used to create a 110 μm corneal flap (250 μm – 140 μm = 110 μm). A 90 μm flap results from a 160 μm spacer. Although the Ziemer laser currently uses Amadeus rings and separate spacers, the transition to disposable rings with built in spacers will occur in 2008. This will further reduce the need for non-disposable instruments and make setup even more efficient.

Early in the release phase of the FEMTO LDV™, Pajic and colleagues concluded that the FEMTO LDV™ produces corneal flaps of a highly predictable quality.[9] Since then, the company has made the FEMTO LDV™ even more precise. In our experience so far using subtraction pachymetry, we are finding a standard deviation in flap thickness of less than 6 μm, much better than with microjoule femtosecond lasers. Our Visante OCT measurements demonstrate even better accuracy, typically within a few microns of the intended depth.

Ziemer's FEMTO LDV™ produces a flap edge at the angle of the cornea as it is released from the applanation plate. This creates an angle of approximately 140 degrees, which has been shown by Dr. John Marshall to cause the least amount of biomechanical weakening.[10] Additionally, since the flap gutter is much narrower with the Ziemer laser, it does not collect blood, mucous, or debris. This reduces the chances of inflammation, infection or sight-threatening conditions such as diffuse lamellar keratitis. Postoperatively, the flap edge is invisible on slit-lamp examination, which is similar to the edge created by a mechanical microkeratome. This is in contrast to flaps made with the IntraLase® laser where the gap commonly fills with fibrocytic epitheloid cells, leaving a characteristic scar around the rim.

Furthermore, centration is less of an issue with Ziemer's FEMTO LDV™. Flap size can be predicted within 0.5 mm by using the average K reading.[11] The surgeon can choose a suction ring size ranging from 8.5 to 11 mm. The programmable, microprocessor-controlled vacuum allows accurate suction and surgeon can view the handpiece assembly directly over the pupil to capture it centrally. We have studied pressure settings and found they do not influence flap thickness or size. Currently, we set the laser suction to 650 millibars of pressure. This level allows for predictable flaps while minimizing patient discomfort and complaints compared with the leur lock/ weighted applanation plate system of the IntraLase®.

Unparalleled Ergonomics and Efficiency

The advanced technology behind Ziemer's FEMTO LDV™ provides both clinical and logistical benefits. The Ziemer laser is compact and mobile because it does not require amplification of the cavity energy, which makes other femtosecond lasers bulky and less stable. Ziemer's FEMTO LDV™ can be moved between rooms on its own wheels and does not require a tightly controlled environment. It can even be transported in a van, completely assembled.

Ziemer's FEMTO LDV™ is usually positioned right beside the excimer laser. The surgeon can use the excimer laser's operating microscope (or any other microscope) to create the corneal flap. The femtosecond laser beam is delivered via an ergometric handpiece, which floats onto the eye via an attached articulated arm (Fig. 28.10). The arm extends over the

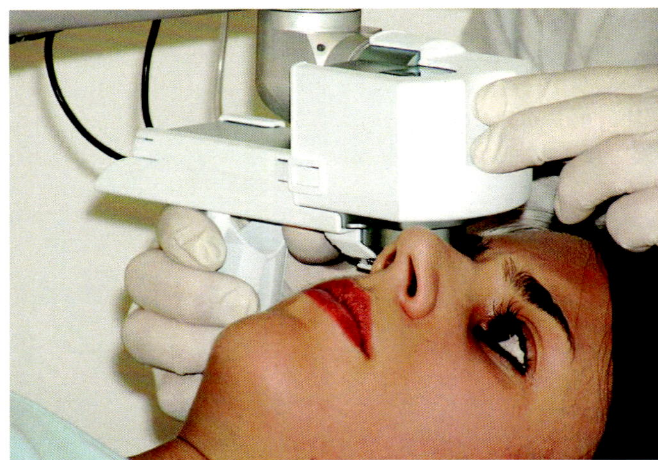

Fig. 28.10: Ziemer's ergonomic handpiece

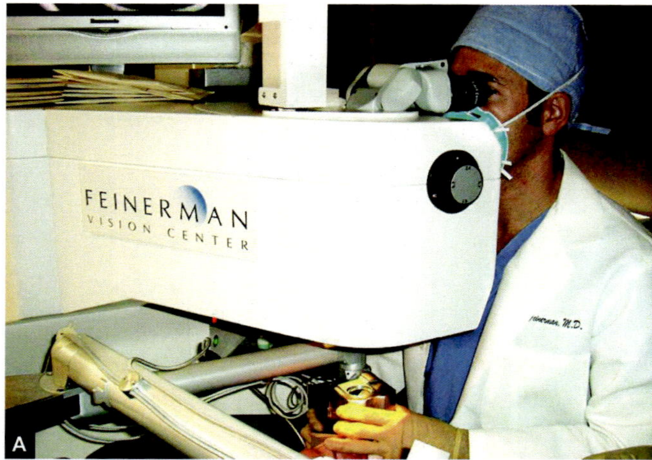

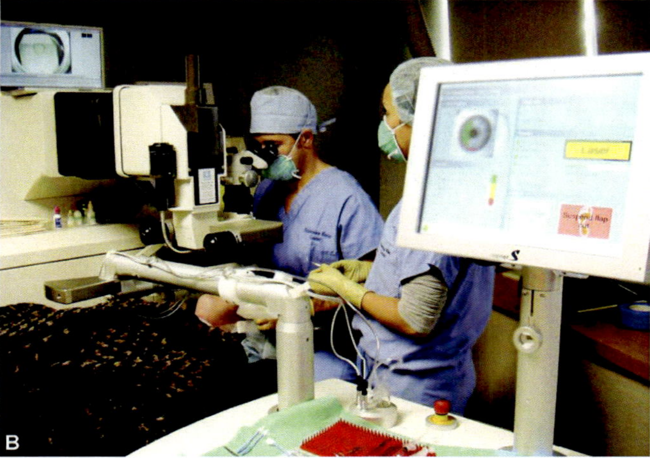

Figs 28.11A and B: FEMTO LDV™ Fits easily under any excimer laser and can be easily rolled between lasers

patient's chest and under the excimer laser's bridge. The surgeon can easily rotate the handpiece 180 degrees to deliver it to the right or left eye. Another significant advantage of the handpiece is its 2 mm focal distance, which increases the laser's numerical aperture.

The entire All-laser LASIK procedure can easily be performed using the Ziemer laser without requiring patients to be transferred between workstations. In fact, the workflow feels familiar for surgeons who previously used a mechanical microkeratome. This cuts down the total treatment time significantly compared to the IntraLase®, which usually must be placed in another room. That scenario leads to double use of anesthetic, additional surgical drapes/disposables, and often more complaints of discomfort. Using Ziemer's FEMTO LDV™ —with the ergometric handpiece and without OBL—the surgeon can remain seated behind the excimer laser. In practices that use more than one excimer laser, the FEMTO LDV™ can be rolled between them. In an ASC or hospital setting the laser can be rolled to the OT for lamellar procedures.

Ziemer's FEMTO LDV™ increases surgical efficiency in many ways. As previously discussed, the few microscopic bubbles formed by the creation of the flap dissipate as soon as the flap is lifted. Thus, the excimer laser ablation can be initiated immediately after completion of the flap, which significantly reduces total procedure time. The lack of OBL also shortens the procedure time and improves accuracy. Furthermore, system startup time is significantly less than with other femtosecond lasers. The FEMTO LDV™ can be cold-started in less than 10 minutes. With a warm start, it is ready to create a flap in less than two minutes. Startup time is less than ten minutes even if laser is transported to another location (Fig. 28.11A and B).

The time it takes to create a flap is approximately 30 seconds. Coupling the device to the patient is accomplished quickly and easily. A sterile handpiece casing, an InterShield spacer for controlling flap thickness, and a suction ring are used to prevent contamination and to change from one patient to the next quickly. These sterile, single-use parts are supplied in procedure packs, which contain all parts required for a bilateral procedure. The cost per pack is significantly less than IntraLase®.

As mentioned previously, the Ziemer laser's suction is microprocessor-controlled. This computer control, along with optimized suction ring geometry, makes suction loss extremely unlikely. Furthermore, if suction is lost during the procedure, the femtosecond procedure can be repeated immediately (as long as the flap is not lifted prior to the second cut). Small patient head movements are also not a concern regarding suction loss. The Ziemer laser treatment is much more controlled than with other femtosecond laser systems, which improves FEMTO LDV™ efficiency. Suction is released automatically after the flap is made. Then the flap edge is gently identified with an edge instrument. The flap is lifted easily with forceps, and the excimer laser treatment can begin immediately.

Efficiency and Benefits of Ziemer FEMTO LDV™

When we consider all of the features and benefits of Ziemer's FEMTO LDV™, it is clear that it provides refractive surgeons with the benefits of mechanical microkeratomes (efficiency, controlled suction, large flaps, and effortless lifting of the flap).[12] Ziemer's laser also provides the benefits of femtosecond technology (accuracy, reproducibility, bladeless, dry and uniform bed surface).

A spacer is currently being released to allow creation of a 90 μm flap for sub-Bowman Keratomileusis (SBK). John Marshall, PhD has referred to SBK as the ultimate flap because it provides the best of both worlds.[13] It allows for the benefits of PRK (maintaining structural integrity of the cornea) with the benefits of LASIK (reducing haze and rapid recovery).

The future use of the FEMTO LDV™ in anterior segment treatments is especially promising. A new handpiece will be released in 2008 for performing a wide variety of corneal procedures, including therapeutic keratoplasty and creation of tunnels for intrastromal rings and insertion of corneal inlays. This head, which currently works at 430 μm, creates glassy-smooth surfaces in stark contrast to the extremely rough surfaces resulting from tissue bridges with microjoule lasers. This allows for insertion of rings and inlays without corneal stromal resistance.

Because the laser does not rely on gas cavitation for tissue dissection, planes of dissection can be immediately placed on top of each other then separated. The tight energy focus means less energy effect from the treatment when compared to microjoule femtosecond lasers, which have been implicated in endothelial cell loss from their long focal length (centimeters). We are continuing to study these additional uses of the FEMTO LDV™ and hope to report on its ability to safely work on top of Descemet's membrane without causing significant cell loss. The development of a computer adjusted z-axis handpiece for the laser is also in development and will further complement the advancements already provided by the Ziemer FEMTO LDV™.

SUMMARY

Based on our experience, the Ziemer laser is a unique advancement in femtosecond technology. Ziemer's FEMTO LDV™ technological improvements will undoubtedly emerge as the best use of femtosecond energy for lamellar dissection procedures.

REFERENCES

1. Vryghem JC, Stodulka P. Flap making in LASIK with the Da Vinci femtosecond laser. April 2007. Paper No. 298778, ASCRS, San Diego, CA, USA.
2. Heisterkamp A, Ripken T, Mamom T, Drommer W, Welling H, Ertmer W, et al. Nonlinear side effects of fs-pulses inside corneal tissue during photodisruption; Appl Phys 2002;B 74:1-7.
3. Lubatschowski H, Maatz G, Heisterkamp, Hetzel U, Drommer W, Welling H, Ertmer W. Application of ultrashort laser pulses for intrastromal refractive surgery. Graefe's Arch Clin Exp Ophthal 2000;238:33-9.
4. Noack J, Vogel A. Laser-Induced Plasma Formation in Water at Nanosecond to Femtosecond Time Scales: Calculation of Thresholds, Absorption Coefficients, and Energy Density. IEEE J. Quantum Electron 1999;35(8): 1156.
5. Vogel A, Noack J. Mechanism of femtosecond laser nanosurgery of cells and tissue. Appl Phys B 2005;81(8):1015.
6. Nguyen C, Pournaras J-AC, Stillitano I, et al. Bubbles disappearing time after LASIK flap creation with the Da Vinci femtolaser device. May 2007. Program 5344/Poster B590, ARVO, Ft. Lauderdale, FL, USA.
7. Krueger R, Thornton I, Van den Berg T. Rainbow glare as an optical side effect of IntraLASIK. Presented at the ASCRS, March 2006, San Francisco, CA.
8. Titzé P, Majo F, Othenin-Girard P. LASIK flap quality study with a new femtolaser on a live human cornea. May 2006. Paper No. 4332, ARVO, Ft. Lauderdale, FL, USA.
9. Pajic B, Boehnke M. *In vivo* performance of a femtosecond surgical laser: first prospective clinical study. April 2007. Paper No. 299626, ASCRS, San Diego, CA, USA.

10. Marshall J. Better Insight of Cornea Ushers in New Generation of Corneal Refractive Surgery. Ocular Surgery News U.S. Edition; January 2008. Slack Publication.
11. Stillitano IG, Nguyen C, Schor P. Flap dimensions and cutting quality of the "Da Vinci" femtosecond laser flap. May 2007. Program 5335/Poster B581, ARVO, Ft. Lauderdale, FL, USA.
12. Ripken T, Bernau W, Oberheide U, et al. Comparison of various femtosecond lasers and conventional microkeratomes for corneal lamellar cuts. May 2006. Poster, 19th Congress of German Ophthalmic Surgeons, Nuremberg, Germany.
13. Marshall J. Wound healing and biomechanics of corneal flap creation. Paper presented at: the XXIV Congress of the ESCRS; September 2006; London, England.

29 Presbyopic LASIK

Amar Agarwal, Athiya Agarwal, Guillermo Avalos

INTRODUCTION

Presbyopia, is the final frontier for an ophthalmologist. In the 21st century the latest developments, which are taking place, are in the field of Presbyopia. In presbyopia, the nearest point that can be focused gradually recedes, leading to the need for optical prosthesis for close work such as reading and eventually even for focus in the middle distance.

PREVIOUS EXCIMER LASER TECHNIQUES

Presbyopic Photorefractive keratectomy (PRK) has been tried. In this using the excimer laser, a mask consisting of a mobile diaphragm formed by two blunt blades was used to ablate a 10-17 micron deep semilunar-shaped zone immediately below the pupillary center, steepening the corneal curvature in that area.

Monofocal vision with LASIK has also been tried to solve the problem of presbyopia. The goal in such cases is to make the patient anisometropic. In this one eye is used for distance vision and the other for near vision. This is obviously not indicated in all subjects. The residual consequences are partial loss of stereopsis, asthenopia, headache, aniseikonia and decreased binocularity.

HISTORY

Guillermo Avalos[1,2] started the idea of Presbyopic LASIK. This is called the PARM technique. He held a live surgical conference in Mexico where he had invited the Agarwals to perform Phakonit and the no-anesthesia cataract surgery technique. There he discussed with them the idea of Presbyopic LASIK and when they came back they started the technique.

PRINCIPLE

The objective is to allow the patient to focus on near objects while retaining his ability to focus on far objects, taking into account the refractive error of the eye when the treatment is performed. With this LASIK technique the corneal curvature is modified, creating a bilateral multifocal cornea in the treated optical zone. A combination of hyperopic and myopic LASIK is done aiming to make a multifocal cornea. We determine if the eye is Presbyopic plano, presbyopic with spherical hyperopia or presbyopia with spherical myopia. These may also have astigmatism in which case the astigmatism is treated at the same time.

PROLATE AND OBLATE CORNEA

It is important for us to understand a prolate and oblate cornea before we progress further on the technique of Presbyopic LASIK. The shape of spheroid (a conoidal surface of revolution) is qualitatively prolate or oblate, depending on whether it is stretched or flattened in its axial dimension. In a prolate cornea the meridional curvature decreases from pole to equator and in an oblate cornea the meridional curvature continually increases. The optical surfaces of the normal human eye both cornea and lens are prolate. This shape has an optical advantage in that spherical aberration can be avoided. Following LASIK the prolateness of the anterior cornea reduces but is insufficient to eliminate its spherical aberration. Thus one should remember the normal cornea is prolate. When myopic LASIK is done the cornea becomes oblate. When hyperopic LASIK is done the cornea becomes prolate.

Every patient treated with an excimer laser is left with an oblate or prolate shaped cornea depending upon the myopia or hyperopia of the patient. The approach to improve visual quality after LASIK is to apply geometric optics and use the patient's refraction, precise preoperative corneal height data and optimal postoperative anterior corneal shape in order to have a customized prolate shape treatment.

TECHNIQUE

First of all a superficial corneal flap is created with the microkeratome. The corneal flap performed with the microkeratome must be between 8.5 to 9.5 mm in order to have an available corneal surface for treatment of at least 8 mm. In this way, the laser beam does not touch the hinge of the flap. In India the Bausch and Lomb Lasik machine is used and in Mexico the Apollo machine is used. Once the flap has been created a hyperopic ablation in an optical zone of 5 mm is done (Fig. 29.1). The treated cornea now has a steepness section. The cornea is thus myopic, prolate. This allows the eye to focus in a range that includes near vision but excludes far vision.

With this myopic-shaped cornea, one now selects a smaller area of the central cornea that is concentric with the previous worked area. The size of the area is a 4 mm optical zone. A myopic LASIK is now done with the 4 mm optical zone (Fig. 29.2). The resulting cornea now has a central area (oblate) that is configured for the eye to focus on far objects and a ring shaped area that allows the eye to focus on near objects (Fig. 29.3). The flap is now cleaned and replaced back in position.

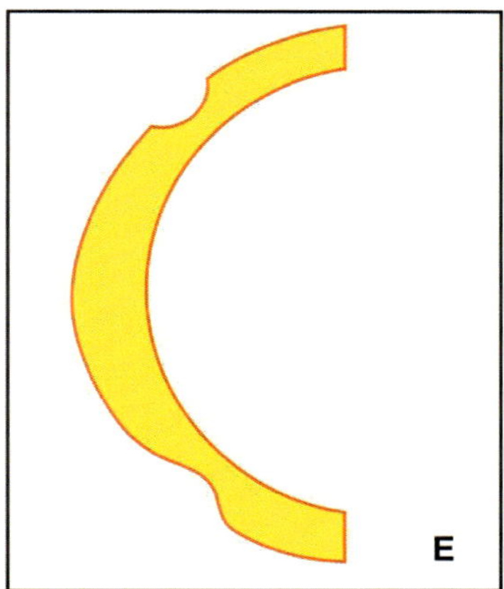

Fig. 29.1: Hyperopic lasik done on the cornea. Myopic prolate cornea produced

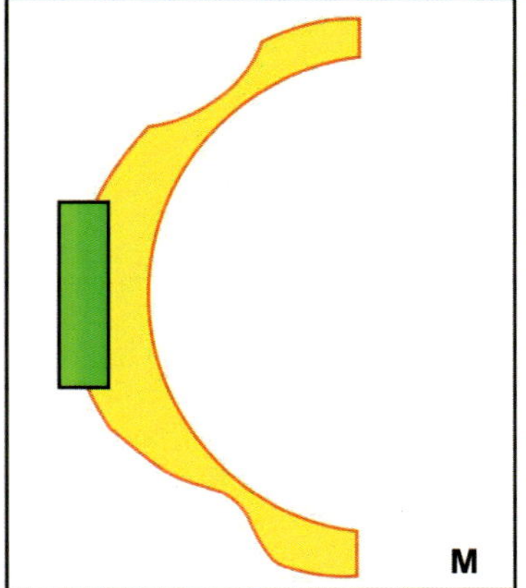

Fig. 29.2: Myopic lasik done. Myopic ablation of 4 mm optical zone performed to create a central oblate cornea

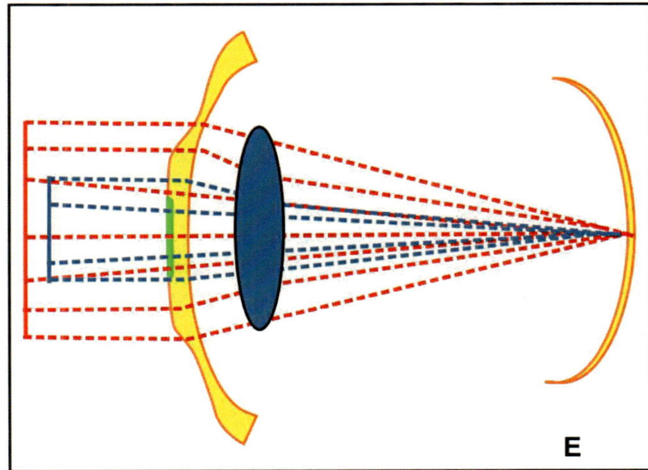

Fig. 29.3: Schematic diagram of a presbyopic cornea in which hyperopic and myopic lasik has been done. The patient can thus focus for near and distance

KERATOMETRY AND PACHYMETRY

Pachymetry is not important for this procedure. The preoperative keratometry reading is extremely important. The postoperative keratometer reading should not exceed 48 D. The keratometer reading should be taken from topography and not from a manual keratometer machine. For each hypermetropic diopter corrected, the corneal curvature increases in 0.89 keratometric diopters as an average. It is recommended to treat patients with keratometry in the range between 41 to 43 D to obtain postoperative curves under 48 D. If the cornea is more than 48 D, it produces undesired optical alterations like glare, halos, decreased visual acuity and decreased contrast sensitivity. The preoperative and postoperative keratometer readings should be nearly the same for the patient to be comfortable.

ASTIGMATISM

If astigmatism is present, it is recommended to use as a limit 2.5 D. One should also remember there is an induced astigmatism of 0.5 to 0.75 D created by the corneal shape after the surgery and this can decrease one or two lines of uncorrected visual acuity.

PLANO EXAMPLES

Now let us look at treating presbyopic patients who are basically plano for distance.

Example 1

Let us take a patient who is plano for distance and is 20/20. For near on addition of + 2 D the patient is J1. The preoperative keratometer let us say is 41 D.

There are three steps in the presbyopic LASIK treatment.

1 step For distance- No treatment is required as the patient is plano 20/20.

2 step For near- Hyperopic LASIK is done of + 2 D. A 5 mm optical zone is taken. We have already mentioned that each diopter of hyperopia corrected changes the corneal curvature by 0.89 D, which is approximately 1 D. So the keratometer changes from 41 to 43 D (approximately).

3 step Myopic LASIK of minus 1 D with a 4 mm optical zone. So keratometer now becomes 42 D.

Regression occurs for hyperopia treatment to about 1 D, so we have done myopic ablation of minus 1 and not minus 2 D. The preoperative keratometer reading was 41 D and postoperative keratometer reading is 42 D, which is nearly the same.

HYPEROPIC EXAMPLES

Now let us look at presbyopic LASIK being performed in a hyperopic eye.

Example 2

Let us take a patient who is hyperopic for distance and is 20/20 with + 1 D. For near on addition of + 3 D the patient is J1. The preoperative keratometer let us say is 42 D.

There are three steps in the presbyopic LASIK treatment.

1 step For distance- Hyperopic LASIK is done of + 1 D with a 5 mm optical zone. So keratometer changes from 42 D to 43 D.

2 step For near- Hyperopic LASIK is done of + 3 D. A 5 mm optical zone is taken. We have already mentioned that each diopter of hyperopia corrected changes the corneal curvature by 0.89 D, which is approximately 1 D. So the keratometer changes from 43 to 46 D (approximately).

3 step Myopic LASIK of minus 2 D with a 4 mm optical zone. So keratometer now becomes 44 D.

Regression occurs for hyperopia treatment to about 1 D, so we have done myopic ablation of minus 2 and not minus 3 D. The preoperative keratometer reading was 42 D but after making the patient plano it is 43 D. The postoperative keratometer reading is 44 D, which is nearly the same.

Though we have to correct totally 4 D for hypermetropia we take it in two steps. One should not do it in one step as that much hyperopia corrected in one step makes the central cornea too steep to perform the myopic ablation.

Example 3

Let us take a patient who is hyperopic for distance and is 20/20 with + 3 D. For near on addition of + 3 D the patient is J1. The preoperative keratometer let us say is 44 D.

The preoperative keratometer reading is 44 D and we have to correct 3 D for distance and 3 D for near. So if we do presbyopic LASIK we will make the keratometer reading 50 D. So, one should not treat such patients with presbyopic LASIK.

MYOPIC EXAMPLE

Now let us look at myopic patients.

Example 4

Let us take a patient who is myopic for distance and is 20/20 with minus 2 D. For near on addition of + 2 D the patient is J1. This means the patient is plano for near. The preoperative keratometer let us say is 43 D.

There are three steps in the presbyopic LASIK treatment.

1 step For distance—Patient is myopic so no treatment is required.

2 step For near- Hyperopic LASIK is done of + 2 D. A 5 mm optical zone is taken. We have already mentioned that each diopter of hyperopia corrected changes the corneal curvature by 0.89 D, which is approximately 1 D. So the keratometer changes from 43 to 45 D (approximately).

3 step Myopic LASIK of minus 3 D with a 4 mm optical zone. So keratometer now becomes 42 D.

Regression occurs for hyperopia treatment to about 1 D, so we have done myopic ablation of minus 3 and not minus 4 D. The preoperative keratometer reading was 43 D but patient was myopic by 2 D, so actually the keratometer reading should be 41 D. The

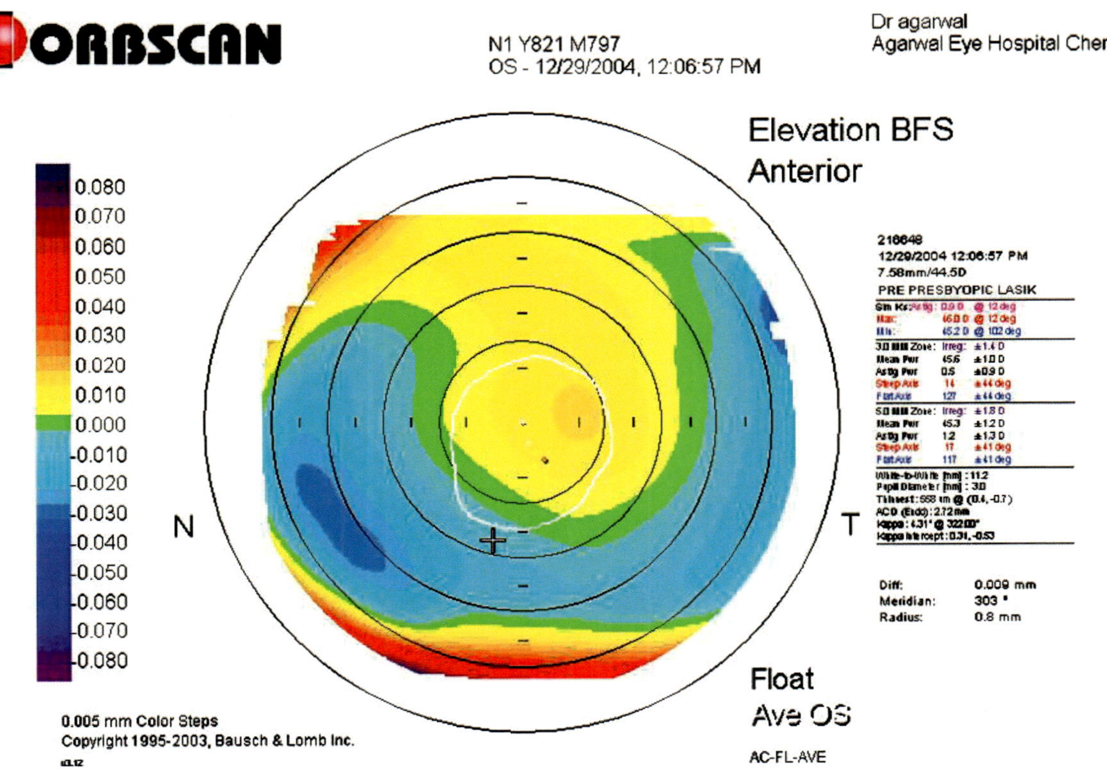

Fig. 29.4: Preoperative topography of a patient before presbyopic LASIK

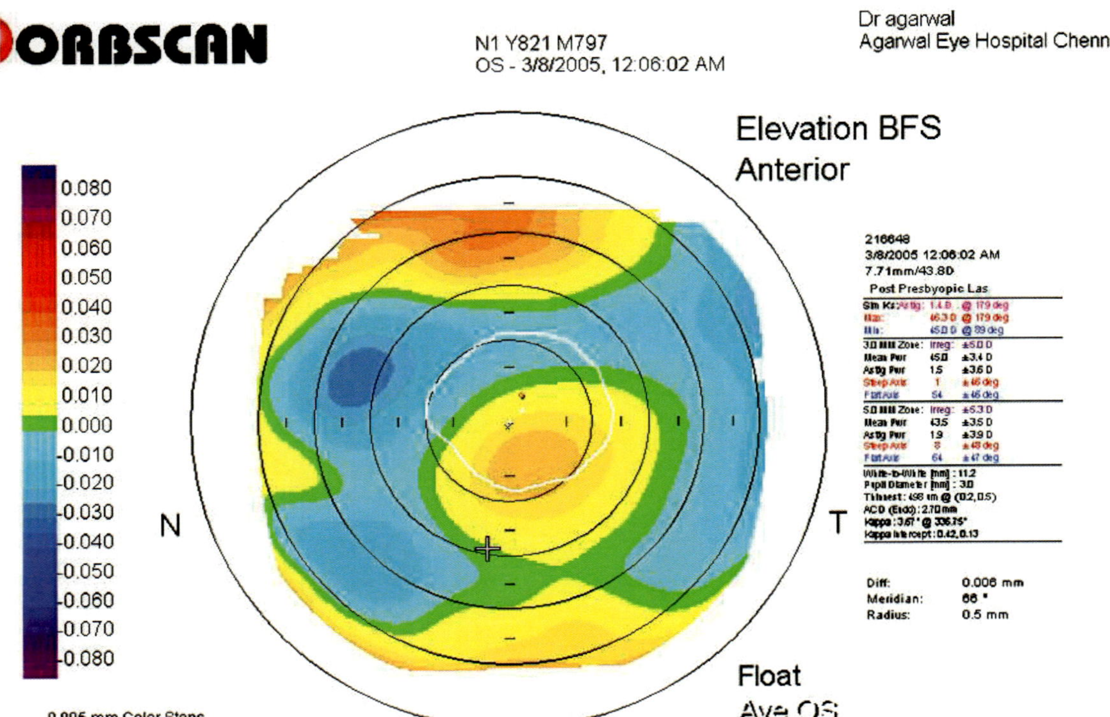

Fig. 29.5: postoperative topography of a patient after presbyopic LASIK

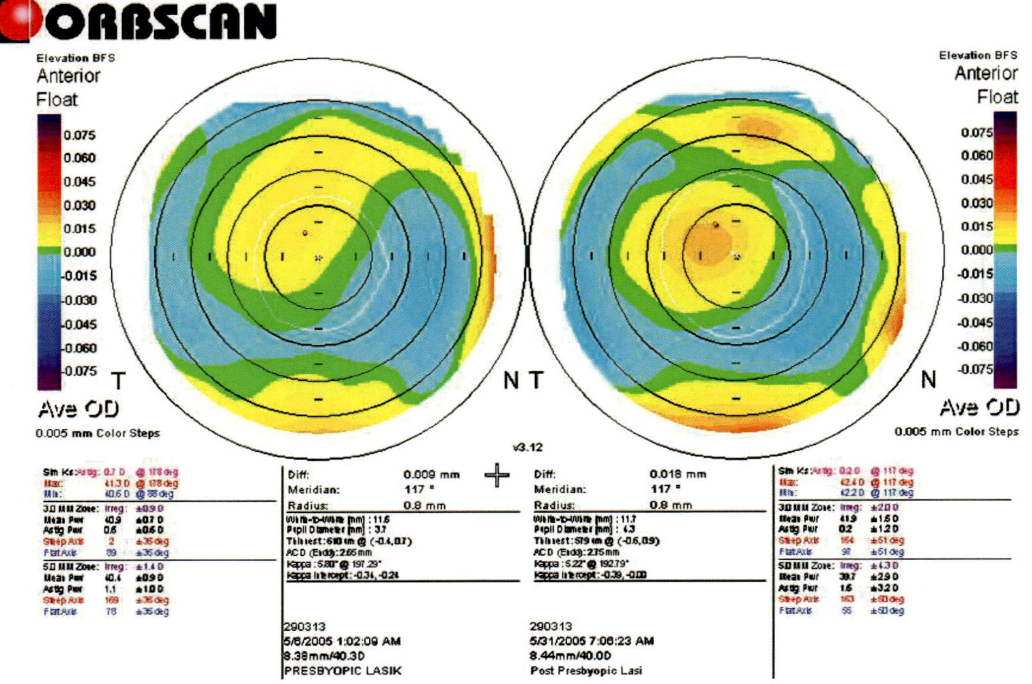

Fig. 29.6: Preoperative topography (picture on the left) of a patient before presbyopic LASIK and picture on the right shows the postoperative topography of the patient after presbyopic LASIK

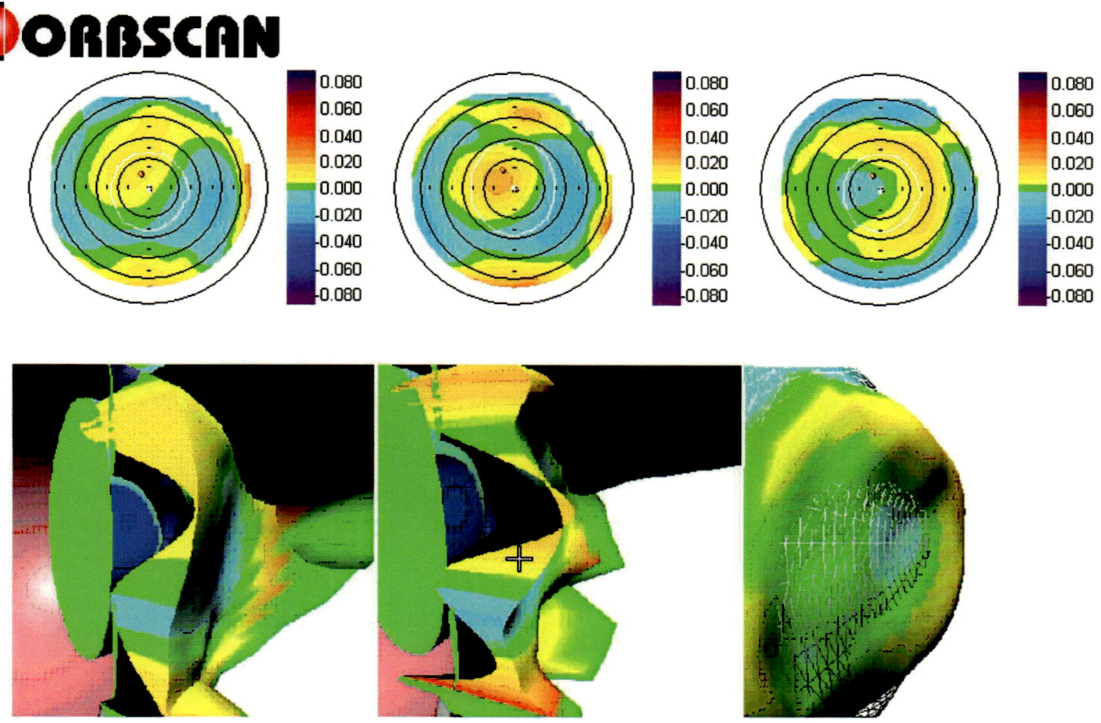

Fig. 29.7: Preoperative and postoperative topography of a patient after presbyopic LASIK shown in a 3 D pattern

postoperative keratometer reading is 42 D, which is nearly the same.

We did myopic ablation of 3 D, as patient is myopic of 2 D and presbyopic of 2 D. Regression factor taken is 1 D.

TOPOGRAPHY

Figures 29.4 and 29.5 show the pre and postoperative corneal topography in a patient in whom presbyopic LASIK has been done. This patient was 20/20 and J1 postoperatively without glasses.

Figure 29.6 shows another case in whom presbyopic LASIK was done. The picture on the left is the preoperative picture and the one on the right is the postoperative picture. Figure 29.7 is the same patients topographic photos showing pre- and post-surgery in a 3 D pattern.

SUMMARY

This idea of presbyopic LASIK is not the end of it all. This technique needs further improvisations to become the technique of choice for one and all.

REFERENCES

1. Guillermo Avalos. Presbyopic LASIK—the PARM technique in Amar Agarwal's Presbyopia : A surgical textbook. Slack Inc, USA, 2002.
2. Agarwal T, et al. Presbyopic LASIK- the Agarwal technique in Amar Agarwal's Presbyopia : A surgical textbook. Slack Inc, USA, 2002.

30 Presbyopia Correction with Central PresbyLASIK Techniques

Dolores Ortiz, Esperanza Sala, Jorge L. Alio

INTRODUCTION

The evidence that presbyopia is correctable by corneal pseudoaccommodation was shown by Artola et al[1] in a study on myopic eyes treated with first-generation PRK lasers. They found that in these patients both measured subjective accommodation and near acuity greater than expected. The corneal aberrations induced by PRK for myopia may reduce the quality of the retinal image for distance but enhance near acuity by way of a multifocal effect that can delay the onset of age-related near vision symptoms. The same finding was first observed and reported by McDonnell et al[2] and others[3] in cases operated for myopia correction by radial keratotomy. However, the first intentional creation of a multifocal ablation profiles designed to correct myopic refractive error and maintain good uncorrected near vision was attempted and reported later by Moreira et al.[4] These authors suggested that the different strategies implemented to create a bifocal effect in particular the strategy to create a central steeper area resulted in a potentially more consistent and safer outcomes.

PresbyLASIK treatment uses the principles of LASIK surgery to create a multifocal corneal surface aimed at reducing near vision spectacle dependence in presbyopic patients. In such techniques, either a central area hyperpositive for near vision is created leaving the midperipheral cornea for far vision[6;7] (central PresbyLASIK) or a central area for distance vision is created with a midpherical corneal area for near[8] (peripheral PresbyLASIK). The first definition and patent of central presbyLASIK technique was developed by Ruiz[5] in 1996. However, to our knowledge, the clinical outcomes of presbyLASIK techniques have been mostly published by means of multiple "podium presentations" but there is a lack of scientific publications on this topic.

PresbyLASIK treatment constitutes the next step in the correction of presbyopia after monovision LASIK.[9-12] Essentially, both groups of techniques create a multifocal corneal surface and so the term "multifocal presbyLASIK" is preferred to differentiate this from other photoablative surgical alternatives developed to reduce spectacle dependence for near vision by increasing the depth of focus based on modifications of the peripheral corneal ablation profile.[13]

The concept of multifocal presbyLASIK is attractive as it uses a well known surgical technique, such as LASIK, that is in widespread use. This technique has also the advantages of being not affected by accommodation fatigue, it is very simple and accessible, i.e not intraocular.

In the evolution of presbyLASIK treatments, the first generation procedures, empirical and intuitive designs based on the previous experience of the surgeon, can be distinguished from the second generation. The first generation treatments were created to achieve multifocality only based on refractive data, whereas the second one imply to perform more scientific treatments, based on corneal geometry and wavefront data.

In this chapter, the objectives are to report the clinical outcomes obtained with the central multifocal presbyLASIK technique in hyperopic patients,[6] and also to show the results when this technique is tested objectively with a light propagation algorithm.[14] At the end, the second generation presbyLASIK treatment, called PresbyMAX, will be introduced.

TECHNOVISION CENTRAL MULTIFOCAL LASIK (PRESBYLASIK)

The central presbyLASIK ablation (Presby-one, Technovision) creates a multifocal corneal profile over a 6 mm diameter (Fig. 30.1). The distance hyperopic correction is applied over the entire 6 mm zone but the central 3 mm of the treatment zone is purposely rendered hyperpositive by a further 1.5 D. A 1.5 mm circumferential transition zone of gradually changing power connects the portion of the cornea corrected for distance with the region corrected for near. The ablation pattern was performed with proprietary software from Technovision (Presby-One, Chaubard) using a H. Eye Tech. Technovision excimer laser platform. This excimer laser uses a flying spot of 0.8 mm with a repetition rate of 50 Hz. It uses an eye tracker system with a mean response time of 10 ms.

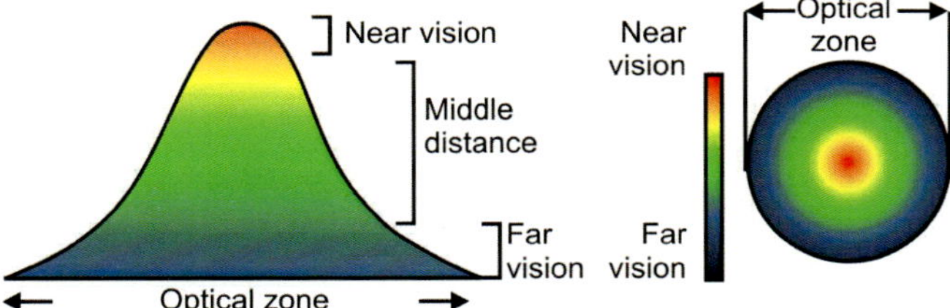

Fig. 30.1: Optical profile of central presbyLASIK (Presby-One, Technovision). (C. Illueca, J.L. Alió, D. Mas, D. Ortiz, J. Pérez, J. Espinosa, E. Sala. "Pseudoaccommodation and visual acuity with Technovision PresbyLASIK and a theoretical simulated Array multifocal intraocular lens". J. Refract. Surg 2007 (In press, On line advance))

A Moria-2 microkeratome (Moria, Paris, France) was used in all cases. A 9.5 mm diameter flap with a 4 mm hinge was targeted in each case depending on the mean keratometric value and corneal diameter according to the algorithm recommended by the company. The hinge was located superiorly for patients under 50 years of age and nasally for those above this age limit. In all cases, flap thickness was pre-set at 160 microns and the excimer laser ablation treatment was centred over the pupil. The cases were all operated by the same surgeon.

CLINICAL STUDY

Patients

A total of 25 patients (50 eyes), were enrolled: 10 female and 15 male, with a mean age of 58 years (range 51 to 68 years). Mean preoperative spherical defect was +1.92 ±0.68 D (range +0.50 D to+3.50 D), mean astigmatism was -0.50±0.94 D (range -1.00D to 0) mean spherical equivalent was +1.69 ± 0.63 D (range +0.50 D to +3.00 D), and mean spectacle near add was +2.27 ± 0.37 (range +1.75 D to +3.00 D). All eyes were hyperopic. Both eyes of each patient were treated.

Inclusion criteria were: 40 to 60 years of age, with hyperopia of less than +4.00D, astigmatism of not more than - 2.00D and a distance best corrected visual acuity of 0.8 or more. All patients were capable of reading J2 to J3 characters of Jaeger charts with an add over the best distance correction of + 1.50D during the preliminary enrollment visit. All patients had a corneal curvature (SimK) between 40 D and 48 D, a horizontal iris diameter (white to white) between 11.5 mm and 12.0 mm, central corneal thickness of no less than 500 microns and no signs of cataract as observed using a slit lamp. Pupil diameter ranged from 2.5mm (photopic conditions) to 6.0mm (mesopic conditions).

Patients with any irregular patterns of corneal topography or history of ocular disease were excluded. Other criteria for exclusion included any clinically relevant opacity of the lens, an ectopic pupil more than 2 mm from the center of the cornea and any signs of binocular vision anomalies at both distance and near.

Measurements

Assessment before presbyLASIK surgery consisted of a complete ophthalmologic examination including topography (CSO topographer, CSO, Florence, Italy), biometry (IOL master), pachymetry (Ophthasonic, Technar, USA), and manifest refraction. Post-operative follow-up examinations took place at 1 day, 1 week and 1, 3 and 6 months after surgery. For the purpose of this study only the 6 months data was used.

Distance visual acuity was tested using the decimal scale visual charts at 4 m; uncorrected distance visual acuity and best corrected distance visual acuity were tested. Near vision was tested using the Holladay contrast acuity test for (CAT; Stereo Optical Co., Chicago, IL); near UCVA at 100% contrast at 40 cm and distance-corrected near visual acuity at 25% and 100% contrast at 40 cm. Near BSCVA was tested using the Lighthouse Reading Test (Lighthouse, NY USA) at 40 cm. All tests were performed monocularly and binocularly. The range of accommodation was measured preoperatively with the EDTRS chart at 40 cm from which the subject has to read a given line (J2) on the chart using the best distance spectacle prescription supplemented with a +2.50D near addition. Plus lenses were added in 0.25 D steps until the line first appears blurred (a). The procedure was repeated again using minus lenses (b). The range of accommodation is the sum, a+b irrespective of sign. This procedure was done under normal light conditions (approximately 90cd/m^2) using 100% contrast optotypes. Contrast sensitivity was tested with best correction using VSRC CST 1800 (Vision Science Research, San Ramon, CA).

Corneal aberrations and point spread function (PSF) values were investigated with the CSO Topographer (CSO, Florence, Italy). Root-mean-square (RMS) and PSF values of corneal aberrations were calculated from the corneal topography. Total ocular aberrations were investigated with the Zywave Hartman Shack aberrometer (Bausch and Lomb, USA) with a pupil diameter of 6 mm.

Results and Conclusions

Safety

Mean amplitude of accommodation (± S.D., range) increased from a preoperative value of 1.43D ± 0.52D (+0.50 to +3.25 D) to 2.12D (± 0.64D, +1.00D to + 3.75D). The change was significant ($p<0.001$).

The distance safety index (ratio of the mean postoperative distance best corrected visual acuity to the mean preoperative distance best corrected visual acuity) was 0.95 monocular and 0.98 binocular. The near vision safety index (ratio of the mean postoperative near best corrected visual acuity to preoperative near best corrected visual acuity) was 0.93 monocular and 0.99 binocular. After presby-LASIK, 7 patients (14%) lost a maximum of 2 lines of best corrected visual acuity for distance and 8 patients (16%) for near vision (Figs 30.2A and B). No patient lost lines of BCVA either for far or near in both eyes simultaneously.

Efficacy

Binocular distance uncorrected visual acuity improved from 0.39 ± 0.19 preoperatively to 0.97 ± 0.14 postoperatively, binocular near uncorrected visual acuity improved significantly from 0.14 ± 0.11 to 0.57 ± 0.20. (Figs 30.3A and B). Binocular distance corrected near visual acuity improved from 0.35 ± 0.21 preoperatively to 0.45 ± 0.22 postoperatively (Fig. 30.3C).

Six months postoperatively, the distance efficacy index (ratio of the mean postoperative distance uncorrected visual acuity to the preoperative distance best corrected visual acuity) was 0.8 monocular and 0.9 binocular. The near vision efficacy index (ratio of the mean postoperative near uncorrected visual acuity to the preoperative near best corrected visual acuity was 0.5 monocular and 0.6 binocular. There is an inverse relationship between uncorrected distance and uncorrected near acuity at 6 months (Pearson correlation coefficient,

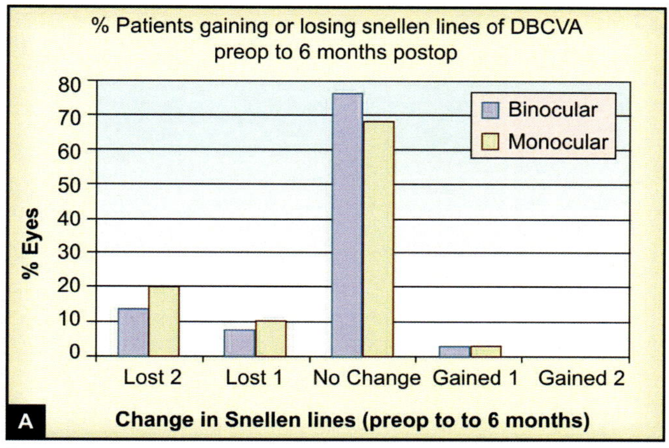

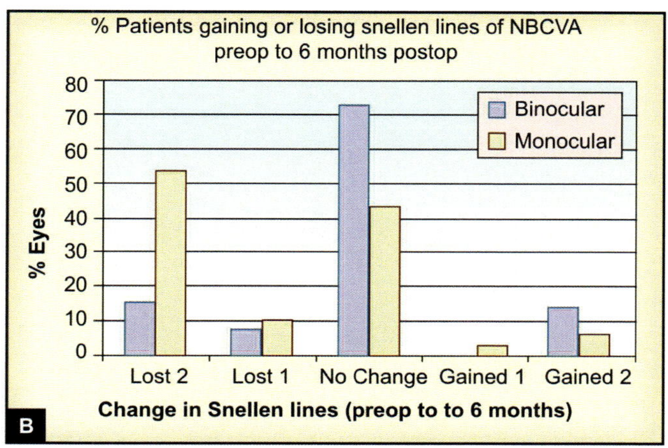

Figs 30.2A and B: Gain and loss of Snellen lines of best-corrected distance and near visual acuity (Alio JL, Chaubard JJ, Caliz A, et al. Correction of presbyopia by technovision central multifocal LASIK (presbyLASIK). J Refract Surg 2006;22:453-60)

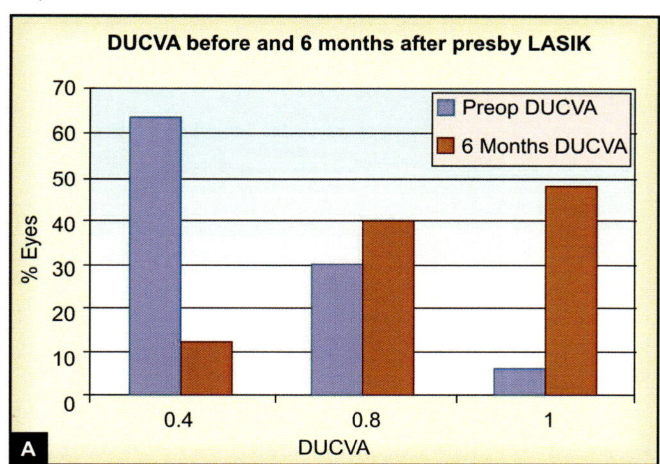

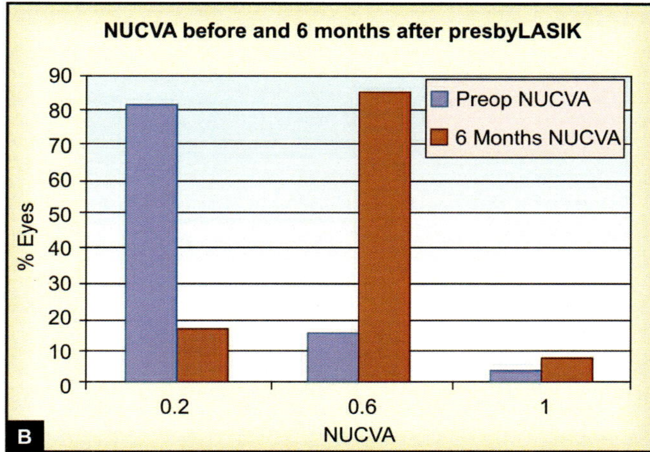

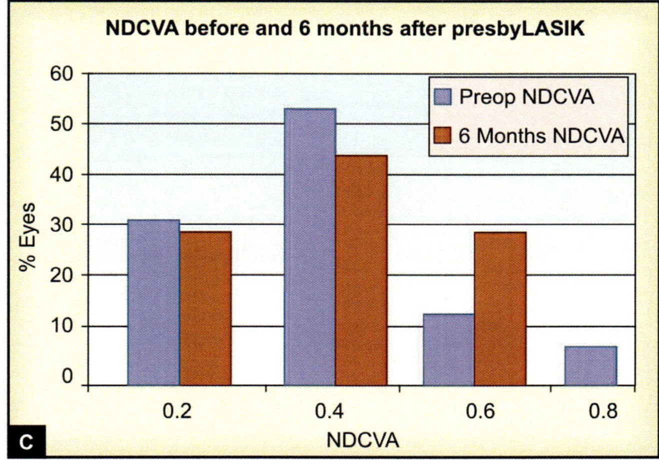

Figs 30.3A to C: Improvements in binocular distance, near uncorrected and distance near corrected visual acuity 6 months after surgery (Alio JL, Chaubard JJ, Caliz A, et al. Correction of presbyopia by technovision central multifocal LASIK (presbyLASIK). J Refract Surg 2006;22:453-60)

(r =-0.474, p=0.0005). After 6 months, only 6 eyes were retreated with a LASIK standard treatment for distance.

Predictability

Six months after presbyLASIK the mean residual refraction was -0.19 ± 0.54 D (range -1.50 to +1.25 D) and the mean spherical equivalent was -0.34 ± 0.55 D (range -1.50 to +1.00 D). The mean astigmatism refraction was -0.42 ± 0.36 D (range -1.25 to 0 D). The percentage of patients with postoperative spherical equivalent within ± 0.5D was 64 % (Fig. 30.4).

Contrast Sensitivity

After 6 months there was no significant change in contrast sensitivity at 1.5 cycles/deg. (Wilcoxon matched pairs test p=0.545). A significant mean reduction was found at spatial frequencies of 3, 6, 12 and 18 cycles/deg (p<0.001). The main results at this regard are shown in Fig. 30.5.

Corneal Aberrations

There was a significant change in corneal aberrations after surgery. The coma coefficients (Z3 + Z5 terms) for a 6 mm. pupil increased from a mean ± S.D of 0.41 μ ±0.17 to 0.54 μ ±0.22 (t-student test, p=0.0018). The coefficients for spherical aberration (Z4 + Z6 terms) decreased from a mean ± S.D of 0.41 μ ±0.4

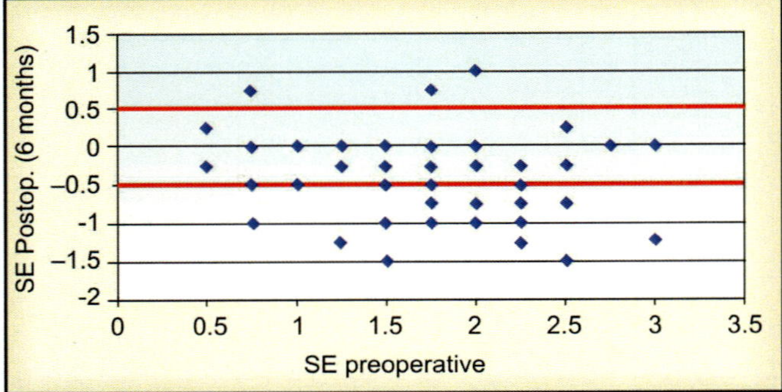

Fig. 30.4: Comparison of spherical equivalent refraction: preoperative vs. 6 months postoperatively (Alio JL, Chaubard JJ, Caliz A, et al. Correction of presbyopia by technovision central multifocal LASIK (presbyLASIK). J Refract Surg 2006;22:453-60)

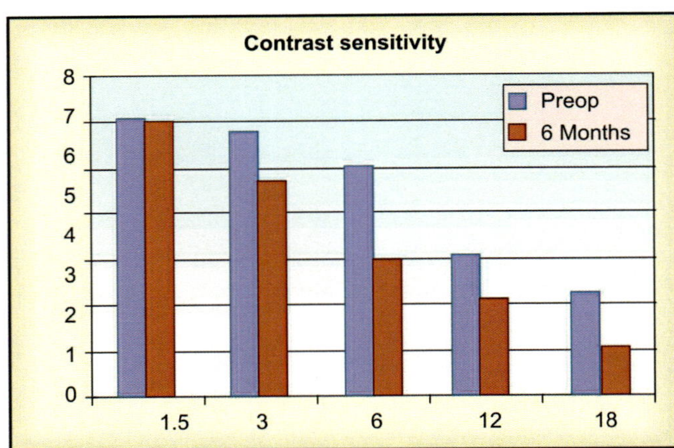

Fig. 30.5: Contrast sensitivity pre and post surgery at 6 months (Alio JL, Chaubard JJ, Caliz A, et al. Correction of presbyopia by technovision central multifocal LASIK (presbyLASIK). J Refract Surg 2006;22:453-60)

to 0.36 μ ±0.14 (t-student test, p = 0.095). A significant correlation was found when comparing the individual changes in spherical aberration and amplitude of accommodation (Pearson correlation coefficient +0.317, n=50, p=0.025). A significant correlation was not found when comparing the individual changes in coma and amplitude of accommodation (Pearson correlation coefficient +0.193, n = 50, p = 0.179).

Point Spread Function

There was a significant change in point spread function values (t-student test, p= 0.0018). The mean ± S.D. reduced from 37.60cd/m^2 ±15.53 to 28.42cd/m^2 ±16.04 suggesting a fall in vision performance. A significant correlation was not found when comparing the individual changes in point spread function with measured accommodation (Pearson correlation coefficient -0.211, n = 50, p = 0.371).

Subjective symptoms

After 6 months, no patient was reporting halos, glare, starburst phenomena or double vision in daylight conditions. Night halos were reported as present but not significant in 3 patients (12%). No patient reported night starburst or double vision at the end of the 6 months follow-up.

Subjectively, 19 patients (76%) reported a high degree of satisfaction, and none of the patients rated the visual outcome at the 6 months visit as low or unsatisfactory. At the end of the 6th month follow up 18 patients (72%) were spectacle independent for all distances.

According to the refractive outcomes of the study, it seems that part of the near vision results are caused by the slight overcorrection associated with the tentative multifocality of the cornea. The change in accommodation was significant but it did not correlate with changes in either coma or the change in point spread function. However, the change in measured accommodation did correlate with the change in spherical aberration. The greater the increase in spherical aberration the greater the expected increase in measured accommodation and vice versa. This would suggest that by purposefully inducing greater fixed amounts of spherical aberration we should increase the measured accommodation for individual cases.

In conclusion, central presbyLASIK using central steepening associated to the correction of low and moderate hyperopia may increase pseudoaccommodation by creating cornea multifocality and significantly improving near vision performance. The ablation profile used resulted in overcorrection and resulting myopia in a significant number of eyes and indicates that a further refinement in the algorithm and ablation is required. A moderate albeit significant loss of contrast sensitivity was observed regarding preoperative levels and some cases may experience moderate loss of BSCVA.

OPTICAL ANALYSIS OF PRESBYLASIK TREATMENT

With the introduction of modern ocular measurements and technical improvements (corneal topography, corneal pachymetry, reliable biometry), calculations made on realistic mathematical models are of great importance for studying the optical performance of the human eye and have become relevant in order to make objective estimates for individuals.[15-17] In order to evaluate the optical quality of the eye after this type of treatment, an eye model can be used to study light distributions at different planes inside the posterior chamber. The cornea can be modeled, using topographical data, as a phase only element and personalized crystalline data can be constructed from each subject using real measures of anterior chamber and axial length, together with the subjective ametropia.[18] With all these elements a mathematical model of each patient's eye can be constructed. Then, applying a propagation algorithm, light patterns can be obtained as they propagate through the eye.

Light propagation algorithm and optical quality parameters

Quality analysis was done as follows: From pre and postsurgical topographies, the morphology of the cornea was determined and by evaluating optical path length differences, the final phase transmittance of this element was obtained. The cornea model consisted of a single surface that separates air from an equivalent keratometric index of $n_k = 1.3375$. Light distributions propagated from the cornea can be numerically evaluated by means of a Fresnel propagation algorithm.[19] Let us consider an input pattern of size Δx_o that has been discretized in N samples. The final expression giving the light field at any distance z from an input field u_0 is:

$$(u_z)_m = DFT^{-1}\left\{\exp\left(i\frac{2\pi}{\lambda}z\sqrt{1-\lambda^2\frac{\tilde{m}^2}{\Delta x_0^2}}\right)DFT\left[u_0\left(m\frac{\Delta x_0}{N}\right)\right]\right\} \quad ...(1)$$

where m, $\tilde{m}$ and μ are discrete indices in space, Fourier and Fresnel domains, respectively, DFT is the acronym of Discrete Fourier Transform, λ is the illuminating wavefront and Δx_o is the size of the object support window.

By introducing the corneal phase transmittance as the input distribution in equation (1), light distribution at the entrance of the crystalline lens was obtained. Data of the crystalline lens was inferred from existing mathematical models[20] together with subjective data of ametropias. Light distribution leaving the crystalline lens can be introduced again in expression (1) as an input function. Then, the final distribution at any distance inside the posterior chamber can be calculated.

The algorithm was applied to obtain light patterns around the retinal plane of the pre and post surgical eye. Several quality parameters that quantify the benefits of the intervention were calculated from light energy distributions: Strehl ratio (SR) in a region around the retina, the spot size on the retina and objective visual acuity. Besides, the improvement of these parameters after presbyLASIK have been evaluated.

The Strehl ratio is defined as the quotient between the maximum intensity of the Fourier transform of the exit pupil function by an aberration free real system. In fact, this corresponds to the quotient between the maximum intensities of the light distribution of both systems at the paraxial focal plane. In the case of a post-presbyLASIK cornea this plane is not well defined, and, in any case, does not provide an accurate method of determining the quality of a pseudo-multifocal system. Thus, we have extended the definition of the Strehl ratio. Since we can access any plane inside the eye, we have calculated the ratio between the maximum intensities of light energies of a real system and an aberration system in a range of distances around a region of interests.

Regarding visual acuity, with our algorithm we can obtain light patterns at any desired plane inside the eye. Thus we have obtained the Full Width at Half Height of the retinal spot. The VA can be defined as the inverse of the subtended angle of this value, in minutes of arc, measured from the image nodal point of the eye. By changing the object distance, we can analyze the variation of the spot size at the retinal plane and thus explore the possibilities of pseudo-accommodation effects.

Results and Conclusions

The study included a total of 8 hyperopic eyes of 8 different patients who underwent central Presby-LASIK surgery with Presby-one software (Chaubard) using a H. Eye Tech. Technovision excimer laser platform. Mean age was 57 years (range 53 to 68). Mean preoperative spherical equivalent was 1.28 ± 0.87 D. The mean value and standard deviation of the distance decimal visual acuity with and without correction were 1.02 ± 0.13 and 0.37 ± 0.15 respectively. The postoperative spherical equivalent refraction was –0.55 ± 0.48 D (range from –1.12 to 0.25 D). Mean distance decimal visual acuity with and without correction was 0.94 ± 0.09 and 0.70 ± 0.20 respectively. Mean pseudoaccommodation range was 1.6 ± 0.4 D.

Visual Acuity

In Figure 30.6, the evolution of the calculated visual acuity without refractive correction for one of the eyes of our study. Calculated VA for different object distances are represented in three different cases. First we have calculated the preoperative case. There we see that, since the eye is hyperopic, no high VA is achieved at any distance. Second, we have depicted the postoperative case. Notice that the VA function stays above 0.5 for object distances from 0.5 to 2.5 m. For further objects the VA shows a soft decay. In order to demonstrate the presence of pseudoaccommodation we have also represented

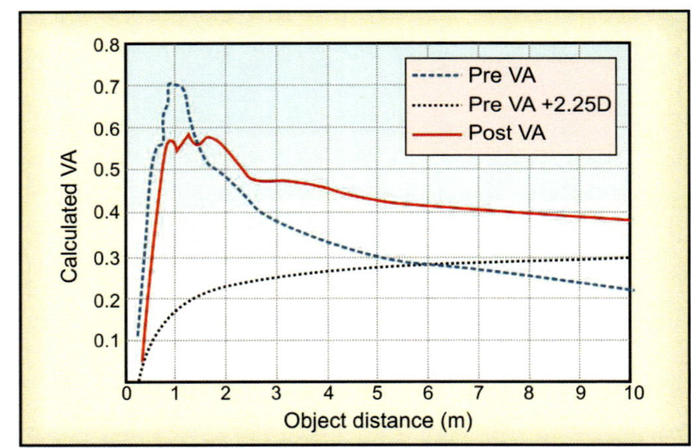

Fig. 30.6: Uncorrected visual acuity for different object distances from the corneal apex for one of the eyes of our study before surgery (dotted line), compensated eye (dashed line) and after surgery (solid line) (Ortiz D, Alio JL, Illueca C, et al. Optical analysis of presbyLASIK treatment by a light propagation algorithm. J Refract Surg 2007;23:39-44)

the preoperative case corrected with an ophthalmic lens free of aberrations, so that we achieve the same refractive status than the post operative case (2.25 D for this case). We can see that in this case, the peak is higher for the corrected distance, but from 1.5 m to far distances, the curve stays lower than the postoperative one.

The analysis of the evolution of the calculated visual acuity for different distance objects (Fig. 30.6) has shown the evidence that presbyLASIK treatment provides a certain degree of pseudoaccommodation. Taking into account visual acuity values of over 0.5 (for this patient the pre-surgical visual acuity was 0.3), this patient would gain approximately 0.5 mm of depth of focus, that is equivalent to 1 D of pseudoaccommodation. These results are consistent with the range of accommodation measured in patients (mean value of 1.6 D). Furthermore, the VA has been increased for far distance objects, when compared with a monofocal lens compensated preoperative eye.

Strehl Ratio

The Strehl ratio value on the retinal plane significantly increased after the surgery for all eyes. We have obtained a mean increase of a factor 4.7. The best case increases its Strehl ratio by factor 9, while the worst experienced an improvement of factor 3, which was also very good.

Energy Distribution

To illustrate this improvement on the optical quality, we have depicted, in (Fig. 30.7) the theoretical light distribution on the retinal plane before (left) and after (right) surgery. Both eyes significantly improve the peak quality, showing a higher and narrower peak after surgery.

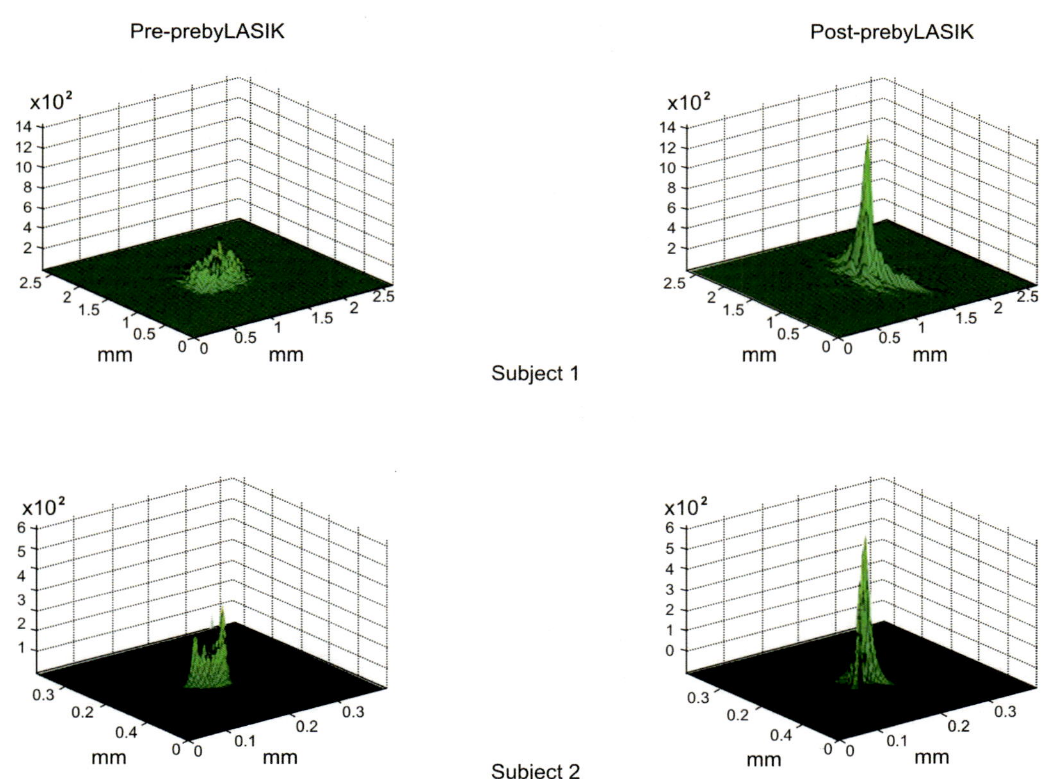

Fig. 30.7: Theoretical light distribution on the retinal plane for two eyes of our study before (left) and after (right) surgery (Ortiz D, Alio JL, Illueca C, et al. Optical analysis of presbyLASIK treatment by a light propagation algorithm. J Refract Surg 2007;23:39-44)

In conclusion, optical analysis models provide an excellent tool to characterize the optical performance of corneal refractive procedures. PresbyLASIK provides an improvement in optical quality, in terms of Strehl ratio, and a certain degree of accommodation. The use of this method for the analysis of other corneal refractive procedures may allow the surgeon to choose the procedure which results in a better optical performance.

PRESBYLASIK VS. MULTIFOCAL REFRACTIVE IOLS: WHAT IS THE BEST FOR VISUAL PERFORMANCE?

Multifocal intraocular lenses (IOLs) can be based on refractive and diffractive technologies.[21] Refractive optics have been extensively used to decrease near vision spectacle dependence of aphakic patients, with the AMO-ARRAY being a typical lens.[22;23]

In an attempt to elucidate the efficacy and validity of laser refractive surgery as a treatment option for presbyopia, we have compared the outcomes achieved in hyperopic patients undergoing central presbyLASIK surgery with the simulated results that they would have obtained from a multifocal IOL implant, such as the AMO Array multifocal IOL.

The Array simulation

The effects of an ideal AMO Array lens on the visual performance of the subject were simulated,by substituting the crystalline lens for an AMO multifocal lens in an eye model. The base power was adjusted for far vision for each individual eye and addition was set to 3.5 D, as established in the AMO specifications. Figure 30.8 shows the refractive structure of the AMO with different zones for near and far vision. The refractive effects of the IOL have been simulated under ideal conditions, under the assumption that no aberrations are induced by surgery. In real cases, however, surgery could induce some higher order aberrations that may decrease quality of vision.

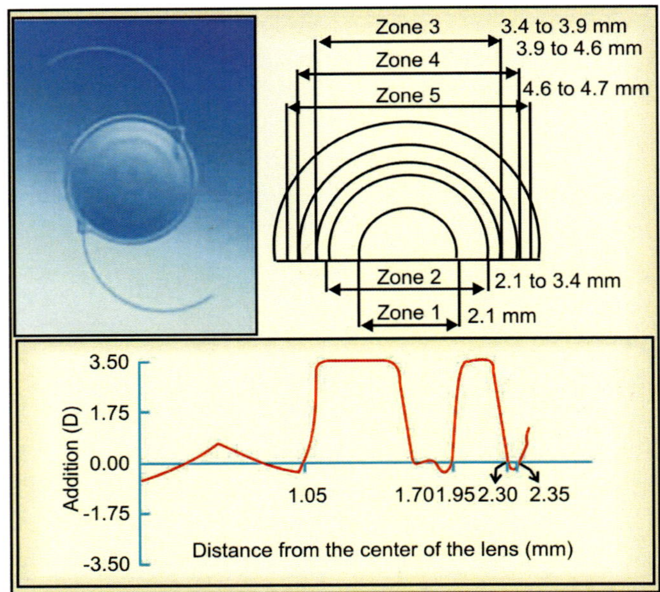

Fig. 30.8: Refractive structure and profile of an AMO Array implant: the odd zones (1, 3 and 5) are adjusted for far vision and the even zones (2 and 4) for near vision, giving an addition of 3.5 D. (C. Illueca, J.L. Alió, D. Mas, D. Ortiz, J. Pérez, J. Espinosa, E. Sala. "Pseudoaccommodation and visual acuity with Technovision PresbyLASIK and a theoretical simulated Array multifocal intraocular lens". J. Refract. Surg 2007 (In press, On line advance))

For this simulation, the crystalline lens was substituted for an adequate IOL and its transmittance was evaluated from its technical specifications.

From the light distribution at the retinal plane, the radial MTF function was calculated and the cut-off frequency was given by the limit of the region that encircles 90% of the volume under the curve. The remaining curve of the MTF is associated with high-frequency background noise, introduced by the calculation method. Let us recall that 30 cycles per degree would correspond to a visual acuity of 1. Hence, from this curve the visual acuity could be estimated for any retinal distribution.

Visual acuity values have been estimated for a range of distances, from near to far vision conditions. For near vision, a pupil diameter of 3 mm was fixed assuming a remaining accommodation of 1 D, whereas far vision conditions consisted of a pupil diameter of 5 mm and no accommodation. For the

Array simulation, only the aperture change was applied when changing from near to far vision.

Results and Conclusions

For the comparison, 10 hyperopic eyes that underwent central PresbyLASIK surgery were analyzed. The mean age was 57 (ranged from 52 to 68). Mean preoperative spherical equivalent was 1.28 0.87 D. The mean value and standard deviation of the distance visual acuity with and without correction were 1.02 ± 0.13 and 0.37 ± 0.15 respectively. For the purpose of this study only the six months data was used. After presbyLASIK treatment, the postsurgical spherical equivalent was -0.55 ± 0.48 D (range from -1.12 to 0.25 D). The mean value and standard deviation of the distance decimal visual acuity with and without correction were 0.94 ± 0.09 and 0.70 ± 0.20 respectively.

For all eyes, the objective visual acuity was studied comparing the values before and after surgery with the visual acuity value that the eye could achieve with its best fitted Array lens. Regarding the visual acuity values, Figure 30.9 shows that the Array-like lens could provide values of visual acuity above 0.5 for object distances ranging from 25 cm to 1 m, achieving a maximum value of 0.9 from 50 to 70 cm (near-intermediate vision). The presbyLASIK treatment also provided good visual responses (VA > 0.5) for distances beyond 45 cm and achieved a maximum value of 0.7 from 70 cm to 1 m.

For far vision (Fig. 30.10), both the Array IOL and the presbyLASIK visual acuities were over 0.5, but the optical performance for Array was lower. These results show that without considering post-implant surgical consequences both procedures could provide comparable visual quality.

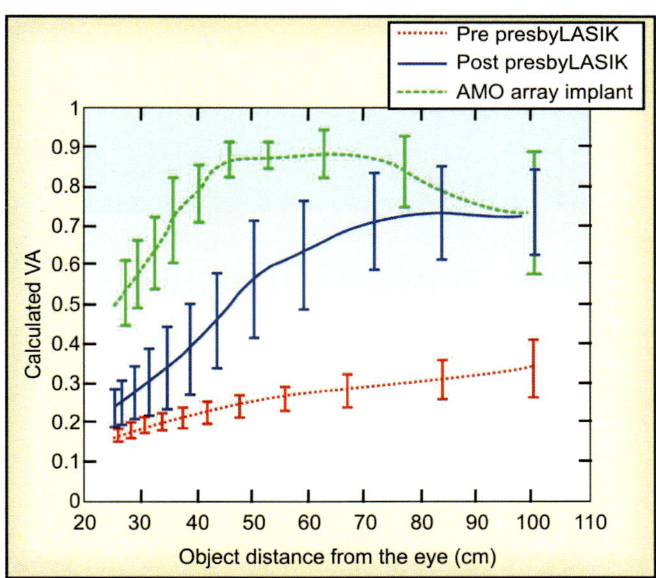

Fig. 30.9: Mean values and standard deviation of the uncorrected visual acuity for near distances for the 10 eyes of our study before presbyLASIK surgery (dotted line), after presbyLASIK surgery (solid line) and with the simulated AMO ARRAY implant (dashed line). Error bar represents ± SD for each distance. (C. Illueca, J.L. Alió, D. Mas, D. Ortiz, J. Pérez, J. Espinosa, E. Sala. "Pseudoaccommodation and visual acuity with Technovision PresbyLASIK and a theoretical simulated Array multifocal intraocular lens". J. Refract. Surg 2007 (In press, On line advance))

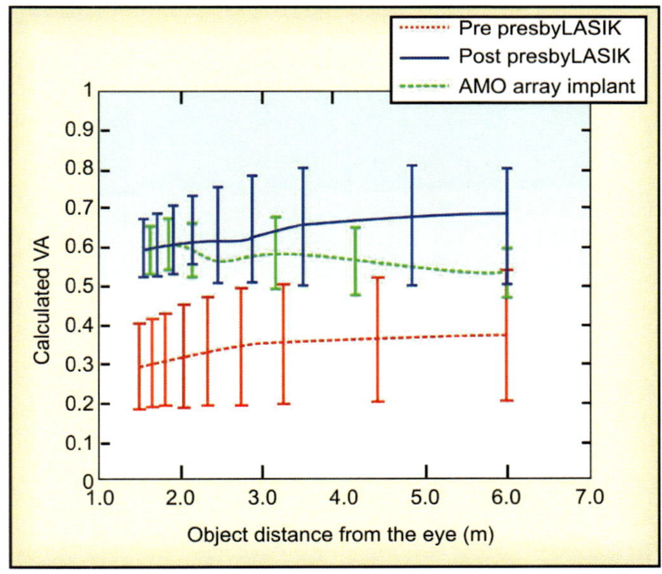

Fig. 30.10: Mean values and standard deviation of the uncorrected visual acuity for far distances for the 10 eyes of our study before presbyLASIK surgery (dotted line), after presbyLASIK surgery (solid line) and with the simulated AMO ARRAY implant (dashed line). Error bar represents SD for each distance. (C. Illueca, J.L. Alió, D. Mas, D. Ortiz, J. Pérez, J. Espinosa, E. Sala. "Pseudoaccommodation and visual acuity with Technovision PresbyLASIK and a theoretical simulated Array multifocal intraocular lens". J. Refract. Surg 2007 (In press, On line advance))

The finding that both the central presbyLASIK technique and a multifocal intraocular lens such as the AMO Array provide similar outcomes for far or near multifocal vision is significant, as both techniques compare favorably with each other. The choice of using one or the other should be based on the age of the patient, individual eye factors, patient desires and clinical judgement. The advantages of corneal multifocal surgery (PresbyLASIK in its different forms), are the ease of accessibility of corneal refractive surgery, its less invasive character than intraocular surgery and its attractive appearance to patients. On the contrary, lens refractive surgery is an intraocular invasive procedure, with a potential for complications that even in expert hands, can lead to complications such as endophthalmitis. Lens intraocular surgery has the advantage of lens multifocality on a stable basis, not affected by corneal wound healing. However, multifocal IOLs do not allow correction of higher order aberrations which are now possible to be corrected with modern excimer laser procedures.

In conclusion, this is the first scientific demonstration that validates presbyLASIK as an alternative to intraocular multifocal surgery such as with the AMO Array design. In the future, this model might allow the ophthalmic surgeon to decide which procedure should be most suitable for a given patient as its predictive capabilities and good clinical correlation provide a scientific basis for the indications of presbyLASIK excimer laser surgery.

SECOND GENERATION TREATMENTS BASED ON CORNEAL WAVEFRONT AND TOPOGRAPHY ANALYSIS: PRESBYMAX® MODEL

Until now, presbyLASIK treatments have been performed by empirical and intuitive designs based on the previous experience of the surgeon. As we have shown during this chapter, these procedures were created to achieve multifocality only based on refractive data. The evolution of presbyLASIK techniques should imply to perform more scientific treatments, based on corneal geometry and wavefront data.

PresbyMAX is a biaspheric excimer laser profile that creates a multifocal cornea to improve near vision. It is the first systematic and scientifically based approach for the correction of presbyopia with excimer laser surgery. It uses the Esiris-Schwind excimer laser and Pendular microkeratome (Schwind, Frankfurt, Germany) or femtosecond technology for a planar flap cut. The software predicts the visual outcome from far and for near in every patient by using a predictive model based on biometrical data of the patient and a light propagation algorithm (previously explained under 'optical analysis of presbyopic LASIC treatment'). The presbyMAX model is pupil predictive, works both in the hyperope and in the myope, is centred on the corneal apex and provides a near vision effect of 1.75 D to 3 D. The adequate patients selection is one of the key factors to be considered in order to obtain a successful presbyMAX.

The following versions of presbyMAX will introduce the concept of multiaspheric profiles. The presbyMAX V02 provide a tri-aspheric profile optimised for the patient's biometrical data in order to maximize the postoperative visual acuity for far and near.

As alternative for monovision, the aspheric presbyMAX V03 is based on the creation of a progressive multifocality across the optical zone with binocular overlap using wavefront diagnosis

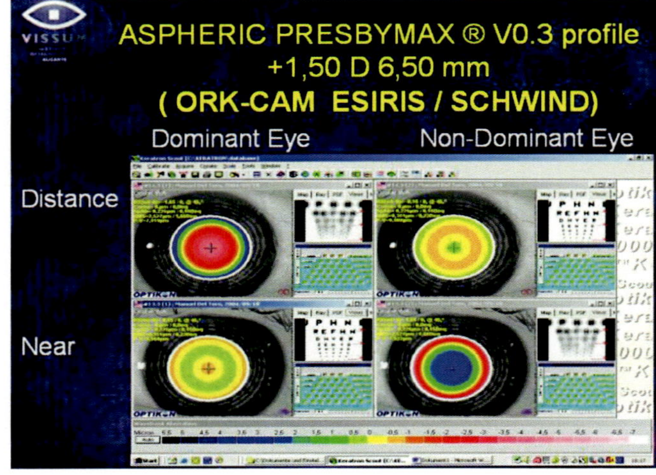

Fig. 30.11: Simulation of the profile of the aspheric presbyMAX V03 for a hyperopic eye with a spherical defect of 1.5 D and 6.5 mm optical zone

data. The idea will be to asymmetrically induce a negative/positive spherical aberration in dominant and no-dominant eye (Fig. 30.11) but with a neutral binocular effect.

REFERENCES

1. Artola A, Patel S, Schimchak P, et al. Evidence for delayed presbyopia after photorefractive keratectomy for myopia. Ophthalmology 2006;113:735-41.
2. McDonnell PJ, Garbus J, Lopez PF. Topographic analysis and visual acuity after radial keratotomy. Am J Ophthalmol 1988;106:692-5.
3. Wilson SE, Klyce SD. Topographic analysis and visual acuity after radial keratotomy. Am J Ophthalmol 1989;107:436-8.
4. Moreira H, Garbus JJ, Lee M, et al. Multifocal corneal topographic changes after radial keratotomy. Ophthalmic Surg 1992;23:85-9.
5. Ruiz LA. Apparatus and method for performing presbyopia corrective surgery. [5,533,997]. 1996. US. 6-1-1994. Ref Type: Patent.
6. Alio JL, Chaubard JJ, Caliz A, et al. Correction of presbyopia by technovision central multifocal LASIK (presbyLASIK). J Refract Surg 2006;22:453-60.
7. Anschutz T. Laser correction of hyperopia and presbyopia. Int Ophthalmol Clin 1994;34:107-37.
8. Cantu R, Rosales MA, Tepichin E, et al. Advanced surface ablation for presbyopia using the Nidek EC-5000 laser. J Refract Surg 2004;20:S711-S713.
9. Cheng AC, Lam DS. Monovision LASIK for pre-presbyopic and presbyopic patients. J Refract Surg 2005;21:411-2.
10. Goldberg DB. Laser in situ keratomileusis monovision. J Cataract Refract Surg 2001;27:1449-55.
11. Jain S, Ou R, Azar DT. Monovision outcomes in presbyopic individuals after refractive surgery. Ophthalmology 2001;108:1430-3.
12. Miranda D, Krueger RR. Monovision laser in situ keratomileusis for pre-presbyopic and presbyopic patients. J Refract Surg 2004;20:325-8.
13. Telandro A. Pseudo-accommodative cornea: a new concept for correction of presbyopia. J Refract Surg 2004;20:S714-S717.
14. Ortiz D, Alio JL, Illueca C, et al. Optical analysis of presbyLASIK treatment by a light propagation algorithm. J Refract Surg 2007;23:39-44.
15. Doshi JB, Sarver EJ, Applegate RA. Schematic eye models for simulation of patient visual performance. J Refract Surg 2001;17:414-9.
16. Ortiz D, Saiz JM, Gonzalez F, et al. Geometric ray tracing for design of customized ablation in laser in situ keratomileusis. J Refract Surg 2002;18:S327-S331.
17. Sarver EJ, Applegate RA. Modeling and predicting visual outcomes with VOL-3D. J Refract Surg 2000;16:S611-S616.
18. Pérez J, Mas D, Illueca C, et al. Complete algorithm for the calculation light patterns inside the ocular media. J Mod Opt 2005;52:1161-76.
19. Mas D, Pérez J, Vázquez C, et al. Near-field light distributions propagated from human corneas: determination of relevant patterns. J Mod Opt 2003;50:1335-52.
20. Pérez J, Mas D, Miret JJ, et al. Fresnel based analysis of Kasprzak's crystalline model: statistical results and individual predictions. Optik 2005;116:49-57.
21. Alio JL, Tavolato M, De la HF, et al. Near vision restoration with refractive lens exchange and pseudoaccommodating and multifocal refractive and diffractive intraocular lenses: comparative clinical study. J Cataract Refract Surg 2004;30:2494-503.
22. Chandhrasri S, Knorz MC. Comparison of higher order aberrations and contrast sensitivity after LASIK, Verisyse phakic IOL, and Array multifocal IOL. J Refract Surg 2006;22:231-6.
23. Montes-Mico R, Alio JL. Distance and near contrast sensitivity function after multifocal intraocular lens implantation. J Cataract Refract Surg 2003;29:703-11.

31 SBK (Sub-Bowman Keratomileusis): Thin Flap LASIK (Technique and Enhancement Procedure)

Roberto Pinelli

INTRODUCTION

SBK (sub-Bowman keratomileusis) is a safe technique to correct all visual defects in patients with pachymetry > 500 microns. It combines the advantages of surface and lamellar procedures, minimal debilitation of corneal biomechanical architecture with the rapid and comfortable visual recovery of lamellar approaches. This technique consists in a natural use of the keratomileusis or LASIK which is spreading even more among the most advance institutes of surgery of vision all over the world. In the past an important problem such as the corneal ectasia was caused especially by the impossibility to catch the flap (which many times was thicker than planned). Today the development of sophisticated microkeratomes and the use of the femtosecond laser allow the surgeons to establish a specific thickness and uniformity of the cornea.

TECHNIQUE DESCRIPTION

The SBK (sub-Bowman keratomileusis) is a technique which is becoming even more popular and consists of the creation of a thin flap (from 80 to 100 microns). The LASIK technique of the last 15 years has been using thicker flaps, up to 160 microns.

Recently, the sub-Bowman keratomileusis has replaced the LASIK at our institute in all cases. A flap between 80 and 100 microns at least has many advantages, which have been already presented in the previous paragraph (Figs 31.1 and 31.2).

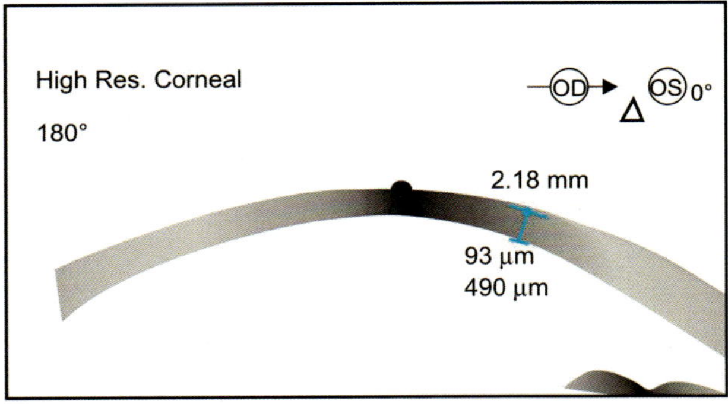

Fig. 31.1: Thin flap LASIK: SBK

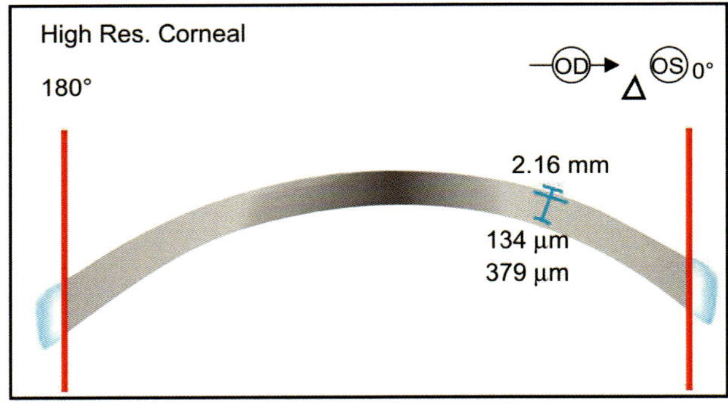

Fig. 31.2: Thicker flap

Today the Visante technology (Zeiss) has been very helpful for the characterization and verification of these thin flaps. In fact, in post-SBK patients we can observe through the Visante that the flap

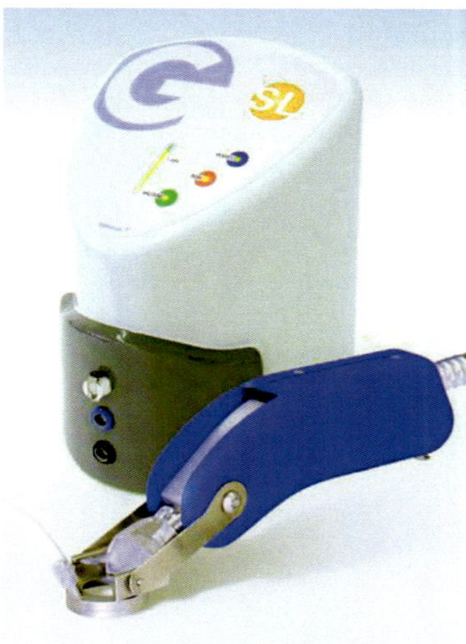

Fig. 31.3: Gebauer SL_PR_03

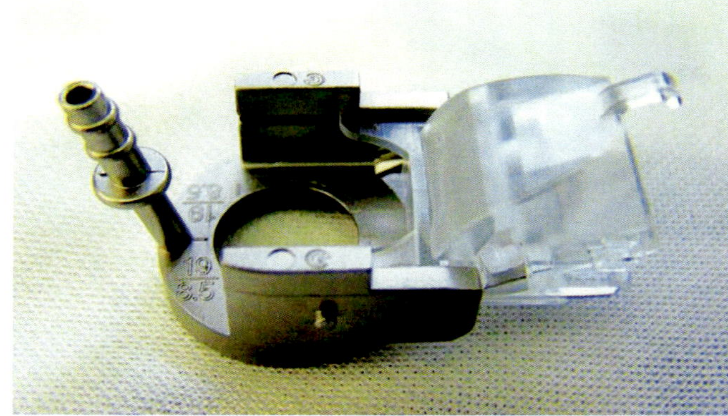

Fig. 31.4: Single-use LASIK set

thickness is very thin and it is barely perceptible, while with other cases with thicker flaps there are surely more evident characteristics also at the Visante. An interesting phenomenon consists in a progressive loss of frequency of late complications (no corneal ectasia cases in 5,000 operations during the last 4 years at our institute). This is because both the new laser programs of tissue saving, then with a reduced ablation for what the tissue is concerned, and the thickness of the flap that consequently gives more tissue in the stroma, allow a limitation of the risk of ectasia and we know that one of the main issues of the corneal ectasia was also the unpredictability of the no-predictivity of the flaps thickness with the microkeratomes of the first generation.

It is possible to perform a sub-Bowman keratomileusis with several instruments: some of them are mechanical microkeratomes (Fig. 31.3), others are femtosecond lasers (Fig. 31.4).[1]

POTENTIAL COMPLICATIONS

Since we have been using the Gebauer product, we have not checked any complication of the flap in more than 5,000 flaps performed in the last years, except for three cases of epithelial shift caused by a loss of suction nevertheless. However, these patients have had a satisfying result in the 4-5 days after the reposition of the contact lens and the reepithelialization.

ENHANCEMENT TECHNIQUES

Enhancement through the sub-Bowman keratomileusis is a very delicate manipulation and potentially more difficult than the lifting of a thicker flap. This is the only characteristic a little more complicated and which requires an advanced trial of the surgeon. In fact, the thin flap is more difficult to handle during the lifting phase and whether it is not manipulated in a soft way, it could be the cause of striae. Then, the enhancement techniques that we use at our institute consist of the flap lifting paying the due attention. In those rare cases (2%) of our treatments in which the flap did not lift, as it was integrated with the stroma, an ASA (Advanced Surface Ablation) was performed as post-SBK retreatment.[2] Our instrument for the SBK retreatment is the Pinelli retreatment spatula (by Janach, Italy).

Finally, the sub-Bowman keratomileusis is a brilliant innovative technique, that we prefer rather than the EpiLASIK because it allows a fast recovery, no pain and a high level of satisfaction of the patient.[3]

The epithelial ingrowth is a rare event yet possible after the enhancement with SBK. We have the 2 percent of retreatment cases and it reveals itself between 3 and 6 months after the operation. In this specific case we can lift the flap once again, clean the epithelium very softly with a spatula, replace the flap and, finally, prescribe steroids therapy in drops for one week.

REFERENCES

1. Chang JS. Complications of sub-Bowman's keratomileusis with a femtosecond laser in 3009 eyes. Journal of Refractive Surgery 2008;24(1):S97-101.
2. Dawson DG, Grossniklaus HE, McCarey BE, Edelhauser HF. Biomechanical and wound healing characteristics of corneas after excimer laser keratorefractive surgery: is there a difference between advanced surface ablation and sub-Bowman's keratomileusis? Journal of Refractive Surgery 2008;24(1):S90-6.
3. Esquenazi S, Bui V, Grunstein L, Esquenazi I. Safety and stability of laser in situ keratomileusis for myopic correction performed under thin flaps. Canadian Journal of Ophthalmology 2007;42(4):592-9.

32 Topographic and Aberrometer-guided Laser

Amar Agarwal, Athiya Agarwal

INTRODUCTION

Since as early as middle of 19th century it has been known that the optical quality of human eye suffers from ocular errors (aberrations) besides the commonly known image errors such as myopia, hyperopia and astigmatism.[1] In early 1970's Fyodorov introduced the anterior radial incisions to flatten the central cornea to correct myopia.[2] Astigmatic keratotomy,[3] keratomileusis and keratophakia, epikeratophakia[4] and currently excimer laser[5] have been used to manage the various refractive errors. These refractive procedures correct lower order aberrations such as spherical and cylindrical refractive errors however higher order aberrations persist, which affect the quality of vision but may not significantly affect the Snellen visual acuity. Refractive corrective procedures are known to induce aberrations.[6] These are subtle deviations from the ideal optical system, which can be corrected by wavefront and topography-guided (customized ablation) LASIK procedures.[7]

ABERRATIONS

Optical aberration customization can be corneal topography guided which measures the ocular aberrations detected by corneal topography and treats the irregularities as an integrated part of the laser treatment plan. The second method of optical aberration customization measures the wavefront errors of the entire eye and treats based on these measurements.[7] Wavefront analysis can be done either using Howland's aberroscope[8] or a Hartmann Shack wavefront sensor [9]. These techniques measure all the eye's aberrations including second-order (sphere and cylindrical), third-order (coma–like), fourth-order (spherical), and higher order wavefront aberrations. Based on this information an ideal ablation plan can be formulated which treats lower order as well as higher order aberrations.

ZYOPTIX LASER

Zyoptix™ (Bausch and Lomb) is a system for Personalized Vision Solutions, which incorporates Zywave™ Hartmann-Shack aberrometer coupled with Orbscan™ IIz multi-dimensional device, which generates the individual ablation profiles to be used with the Technolas® 217 Excimer Laser system. Thus this system utilizes combination of wavefront analysis and corneal topography for optical aberration customization.

ORBSCAN

The Orbscan (Bausch and Lomb) corneal topography system uses a scanning optical slit scan that is fundamentally different than the corneal topography that analyses the reflected images from the anterior corneal surface. The high-resolution video camera captures 40 light slits at 45 degrees angle projected through the cornea similarly as seen during slit lamp examination. The slits are projected on to the anterior segment of the eye: the anterior cornea, the posterior cornea, the anterior iris and anterior lens. The data collected from these four surfaces are used to create a topographic map. This technique provides more information about anterior segment of the eye, such as anterior and posterior corneal curvature and corneal thickness.[10] It improves the diagnostic accuracy and it has passive eye-tracker from frame to frame, 43 frames are taken to ensure accuracy. It is easy to interpret and has good repeatability. Three different maps are taken, and the one featuring the least eye movements is used. The maximum movements considered acceptable are 200 μ.

ABERROMETER

Zywave™ is based on Hartmann –Shack aberrometry (Fig. 32.1) in which a laser diode (780 nm) generates a laser beam that is focused on the retina of the patient's eye (Fig. 32.2). An adjustable collimation system compensates for the spherical portion of the refractive error of the eye. Laser diode is turned on for approximately 100 milliseconds. The light reflected from the focal point on the retina (source of wavefront) is directed through an array of small lenses (lenslet) generating a grid like pattern (array) of focal points (Fig. 32.3). The position of the focal points are detected by Zywave™. Due to deviation of the points from their ideal position, the wavefront can be reconstructed. Wavefront display shows

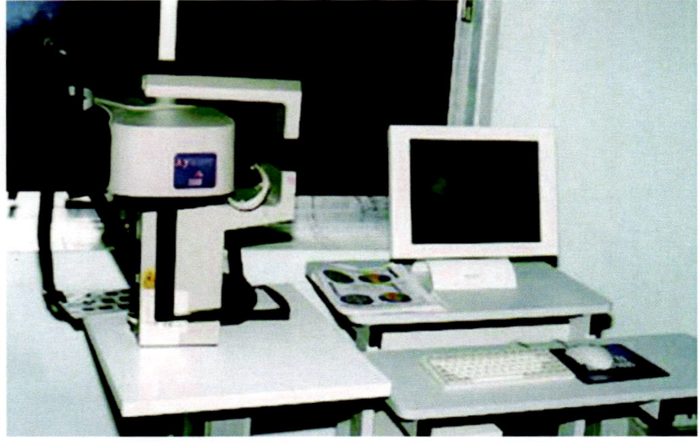

Fig. 32.1: Hartmann-Shack aberrometer

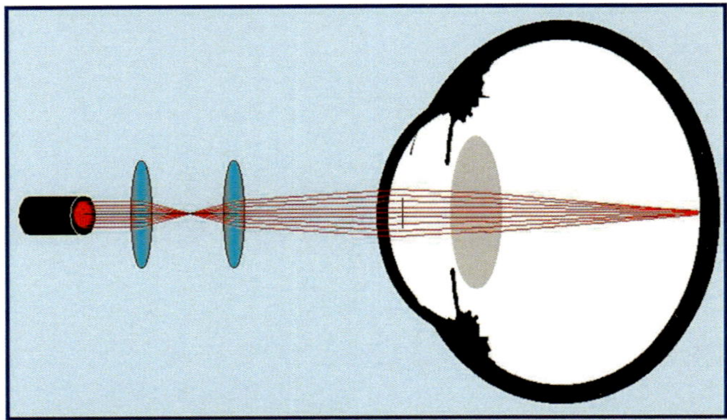

Fig. 32.2: Zywave projects low-intensity HeNe infrared light into the eye and use the diffuse reflection from the retina

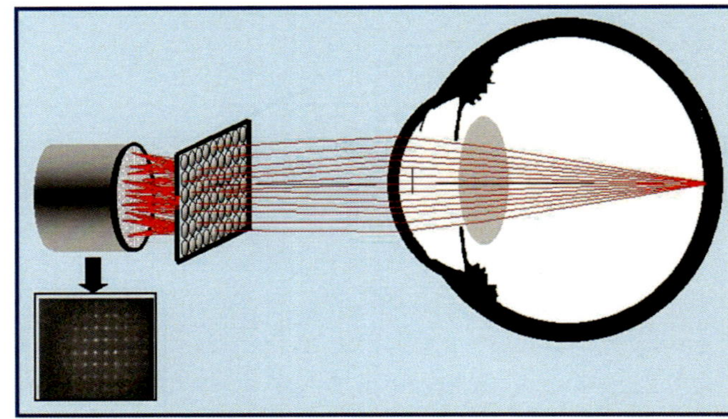

Fig. 32.3: Schematic illustration of the Bausch and Lomb Zywave aberrometer. A low-intensity HeNe infrared light is shone into the eye; the reflected light is focused by a number of small lenses (lenslet-array), and pictured by a CCD-camera. The capture image is shown on the bottom left

(a) higher order aberrations, (b) predicted phoropter refraction (PPR) calculated for a back vertex correction of 15 mm and (c) simulated point spread function (PSF). Zywave™ examinations are done with (a) single examination with undilated pupil and (b) five examinations with dilated pupil (mydriasis) non-cycloplegic, using 5 percent phenylephrine drops. One of these five measurements, which matched best with the manifest refraction of the undilated pupil, is chosen for the treatment.

ZYLINK

Information gathered from Orbscan and Zywave are then translated into treatment plan using Zylink™

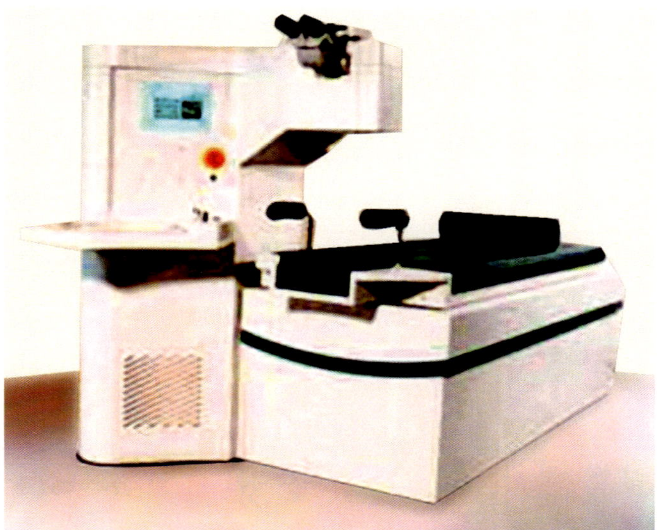

Fig. 32.4: Technolas 217 z excimer laser system

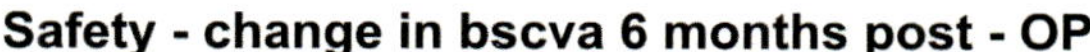

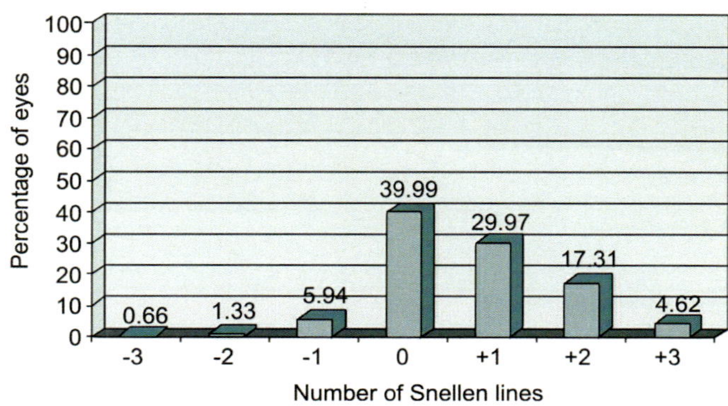

Fig. 32.5: Changes in BSCVA 6 months postoperatively (Safety)

software and copied to a floppy disk. The floppy disk is then inserted into the Technolas 217 system (Fig. 32.4), fluence test carried out and a Zyoptix treatment card was inserted. A standard LASIK procedure is then performed with a superiorly hinged flap. A Hansatome™ microkeratome is used to create a flap. Flap thickness varied from 160 to 200 μm. A residual stromal bed of 250 μm or more is left in all eyes. Optical zone varied from 6 to 7 mm depending upon the pupil size and ablation required. Eye tracker is kept on during laser ablation. Postoperatively all patients are followed up for at least 6 months.

RESULTS

We did a study comprising 150 eyes with myopia and compound myopic astigmatism. Preoperatively, the patients underwent corneal topography with Orbscan II z™ and wavefront analysis with Zywave™ in addition to the routine pre-LASIK work-up. The results were assimilated using Zylink™ and a customized treatment plan was formulated. LASIK was then performed with Technolas® 217 system. All the patients were followed up for at least six months.

Mean preoperative BCVA (in decimal) was 0.83 ± 0.18 (Range 0.33-1.00). Mean postoperative (6 months) BCVA was 1.00 ± 0.23 (Range 0.33-1.50). Difference was statistically significant (p = 0.0003).

Out of 150 eyes that underwent customized ablation, 3 eyes (2%) lost two or more lines of best spectacle corrected visual acuity (BSCVA).

Safety index = Mean postoperative BSCVA / Mean preoperative BSCVA = 1.20 (Fig. 32.5). Mean preoperative UCVA was 0.06 ± 0.02 (Range 0.01-0.50). Mean postoperative UCVA was 0.88 ± 0.36 (Range 0.08-1.50). Difference was statistically significant (p = 0.0001).

Efficacy index = Mean postoperative UCVA / Mean preoperative UCVA = 14.66 (Fig. 32.6). Preoperatively, none of the eyes had UCVA of 6\6 or more and one eye (0.66%) had UCVA of 6/12 or more. At 6 months postoperatively, 105 eyes (69.93%) had UCVA of 6\6 or more and 126 eyes (83.91%) had UCVA of 6/12 or more.

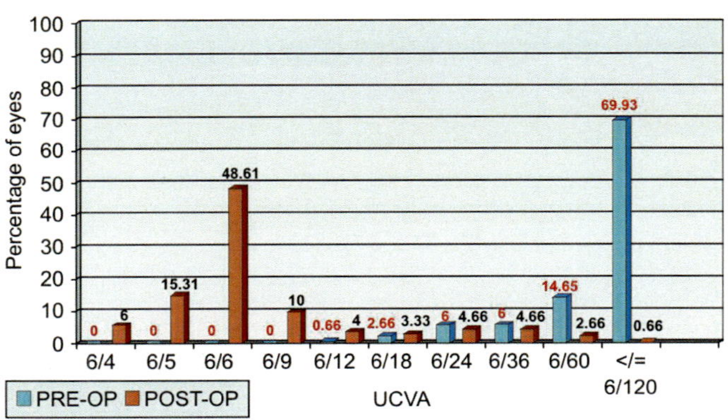

Fig. 32.6: Compares pre- and postoperative UCVA (Efficacy)

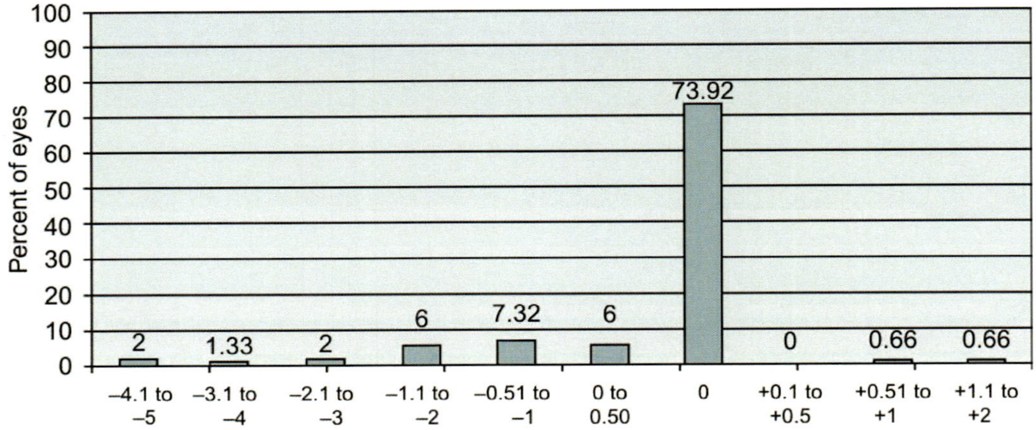

Fig. 32.7: The refractive results postoperatively after 6 months

Mean preoperative spherical equivalent was –5.25 D ± 1.68 D (Range –0.87 D to –15 D). Mean postoperative spherical equivalent (6 months) was –0.36 D ± 0.931 D (Range –4.25 D to +1.25). Difference between the two was statistically significant ($p< 0.05$) (Fig. 32.7). 132 eyes (87.91%) were within ±1.00 D of emmetropia while 120 eyes (79.92%) were within ± 0.05 D of emmetropia. 1 eye (0.66%) was overcorrected by > 0.5 D and 1 eye (0.66%) was overcorrected by >1D. The mean pupil diameter was 5.1 mm ± 0.62 mm. Preoperatively, 95 eyes (63.27%) had third order aberrations. 42 eyes (28%) had second order aberration alone, while 13 eyes (8.65%) had fourth and fifth order aberrations. Postoperatively, 60 eyes (40%) had third order aberration.75 eyes (50%) had second order alone while 15 eyes (10%) had higher order aberrations.

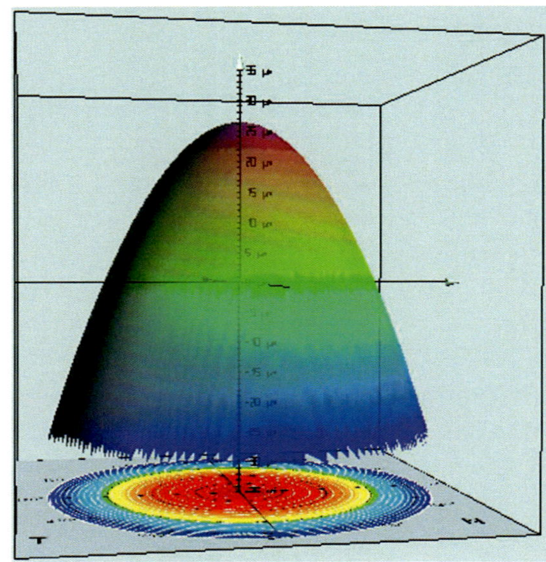

Fig. 32.8: Second order sphere

DISCUSSION

Hartmann–Shack wavefront sensor was first used by Liang and colleagues to detect ocular aberrations.[11] They applied an adaptive optics deformable mirror to correct the lower and higher order aberrations of the eye. They reported a 6 times increase in contrast sensitivity to high spatial frequency when the pupil was large. This study demonstrated that correction of higher order aberrations could lead to supernormal vision in normal eyes. Figures 32.8 to 32.10 show various aberrations.

In our series, using Zyoptix and Technolas 217 system, which is wavefront and corneal topography guided, we yielded results that are comparable to standard LASIK procedure[12]. In a series of 347 eyes, McDonald et al [12] reported a postoperative refraction of –0.29 ± 0.45 D (–0.36 ± 0.93 D in our series) with standard LASIK. 57 percent of the eyes in their series had postoperative UCVA of ≥ 6/6. In our study, 70 percent of the eyes had UCVA of ≥ 6/6, six months postoperatively.

Higher order aberrations were reduced postoperatively in our study. Third-order aberration

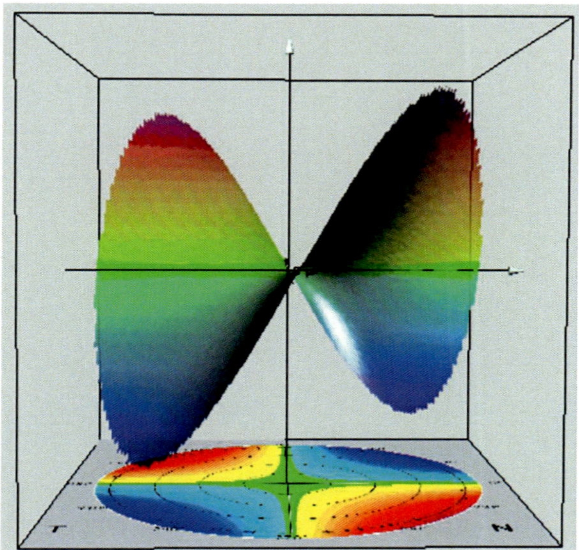

Fig. 32.9: Second order astigmatism

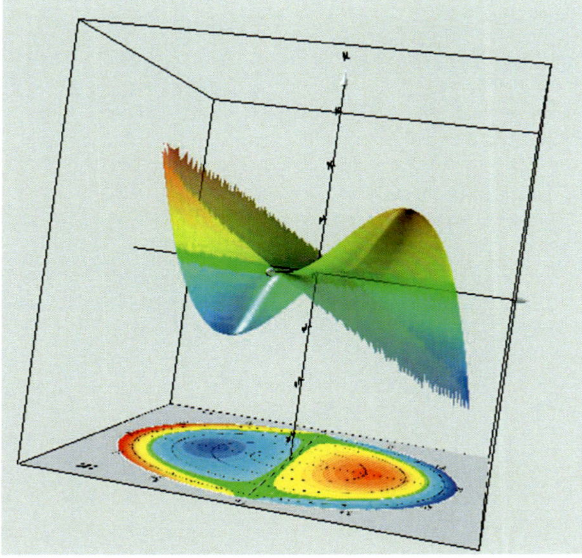

Fig. 32.10: Third order coma

(coma) was most common in our series, followed by second-order (defocus and astigmatism) and fourth-order (spherical aberration). Postoperatively, after 6 months, there was considerable decrease in third-order and fourth-order aberrations. While most of the eyes had only defocus and astigmatism (i.e. second-order aberration). A slight increase in fourth-order aberration (spherical) was noted. Spherical aberration is known to increase after LASIK.[13-15] Roberts has reported that cornea changes its shape in response to ablation and this change, along with wound healing effects have to be taken into account before customized correction can nullify higher-order aberrations. Roberts and coworkers suggest that increase in spherical aberrations following LASIK may be caused by a biomechanically induced steepening and thickening that may occur in mid periphery of the cornea.[13] MacRae and coworkers have reported that simply creating a LASIK flap increases higher-order aberrations in unpredictable manner.[14] They suggest that improved results can be obtained using a surface ablation such as PRK or LASEK, or by doing a two-stage LASIK, with the second stage adjusting for the aberration created by the flap and initial ablation.

Scotopic visual complaints have been the bugbear of LASIK procedures, ranging from mild annoyance to server optical disability.[16,17] Nighttime starbursts, reduced contrast sensitivity and haloes are the most common complaints. [16,17] Spherical aberration that is induced during LASIK may account for this scotopic complaints.[14] Pupil diameter is another factor that is important. When pupil diameter is large, as in young patients, dim light vision is improved after customized correction.[18,19] In our series, 11 percent of the patients complained of haloes around light at night and difficult night driving. In dim light, the mean pupil diameter in these patients was 4.2 mm while it was 5.9 mm in other patients. Smaller pupil diameter and induced higher-order aberration may account for these scotopic visual complaints.

Twenty-five percent of the patients in our series reported improvement in bright light vision, while 40 percent showed improvement in dim light vision. A similar improvement was noted by Cox and co-workers (presentation by Cox IG at Zyoptix Alliance meeting, 2002 reported in *Ocular Surgery News*, July 2002 volume 13, number 7). In our series, treatment optical zone ranged from 6 to 7 mm. Treatment with larger optical zones and transition zones as compared to conventional LASIK may be possible since entire corneal topography and not just the central cornea overlying pupil along with wavefront ablation in dilated pupil are considered during treatment. This may induce lesser spherical aberration post-LASIK and account for improved scotopic vision.

Though we did not measure contrast sensitivity and glare acuity postoperatively, our results suggest improved quality of vision and fewer glare problems with Zyoptix treatment. A more temporal appraisal of the procedure has to be carried out with comparison to standard LASIK. Short-term results suggest wavefront and topography guided LASIK may be a safe and effective procedure which improves the visual performance.

CONCLUSION

Wavefront and topography guided LASIK procedure leads to better visual performance by decreasing higher order aberration. Scotopic visual complaints may be reduced with this method.

REFERENCES

1. Helmholtz H. Handbuch der physiologischen optik. Leipzig: Leopold Voss 1867;137-47.
2. Fyodorov SN, Durnev VV. Operation of dosaged dissection of corneal circular ligament.
3. Binder PS, Waring GO III. Keratotomy for astigmatism. In Waring GO III (Ed): Refractive Keratotomy for Myopia and Astigmatism. Mosby Year Book 1085-1198, 1992. in cases of myopia of mild degree. Ann Ophthalmol II 1979;1885-90.
4. Kaufmann HE. Correction of aphakia. Am J Ophthalmol 1980;89:1.
5. McGhee CNJ, Taylor HR, Garty DS, et al. Excimer Lasers in Ophthalmology: Principles and Practice. Martin Duntz: London, 1997.
6. MacRae S, Porter J, Cox IG, et al. Higher-order aberrations after conventional LASIK. ISRS: Dallas, Texas, 2000.
7. MacRae SM. Supernormal vision, hypervision, and customized corneal ablation. Guest Editorial J Cat Refract Surg 2000;26(2).
8. Howland HC, Howland B. A subjective method for the measurement of monochromatic aberrations of the eye. J Opt Soc Am 1977;67:1508-18.
9. Liang J, Williams DR, Miller DT. Supernormal vision and high-resolution retinal imaging through adaptive optics. J Opt Soc Am 1997;2884-92.
10. Fedor P, Kaufman S. Corneal topography and imaging. eMedicine Journal 2001;2(6).
11. Liang J, Williams D. Aberrations and retinal image quality of the normal human eye. J Opt Soc AM A 1997;14:2884-92.
12. McDonald MB, Carr JD, Frantz JM, et al. Laser in situ keratomilieusis for myopia up to –11 diopters with up to –5 diopters of astigmatism with summit autonomous LADARVision excimer laser system. Ophthalmology 2001;108:309-16.
13. Roberts C. The cornea is not a piece of plastic. J Refract Surg 2000;16:407-13.
14. MacRae SM, Roberts C, Porter J, et al. The biomechanics of a LASIK flap. ISRS Mid –Summer Meeting: Orlando, Florida, 2001.
15. Applegate RA, Howland HC, Klyce SD. Corneal aberration and refractive surgery. In MacRae S (Ed). Customized Corneal Ablation. Thorofare NJ: Slack, Inc., 2001.
16. Holladay JT, Dudeja DR, Chang J. Functional vision and corneal changes after laser in situ keratomileusis determined by contrast sensitivity, glare testing, and corneal topography. J Cataract Refract Surg 1999;25:663-9.
17. Perez-Santonja JJ, Sakla HF, Alio JL. Contrast sensitivity after laser in situ keratomileusis. J Cataract Refract Surg 1998;24:183-9.
18. Applegate R, Howland H, Sharp R, et al. Corneal aberrations and visual performance after refractive keratectomy. J Refract Surg 1998;14:397-407.
19. Oshika T, Klyce S, Applegate R, et al. Comparison of corneal wavefront aberrations after photorefractive keratectomy and laser in situ keratomileusis. Am J Ophthal 1999;127:1-7.

NAVWave: Nidek Technique for Customised Ablation

Masanao Fujieda, Mukesh Jain, Peter Keller

INTRODUCTION

NAVWave is a coupling of two brilliant technologies, to deliver customized ablation for the correction of refractive error. The OPD-Scan® system, combining wavefront analysis with corneal topography to map the aberrations of the entire optical system, is linked with Nidek's unique Final Fit Software to evaluate and convert the data to produce the precise ablation parameters for customized excimer laser ablation of the cornea.

OPD-Scan

The OPD-Scan (Optical Path Difference Scanning System) is equipped with corneal topography, aberrometry, refractometry, keratometry and pupilometry functions within a single device overcoming the potential problems of inter-device misalignment. The OPD-Scan® measures both corneal topography using Placido disk reflection method as well as total ocular aberrations using dynamic skiascopy technology. Dynamic skiascopy currently provides the most direct measurement of any wavefront system without using a lenslet array or the projection of a grid target onto the retina. The technique of skiascopy has been successfully used in auto-refractometers but has now been modified to permit the additional measurement of higher order aberrations. The major difference between the dynamic skiascopy based OPD-Scan® and other skiascopy based auto-refractometers is that the OPD-Scan® can measure the distribution of refractive error in a wider corneal zone as it provides internally with a photo diode array at a conjugate position with the cornea.

A constant-speed single direction slit-shaped infrared ray is projected towards the entrance pupil center as a thin beam and onwards to strike the retina. An aperture and a photo diode array that is conjugate with the retina for emmetropia collect the reflected light from the retina. There are four photodetectors above and four photodetectors below the optical axis. There are also two photodetectors, one of each side, which detect the center of the photodetector pairs. The basic principle is in many ways similar to confocal microscopy in that only the light reflected from the retina that passes through the aperture would reach the photodiode array. How the reflected light reaches the photo diode array depends on the positional relationship between the retina and aperture. We have just said only the reflected light that passes through the aperture will be collected. In case of emmetropic eye, the aperture is positioned on the retina, and when the slit shape light goes across the aperture, the reflected light hits all photo-diode cells simultaneously. Therefore, there is no time lag between different detection time and the time difference should be zero. In hyperopia, the aperture is positioned behind the retina and hence there is a time lag between different diodes detection time.

In the myopic eye, the aperture stop is located in front of the retina. The incoming slit-shaped light bundle bounces off the retina and the reflecting slit moves in an opposite direction compared to the incoming slit. This causes some photodetectors cells to stimulate earlier that the others. By correlating the time differences with refractive errors, a refractive error at each position on the cornea (photo diode position) with respect to the corneal center can be derived. By simple rotation of the measurement system through 180 degrees, the distribution of refractive errors can be obtained through 360-degree meridians.[1-2] The OPD scan also measures corneal topography using a Placido ring method and which has been widely utilized for almost two decades.

Topography and Wavefront Analyzer

The OPD-Scan is a combined corneal topography device and wavefront analyzer. The purpose of laser keratorefractive surgery is to photo ablate the cornea to alter its refracting power, and thereby improve unaided vision. The early systems were effective at reducing primary defocus and astigmatism but often led to increased higher order aberrations. Customized ablation now offers the potential to correct not just the lower order errors but also the majority of significant higher-order aberrations to achieve better vision. Generally, the treatment area consists of an Optical Zone (OZ) and a Transition Zone (TZ). The optical zone plays the largest role in optical performance and should be larger than the pupil diameter whereas the transition zone blends the OZ with the untreated cornea to avoid abrupt changes in shape that are thought to trigger unwanted healing effects. The transition zone is also thought to play an important role in improving visual performance under scotopic conditions as the pupil enlarges, however, it is impossible to design the transition zone from wavefront analyzer information alone without thought to the cornea over relying areas outside the entrance pupil.

A major functional difference between dynamic-skiascopy and Hartmann-Shack type devices lies in the range of measurements capability:

OPD-Scan principle:	Sphere: –20 to +22D,	Cylinder: 0 to ±12D
Hartmann-Shack principle	Sphere: –15D to +7D,	Cylinder: 0 to ±6D

OPD Power Map

The data generated by the OPD are typically displayed in map form showing the distribution of wavefront errors of the entire eye (D). Figure 33.1A illustrates the OPD map of a –4.75 D spherical model eye. In this map, the refractive error at a desired position on the cornea within a 6 mm diameter is displayed. Since the map is of a spherical model eye uncorrected for spherical aberration, the measured errors vary with each concentric zone; the outermost concentric zone being more negative (reddish) than the central zone. In this figure, the terms, Sphere, Cylinder, and Axis have their conventional meaning and are displayed in the middle left for the central zone as: S: –4.75, C: –0.00,

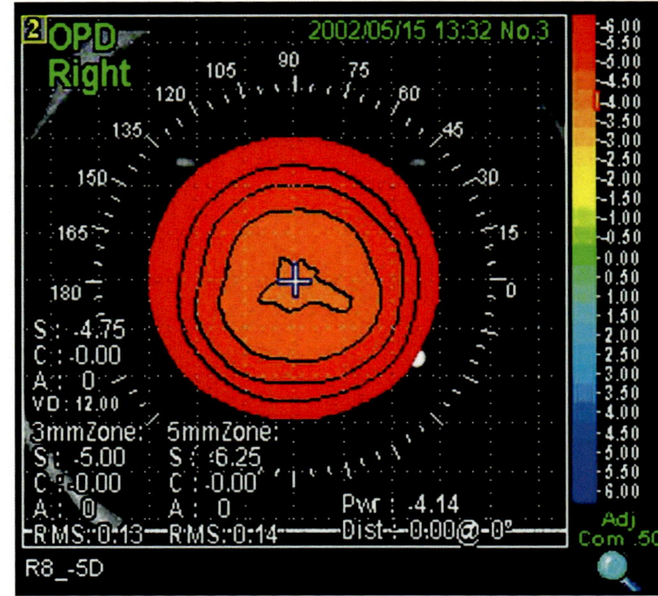

Fig. 33.1A: OPD map of a –4.75 D spherical model eye

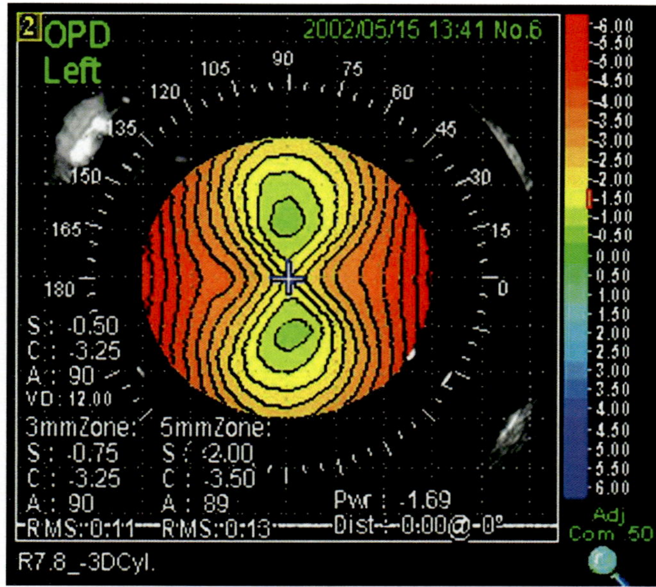

Fig. 33.1B: OPD map of a 3 D cylindrical model eye

A: 0.0. This is repeated for 3 mm and 5 mm annulus zones immediately below the central data and show increasingly negative defocus errors in the periphery. Figure 33.1B illustrates the OPD map of a 3D cylindrical model eye. In this map of with-the-rule astigmatism the steeper meridian (in the 0° to 180° direction) and flatter meridian (in the 90° to 270° direction) are observed as a color-coded butterfly pattern. It is also clear from the map that even in this cylindrical model eye there is significant spherical aberration.

The OPD-Scan® also allows the mapping of various individual aberrations described in terms of Zernike coefficients from the wavefront data. The low-order components (up to 5) that can be corrected with spectacle lenses and some high-order components (6 and higher) can be displayed. Figure 33.2A illustrates an OPD map of an emmetropic human eye. This map is color-coded in three greenish colors for simple pattern recognition. Figure 33.2B shows an eye with myopic astigmatism and Figure 33.2C shows a hyperopic astigmatism eye. The OPD-Scan® produces maps that are easily interpreted, using display techniques familiar to corneal topography maps. Just as computer assisted

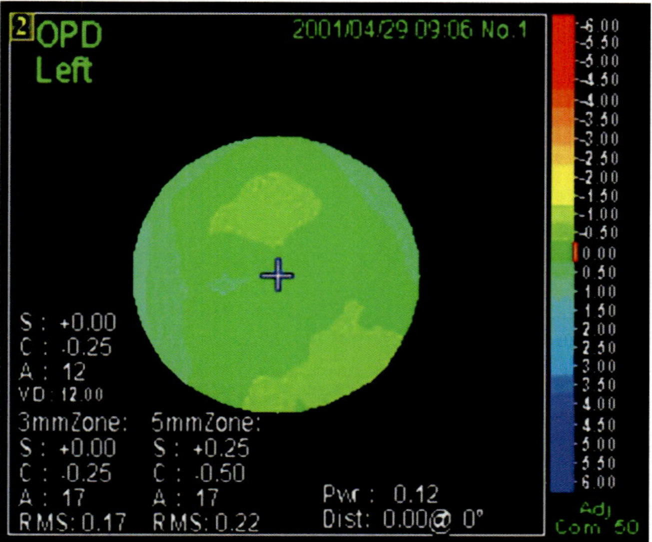

Fig. 33.2A: OPD map of an emmetropic human eye

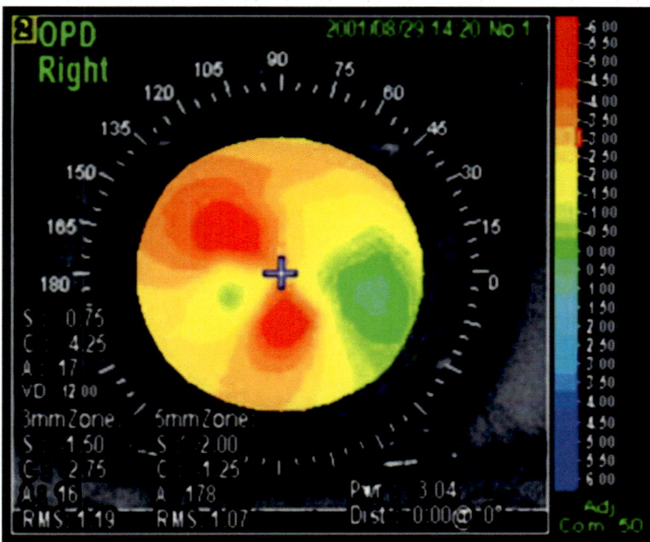

Fig. 33.2B: OPD map of a myopic astigmatism eye

corneal topography devices raised the standard of keratometry, so too do wavefront devices provide us with a wealth of information over and above sphere, cylinder and axis.

In addition, it is easily perceived whether the map has a butterfly pattern and illustrates symmetric or asymmetric astigmatism from the symmetry of the butterfly pattern. The OPD map provides us with more visual and multifactorial refractive information

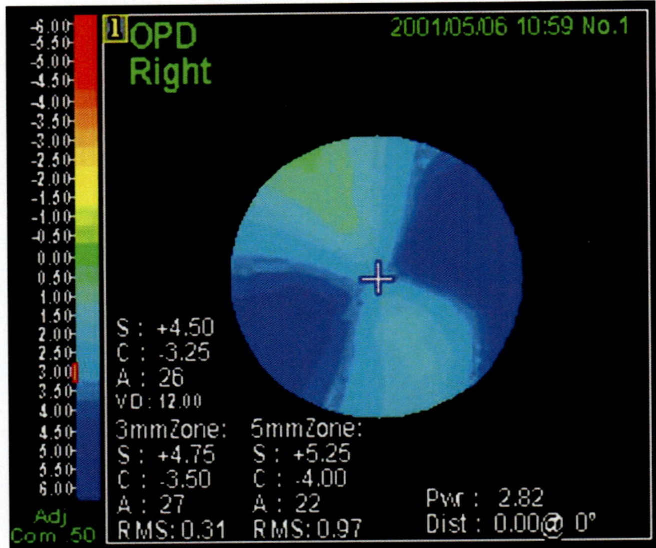

Fig. 33.2C: OPD map of a hyperopic astigmatism eye

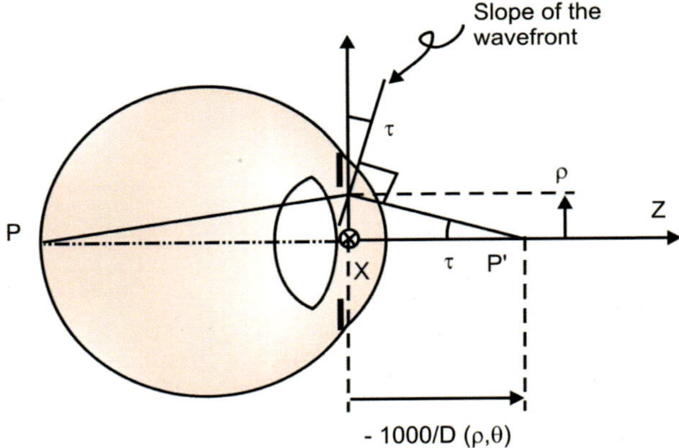

$$W(\rho,\theta)=\int_{\theta}^{\rho}\frac{\partial W(\rho,\theta)}{\partial\rho}\,d\rho=-\int_{\theta}^{\rho}\frac{\rho D(\rho,\theta)}{1000}\,d\rho$$

Fig. 33.3: Conversion between wavefront aberration and refractive errors

compared to a conventional auto refractometer that provides S, C and A data only.

OPD Power Map and Wavefront Map

To explain how the OPD-Scan® measures optical aberrations begins with the duality of light, and that light can be thought to propagate in waves. The wavefront is defined as a plane perpendicular to the direction in which light travels and deviations from the ideal wavefront are termed wavefront errors and these errors tell us about the optical properties of the system. To illustrate this point consider the following diagram, Figure 33.3, of a simplified schematic eye with light reflected back out of the eye from a single point P on the retina. For a perfectly emmetropic eye the exiting wavefront will be a plane wave perpendicular to the Z-axis. However in this case the eye is myopic so the wavefront converges to a point P′ where it intersects the reference axis. The difference in slope between the wavefront and the ideal wavefront allows the construction of the wavefront error map for multiple discrete points. The difference is often described using Zernike polynomials with each coefficient relating to a particular type of aberration such as Defocus, Astigmatism, Coma, Trefoil and so on.[4] Thus, one can tell the type and amount of aberrations that the eye produces. This information is useful for comparing preoperative and post-operative changes in ocular aberration quantitatively.

OPD Map and Cornea Topography Map

This section describes one example in which a comparison between corneal topography and OPD map provides new information. Figure 33.4 illustrates the OPD map of total ocular refraction and the corneal refractive power map among corneal topographic maps for the same eye. The Corneal refractive map illustrates the distribution of corneal refractive powers calculated by Snell's law showing corneal astigmatism of about 2D. The OPD map on the left reveals total refractive astigmatism of 0.5 D at most with the difference being most likely due to crystalline lens astigmatism perpendicular to and therefore canceling the corneal astigmatism of 2D. Quite clearly the full corneal astigmatism of 2D should not be corrected whether it be by contact lenses or refractive surgery. To surgically correct refractive error demands an understanding of both the total ocular refractive status and the corneal surface ensuring a quick and

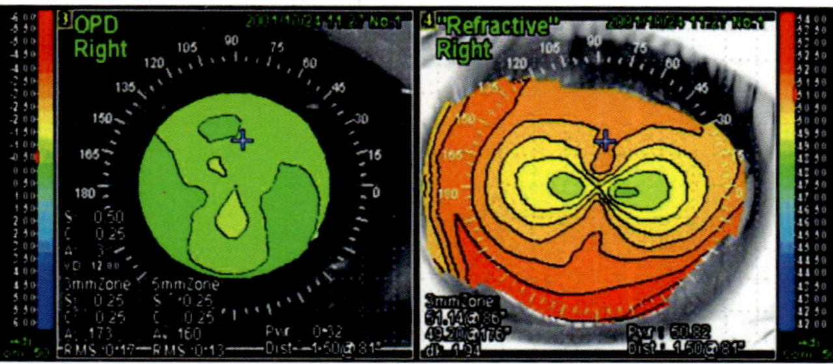

Fig. 33.4: OPD map of total ocular refraction and corneal topography map for the same eye

correct diagnosis. The change in total refraction can be converted into an equivalent change in corneal surface shape and power. The Target Refractive map, method of calculating a shape of ablation, is obtained by adding the ocular refractive error map as measured by the OPD, to the corneal refractive power map. Either of them can be optically calculated from each other, but Axial and Instantaneous maps among topography maps cannot be calculated directly from the OPD map.

Relational expression: Refractive + OPD ≈ Target Refractive

Aligning Topography Data with OPD Data

The abovementioned Target Refractive maps merge corneal information (Refractive) and total refractive information (OPD). It is important to avoid problems due to any change in eye alignment when moving from one device to another when collecting total ocular refraction data and corneal topography data. This potential problem is overcome with the OPD-scan by incorporating the two devices within one instrument. The OPD-Scan® compensates for any positional shift between the refractive map and OPD map by determining the location of the first Purkinje images its reference point.

Measurement of Pupillary Diameter

The OPD-Scan® can measure the diameter and center position for both photopic and scotopic pupils as shown in Figure 33.5. To prevent halos and glare, the ablated area should be outside the nighttime dilated pupil. It would be ideal to compare a pupil image exposed to the laser with photopic and scotopic pupil diameters and respective pupil centers, and to align the laser axis with scotopic pupil center. To avoid halo and glare due to poorly sized optical zones, the ablated area should be larger than the pupil under scotopic conditions.

Final Fit Software: Outline and Features

The Final Fit Software is designed to calculate ablation profile through analysis of both topography and OPD data obtained by the OPD-Scan® and generation of exact laser pulse shot data that control the laser delivery system such as the movable

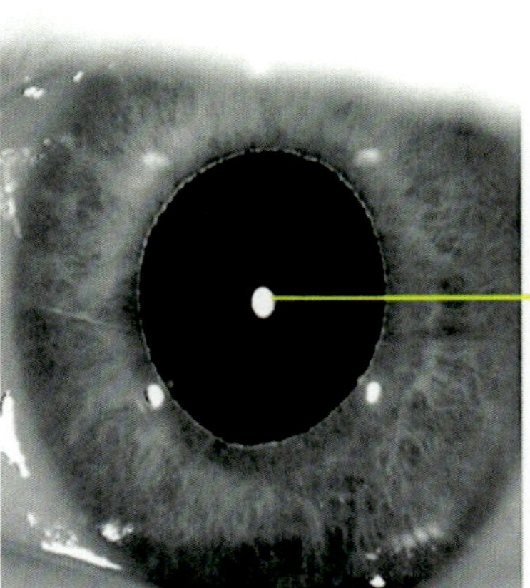

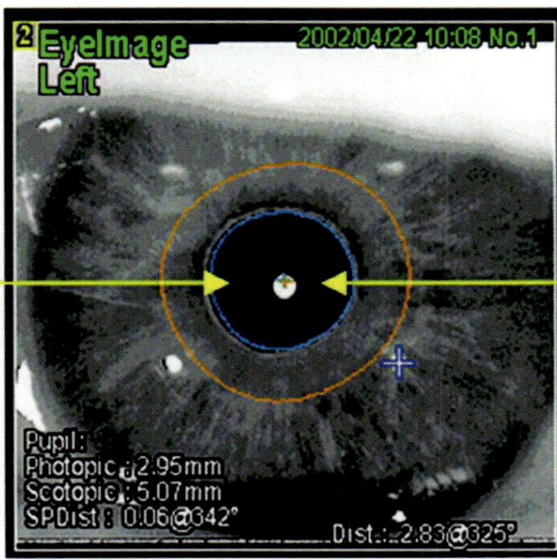

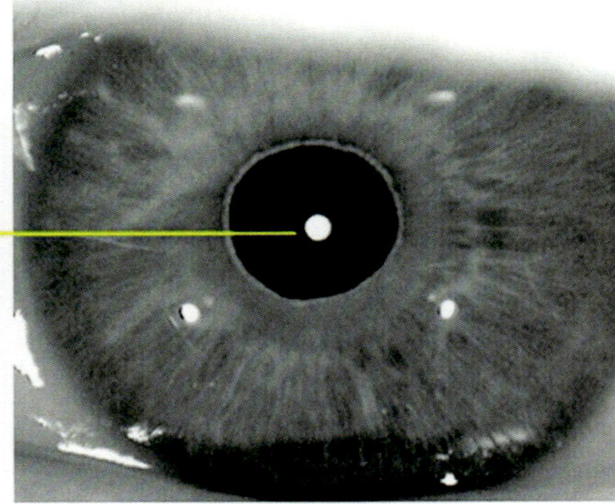

Fig. 33.5: By aligning a bright corneal reflex of photopic pupil image with that of scotopic pupil image, it is possible to display the each pupil diameter, pupil center, and the distance between both pupil centers

apertures with the Nidek EC5000CX II refractive laser. With the Final Fit Software, the ablation profile data are divided into three components, as shown in Figure 33.6, so that they correspond to the ablation mechanism of the EC-5000CXII. Radially symmetric components are ablated by scanning and rotating the rectangular laser beam controlled by the opening and closing of a diaphragm, linearly symmetric components are ablated by the laser beam controlled by the opening and closing of a slit mask, and irregular components are divided into small spots of 1 mm in diameter and ablated respectively, Multi Point Ablation.

The Final Fit software also displays preoperative and postoperative topography maps at the upper part of the screen, allowing the operator to optimize the conditions for operation such as the amount of correction, optical zone (OZ) and transition zone (TZ) for each eye (Fig. 33.6).

Customized Ablation

With the Final Fit software, the following ablation modes are available:

	OZ	*TZ*
1.	Spherical	OATZ * OATZ (Optimized Aspherical Transition Zone)
2.	Topo-guided	OATZ
3.	Wavefront-guided	OATZ

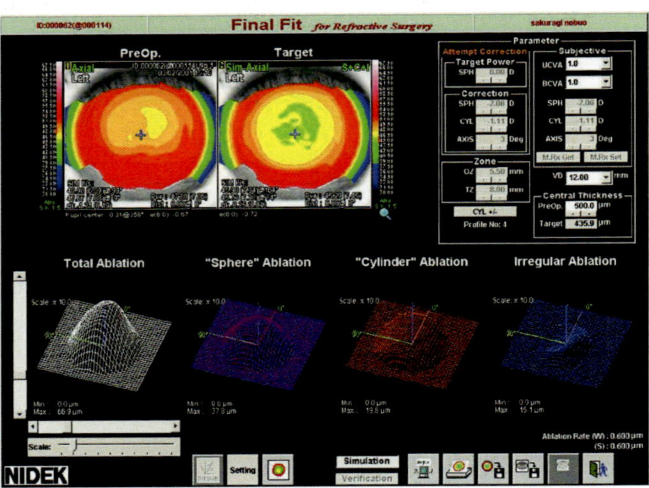

Fig. 33.6: Final fit software divides ablation profile data into three components; sphere ablation, cylinder ablation and irregular ablation

Spherical with OATZ Ablation

Spherical with OATZ ablation allows for customized ablation surgery in the periphery of the cornea to reduce nighttime halo, glare and the possible resultant decrease in contrast sensitivity. With the customized ablation method, spherical lenses and cylindrical lenses are ablated in accordance with the amount of correction in the optical zone (OZ), and the ablated surface is smoothly connected with the non-ablated periphery of the cornea through the transition zone (TZ), This is to reduce nighttime halo, glare and a decrease in contrast sensitivity thought to be caused by abrupt changes in shape in the TZ.[5] The TZ shape can be determined by selecting the appropriate profile in Final Fit Software.

The instantaneous corneal topography map is ideal for grasping subtle changes in corneal shape because the map better represents local corneal shape. Figure 33.7 shows that the position of the red ring representing the area with abrupt change in curvature changes with each power profile. As the profile moves up from a to c, the red ring moves to the periphery of the cornea, increasing the OZ and increasing the depth of ablation.

Topo-guided Customized Ablation

Topo-guided with OATZ ablation allows customized ablation for correcting pathological or postoperative corneal irregularities, such as decentered ablations. With the Topo-guided ablation method the larger irregularities are removed first. This ablation method allows the operator to ablate corneal irregularities with the minimum ablation depth. In these cases manifest refraction results can be unreliable but by removing much of the irregularities and then re-measuring and re-analyze the eye with the OPD-Scan superior results can be achieved.

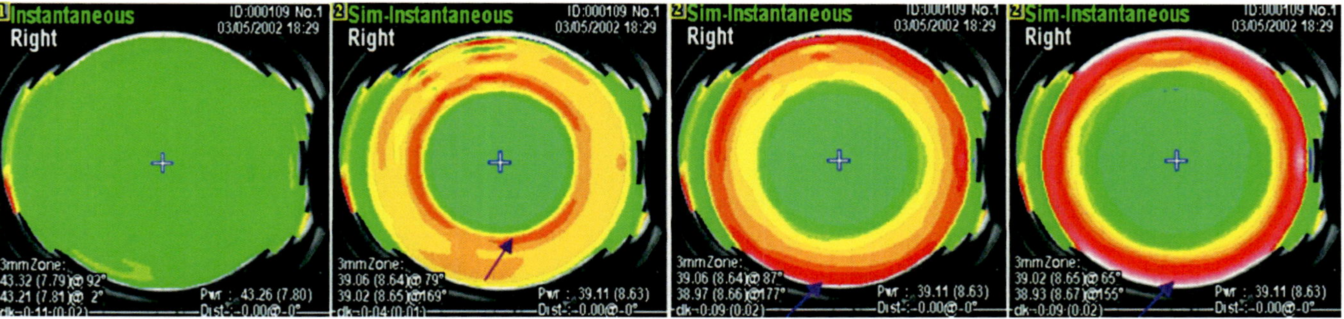

Fig. 33.7: As the profile moves up from a to c, the red ring (indicated by "!") moves outward, the OZ and ablation depth increase. PMMA model eye; Hemisphere, 43.27D (7.8 mm), Parameter; Sph: –5D, Cyl: 0D, OZ: 5.0 mm, TZ: 9.0 mm, Ablation rate: 0.3 μm/shot

Wavefront-guided Customized Ablation

Unlike some other wavefront analyzers, which calculate ablation depth directly from the amount of aberration, the OPD-Scan calculates ablation depth from what is required to change corneal surface power. As mentioned earlier, the preoperative refractive map and OPD map are used to generate the target refractive map, as well as corneal elevation data and the difference between the data used to determine the shape of ablation.

Wavefront-guided ablation allows for the display of an aberration-free area (0D) and to optimize the transition zone. The wavefront-guided ablation method is intended to reduce the amount of aberrations in the entire treatment zone (OZ + TZ). Although the above explanation presumes a target refractive endpoint of emmetropia this can be programmed to achieve various levels of emmetropia as desired, for example –1 D of myopia.

OPD Scan image **EC5000 image**

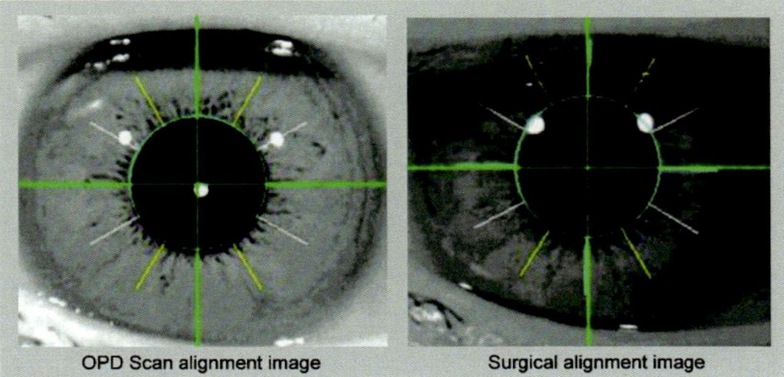

Fig. 33.8: Torsion offset measurement (–12°) calculated from eye images taken by OPD Scan and EC-5000CXII

Features of the Final Fit Software

The features of the Final Fit are listed below:

- Preoperative and postoperative simulated topography data allow an estimation of postoperative outcome (Safety)
- The three ablation modes, Normal (Spherical lens)/Topo-guided/ Wavefront-guided ablation are selectable according to the eye to be operated on (Quality of vision)
- Vision quality can be enhanced by a smooth TZ with an OATZ (Optimized Aspherical Transition Zone) (Quality of vision)
- The comparison function allows the operator to display preoperative, and postoperative topography map, the OPD map, and differential maps (Evaluation of postoperative outcome)
- The topography data of the entire cornea and pupil contour displayed allows the operator to easily check the positional relationship between the treatment area and pupil, and distribution of powers. In addition, the OPD map allows the operator to check the distribution of refractive errors within a pupil. (This is also available with the OPD-Scan) (Evaluation of postoperative outcome).

Correction of Cyclotorsion

Little attention has been previously given to the possible shift of cylinder axis due to cyclotorsional rotation of the eye and many ophthalmic devices measure patients in the upright sitting position whereas during refractive surgery, the patient is in a recumbent position[6]. For this reason, when using the data obtained by the OPD-Scan in corneal refractive surgery, the eye rotation caused by this counter-rolling of the eyeball must be compensated. The OPD-Scan® analyzes iris pattern, pupil contour, pupil center and pupil size by capturing anterior eye images just after topography measurement. The pupil position information is then used for image registration and alignment as part of the Final Fit calculations. The Final Fit Software generates ablation profiles and sends this together with the iris image registration data to the excimer laser system.

The iris image of the patient's eye lying on a bed will be captured by CCD camera installed in EC-5000CXII laser system and then pupil center is calculated. Pupil center will also be determined against the iris image obtained by OPD Scan. Similar distinctive iris patterns will be detected from both iris images. The angle for some distinctive iris pattern will be measured from the baseline, which will go through each Pupil center and the angle difference between both images will be torsional angle error for as shown in Figure 33.8.

REFERENCES

1. MacRae S, Fujieda M. Customized Ablation using the NIDEK Laser, Customized Corneal Ablation. Slack 2001; 17:211-217.
2. Campbell CE, Benjamin WJ, Howland HC. Objective refraction: retinoscopy, autorefraction and photo-refraction. In Benjamin WJ, Borlish IM (Ed): Borish's Clinical Refraction. Saunders 1998;18:594-600.
3. Thibos LN, Applegate RA. "Assessment of Optical Quality" in Customized Corneal Ablation: The Quest for SuperVision. Chapter 6, Slack Incorporated, New Jersey, USA, 2001.
4. Thibos LN, Applegate RA, Schwiegerling JT, Webb R, et al. "Standards for Reporting the Optical Aberrations of Eyes", Vision Science and Its Applications (OSA Trends in Optics and Photonics, Optical Society of America, Washington DC, 2000;35:232-44.
5. Wachler BS, Durrie DS, Assil KK, Krueger RR. Role of clearance and treatment zones in contrast sensitivity: significance in refractive surgery. J Cataract Refract Surg 1999;25(1):16-23.
6. Miller EF. Counter-rolling of the human eyes produced by head tilt with respect to gravity. Acta Otolaryngol 1962;54:479-501.
7. Wachler BS, Krueger RR. Agreement and repeatability of pupillometry using videokeratography and infrared devices. J Cataract Refract Surg 2000;26(1):35-40.

34 Pearls for Successful Refractive Surgery

Guillermo L Simon-Castellvi, Sarabel Simon-Castellvi,
José Mª Simon-Castellvi, Demetrio Pita-Salorio

INTRODUCTION

Pearls for successful refractive surgery may well be one of the most important chapters of all as it intends to outline some fundamental helpful hints and skillful acts in refractive surgery that may improve the result of the procedures previously described, and may help to avoid the most common complications. The authors have included those little secret details that can make the difference between two well-executed procedures, your demanding patient will appreciate.

This chapter has been written keeping in mind that patients always ask for the utmost, specially in the refractive field. They demand for rapid recovery of vision and complete satisfaction. We have learned from our mistakes, and modified our techniques as experience has been gained: we have tried to summarize an experience of more than 12 years in refractive surgery. Most of our tips and tricks are applicable to the most often used techniques, but we will emphasize on the ones that—in our hands—have the best results, i.e. photorefractive keratectomy (PRK), laser-in-situ keratomileusis (LASIK) and radial keratotomy (RK) or astigmatic keratotomies. We will not refer to techniques like epikeratoplasty, surgical keratomileusis, intrastromal rings or intracorneal lenses, epicapsular phakic lenses, and others, since some are too old and others are still too new.

We hope that novice refractive surgeons will benefit from our extended experience, beyond what they can learn at instructing courses. We do not forget that refractive procedures have a definite learning curve, and that we are still on it—things may well change in the close future.

PATIENT SELECTION

Patient selection is the most often underestimated aspect in refractive surgery though it may be the most important one. The main rule is to avoid potentially problematic patients (Figs 34.1 to 34.4). We all know who they are, don't we ? **Whatever the patient pays for the refractive surgery, it is never worth a legal**

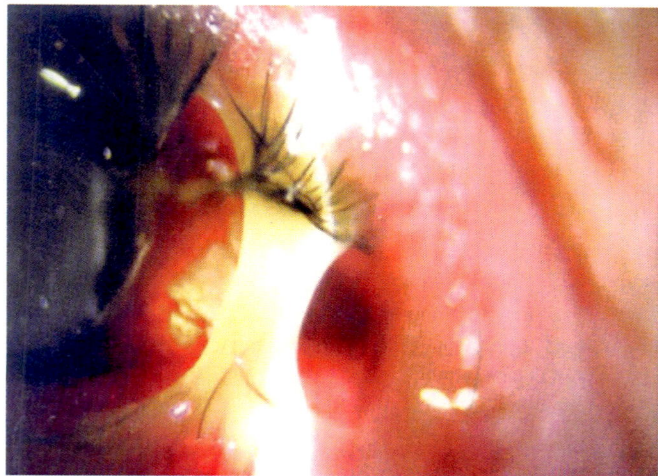

Fig. 34.1: Shows a patient with an acute infection of the eye—infections have to be successfully treated prior to refractive surgery, and conjunctival cultures are strongly recommended before undergoing refractive surgery

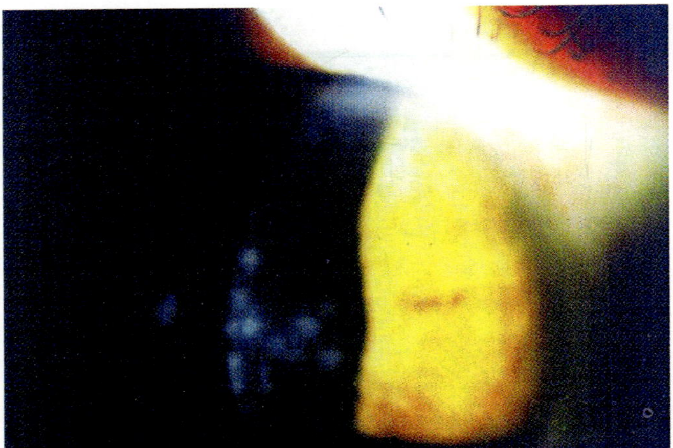

Fig. 34.2: Shows the sequelae of an adenoviral acute keratitis—subepithelial infiltrates will last for months, and refractive surgery is not advisable at this stage

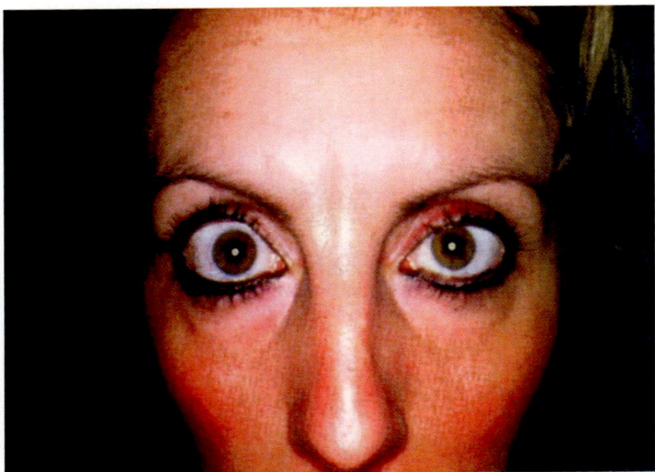

Fig. 34.3: A case of lid retraction: be extremely careful with patients suffering from this disease

process. Keep this important rule in mind, and you will certainly avoid headaches. Obviously, an assessment of motivations and expectations has to be done to determine whether the patient's objectives will be satisfactorily addressed by the surgical technique you suggest. We do not operate a patient before, at least, three consultations. During the consultations, we make sure, and write so, that the patient has well understood every aspect of the surgical technique he or she demands for.

- *Do not operate on patients before detailed instruction and discussion, or without written consent.*
- *Do not operate on patients younger than 18 to 20*—they are often not cooperative enough, the refraction is not stable and may vary with growth. Patients older than 18 do not require, in Europe, parent's permission to sign surgery acceptance.
- *Do not operate on patients with unstable refraction*—should the diopters increase soon after surgery, the patient will imagine his or her surgical procedure was not correctly performed. We always wait for at least 6 months of stable refraction.
- *Do not operate on pregnant women*—their cornea and refraction may vary during pregnancy. You will also avoid accusations if pregnancy problems appear. Wait at least six months after delivery.
- *Do not operate on patients with past history of herpes simplex virus keratitis.* They are like clock bombs—one day, they blast. If necessary start oral antiviral medication a few days before surgery (Famciclovir, 250 mg/8 h, 10 days, PO).
- Try not to operate patients with:
  - *collagen vascular diseases (lupus, rheumatoid arthritis) or severe atopic disease*—corneal healing process may be affected by the illness, and unwanted scars may lower visual acuity.
  - *previous refractive surgery*—cornea may become unstable and ulcers (recurrent or not) may appear. LASIK procedure may be applied on the same eye more than twice.
  - *people in poor health or immunocompromised*—they have a greater risk of severe infection.

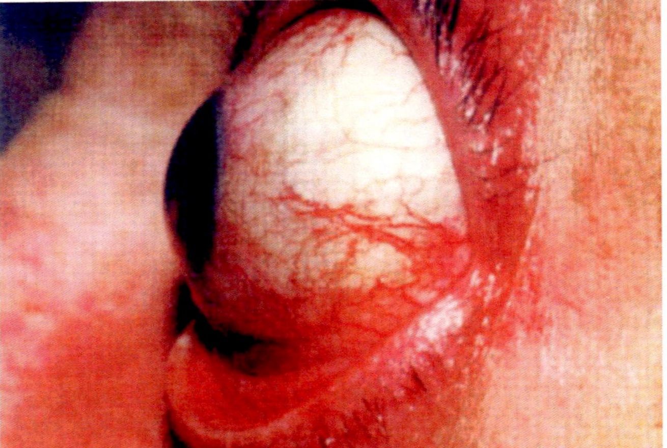

Fig. 34.4: A case of thyroid disease exophthalmos: be extremely careful with patients suffering from thyroid disease exophthalmos—those patients will require extracare, and extra-artificial tear solutions before and after surgery

Wait until they are in good health, if possible. Vitamin and mineral supplementation may help.
  - patients with acute or chronic *dacryocystitis*—make a dacryocystorhinostomy surgery prior to refractive surgery.
  - patients with *severe Sjögren syndrome*. Cornea might never heal.
  - patients with *marked corneal vascularization*.
- Be extremely careful with patients suffering from
  - lagophthalmos
  - blepharitis
  - lid retraction or exophthalmos (thyroid disease)
  - poor blinking.

Those patients will require extracare, and extra-artificial tear solutions before and after surgery.

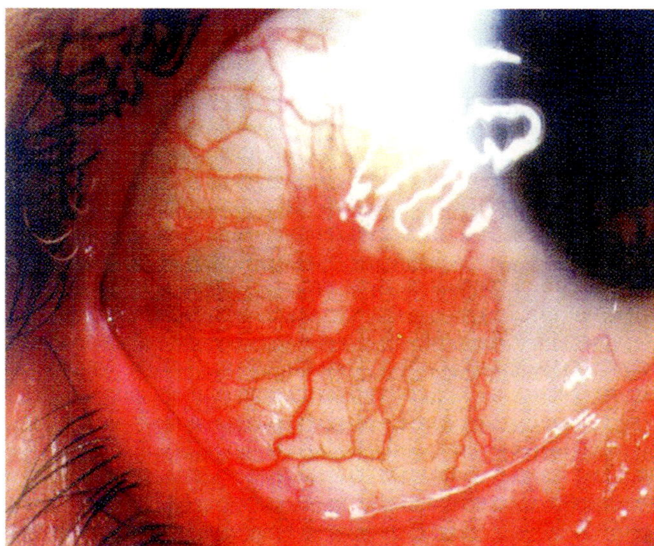

Fig. 34.5: A patient with episcleritis: the disease must be clearly addressed prior to elective refractive surgery

Specials for Autoimmune Disorders

Should you finally decide to treat refractive errors in patients with autoimmune disorders (like lupus, rheumatoid arthritis, scleroderma, Wegner's granulomatosis, polyarteritis nodosa and others), caution is the word to bear in mind. A close follow-up is mandatory.

Patients with low-grade disease may be treated—in an inactive phase of the illness—but bearing in mind that these are systemic diseases, and that ocular tissues are also affected, in various degrees. *Patients who have ocular complications are not good candidates for elective refractive surgery.*

A relatively inactive disease at one point can turn into a fulminating process requiring massive treatment for stabilization—it sometimes occurs just after refractive surgery. In autoimmune disorders (Figs 34.5 to 34.7), the most common ocular diseases are dry eye (secondary Sjögren syndrome), uveitis, scleritis or periscleritis, interstitial keratitis with or without corneal thinning and, more rarely, retinal vasculitis. Corneal thinning in such patients may predispose the eye to a greater chance of perforation—*try to under-correct*, and never go too deep inside corneal stroma. Try to stop topical steroid therapy the sooner the better, to enhance wound healing.

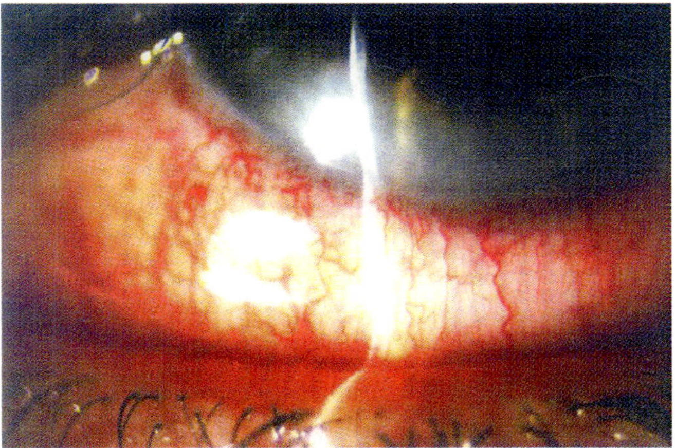

Fig. 34.6: A patient with uveitis: the disease must be clearly addressed prior to elective refractive surgery

Before undertaking a refractive procedure in one such patient, the ophthalmologist must check for all these, and must be aware of the drugs being used to treat the patient, mostly immunosuppressors. *Patients taking strong medication are not good candidates to refractive surgery.* We have to check the posterior capsule of the lens, a subcapsular posterior cataract may have developed as a result of systemic steroid therapy.

Patients with high-dose *steroid therapy* are more prone to ocular infections and their healing is delayed (wound healing is unpredictable). Another drug commonly used to treat rheumatoid disorders is *hydroxy-*

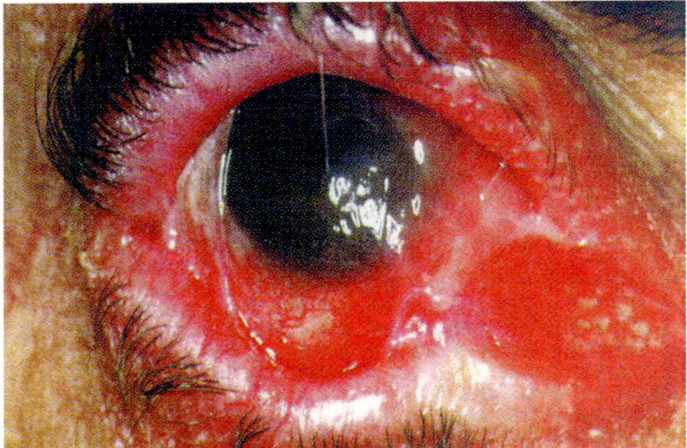

Fig. 34.7: Cicatricial pemphigoid is a chronic disease affecting mucous membranes and is an absolute contraindication for elective refractive surgery

chloroquine—it can cause reversible corneal deposits and macular problems.

Performing LASIK in a controlled lupus patient is relatively safe due to effective current therapies. Discard dry eye, and make a consultation to a rheumatologist to assess disease activity on sedimentation rate, C3 and C4 levels and systemic involvement. Make sure that the patient knows and accepts the risk of an increased inflammatory ocular response. A close follow-up is also mandatory to handle possible complications—try not to operate a patient who lives too far away from your office.

GENERAL RECOMMENDATIONS

- Ask your patient to leave *soft contact lenses (any kind) at least 2 weeks before refraction, and 2 weeks before surgery*. Gas-permeable wearers and *hard contact lens wearers should be out of these lenses a minimum of four to six weeks before measurements and surgery*. Some surgeons ask the patient to leave soft contact lenses only 48 to 72 hours before surgery—we have experienced that 48 to 72 hours may not be enough for some patients. Corneal topography might still change, and so might refraction. We have observed significant changes in corneal topography even more than one month after leaving contacts...
- Do always perform the following tests before surgery:
  - Visual acuity, with and without correction
  - Lensometry
  - Refractometry *with and without cycloplegia—we always correct in between both measurements, and have an increased postoperative patient satisfaction.*
  - Keratometry (manual and automated, if possible), to better assess astigmatism axis.
  - Corneal topography or videokeratography, to *rule out keratoconus*. Patients with keratoconus should not undergo refractive surgery. Flat corneas (< 41 D) make it difficult to perform keratotomy—avoid them, your patient will not be satisfied when reading. Convex corneas (> 47 D) ease the blocking of the keratome pass—test your keratome carefully before the procedure.
  - Measurement of pupil diameter in normal and dim light (using a pupilloscope or a pupillometer). Patients with wide pupils under dim light (more than 7-8 mm, mainly high myopes) should be discouraged from having laser refractive surgery if night vision is essential (like professional night drivers). Their risk for glare disability is increased. In patients with pupils under 7 mm in dim light, we choose flap diameter and ablation zone according to the dim light pupillary measurements—*the wider the pupil, the wider the ablation zone and flap diameter.*
  - Measurement of intraocular pressure (IOP). Any case of increased IOP (glaucoma) should be addressed before refractive surgery, specially before LASIK. *LASIK corneal thinning may artificially lower IOP measurements and make postoperative glaucoma follow-up very difficult...*
  - Pachymetry—take measurements at the visual axis and periphery. Mandatory for LASIK, and for PRK. *We do not perform LASIK to patients with one measurement lower than 500 microns, if myopia is more than 6 diopters. Refuse to treat any patient with corneal readings of 480 microns or*

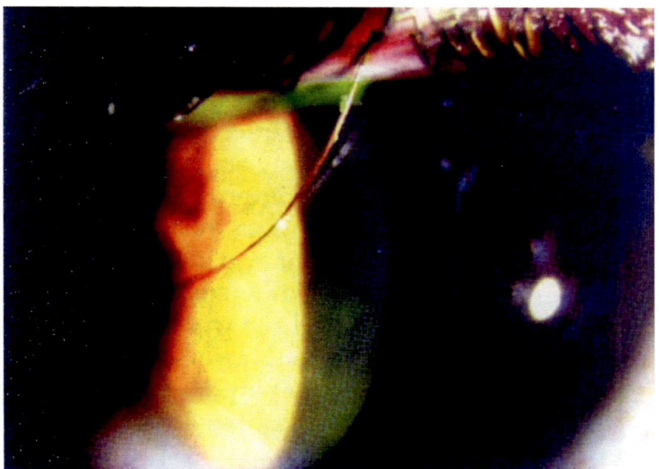

Fig. 34.8: Trichiasis is a condition in which the eyelashes are directed towards the globe and irritating the cornea and the conjunctiva. Epilation provides relief of trichiasis, though may be only temporary. This condition must be successfully addressed prior to elective refractive surgery

less—chances are that the patient develops induced keratoconus in the future (corneal ectasia).

- Slit-lamp examination—rule out any pathology (Fig. 34.8) that may affect or endanger visual recovery or postoperative evolution (postherpetic scars, corneal new vessels, blepharitis, conjunctivitis, ...peripheral corneal new vessels (pannus) secondary to long-term contact lens wearing may increase the risk of a small hemorrhage—stop the use of contacts a few months before surgery: some vessels will disappear and the remaining vessels will be less likely to bleed. Assessment of tear film is also important. Any punctate keratopathy can interfere with the refractive measurements—treat it with artificial eyedrops, and do not perform measurements until the cornea is clear.
- Mydriatic fundus examination, including peripheral retina—most of our refractive patients are myopes, and therefore have increased risk of *retinal peripheral degenerations, that must be prophylactically treated (laser photocoagulation) at least one month (better 6 weeks) before refractive surgery.*

ANTIBIOTIC PROPHYLAXIS: PREOPERATIVE HYGIENIC MEASURES

With the use of different antibiotic drugs and pre- and postoperative preparations and treatment, we can now play an active role in preventing infections before and after refractive surgery. We believe the most important part of any regimen is to prevent the pathogen getting into the tissue or kill it before it grows in it.

As doctors we are treating one patient, and this means that if the patient develops an infection, he or she may have a lifetime of reduced vision, or loss of that eye.

The most common source of infection is the patient's own flora, so we must effectively act over the skin, the lids and ocular surface before compromising the surface of the eye. The eye has a tremendous inherent antimicrobial capability. Nevertheless, if you follow these easy steps, your infection rate will dramatically decrease.

- Instruct your patients (men and women) not to wear *facial make-up* from at least two weeks prior to surgery. Granules in the tear film can create problems such as infections, irregularities of the cornea in PRK, or debris beneath the corneal flap in LASIK. Do not forget that some men are also using make-up!
- Always use pre-intraoperative and postoperative antibiotics. Our current regimen includes *preoperative ciprofloxacin eyedrops,* four times a day, starting three days before surgery. Just before and just after surgery, we use topical *dexamethasone, ciprofloxacin and tobramycin* (aminoglycoside). After surgery, we prescribe topical *tobramycin and fluorometholone,* four times a day. Antibiotics are discontinued one week after surgery, while fluorometholone is progressively reduced. Two weeks after surgery, our patients only use artificial tears. If epithelial toxicity is observed, we do not discontinue antibiotic until the epithelium has healed, specially because of the simultaneous use of topical steroids. We usually prescribe fluorometholone because it has a lower risk of IOP

increase, and does penetrate the eye less than dexamethasone. If dexamethasone extrapower is needed, we also prescribe it.

- We do not regularly use povidone-iodine 5 percent solution into the cul-de-sac immediately before surgery. Although it theoretically makes sense, it also increases the risk of povidone-iodine remnants under the corneal flap in LASIK, and inside the grooves of keratotomies. Povidone-iodine may be irritating to the eye, even at the commonly used dilutions. We do only skin preparation and instill povidone-iodine into the cul-de-sac in patients at higher risk of infections (like patients with chronic blepharitis, and always after treating it). *Avoid the use of povidone-iodine in LASIK surgery except for patients at higher risk of infection.*
- We only use *lid scrubs* in patients with blepharitis. We do not prescribe them on a regular basis, since we believe that bad lid cleaning may "awake" lid bacteria that, otherwise would not lead to an increased risk of infection.
- If there are any mucous or greasy debris in the tear film, *irrigate* this always prior to the surgery, *gently*, making sure you do not damage corneal epithelium. Intensive irrigation creates more potential problems with the epithelium, with corneal healing and with postoperative patient comfort.
- *Draping the lid* may be the most important factor, not only from a visualization standpoint, but also in isolating any bacteria on the lid. We use wide SteriStrips™ to get the eyelashes out of the way. Insert the speculum carefully, to avoid carrying bacteria to the eye. Always *use lint-free plastic dressing*, to avoid contaminant particles. Do not use cotton drapes, since they are not particle-free.
- Do not use *antibiotic ointments* as prophylaxis—its antibiotic component does not penetrate the cornea enough, and they may interfere with healing in LASIK and RK. In LASIK, ointments may induce dislodging of the flap, as they may reach the space under the corneal flap. Steroid plus antibiotic ointments can be safely used after photorefractive keratectomy (PRK)—we have been safely using them in hundreds of patients at the end of laser application, and before applying an eye bandage.
- Everyone in the operating room, should wear a gown, cap, mask and sterile lint-free gloves. For LASIK, we prefer not using gloves.
- We always try to use *the least toxic products*, and to keep the corneal epithelium in the best condition. The overuse of anesthetic drugs may soften the corneal epithelium, that may be easily torn during the procedure, producing patient's discomfort. To keep the corneal epithelium in good condition, in some patients with specially fragile epithelium we prescribe treatment with a *0.18 percent sodium hyaluronate solution* (Vislube,™ Lab. Chemedica,™—Germany, distributed by Thea™ in Spain), two or three times a day, a few days prior to surgery. The drops are discontinued after surgery, until complete reepithelialization. The treatment is then restarted for 1 to 2 months—these patients have a higher degree of satisfaction and comfort.
- One drop of diluted *pilocarpine* 0.5 to 1 percent half an hour before surgery constricts the pupil, easing the centration of suction ring in LASIK, and making the patient less sensitive to the microscope lights.

HOW MUCH SHOULD I CORRECT

The software installed in most of the refractive lasers outside Europe is calibrated for PRK—a personal nomogram has to be calibrated for LASIK. In Europe, the rapid emergence and huge experience with LASIK procedures is summarized in very reliable nomograms for LASIK, installed in the software of our lasers.

For LASIK

After performing accurate refractometry—with and without cycloplegia—*correct in between both measurements*. With our excimer laser, a LASIK procedure can correct up to 16 D of myopia, up to 5 D of astigmatism and up to 5 D of hyperopia, in a safe way. The number of diopters you can correct, mainly depends on the nomograms of your excimer laser.

For PRK

- In mild myopias (< 6 D), we tend to overcorrect 0.25 D.
- On the contrary we slightly undercorrect (–0.5 D) high myopias, to ease near vision. These patients are used to see quite well for short distances.

Experience shows that corneal healing varies with age—we learned this from our cataract patients. Tend to overcorrect (0.25-0.5 D) in young people (20-35 years), and undercorrect (about 0.5 D) in your older patients (35-45 years). Our impression is that the process of healing is somewhat faster in males than in females, though it does not seem to influence refractive results.

LASER CORRECTION OF ASTIGMATISM

Excimer laser correction of low astigmatism is not easy. A LASIK procedure can correct up to 5 D of astigmatism. The following rules may help you.

- *Neglect lens-induced astigmatism* (always very low, except for some cases of cataract, where refractive surgery is not indicated and cataract surgery should be done)
- *Correct corneal astigmatism.*
- *Trust the value and axis of your computerized corneal topographer*, specially if it is in accordance to your subjective readings.
- The software included in excimer lasers in Europe eases correction without having to calculate the spherical component—this step is automatically done by the laser.
- For mild astigmatisms (up to 1 D) we slightly undercorrect, for high astigmatisms we correct 100 percent. Low residual astigmatism is very well tolerated.

LASIK SPECIALS

- The rapid visual recovery and low incidence of eye-threatening complications with the LASIK procedure provides an opportunity to perform simultaneous bilateral surgery. Most of our patients prefer bilateral surgery.
- When you give a LASIK patient a medication, you are going to have a greater likelihood of compromising the epithelium either during or after the procedure. Try always to use *the least toxic products*, and keep corneal epithelium in good condition. Choose fluoroquinolones rather than aminoglycosides and low-toxicity topical anesthetics.
- Start the administration of *topical anesthetic* (three times in 10 minutes) about 10 minutes before surgery—excessive dosing may induce toxic epithelial damage that will produce discomfort after the surgery.
- All of our patients are given *5 to 10 mg of diazepam orally*, 30 minutes before the procedure. Anxiety is dangerous—we need perfect patient cooperation, to look at the fixation light and to be steady during the operation. Hypnotic suggestion to calm the patient is always useful.
- Do always verify the information to be entered into the laser's computer, and also verify it once entered. This point is specially important if you treat large series of cases.
- *Do not completely trust the autotracking* mechanism of your excimer laser (if yours has got it). The low frequency of tracking makes it possible for the patient to do small movements. Good previous instruction is the best way to achieve perfect patient steadiness. This is about to change with the new eye trackers working at frequencies higher than 100 (i.e. 200). When performing ablation, if centration is lost, stop immediately, have the patient refixate, and then complete ablation.
- *Use always the same microkeratome, with new blades*—the keratomes are adjusted manualy, and they are all different. Your jeweller may have to polish the riels of your translational keratome to allow a perfect and smooth pass of the blade. New *rotational keratomes* are better adjusted.
- *Rotational devices*, like Moria's Barraquer-Carriazo microkeratome, *allow the surgeon to select any hinge position and to vary the flap size*. We believe that

disposable microkeratomes will play an important role in the close future as they become truly reliable and safe.

- You need to become familiar with your microkeratome—do not perform LASIK on humans before you have done dozens of keratectomies in bank or animal eyeballs. We suggest the novice to practice the insertion of the microkeratome head into the suction ring.
- Adjust your instruments to have a *corneal flap of 160 microns*—verify that the thickness plate is number 160. Thin flaps may lead to irregular astigmatism, and are more prone to wrinkles and malposition. *For corrections greater than 15 D, use a plate of 130 microns*. Some keratomes are adjustable (like Eye Technology MicroPrecision that may be adjusted by 1 micron steps).
- *LASIK requires a special speculum*. Do not use the speculums you have for cataract surgery—these may force microkeratome malposition and therefore make difficult the full pass of the blade. Choose a speculum that allows easy application of the suction ring, and that does not stand in the way of the blade. Speculum design and lid draping are essential elements to obtain good exposure.
- The list of contaminants—and the way they can reach the eye—is endless. Even when you try to get them out with irrigation, there will be missed pockets of fluid or particles. *We do not use gloves to perform LASIK*—instead, we thoroughly rinse our hands with an antiseptic agent (with no iodine), and alcohol. We use gloves when operating on hepatitic patients, and—at the moment—we do not operate AIDS. *Use only Merocel™ sponges, since they are particle-free*.
- Your excimer laser room should always have the same *humidity rate* and *temperature*, in order to make results predictable. Install an air-conditioner in the room to regulate those parameters—it must have a particle filter to filter particles and bacteria from the outside.
- To preserve epithelium, moisten the cornea with balanced salt solution (BSS) before applying the suction ring and *never do so before performing the keratectomy. Dry the cornea just before applying the ring*. If you have superficial punctate keratitis or hypoxia, the cornea will be thickened, and this will have an influence on your results (with any kind of LASIK procedure).
- We prefer the use of *cold* BSS during the whole extent of LASIK procedures. We keep BSS refrigerated at 5 to 6°C. We believe this lowers postoperative inflammation and flap edema.
- After applying the suction ring, always dry the cornea before measuring the IOP intraoperatively (glass *intraoperative Barraquer applanation tonometer*), make sure that IOP is greater than 65 mm Hg, with meniscus well within the circle of the applanation tonometer. If suction is good, the patient will loose the fixation light—a temporary and reversible blindness indicates the suction is good enough, and IOP is higher than 50 mm Hg. The patient will see the fixation light short after the blade pass (after the end of suction). Never move the suction ring after you start suctioning—if necessary, stop everything, reverse suction and start again. Inadequate IOP rise during suction may result in an inadequate flap.
- Intraoperative surgical events include *subconjunctival hemorrhages* (Figs 34.9 and 34.10) we use strong *decongestants* (naphazoline or oxymetazoline) prior to surgery, starting 10 to 20 minutes before the procedure is done as we drop pilocarpine. They produce constriction of conjunctival blood vessels, decreasing the risk of bleeding (like the bleeding from the pannus vessels). Patient satisfaction is greater if the eye keeps "white" after surgery. These drops are specially useful in long contact lens wearers, where tremendous pannus vessels are present at the limbus.
- *Apply excimer laser on a dry stromal bed*, to avoid variability of the results due to tissue drying.
- One of the most critical steps in LASIK is accurate flap repositioning. After replacing the flap, *thoroughly clean the interface* with *cold* BSS™ and *remove any air-bubble*. Too much irrigation may bring debris from the cul-de-sac into the interface and cause tissue swelling and retraction.

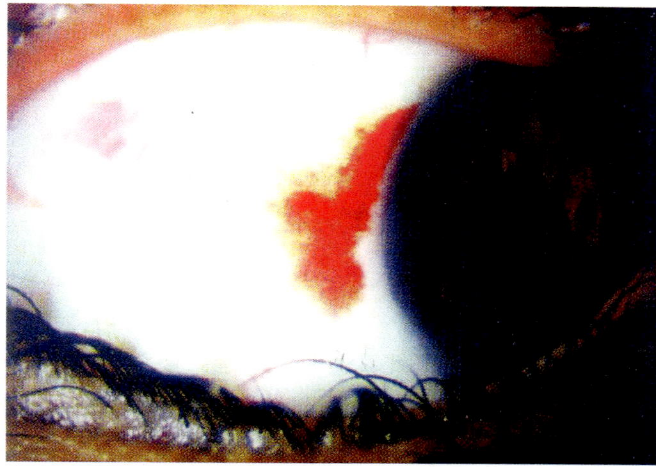

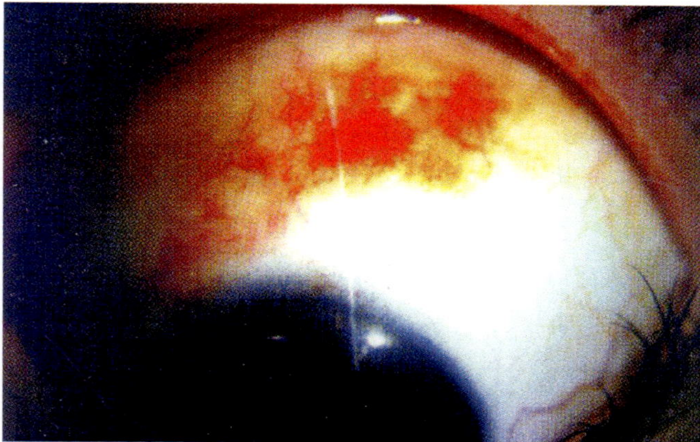

Figs 34.9 and 34.10: Show small hemorrhages as a result of the suction applied with the suction ring of the keratome—notice their localization, close to the limbus, where the ring was placed

After doing so, we use an antibiotic wet Merocel™ sponge to gently *express any fluid from the interface* to increase adherence and avoid microwrinkles. To increase flap adherence, after irrigating the flap we *carefully dry the cornea* with canned Millipore filtered air. By doing so, the flap adheres almost instantly. We wait a couple of minutes for the flap to dry in place, and we verify the flap adhesion by depressing the peripheral cornea with a dry Merocel™ sponge.

- We recommend *minimal exposure of the stromal bed* to external contaminants like debris, foreign materials or contaminants.
- Ophthalmic surgeons should not be averse to delay the completion of the surgery when appropriate—the rule is "safety prevails over business". To avoid patient's anger, instruct your patients that surgery can be delayed at any stage if the surgeon thinks it is best.
- After the LASIK procedure, the patient has to be inspected at a slit lamp to check for flap wrinkles and stromal debris, and to ensure good flap position after resumption of normal blinking. Do so about 30 to 40 minutes after the end of the surgery. Should the flap become dislodged within the first hours after surgery, it can be easily repositioned. These patients have a higher risk of having complications and must be followed more closely than other routine cases. In those exceptional cases, you can use a *soft bandage contact lens* to obtain good apposition of the flap. If the flap dislocation is not reported until the first day after surgery, you must clear the epithelium from the edge of the flap and stromal bed that has been exposed.
- We always examine the LASIK patients about ½ an hour and 4 to 5 hours after surgery, and daily during the first 5 days after surgery. We do control examinations after 1 week, 2 weeks, 1 month, and then every month during six months. The earlier you detect complications, the easier they are to solve.
- If you ever encounter an infection under a flap or in an incision, you must open the epithelium to allow good antibiotic penetration. If the infection is under a flap, we suggest you turn up the flap to obtain cultures and clean the corneal stroma with antibiotics.
- In case of significant over- or undercorrection, a new LASIK procedure can be done reopening the same flap, *two months after the first procedure*. If you wait more, chances are that you may have to perform a new keratectomy, a new flap. Visual and refractive results are to be considered stable one to two months after LASIK. The most frequent reasons for retreatment are: undercorrection, overcorrection, wrinkles of the flap, epithelial ingrowth and shifted flap. If retreatment is needed, do not wait more than three months—the more you wait, the more difficult it will be to treat.

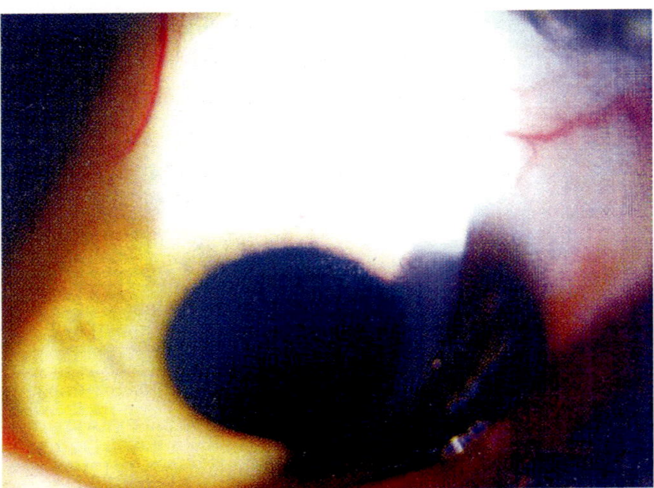

Fig. 34.11: Shows reepithelialization defect at the flap's border (superiorly), that disappeared with good lubrication

- A good LASIK procedure does not either decrease or increase visual acuity—nevertheless *some patients may experience a "one-line" decrease of visual acuity with no apparent cause.*
- After a LASIK procedure, *patient's comfort is increased by the use of artificial tear solution up to two months after surgery.* We prescribe preservative-free drops, for increased degree of comfort. After LASIK, good corneal lubrication is essential to help alleviate discomfort and maintain integrity of the surface epithelium, thus, avoiding complications (Figs 34.11 and 34.12). Our best experience is with polyvinyl alcohol (PVA) 1.4 percent, although any of the currently available commercial preparations may help.

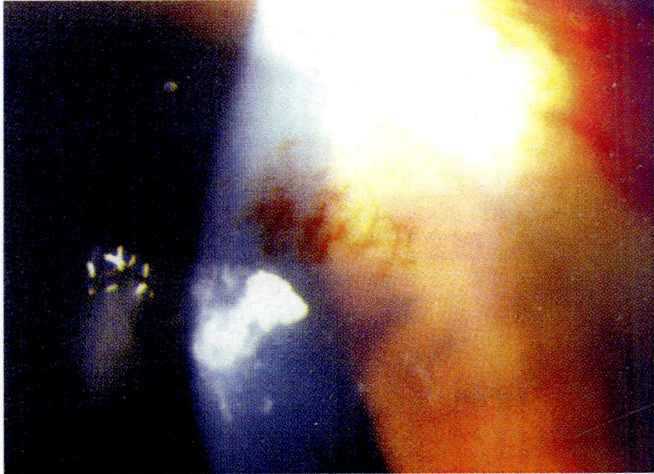

Fig. 34.12: Shows calcium deposits on an ulceration of the flap and new vessels growing towards the flap edge, very uncomfortable to the patient

- *Epithelial ingrowth* is very rare, but may happen, specially in dislocated flaps or in cases with not uniform keratome blade pass. This epithelium has to be removed successfully to avoid further complications. Since most complications of LASIK are related to the use of the keratome, the ophthalmic refractive surgeon needs to develop skills and expertise in the use of this instrument.
- Change the gas bottle as soon as your laser requests it, or when calibration of the laser shows the need to do so—trying to artificially extend gas bottle life may lead to undercorrections. A better visual result is worth the extra cost.
- We suggest you to have a *spare bottle* in the operating room—one never knows when the gas will be over.
- *Which excimer laser should I buy for LASIK?* Not an easy question to answer. No excimer laser is ideal. Some are better suited for low myopias (like Chiron Technolas^{TM}), others for high myopias (like Keratom Schwind^{TM}), some can treat far-sightedness, others cannot, some are really good at treating astigmatism, others cannot do it at all. We would choose a flying spot laser, with a high-frequency eye tracker, not very expensive and with an excellent technical service. Be suspicious of the salesman, and always compare.

Special Care of LASIK Instrumentation

- Follow your manufacturer's instructions for proper assembly of your instrumentation. The microkeratome should be disassembled after any bilateral procedure. We always personally assemble the keratome and test it before each procedure, after laser calibration.
- Carefully *clean and inspect your instruments* before sterilization. Get rid of debris by thoroughly rinsing them with double-distilled sterile water. Any deposit on your keratome surface may prevent its smooth operation.

- Use only soft wipes for head cleaning, like lint-free polyvinyl alcohol (PVA) or Acetal surgical instruments wipes. You can also use a soft toothbrush.
- After careful double cleaning (clean twice), *instruments should be dried quickly* with filtered canned air to prevent water spots and mineral stains (that may suprisingly appear despite the use of double-distilled water).
- Instruments should preferably be made sterile with *ethylene oxide*, to avoid rust from autoclave. You may have experienced that even rust-free instruments are not really free of rust—they also become rusty with time if autoclaved. At the end of each procedure, clean the microkeratome and the suction ring meticulously, with double-distilled water to prevent debris and possible future malfunction. Proper care and cleaning is one of the secrets of correct and safe function of the microkeratome. We do not trust anyone for our instruments care. In our cabin, we use steam sterilization (Statim™) with automated instrument drying between patients (cycles of 9 minutes at 135 °C and high pressure), and ethylene oxide cold sterilization between surgical sessions. Do not forget (or artificially shorten) instrument aeration needed for gas sterilization.
- If you *autoclave*, autoclave fluids should be emptied daily. Use only double-distilled deionized water.
- Remember that the use of germicides (like Instrunet™) is possible though may result in corrosion of the instrument's surface. If you use them, make sure to rinse very thoroughly after taking the instrument out of the germicide bath.
- *Never recycle the blades*—the same blade can be used for both eyes of a same patient, if a bilateral procedure is done. After using the blades, throw them away in a special needle container. Recycled blades increase the risk of infections, and the risk of intrastromal corneal metallic debris. Recycled blades are never sharp. A better visual result is worth the extra-cost.
- *Inspect the edge of the blade* under the microscope to detect any irregularity.
- *Calibrate* your excimer laser *before every procedure*—ablate the Kodak Wratten filter and/or PMMA (Polymethylmethacrylate) disk as taught by the manufacturer of your laser. Remember that each laser manufacturer has its specific technique to calibrate the laser (refer to the manufacturer's instructions).
- During your training period, do not use the keratome on any material other than ocular tissue. Harder material may seriously damage your expensive microkeratome.
- Do not forget that your surgical *applanation tonometer can only be made sterile by using disinfecting soap*—applanator lenses neither do admit steam sterilization nor surface alcohol wipe!
- After cleaning, sterilizing and packaging, carefully *store your instruments in a moisture-free area*.

PRK AND LASIK SPECIALS

- *Have your laser checked on a regular basis*—the effects of a noncalibrated laser may be catastrophic. Technicians are responsible for the cleaning of the mirrors inside your laser and for the energy delivered.
- We always do LASIK in refractions above 2 diopters. PRK is being progressively abandoned in favor of LASIK.
- The word "fluence" stands for the amount of energy on a surface (density of energy). A third generation laser should work with energy fluence of about 80 to 130 mJ. Low fluence means less heat damage to the cornea whereas high fluence means higher risk of haze in PRK.
- Try to work at high frequency—the higher the frequency, the shorter the pulses and the lesser the thermal damage.
- Night vision comfort directly depends on the optic zone and the transition zone. The wider the optic zone, the deeper the ablation. *Never choose a large optic zone without a transition zone*—you will only favor night blindness and discomfort for the patient. The optic zone and the transition zone can be established according to pupillometry in dim light. To avoid symptomatic halos, choose a wide

Table 34.1: Optic and transition zone in PRK

PRK	Degree of myopia	Optic zone	Transition zone
	–1 to –4 D	5.5 mm	5.5 mm
	–4 to –5.5 D	5.25 mm	5.25 mm
	–5.5 to –8 D	5 mm	7 mm

ablation zone with wide transition zone. Nevertheless, the following values will suit most patients (Table 34.1).

- *For LASIK, do not use an optic zone lower than 5 mm*—an optic zone lower than 5 mm means high risk of uncomfortable day and night vision, with symptomatic halos. The optic zone and transition zone will depend on your pachymetry readings, in order to avoid going too deep into the corneal stroma. Use the widest optic zone you can (using the new rotational microkeratomes that allow wider optic and transition zones), without going too deep. The wider the optic zone, the better will be the night vision.
- *For PRK never go deeper than 110 to 115 microns.*
- *For LASIK, never ablate more than 50 percent of the smallest pachymetry reading, bearing in mind that the flap is about 160 microns*, i.e. 50 percent of (smallest pachymetry reading minus 160 microns). In some cases, like thin corneas, it is advisable to lower the size of ablation and transition zones to lower the depth of the corneal ablation.

PRK SPECIALS

- PRK was an excellent technique a few years ago, but it is painful, visual recovery is slow and there are many complications. *Try to convert to LASIK*—it is almost painless and visual recovery is very fast.
- Prescribe topical steroids for weeks in:
  - young patients—their healing is aggressive and they are more prone to haze
  - high myopias, where high fluence is used. Thermal damage is high.
  - patients with high ablation depth
  - patients with visible haze
  - patients that will be exposed to UV rays (patients on holidays)
  - retreatments.
- You may lower or stop topical steroids in:
  - old patients
  - low myopia
  - low fluence during surgery
  - overcorrected patient
  - clear cornea
  - raising IOP (try to use 0.25 percent fluorometholone or nonsteroidal antiinflammatory agents)
  - autoimmune diseases with no extraordinary ocular inflammation after refractive surgery
- We prescribe *diclophenac* (Colirio Voltaren™ or Colirio Diclofenaco-Lepori™) eyedrops, three/four times a day to increase patient comfort and control postoperative pain.
- Some patients suffer from a visual acuity loss months or years after PRK, with no apparent anatomic cause. Prescribe strong steroid topical therapy (we use betamethasone, four times a day), and your patient will probably recover visual acuity in a few days. Discontinue the drops progressively. *Corticosteroids are a good immediate treatment for regression*—most times they solve the problem. If regression persists and becomes stable, you will have to decide whether to reoperate or not. *If topical steroid therapy does not work, try manual corneal epithelial debridement* (sometimes it works), and be ready to assume that retreatment may be needed if the degree of residual myopia is unacceptable for your patient.
- Do not be afraid of central islands—they are frequently transient. They may also be effectively treated with a second ablation.
- **Do not be afraid of minor degrees of decentration—they are often asymptomatic. In fact, why do you do topography after PRK if your patient is satisfied?**

ASTIGMATIC AND REFRACTIVE KERATOTOMIES SPECIALS

- Unfortunately, we cannot faithfully trust any published nomogram (optic zone, number of cuts, depth of the cuts,...)—you will have to build your own one, according to your own experience. There are too many factors influencing the final refractive result (sex, age, number of diopters, size and thickness of the blade, sharpness of the blade, corneal depression, IOP, ...). The published nomograms will be a good guide for you when you start. Unfortunately, radial keratotomies (RK) and astigmatic keratotomies (AK) are to be considered unpredictable when compared to the precision of LASIK. RK is being abandoned in favor of LASIK.
- *RK is not an advisable technique for the elderly*—despite the fact that you will treat a larger optic zone and that they need a lower number of cuts when compared to young people, the refractive result is quite unstable due to the lower degree of healing.
- *RK is not an advisable technique for myopias higher than –4 D*. The optic zone will be quite small, thus, compromising quality of vision by favoring glare and halos, specially at night.
- *RK tends to overcorrect*—the most frequent refractive complication is a residual hyperopia. Lindstrom's mini-RK seems to be a better technique, though not the definite one. Short incisions have a higher risk of induced astigmatism.
- *In case of residual hyperopia after refractive keratotomy*, the success rate of reopening incisions and suturing them is about 50 percent, i.e. too low to be satisfactory. In one of such cases, we would do LASIK, not sutures, despite the fact that we do not like the idea of doing LASIK after keratotomies—at this moment of our experience. Nevertheless, our satisfaction is increasing when doing LASIK after keratotomies. In fact we do not like, but do it.
- *In case of undercorrection of myopia with RK*, we prefer to reduce the optic zone (always keeping it larger than 3 mm). Enlarging incisions while making them deeper may be effective from a refractive point of view in the short, but become unstable and tend to overcorrect (residual hyperopia) with time. If possible "enlarge", do not "deepen".
- Use diamond knives—they provide better clean predictable incisions.
- Perform incisions on *dry cornea*.
- Blood should not enter the incision. *Carefully clean incisions with cold BSS at the end of surgery* and do not apply a compressive bandage to avoid corneal edema.

SECTION FIVE

Lens-based Refractive Surgery

35 Mirlex: Bimanual Phaco/Phakonit/MICS: Surgical Technique

Amar Agarwal

HISTORY

On August 15th 1998 the author (Amar Agarwal) performed the first 1 mm cataract surgery by a technique called PHAKONIT.[1,2] In this the cataract was removed through a bimanual phaco technique. It was performed without any anesthesia. The first live surgery in the world of Phakonit was performed on August 22nd 1998 at Pune, India by the author (Amar Agarwal) at the Phako and Refractive surgery conference. This was done in front of 350 ophthalmologists.

The problem with this technique was to find an IOL, which would pass through such a small incision. Then on October 2nd 2001 the author (Amar Agarwal) did a case of Phakonit with the implantation of a Rollable IOL. This was done in his Chennai (India) hospital. The lens used was a special lens from Thinoptx. This lens used a Fresnel principle and was designed by Wayne Callahan from USA. The first such ultrathin lens was implanted by Jairo Hoyos from Spain. One of the authors (Am A) then modified this into a special 5 mm optic rollable IOL.

TERMINOLOGY

The name PHAKONIT has been given because it shows phaco (PHAKO) being done with a needle (N) opening via an incision (I) and with the phako tip (T). This is also because it is Phako being done with a Needle Incision Technology. In Mirlex we are doing microincisional refractive lens exchange.

SYNONYMS

1. Bimanual phaco
2. Microincision cataract surgery
3. Microphaco
4. Bimanual microphaco
5. Sleeveless phaco.

TECHNIQUE OF PHAKONIT FOR CATARACTS

Anesthesia

The technique of Phakonit can be done under any type of anesthesia. In the cases done by the author no anesthetic drops were instilled in the eye nor was any intracameral anesthetic injected inside the eye. This was *No Anesthesia Cataract Surgery*. The author have analyzed that there is no difference between Topical Anesthesia Cataract Surgery and No Anesthesia Cataract Surgery. If there is a difficult case the authors use a peribulbar block.

Incision

In the first step a needle with viscoelastic is taken and pierced in the eye in the area where the side port has to be made . The viscoelastic is then injected inside the eye. This will distend the eye so that the clear corneal incision can be made. Now a temporal

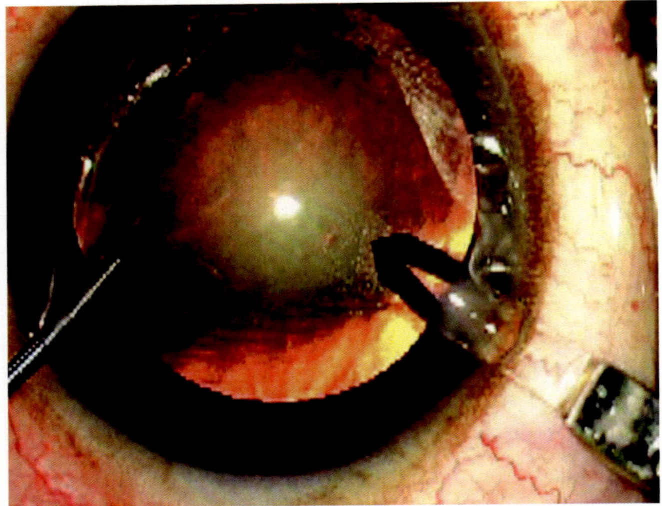

Fig. 35.1: Clear corneal incision made with a special knife (MST, USA). Note the left hand has a globe stabilization rod to stabilize the eye (Geuder, Germany). This knife can create an incision from sub-1 mm to 1.2 mm

clear corneal incision is made. A special knife can be used for this purpose (Fig. 35.1). Note in Figure 35.1 the left hand holds a globe stabilization rod (Geuder, Germany). This helps stabilize the eye while creating the clear corneal incision. The special knife is held in the dominant hand. This knife has been designed by Mateen Amin. It creates an incision of either sub-1 mm or 1.2 mm depending on which size knife is chosen by the surgeon. If one is using a sub-1 mm knife then one should use a 21 gauge irrigating chopper and a 0.8 mm phaco needle. This keratome and other instruments for Phakonit are made by Huco (Switzerland) ,Gueder (Europe) and Microsurgical technology (MST-USA).

Rhexis

The rhexis is then performed of about 5-6 mm. This is done with a needle (Fig. 35.2). In the left hand a straight rod is held to stabilize the eye. This is the Globe stabilization rod. The advantage of this is that the movements of the eye can get controlled as one is working without any anesthesia. Microsurgical Technology (USA) have designed an excellent rhexis forceps for Phakonit (Fig. 35.3). This goes through a 1 mm incison. Those comfortable with a forceps in Phako can use this special forceps in Phakonit

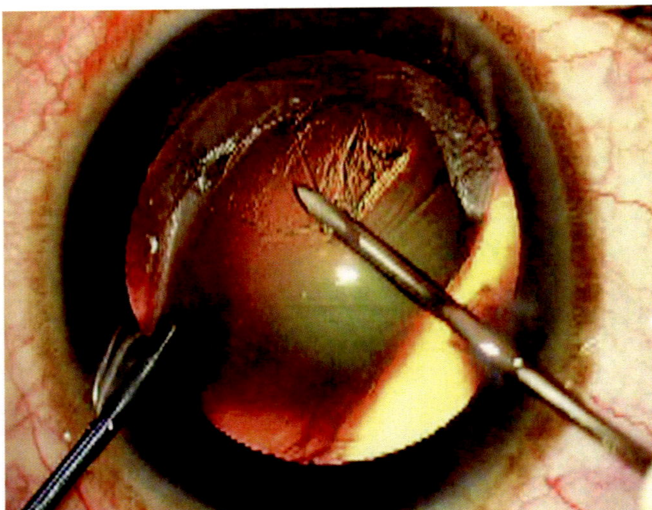

Fig. 35.2: Rhexis started with a needle

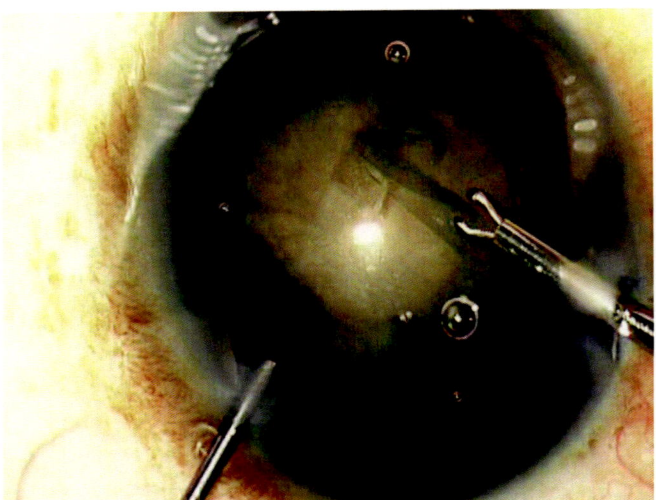

Fig. 35.3: MST rhexis forceps used to perform the rhexis in a mature cataract. Note the trypan blue (Blurhex—Dr. Agarwal pharma) staining the anterior capsule

Hydrodissection

Hydrodissection is performed and the fluid wave passing under the nucleus checked. Check for rotation of the nucleus.

Phakonit

After enlarging the side port a 20 or 21 gauge irrigating chopper connected to the infusion line of the phaco machine is introduced with foot pedal on position 1. There are various irrigating choppers. In

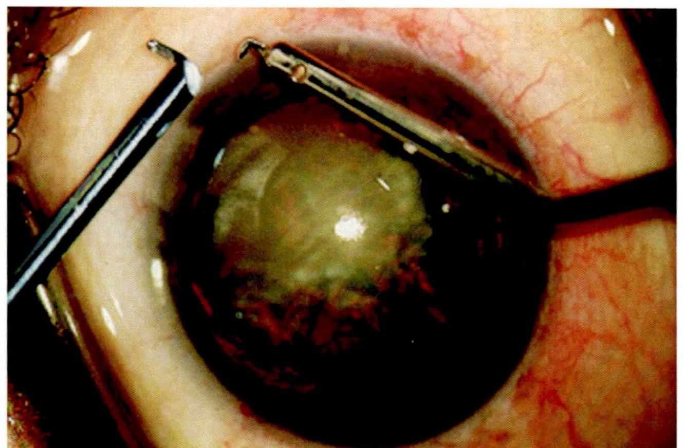

Fig. 35.4: Two designs of Agarwal irrigating choppers. The one on the left has an end opening for fluid (Microsurgical Technology). The one on the right has two openings on the sides (Geuder—Germany)

Figure 35.4 you will notice two designs of irrigating choppers which we have designed. On the left is the Agarwal irrigating chopper made by the MST (Microsurgical Technology) company. This is incorporated in the Duet system. The irrigating chopper on the right is made by Geuder, Germany. Notice in the left figure the opening for the fluid is end opening, whereas the one on the right has two openings in the side. Depending on the convenience of the surgeon, the surgeon can decide which design of irrigating chopper they would like to use.

The Agarwal irrigating chopper with a special design of Larry Laks from USA has been made by the MST (Microsurgical Technology) company. This is incorporated in the Duet system (Fig. 35.5). Other excellent irrigating choppers by various surgeons are present with the same company (Fig. 35.6).

The phaco probe is connected to the aspiration line and the phaco tip without an infusion sleeve is

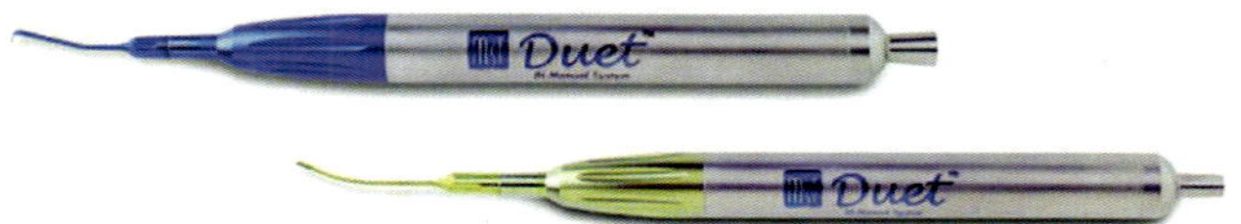

Fig. 35.5: Duet handles from MST, USA. The advantage of these handles is that one can change the irrigating chopper tips

introduced through the clear corneal incision (Figs 35.7 and 35.8). Using the phaco tip with moderate ultrasound power, the center of the nucleus is directly embedded starting from the superior edge of rhexis with the phaco probe directed obliquely downwards towards the vitreous. The settings at this stage is 50 percent phaco power, flow rate 24 ml/min and 110 mm Hg vacuum. When nearly half of the center of nucleus is embedded, the foot pedal is moved to position 2 as it helps hold the nucleus due to vacuum rise. To avoid undue pressure on the posterior capsule the nucleus is lifted a bit and with the irrigating chopper in the left hand the nucleus chopped. This is done with a straight downward motion from the inner edge of the rhexis to the center of the nucleus and then to the left in the form of a laterally reversed L shape. Once the crack is created, the nucleus is split till the center. The nucleus is then rotated 180° and cracked again so that the nucleus is completely split into two halves.

The nucleus is then rotated 90° and embedding done in one half of the nucleus with the probe directed horizontally . With the previously described technique, 3 pie-shaped quadrants are created in one half of the nucleus. Similarly 3 pie-shaped fragments are created in the other half of the nucleus. With a short burst of energy at pulse mode, each pie shaped fragment is lifted and brought at the level of iris where it is further emulsified and aspirated sequen-

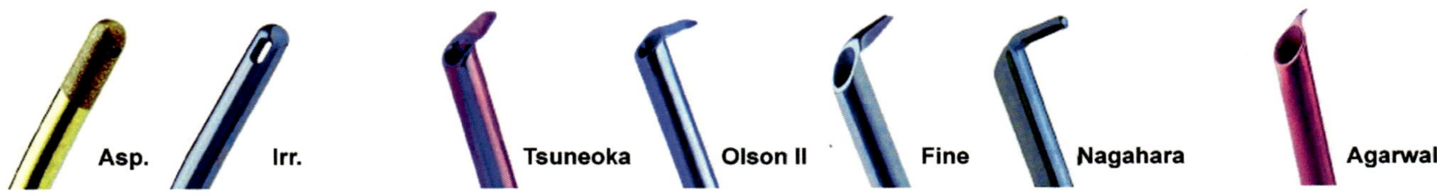

Fig. 35.6: Various irrigating chopper tips designed by various surgeons. These can be fixed onto the duet handles (MST, USA)

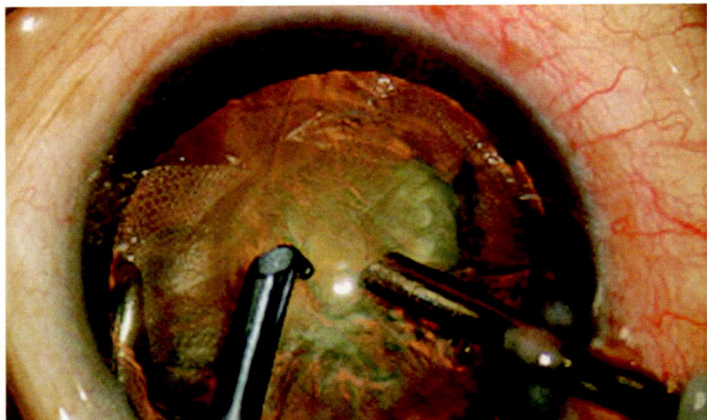

Fig. 35.7: Phakonit irrigating chopper and phako probe without the sleeve inside the eye

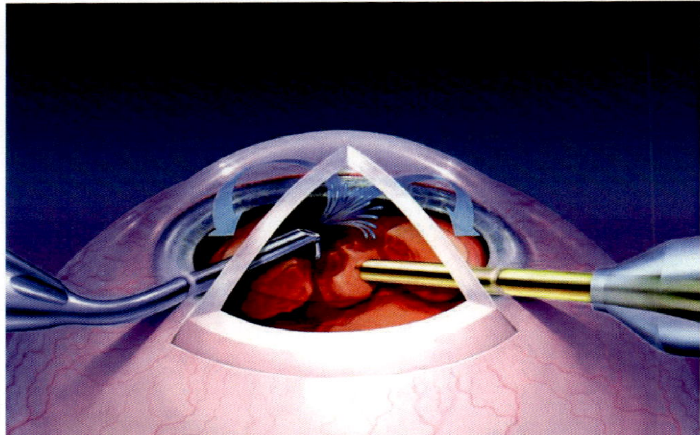

Fig. 35.8: Phakonit done. Notice the irrigating chopper with an end opening *(Courtesy* Larry Laks, MST, USA)

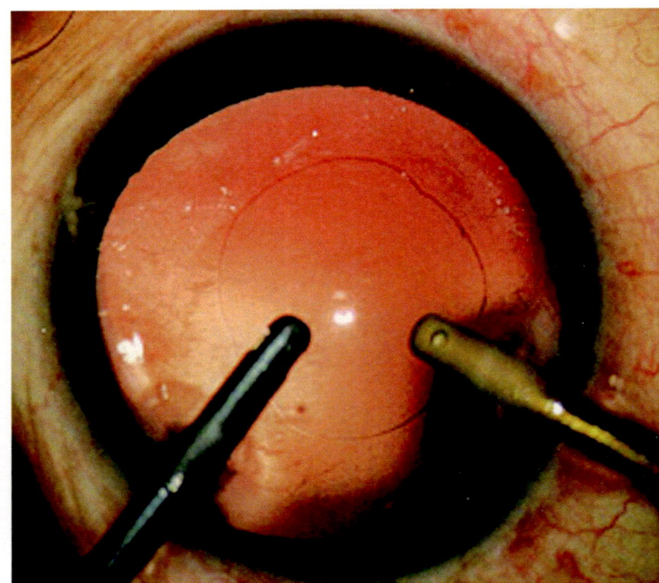

Fig. 35.9: Bimanual irrigation aspiration completed

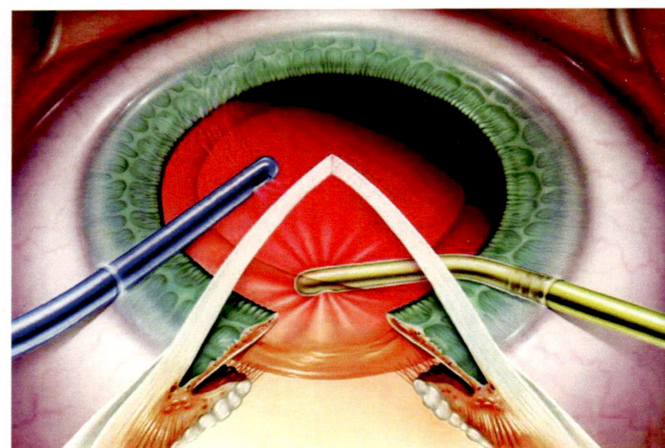

Fig. 35.10: Soft tip I/A from MST, USA (*Courtesy,* Larry Laks, MST, USA)

tially in pulse mode. Thus the whole nucleus is removed. Cortical wash-up is then done with the bimanual irrigation aspiration technique (Fig. 35.9). Microsurgical Technology (USA) have also designed a soft tip IA which is very safe for the posterior capsule (Fig. 35.10).

PHAKONIT WITH CUT SLEEVE

During phakonit another unique problem faced was that of splashing of the fluid from the base of the phaco needle outside the incision during emulsification. This splashing of fluid is due to the fact that the fluid in contact with the base of the vibrating phaco needle during emulsification was churned thus releasing droplets of fluid. These fluid droplets could hamper the surgeons view directly or by getting deposited on the microscope objective.

To eliminate wound burns we should have some way of cooling the corneal wound of entry. This is usually taken care by the fluid that leaks out of the eye from the main wound as the naked phaco needle without the sleeve does not provide a water tight wound. To provide irrigation into the anterior

chamber we use the irrigating chopper through the side port connected to the irrigating bottle along with an air pump specially devised for this purpose. To prevent the splashing of fluid during emulsification from the base of the phaco needle we use the cut sleeve around the base of the phaco needle . We cut the sleeve in such a manner that it covers only the base of the phaco needle and does not enter the eye. Thus we are able to prevent the splashing of fluid during emulsification.

During phakonit surgery fluid is constantly leaking out of the eye from the main wound of entry, as the incision around the phaco needle without the sleeve is not watertight. This fluid is coming from the irrigating chopper connected to the air injector. If we connect another fluid irrigating line the phaco needle with cut sleeve, fluid travels from the base of the phaco needle towards the wound of entry from outside. This stream of fluid meets the stream coming from inside eye at the corneal entry wound causing turbulence and fluid collection in the operating field. This reduces visibility during surgery. Moreover since the wound is cooled internally by the fluid leaking from the eye outwards there is no need for this second irrigation line. More importantly when we connect the second irrigation line to the phaco hand piece with the cut sleeve, the irrigation is always on but we need it only during emulsification. Hence, it is better to use an assistant who could drop cooled BSS at the external wound only during emulsification. So we advocate *"Phakonit with Cut Sleeve with out Irrigation"* to eliminate water splashing during phakonit to improve visibility during the surgery.

AIR PUMP

One of the real bugbears in Phakonit when we started it was about the problem of destabilization of the anterior chamber during surgery. This was solved to a certain extent by using an 18 gauge irrigating chopper. A development made by us (Sunita Agarwal) was to use an anti-chamber collapser[4,5] which injects air into the infusion bottle (Read Air pump chapter). This is an air pump. This pushes in more fluid into the eye through the irrigating chopper and also prevents surge. Thus we were not only able to use a 20 gauge irrigating chopper but also solve the problem of destabilization of the anterior chamber during surgery. This increases the steady-state pressure of the eye making the anterior chamber deep and well maintained during the entire procedure. It even makes phacoemulsification a relatively safe procedure by reducing surge even at high vacuum levels. Thus this can be used not only in Phakonit but also in Phaco-emulsification.

CRUISE CONTROL

The Cruise Control is a disposable, flow-restricting (0.3 mm internal diameter) device that is placed in between the phaco handpiece and the aspiration tubing of any phaco machine. The goal is very similar to that of the flare tip (Alcon): combining a standard phaco tip opening with a narrower shaft to provide more grip with less surge. This has been popularized by David Chang and I Howard Fine (USA) for phakonit surgery. STAAR Surgical introduced this disposable Cruise Control device, which can be used with any phaco machine.

PHAKONIT CAN BE DONE WITH ANY PHACO MACHINE

It is not necessary that only a top end phaco machine is required. The key is to use any machine already present and start Phakonit. The Parameters are:

Power 50 percent phaco power. Start in the continuous mode and once chopping has been done then shift to the pulse mode.

Suction 100 mm of Hg. One has to use the air pump or anti chamber collapser so that no surge occurs. In other words some sort of forced gas infusion has to be used. One can do without it but the problem will come in difficult cases and one has to go slower.

Flow rate 20-24 ml/min

This is what we use for an Alcon or AMO machine.

Phaco needle if one uses a 0.8 mm phaco needle with a 21 gauge irrigating chopper then one can do a sub -1 mm cataract surgery.

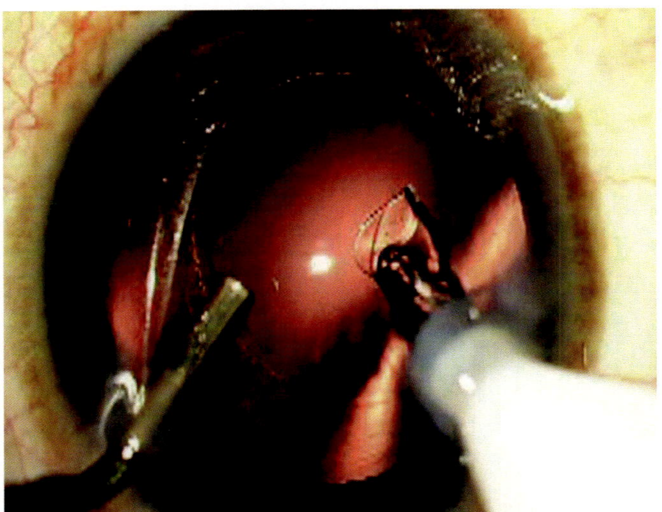

Fig. 35.11: Thinoptx roller cum injector inserting the IOL in the capsular bag

Irrigation over corneal incision. It is better than not applying it. You can feel very safe with it as it negates the possibility of a corneal burn.

THINOPTX ROLLABLE IOL

Thinoptx the company that manufactures these lenses has patented technology that allows the manufacture of lenses with plus or minus 30 diopters of correction on the thickness of 100 microns. The Thinoptx technology developed by Wayne Callahan, Scott Callahan and Joe Callahan is not limited to material choice, but is achieved instead of an evolutionary optic and unprecedented nano-scale manufacturing process. The lens is made from off-the-shelf hydrophilic material, which is similar to several IOL materials already on the market. The key to the Thinoptx lens is the optic design and nano-precision manufacturing. The basic advantage of this lens is that they are Ultra-Thin lenses. One of the authors (Am A) modified this lens to make a special 5 mm optic rollable IOL.

Thinoptx have made a special injector which not only rolls the lens but also inserts the lens. This way we do not need to use our fingers for rolling the lens. In Figure 35.11 you will notice this special injector injecting the IOL in the capsular bag. The tip of the noozle is kept at the edge of the incision.

TOPOGRAPHY

We also perfomed topography with the Orbscan to compare cases of phakonit and phaco and we found that the astigmatism in phakonit cases is much less compared to phaco (Fig. 35.12). Stabilization of

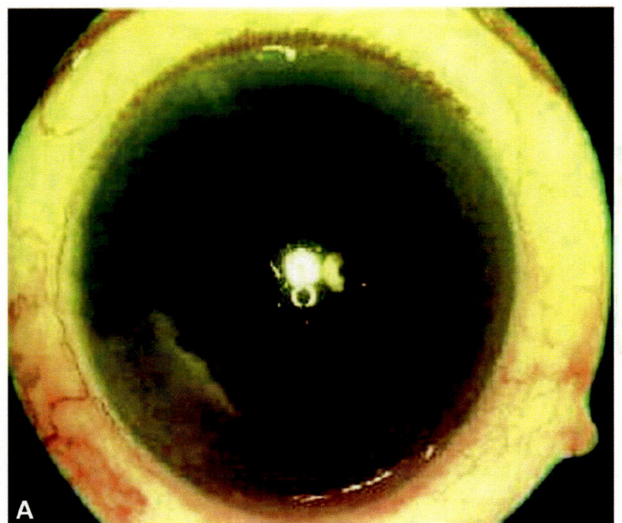

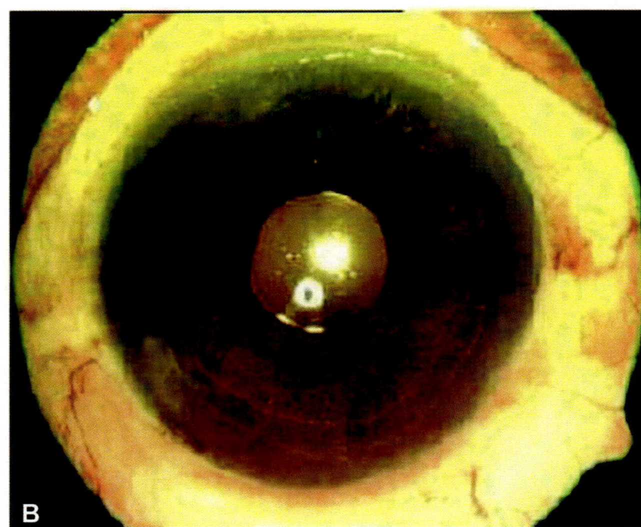

Fig. 35.12: Comparision between phako foldable and phakonit thinoptx IOL
(A) Shows a case of phako with a foldable IOL (B) Shows phakonit with a thinoptx rollable IOL
(*Source:* Dr Agarwal's eye hospital)

Table 35.1: Phaco vs phakonit

Features	Phaco	Phakonit
1. Incision size	3 mm	sub 1.4 mm
2. Air pump	Not mandatory	Mandatory
3. Hand usage	Single handed phaco possible	Two hands (bimanual)
4. Nondominant hand entry and exit	Last to enter and first to exit	First to enter and last to exit
5. Capsulorhexis	Needle or forceps	Better with needle
6. IOL	Foldable IOL	Rollable IOL
7. Astigmatism	Two unequal incisions create astigmatism	Two equal ultrasmall incisions negate the induced astigmatism
8. Stability of refraction	Later than phakonit	Earlier than phaco
9. Iris prolapse-intraoperative	More chances	Less chances due to smaller incision

refraction is also faster with Phakonit compared to phaco surgery. Table 35.1 compares the differences between phaco and phakonit.

ACRITEC IOL

The Acry.Lyc IOL is manufactured by the Acri.Tec company in Berlin, Germany. This lens is a sterile foldable intraocular lens made of hydrophobic acrylate. The intraocular lens consists of highly purified biocompatible hydrophobic acrylate with chemically bonded UV-absorber. It is a single piece foldable IOL like a plate-haptic IOL. The lens is sterilized by autoclaving. The lens comes in a sterile vial, filled with water and wrapped in a sterile pouch.

INTRAOPERATIVE PROTOCOL FOR VANCOMYCIN PROPHYLAXIS

One can inject vancomycin inside the eye at the end of the surgery to prevent endophthalmitis from occurring. For this the intraoperative protocol is:

1. 250 mg vial of vancomycin is taken to be dissolved in 25 ml of Ringer lactate (RL) or balanced salt solution (BSS).
2. This will give a concentration of 1 mg in 0.1 ml.
3. At the end of the surgery, insert 0.1 ml of vancomycin containing 1 mg into the capsular bag behind the IOL. If need be additional BSS/RL can be injected into the eye to make the eye firm.

CONVERSION TO PHACO OR ECCE

While performing phakonit if the surgeon experiences difficulties like corneal edema on table or continuous destabilization of the anterior chamber, one should convert to phaco or extracapsular cataract extraction (ECCE). One should not be egoistic about this as the patient's vision is of utmost importance.

There will be slight difficulty in doing phaco as the side port incision is 1 mm and while doing phaco there will be fluid leakage. In such a case one can suture the side port incision to make things easy. The normal chopper will be able to pass through a sutured side port and there will not be a leakage. While converting to ECCE, suturing of the clear corneal incisions should be done. The ECCE should then be performed as usual from the superior end through a scleral incision after cutting the conjunctiva.

If phakonit is continued with destabilization of the anterior chamber, there can be permanent endothelial damage. Therefore, it is more prudent to convert in such cases.

SUMMARY

There are various problems, which are encountered, in any new technique and so also with Phakonit. With time these will have to be solved. The important point is that today we have broken the 1 mm barrier for cataract removals. This can be done easily by separating the phaco needle from the infusion sleeve. As the saying goes—

"We have miles to go before we can sleep".

REFERENCES

1. Agarwal S, Agarwal A, Sachdev MS, Mehta KR, Fine IH, Agarwal A. Phacoemulsification, Laser Cataract Surgery and Foldable IOL's; 2nd edition Jaypee Brothers 2000; Delhi, India

2. Benjamin F Boyd, Agarwal S, Agarwal A, Agarwal A. Lasik and beyond lasik. Highlights of Ophthalmology 2000, Panama
3. Laura J Ronge: Clinical Update; Five Ways to avoid Phaco Burns; February 1999.
4. Fishkind WJ. The phaco machine: How and why it acts and reacts? In Agarwal's Four volume textbook of Ophthalmology. Jaypee Brothers: New Delhi; 2000.
5. Seibel SB. The fluidics and physics of phaco. In: Agarwal's et al (Eds). Phacoemulsification, Laser cataract surgery and Foldable IOLs (Second edition). Jaypee Brothers: New Delhi; 2000;45-54.
6. Agarwal, et al. No anesthesia cataract surgery with karate chop; In Agarwal's Phacoemulsification, Laser cataract surgery and foldable IOLs (Second Edition). Jaypee Brothers: New Delhi; 2000;217-26.

36 Microphakonit Cataract Surgery with A 0.7 mm Tip

Amar Agarwal

HISTORY

On August 15th 1998, the author (Amar Agarwal) performed 1 mm cataract surgery by a technique called PHAKONIT[1-13] (Phako being done with a Needle Incision Technology). Dr. Jorge Alio (Spain), coined the term MICS or Microincision Cataract Surgery[14] for all surgeries including laser cataract surgery and Phakonit. Dr. Randall Olson (USA), first used a 0.8 mm phaco needle and a 21 gauge irrigating chopper and called it Microphaco.[15-18]

On May 21st 2005, for the first time a 0.7 mm phaco needle tip with a 0.7 mm irrigating chopper was used by the author to remove cataracts through the smallest incision possible as of now. This is called Microphakonit.

MICROPHAKONIT (0.7 MM) NEEDLE TIP

When we wanted to go for a 0.7 mm phaco needle the point which we wondered was whether the needle would be able to hold the energy of the ultrasound. We gave this problem to Larry Laks from MST, USA to work on. He then made this special 0.7 mm phaco needle (Fig. 36.1). As you will understand if we go smaller from a 0.9 mm phaco needle to a 0.7 mm phaco needle the speed of the surgery would go down. This is because the amount of aspiration flow rate would be less.

It was decided to solve this problem by working on the wall of the 0.7 mm phaco needle. There is a standard wall thickness for all phaco tips. If we say the outer diameter is a constant, the resultant inner diameter is an area of the outer diameter minus the area of the wall.

The inner diameter will regulate the flow rate/ perceived efficiency (which can be good or bad, depending on how you look at it). In order to increase the allowed aspiration flow rate from what a standard 0.7 mm tip would be, MST (Larry Laks) had the walls made thinner, thus increasing the inner diameter. This would allow a case to go, speedwise, closer to what a 0.9 mm tip would go (not exactly the same, but closer). With the gas forced infusion it would work very well. Finally, we

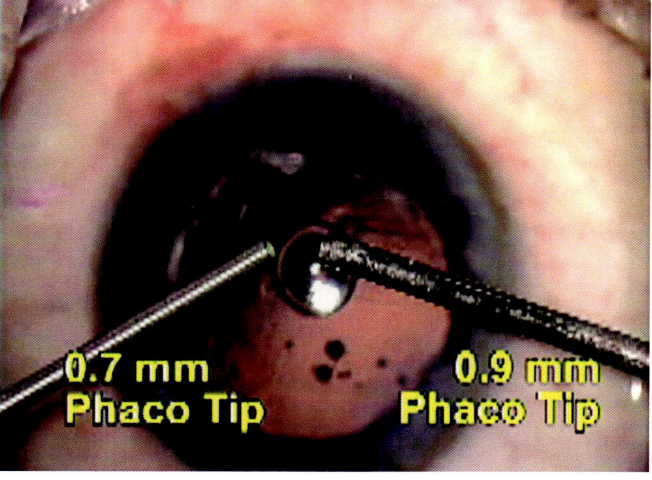

Fig. 36.1: 0.7 mm phaco tip (microphakonit) as compared to a 0.9 mm phaco tip (phakonit)

decided to go for a 30 degree tip to make it even better.

MICROPHAKONIT (0.7 MM) IRRIGATING CHOPPER

There are two designs of 20 gauge (0.9 mm) irrigating choppers which we have designed. One is the Agarwal irrigating chopper made by the MST (Microsurgical Technology) company. The opening for the fluid in this are end opening. This is incorporated in the Duet system. The other irrigating chopper is made by Geuder, Germany. This has two openings in the side. Depending on the convenience of the surgeon, the surgeon can decide which design of irrigating chopper they would like to use. There are advantages and disadvantages of both types of irrigating choppers. The end opening chopper has an advantage of more fluid coming out of the chopper. The disadvantage is that there is a gush of fluid which might push the nuclear pieces away. The advantage of the side opening irrigating chopper is that there is good control as the nuclear pieces are not pushed away but the disadvantage is that the amount of fluid coming out of it is much less. That is why, if one is using the side opening irrigating chopper one should use an air pump or gas forced infusion.

The MST in their irrigating chopper increased flow by removing the flow restrictions incorporated in other irrigating choppers as a bi-product of their attachment method. They also had control of incisional outflow by having all the instruments to be of one size and created a matching knife of the proper size and geometry.

When we decided to go smaller to using a 0.7 mm irrigating chopper (Fig. 36.2) we decided to go for an end-opening irrigating chopper. The reason is as the bore of the irrigating chopper was smaller the amount of fluid coming out of it would be less and so an end-opening chopper would maintain the fluidics better. With gas forced infusion we thought we would be able to balance the entry and exit of fluid into the anterior chamber and that is what happened.

We measured the amount of fluid coming out of the various irrigating choppers with and without an air pump (Table 36.1). We also measured the values using the simple aquarium air pump (external gas forced infusion) and the accurus machine giving internal gas forced infusion.

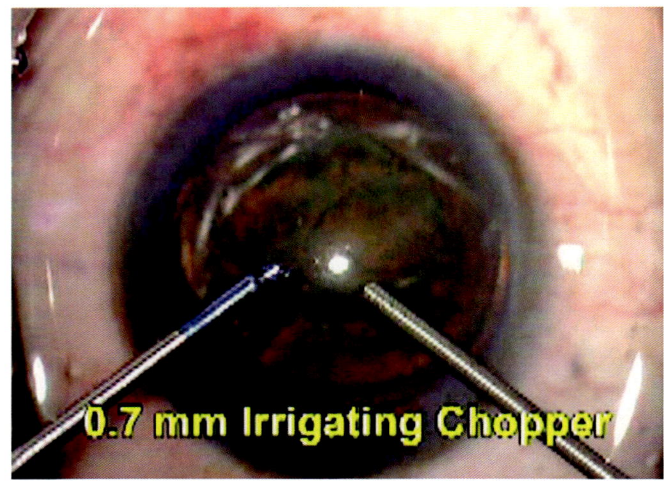

Fig. 36.2: 0.7 mm irrigating chopper

Table 36.1: Fluid exiting from various irrigating choppers (Values in ml/minute)

Irrigating chopper	*Without gas forced infusion*	*With gas forced infusion using the Accurus machine at 50 mm Hg*	*With gas forced infusion using the Accurus machine at 75 mm Hg*	*With gas forced infusion using the Accurus machine at 100 mm Hg*	*Air pump with regulator at low*	*Air pump with regulator at high*
0.9 mm Side opening	25	36	42	48	37	51
0.9 mm End opening	34	51	57	65	52	68
0.7 mm End opening	27	39	44	51	41	54

The microphakonit irrigating chopper which we have designed is basically a sharp chopper which has a sharp cutting edge and helps in karate chopping or quick chopping. It can chop any type of cataract.

AIR PUMP AND GAS FORCED INFUSION

The main problem in phakonit we had was the destabilization of the anterior chamber during surgery. We solved it to a certain extent by using an 18 gauge irrigating chopper. Then Sunita Agarwal suggested the use of an antichamber collapser,[19] which injects air into the infusion bottle. This pushes more fluid into the eye through the irrigating chopper and also prevents surge (Figs 36.3 and 36.4). Thus, we were able to use a 20/21 gauge irrigating chopper as well as solve the problem of destabilization of the anterior chamber during surgery. Now with a 22 gauge (0.7 mm) irrigating chopper it is extremely essential that gas forced infusion be used in the surgery. This is also called external gas forced infusion.

When the surgeon uses the air pump contained in the same phaco machine, it is called internal gas forced infusion (IFI). To solve the problem of infection we use a millipore filter connected to the machine. The advantages of the Internal Forced Infusion over the External are:

1. The surgeon does not have to incorporate an external air pump to the surgical system to obtain the advantages of the forced infusion.

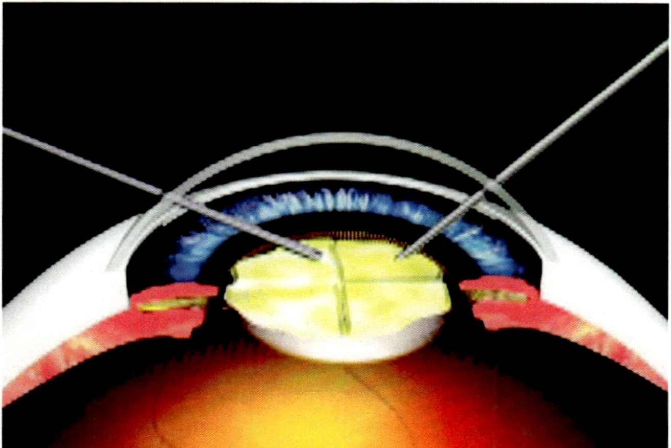

Fig. 36.3: Normal anterior chamber when case is started. Air pump is not used

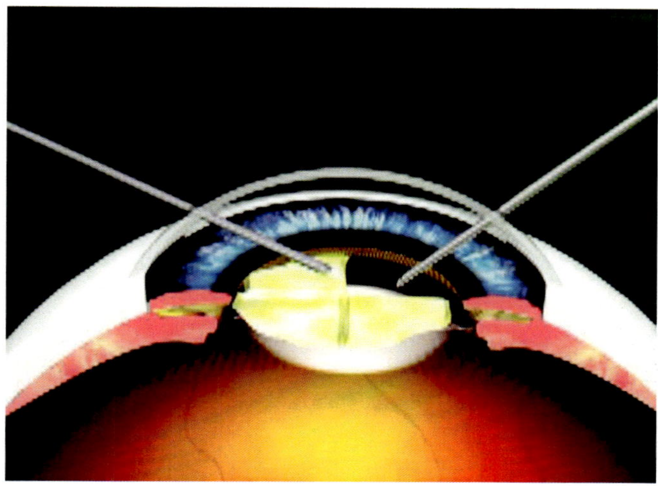

Fig. 36.4: Surge and chamber collapse when nucleus is being removed. Air pump is not used. Note the chamber depth has come down. When we use the air pump this problem does not occur

2. The surgeon can control all the parameters (forced infusion rate, ultrasonic power modulations and vacuum settings) in the same panel of the surgical system he or she is working with.
3. The forced infusion rate can be actively and digitally controlled during the surgery, adjusting the parameters to the conditions and/or the surgical steps of each individual case.

When we decided to use the 0.7 mm MST Duet set we decided to use the internal gas forced infusion of the Accurus machine to measure the pressure of air exactly. This is from Alcon. The advantage by this was that we could regulate the amount of air entering into the infusion bottle and thus titrate the system in such a way that there is no surge or collapse of the anterior chamber. When we are using a 0.7 mm irrigating chopper the problem is that the amount of fluid entering the eye is not enough. To solve this problem gas forced infusion is a must.

The anterior vented gas forced infusion system (AVGFI) of the Accurus surgical system helps in the performance of phakonit. This was started by Arturo Pérez-Arteaga from Mexico. The AVGFI is a system incorporated in the Accurus machine that creates a positive infusion pressure inside the eye.

It consists of an air pump and a regulator which are inside the machine; then the air is pushed inside the bottle of intraocular solution, and so the fluid is actively pushed inside the eye without raising or lowering the bottle. The control of the air pump is digitally integrated in the Accurus panel. We preset the infusion pump at 100 mm Hg when we are operating microphakonit.

As you will notice in Table 36.1, if we use the air pump at high it is equal to using the Accurus machine at about 100 mm Hg pressure and if we use the air pump at low it is equal to using the Accurus machine at 50 mm Hg pressure. Some air pumps come with such a regulator so that one can have more air coming out of them. The regulator has a switch for low and high pressure. The cost of the air pump is about US $ 2 to US $ 10/- depending on the country. This can be got from an aquarium shop. If one uses an air pump one can connect a millipore filter to it to prevent any infection. Alternatively, one can use a gas forced internal infusion system using the Accurus machine. In such a case preset the pump at 100 mm Hg.

BIMANUAL 0.7 MM IRRIGATION ASPIRATION SYSTEM

Bimanual irrigation aspiration is done with the bimanual irrigation aspiration instruments. These instruments are also designed by Microsurgical Technology (USA). The previous set we used was the 0.9 mm set. Now with microphakonit we use the new 0.7 mm bimanual I/A set (Figs 36.5 and 36.6) so that after the nucleus removal we need not enlarge the incision.

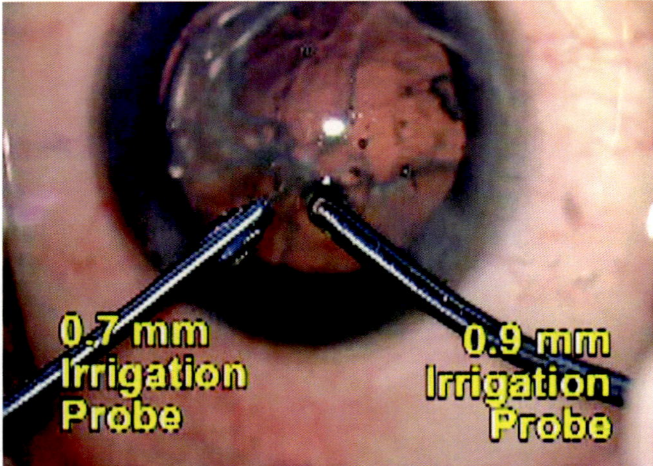

Fig. 36.5: 0.7 mm irrigation probe used for bimanual i/a compared to the 0.9 mm irrigation probe

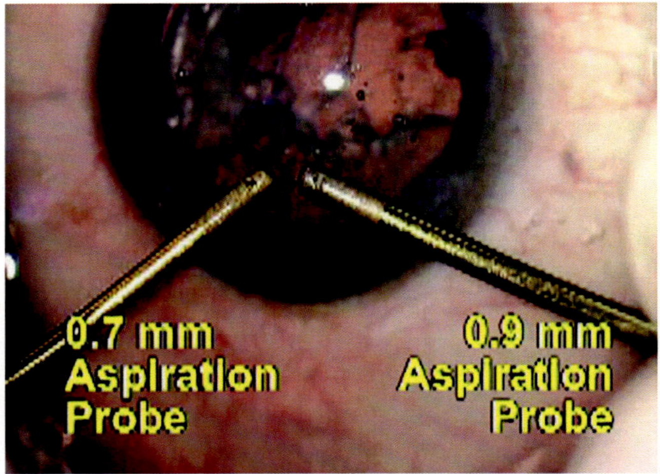

Fig. 36.6: 0.7 mm aspiration probe used for bimanual i/a compared to the 0.9 mm aspiration probe

DUET HANDLES

All these instruments of the 0.7 mm set fit onto the handles of the Duet system. So if a surgeon has already got the handles and is using it for phakonit they need to get only the tips and can use the same handles for microphakonit.

DIFFERENCES BETWEEN 0.9 MM AND 0.7 MM SETS IN CATARACT SURGERY

Table 36.2 indicates the differences between the two techniques.

TECHNIQUE

Incision

The incision is made with a keratome. This can be done using a sapphire knife or a stainless steel knife. One should be careful when one is making the incision so that the incision is a bit long as one would be using gas forced infusion in microphakonit. Before making the incision, a needle with

Table 36.2: Differences between phakonit and microphakonit

Features	*Phakonit*	*Microphakonit*
Irrigating chopper	0.9 mm	0.7 mm
Phaco needle	0.9 mm	0.7 mm
Control in surgery	Good	Better control
Valve construction	Extremely important	Not very important as incision is much smaller
Iris prolapse	Can occur if valve is bad	Very rare
Intraoperative floppy iris syndrome	Can be managed	Much better to manage as incision is much smaller and there is better control
Hydrodissection	Can be done from both incisions	To be careful as very little space is there for escape of fluid
Air pump (Gas Forced Infusion, GFI)	Can be done without it though better with it	Mandatory. 0.7 mm irrigating choppers even with higher end machines need GFI
Flow rate	Can keep any value	Do not keep it very high 20-24 ml/min
Bimanual I/A	0.9 mm	0.7 mm

viscoelastic is taken and pierced in the eye in the area where the side port has to be made. The viscoelastic is then injected inside the eye. This will distend the eye so that the clear corneal incision can be made easily. Make one clear corneal incision between the lateral rectus and inferior rectus and the other between the lateral rectus and superior rectus. This way one is able to control the movements of the eye during surgery.

Rhexis

The rhexis is then performed of about 5-6 mm. This is done with a needle. In the left hand a straight rod is held to stabilize the eye. This is the Globe stabilization rod. The advantage of this is that the movements of the eye can get controlled if one is working without any anesthesia or under topical anesthesia.

Hydrodissection

Hydrodissection is performed and the fluid wave passing under the nucleus checked. Check for rotation of the nucleus. The advantage of microphakonit is that one can do hydrodissection from both incisions so that even the subincisional areas can get easily hydrodissected. The problem is as there is not much escape of fluid one should be careful in hydrodissection as if too much fluid is passed into the eye one can get a complication.

Microphakonit

The 22 (0.7 mm) gauge irrigating chopper connected to the infusion line of the phaco machine is introduced with foot pedal on position 1. The phaco probe is connected to the aspiration line and the 0.7 mm phaco tip without an infusion sleeve is introduced through the clear corneal incision (Fig. 36.7). Using the phaco tip with moderate ultrasound power, the center of the nucleus is directly embedded starting from the superior edge of rhexis with the phaco probe directed obliquely

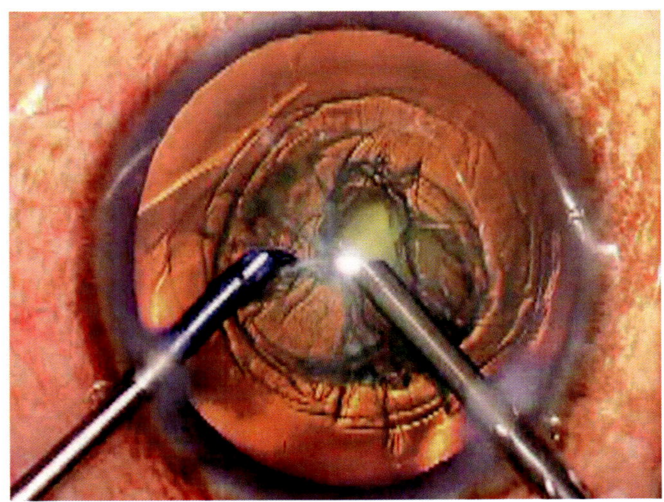

Fig. 36.7: Microphakonit started. 0.7 mm irrigating chopper and 0.7 mm phako tip without the sleeve inside the eye. All instruments are made by MST, USA. The assistant continuously irrigates the phaco probe area from outside to prevent corneal burns

downwards towards the vitreous. The settings at this stage are 50% phaco power, flow rate 20 ml/ min and 100-200 mm Hg vacuum. Using the karate chop technique the nucleus is chopped (Figs 36.8A to D). Thus, the whole nucleus is removed (Fig. 36.9). Cortical wash-up is then done with the bimanual irrigation aspiration (0.7 mm set) technique (Figs 36.10 and 36.11). During this whole procedure of microphakonit gas forced infusion is used.

SUMMARY

With microphakonit a 0.7 mm set is used to remove the cataract. At present this is the smallest one can use for cataract surgery. With time one would be able to go smaller with better and better instruments and devices. The problem at present is the IOL. We have to get good quality IOL's going through sub 1mm cataract surgical incisions so that the real benefit of microphakonit can be given to the patient.

KEY POINTS

1. On May 21st 2005, for the first time a 0.7 mm phaco needle tip with a 0.7 mm irrigating chopper was used to remove cataracts through the smallest incision possible as of now. This is called Microphakonit.
2. To increase the allowed aspiration flow rate from what a standard 0.7 mm tip would be, MST (Larry Laks) had the walls made thinner, thus increasing the inner diameter. This would allow a case to go, speed-wise, closer to what a 0.9 mm tip would go (not exactly the same, but closer).

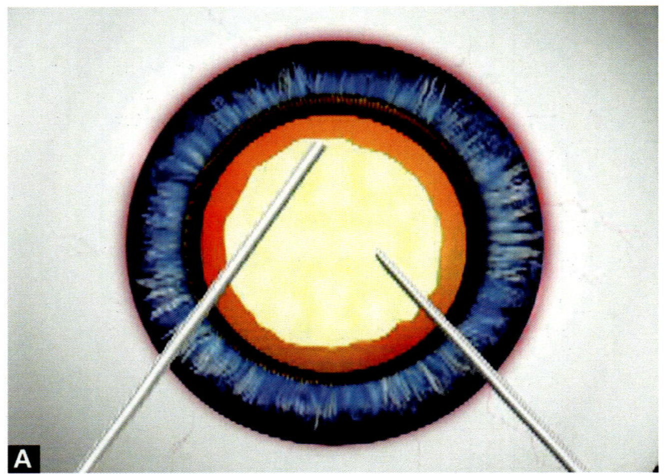

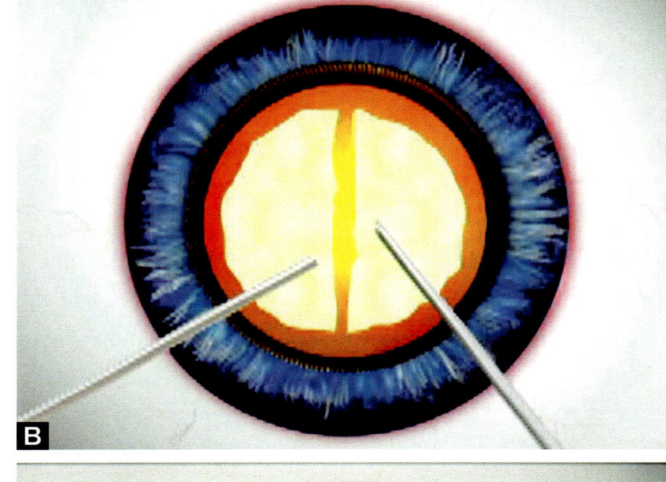

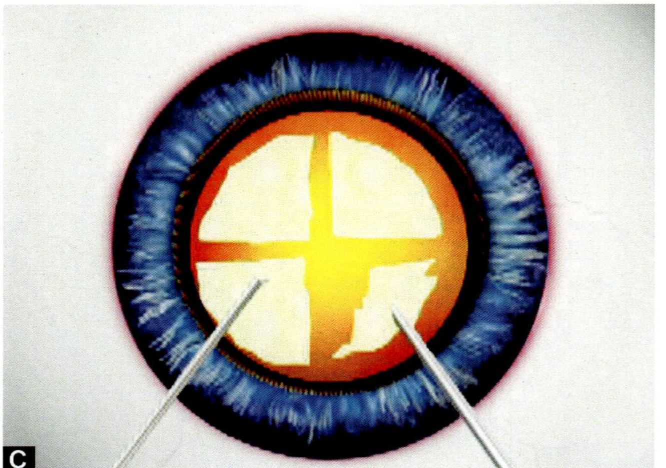

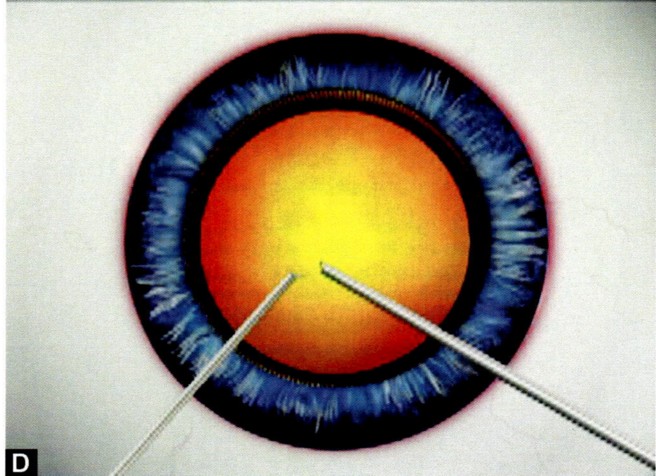

Figs 36.8A to D: Nucleus removal

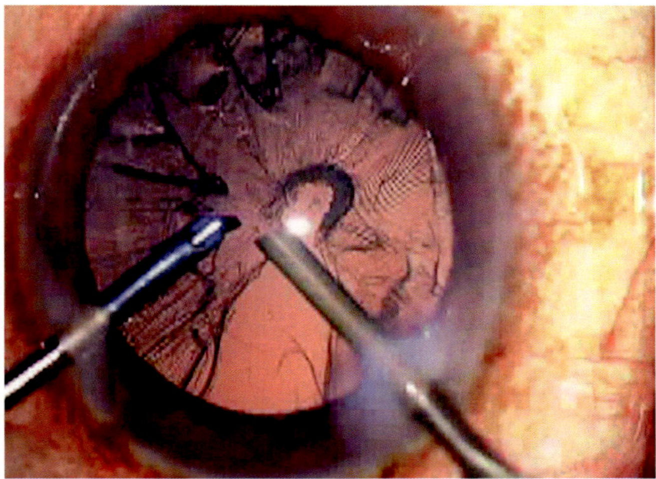

Fig. 36.9: Microphakonit completed. The nucleus has been removed

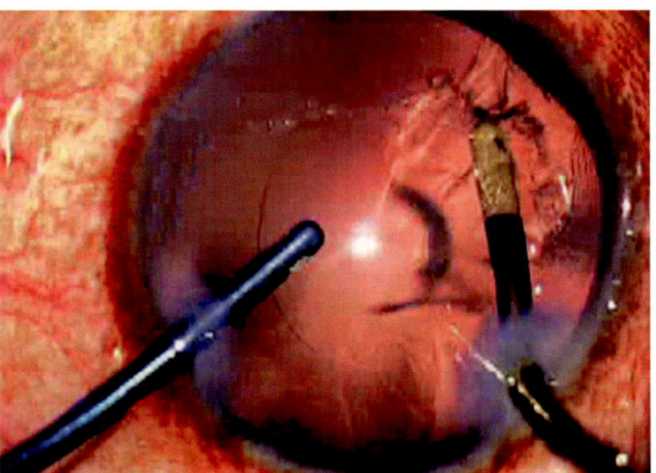

Fig. 36.10: Bimanual irrigation aspiration started with the 0.7 mm set

3. The microphakonit irrigating chopper is basically a sharp chopper which has a sharp cutting edge and helps in karate chopping or quick chopping. It can chop any type of cataract.
4. The advantage of microphakonit is that one can do hydrodissection from both incisions so that even the subincisional areas can get easily hydrodissected.
5. With microphakonit a 0.7 mm set is used to remove the cataract. At present this is the smallest one can use for cataract surgery. With time one would be able to go smaller with better and better instruments and devices.

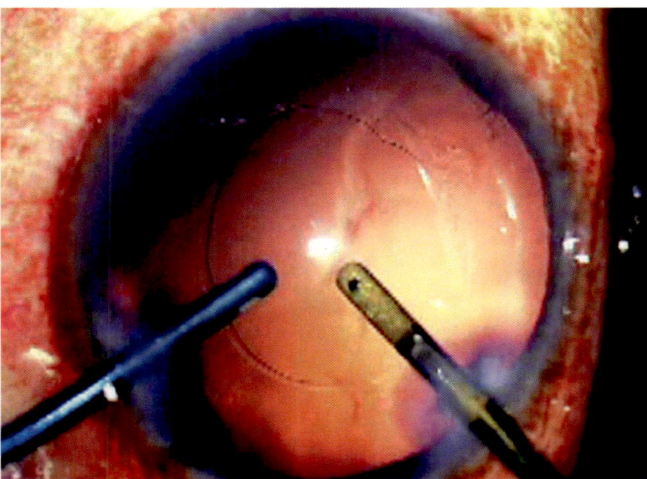

Fig. 36.11: Bimanual irrigation aspiration completed.

REFERENCES

1. Agarwal A, Agarwal S, Agarwal A: No anesthesia cataract surgery; In Agarwal et al. Textbook Phacoemulsification, Laser cataract surgery and foldable IOL's, First edition; Jaypee, India, 1998;144-54.
2. Pandey S, Wener L, Agarwal A, Agarwal S, Agarwal AT, Apple D. No anesthesia cataract surgery. J Cataract and Refractive Surgery 2001;28:1710.
3. Agarwal A, Agarwal S, Agarwal AT. Phakonit: A new technique of removing cataracts through a 0.9 mm incision; In Agarwal et al. Textbook Phacoemulsification, Laser cataract surgery and foldable IOL's, First edition; Jaypee, India, 1998;139-43.
4. Agarwal A, Agarwal S, Agarwal AT. Phakonit and laser phakonit: Lens surgery through a 0.9 mm incision; In Agarwal et al. Textbook Phacoemulsification, Laser cataract surgery and foldable IOL's, Second edition; Jaypee, India, 2000;204-16.
5. Agarwal A, Agarwal S, Agarwal AT. Phakonit; In Agarwal et al. Textbook Phacoemulsification, Laser cataract surgery and foldable IOL's, Third edition; Jaypee, India, 2003; 317-29.
6. Agarwal A, Agarwal S, Agarwal AT. Phakonit and laser phakonit; In Boyd/Agarwal et al. Textbook Lasik and Beyond Lasik, Higlights of Ophthalmology, Panama, 2000;463-8.
7. Agarwal A, Agarwal S, Agarwal AT. Phakonit and laser phakonit- Cataract surgery through a 0.9 mm incision; In Boyd/Agarwal et al. Textbook Phako, Phakonit and Laser Phako, Higlights of Ophthalmology, Panama, 2000;327-34.
8. Agarwal A, Agarwal S, Agarwal AT: The Phakonit Thinoptx IOL; In Agarwals textbook Presbyopia, Slack, USA, 2002; 187-94.
9. Agarwal A, Agarwal S, Agarwal AT. Antichamber collapser; J Cataract and Refractive Surgery 2002;28:1085.

10. Pandey S, Wener L,Agarwal A, Agarwal S, Agarwal AT, Hoyos J. Phakonit: Cataract removal through a sub 1.0 mm incision with implantation of the Thinoptx rollable IOL; J Cataract and Refractive Surgery 2002;28:1710.
11. Agarwal A, Agarwal S, Agarwal AT. Phakonit: Phacoemulsification through a 0.9 mm incision. J Cataract and Refractive Surgery 2001;27:1548-52.
12. Agarwal A, Agarwal S, Agarwal AT. Phakonit with an acritec IOL. J Cataract and Refractive Surgery 2003;29:854-55.
13. Agarwal S, Agarwal A, Agarwal AT. Phakonit with Acritec IOL. Highlights of Ophthalmology 2000.
14. Jorge Alio. What does MICS require in Alios textbook MICS; Highlights of Ophthalmology 2004;1-4.
15. Soscia W, Howard JG, Olson RJ. Microphacoemulsification with Whitestar. A wound-temperature study; J Cataract and Refractive Surgery 2002,28:1044-6.
16. Soscia W, Howard JG, Olson RJ. Bimanual phacoemulsification through two stab incisions. A wound-temperature study. J Cataract and Refractive Surgery 2002,28:1039-43.
17. Randall Olson. Microphaco chop in David Changs textbook on Phaco Chop; Slack, USA 2004;227-37.
18. David Chang. Bimanual phaco chop in David Changs textbook on Phaco Chop; Slack, USA, 2004;239-50.
19. Agarwal A. Air pump in Agarwal's textbook on Bimanual phaco: Mastering the phakonit/MICS technique; Slack, USA 2005.

Correcting Astigmatism Through the Use of Limbal Relaxing Incisions

Louis D "Skip" Nichamin

INTRODUCTION

In recent years the concept of "refractive cataract surgery" has received increased attention from surgeons, and the need for its adoption has recently been made more urgent by the increased availability of new presbyopia-correcting intraocular lenses. As such, the need to manage pre-existing astigmatism has become a requisite aspect of modern phaco surgery. Experience with keratorefractive surgery has proven that astigmatism of as little as 0.75 diopters (D) may leave a patient symptomatic with visual blur, ghosting and halos. To fully embrace this notion of refractive cataract surgery, the dedicated surgeon must aspire to a level of accuracy that one would equate with corneal-based refractive surgery. The most popular approach to achieve this goal is through the use of corneal, and specifically, limbal relaxing incisions (LRIs).

LIMBAL RELAXING INCISIONS

The modern era of cataract and astigmatism surgery began in the mid-1980's when several pioneering surgeons first suggested that astigmatic keratotomy might be combined with cataract and implant surgery.[1,2] Overtime, other innovators began to recognize the benefit of moving these incisions out to a more peripheral, limbal location.[3-5] Indeed, experience has shown us that LRIs possess several advantages over astigmatic keratotomy incisions placed at a more central optical zone. These would include less of a tendency to cause a shift in the resultant cylinder axis and less likelihood of inducing irregular astigmatism. These incisions are easier to create, and overall are simply more forgiving. Another important advantage gained by moving out to the limbus involves the "coupling ratio" which describes the amount of flattening that occurs in the incised meridian relative to the amount of steepening that results 90 degrees away; paired LRI's (when kept at or under 90 degrees of arc length) exhibit a very consistent 1:1 ratio, and therefore elicit little change in spheroequivalent, obviating the need to make any change in implant power.

THE PLAN

Perhaps the most challenging aspect of astigmatism surgery involves the determination of the quantity and exact location of the cylinder that is to be corrected, and thereby formulating a surgical plan. Unfortunately, preoperative measurements—keratometry, refraction, and corneal topography—do not always correlate. Lenticular astigmatism may account for some of this disparity, particularly in cases where there is a wide variance between refraction and corneal measurements; however, some discrepancies are likely due to the inherent shortcomings of traditional measurements of astigmatism. Standard keratometry, for example, measures only two points in each meridian at a single optical zone of approximately 3 mm.

When confounding measurements do arise, one may compromise and average the disparate readings; for example, if refraction shows 2 D of astigmatism and keratometry reveals only 1 D, it would be reasonable to correct for 1.5 D. Alternatively, if preoperative calculations vary widely, one may defer placing the relaxing incisions until a stable refraction post-implantation is obtained, and then correct the astigmatism; LRI's may be safely performed in the office in an appropriate treatment-room setting. Corneal topography can be very helpful when refraction and keratometry do not agree, and it is ***increasingly*** becoming the overall guiding measurement upon which the surgical plan is based. Topography is also helpful in detecting subtle corneal pathology such as keratoconus fruste which would likely negate the use of LRI's, or subtle irregular astigmatism such as that caused by epithelial basement membrane dystrophy.

NOMOGRAMS

Once the amount of astigmatism to be corrected has been determined, a nomogram must be consulted to determine the appropriate arc length of the incisions. A number of popular nomograms are currently available.[6] Our nomogram of choice originated from the work of Dr Stephen Hollis and incorporates concepts taught by Spencer Thornton, particularly his age modifiers.[7] As seen in Table 37.1, astigmatism is considered to be with-the-rule if the steep axis (plus cylinder) is between 45-135 degrees. Against-the-rule astigmatism is considered to fall between 0-44 and 136-180 degrees. One aligns the patient's age with the amount of preoperative cylinder to be corrected and finds the suggested arc length that the incisions should subtend.

An empiric blade depth setting is commonly used when performing LRI's, typically at 600 microns. This would seem to be a reasonable practice when treating cataract patients; however, in the setting of refractive lens exchange surgery or when employing presbyopia correcting IOLs—where ultimate precision is required—it is our preference to perform pachymetry and utilize adjusted blade depth settings. Pachymetry may be performed either preoperatively or at the time of surgery. Readings are taken over the entire arc length of the intended incision, and an adjustable micrometer diamond blade is then set to approximately 90 percent of the thinnest reading obtained. Refinements to the blade depth setting as well as nomogram adjustments may be necessary depending upon individual surgeon technique, the instruments used and, in particular, the style of the blade (Figs 37.1A and B). It should also be noted that in eyes that have previously undergone radial keratotomy, the length of the incisions should be reduced by approximately 50 percent, and in eyes that have undergone "significant" prior keratotomy surgery, it may be best to avoid additional incisional surgery and employ a toric IOL or laser technology instead.

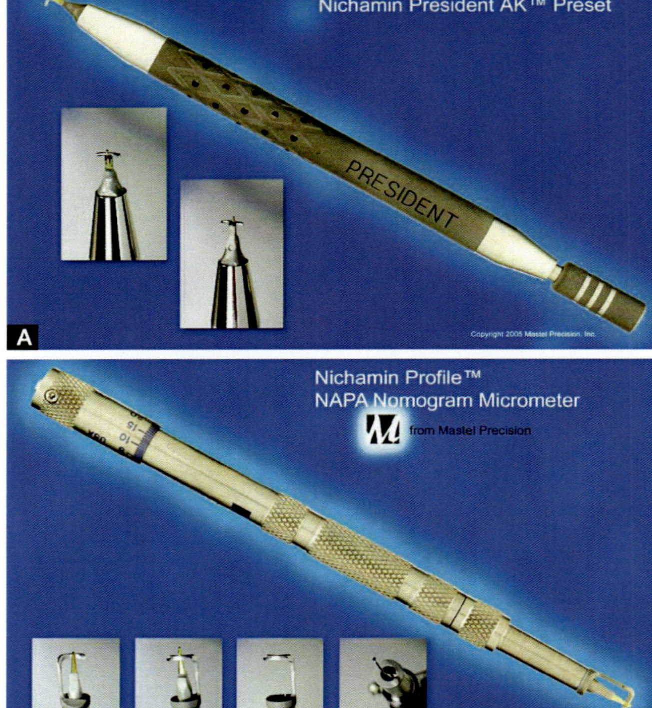

Figs 37.1A and B: Preset and adjustable micrometer (for use with the NAPA Nomogram) diamond knives by Mastel Precision. Similar designs are available from Storz Instruments and other manufacturers

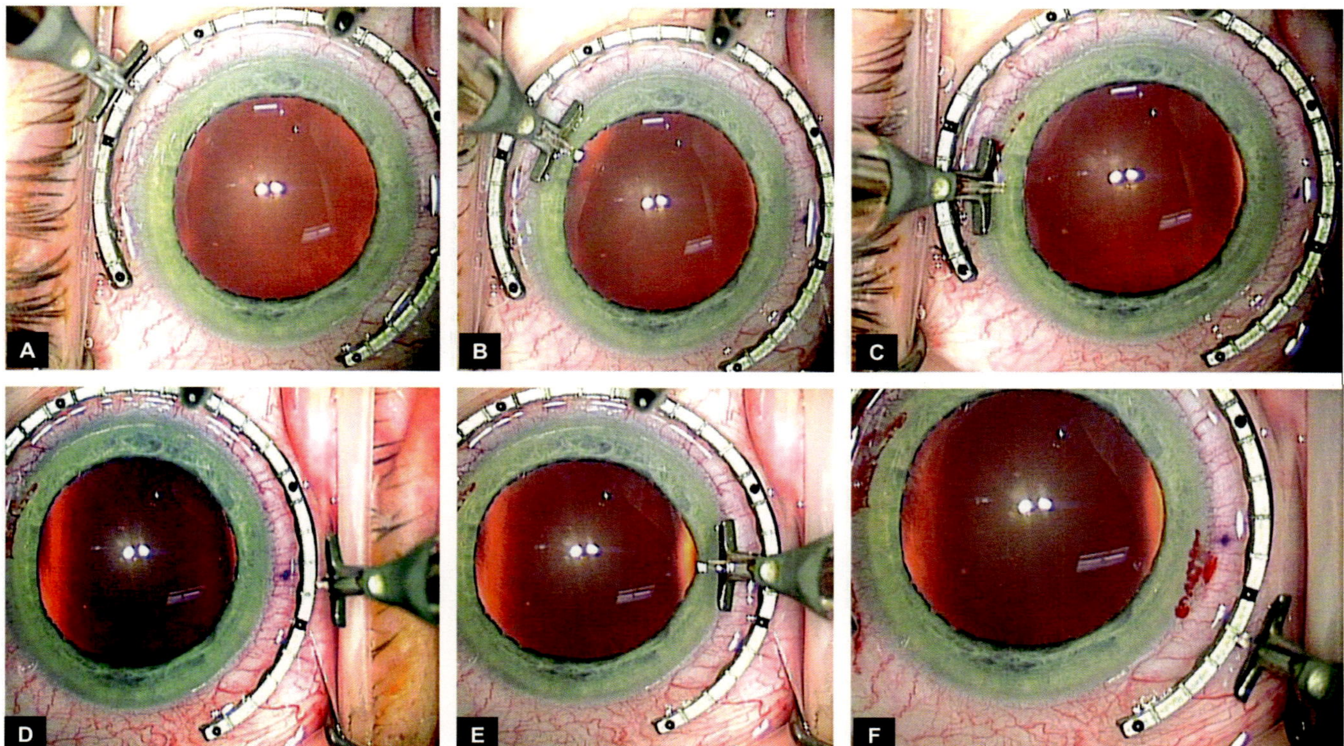

Figs 37.2A to F: A pair of limbal relaxing incisions delineating 40° of arc are shown placed over the steep 77° meridian. Note faint 6 O'clock ink orientation mark in this right eye. Surgeon is seated temporally

SURGICAL TECHNIQUE

In most cases, the relaxing incisions are placed at the outset of surgery in order to minimize epithelial disruption (Figs 37.2A to F). The one exception to this rule occurs when the phaco incision intersects or is encompassed within an LRI of greater than 40 degrees of arc; if it is extended to its full arc length at the start of surgery, significant gaping and edema may result secondary to intraoperative wound manipulation. In this setting, the phaco incision is first made by creating a shortened LRI whose arc length corresponds to the width of the phaco and IOL incision. This amounts to a two-plane grooved phaco incision whose depth is either 600 microns or has been determined by pachymetry as described above. Following IOL implantation and prior to viscoelastic removal, while the globe is still firm, the relaxing incision is extended to its full arc length as dictated by the nomogram. When an LRI is superimposed upon the phaco tunnel, the keratome entry is accomplished by pressing the bottom surface of the keratome blade downward upon the outer or posterior edge of the LRI. The keratome is then advanced into the LRI at an iris-parallel plane. This angulation will promote a dissection that takes place at mid-stromal depth which will help assure adequate tunnel length and a self-sealing closure.

Proper centration of the incisions over the steep corneal meridian is of utmost importance. According to Euler's theorem, an axis deviation of 5, 10 or 15 degrees will result in 17 percent, 33 percent and 50 percent reduction, respectively, in effect.[8] This reduction in effect holds true for both relaxing incisions and toric IOL's. Also, increasing evidence supports the notion that significant cyclotorsion may occur when assuming a supine position.[9] For this reason, most surgeons advocate placing an orientation mark at the 12:00 or 6:00 limbus while the patient is in an upright position. This is particularly impor-

Table 37.1: The "NAPA" nomogram Nichamin Age and Pachymetry-Adjusted Intralimbal Arcuate Astigmatic Nomogram

Louis D "Skip" Nichamin, The Laurel Eye Clinic, Brookville, PA

Preoperative cylinder (Diopters)	*Paired Incisions in Degrees of Arc*					
	20-30 years	*31-40 years*	*41-50 years*	*51-60 years*	*61-70 years*	*71-80 years*
With-the-rule (Steep Axis 45°-135°)						
0.75	40	35	35	30	30	
1.00	45	40	40	35	35	30
1.25	55	50	45	40	35	35
1.50	60	55	50	45	40	40
1.75	65	60	55	50	45	45
2.00	70	65	60	55	50	45
2.25	75	70	65	60	55	50
2.50	80	75	70	65	60	55
2.75	85	80	75	70	65	60
3.00	90	90	85	80	70	65
Against-the-rule (Steep Axis 0-44°/136-180°)						
Preoperative cylinder (Diopters)	*20-30 years*	*31-40 years*	*41-50 years*	*51-60 years*	*61-70 years*	*71-80 years*
0.75	45	40	40	35	35	30
1.00	50	45	45	40	40	35
1.25	55	55	50	45	40	35
1.50	60	60	55	50	45	40
1.75	65	65	60	55	50	45
2.00	70	70	65	60	55	50
2.25	75	75	70	65	60	55
2.50	80	80	75	70	65	60
2.75	85	85	80	75	70	65
3.00	90	90	85	80	75	70

Blade depth setting is at 90 percent of the thinnest pachymetry.

tant when employing injection anesthesia wherein unpredictable ocular rotation may occur. An additional measure that may be used to help center the relaxing incisions is to identify the steep meridian (plus cylinder axis) intraoperatively using some form of keratoscopy. The steep meridian over which the incisions are to be placed corresponds to the shorter axis of the reflected corneal mire. Another common way in which the steep meridian is marked utilizes a Mendez Ring or similar degree gauge which is aligned with the previously placed limbal orientation mark, and then locating the cylinder axis on the 360 degree gauge.

The LRI should be placed at the most peripheral extent of clear corneal tissue, just inside of the true surgical limbus. This holds true irrespective of the presence of pannus. If bleeding does occur, it may be ignored and will cease spontaneously. One must avoid placing the incisions further out at the true

Table 37.2: Potential problems

- Infection
- Weakening of the globe
- Perforation
- Decreased corneal sensation
- Induced irregular astigmatism
- Misalignment/axis shift
- Wound gape and discomfort
- Operating upon the wrong (opposite) axis!

surgical limbus in that a significant reduction of effect will likely occur due to both increased tissue thickness and a variation in tissue composition; these incisions are, therefore, really intralimbal in nature. In creating the incision, it is important to hold the knife perpendicular to the corneal surface in order to achieve consistent depth and effect, and will help to avoid gaping of the incision. Good hand and wrist support is important, and the blade ought to be held as if one were throwing a dart such that the instrument may be rotated between thumb and index finger as it is being advanced, thus leading to smooth arcuate incisions. Typically, the right hand is used to create incisions on the right side of the globe, and the left hand for incisions on the left side. In most cases it is more efficient to pull the blade toward oneself, as opposed to pushing it away.

COMPLICATIONS

LRI's have without question become a very safe and effective way of managing astigmatism at the time of cataract surgery. Nonetheless, as with any surgical technique, potential complications exist, and several are listed in Table 37.2. Of these, the most likely to be encountered is the placement of incisions upon the wrong axis. When this occurs, it typically takes the form of a 90 degree error with positioning upon the opposite, flat meridian. This, of course, results in an increase and likely doubling of the patient's pre-existing cylinder. Compulsive attention is required in this regard. The surgeon ought to consider employing safety checks to prevent this frustrating complication from occurring such as having a written plan that is brought into the OR and is kept visible and properly oriented. Incisions are always placed upon the plus (+) cylinder axis, and opposite to the minus (–) cylinder axis.

Although very rare, corneal perforation is possible. This may be due to improper setting of the blade depth, or as a result of a defect in the micrometer mechanism. This latter problem may arise after repeated autoclaving and many sterilization runs. Periodic inspection and calibration is therefore warranted, even with pre-set single depth knives. When encountered, unlike radial microperforations, these circumferential perforations will rarely self-seal and will likely require placement of temporary sutures.

SUMMARY

Refinement of the refractive outcome may arguably be the single most pressing challenge faced by today's cataract surgeon. Along with spherical error, pre-existing astigmatism may now be safely and effectively reduced at the time of cataract surgery. Astigmatic relaxing incisions are the most common method used to accomplish this goal. By moving these incisions out to an intralimbal location, the complications and difficulties associated with astigmatic keratotomy have been greatly reduced.

REFERENCES

1. Osher RH. Combining phacoemulsification with corneal relaxing incisions for reduction of pre-existing astigmatism. Paper presented at the annual meeting of the American Intraocular Implant Society. Los Angeles: 1984.
2. Maloney WF. Refractive cataract replacement: a comprehensive approach to maximize the refractive benefits of cataract extraction. Paper presented at the annual meeting of the American Society of Cataract and Refractive Surgery. Los Angeles 1986.
3. Budak K, Friedman NF, Koch DD. Limbal relaxing incisions with cataract surgery. J Cat Refract Surg 1998; 24(4):503-8.
4. Muller-Jensen K, Fischer P, Siepe U. Limbal relaxing incisions to correct astigmatism in clear corneal cataract surgery. J Refract Surg 1999;15(5):586-9.
5. Nichamin LD. Changing approach to astigmatism management during phacoemulsification: peripheral

arcuate astigmatic relaxing incisions. Paper presented at the annual meeting of the American Society of Cataract and Refractive Surgery. Boston: 2000.

6. Gills, JP. A complete guide to astigmatism management. Thorofare, SLACK, Inc.; 2003.
7. Thornton SP. Radial and astigmatic keratotomy: the American system of precise, predictable refractive surgery. Thorofare, SLACK, Inc.; 1994.
8. Abrams D. Ophthalmic optics and refraction. In: Duke-Elder SS, (Ed). System of Ophthalmology. St. Louis, Mosby, 1970;671-4.
9. Swami AU, Steinert RF, Osborne WE., et al. Rotational malposition during laser *in situ* keratomileusis. Am J Ophthal 2002;133(4)561-2.

38 Refractive Cataract Surgery

R Bruce Wallace III

Over the past twenty years, the safety profile for cataract surgery has improved dramatically. Small incision procedures have led to much better surgical predictability with reduced risk and rapid visual recovery. And what was once considered a serendipitous benefit, reduced spectacle dependency, has now become commonplace; even expected by most patients. The evolution of refractive cataract surgery has involved many technological breakthroughs championed by a large group of innovators. What stands before us now is a formula for success. By implementing refractive cataract surgery "systems" we can greatly improve our opportunity to achieve the results our patients have learned to expect. These treatment systems include more precise biometry, better anesthesia, safer lens removal and the proper use of newer presbyopia correcting intraocular lenses.

- Preoperative biometry and IOL selection and power calculation
- Patient selection and patient counseling for presbyopia correcting IOLs
- Refractive lens surgery techniques, inflammation and infection prophylaxis
- Reducing astigmatism
- Postoperative patient management and maximizing results

Preoperative Biometry and Intraocular Lens Calculation

Better biometry techniques combined with computerized fourth generation theoretic formulas have led to a higher level of accuracy for IOL power calculation. Our goal is to be within 0.50D of our spherical target for over 90% of eyes undergoing a cataract or refractive lens surgery. Inaccurate axial length measurements remain the most common cause for errors in IOL power selection.[1] For most cataract surgeons, contact A-scan ultrasonography has been the chosen method to measure postoperative axial lengths. However, the lower level of accuracy of this technique compared to immersion A-scan and partial coherence interferometry makes contact ultrasound scans less attractive.[2] Immersion A-scan, once mastered, is more accurate without necessarily requiring more time or effort.

But, in my opinion when it comes to user friendliness and the most dependable measurement, partial coherence interferometry with the Zeiss Meditec IOLMaster version 5.0 is unsurpassed. The 5.0 IOLMaster upgrade in many ways represents a whole new device capable of achieving much faster readings. We have found more reproducibility and dependability for preoperative axial length measurements and keratometry. (The upgrade also provides technicians a safety net of computer prompts to alert them to questionable readings and signals endpoints to acceptable readings.) The keratometry has become so dependable that many surgeons rely more on these readings than corneal topography when planning peripheral corneal relaxing incisions or toric IOL implantation.

Using the latest IOL formulas such as the[6,7] Holladay II, Hoffer Q and Haigis II is important to achieve the best refractive results.[3] These formulas are available on computer programs with the ability to provide outcomes analysis and ongoing personalization of lens constants, a valuable asset to better IOL power calculation. Preferably, a high level of refractive accuracy should be established with these tools when implanting monofocal IOLs during cataract surgery before a surgeon can confidently enter the refractive lens arena.

A growing challenge is the ability to accurately measure the correct central corneal power for post corneal refractive patients.[4] New instrumentation, such as the Oculus Pentacam and contact lens fitting software available on the latest corneal topographers, may provide more reliable keratometric measurements for these frequently demanding patients.

Monovision and Presbyopia Correcting IOLs

A number of intraocular lenses (IOLs) are available for the surgical correction of presbyopia. Blended vision or monovision can be created with standard monofocal IOLs. Similar to contact lens monovision, not all patients will be happy with this choice, especially if they were unsuccessful with monovision contact lens trials. However, for the successful monovision contact lens wearer who has become contact lens intolerant, monovision with monofocal IOLs makes sense. We usually target plano to –0.50D for the dominant distance eye and –1.75D for the nondominant near eye. (However, there remains surprisingly limited evidence that ocular dominancy really matters for many monovision patients.) This combination can result in surprisingly good uncorrected near vision without sacrificing intermediate vision. Success with lower levels of myopia in the near eye compared to contact lens fitting may be due to a pseudoaccommodative effect of monofocal IOLs.[5]

However, most cataract surgeons are choosing a PC-IOL over monovision monofocal IOLs. Even though more costly, this method maintains binocularity and stereopsis.[9,10] Multifocal and accommodative IOLs are the PC-IOLs available today. Similar to the early days of monofocal IOLs, multifocal IOLs have experienced a relatively slow acceptance. Clinical investigation for almost two decades has shown significantly better uncorrected near vision with multifocal IOLs compared to monofocal IOLs, yet unwanted visual sensations delayed their popularity.[8-11]

One of the first successful multifocal IOLs was the Allergan Array IOL. The Array is a zonal progressive refractive IOL with five blended power zones of alternating distance and near that provide distance (50%), near (37%) and intermediate (13%). Many clinical studies demonstrated the refractive benefit of the Array IOL over monofocal IOL controls.[12-14] Fortunately, most patients learned to ignore halos and glare after a period of visual cortical adaptation.[15] Another concern about multifocal IOLs has been the potential for loss of contrast sensitivity. Even though some measurable loss of contrast has been detected in clinical studies, patients have not found contrast sensitivity loss with multifocal IOLs, like the Array, to be problematic.[16]

Recently the Array IOL was replaced with the AMO ReZoom refractive IOL. The ReZoom is a second generation zonal refractive IOL manufactured on the acrylic 3-piece AR-40 Sensar monofocal platform. This lens is the result of extensive study of the optical changes necessary to reduce halos and glare occasionally experienced after Array IOL implantation. By altering zone diameters, there was found to be less of an incidence of unwanted visual sensations. Another advantage includes a round, square "Optiedge" to reduce posterior capsular opacification while at the same time avoiding dysphotopsia associated with peripheral retinal reflections from squared edges. Because of its three-piece design, the ReZoom can be implanted in the ciliary sulcus if a posterior capsular tear is encountered. Yet a power adjustment will be necessary due to relative anterior insertion compared to capsular bag placement. Because it has a refractive optic, all light is transmitted, which is an advantage over diffractive multifocal IOLs. Experience with the ReZoom has been encouraging with a large majority of patients never or almost never needing glasses after surgery. Compared to the Array, the ReZoom appears to offer better near vision and less halo and glare with early clinical use showing great promise.[17]

Another multifocal IOL available today is the Alcon ReStor (Fig. 38.1). Originally designed by 3M with a posterior diffractive surface, the ReStor's diffractive component is on the central anterior surface of the IOL. The apodized diffractive-refractive Alcon ReStor IOL has rapidly become popular. The anterior optical surface of the monofocal Acrysof was modified by adding diffractive rings to the anterior central 3.6 mm of the 6.0 mm optic of the Acrysof IOL, which vary in step height and spacing in order to maximize multifocality and, at the same time, reduce halo and glare. As the pupil enlarges in scotopic conditions, there is more light for the distance vision and less light for near. This special modification of a diffractive optic has been termed apodization. Half of the 82 percent of light transmission is for distance and half for near with the remaining 18 percent lost to higher orders. This one-piece acrylic IOL with frosted square edges is also available in a three-piece version if sulcus implantation is indicated. FDA submitted data in the US showed that 80 percent of bilaterally implanted ReStor patients never wore glasses after surgery.[18] The newer aspheric ReSTOR may offer better quality of vision at all distances.

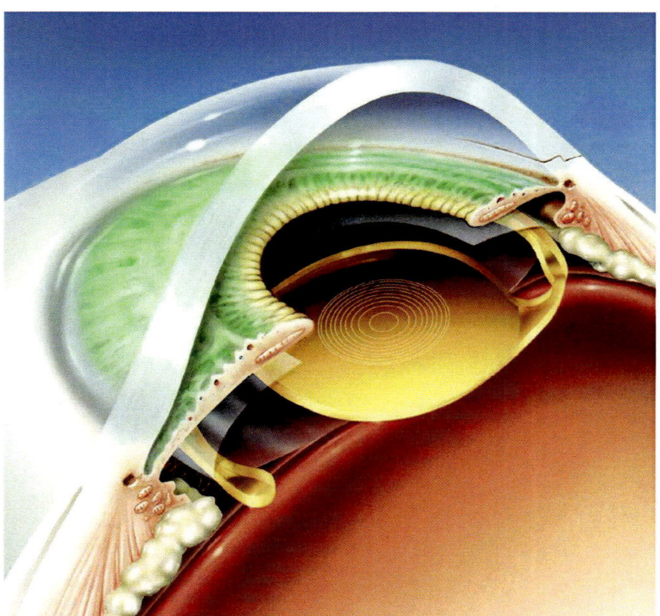

Fig. 38.1: Restor implant (Courtesy: Dr.Robert Weinstock)

A more recent diffractive aspheric lens, the AMO Tecnis MIOL, has been gaining widespread popularity. The diffractive portion covers the entire posterior surface of the optic, making the Tecnis MIOL less pupil dependent. There appears to be surprisingly good intermediate vision with this PC-IOL.

Another category of PC-IOLs includes accommodating IOLs. These IOLs attempt to mimic natural accommodation of the crystalline lens.[19] The current accommodative IOLs include the eyeonics crystalens and the HumanOptics 1CU. The most often implanted accommodative IOL is the eyeonics crystalens. This single piece silicone IOL has hinged haptics to allow for posterior vaulting and anterior-posterior movement of the 4.5 mm optic (Fig. 38.2). FDA trials demonstrated impressive results with this lens design.[20] A recent study has shown that some patients' vision appears to improve during the first three years after implantation.[21]

The Akkomodative 1CU is a hydrophilic, acrylic, foldable IOL with four flexible haptics attached to a 5.5 mm optic. The lens can be implanted with folding forceps or by injector. A multicenter study in Italy of approximately 30 IOLs showed greater than 85% achieving uncorrected vision of 20/25 and J2.[24] The 1CU, which is known mostly in Europe, is under further study in Europe and trials in the United States are likely. Mixing different PC-IOLS has been shown to offer the relative advantages of

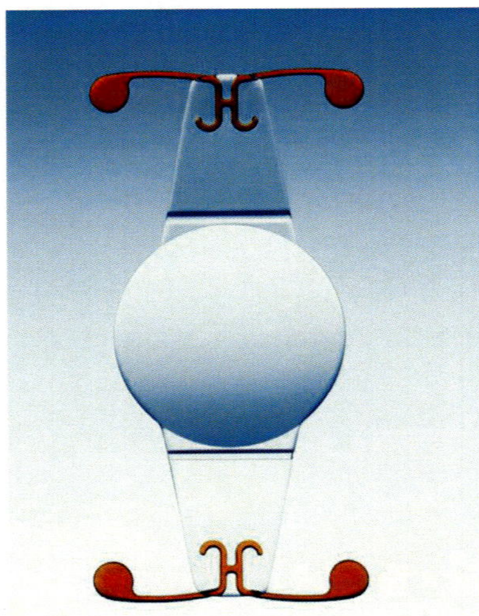

Fig. 38.2: Crystalens (Courtesy-Dr. Robert Weinstock)

separate technologies without apparent confusion to the patient (Bucci reference).

Also under clinical investigation are a number of dual optic accommodative IOLs. The dual optic arrangement involves two attached lenses with one lens having a high minus power which remains fixed posteriorly and an anterior high plus lens that can travel anterior-posterior during accommodation. The Visiogen Synchrony and Bausch and Lomb Safarazzi IOLs are undergoing FDA trials. The Visiogen Synchrony has shown impressive accommodative amplitude.[25]

Patient Selection and Patient Counseling for Presbyopia Correcting IOLs

The best candidates for Presbyopia Correcting IOLs (PC-IOLs) are hyperopic presbyopes over the age of 50 who have a strong desire to reduce their dependency on spectacles. Like many LASIK surgeons, Dr. Kurt Buzard prefers refractive lens exchange over LASIK for older hyperopes in order to achieve better quality and longer lasting multifocal vision.[27] Certainly older myopes, especially those with greater than 3.0D, can also benefit from PC-IOLs. However, the risk of postoperative retinal detachment is greater for high myopes.[28] Fortunately, with improvements in phacoemulsification fluidics allowing for more stable anterior and posterior segments, this is likely to become less of a concern. Patients with over 2.5D of preoperative astigmatism can still achieve acceptable outcomes with astigmatic surgery, yet less predictably.

When discussing PC-IOLs, surgeons develop a sixth sense as to a patient's level of understanding and their expectations. A demanding, unforgiving personality is not the best profile for a PC-IOL candidate. Potential PC-IOL patients are advised by surgeons and staff members of the benefits and limitations of various PC-IOLs. Brochures and educational videos can offer additional information to bring the patient to a proper level of realistic expectation. By emphasizing that PC-IOLs require adjusting to a new visual system and that many people will need to allow time for this adjustment, most PC-IOL patients will be tolerant in the first few months as visual cortical neuroadaptation yields better multifocality and unwanted visual sensations become less noticeable.

Refractive Cataract Surgery Techniques, Inflammation and Infection Prophylaxis

When it comes to Refractive Cataract Surgery (RCS) surgery, every effort should be made to perform a precise, painless and predictable procedure. For infection and inflammation prophylaxis, our patients receive topical fourth generation fluoroquinolones, prednisolone acetate and nonsteroidal anti-inflammatory topical medications beginning three days prior to surgery and continued postoperatively. Topical povidone iodine is instilled immediately before and after the procedure. Topical anesthesia with light IV sedation contributes to rapid visual recovery. When preparing the eye for surgery, care is taken to isolate the lashes and lid margins with an adhesive eye drape. The lid speculum is placed carefully in order to avoid corneal contact. Both dispersive and retentive ophthalmic viscodevices (OVDs) are injected in order to protect the corneal endothelium. Prior to anterior capsulotomy, a 6.0 mm optical zone marker is placed on the central cornea to offer a template in order to consistently create a

5.0 to 5.5 mm capsular opening to allow for overlap of the peripheral anterior capsule onto the anterior surface of the IOL.[29] Anterior capsular overlap has been shown to reduce the incidence of posterior capsular opacification (PCO).[30]

Utilizing the latest phacoemulsification technology contributes to improved surgical predictability and competence. Better fluidics, less surge and less heat reduce complications and help to hasten visual recovery.[31] Most cataract surgeons are familiar with nuclear cracking and chopping phaco techniques. However, for softer nuclei, nuclear flipping techniques are usually more effective. For most eyes, I bisect the nucleus and flip each half into the pupillary plane before emulsifying.[32] The "Burst Hemi-flip" method is a surgeon friendly method of nuclear removal that takes advantage of newer phaco technology and has universal application even for softer nuclei. (i.e. refractive lens exchange). And, as we move toward pure refractive lens procedures, we should look for surgical protocols for true cataractous nuclei that can be reliably applied to precataractous lenses.

After PC-IOL insertion through an injector, it is best to remove all the OVD, including under the IOL optic, to avoid postoperative pressure spikes and provide faster visual recovery. Thanks to improvements in technique, most RCS patients can be visually functional minutes after their procedure.

Reducing Astigmatism

Until toric IOLs become more widely available, quality vision after RCS will depend on the ability to surgically create a relatively astigmatic free cornea. The goal for astigmatism control should be the creation of a resultant cylinder of less than 1D at any axis. Most patients enjoy good unaided visual acuity with this degree of astigmatism. Some studies suggest a benefit to leaving some amount of residual against-the-rule cylinder so that uncorrected near vision after cataract surgery is improved.[33] However, surgical practices utilizing multifocal IOLs and/or monovision will not find this to be an advantage because of the compromise of the loss of distance visual acuity with amounts over 1D of cylinder.

Today's small incision phaco procedures (utilizing 3.0 mm and smaller) have a relatively astigmatic neutral effect on the cornea. If we are to reduce cylinder, additional corneal surgery will be required – either by a peripheral incision on the steep axis, peripheral intrastromal shrinking on the flat axis or excimer laser on the central cornea. For cataract surgeons, the most frequently performed procedure to reduce astigmatism has been peripheral arcuate corneal incisions placed on the steep axis termed limbal relaxing incisions (LRIs). These incisions are not limbal but are placed 1.0 to 1.5 mm inside the limbus in clear cornea. LRIs can provide a safe, effective and long lasting solution to vision degrading cylinder.

A stumbling block to acceptance of LRIs is the confusion surrounding the term "limbal relaxing incision". As Doug Koch has emphasized, these are really peripheral corneal relaxing incision (PCRIs). Paul Arnold likes the name peripheral astigmatic keratometry (PAK). It makes sense to consider renaming the LRI procedure, because if these incisions are placed at the surgical limbus, they will offer little astigmatic correction.

One of the more challenging tasks that the surgeon faces is deciding which astigmatism preoperative measurements should be used when planning a surgical correction. Do we depend on the cylinder diopters and axis from the refraction, the keratometry, or do we always need to perform corneal topography? One study showed the frequency of poor correlation of all three methods of measurement, especially with less than 2D of astigmatism. Fortunately, unlike correction of spherical refractive errors, astigmatism correction is more forgiving, especially when treating moderate to low levels.

One way to plan surgical correction of astigmatism is to initially assess the refraction and the keratometry simultaneously. If good correlation exists as to the amount of cylinder and axis, planning astigmatism correction during lens surgery is fairly straightforward. If, however, there is poor correlation (even though keratometry should be more reliable), surgical correction can be less predictable, even when corneal topography is performed. This is where the "art" of astigmatism correction applies. The surgeon needs to also judge the relative reliability of the astigmatic information. If after careful consideration there is doubt as to a reasonable surgical plan, the astigmatism correction should be postponed until after cataract surgery and an adequate time for incision healing has taken place.

After deciding on just how much cylinder needs treatment and its location (axis), a nomogram is used that will lead the surgeon to the best choice of incision(s) based on axis location, type of phaco incision and age of patient. The nomograms I have used most frequently are mine and another developed by Nichamin (Tables 38.1 and 38.2).

LRI Surgical Technique

After choosing a nomogram, LRI surgeons need to decide what instrumentation to use. LRI instruments come in many shapes and styles. I designed for Duckworth and Kent the Wallace LRI kit. The kit includes a Mendez axis marker, a thin profile knife with a single footplate trifacet 600 mm diamond blade and a caliber 0.12 mm curved forceps (Fig. 38.3). The 360 degrees ring of the Mendez marker has visible numbers that are helpful to guide the surgeon to the correct axis. After placing the axis mark inside the Mendez marker with the 0.12 forceps, a mark is placed on each side of the axis mark to outline the length of the intended incision. Then the surgeon fixates the globe with the same 0.12 mm forceps and places the knife in the distal corneal mark. The diamond blade, placed vertical to the corneal surface, is then advanced toward fixation, "connecting the dots" in the peripheral cornea in an arcuate fashion. I usually perform these incisions before the phaco incision is made. I have never experienced a corneal perforation requiring a suture after an LRI procedure.

Another surgical option to reduce astigmatism involves corneal steepening rather than flattening the corneal periphery. Conductive keratoplasty (CK), originally designed to treat hyperopia, can also treat cylindrical refractive errors. A nomogram has been developed by Matos to treat cylinder with CK at the 9 mm optical zone for 1D, 2D and 3D of cylinder.

Bioptics with laser vision correction (LVC) can also treat postoperative astigmatism along with problem myopia or hyperopia after RCS (Ref to enhancement section).

Improvements in toric IOLs provide another option for astigmatic reduction. Currently available are the one piece IOLs, Alcon Toric and Staar Toric. The Alcon Toric is an acrylic lens that provides a "stickier" surface on the optic and less tendency to "propeller", or shift the axis once implanted. With Alcon's Toric IOL planner on line, surgeons can better place the recommended IOL axis for the best results.

Postoperative Patient Management: Maximizing Results

The two most frequent patient complaints after RCS with PC-IOLs revolve around halos and glare and less than desirable uncorrected near vision. Multifocal PC-IOLs are known to be more likely than accommodative IOLs to cause halos and glare, especially under mesopic conditions such as night-time driving. Most patients will learn to ignore these unwanted visual sensations, similar to adjusting to the wearing of a watch, a ring or a seatbelt. Visual cortical neuroadaptation gradually allows patients to more quickly and seamlessly use distance, intermediate and near vision and ignore other visual imagery. Since multifocal optics split light, patients with postoperative dry eye syndrome may notice more visual disturbances than monofocal IOL patients. Liberal use of ocular lubricants, punctual occlusion and topical cyclosporine (Restasis) can improve visual function.

Similarly, even mild PCO can disturb the quality of vision with PC-IOLs. YAG laser posterior capsulotomy may need to be performed earlier to restore multifocal vision (especially near).

Residual refractive errors may need to be addressed with laser vision correction (LVC) or LRI. For problem hyperopia, CK and LVC can help to enhance uncorrected vision. Many low level myopic eyes, especially unilateral, may not need enhancement due to the benefit of better near acuity. Intolerable low myopia can be corrected with LVC or mini-RK. Because RCS patients commonly have dry eyes and are not the best candidates for LVC, we have performed mini-RK for a number of these patients, usually to the 5.0 mm OZ, with great success. For higher levels of spherical error (>1.5D) piggyback IOLs or even IOL exchange may be a better option.

SUMMARY

Safer, more predictable cataract surgery and the growing demand to surgically correct presbyopia have increased the interest in RCS. The challenge for the RCS surgeon is to bring to their practice the necessary technology and surgical skills necessary to achieve consistent refractive results. Also important is the need to constantly upgrade equipment, pharmaceuticals, PC-IOLs and fine-tuning modalities as the art and science of RCS continues to evolve.

REFERENCES

1. Olsen T. Sources of error in IOL power calculations.
2. Ref BD on pp/16 c 3, 3& 4/11,6
3. Hoffer KJ. The Hoffer Q. Formula: a comparison of theoretic and regression formulas. J Cataract Refract Surg 1993;19:700-712. Errata: 1994;20:677.
4. Byrne SF. A-Scan Axial Eye Length Measurements: A Handbook for IOL Calculations. Mars Hill, NC: Grov Publisher, 1995.
5. Ravalico G, Baccara F. Apparent accommodation in pseudophakic eyes. Acta Ophthalol 1990;68:604-06.
6. Brooks SE, Johnson D, Fischer N. Anisometropia and Binocularity. Ophthalmology 1996;103:1139-43.
7. Jain S, aurora I, Asar DT. Success of monovision in presbyopes: review of literature and potential applications to refractive surgery. Surv Ophthalmol 1996;40:491-99.
8. Keates R, Pearce J, Schneider R. Clinical results of the multifocal lens. J Cataract Refract Surg 1987;13:557-60.
9. Lindstrom R. Food and Drug Administration study update-one year results from 671 patients with the 3M multifocal intraocular lens. Ophthalmology 1993;100:91-97.
10. Gimbel H, Sanders D, Raanan M. Visual and refractive results of multifocal intraocular lenses. Ophthalmology 1991;98: 881-88.
11. Knorz M, Aron-Rosa D, Claessens D, et al. Vision with the True Vista bifocal IOL. European J Implant Ref Surg 1992;4:95-98.
12. Javitt KC, Wang F, Trentacost D, et al. Outcomes of cataract extraction with multifocal intraocular lens implantation. Ophthalmology 1997;104:589-99.
13. Steinert R, Post C, Brint S, et al. A prospective, randomized, double-masked comparison of a zonal-progressive multifocal intraocular lens and a monofocal intraocular lens. Ophthalmology 1992;99:853-860.
14. Steinert R, Aker B, Trentacost D, et al. A prospective comparative study of the AMO array zonal-progressive multifocal silicone intraocular lens and a monofocal intraocular lens. Ophthalmology 1999;106:1243-55.
15. Hunkeler JD, Coffman TM, Paugh J, et al. Characterization of visual phenomena with the array multifocal intraocular lens. J Cataract Refract Surg 2002;28:1195-1204.
16. Pieh S, Weghaupt H, Skorpik C. Contrast sensitivity and glare disability with diffractive and refractive multifocal intraocular lenses. J Cataract Refract Surg 1998;24:659-62.
17. O'Heineachain R. Good initial results with two new multifocals. Eurotimes 2005;10:Issue10:10.
18. Davison JA, Simpson MJ. History and Development of the Apodized Diffractive Intraocular Lens. Accepted for publication by the Journal of Cataract and Refractive Surgery, November 2005.
19. Glasser A, Campbell MCW. Presbyopia and the optical changes in the human crystalline lens with age. Vision Res 1998;38:209-29.
20. Cummings JS, Slade SG, Chayet A, et al. Clinical evaluation of the model AT-45 silicone accommodating intraocular lens: result of the feasibility and initial study of a Food and Drug Administration clinical trial; the AT-45 study group. Ophthalmology 2001;108:2005-2009.
21. Mark Boren Reference.
22. Picardo V. Getting to know the 1CU. J Cataract Refract Surg Today 2002;2:21.
23. Dan McWard Reference.
24. Buzard KA. Clear Lensectomy for Refractive Errors. In: Wallace RB (Ed): Refractive Cataract Surgery and Multifocal IOLs. Thorofare, NJ: SLACK Incorporated; 2001:59-72.
25. Retzlaff J, Sanders DR, Kraff MC. Lens Implant Power Calculation. Thorofare, NJ: SLACK Incorporated; 1990.
26. Wallace RB. Capsulotomy Diameter Mark. J Cataract Refract Surg 2003;29:1866-68.
27. Apple DJ, Peng Q, Visessook N, et al. Eradication of posterior capsule opacification; documentation of a marked decrease in Nd:YAG laser posterior capsulotomy rates noted in an analysis of 5416 pseudophakic human eyes obtained postmortem. Ophthalmology 2001;108:505-18.
28. AMO Reference for phaco fluidics.
29. Burst Hemi-flip.
30. Verzella F, Calossi A. Multifocal effect of against-the-rule myopic astigmatism in pseudophakic eyes. J Refract Corneal Surg 1993;9:58-61.
31. Sawusch M, Guyton D. Optimal astigmatism to enhance depth of focus after cataract surgery. Ophthalmology. 1991;98:1025-29.
32. Masket S, Tennen D. Astigmatic stabilization of 3.0mm temporal clear corneal cataract incisions. J Cataract Refract Surg 1996;22:1451-55.
33. Wallace RB. On-axis cataract incisions: where is the axis? 1995 ASCRS Symposium of Cataract, IOL and Refractive Surgery Best Papers of Sessions. 1995;67-72.

39 IOL Power Calculation in Standard and Refractive Surgery Cases

Samuel Boyd, Luis W Lu

Selecting the proper intraocular lens (IOL) power is an important process, and is best performed few days prior to surgery. Also of importance, is the physician's ability to communicate with the patient. Among the basic ingredients of developing that strong trusting relationship between physician and patient, is our ability to articulate and discuss the course of treatment through the spoken word.[1]

EVALUATING THE PATIENT PRIOR TO SURGERY

Prior to explaining the patient about the cataract surgical procedure, a full ocular evaluation is performed, the type of cataract is determined (Fig. 39.1). A Potential Acuity Meter (PAM) will predetermine the expected outcome in the majority of surgical cases. Certain tests are performed if indicated if questions arise from patient of family members as well. These will include slit lamp digital photography, retinal digital photography, Optical Coherence Tomography (OCT). Endothelial cell count, Optical or Contact Corneal Pachymetry (CCP), or any other specific test is done if indicated.

Once the surgery is to be performed, the risks, complications and alternatives are explained. The expected postoperative refraction is determined. Careful discussion with the patient will enlighten the surgeon as to the patient's expectations. Some patients know exactly what they want regarding the postoperative visual acuity, while others will leave the decision up to their surgeon.[2,3]

PATIENT'S EXPECTATIONS

It is essential to clarify to the patient what he/she may expect and what not to expect from surgery. Postoperative patient satisfaction is based on this pre-op surgeon-patient communication and understanding. What are the patient's daily needs and what final uncorrected visual acuity for distance and near he would prefer? Does he want to read without glasses? If so, he must understand he will not see clear at distance unless the patient will be informed of the alternative of a multifocal IOL. Myopic patients prefer to be myopes. Hyperopes do better by performing eventual bilateral surgery. Slight myopia might be desirable.

In certain patients the availability of foldable multifocal IOLs, accommodative implants, monovision, toric, and piggyback implantation have to be explained. Final visual satisfaction with these methods will depend a great deal on the selection by the surgeon of the right patient with reasonable expectations for these alternatives.

Some surgeons advocate emmetropia for all their patients, while others advocate a slight myopia. Studies have shown that a small amount of myopic astigmatism can enhance the depth of focus of the pseudophakic eye, with adequate 20/30 visual acuity

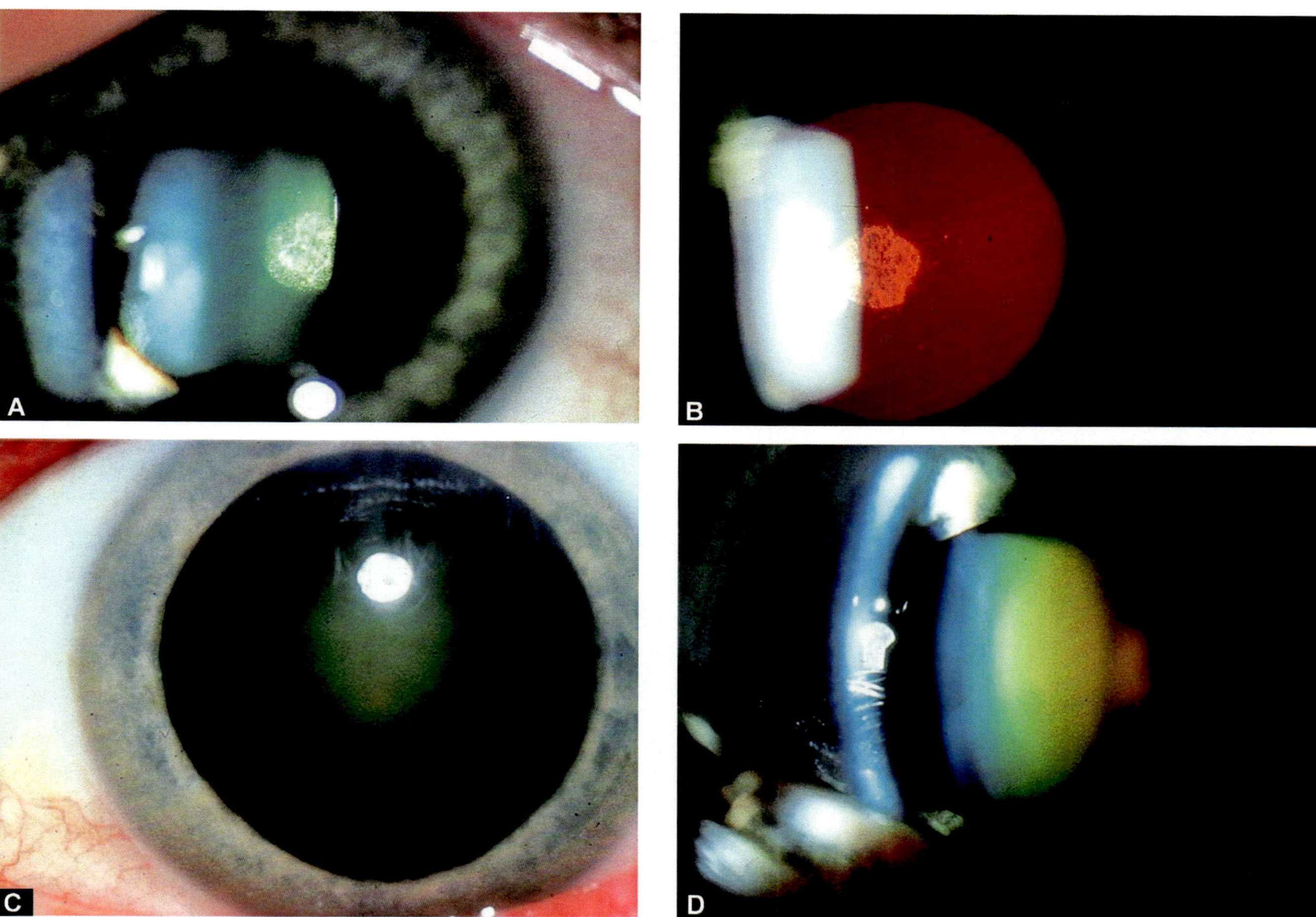

Figs 39.1 A to D: Posterior Subcapsular Cataract (top, left and right). Cataract with Nuclear Sclerosis (bottom, left and right). Figures 1A and B are three dimensional photographs of a characteristic posterior subcapsular cataract, seen with the slit lamp (top-left) and with indirect illumination also using the slit lamp (top-right). Figures 1C and D are three dimensional photos of nuclear sclerotic cataract, viewed with diffuse illumination (left) and with the slit lamp beam (right). This is the most common form of cataract. Patients tend to be hindered more by loss of contrast sensitivity rather than glare. (Reproduced with permission from AAO's Basic and Clinical Science Course, Lens and Cataract 2003, enhanced by Highlights of Ophthalmology)

for both near and distance fixation, thus providing spectacle independence. However not all eyes, or all patients, are the same. The surgeon has to review the patient's needs and expectations, the status of the fellow eye, the IOL power for emmetropia, and then choose the IOL power accordingly. Keep in mind that patients can easily tolerate a 1.5 to 2.0 D difference in refractive error between the two eyes (anisometropia), with no risks of asthenopia and/or diplopia.

The surgeon has also to remember that emmetropic patients do not tolerate any error in IOL power calculations; they might reluctantly accept induced myopia, but they will rarely accept induced hyperopia. In certain cases, in which both eyes eventually have to be operated on, it is recommended to perform cataract surgery in the non-dominant eye first, to make the proper final adjustments for the second eye at the time of the surgery.

DETERMINING CORNEAL POWER

According to the Gullstrand eye model, total corneal power is 43.00D, which is the sum of the anterior corneal surface (49.00D) and the posterior corneal surface (-6.00D). Corneal power measurements using conventional manual keratometers are estimates based on the curvature of the anterior corneal surface in the paracentral 3 mm and a conversion to a total corneal power using the keratometric index of refraction, which assumes Gullstrand proportions between the anterior and posterior corneal curvatures. However, changes in corneal shape after refractive surgery alter these relationships and render incorrect the assumptions necessary for the accurate use of conventional keratometers. Furthermore, normal corneal curvature is prolate, not spherical, and the validity of using the paracentral cornea to determine the effective anterior corneal curvature once the aspheric shape has been altered by refractive surgery has not been confirmed.[4]

DETERMINING IOL POWER (BIOMETRY)

Ocular biometry must be performed prior to cataract surgery. Biometry is the discipline in charge of the physical parameters of the eyeball, and includes two fundamental explorations, keratometry and the axial length measurement of the eye. However, in clinical practice, the term biometry refers to the latter and considers keratometry to be a separate process.

There is no question that when well selected and properly done the modern methods of Partial Coherence Interferometry (now known as Optical Coherence Biometry) and Advanced Ultrasonic Contact and Immersion Ultrasonography afford us the best way of achieving the desired postoperative refraction. Determination of intraocular lens power through meaningful keratometric readings and axial length measurements, have become a "standard of care". A challenging technique to obtain good visual results and patient satisfaction.[5]

AVOIDING POSTOPERATIVE REFRACTIVE ERRORS

This is particularly true considering the high patient's expectations and the minimal astigmatism created by small incision cataract surgery, particularly phacoemulsification. Patients look forward to wearing spectacles postoperatively only under special circumstances. As 70 percent of cataract patients have less than 1 diopter of astigmatism, it is expected that at least these amount of patients should obtain the desired expected refraction after surgery. Another 20 percent of patients have between 1 and 2 diopters and those might require the addition of additional astigmatism surgery. The remaining 10 percent of patients have astigmatism higher than 2 diopters and perhaps the addition of Toric IOL implantation and Bioptics might produce the desired results. In other words, the surgeon should deliver refractive surgical expectations based upon the preoperative biomicroscopic exam, biometric readings, IOL power formulas selected, and the surgical experience to deliver a flawless result.[6]

Therefore, exact determination of the IOL power to match the specific planned postoperative refraction is essential. The advent of foldable multifocal IOL and accommodative IOL make this even more of an important, though complex subject, as well as performing surgery on eyes with different axial lengths: normal (Fig. 39.2), short as in hyperopia (Fig. 39.3), long as in myopia (Fig. 39.4).[7]

THE CHALLENGE OF THE COMPLEX CASES

Corneal refractive surgery with its variety of procedures including excimer refractive laser surgery (Fig. 39.6), radial keratotomy (Fig. 39.7), and intracorneal ring segments (Fig. 39.8) can make the IOL power calculation more difficult by making more complex the calculation of the actual corneal power. In these particular cases, Computerized Videokeratography provides additional important data in the solution of these particular problems.

IOL power calculation in pediatric cataract patients (Fig. 39.10), in eyes with previous vitreoretinal surgery and use of silicone oil, in very short eyes (Figs 39.3A and B), in extremely long eyes (Fig. 39.4), in previous corneal transplant patients, secondary implantations, IOL exchange, previous vitrectomy, or when planning multifocal IOL implantation are some of the cases considered to be challenging for calculations.[8,9]

In clinical practice, the axial length (AL) is measured with the **IOL Master** (Partial Coherence Inter-

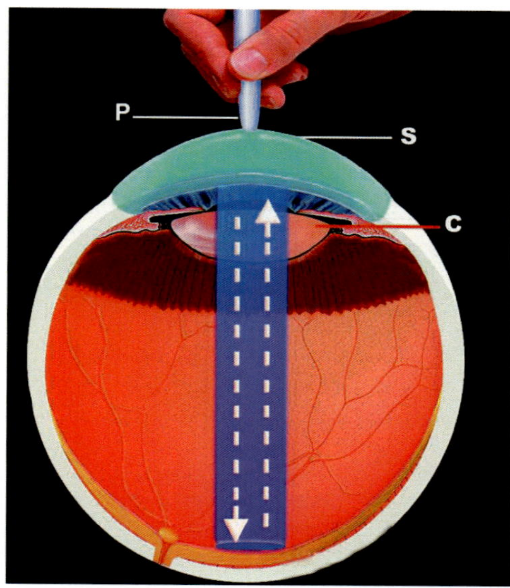

Fig. 39.2: Determination of IOL Power in Patients with Normal Axial Length (Normal Eyes). The use of ultrasound to calculate the intraocular lens power takes into account the variants that may occur in the axial length of the eye and the curvature of the cornea. The ultrasound probe (P) emits and receives high frequency sound waves. The sound waves travel through the eye until they are reflected back by any structure that stands perpendicularly in their way (represented by arrows). The speed of the ultrasound waves (arrows) is higher through a dense lens (C) than through a clear lens. Soft tipped transductors (P) are recommended to avoid errors when touching the corneal surface (S). The computer of the ultrasound unit can automatically multiply the time by the sound velocity to obtain the axial length. (Art from Highlights of Ophthalmology)

ferometry) when possible and with ultrasonography, using a biometry unit. Measurement of the AL is achieved using an immersion or a contact technique. It is always advisable to have both eyes measured for comparison purposes.

When using ultrasound, the axial length is determined by measurements obtained from the eye tissue interfaces with the ultrasound beam (Fig. 39.2 arrows). The A- scan must be carefully calibrated and the velocity must correspond to whether or not the patient is phakic, pseudophakic, or aphakic and may need to be modified in some of the special cases previously described. When using an A-Scan Biometer there are components that the user must understand as the probe configuration, the transducer, the

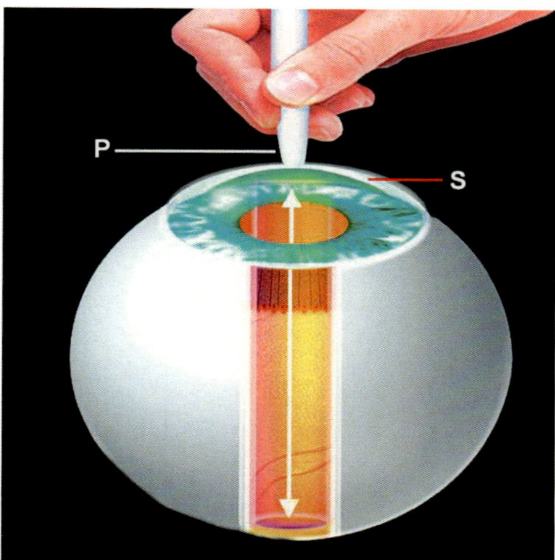

Fig. 39.3: IOL Power Calculation in Patients With Very Short Axial Length (Hyperopia). In eyes with short axial lengths, the third generation formulas such as the Holladay 2 and Hoffer-Q seem to provide the best results. Holladay found that the size of the anterior and posterior segments is not necessarily proportional in extremely short eyes (< 20.0 mm). Only 20 percent of short eyes present a small anterior segment (nanophthalmic eyes); as 80 percent present a normal anterior segment and an abnormally short posterior segment as shown here. (P) represents probe, (S) represents corneal surface. (Art from Highlights of Ophthalmology)

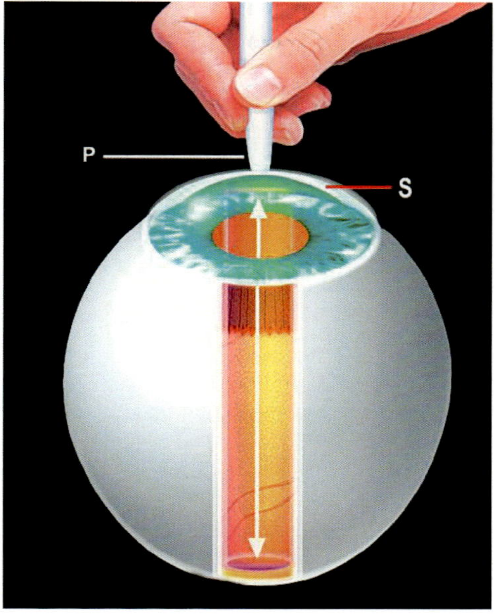

Fig. 39.4: IOL Power Calculation in High Myopia. In high myopia with axial lengths higher than 27.0 mm the use of the SRK/T formula has shown good predictability. Probe (P), corneal surface (S). (Art from Highlights of Ophthalmology)

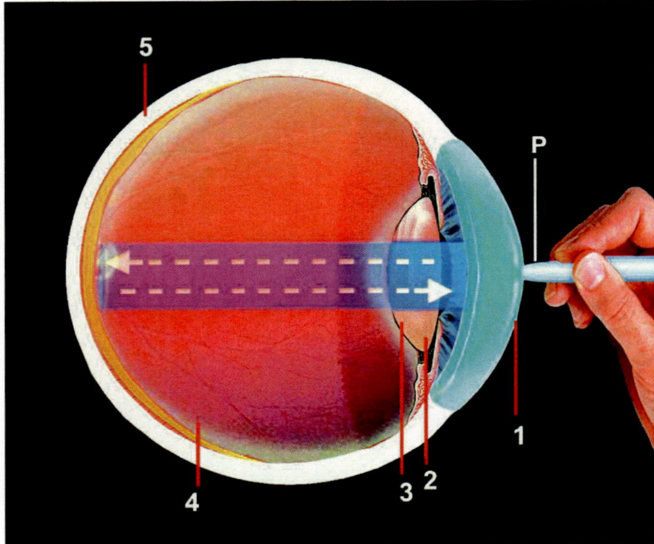

Fig. 39.5: A scan of a normal eye (1) Cornea; (2) Anterior lens capsule; (3) Posterior lens capsule; (4) Retina; (5) Sclera. P. A-Scan probe

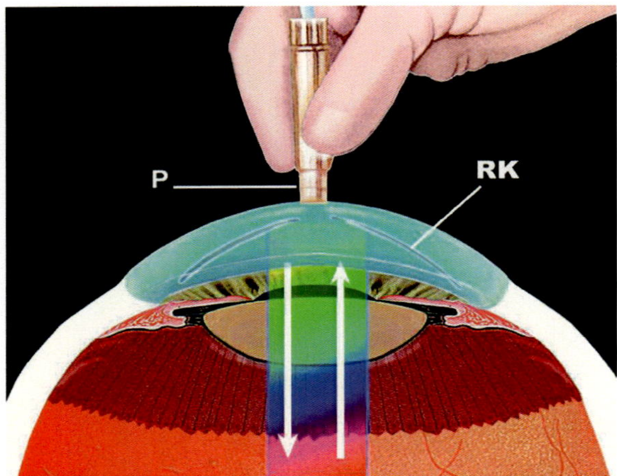

Fig. 39.7: IOL Power Calculation in Patients After Radial Keratotomy. Patients who have undergone previous radial keratotomy using an optical zone smaller than 4.0 mm, cannot have their central corneal curvature measured reliably with the standard keratometric methods. Axial length measurement may be done with the standard A scan ultrasonographic technique (Art from Highlights of Ophthalmology)

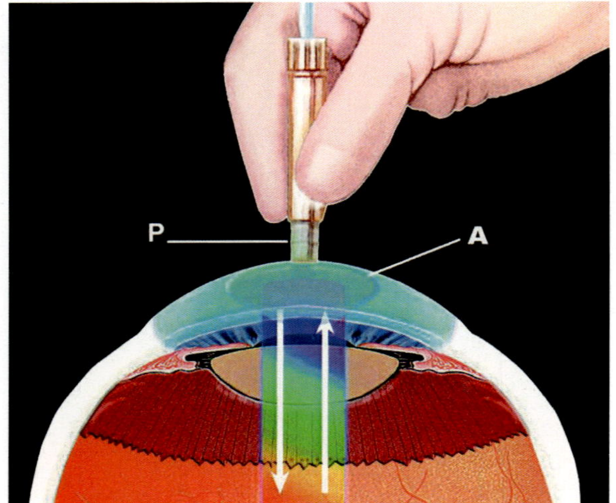

Fig. 39.6: IOL Power Calculation After Excimer Laser Procedure. In this group of patients there is a degree of variation in the results of the IOL power calculation. This is the result of the varying modification in the central curvature of the cornea after the central excimer laser ablation (A). (Art from Highlights of Ophthalmology)

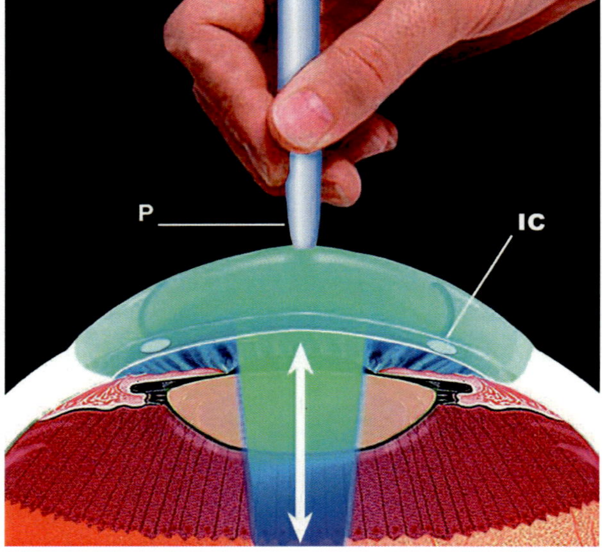

Fig. 39.8: IOL Power Calculation After an Intracorneal Ring Segment Procedure. As with other refractive procedures on the cornea, this technique for correction of low myopia also modifies the corneal curvature. When the preoperative data is not available for the IOL power calculation by the history method, the central flattest K obtained by corneal topography is utilized for the IOL power calculation as the central corneal power. In this illustration we can see the ultrasound transducer (P) on the central cornea inside the area in which the Intracorneal Rings (IC) are placed. (Art from Highlights of Ophthalmology)

emitted ultrasound beam, the oscilloscope, the sensitivity setting, the velocity setting, the electronic gates, and the biometer's report (Fig. 39.5).[10,11]

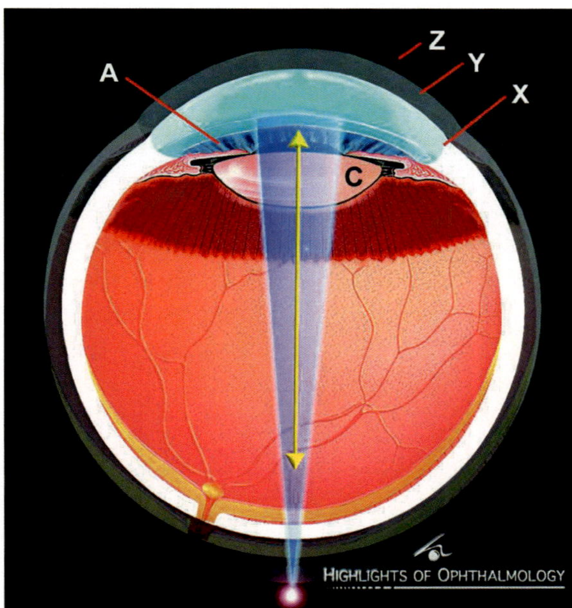

Fig. 39.9: IOL Power Calculation in Pediatric Cataract. The growth of the globe is ecographically registered until young ages. However, the lens continues growing throughout the life of the individual. In normal circumstances, the anterior chamber (A) depth is reduced as the lens (C) increases in size. In this illustration we can see the changes in the size of the globe through the shaded images that outline the growth of the eye by stages. At birth, the eye measures approximately 17.5 mm; at three years of age it measures 21.8 mm (X), at ten years 22.5 mm identified in (Y), and in normal adulthood nearly 24-mm (Z). During IOL power selection, some surgeons do prefer to leave the child in a hyperopic stage (arrows) as emmetropia will be accomplished with the expected growth of the eye. Other surgeons prefer to aim for emmetropia for the prompt treatment of the associated amblyopia. (Art from Highlights of Ophthalmology)

COMMONLY USED FORMULAS

There are different basic groups of formulas, the Theoretical and the Empirics or Regression Formulas. The Theoretical Formulas are based on geometrical optics. The different theoretical formulas differ in the method they calculate the ELP (Estimated Lens Position), the IOL position related to the cornea. The only variable that cannot be measured preoperatively and that the formula must estimate. In the First Generation Theoretical formulas, the ELP (then ACD) was a constant factor depending of the IOL position (Fyodorov, Colenbrander, Hoffer, Thijssen, Van Der Heijde, and Binkhorst). The Second

Table 39.1: The "average" formula is obtained calculating the mean of the three formulas: Hoffer, Holladay and SKR/T

AL	< 22.0	22.0-24.0	> 24.0
Formula	Holladay II Modified Hoffer Q	Average Holladay I	SRK/T Holladay I

Generation related the ELP to the AL (Binkhorst, Shammas, and Hoffer). In the Third Generation the ELP varies in function of the AL and Keratometry (Holladay 1 in 1988, SRK/T in 1990, Hoffer Q in 1993). The Fourth Generation Theoretic Formulas are based on the ELP calculation in more than two variables (Olsen in 1990, Holladay II in 1996).The Holladay II formula is included in the Holladay IOL Consultant^{TM} software.[12,13]

The Regression or Empiric Formulas are based on the retrospective statistical analysis of refractive results of multiple surgical procedures. Sanders, Retzlaff and Kraff described the most utilized formula SRK (in 1980) P = A-2.5 AL–0.9 K. Modifications were added to the formula for eyes with AL >24.5-mm and < 22-mm .The new formula was called SRK II. In the last few years the Regression Formulas has been considered less predictable than the latest generation of Theoretic Formulas. The Hoffer Q, Holladay I and SRK/T are available in the Hoffer 2.5 software.

In conclusion, the recommended formulas are given in Table 39.1.

MAIN CAUSES OF ERROR

The most common cause of postoperative refractive error is due to the imprecise preoperative biometric measurements. From these causal errors in IOL power calculations, fully 68 percent are due to errors in axial length (AL) measurement, 22 percent are due to not using the appropriate formula, and 10 percent are attributed to keratometric readings (Olsen).[14]

Mendicute's 1998 short series concluded that 73.68 percent of the cause was faulty AL measurement, 15.78 percent were due to an error in data transcription to the software, and 5.26 percent an error in keratometric readings.

AL measurements have improved by the increasing number of immersion procedures, and the usage of the Partial Coherence Interferometry (IOL Master) to the point that we can now state that 85 to 90 percent cases will result to within 1 diopter of the desired postoperative refraction.

With the increased usage of the Holladay Consultant software containing the Holladay II formula and the recently released Hoffer 2.5 software, which utilizes the latest versions of the Average Formula, Hoffer Q, Holladay I, and SRK/T, (Table 39.1) and the incorporation of the Haigis formula within the IOL Master, we are certainly using the most advanced theoretical formulas in the market.[15,16]

And finally, I would like to emphasize that keratometry must be performed in an automated as well as in a calibrated manual keratometer, and it is probably most accurate when performed more than once prior to surgery.

TARGETING POSTOPERATIVE REFRACTION

This is a parameter that has to be decided by the treating physician and inputted into the software for the IOL power calculation. All the other parameters, except the ELP, are measured or assumed values, over which the physician has no control.

When selecting a lens implant power, Dr. Luis Lu, generally recommend that the surgeon targets mild myopia of -0.25 to -0.50 D in a previous emmetropic or previous hyperopic patient. The second eye is targeted to have the same postoperative refraction or aims for monovision if the patient requests this alternative and the second eye is the non-dominant eye. In myopic patients, we always aim for myopia, and the degree of postoperative negative lens depends of the needs of each patient. A common request is a –0.5 to –0.75 D in the dominant eye and –2.25 to –2.50 D in the non-dominant eye. These patients will wear corrective lenses after surgery as they are so used to.

In patients who have no desire in wearing postoperative corrective glasses, a slight myopic astigmatism is to be accomplished.

Also, patients need to be counseled in regard to expectations of refractive changes and that they will generally need reading glasses or bifocals as the implant has no power of accommodation. Patients that will be candidates for multifocal IOL implantation, accommodative IOL implantation or monovision, need extra time to thoroughly explain the expected results to these patients. If realistic expectations are not present, the surgeon should suggest another alternative instead of facing an eventually dissatisfied patient.

IOL POWER CALCULATION IN COMPLEX CASES

Specific Methods to Use in Complex Cases

Considering that there are no specific methods on which there is full agreement as to what to do in these patients, **we hereby recommend** the use of third/ fourth generation of the theoretical formulas, preferably more than one and that the highest resulting IOL power should be considered to be used for the implantation. These preferred formulas include the Holladay 2, SRK/T, and the Hoffer Q. The regression formulas will induce undercorrection (e.g. SRK I or SRK II). We also recommend that in certain complex cases you should consider the use of the central 3.0-mm corneal topography's flattest curve as a keratometric method unless you are fortunate to have all the information needed for the "refractive history method." This reading is fed to the computer utilizing the selected formulas. The computer will then provide you with the power of the IOL to be utilized.[17]

DETERMINING IOL POWER IN PATIENTS WITH PREVIOUS REFRACTIVE SURGERY

Patients who have undergone excimer laser procedures, radial keratotomy or intracorneal segment rings, have had modifications to their corneal curvatures (Figs 39.6 to 39.8). Accurate keratometric readings are fundamental in calculating IOL power. IOL power calculation for cataract surgery in patients previously submitted to refractive surgery by modification of the corneal curvature is a new challenge for the cataract surgeon because (1) Patients who previously decided to undergo refractive surgery are more psychologically resistant to wearing spectacles to correct residual ametropia and consequently, their expectations for cataract surgery are unusually high. (2) So far there is no universally accepted formula to calculate these patients' IOL power accurately. Routine keratometry readings do not reflect the true central corneal curvature in these cases and may result in errors if used for IOL calculations. Standard keratometric readings should not be used for IOL power calculations in these patients. If done, the standard IOL power-predictive formulas based on such readings will result in a very undesirable and substantial undercorrection.[18-20]

To better understand the issue of IOL power calculations in ablative refractive surgery, it is wise to look first for the reasons leading to miscalculation. Errors mainly depend on two factors. First, current keratometers and videokeratography systems do not correctly measure central corneal power in these eyes, because they instead measure the curvature of the anterior corneal surface. This measurement is converted into keratometric diopters, with a standardized keratometric index of refraction (usually 1.3375) on the basis of the paraxial equation $P = (n-1)/r$, where P is the corneal power (diopters), n is the standardized keratometric index of refraction, and r is the radius of the anterior corneal surface (meters). The keratometric index of refraction refers to a theoretical single refractive lens—representing the anterior and posterior corneal surfaces—and assumes a stable ratio of anterior-to-posterior corneal curvature. Of course, LASIK and PRK disrupt this ratio, making the standard keratometric index of refraction invalid. The second problem is that most IOL power calculation formulas incorrectly predict the effective lens position. Using the postrefractive surgery K-value causes effective lens position underestimation and contributes to IOL underestimation. Aramberri solved this problem by introducing the double-K method. The prerefractive surgery K is used to calculate the effective lens position, and the postrefractive surgery K produces the IOL power using the vergence formula.[21-23]

METHODS MOST OFTEN USED

This section reviews the methods proposed to estimate the true power of the central cornea in eyes that have undergone corneal refractive surgery. The clinical history method and the contact lens method have been well discussed during the past decade. Hoffer states that the problem we have is determining the true optical central power of the cornea using the present instrumentation available. Keratometers and topographers measure the cornea too peripherally and miss the central, flat part of the cornea. The result is an overestimation of the corneal power that, when entered into the IOL power formula, produces an overly weak IOL power and thus a hyperopic refractive result. The methods described herein are intended to better estimate the true power of the altered cornea.[24, 25]

CLINICAL HISTORY METHOD

Holladay proposed this method based on the idea that refractive surgery has changed the corneal power and that this refractive change must be substracted to the presurgical power of the cornea in order to estimate its present power. You need to obtain:

- A preoperative average K reading (Kp)
- A preoperative spherical equivalent refractive error (Rp, before refractive corneal surgery)
- A postoperative spherical equivalent refractive error (Ro, after the eye has healed following refractive surgery and visual acuity has stabilized but before cataract formation)

  To calculate the eye's estimated corneal power (K), use the Hoffer formula:

  $$K = Kp + (Rp) - (Ro)$$

  Remember to add algebraically and to change the sign when opening the second parenthesis.

  Vertex-correcting the refractions is no longer recommended.

CONTACT LENS METHOD

Contact lens method was first described by Ridley, later by Soper, and more recently published by Holladay. It was transformed into a formula by Hoffer. The method is based on the concept that, if a hard PMMA contact lens of known base curve (i.e. 36.00D) and known power (i.e. Plano) is placed on the cornea and the refraction does not change, the effective power of the cornea must be 36.00 D. If the power is different from plano and/or the difference in refraction is not zero, the formula will calculate the power. This method is limited to those cataractous eyes with a minimum best corrected visual acuity of 20/80. The method will not work in eyes that are not able to be refracted.

You need to obtain:

- A hard PMMA (not RGP) contact lens with a base curve (B) close to the estimated K reading and with a known power (P, easier if plano).
- A bare manifest refraction without a contact lens (Rb).
- A manifest overrefraction with a contact lens (Rc). To calculate the eye's estimated corneal power (K), use the formula:

  $$K = B + P + Rc - Rb$$

  Remember to add algebraically and that is not longer recommended to vertex-correcting the refractions.

MALONEY TOPOGRAPHY METHOD

Maloney, in Los Angeles has been using a formula that Hoffer calls the Maloney Topographic Method. You only need to obtain the postoperative simulated central K reading from the topographic unit (Kt). To calculate the eye's estimated corneal power (K), use the formula: $K = 376/\ (337.5/Kt) - 5.5$

THE TOPOGRAPHY METHOD

When information is not available for the Clinical History Method, it has been recommended by Zacharias and Centurion, as well as by Torres and Suarez, that the keratometric reading be taken with the topography unit, using the flattest K found in the central 3 mm of the corneal mapping.

Hoffer has suggested that after looking at the preceding methods, we should choose the lowest K reading from those you have calculated to use in the formula and then employ the Aramberri Double-K Method.

ARAMBERRI DOUBLE-K METHOD

In 2001, Dr Jaime Aramberri had the idea that the postsurgical flatter K reading should not be used in modern, theoretic formulas to calculate the estimated position of the IOL (estimated lens position, ELP, the visual axial distance from the apex of the cornea to the principal plane of the IOL, or anterior chamber depth). This concept is based on the fact that the flattening and thinning of the cornea has not changed the biometric measurements of the anterior chamber structures; that is, the cornea has not changed its distance relationship with the crystalline lens and iris. Hoffer calls it the Aramberri Double-K Method.[26]

What you need to do is:

- Use the preoperative K reading (Kp. e.g. 43.50 D) in the part of the formula that predicts the estimated lens position (anterior chamber depth)
- Use the postoperative (Ko, e.g. 35.00 D) in the part of the formula that calculates the IOL power.

Presently this option is only available on the Hoffer Programs version 2.5. This method has not been tested for accuracy on a large reported series.

K-Method in Previous Radial Keratotomy

For patients with previous RK with optical zone (OZ) of less than 4.0 mm, use the clinical history method if possible, otherwise use the flattest K of the central 3.0 mm in the topographic map, or both. Check the IOL power with the SRK/T formula of the Hoffer 2.5 software. If the OZ is larger than 4.0 mm, use the measured K obtained with the keratometer as it will not be affected.

In conclusion, in patients with previous Myopic LASIK/LASEK/PRK, use the clinical history method if possible, otherwise use the flattest K of the central 3.0 mm of the topographic map. In Hyperopic Lasik/

PRK, Conductive Keratoplasty (CK), and intracorneal rings, the central corneal thickness is basically unaffected. In these cases the K readings obtained can be used for the IOL power calculation. The clinical history method is utilized to double-check the corneal power (Figs 39.6 to 39.8).

THE ESCAF APHAKIC OR REFRACTION METHOD

In 2002, Dr Luis Escaf from Colombia proposed a method of calculating the IOL power for postrefractive surgery eyes that does not require the axial length or average K reading, presented at the Pan-American Congress of Ophthalmology. It is based on the concept of manually determining the aphakic refraction of the eye immediately after surgery. Soon after, the use of a handheld autorefraction device (Ianchulev 2003) was utilized based upon the same concept and right after cataract removal in the operating room (OR). After using this method in a series of eyes, both proposed a formula to convert the refraction obtained into an IOL power (P) of a given A constant (A). This method could also be used for normal eyes but could require a clear cornea after cataract removal and the availability of a full inventory of lens powers in the OR.

Escaf $P = [(2.0 \times Rx) - 2.00\ D] + (A - 118.0)$

Ianchulev $P = (2.02 \times Rx) + (A-118.4)$

IOL POWER CALCULATION IN PEDIATRIC CATARACTS

Once a decision has been made to perform cataract surgery in a pediatric patient, the next consideration is the selection of optical rehabilitation that will be used for that particular patient.

For patients with monocular cataracts, aphakic spectacles are not practical. Before one year of age, use of contact lens rehabilitation is suggested, after age 1 year, an IOL should be considered.

In patients with bilateral cataracts, contact lens rehabilitation is recommended before 1 year of age. The unpredictable response and growth of an eye in a child less than one year of age may preclude selection of an IOL as a primary procedure in children (Fig. 39.9).

The situation has now changed significantly. The previous failures with spectacles and contact lenses, the new developments in technology and surgical techniques, and the positive thinking of a new generation of surgeons has led us to implant posterior chamber IOLs in children. The development of improved medications to prevent and control inflammation, the introduction of posterior capsulorhexis, and better viscoelastics and IOLs, has allowed us to become more successful with IOL implantation in children.[27-32]

Measures should be taken to select a lens of appropriate power for the age of the child. Replacement of an IOL that has been placed in the eye of a child is difficult because the adhesions formed. The power selection should be one that is appropriate for a lifetime. The surgeon should attempt to anticipate the refractive error at maturity. Some of the considerations in selecting a lens power are the age of the child, the refractive error of the fellow eye and the refractive error of the parents. Biglan calculates the lens power for the eye to achieve emmetropia using a SRK II formula. Aramberri recommends the use of the Third generation theoretical formulas. Biometric readings may be difficult to obtain in children. If the child has not had axial length determination or is uncooperative for preoperative studies, the axial length determination and keratometry are performed in the operating room after the child has been anesthetized. Lens power calculations are performed while the patient is being prepared and draped and the surgical microscope has been positioned.

REFERENCES

1. Lu L. IOL power calculation in standard and complex cases. In: Boyd S (Ed): New Outcomes in Cataract Surgery. Highlights of Ophthalmology 2005;29-53.
2. Boyd BF. The Art and Science of Cataract Surgery, 2001; 36-59.
3. Boyd BF. Undergoing cataract surgery with a master surgeon: a personal experience. Highlights of Ophthalmol. Bi-monthly Journal, 1999;27(1):3.
4. Chu R, Goyal N, Jiang W, Khan B, Pepose J, Sanguhera P. Calculating IOL power after refractive surgery: peer reviewed literature. Cataract and refractive surgery today 2005;4:1-3.

5. Celikkol L, Pavlopoulos G, Weinstein B, et al. Calculation of intraocular lens power after radial keratotomy with computerized videokeratography. Am J Ophthalmol 1995;120:739-50.
6. Chen L, Mannis MJ, Salz JJ, et al. Analysis of intraocular lens power calculation in post-radial keratotomy eyes. J Cataract Refract Surg 2003;29:65-70.
7. Hoffer KJ. Intraocular lens power calculation for eyes after refractive keratotomy. J Refract Surg 1995;11:490-3.
8. Grinbaum A, Treister G, Moisseiev J. Predicted and actual refraction after intraocular lens implantation in eyes with silicone oil. J Cataract Refract Surg 1996;22:726-9.
9. Grusha YO, Masket S, Miller KM. Phacoemulsification and lens implantation after pars plana vitrectomy. Ophthalmology 1998;105:287-94.
10. Holladay JT, Gills JP, Leidlein J, Cherchio M. Achieving emmetropia in extremely short eyes with two piggyback posterior chamber intraocular lenses. Ophthalmology 1996;103:1118-23.
11. Holladay JT. Standardizing constants for ultrasonic biometry, keratometry and intraocular lens power calculations. J Cataract Refract Surg 1997;23:1356-70.
12. Hoffer KJ: The Hoffer Q formula: A comparison of theoretic and regression formulas. J Cataract Surg 1993; 19:700-11.
13. Koch D, Wang I. Calculating IOL power in eyes that have had refractive surgery. J Cataract Refract Surg 2003;29: 2039-42.
14. Olsen T, Thim K, Corydon L. Theoretical versus SRK I and SRK II calculation of intraocular lens power. J Cataract Refract Surg 1990;16:217-25.
15. Holladay JT. Consultations in refractive surgery. Refract Corneal Surg 1989;5:203.
16. Hoffer KJ. Ultrasound velocities for axial length measurement. J Cat Refract Surg 1994;20:554-62.
17. Holladay JT. Intraocular lens power in difficult cases. In: Masket S, Crandall A (Eds): Atlas of Cataract Surgery. Martin Dunitz, 1999;19:147-58.
18. Lyle WA, Jin GJC. Intraocular lens power prediction in patients who undergo cataract surgery following previous radial keratotomy. Arch Ophthalmol 1997; 115:457-61.
19. Maeda N, Klyce SD, Smolek MK, McDonald MB. Disparity between keratometry-style reading and corneal power within the pupil after refractive surgery for myopia. Cornea 1997;16:517-24.
20. Olsen T, Nielsen PJ. Immersion vs contact in the measurement of axial length by ultrasound. Acta Ophthalmol 1989;67:101-2.
21. Aramberri J. Intraocular lens power calculation after corneal refractive surgery: double-K method. J Cataract Refract Surg 2003;29:2063-8.
22. Rosa N, Capasso L, Lanza M. Double-K method to calculate IOL power after refractive surgery. J Cataract Refract Surg 2005;31:254-6.
23. Savini G, Hoffer K, Zanini M. IOL Power calculations after LASIK and PRK. Cataract and Refractive Surgery Today—Europe 2007;4:1-7.
24. Zacharias W, Centurion V. Biometry and the IOL calculation for the cataract surgeon: Its importance. Faco Total 2000;66-88.
25. Zaldivar R, Schultz MC, Davidorf JM, et al. Intraocular lens power calculations in patients with extreme myopia. J Cataract Refract Surg 2000;26:668-74.
26. Aramberri J. Intraocular lens power calculation after corneal refractive surgery: Double K method. J Cataract Refract Surg 2003;29:2063-8.
27. Brady KM, Atkinson CS, Kilty LA, Hiles DA. Cataract surgery and intraocular lens implantation in children. Am J Ophthalmol 1995;120:1-9.
28. Dahan E, Drusedan MUH. Choice of lens and dioptric power in pediatric pseudophakia. J Cataract Refract Surg 1997;23:618-23.
29. Gayton JL, Apple DJ, Peng Q, et al. Interlenticular opacification: Clinicopathological correlation of a complication of posterior chamber piggyback intraocular lenses. J Cataract Refract Surg 2000;26:300-36.
30. Gimbel HV. Posterior continuous curvilinear capsulorhexis and optic capture of the intraocular lens to prevent secondary opacification in pediatric cataract surgery. J Cataract Refract Surg 1997;23:652-6.
31. Gimbel HV, Basti S, Ferensowicz MA, DeBroff BM. Results of bilateral cataract extraction with posterior chamber intraocular lens implantation in children. Ophthalmology 1997;104:1737-43.
32. Kora Y, Shimizu K, Inatomi M, et al. Eye growth after cataract extraction and intraocular lens implantation in children. Ophthalmic Surg 1993;24:467-75.

RECOMMENDED READING

1. Boyd S. New Outcomes in Cataract Surgery. Highlights of Ophthalmology 2005.
2. Lu LW, Fine IH. Phacoemulsification in Difficult and Challenging Cases. New York: Thieme 1999.
3. Mendicute J, Aramberri J, Cadarso L, Ruiz M. Biometria, Formulas and Manejo de la sorpresa refractiva en la cirugia de catarata. España. Tecnimedia Editorial 2000.

40 No Anesthesia Cataract/ Clear Lens Extraction

Athiya Agarwal, Amar Agarwal

INTRODUCTION

On June 13th 1998 at Ahmedabad, India the first no anesthesia cataract surgery was done by the authors (Amar Agarwal) at the Phako and Refractive Surgery conference. This was performed as a live surgery in front of 250 delegates. This has opened up various new concepts in cataract surgery.[1] In this surgery, the technique of karate chop was used.

For high refractive errors, clear lens extraction with phacoemulsification is a very good alternative. In such cases, if necessary one can implant an IOL or leave the patient aphakic if the myopia is very high and does not warrant an IOL. This technique is very useful in hypermetropes, as LASIK does not give excellent results in such cases. The most commonly done refractive surgery in the world is not PRK or LASIK, it is cataract surgery. This is why this chapter will discuss phacoemulsification techniques for removal of cataract as well as clear lens extraction.

NUCLEUS REMOVAL TECHNIQUES

Since the introduction of Phacoemulsification as an alternative to standard cataract extraction techniques surgeons throughout the world have been attempting to make this new procedure safer and easier to perform while assuring good visual outcome and patient recovery. The fundamental goal of phaco is to remove the cataract with minimal disturbance to the eye using the least number of surgical manipulations. Each maneuver should be performed with minimal force and maximal efficiency should be obtained.

The latest generation phaco procedures began with Dr Howard Gimbel's "divide and conquer" nuclear fracture technique in which he simply split apart the nuclear rim. Since then, the authors have evolved through the various techniques, namely four quadrant cracking, chip and flip, spring surgery, stop and chop and phaco chop.

Clear lens removal by phacoemulsification is a very good alternative to manage refractive errors. In these cases, as the nucleus is soft one can use only Phacoaspiration to remove the nuclei, rather than use ultrasound power.

KARATE CHOP

Unlike the peripheral chopping of Nagahara or other stop and chop techniques, the authors have developed a safer technique called "central anterior chopping" or "karate chop". In this method the phaco tip is embedded by a single burst of power in the central safe zone and after lifting the nucleus a little bit (to lessen the pressure on the posterior capsule) the chopper is used to chop the nucleus. In soft nuclei, it is very difficult to chop the nucleus.

In most cases, one can take it out in toto. But if the patient is about 40 years of age then one might have to chop the nucleus.

SOFT CATARACTS

In soft cataracts, the technique is a bit different. The authors embed the phaco tip and then cut the nucleus as if they are cutting a piece of cake. This should be done 2 to 3 times in the same area so that the cataract gets cut. It is very tough to chop a soft cataract, so, this technique helps in splitting the cataract.

AGARWAL CHOPPER

The authors have devised their own chopper. Other choppers, which cut from the periphery, are blunt choppers. Their chopper is a sharp chopper. It has a sharp cutting edge. It also has a sharp point. The advantage of such a chopper is that you can chop in the center and need not go to the periphery.

In this method by going directly into the center of the nucleus without any sculpting, ultrasound energy required is reduced. The chopper always remains within the rhexis margin and never goes underneath the anterior capsule. Hence, it is easy to work with even small pupils or glaucomatous eyes. Since the authors do not have to widen the pupil, there is little likelihood of tearing the sphincter and allowing prostaglandins to leak out and cause inflammation or Cystoid Macular Edema (CME). In this technique the authors can easily go into even hard nuclei on the first attempt.

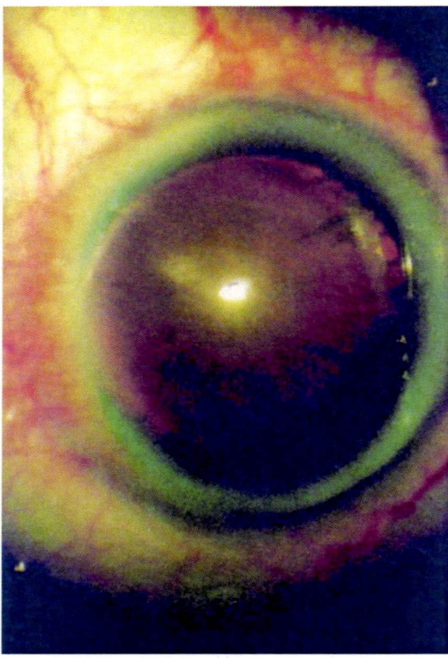

Fig. 40.1: Eye with cataract

THE AUTHORS' KARATE CHOP TECHNIQUE

Incision

A temporal clear corneal section is made. If the astigmatism is plus at 90 degrees then the incision is made superiorly (Read Chapter-2 on Corneal Topography).

First of all, a needle with viscoelastic is injected inside the eye (Fig. 40.1) in the area where the second site is made (Fig. 40.2). This will distend the eye so that when you make a clear corneal

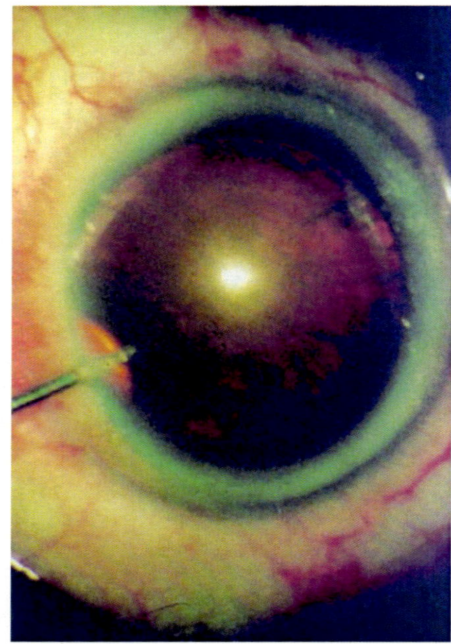

Fig. 40.2: Needle with viscoelastic entering the eye to inject the viscoelastic. **This is the most important step in no anesthesia cataract/clear lens surgery. This gives an entry into the eye through which a straight rod can be passed to stabilize the eye. Note no forceps holds the eye**

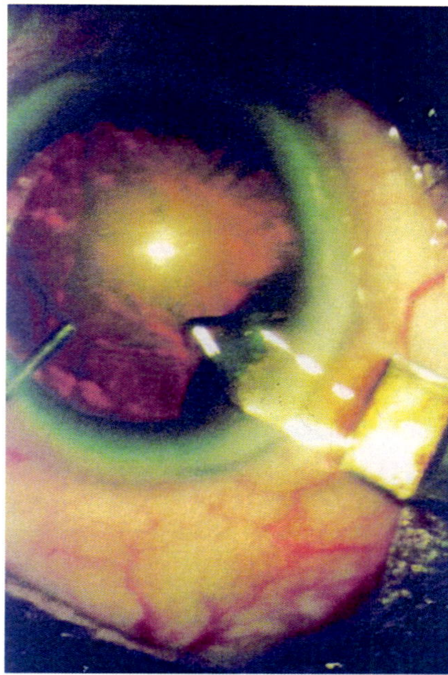

Fig. 40.3: Clear corneal incision. Note the straight rod inside the eye in the left hand. The right hand is performing the clear corneal incision. This is a temporal incision and the surgeon is sitting temporally

incision, the eye will be tense and one can create a good valve. Now use a straight rod to stabilize the eye with the left hand. With the right hand make the clear corneal incision (Fig. 40.3).

When the authors started making the temporal incisions, they positioned themselves temporally. The problem by this method is that, every time the microscope has to be turned which in turn would affect the cables connected to the video camera. Further the theater staff would get confused between right eye and left eye. To solve this problem, the authors then decided on a different strategy. They have operating trolleys on wheels. The patient is wheeled inside the operation theater and for the right eye the trolley is placed slightly obliquely so that the surgeon does not change his or her position. The surgeon stays at the 12 o'clock position. For the left eye, the trolley with the patient is rotated horizontally so that the temporal portion of the left eye comes at 12 o'clock. This way the patient is moved and not the surgeon.

Rhexis

Capsulorrhexis is then performed through the same incision (Fig. 40.4). **While performing the rhexis it is important to note that the rhexis is started from the centre and the needle moved to the right and then downward.** This is important because today concepts have changed of temporal and nasal. It is better to remember it as superior, inferior, right or left. If we would start the rhexis from the center and move it to the left then the weakest point of the rhexis is generally where you finish it. In other words, the point where you tend to lose the rhexis is near its completion. If you have done the rhexis from the center and moved to the left, then you might have an incomplete rhexis on the left-hand side either inferiorly or superiorly. Now, the phaco probe is always moved down and to the left. So, every stroke of your hand can extend the rhexis posteriorly creating a posterior capsular rupture. Now, if we perform the rhexis from the center and move to the right and then push the flap inferiorly—then if we have an incomplete rhexis near the end of the rhexis, it will be superiorly and

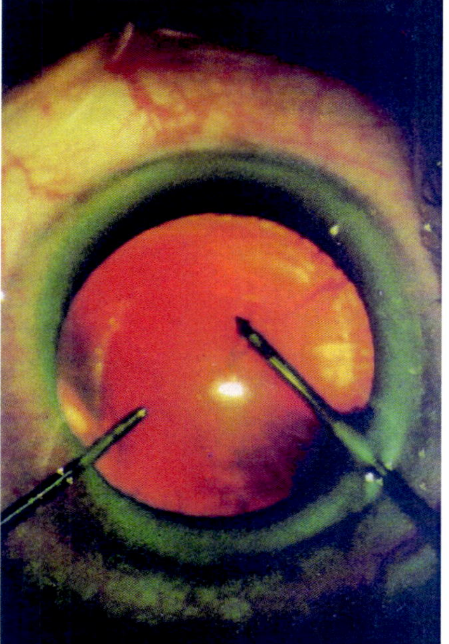

Fig. 40.4: Rhexis being done with a needle

to the right. Any incomplete rhexis can extend and create a posterior capsular tear. But in this case, the chances of survival are better. This is because we are moving the phaco probe down and to the left, but the rhexis is incomplete up and to the right.

If you are a left handed person start the rhexis from the center and move to the left and then down.

Hydrodissection

Hydrodissection is then performed (Fig. 40.5). Watch for the fluid wave to see that hydrodissection is complete. There is no need to perform hydrodelineation. Viscoelastic is then introduced before inserting the phaco probe.

Karate Chop: Two Halves

We then insert the phaco probe through the incision slightly superior to the center of the nucleus (Fig. 40.6). At that point apply ultrasound and see that the phaco tip gets embedded in the nucleus (Fig. 40.7). **The direction of the phaco probe should be obliquely downwards toward the vitreous and not horizontally towards the iris. Then only the nucleus will get embedded.** The settings at this stage are 70 percent phaco power, 24 ml/minute flow rate and 101 mm of Hg suction. By the time the phaco tip gets embedded in the nucleus, the tip would have reached the middle of the nucleus. Do not turn the bevel of the phaco tip downwards as the embedding is better the other way. The authors prefer a zero or 15-degree tip but any tip can be used.

Now stop phaco ultrasound and bring your foot to position 2 so that only suction is being used. Now lift the nucleus. When the authors say lift it does not mean lift a lot but just a little so that when the pressure is applied on the nucleus with the chopper the direction of the pressure is downwards. If the capsule is a bit thin like in hypermature cataracts you might rupture the posterior capsule and create a nucleus drop. So when we lift the nucleus the pressure on the posterior capsule is lessened. Now, with the chopper cut the nucleus with a straight downward motion (Fig. 40.8) and then move the chopper to the left when you reach the center of the nucleus. In other words, your left hand moves the chopper like a laterally reversed L.

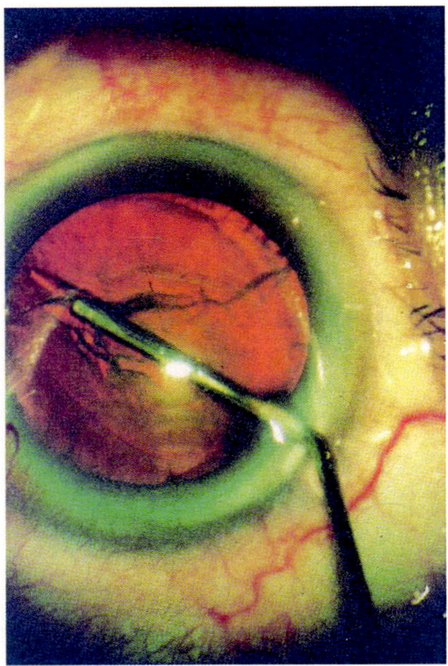

Fig. 40.5: Hydrodissection

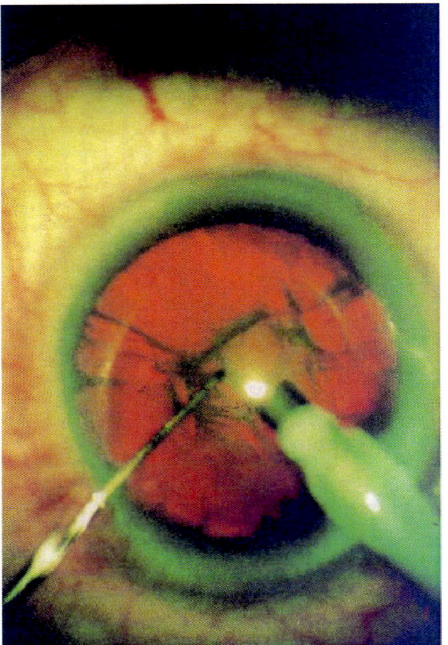

Fig. 40.6: Phaco probe placed at the superior end of the rhexis

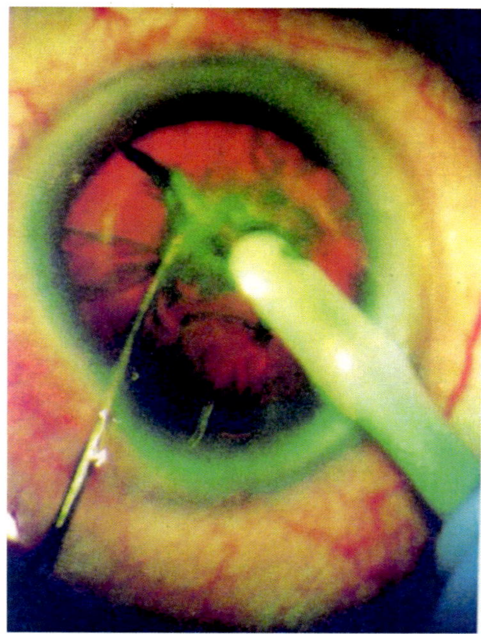

Fig. 40.7: Phaco probe embedded in the nucleus. **We started from the superior end of the rhexis and note it has got embedded in the middle of the nucleus.** If we had started in the middle then we would have embedded only inferiorly that is at the edge of the rhexis and chopping would be difficult

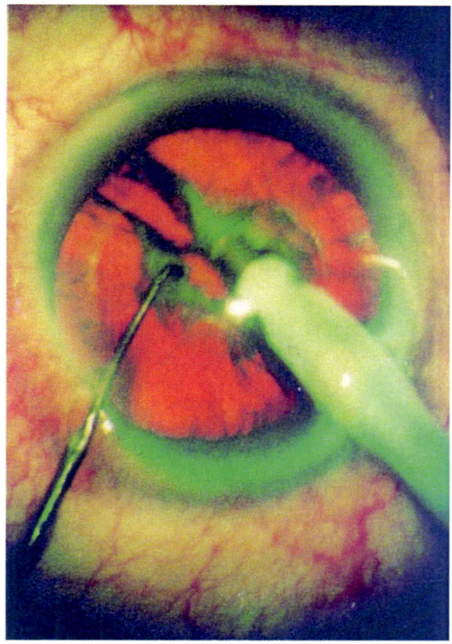

Fig. 40.8: Left hand chops the nucleus and splits like a laterally reversed L, that is downwards and to the left

Remember, do not go to the periphery for chopping but do it at the center.

Once you have created a crack, split the nucleus till the center. Then rotate the nucleus 180 degrees and crack again so that you get two halves of the nucleus. In brown cataracts, the nucleus will crack but sometimes in the center the nucleus will still be attached. You have to split the nucleus totally in two halves and you should see the posterior capsule throughout.

Karate Chop: Further Chopping

Now that you have two halves, you have a shelf to embed the probe. So, now place the probe with ultrasound into one-half of the nucleus (Fig. 40.9). You can pass the direction of the probe horizontally as now you have a shelf. Embed the probe, then pull it a little bit. This step is important so that you get an extra bit of space for chopping. This will prevent you from chopping the rhexis margin. Apply the force of the chopper downwards. Then move the chopper to the left so that the nucleus gets split. The chopper moves like a laterally reversed "L" in other words down to the left. Again, you should see posterior capsule throughout so that you know the nucleus is totally split. Then release the probe, as the probe will still be embedded into the nucleus. Like this, create three quadrants in one-half of the nucleus. Then make another three halves with the second half of the nucleus. Thus, you now have 6 quadrants or pie-shaped fragments. **The settings at this stage are 50 percent phaco power, 24 ml/minute flow rate and 101 mm of Hg suction.**

Remember 5 words: Embed, pull, chop, split and release.

Pulse Phaco

Once all the pieces have been chopped, take out each piece one by one and in pulse phaco mode aspirate the pieces at the level of the iris. Do not work in the bag unless the cornea is preoperatively bad or the patient is very elderly. **The setting at this stage can be phaco power 50 to 30 percent, flow rate 24 ml and suction 101 mm of Hg.**

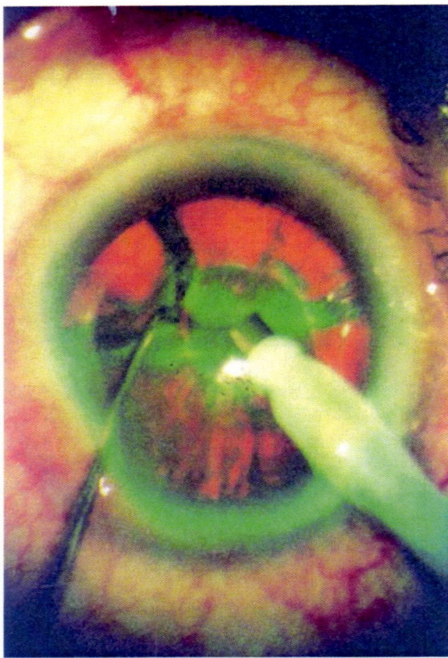

Fig. 40.9: Phaco probe embedded in one half of the nucleus. Go horizontally and not vertically as you have now a shelf of nucleus to embed. Chop and then split the nucleus

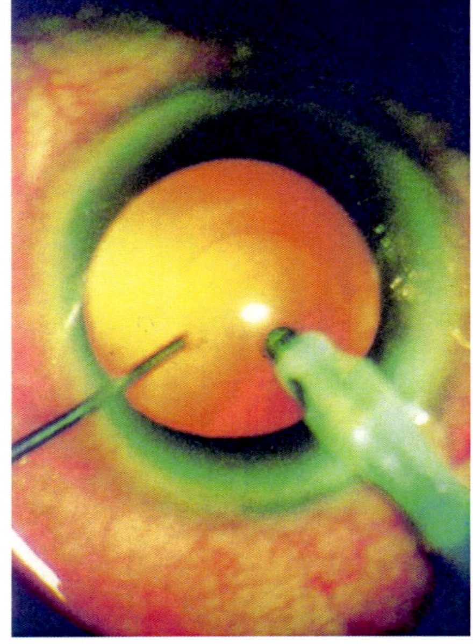

Fig. 40.10: Cortical aspiration completed. Note the straight rod in the left hand which helps to control the movements of the eye

Remember, it is better to have striate keratitis than posterior capsular rupture

Cortical Washing and Foldable IOL Implantation

The next step is to do cortical washing (Fig. 40.10). Always try to remove the subincisional cortex first, as that is the most difficult. In Figure 40.11 note the cortical aspiration is complete. Note also the rhexis margins. Everytime the left hand has the straight rod controlling the movements of the eye. If necessary use a bimanual irrigation-aspiration technique. Then inject viscoelastic and implant the foldable IOL. The authors use the plate haptic foldable IOL (Fig. 40.12) with large fenestrations generally as they find them superior (Fig. 40.13). Take out the viscoelastic with the irrigation-aspiration probe (Fig. 40.14).

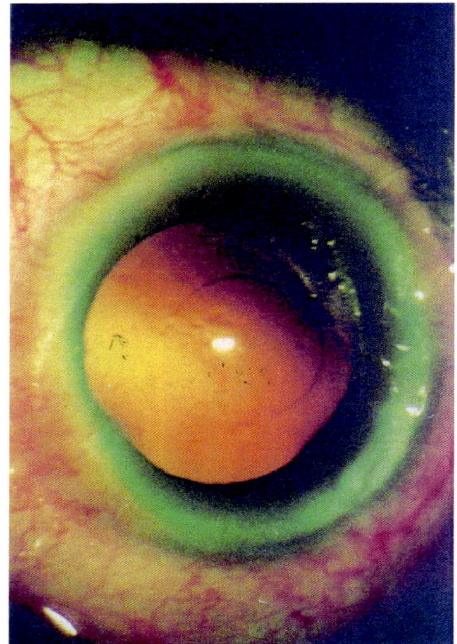

Fig. 40.11: Eye distended with viscoelastic. Note the rhexis margins

Stromal Hydration

At the end of the procedure, inject balanced salt solution (BSS) inside the lips of the clear corneal incision (Fig. 40.15). This will create a stromal hydration at the wound. This will create a

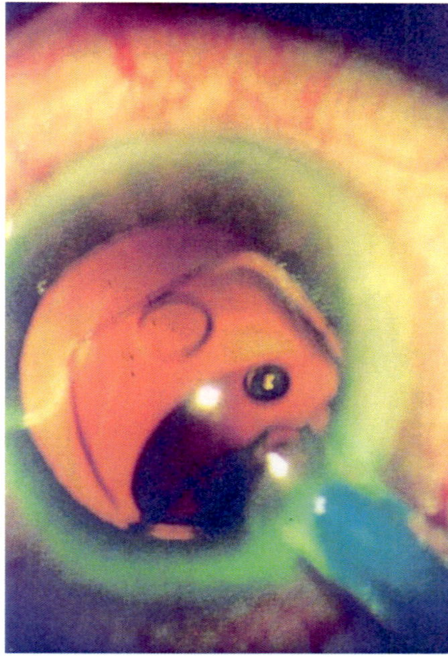

Fig. 40.12: Plate haptic foldable IOL with large fenestrations being implanted

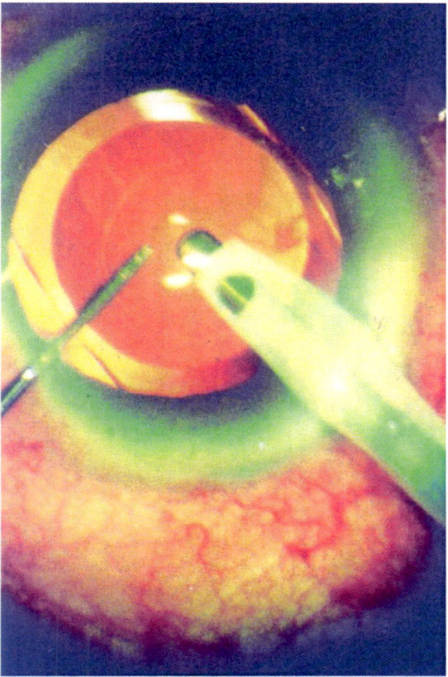

Fig. 40.14: Viscoelastic removed with the irrigation-aspiration probe

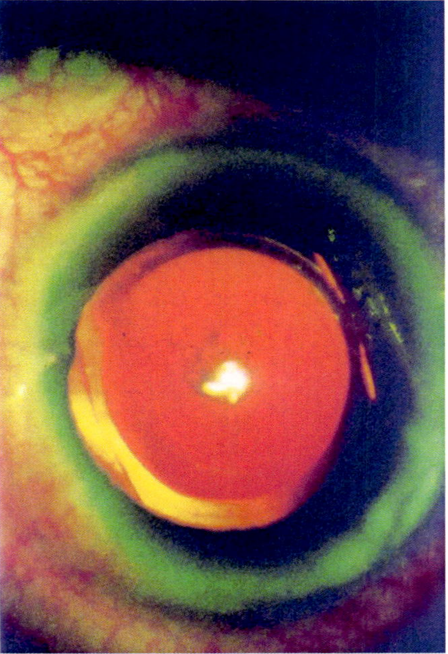

Fig. 40.13: Foldable IOL in capsular bag

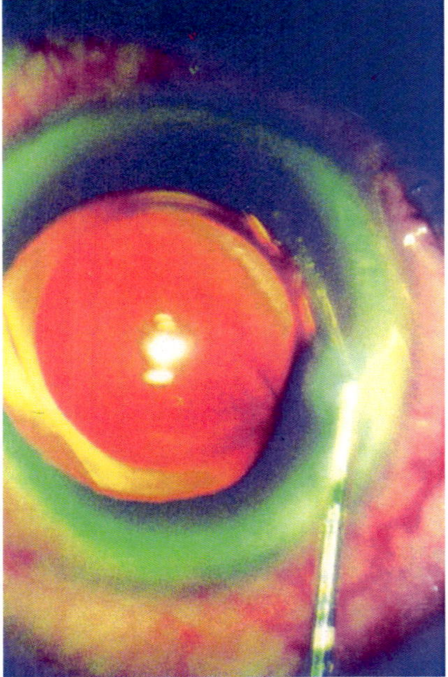

Fig. 40.15: Stromal hydration

whiteness, which will disappear after 4 to 5 hours. The advantage of this is that the wound gets sealed better.

No Pad, Subconjunctival Injections

No subconjunctival injection is given or pad applied to the eye. The patient walks out of the theater and goes home. The patient is seen the next day and after a month glasses are prescribed.

NO ANESTHESIA CLEAR LENS EXTRACTION

In cases of clear lens removals, the same technique is followed. No anesthesia is used. If one is not good then it is advisable to use a parabulbar anesthesia (pinpoint anesthesia) rather than a peribulbar block. The reason is that, in such cases one could perforate the globe with the needle. Once the patient is draped, the syringe with viscoelastic is taken and the viscoelastic injected inside the eye using a 26-gauge needle. Then the temporal clear corneal incision is made. If the astigmatism is + at 90 degrees then a superior incision is made.

The rhexis is then done using a needle. This is followed by hydrodissection. The phaco probe is passed into the eye and using phaco aspiration the soft nucleus removed. One does not have to use ultrasound, as the nucleus in such cases is very soft. This is followed by cortical aspiration. Depending on the biometry a foldable IOL is implanted in the eye. If the patient has high myopia and an IOL is not required then an IOL is not implanted. The authors have realized, that, chances of retinal detachment do not increase just because the eye is aphakic. The authors prefer to keep one eye emmetropic and the other slightly myopic to about 1 to 1.5 D so that the patient can see without glasses for distance and near with both eyes open.

Compared to LASIK this is a very good alternative, as LASIK does not help much in hyperopes and in high myopes (powers above –15 D).

PHACODYNAMICS OF THE PHACO CHOP TECHNIQUE

We should take full advantage of the phaco machine's capability thereby decreasing physical manipulation of the intraocular tissues. In this phaco chop technique, the authors use a vacuum of 101 mm of Hg, about 50-70 percent phaco power and the flow rate 24 ml/minute.

In this phaco chop technique, the most important parameter is the vacuum, which needs to be sufficient to stabilize the nucleus while the chopper is splitting it. If the action of the chopper is dislodging the vacuum seal on the phaco tip, it is said that the vacuum can be raised from 120 to 200 mm of Hg. After embedding the phaco needle with mild linear ultrasound power in foot switch position 3, it is important to raise the pedal back to foot switch position 2, while the vacuum builds up. This is because the purpose of ultrasound was to completely embed the aspiration port into the nucleus to obtain good vacuum seal. In foot switch 3, there is risk of adverse heat build-up because the occluded tip prohibits any flow of cooling. Also, when manipulating the nucleus by pulling with the embedded tip, the vacuum seal is likely to be compromised by the vibrating needle if it is in foot switch position 3.

ADVANTAGES

The phacoemulsification procedure has been proved to be reasonably safe to the endothelium. As compared to the "divide and conquer" technique, this phaco karate chop technique eliminates the need for trenching thereby producing significant reduction in phaco time and power consumed which in turn decreases endothelial cell damage. Even with increased density of cataract, there is a less pronounced increase in phaco time. Here we utilize the "Chop" to divide the nucleus by mechanical energy. It is safe and effective in nuclear handling during phacoemulsification.

In conventional chop, the disadvantage is that, the chopper is placed underneath the anterior capsule and then pulled towards the center. This can potentially damage the capsule and the zonules. In phaco chop, the authors do not go under the rhexis, the vertical element of the chopper remains within the rhexis margin and is visible at all stages. Hence it is very easy to work with even in small pupils or glaucomatous eyes. The stress is taken by the impacted phaco tip and the chopper rather than transmitting it to the fragile capsule.

By going directly into the center of the nucleus with the phaco tip and not doing any sculpting, the authors do not need as much ultrasound energy as is usually required. It is safe and easy to perform and the authors do not have to pass so much BSS (irrigating fluid) into the eye.

DISADVANTAGES

This technique demands continuous use of the left hand and hence requires practice to master it.

TOPICAL ANESTHESIA CATARACT/CLEAR LENS SURGERY

All cases done by the authors were previously done under topical anesthesia. 4 percent xylocaine drops were instilled in the eye about 3 times, 10 to 15 minutes before surgery. No intracameral anesthesia was used. It is not advisable to use xylocaine drops while operating. This can damage the epithelium and create more trouble in visualization. No stitches and no pad are applied. This is called the—no injection, no stitch, no pad cataract surgery technique. Now the authors have shifted all their cases to the no anesthesia technique. This is done in both their hospitals in India (Chennai and Bangalore).

NO ANESTHESIA CATARACT/CLEAR LENS SURGERY

The authors had been wondering whether any topical anesthesia is required or not. So, they then operated patients without any anesthesia. In these patients no xylocaine drops were instilled. The patients did not have any pain. It is paradoxical because we have been taught from the beginning that we should apply xylocaine. This is possible because the authors do not touch the conjunctiva or sclera. They never use any one-tooth forceps to stabilize the eye. Instead what the authors use is a straight rod which is passed inside the eye to stabilize it when they are performing rhexis, etc. **The first step is very important. In this they first enter the eye with a needle having viscoelastic and inject the viscoelastic inside the eye.** This is done in the area of the side port. Now, they have an opening in the eye through which a straight rod can be passed to stabilize the eye. The anterior chamber should be well maintained and the amount of ultrasound power used very less. If you tend to use the techniques like trenching then the ultrasound power generated is high, which in turn generates heat. This causes pain to the patient. If you follow these rules one can perform no anesthesia cataract or clear lens extraction surgery. It is not necessary to do this, as there is no harm in instilling some drops of xylocaine in the eye. The point that there is always a discussion which anesthetic drop to use. It does not matter. The technique, which you perform, should not produce pain to the patient.

SUMMARY

As in any other field, progress is inevitable in ophthalmology more so in refractive surgery. The authors have started to look on refractive surgery as a craft and one should constantly try to improve their craft and become better every day. By this, we will be able to provide good vision to more people than any one dared dreaming a few decades ago. It also goes without saying that we are and will be forever grateful to all our patients because without their faith, the authors would never have had the courage to proceed.

Keeping this in mind, the authors hope and wish that the effectiveness and the advantages of this "No anesthesia cataract and clear lens extraction technique" be realized and practiced, thereby, making the technique of phacoemulsification safer and easier providing good visual outcome and patient recovery.

REFERENCE

1. Agarwal S, Agarwal A, Sachdev M et al. Phacoemulsification, Laser Cataract Surgery and Foldable IOLs. Jaypee Brothers: New Delhi 1998;144-54.

41 Phakic IOL

Benjamin F Boyd, Samuel Boyd, Amar Agarwal

INTRODUCTION

Phakic IOLs[1-60] have recently gained popularity for the management of high refractive errors. This has been partly due to the inability of corneal refractive procedures to satisfactorily correct higher refractive errors due to the problems associated with regression,[1] ectasia and poor quality of the corneal refractive surface[2,3] after ablation for higher powers.

The increasing use of phakic IOLs has also been due to tremendous improvements in the designs and materials used for these IOLs and also due to better microsurgical techniques and vastly improved surgical skills as also due to better viscoelastic devices. Major advantages associated with the use of phakic IOLs include ability to correct higher amounts of ametropia, fast visual recovery, better quality of vision with lesser induction of higher order aberrations and preservation of accommodation. All these factors combined with the ease for the regular cataract surgeon to also enter the field of refractive surgery have contributed to the rapidly gaining popularity of phakic IOLs.

Phakic IOLs can be classified into anterior chamber phakic IOLs (ACPIOLs) and posterior chamber phakic IOLs (PCPIOLs). ACPIOLs can be subclassified as angle-supported or iris-supported. These can be implanted for both myopia and hypermetropia as well as for astigmatism and presbyopia. Despite the popularity and success that they are enjoying, phakic IOLs may still be associated with complications and these patients need to be under constant surveillance for early detection of any possible complications.

ANGLE-SUPPORTED PHAKIC IOLs

The haptics of an appropriately sized angle-supported phakic IOL is supposed to rest on the scleral spur. Perfect sizing of the IOL is difficult and not always possible. The haptics of an excessively large IOL may press on the corneoscleral trabeculae, Schlemm's canal and the blood vessels and nerves in the angle. This pressure may lead to the erosion of angle tissues with displacement of the haptics onto the ciliary body and iris ischemia and atrophy with progressive pupillary ovalization. An excessively small IOL may damage the corneal endothelium due to its moving around in the anterior chamber.

IOL size, design and positioning are important in the prevention of complications. The patient must undergo thorough examination of the eye and its anatomy before implanting a phakic IOL. The fifth-generation ZSAL-4/plus phakic lens is an angle-supported lens, which has been modified to have a larger optic diameter, and a new haptic geometry. This increases haptic flexibility and disperses compression forces equally against the angle structures.[4]

The ZB5M generation of the Baikoff angle-supported lenses also have better efficacy and predictability and the potential risk for damage to the

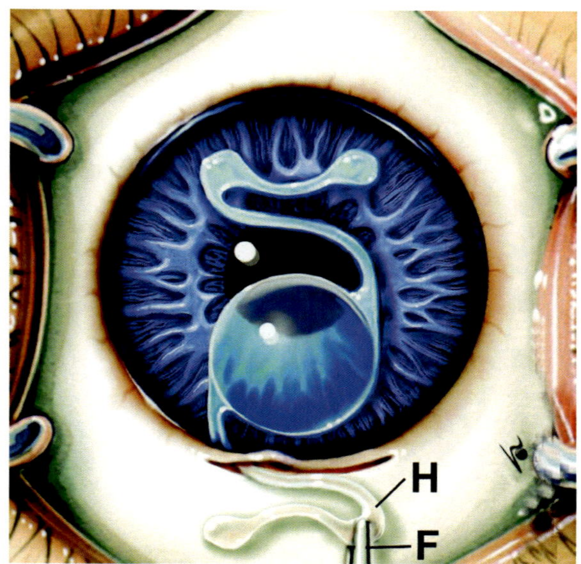

Fig. 41.1: Insertion technique of the anterior phakic chamber intraocular lens.

The forceps retain a grasp on the optic and the IOL is placed into the anterior chamber (arrow). The forceps (F) are repositioned to grasp the elbow (H) of the proximal haptic and the IOL is continued into the anterior chamber (arrow). This technique avoids the insertion of an instrument into a phakic eye all the way into the pupillary area. The distal footplates are directed toward the angle. The proximal haptic is then placed in the incision, but the proximal footplates remain outside the eye *(After Boyd's* **"Atlas of Refractive Surgery"***)*

corneal endothelium has been greatly reduced.[5,6] Problems like night halos with pupillary dilation exceeding the optic size, and pupillary ovalization in the meridian of the haptics are still present. The designs are being continuously modified and upgraded to avoid these problems.

The Nu-Vita lens, formerly the Baikoff AC-IOL is based on the Kelman Multiflex style. The one style of aphakic anterior chamber lens that has survived during the last 15 years is the Kelman Multiflex style (Fig. 41.1). This technology takes advantage of the fact that most surgeons can place an anterior chamber lens more easily than the other styles.

IRIS SUPPORTED PHAKIC IOLs

Worst introduced the iris claw lens in 1977 and implanted an opaque iris claw lens in the phakic eye

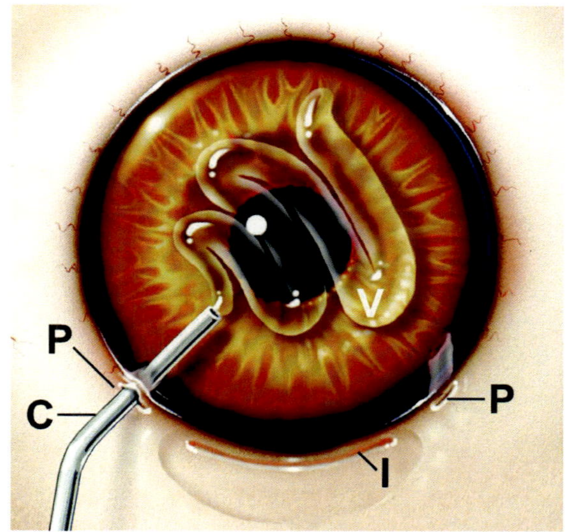

Fig. 41.2: Artisan IOL surgical implantation technique—incisions.

One or two paracentesis stab incisions (P) are made according to the technique to be used. The anterior chamber is filled with a high molecular weight viscoelastic via a cannula (C) placed through one of the paracentesis. A 5-6 mm incision (I) is then made. A peripheral iridotomy must be made now or at the end of the procedure. *(After Boyd's* **"Atlas of Refractive Surgery"***)*

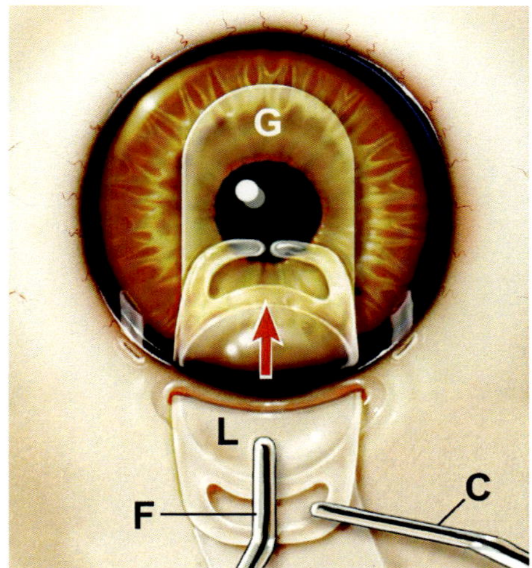

Fig. 41.3: Artisan IOL surgical implantation technique—insertion.

A lens glide (G) is placed through the incision and across the anterior chamber. With viscoelastic filling the anterior chamber, the Artisan lens (L) is grasped with a special forceps (F) and inserted into the wound on the lens glide. A second instrument, an irrigating cannula (C), is placed inside the haptic loop and serves to push the lens (arrow) inside the anterior chamber. *(After Boyd's* **"Atlas of Refractive Surgery"***)*

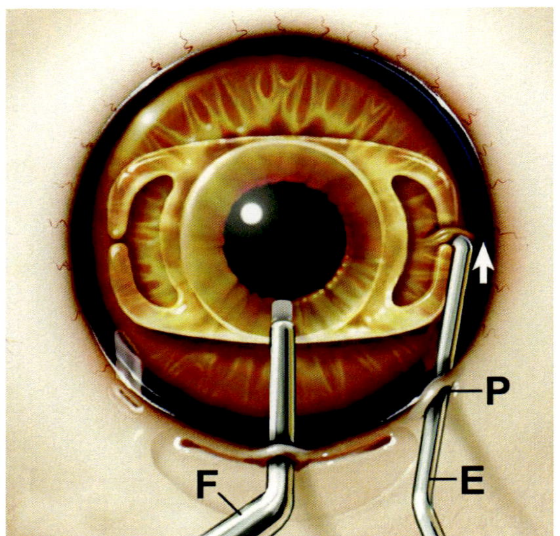

Fig. 41.4: Artisan IOL surgical implantation technique—enclavation.

The special Operaid irrigating enclavation instrument (E) is introduced through the stab incision (P) or through the main incision under the Artisan loop tip. Using the instrument, a fold of iris is lifted (arrow) through the slot in the tip of the lens haptic. The instrument is withdrawn slowly, being careful that it does not catch the iris. The Artisan forceps (F) stabilizes the lens during this maneuver *(After Boyd´s* **"Atlas of Refractive Surgery"***)*

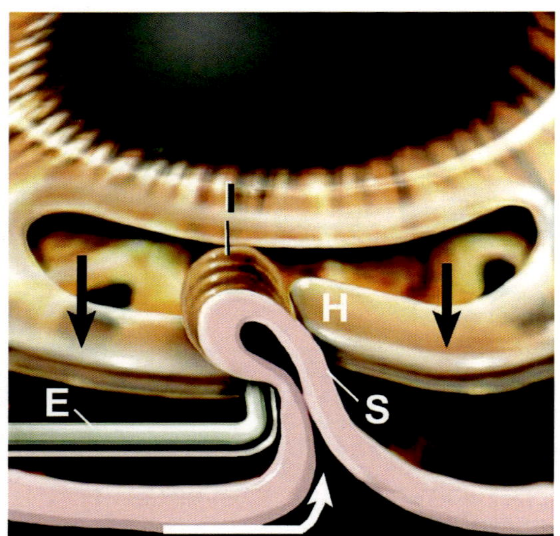

Fig. 41.5: Artisan IOL surgical implantation technique—enclavation detail.

This magnified portion of the lens haptics shows how the enclavation instrument (E) engages a small fold of the iris (I) beneath the distal haptic (H). The iris fold is "snow-plowed" forward (white arrow) and gently captured in the slot (S) of the haptics. The IOL and its haptics are pushed posteirorly (black arrows) to assist this enclavation of the iris *(After Boyd´s* **"Atlas of Refractive Surgery"***)*

of a patient who had unbearable diplopia in 1979. In 1986, Fechner and Worst introduced the iris claw phakic myopic lens. These have become popular now as the Artisan and the Verisyse lenses. These remain in place due to iris enclavation and so no angle complications are generally encountered, though they may be associated with various other complications.

The pupil should be kept moderately constricted. One or two stab incisions are made according to the technique to be used (Fig. 41.2), and the anterior chamber filled with high molecular weight viscoelastic. A 5-6 mm incision is made (Fig. 41.3). A peripheral iridotomy must be made, now or at the end

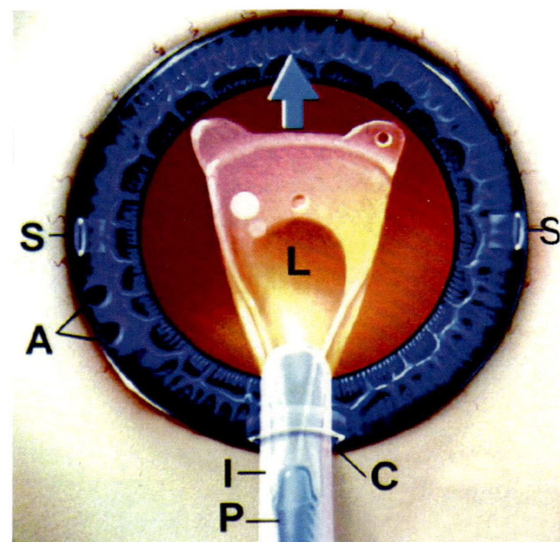

Fig. 41.6: Foldable posterior chamber phakic lens (ICL) - insertion technique - step 1.

A double YAG laser peripheral iridotomy (A) to avoid iris blockage, is performed the week prior to lens implantation in order to avoid iris pigment deposition on the lens. Iridotomies would be very difficult to do intraoperatively because of the widely dilated pupil. First, a 3.0 mm temporal clear corneal incision (C) is performed, as well as two side port incisions (S) 90 degrees away from the main incision and 180 degrees away from each other. The chamber is filled with viscoelastic material (not shown). The foldable posterior chamber lens will be placed between the iris and natural lens. The folded lens (L) is inserted into the eye via the special inserter (I) which has been placed through the corneal incision. A plunger (P) inside the inserter pushes the distal haptics of the ICL into the anterior chamber (arrow) while unfolding as shown. The lens haptics will be placed in the posterior chamber later. This illustration is shown from the surgeon's point of view as he/she is operating. The lens is implanted from the temporal side of the eye *(After Boyd´s* **"Atlas of Refractive Surgery"***)* of the procedure, and the iris reposited completely. The lens is gently and slowly nudged into the eye (Fig. 41.4), rotated into the 3 to 9 o'clock axis and centered over the pupil. The wound is partially sutured, leaving an opening sufficient to introduce a forceps.

The lens is centered over the pupil and gently pressed onto the iris with an artisan forceps. The longer inferior blade of this forceps is an important feature, ensuring stability of the lens while it is attached to the iris. An Operaid Enclavation Instrument is introduced through the stab incision superior to the Artisan loop tip. This instrument comes double armed, in right and left hand configurations, to use depending on which loop of the IOL the iris is being attached.

Using the enclavation instrument, a fold of iris is lifted through the slot in the tip of the lens haptic (Fig. 41.4 and detail in Fig. 41.5). The instrument is withdrawn slowly, being careful that it does not catch the iris. The maneuver is repeated for the other tip of the lens. If a peripheral iridotomy has not already been made, it must be made now. The iridotomy is a vital part of the procedure and must not be omitted. Lens position and fixation are inspected. When perfect, the wound is closed carefully. All viscoelastic is patiently removed while maintaining the depth of the anterior chamber with balanced salt. Steroid and antibiotic drops are placed. If there might be residual viscoelastic, prophylactic iopidine or latanoprost may be used to control any rise in pressure.

POSTERIOR CHAMBER PHAKIC IOLs

The initial posterior chamber phakic IOLs (PCPIOL) were made of silicone[7,8] but they lead to complications such as development of cataract, endothelial loss and chronic uveitis. The new generation of PCPIOLs are made of Collamer,[9] a copolymer of hydroxyethylmethacrylate and porcine collagen (ICL-Staar, Switzerland) (Figs 41.6 to 41.8).

IOL-iris touch, IOL-crystalline lens touch, and anterior chamber shallowing,[10] may cause pigmentary dispersion,[11,12] cataract formation,[13-15] and shallowing of the iridocorneal angle.[16] IOL decentration[14] has also frequently been described. The ideal position of the PCPIOL is for the haptics to rest on the zonules with an appropriate vault over the anterior lens capsule. Positioning in the sulcus can lead to pigment dispersion[17] and inflammation and is therefore not desirable. The PCPIOL produces resistance to the flow of aqueous across the pupil and this situation is worsened with the increase in size of the crystalline lens with age. Proper sizing of the IOL is of great importance. A small size IOL applies pressure against the natural lens, the ciliary body and the posterior surface of the iris causing cataract, uveitis and pigment dispersion respectively.

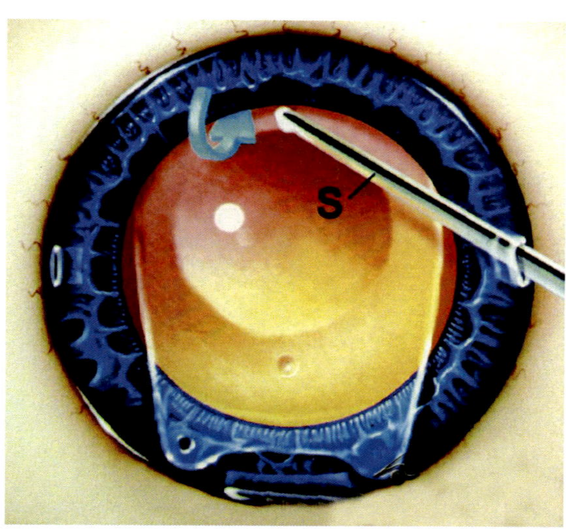

Fig. 41.7: Foldable posterior chamber phakic lens (ICL)—insertion technique of the haptics.

The distal haptics of the ICL are placed in behind the iris before the proximal haptics. With a spatula (S), inserted through one of the side ports, the distal extremity of the ICL is gently pushed (arrow) into the posterior chamber, to the ciliary sulcus. The same movement is used to place the proximal haptics into the posterior chamber. This illustration is shown from the surgeon's point of view as he/she is operating *(After Boyd's* **"Atlas of Refractive Surgery"***)*

RECENT ADVANCES

Latest models of all types of phakic IOLs[60] including the Artisan lenses, the Baikoff and NuVita angle supported IOLs, the ICL, the Medenium silicone PCPIOL etc., have all improved vastly over the previous prototypes and recent data for most of them are encouraging.

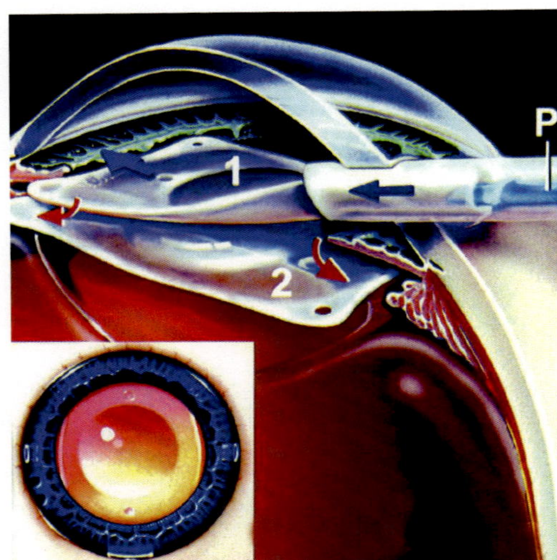

Fig. 41.8: Conceptual cross section of all stages for implantation of a foldable posterior chamber phakic lens (ICL). This conceptual cross section shows the insertion and unfolding of the (ICL) compared to the final configuration of the ICL in position behind the iris and in front of the crystalline lens. (1) The plunger (P) inside the inserter pushes the distal haptics of the ICL into the anterior chamber (blue arrows) while unfolding as shown. (2) In separate maneuvers, the haptics are then placed (red arrows) into the posterior chamber behind the iris and into the ciliary sulcus. The iris will then be constricted. The inset shows a surgeon's view of this final configuration.

This illustration is a section of the eye taken from 3 to 9 o'clock, as the ICL is inserted through the temporal approach. *(After Boyd´s* **"Atlas of Refractive Surgery"***)*

REFERENCES

1. Pérez-Santonja JJ, Bellot JJ, Claramonte P, et al. Laser in situ keratomileusis to correct high myopia. J Cataract Refract Surg. 1997;23:372-85.
2. Applegate RA, Howland HC. Refractive surgery, optical aberrations, and visual performance. J Refract Surg 1997;13:295-9.
3. Oliver KM, Hemenger RP, Corbett MC, et al. Corneal optical aberrations induced by photorefractive keratectomy. J Refract Surg 1997;13:246-54.
4. Pérez-Santonja JJ, Alió JL, Jiménez-Alfaro I, Zato MA. Surgical correction of severe myopia with an angle-supported phakic intraocular lens. J Cataract Refract Surg 2000;26:1288-302.
5. Baikoff G, Arne JL, Bokobza Y, et al. Angle-fixated anterior chamber phakic intraocular lens for myopia of –7 to –19 diopters. J Refract Surg 1998;14:282-93.
6. Alió JL, de la Hoz F, Pérez-Santonja JJ, et al. Phakic anterior chamber lenses for the correction of myopia. A 7-year cumulative analysis of complications in 263 cases. Ophthalmology 1999;106:458-66.
7. Fechner PU, Haigis W, Wichmann W. Posterior chamber myopia lenses in phakic eyes. J Cataract Refract Surg 1996;22:178-82.
8. Zaldivar R, Davidorf JM, Oscherow S. Posterior chamber phakic intraocular lens for myopia of –8 to –19 diopters. J Refract Surg 1998;14:294-305.
9. Assetto V, Benedetti S, Pesando P. Collamer intraocular contact lens to correct high myopia. J Cataract Refract Surg 1996;22:551-6.
10. Trindade F, Pereira F, Cronemberger S. Ultrasound biomicroscopic imaging of posterior chamber phakic intraocular lens. J Refract Surg 1998;14:497-503.
11. Maden A, Gunenc U, Erkin E. Gonioscopic changes in eyes with posterior chamber intraocular lenses. Doc Ophthalmol 1992;82:231-8.
12. Abela-Formanek C, Kruger AJ, Dejaco-Ruhswurm I, et al. Gonioscopic changes after implantation of a posterior chamber lens in phakic myopic eyes. J Cataract Refract Surg 2001;27:1919-25.
13. Brauweiler PH, Wehler T, Busin M. High incidence of cataract formation after implantation of a silicone posterior chamber lens in phakic, highly myopic eyes. Ophthalmology 1999;106:1651-5.
14. Menezo JL, Peris-Martinez C, Cisneros A, Martínez-Costa R. Posterior chamber phakic intraocular lenses to correct high myopia: a comparative study between Staar and Adatomed models. J Refract Surg 2001;17:32-42.
15. Fink AM, Gore C, Rosen E. Cataract development after implantation of the Staar Collamer posterior chamber phakic lens. J Cataract Refract Surg 1999;25:278-82.
16. Arne JL, Lesueur LC. Phakic posterior chamber lenses for high myopia: functional and anatomical outcomes. J Cataract Refract Surg 2000;26:369-74.
17. Brandt JD, Mockovak ME, Chayet A. Pigmentary dispersion syndrome induced by a posterior chamber phakic refractive lens. Am J Ophthalmol 2001;131:260-3.
18. Mimouni F, Colin J, Koffi V, Bonnet P. Damage to the corneal endothelium from anterior chamber intraocular lenses in phakic myopic eyes. Refract Corneal Surg 1991;7:277-81.
19. Saragoussi JJ, Cotinat J, Renard G, et al. Damage to the corneal endothelium by minus power anterior chamber intraocular lenses. Refract Corneal Surg 1991;7:282-5.
20. Rao GN, Stevens RE, Harris JK, Aquavella JV. Long-term changes in corneal endothelium following intraocular lens implantation. Ophthalmology 1981;88:386-97.
21. Long-term corneal endothelial cell loss after cataract surgery. Results of a randomized controlled trial. Oxford Cataract Treatment and Evaluation Team (OCTET). Arch Ophthalmol 1986;104:1170-5.
22. Matsuda M, Miyake K, Inaba M. Long-term corneal endothelial changes after intraocular lens implantation. Am J Ophthalmol 1988;105:248-52.

23. Baikoff G. The refractive IOL in a phakic eye. Ophthalmic Pract 1991;9:58-61, 80.
24. Iradier MT, Hernandez JL, Estrella J, et al. Lente de Baikoff: estudio de los resultados refractivos. Arch Soc Esp Oftalmol 1992;62:259-65.
25. Bour T, Piquot X, Pospisil A, Montard M. Répercussions endothéliales de l'implant myopique de chambre antérieure ZB au cours de la première année. Etude prospective avec analyse statistique. J Fr Ophtalmol 1991;14:633-41.
26. Alió JL, Pérez-Santonja JJ, Artola A. Surgical correction of myopia. In Nema HV, Nema N, (Eds): Recent Advances in Ophthalmology. New Delhi: Jaypee Brothers Medical Publishers (P) Ltd 1996;1-28.
27. Saragoussi J-J, Puech M, Assouline M, et al. Ultrasound biomicroscopy of Baikoff anterior chamber phakic intraocular lenses. J Refract Surg 1997;13:135-41.
28. Bourne WM, Nelson LR, Hodge DO. Continued endothelial cell loss ten years after lens implantation. Ophthalmology 1994;101:1014-23.
29. Jiménez-Alfaro I, García-Feijoó J, Pérez-Santonja JJ, et al. Ultrasound biomicroscopy of ZSAL-4 anterior chamber phakic intraocular lens for high myopia. JCRS 2001;27(10):1567-730.
30. Pérez-Santonja JJ, Iradier MT, Sanz-Iglesias L, et al. Endothelial changes in phakic eyes with anterior chamber intraocular lenses to correct high myopia. J Cataract Refract Surg 1996;22:1017-22.
31. Fechner PU, Haubitz I, Wichmann W, Wulff K. Worst-Fechner biconcave minus power phakic iris-claw lens. J Refract Surg 1999;15:93-105.
32. Menezo JL, Cisneros AL, Rodriguez-Salvador V, et al. Endothelial study of iris-claw phakic lens: four-year follow-up. J Cataract Refract Surg 1998;24:1039-49.
33. Jiménez-AlfaroI, Benítez del Castillo JM, García Feijoó J, et al. Safety of posterior chamber phakic intraocular lenses for the correction of high myopia : anterior segment changes after posterior chamber phakic intraocular lens implantation. Ophthalmology 2001;108(1):90-9.
34. Zaldivar R, Davidorf JM, Oscherow S, et al. Combined posterior chamber phakic intraocular lens and laser in situ keratomileusis: bioptics for extreme myopia. J Refract Surg 1999;15:299-308.
35. Apple DJ, Werner L. Complications of cataract and refractive surgery: a clinicopathological documentation. Trans Am Ophthalmol Soc. 2001;99:95-107discussion, 107-9.
36. Kashani AA. Phakic intraocular lens. J Cataract Refract Surg 1999;25:1033-4 [letter].
37. Pérez-Santonja JJ, Bueno JL, Zato MA. Surgical correction of high myopia in phakic eyes with Worst-Fechner myopia intraocular lenses. J Refract Surg 1997;13:268-84.
38. Pérez-Santonja JJ, Iradier MT, Benítez del Castillo JM, et al. Chronic subclinical inflammation in phakic eyes with intraocular lenses to correct myopia. J Cataract Refract Surg 1996;22:183-7.
39. Pérez-Santonja JJ, Hernandez JL, Benítez del Castillo JM, et al. Fluorophotometry in myopic phakic eyes with anterior chamber intraocular lenses to correct severe myopia. Am J Ophthalmol 1994;118:316-21.
40. Benítez del Castillo JM, Hernandez JL, Iradier MT, et al. Fluorophotometry in phakic eyes with anterior chamber intraocular lens implantation to correct myopia. J Cataract Refract Surg 1993;19:607-9.
41. Alió JL, de la Hoz F, Ismail MM. Subclinical inflammatory reaction induced by phakic anterior chamber lenses for the correction of high myopia. Ocular Inmunol Inflam 1993;1:219-23.
42. Miyake K, Asakura M, Kobayashi H. Effect of intraocular lens fixation on the blood-aqueous barrier. Am J Ophthalmol 1984;98:451-5.
43. Othenin-Girard P, Pittet N, Herbort CP. La barriére hémato-aqueuse aprés opération de cataracte: comparaison de l'implantation dans le sac capsulaire et dans le sulcus. Can J Ophthalmol 1993;28:55-7.
44. Brown DC, Grabow HB, Martin G, et al. Staar Collamer intraocular lens: clinical results from the phase I FDA core study. J Cataract Refract Surg 1998;24:1032-8.
45. Rosen E, Gore C. Staar Collamer posterior chamber phakic intraocular lens to correct myopia and hyperopia. J Cataract Refract Surg 1998;24:596-606.
46. Davidorf JM, Zaldivar R, Oscherow S. Posterior chamber phakic intraocular lens for hyperopia of +4 to +11 diopters. J Refract Surg 1998;14:306-11.
47. Pesando PM, Ghiringhello MP, Tagliavacche P. Posterior chamber collamer phakic intraocular lens for myopia and hyperopia. J Refract Surg 1999;15:415-23.
48. Bylsma SS, Zalta AH, Foley E et al. Phakic posterior chamber intraocular lens pupillary block. JCRS 2002; 28(12):2222-8.
49. Fellner P, Vidic B, Ramkissoon Y, et al. Pupil ovalization after phakic intraocular lens implantation is associated with sectorial iris hypoperfusion. Arch Ophthalmol 2005; 123(8):1061-5.
50. Baikoff G. Phakic anterior chamber intraocular lenses. Int Ophthalmol Clin 1991;31:75-86.
51. Foss AJ, Rosen PH, Cooling RJ. Retinal detachment following anterior chamber lens implantation for the correction of ultra-high myopia in phakic eyes. Br J Ophthalmol 1993;77:212-3.
52. Ruiz-Moreno JM, Alió JL, Pérez-Santonja JJ, de la Hoz F. Retinal detachment in phakic eyes with anterior chamber lenses to correct severe myopia. Am J Ophthalmol 1999; 127:270-5.
53. Alió JL, Ruiz-Moreno JM, Artola A. Retinal detachment as a potential hazard in surgical correction of severe myopia with phakic anterior chamber lenses. Am J Ophthalmol 1993;115:145-8.
54. Martínez-Castillo V, Boixadera A, Verdugo A, et al. Rhegmatogenous Retinal Detachment in Phakic Eyes After Posterior Chamber Phakic Intraocular Lens Implantation for Severe Myopia. Ophthalmology 2005;112(4):580-5.

55. Panozzo G, Parolini B. Relationships between vitreoretinal and refractive surgery. Ophthalmology 2001;108: 1663-8.
56. Arevalo JF, Azar-Arevalo O. Retinal detachment in phakic eyes with anterior chamber intraocular lenses to correct severe myopia. [letter]Am J Ophthalmol 1999; 128:661-2.
57. Kwok AK, Young AL, Bhende P, Lam DS. Retinal detachment in phakic eyes with anterior chamber intraocular lenses to correct severe myopia [letter]. Am J Ophthalmol 1999;128:395-6.
58. Melberg NS, Thomas MA. Nuclear sclerotic cataract after vitrectomy in patients younger than 50 years of age. Ophthalmology 1995;102:1466-71.
59. Blodi BA, Paluska SA. Cataract after vitrectomy in young patients. Ophthalmology 1997;104:1092-5.
60. Boyd B. Atlas of Refractive Surgery; Highlights of Ophthalmology, Panama.

42 Posterior Chamber Implantable Collamer Lens ICL and Toric ICL

Alaa El-Danasoury

Since 1983, many phakic intraocular lens (IOLs) have emerged; they can be classified into 3 major categories; anterior chamber angle fixated lenses, originally introduced by Baikoff and Joly,[1,2] the iris-fixated lens introduced by Fechner and Worst,[3] and the posterior chamber, sulcus-fixated lens introduced by Fyodorov,[4] and modified by Staar company.[5] The penetration of phakic IOLs in the refractive surgery practice was relatively slow during the last 2 decades of the last century due to many factors including the potential complications of intraocular surgery, the poor early designs, the underdeveloped techniques of implantation, the relatively high incidence of complications in the early reports and above all the lack of long-term published results in peer reviewed literature; also, the introduction of excimer laser refractive surgery and the booming of LASIK in its early years as "the one procedure" that can correct all refractive errors added to the factors that delayed the wide spread use of phakic IOLs.

Over the last decade, phakic IOLs passed through many stages of innovation and development; surgical techniques were made better and more information became available on the long term results. Refractive surgeons around the world became more interested in phakic IOLs. Also the better understanding of the biomechanical effect of LASIK on the cornea especially in high amounts of myopia, the increasing number of reported corneal ectasia after LASIK and the development of sophisticated wave front analyzers that objectively measured the negative effect of LASIK on the quality of vision especially to surgically induced high order aberrations made many refractive surgeons reconsider the assumption that alteration of the natural corneal shape is the best way to address myopic and astigmatic refractive errors.[6]

The introduction of the toric phakic IOLs was a great step towards improving the clinical results and widening the range of correction provided by the toric IOLs. To date only 2 toric phakic IOLs are available; the iris fixated toric Artisan lens and the posterior chamber toric implantable collamer lens (ICL).

This chapter summarizes the evolution, indications, patients' selection criteria, surgical techniques, clinical results and possible complications of the posterior chamber implantable collamer lens.

Evolution

The original design of posterior chamber phakic IOL was introduced by Fyodorov in 1986, it had a collar-button optic and a posterior chamber haptic; the lens was made of silicone and was partially implanted in the posterior chamber through fixation wings with the optic at the pupillary plane (Fig. 42.1). The prototype of modern ICL was introduced

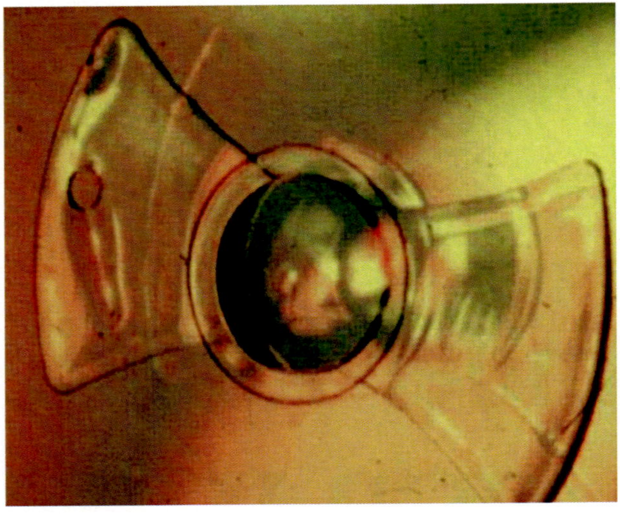

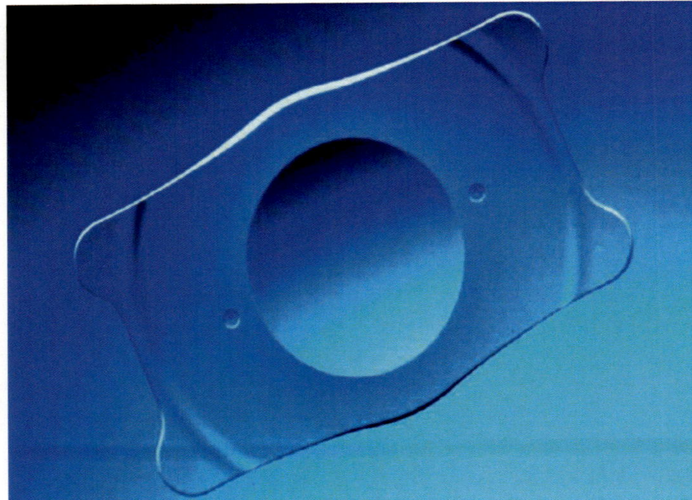

Fig. 42.1: (A) Original design of phakic posterior chamber lenses (Fyodorov, 1986); fixation wings were implanted in the posterior chamber between the iris and the anterior capsule of the crystalline lens and the collar-button optic was positioned at the pupillary plane. (B) Currently used ICL (model V4); note the 4 laser marks engraved on the haptic: 2 orientation marks on the leading right and trailing left foot plates and 2 alignment marks on either sides of the optic. Courtesy of Staar Surgical

in 1990 in Russia; the fixation wings were replaced with a plate haptic with square edges. In 1993, Pesando implanted the first ICL prototype (IC2020) in Torino, followed by Skorpik in Vienna and Zaldivar in Argentina.[5,7,8]

ICL is manufactured by Staar Surgical (Nidau, Switzerland). It is a single-piece, plate-haptic lens, designed to vault anteriorly to the crystalline lens and intended to have minimal contact with the natural lens. The lens material is a proprietary hydrophilic collagen polymer (copolymer of 63% hydroxy-ethyl-methyl-acrylate, 0.2% collagen and 3.4% of a benzofenone for UV absorption) known as Collamer, with a water content of 34%, a light transmission of 99%, and a refractive index of 1.45 at 35° C. According to the manufacturer, the Collamer material is biologically quiet, as collagen has an affinity for fibronectin; upon implantation, a monolayer of fibronectin would coat the IOL surface, inhibiting deposition of other proteins. Therefore, the material would not be recognized as a foreign body, and flare, cell deposition, and inflammation would be minimized.

The design of the ICL progressively evolved from the initial prototypes first implanted in 1993 (models IC2020, and IC2020-M) to the currently used model (V4). The optic diameter progressively increased, from 3.5 to 4.5 mm in the myopic IC2020, to 4.65 to 5.50 mm in the myopic V4, and the lens became progressively thinner. Until the second half of 1996, the ICL had no marks to help identify the anterior optic surface. It was therefore difficult to confirm if the lens was in an upside-down position after its injection. The V2 version of the ICL started to be manufactured with orientation marks on the haptics, which lead to an increase in popularity of ICL implantation by injection. Throughout the evolution of the ICL, one of the major changes in the design features was implemented in the lens vaulting; the currently available model (V4) has steeper radius of curvature, this allowed an additional 0.13 to 0.21 mm of anterior vaulting in comparison to its predecessor, the V3 depending on the diopteric power of the lens.[9]

Current ICL Models and Powers

Today, three ICL versions are available for use, a myopic, a hyperopic and a toric versions.

Myopic ICL

The myopic version of the ICL (V4) is plano-concave with the anterior surface being plano, the optic diameter ranges from 4.65 to 5.50 mm. The thickness of the lens is less than 50 μm at the center of the optic, and less than 100 μm at the haptic plate. The thickest part of the myopic ICL is the junction between the optic and the haptic and ranges from 300 to 700 μm. The overall length of myopic ICL ranges from 11.50 to 13.00 mm in 0.50 mm increments. Power ranges from -23.00 to -3.00 diopters (D) in half-diopter increments.

Hyperopic ICL

The hyperopic ICL (V3) is concave-convex, with the anterior surface being convex. Optic diameter is fixed at 5.50 mm for all powers; the thickest part is the center of the optic. Overall lengths of hyperopic ICL range from 11.00 to 12.50 mm in 0.50 mm increments. Power ranges from 3.00 to 21.50 D in half-diopter increments.

Toric ICL

The toric ICL (V4) has a toric convex-concave optic that incorporates the desired cylindrical power in a specific axis as required to correct a given patient's astigmatic condition. It is manufactured using the platform of the non-toric design and is similar to the spherical ICL in terms of size, thickness and configuration, with the addition of a toric optic to correct myopia with astigmatism. To minimize rotation required by the surgeon during implantation, the toric ICL is custom made to be implanted on the horizontal axis. The order-delivery time for a toric ICL is between 4 and 6 weeks; to shorten this time, the surgeon has the option to use a ready made toric ICL of the same required power with an axis of the cylinder within 22.5° of the required, in such case the "alternative" toric ICL will have to be rotated inside the eye to compensate for the difference in axis orientation. Each toric ICL is sent to the surgeon with a guide demonstrating the amount and direction of rotation from the horizontal axis required to align the toric ICL cylinder axis to correct the patient's astigmatism. It is recommended that rotation is less than 22.5° from the horizontal.[10] The cylindrical power ranges from 1.0 to 6.0 D with the same range of spherical power as the myopic ICL.

Myopic ICL (V4) was approved by the FDA in 1995 for the full range of powers between –20.00 and –3.00 D. FDA studies for toric and hyperopic ICL are in process. Table 42.1 summarizes the characteristics and the power ranges for the currently available 3 ICL models. Besides the refractive powers described in Table 42.1, which are currently available in international markets, Staar can also manufacture customized lenses upon request from surgeons; this includes myopic ICLs from as low as -0.50 D to as high as –23.00 D, hyperopic ICLs from as low as +0.50 D to as high as +21.50 D, as

Table 42.1: Characteristics of the currently available myopic (V4), hyperopic (V3) and toric ICL (V4) models

ICL	*Spherical Power*	*Cylindrical Power*	*Optic Diameter*	*Optic/Haptic Thickness*	*Overall Height*
Myopic model (V4)	-3.0 to -12.0 D	0.0	5.50 mm	0.3 to 0.5 mm	1.15 to 1.77 mm
	-12.5 to -13.5 D	0.0	5.25 mm	0.5 mm	1.08 to 1.78 mm
	-14.0 to -16.5 D	0.0	5.00 mm	0.5 to 0.6 mm	1.12 to 1.89 mm
	-17.0 to -23.0 D	0.0	4.65 mm	0.5 to 0.7 mm	1.19 to 2.05 mm
Hyperopic model (V3)	+3.0 to +12.0 D	0.0	5.50 mm	0.2 mm	1.25 to 2.29 mm
	+12.5 to +13.5 D	0.0	5.50 mm	0.2 mm	1.61 to 2.36 mm
	+14.0 to +16.5 D	0.0	5.50 mm	0.2 mm	1.68 to 2.49 mm
	+17.0 to +21.5 D	0.0	5.50 mm	0.2 mm	1.82 to 2.79 mm
Toric model (V4)	-3.0 to -12.0 D	+1.0 to +6.0 D	5.50 mm	0.3 to 0.5 mm	1.5 mm
	-12.5 to -13.5 D	+1.0 to +6.0 D	5.25 mm	0.5 mm	1.5 mm
	-14.0 to -16.5 D	+1.0 to +6.0 D	5.0 mm	0.5 to 0.6 mm	1.5 to 1.6 mm
	-17.0 to -23.0 D	+1.0 to +6.0 D	4.65 mm	0.5 to 0.7 mm	1.6 to 1.7 mm

well as toric ICLs with spherical power from -23.00 to +20.00 D, and cylinders from +0.50 to +10.00 D at any axis from 0 to 180°. In addition to these, any combination of the myopic and hyperopic versions with cylinder corrections can be customized.

INDICATIONS OF ICL AND T-ICL

High myopia and high myopic astigmatism remain the most common indications for ICL and toric ICL; LASIK being more commonly performed for low and moderate amounts of myopia. Patients who suffer from high astigmatism and high myopia are usually not suitable candidates for corneal-reshaping procedures because there is an increased risk of corneal ectasia, associated with low visual quality and unpredictability.[11] These cases of high myopia or high compound myopic astigmatism are better candidates for ICL or toric ICL. There is no clear cut as for the upper limit for safe LASIK, however there is general agreement to be somewhere between 7.00 and 9.00 D of myopia. In a prospective bilateral randomized study we showed that phakic IOLs are more effective, more predictable and safer than LASIK for myopia above 9.00 D; also a subgroup of patients who had LASIK in one eye and phakic IOL in the other eye preferred the phakic IOL eye, better quality of vision was the main reason for their preference,[12] for this reason we routinely perform ICL / toric ICL for correction of myopia of 8.00 D or more, even if there is no contraindication for LASIK.

In lower amounts of myopia we implant ICL / toric ICL for any case that carries any risk of post-LASIK ectasia or flap complications, these include eyes with relatively thin corneas that do not allow leaving 300 µm of stromal bed, corneas steeper than 48.00 D or flat corneas with expected post-LASIK K reading flatter than 35.00 D and corneas with suspicious topography including forme fruste keratoconus or keratoconus suspect cases.

Stable keratoconus is another growing indication for ICL and toric ICL, in the last 2 years we performed more than 80 ICL / toric ICL for cases with stable keratoconus with very good results that will be discussed later in the report section.

Other indications of ICL and toric ICL include correction of residual refractive errors after LASIK, corneal grafting, intracorneal ring segments implantation, corneal collagen crosslinking and pseudophakia.

The excellent quality of vision and the high predictability of ICL / toric ICL as compared to excimer laser procedures carry the possibility of reducing the upper limit of keratorefractive procedures in the near future.

Hyperopic ICL are indicated to correct hyperopia up to 10.00 D provided the anterior chamber depth is adequate, since hyperopes usually have shallower anterior chamber and narrower angle compared to myopes, hyperopic ICLs are less commonly used compared to myopic and toric ICLs.

SELECTION CRITERIA AND PREOPERATIVE ASSESSMENT

To be considered a good candidate for ICL implantation a patient should have a stable manifest refraction, an anterior chamber depth of at least 2.7 mm calculated from the endothelium, a central endothelial count of more than 2200 cells/mm^2, and an open angle of the anterior chamber.

Refraction

Manifest refraction is usually sufficient for low and moderately high myopes, however in extreme myopia contact lens over-refraction is recommended. In hyperopes, a cycloplegic refraction is advisable especially in younger subjects to eliminate the possible effect of accommodation. We perform manifest refraction for myopia less than 15.00 D, contact lens overrefraction for myopia of 15.00 D and above and cycloplegic refraction for all hyperopes. In all cases, the vertex distance of the refraction should be recorded to be used in calculation of the ICL power. A 1.00 mm error in vertex distance was found to correspond to a 1% miscalculation of ICL power.[13]

Stability of refraction

Simple refractive errors usually stabilize between 18 and 21 years of age. A documented stable refraction for at least one year is advisable if the patient is not to be subjected to a secondary procedure later in his life. There is no published data on ICL implantation in children, however due to the exchangeability of the ICL it might be a good option for children with anisometropia. A long term prospective clinical trial is needed to study the efficacy, predictability and safety of ICL implantation in children.

Anterior Chamber Depth

A sufficient anterior chamber depth (ACD) is an important factor to prevent endothelial cell loss after phakic IOLs implantation. ICL is the farthest phakic IOL from the endothelium; it is estimated that an anterior chamber depth of 2.7 mm from the endothelium to the anterior surface of the crystalline lens is the lower limit for safe ICL implantation.

ACD can be measured using optical devices (IOL Master, Carl Zeiss, Thornwood, NY, USA), anterior segment imaging devices (Pentacam, Oculus, Dutenhofen, Germany and Orbscan; Bausch and Lomb, Rochester, NY, USA) or an A-scan ultrasound. The IOL Master measures the anterior chamber depth via a 0.7-mm wide light section and gives accurate measurements of the ACD. We compared ACD measured with both IOL Master and Orbscan II in 100 consecutive eyes and we found no statistically significant difference between both devices. Reuland et al reported similar results comparing anterior chamber depth values determined by Pentacam and IOL Master.[14] Contact ultrasound can also be used but it has to be noted that it leads to an impression on the cornea, which influences the true anterior chamber depth. Immersion ultrasound gives accurate measures but it is not widely used because of the complicated and time consumed technique.

Pupil Size

ICL optic diameter ranges from 4.65 to 5.50 mm depending on the power of the lens. Since the ICL is implanted in the posterior chamber, the effective optic diameter at the corneal plane is larger than the actual diameter; it ranges from 6.17 to 7.30 mm at the corneal plane for the same power range. Patients with scotopic pupil diameter larger than the effective lens optic diameter might experience night glare or haloes around light.

Corneal Topography

Topography is essential for all patients undergoing refractive surgery mainly to help diagnosis early and moderate cases of keratoconus. Abnormal topography is not an absolute contraindication for ICL surgery. Many cases that are not good candidates for excimer laser refractive surgery can safely have ICL; these include steep corneas, flat corneas and keratoconus suspect. Cases with stable keratoconus and good spectacle corrected visual acuity can also benefit from ICL surgery.

Gonioscopy

Gonioscopy is important to exclude patients with narrow or abnormal angle as ICL implantation in such cases may lead to narrowing of the angle of the anterior chamber with secondary glaucoma.

A comprehensive ophthalmic examination has to be performed for all patients before undergoing ICL surgery including but not limited to slit-lamp biomicroscopy, IOP measurement and dilated fundus examination.

ICL Sizing

Estimating the proper size and power for the ICL to be implanted in a given eye is key factor for successful ICL surgery.

Since the ICL was designed so that its haptic plate rests horizontally on the ciliary sulcus, the length of the ICL should ideally be equal to the horizontal sulcus diameter. Nowadays there are 2 main methods to determine the length of the ICL before implantation; the widely used conventional method based on white-to-white measurement and the relatively new method using high frequency ultrasound imaging devices to measure the actual sulcus diameter.

The conventional method for sizing of myopic ICL is based on adding 0.50 mm to the horizontal white-to-white measurement for anterior chamber depth < 3.5 mm and 1.0 mm to the horizontal white-to-white measurement for anterior chamber depth > 3.5 mm for the myopic ICL model. In Asian eyes and due to some anatomical differences from Caucasian eyes, Chang et al recommended adding 0.5 mm to the horizontal white-to-white measurement for eyes with anterior chamber depth ≤ 3.0 m, and adding 1.0 mm for anterior chamber depth > 3.0 mm.[15]

The white-to-white corneal diameter can be measured manually with calipers, IOL master or Orbscan. The conventional method is more widely used than the high frequency ultrasound method because it is simple and cost effective. In 100 consecutive ICL surgeries we found no statistically significant difference in the white-to-white measurements using calipers and Orbscan II. The same finding was also reported by Choi and co-workers.[16] In cases with limbal pigmentation it should be noted that Orbscan may overestimate the white-to-white measurement; and in this particular case, calipers measurements are more reliable. Fig. 42.2 shows an eye with limbal pigmentation that received an oversized ICL based on an Orbscan II white-to-white measurement resulting in a high vault.

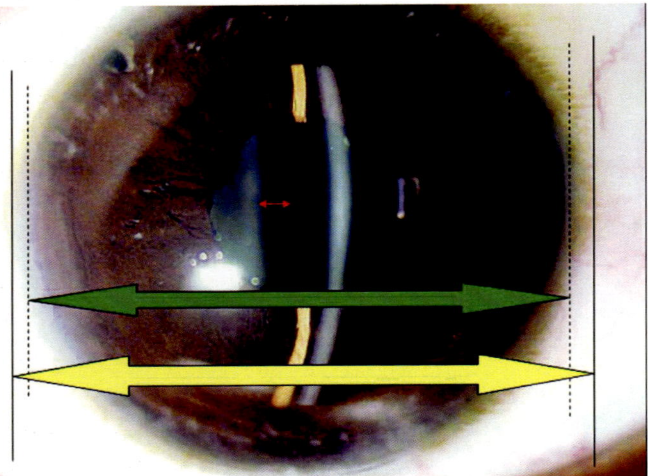

Fig. 42.2: shows an eye with limbal pigmentation and high ICL vault (about 800 μm, red arrow); the ICL was oversized because the actual white-to-white measurement (green arrow) was overestimated by the Orbscan II as Orbscan measurement included the limbal pigmentation (yellow arrow)

Choi et al,[16] described a method to calculate the sulcus-to-sulcus horizontal diameter using an ultrasound biomicroscope (UBM) with a 50 MHz probe; they evaluated the vault results of ICL length determined using UBM method and compared the results to those of the conventional method. The UBM used in their study had the limitation of producing only 5 x 5 mm fields per scan making measurement of the direct sulcus-to-sulcus horizontal diameter not possible. In their series, all 13 eyes that had ICL implantation based on the UBM sizing method showed ideal vault, whereas among 17 eyes who received ICL based on the conventional sizing methods; 10 (58.8%) eyes showed ideal vault, 3 (17.6%) eyes showed excessive vault, and 4 (23.6%) eyes showed insufficient vault at 1 month after operation. They concluded that, in their hands, the UBM method, achieved significantly better ICL vaults than the conventional white-to-white method. They also evaluated the ICL foot plate locations and found no statistically significant differences between cases where ICL length was determined based on UBM method and the cases where they used the conventional white-to-white measurement.

The introduction of the modern high frequency ultrasound measuring tools was very valuable for understanding the anatomy of the ciliary sulcus and carries a promise to improve the determination of the ICL length. Few of these devices are now commercially available as the Artemis (Ultralink LCC, ST Petersburg, Fla), HiScan (Opticon, Rome, Italy) and the Vumax (Sonomed, NY, USA).

The conventional method for ICL sizing may not be ideal because the correlation between the white-to-white measurement and the sulcus diameter is proven not be accurate,[17] the amount of scleral overriding on the anterior corneal surface is variable and the point selected for measurement varies among surgeons. However white-to-white although not ideal is good enough; the rate of ICL replacement for long or short size is extremely low (less than 0.8%).[7] This low rate of incorrect ICL sizing using the conventional white-white method may be at least partly explained by the assumption that the haptic might safely sit in the sulcus, on the zonules or on the ciliary processes with no adverse effects. Vukich and coworkers studied the position of the foot plates after ICL implantation and showed that in about 40% of cases the ICL foot plates rest on the zonules without causing side effects (Vukich J, personal communication). We believe that the conventional white-to- white measurement will remain widely used at least till high frequency ultrasound technology that measures the sulcus diameter reaches maturity and becomes friendly to use and reproducible. A surgeon using the conventional method needs to ensure proper calibration of his instruments, look for scleral overriding and watch limbal pigmentation in case of using an Orbscan for white-to-white measurement.

ICL Power Calculation

Compared to cataract patients, refractive surgery patients are younger, more demanding and less willing to use spectacles; this entails a very accurate power calculation for ICL. Fortunately this is made more feasible because the position of ICL in the eye is less variable than that of aphakic IOL after cataract surgery.[7]

Two calculation softwares are provided by the company, one is for spheric and the other for toric ICL power calculation. Calculation softwares provide the surgeon with the ability to calculate the power of the ICL and also the lens size for given preoperative measurements. The software incorporates a formula that derives from a standard IOL power calculation for phakic eyes, described by Holladay in 1993.[18] The only measurements necessary for the calculation are the corneal power, the preoperative refraction, the anterior chamber depth and the vertex distance of the refraction. The power of the lens is calculated based on the desired postoperative refraction. It is not necessary to determine the biometric dimensions of the globe (axial length, crystalline lens thickness, and vitreous chamber), as they remain completely unchanged.

Basically,

$$IOL = \frac{1336}{\dfrac{1336}{\dfrac{1000}{\dfrac{1000}{PreRx} - V} + K} - ELP} - \frac{1336}{\dfrac{1336}{\dfrac{1000}{\dfrac{1000}{DPostRx} - V} + K} - ELP}$$

where ELP is the expected lens position in mm (distance from corneal vertex to principal plane of IOL), IOL is the intraocular lens power in D, K is the net corneal power in D, PreRx is the preoperative refraction in D, DPostRx is the desired postoperative refraction in D, and V is the vertex distance in mm of refractions. The ELP = AA + SF, where AA is the anatomic anterior chamber depth in mm (distance from corneal vertex to plane of iris root), and SF is the surgeon factor in mm (distance from plane of iris root to principal plane of lens, negative in anterior chamber).

The Toric ICL Power Calculation Software incorporates mathematical operations described by Sarver and Sanders in 2004 and used to convert standard toric parameters of sphere, cylinder, and axis to astigmatic decomposition components and vice-versa.[19] These operations can be used to derive equations to calculate the ideal toric IOL power for a phakic or aphakic astigmatic eye, predict the postoperative spectacle correction for a selected toric IOL with power other than the ideal power, and back calculate a parameter to be used to optimize predictability of the calculations based on clinical data. The software also provides a guide for achieving proper alignment of the toric ICL. As described before, a customized lens is manufactured to be implanted on the horizontal meridian while an alternative lens with the same power and different axis can be implanted on a different axis to achieve the desired refractive correction. Example of customized and alternative toric ICL powers is shown in Fig. 42.3.

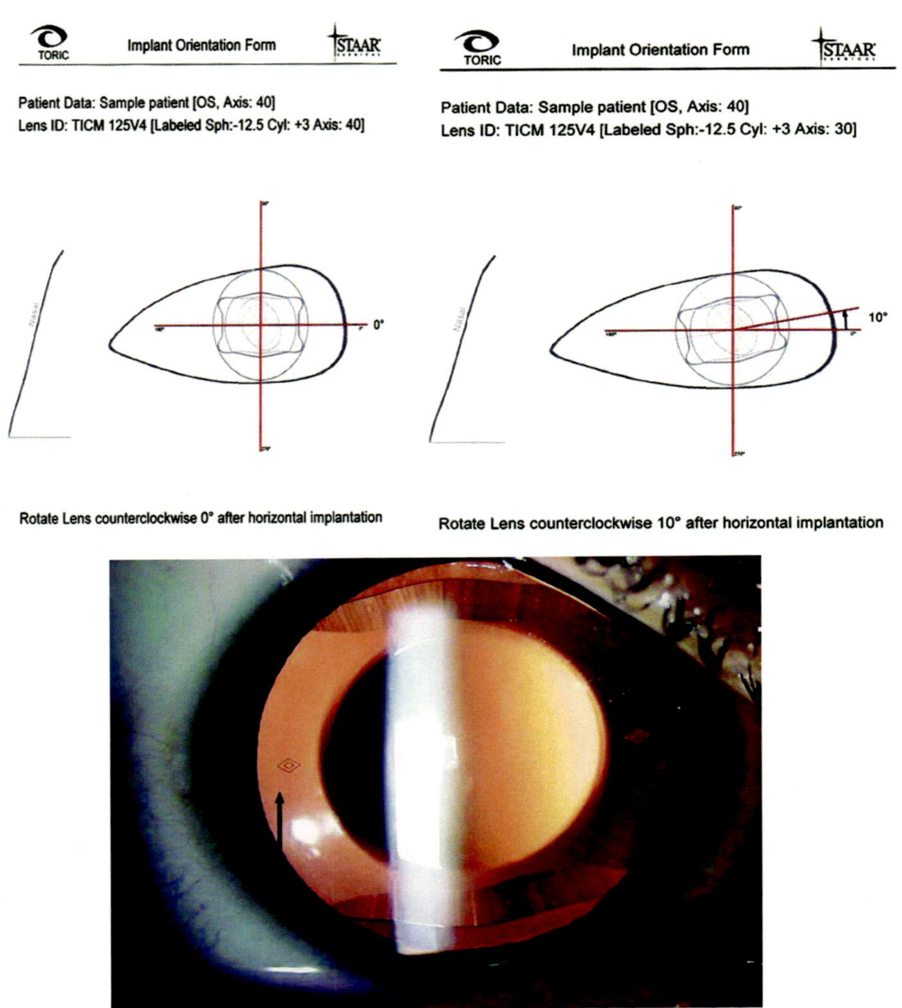

Fig. 42.3: Examples of a customized lens (top left) and an alternative toric ICL (top right) for a same preoperative refraction. Note the power calculated for a customized lens is -12.50 +3.00 x 40°, a toric ICL with this power would be implanted at the horizontal meridian (180°); an alternative lens with same power and different axis (-12.50 +3.00 x 30°) can also be used but it will need to be rotated 10° counterclockwise to compensate the difference in axis orientation. The alternative was used in this case and shown after implantation. Note the alignment marks (arrows) are aligned at 10° counterclockwise from the horizontal meridian

SURGICAL TECHNIQUES

Many surgeons prefer to perform two peripheral iridotomies one or two weeks before the surgery using a ND:YAG laser to prevent postoperative pupillary block. Peripheral iridotomies are performed superiorly 90° apart.[7,15,16] Before surgery pupil must be widely dilated; in our practice; 1% cyclopentolate hydrochloride (Cyclogyl; Alcon labs, Inc. Fortworth, TX, USA) and 2.5% phenylepherine hydrochloride (Mydfrin; Alcon labs) instilled every 15 minutes for 1 hour before surgery usually result in efficient pupillary dilation. We routinely perform ICL surgery performed under topical anesthesia (0.5% bupivacaine hydrochloride). It is advisable to double check the white-to-white measurement with calipers before starting the surgery.

ICL Loading

The inside of the insertion cartridge is lubricated with a viscoelastic material (sodium hyaluronate or methyl cellulose). The lens is removed from the sealed glass container and is loaded inside the cartridge preferably under the surgical microscope. For smooth injection of the lens, it is important to load the lens with both longitudinal edges of the haptic symmetrically tucked under the edge of the cartridge with the lens vaulted anteriorly, it is also helpful to align the two holes located on the haptic of the ICL (or the laser engraved axis marks on the toric ICL) with the longitudinal axis of the cartridge. The coaxial forceps designed by Aus Der Au for ICL loading (E. Janach, Como, Italy) is used to pull the lens through the cartridge tunnel. Inspection of the lens inside the tunnel to exclude twisting of the lens helps making the injection inside the anterior chamber symmetrical, smooth and reproducible. If the lens is noticed to be twisted in the cartridge tunnel it is preferable to take it out and reload properly.

ICL Implantation

A clear corneal temporal incision is made with a diamond knife or a metal disposable keratome. The size of the incision can vary from 2.6 to 3.2 mm depending on the surgeon preference; in our first cases we used a 3.2 mm incision; today we are using a 2.8 mm incision; this enables a smooth injection and shown to have negligible effect on postoperative astigmatism.[20]

The anterior chamber is filled with viscoelastic before the lens is slowly injected using the MicroSTAAR injector, (Staar, Nidau, Switzerland). It is worth mentioning that the injection should be slow enough to allow the leading foot plate to unfold in the anterior chamber before the trailing foot plate is injected out of the cartridge, (Fig. 42.4). This will prevent the lens from unfolding upside down in the anterior chamber. Once the lens unfolds in the anterior chamber the marks on the distal and proximal foot plates are checked for proper orientation. The foot plates near the main incision are then tucked under the iris using an ICL manipulator; we use a Battle ICL manipulator (Rhein medical, Inc. Tampa, Fl, USA) that has a small oval tip with a rough lower surface that gives the surgeon good control on the foot plate. Keeping the lower surface of the manipulator tip flat on the foot plate makes manipulation easier. All manipulations should be as peripheral as possible with no instruments touching the optic or crossing the pupillary zone.

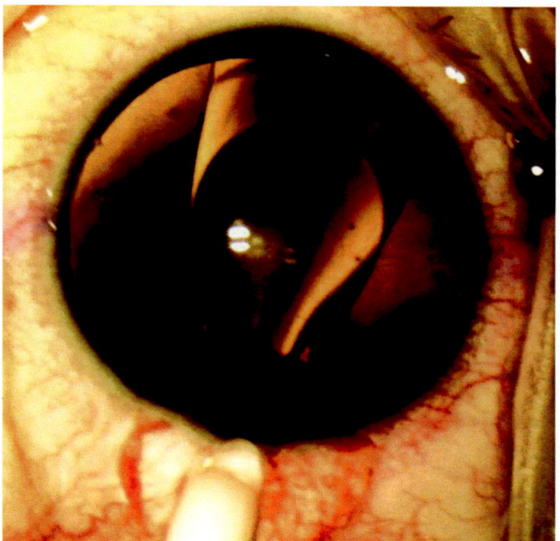

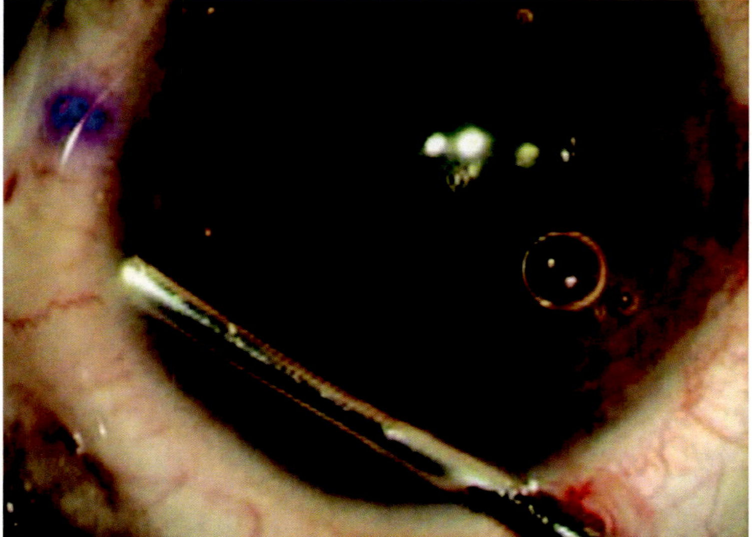

Fig. 42.4: Allowing the leading foot plates to unfold before the trailing foot plates are injected to prevents the lens from unfolding upside down in the anterior chamber (left). Using a vitreous cutter helps obtaining a small, patent and reproducible peripheral iridectomy (right)

The distal foot plates are tucked under the iris through a side port. Correct position of the ICL is verified. If laser iridotomies were not done before surgery then a freshly prepared miotic agent (Carbachol 0.01%, Alcon labs, Inc.) is injected to constrict the pupil and surgical iridectomies are performed. We routinely use a vitrector to perform peripheral surgical iridectomy; the tip of the vitrector is inserted, under viscoelastic, through the main incision to touch the peripheral superior iris tissue, vacuum (300 mmHg) is activated and once the iris tissue is aspirated in the vitrector tip, cutting is activated; one cut is enough to perform a small patent peripheral iridectomy. Alternatively iridectomy can be performed with forceps and scissors.

In our experience laser iridotomies although effective are sometimes difficult to perform especially on eyes with thick brown irides, we prefer surgical iridectomy with the vitrector over scissors as the size and the site of the iridectomy is more controllable. Once the iridectomy is performed, a thorough irrigation and aspiration of the remaining viscoelastic is performed meticulously to prevent postoperative high intraocular spikes.

At the completion of the procedure we inject intracameral preservative free antibiotic (vancomycin 1mg/ml).

Implantation of toric ICL is basically the same as spheric ICL with the exception that the axis of the cylinder of the lens has to be aligned correctly to correct the preoperative astigmatism. If the surgeon is using a custom made lens; the longitudinal axis of toric ICL, marked with laser marks has to be aligned horizontally (0° rotation from the horizontal meridian), in case the surgeon is using an alternative lens that has the same spherocylindrical power and different axis orientation, the lens will need to be rotated to compensate for this axis difference, the manufacturer recommends the rotation to be less than 22.5° from the horizontal axis. In our practice we use alternative lenses with axis difference less than 15° and we center our incision on the axis of implantation to minimize rotation of the toric ICL inside the eye. More than half of toric ICLs we implanted over the last year were alternative lenses to speed the delivery time.

Marking the horizontal axis is best done while the patient is sitting at the slit lamp biomicroscope prior to surgery. During surgery a Mendez ring (Katena Products, Inc. Denville, New Jersey, USA) can be used to measure the required rotation from horizontal. It is also advisable to recheck the alignment of the laser marks that mark the axis of the cylindrical power on the lens haptic after implantation and before constricting the pupil.

There is a growing interest in performing bilateral surgeries on the same surgical session; we perform bilateral ICL surgery on most of our patients on the same surgical session; each eye is treated as a separate case and separate sets of instruments are used for each procedure.

POSTOPERATIVE CARE

Patients are usually discharged few hours after ICL surgery. Before discharge, it is recommended to measure the intraocular pressure, to ensure patency of the peripheral iridectomy and to assess centration and vaulting of ICL and the depth of the anterior chamber. We prescribe topical antibiotics; maxifloxacin hydrochloride 0.5% (Vigamox; Alcon labs, Inc.) four times a day for 1 week and topical steroids; prednisolone acetate 1% (Predforte; Allergan, Mayo, Ireland) four times a day for 3 weeks.

During subsequent postoperative examinations, a routine ophthalmologic assessment is performed, including corrected and uncorrected visual acuity, refraction, intraocular pressure, etc. ICL vault is important to be assessed on each postoperative examination. Vault is defined as the distance between anterior capsule of the crystalline lens and the posterior surface of the ICL; a vault between 200 and 700 µm is considered safe. There is no clinical evidence as to what is the "Ideal vault for an ICL" however there is a general agreement that it is somewhere between 250 and 500 µm. The ICL length is the major determinant of vault; Choi et al, showed that the ICL power had no statistically significant correlation with the ICL vault if the foot plates were located in the ciliary sulcus.[16] The ICL vault can be clinically assessed on the slit lamp biomicroscope by comparing the vault with the cornea thickness; usually a vault equal to ½ to 1 ½ corneal thickness is considered acceptable.[7] We recently used the Anterior Segment Analysis System (EAS-1000, Nidek, Gamagori, Japan) to objectively measure the vault of the ICL inside the eye (Fig. 42.5) shows a postoperative image captured from the EAS-1000 allowing objective measurement of the vault.

CLINICAL RESULTS

Clinical results published in literature,[5,8,13,20-27] as well as reports from FDA studies,[7,28] demonstrated impressive results, including a high predictability, efficacy, safety, stability as well as very high level of patients' satisfaction after ICL and toric ICL implantation. Long term follow-up on a large series already established the safety of spherical ICL.[19] In this section we shall report our results with ICL and toric ICL for different indications over the last 2 years and review some of the results published in the literature.

Over the last 2 years we performed more than 270 cases of spheric ICL and more than 230 cases of toric ICL. ICL is our procedure of choice for all eyes with myopia higher than 8.00 D. We use toric ICL in cases with compound myopic astigmatism when the cylindrical component of the refraction is above 1.00 D. In myopia of 8.00 D or less we perform LASIK provided the corneal topography carries no suspicion and the corneal thickness allows leaving at least 300 microns after an ablation of at least 6.0 mm diameter.

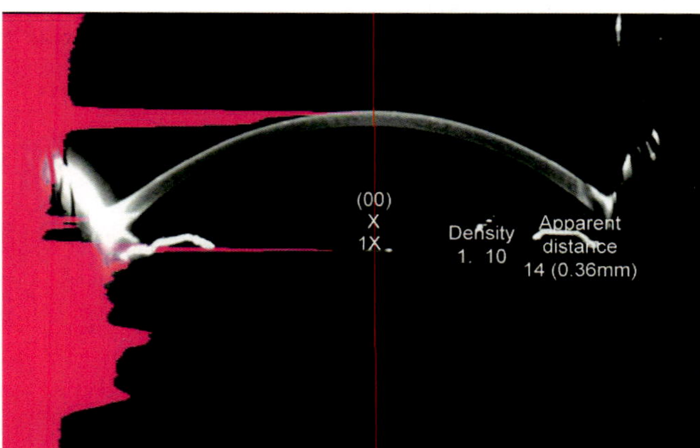

Fig. 42.5: Anterior segment image using the Scheimpflug principle (EAS-1000, Nidek, Gamagori, Japan) allows objective measurement of the ICL vault; 360 μm in this case

ICL in Myopia above 8.00 D

A series of 42 consecutive eyes of 25 patients received spherical ICL for correction of myopia above 8.00 D; the mean age of this group was 27 yrs (range; 18 to 40 yrs) and the follow-up rate at 12 months was 81% (34 eyes).

Refractive outcome

At baseline; the mean MRSE was -10.50 ± 2.19 (range; -17.25 to -8.38 D) and the mean refractive cylinder was 0.73 ± 0.29 D (range; 0.00 to 1.00 D). Emmetropia was the refractive target in all eyes. At one year, the mean MRSE was -0.07 ± 0.34 D (range; -0.63 to 0.38 D), the mean manifest refractive cylinder was 0.65 ± 0.43 D (range, 0.00 to 1.25 D). Of the 34 eyes examined at 1 year, 27 eyes (79%) were between ± 0.50 D, 4 eyes (12%) between -0.51 and -1.00 D, 1 eye (3%) between -1.01 and -2.00 D and 2 eyes (6%) between 0.51 and 1.00 D (Fig. 42.6A), shows the attempted versus achieved spherical equivalent correction 12 months after operation in this group.

Visual outcome

At baseline, 2 eyes (4.8%) could see 20/16, 31 eyes (73.8%) saw 20/20 or better and 41 eyes (97.6%) saw 20/40 or better. One eye had a SCVA worse than 20/50. Twelve months after the operation; 4 eyes (11.8%) saw 20/16 or better, 29 eyes (85.3%) saw 20/20 or better and all eyes could see 20/40 or better without correction (Fig. 42.7A), shows a comparison between preoperative SCVA and postoperative UCVA in the 34 eyes who completed the 1 year examination. Three eyes (8.8%) lost 1 line

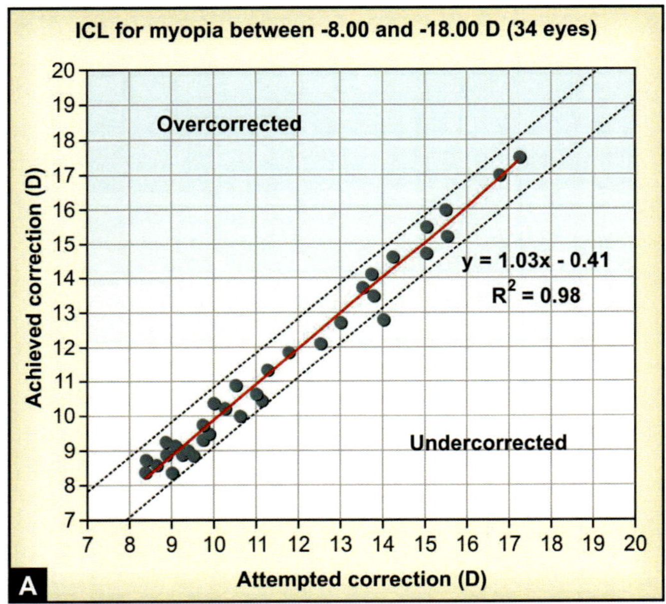

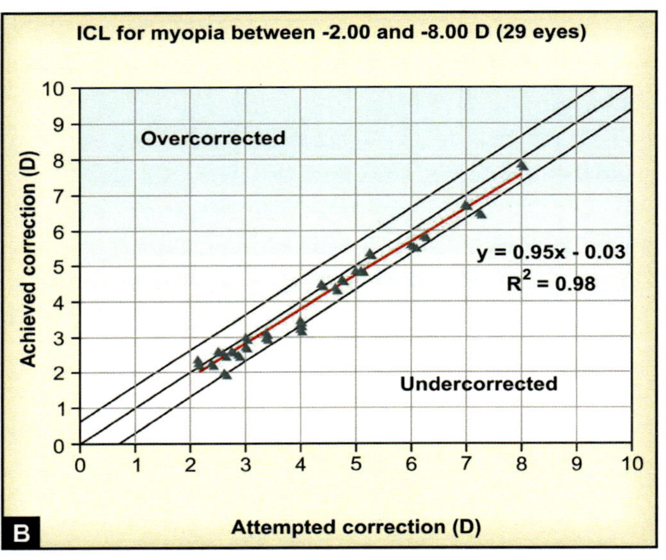

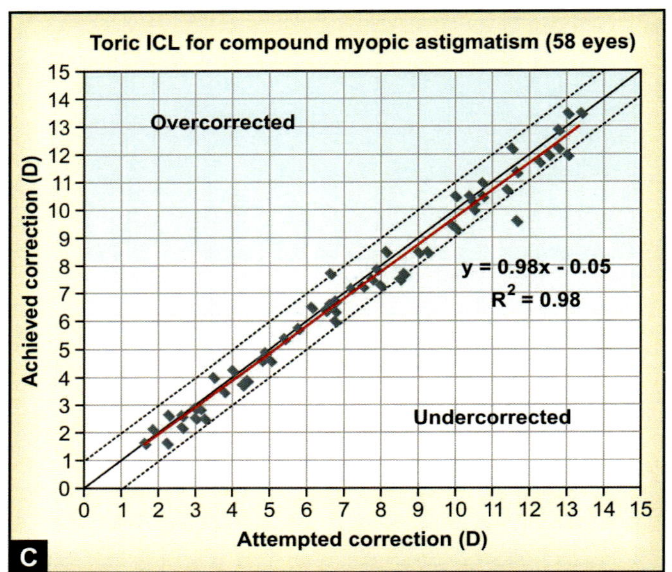

Figs. 42.6A to C: Scattergrams showing the attempted versus achieved spherical equivalent correction (predictability) 12 months after surgery in 3 different groups. The predictability of ICL for correction of myopia between -8.00 and -18.00 D in shown is graph A and between -2.00 and -8.00 D in graph B. Graph C shows the predictability of toric ICL for correction of compound myopic astigmatism with a spherical equivalent refraction between -2:00 and -14:00 D

of SCVA, 9 eyes (26.5%) did not loose or gain lines, 16 eyes (47.1%) gained 1 line and 6 eyes (17.6%) gained 2 lines or more lines of spectacle corrected visual acuity. After the 1 month examination, the mean change of MRSE was less than 0.50 D at each examination interval.

ICL in Myopia between -2.00 and -8.00 D

As we described earlier, we use ICL as our procedure of choice for correction of myopia less than 8.00 D in cases that are risks for LASIK. In a series of 35 consecutive eyes that received ICL for myopia between -2.00 and -8.00D; the mean age was

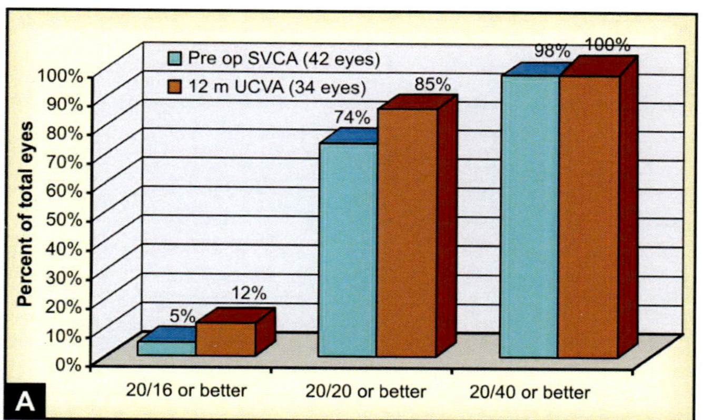

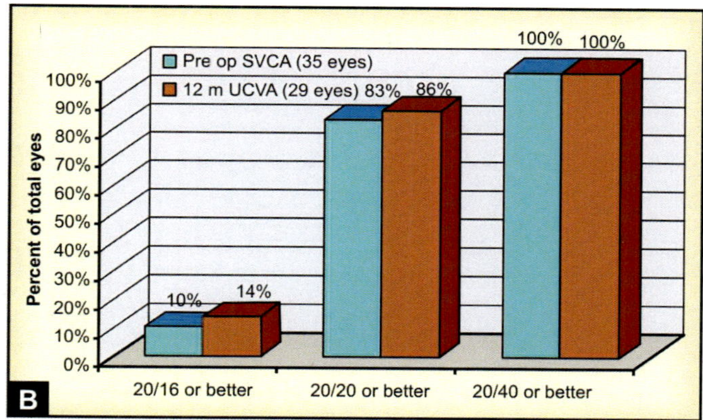

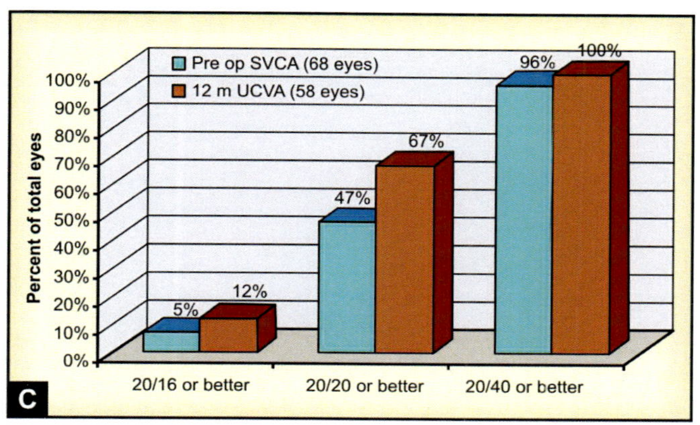

Fig. 42.7: Postoperative uncorrected visual acuity at 12 months compared to preoperative best spectacle-corrected visual acuity (efficacy) of the same 3 groups shown in Fig. 42.6

28 years, the mean baseline MRSE was -4.69 ± 1.59 D (range; -8.00 to -2.13 D), the mean refractive cylinder was 0.42 ± 0.26 D (range; 0.00 to 1.00 D). Emmetropia was the target in all eyes.

Refractive outcome

One year after operation; 29 eyes (82.9%) were examined, the mean baseline MRSE was -0.14 ± 0.27 D (range; -0.75 to 0.25 D); 86.2% eyes were between ± 0.50 D and all eyes were between ± 1.00 D of emmetropia. The mean refractive cylinder was 0.43 ± 0.28 D (range; 0.00 to 1.25 D); 25 eyes (86.2%) were between ± 0.50 D and, 4 eyes (13.8%) between -0.51 and -1.00 D (Fig. 42.6B) shows the predictability of refractive correction in these 29 eyes.

Visual outcome

Of the 29 eyes that completed the 1 year examination, baseline spectacle-corrected visual acuity was 20/16 or better in 3 eyes (10.3%), 20/20 or better in 24 eyes (82.8%) eyes and 20/32 or better in 28 eyes (96.6%) eyes. One year after operation; 4 eyes (13.8%) saw 20/16 or better, 25 eyes (86%) saw 20/20 or better and all eyes saw 20/32 or better without correction.

Two eyes (6.9%) lost 1 line of SCVA, 14 eyes (48.3%) did not loose or gain any lines, 10 eyes (34.5%) gained 1 line and 3 eyes (10.3%) gained 2 or more lines of SCVA (Fig. 42.7B) shows a comparison between the baseline SCVA and the one year UCVA in this group.

Toric ICL

We analyzed the results of toric ICL implantation in a series of 68 consecutive eyes. The mean age was 26 yrs (range; 19 to 45 yrs). The baseline mean MRSE was -7.07 ± 3.35 D (range; -13.38 to -2.25 D), mean refractive cylinder was 2.34 ± 0.81 D (range; 1.25 to 4.75 D).

Refractive outcome

At 12 months, 58 eyes (85.3%) were examined; mean MRSE was -0.16 ± 0.41 D (range; -1.75 to 1.13 D); 49 eyes (84.5%) were between ± 0.50 D of emmetropia, 5 eyes (8.6%) between -1.00 and -0.51 D, 3 eyes (5.2%) between -2.00 and -1.10 D. One eye (1.7%) was overcorrected by 1.13 D (Fig. 42.6C) shows the attempted versus achieved correction of MRSE for this group of 58 eyes with toric ICL.

Refractive stability was reached at 1 month after operation; mean change in MRSE was less than 0.50 D at all postoperative examination intervals.

Mean refractive cylinder at 12 months was 0.38 ± 0.66 D (range; 0.00 to 1.75 D). The stability of the refractive cylinder was documented from the one month examination and afterwards; refractive cylinder changed by less than 1.00 D in all cases and by less than 0.50 D in more than 95.5% of cases. The mean difference was less than 0.05 D at each reporting interval. Sanders and Sarver reported similar stability of the refractive cylinder.[29]

Analysis of the vector stability of cylinder showed that the cylinder is stable from the first month examination and it changed by less than 1.00 D in more than 98.3% of cases and by less than 0.5 D in more than 94.8% of cases at each interval. The mean difference was between 0.20 and 0.28 D at each reporting interval. This shows the stability of the cylindrical correction and supports the data published by Sanders et al who reported a change of ≤ 1.00 D in between 96.8% and 97.4% and ≤ 0.50% in between 85.3% and 87.2% of cases.[10] Vector analysis using the double angle minus cylinder method is shown in Fig. 42.8.

Visual outcome

At base line, best spectacle-corrected visual acuity was 20/16 or better in 4 eyes (6.9%) eyes, 20/20 or better in 28 eyes (46.6%), 20/32 or better in 52 eyes (89%) eyes, all eyes could see 20/50 or better with spectacles. One year after surgery, uncorrected visual acuity was 20/16 or better in 7 eyes (12.1%), 20/20 or better in 39 eyes (67.2%) and 20/32 or better in 50 eyes (86.2%). All eyes could see 20/40 or better without correction.

21 eyes (36.1%) maintained their baseline spectacle-corrected visual acuity, 1 eye (1.7%) lost 1 line, 29 eyes (43.1%) gained 1 line and 11 eyes (19%) gained 2 or more lines of spectacle-corrected visual acuity.

Stability of toric ICL alignment after implantation

We evaluated the stability of the toric ICL alignment after implantation using the OPD-scan (NIDEK, Gamagori, Japan). The OPD (optical path difference) map measures the objective refraction of the entire

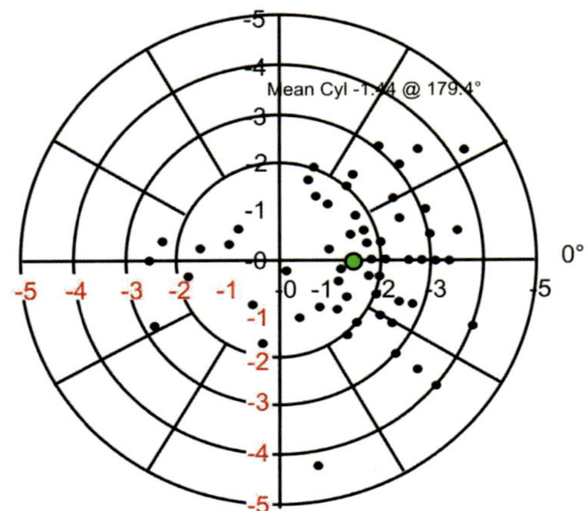

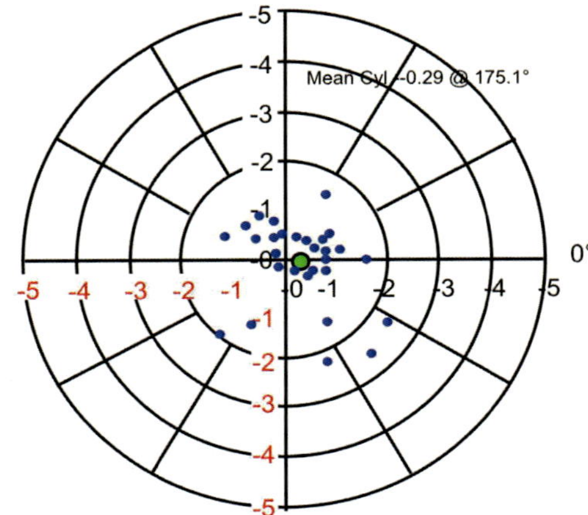

Fig. 42.8: Double angle minus cylinder scatter plot at base line (left) and at 12 months after implantation of toric ICL. Mean vector cylinder changed from -1.44 D at 180° to -0.29 at 175.1°

eye over a 6 mm pupil while the internal OPD map measures the objective refraction of the entire eye minus the anterior corneal surface over the same pupil diameter. Subtracting the preoperative from the postoperative OPD map of a given eye can reveal the effective power of the implanted ICL at any point within the 6 mm pupil (Fig. 42.9) shows preoperative and postoperative OPD maps of an eye that received toric ICL documenting the stability of the refractive correction over 1 year. Also, comparing the axis and power of the cylinder using the internal OPD map at each postoperative examination is a sensitive objective method to detect any late rotation of a toric ICL after implantation (Fig. 42.10) shows baseline and postoperative internal OPD maps of an eye that received toric ICL.

The mean value of rotation of the axis of the cylinder in our series was between 0.06 and 0.9° for all time intervals. Axis misalignment was ≤ 5° at 1 year follow up in 89.6% of eyes, ≤ 10° in 98.3% and ≤ 20° in all eyes.

One eye had axis misalignment more than 20°, was diagnosed at the end of the first week after operation and was most probably due to misalignment during implantation as the pupil got smaller than the optic diameter during alignment of the axis; realignment was performed on the 8th postoperative day and no rotation was observed afterwards, and at 1 year the axis misalignment of this eye was 2.0°. Table 42.2 compares our refractive and visual results with similar studies published in the literature.

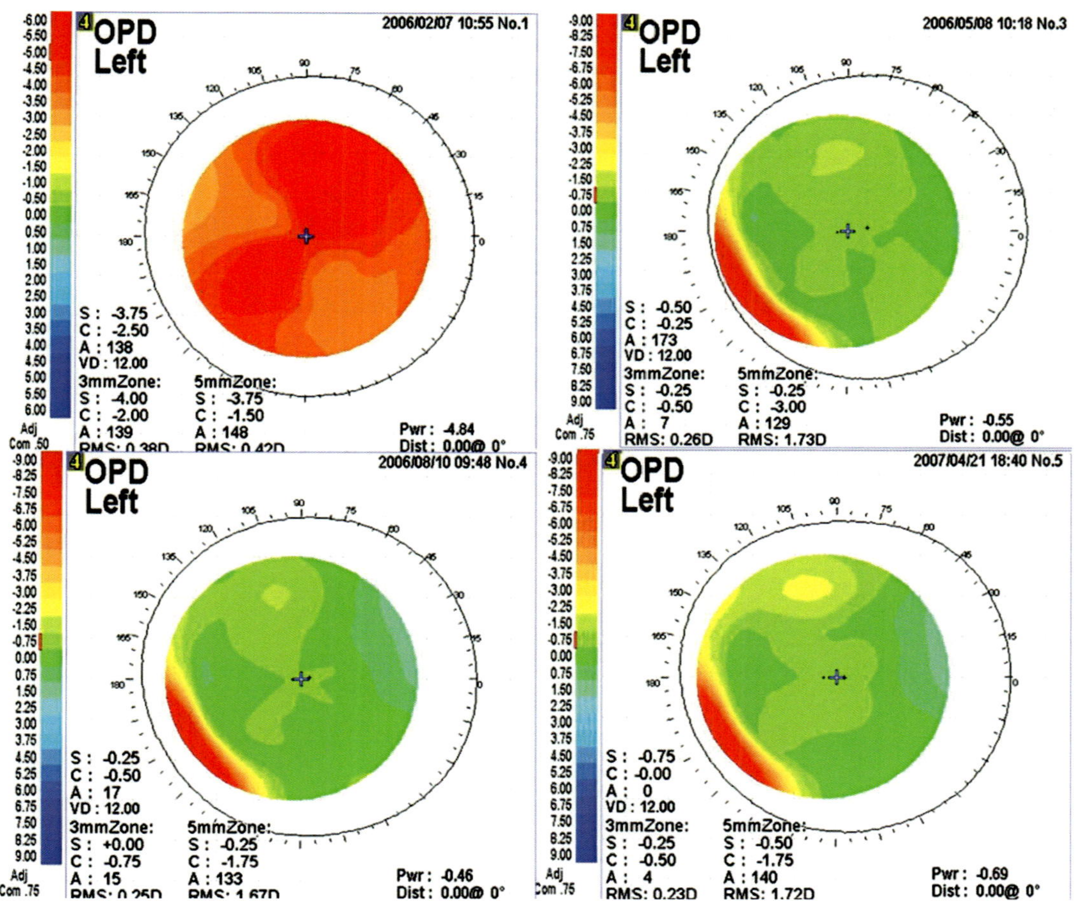

Fig. 42.9: shows the total optical path difference (OPD) of an eye with preoperative refraction of -3.75 -2.50 x 138° (top left), a toric ICL was implanted, the OPD map 3 months after the operation (top right) shows an objective refraction of -0.50 -0.25 x 173. OPD map was stable in the following exams; 6 and 12 months after surgery (bottom)

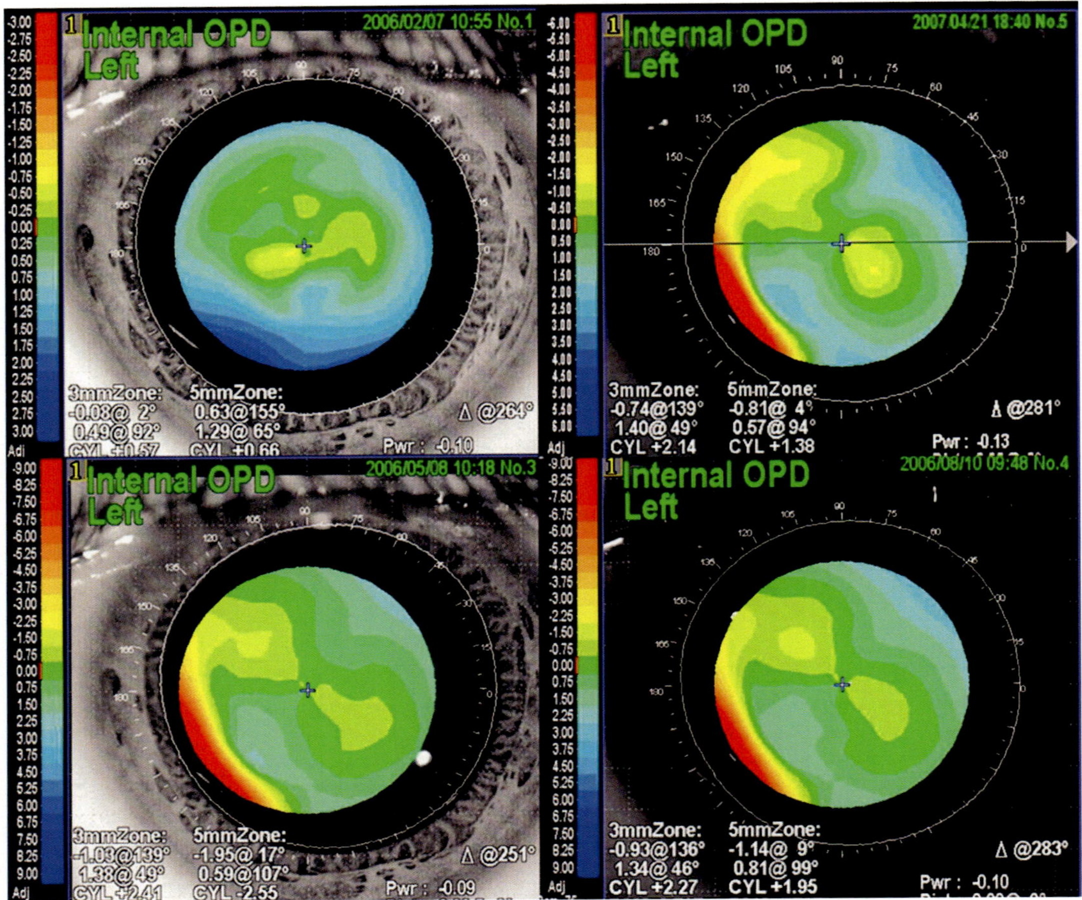

Fig. 42.10: Demonstrates the internal optical path difference (internal OPD) in the same eye shown in Fig. 42.11. Note the stability of the axis of the internal astigmatism (equivalent to the astigmatic axis of the toric ICL) overtime.

ICL in stable keratoconus

Keratoconus commonly presents during the second decade of life. Many of the cases slowly and gradually progress in severity, but the rate of progression and the length of time that the disease remains actively progressive vary considerably. The ectasia may progress slowly but continuously for years and then stabilizes permanently, or periods of progression may alternate with period during which the ectatic process appears to have arrested. In some cases the ectasia remains stable after its initial appearance. It is uncommon for the condition to progress after the age of 40 years, but exceptions do occur.[30] ICL and toric ICL can be used to correct myopia and compound myopic astigmatism in eyes with stable keratoconus. Bartels et al used a toric phakic lens to correct high astigmatism in an eye with pellucid marginal degeneration.[31]

We are conducting a prospective randomized clinical trial to assess the efficacy, predictability and safety of toric ICL for correction of compound myopic astigmatism associated with stable keratoconus. We included 23 eyes of 17 patients. All eyes had stable keratoconus documented by videokeratography, clear central cornea, MRSE between -4.00 and -15.00 D, spectacle-corrected visual acuity of 20/40 or better, stable manifest refraction for at least 1 year together with the other previously mentioned selection criteria for ICL implantation including an endothelial cell count above 2200 cell/mm^2 and anterior chamber depth of 2.7 mm or more calculated from the endothelium.

Table 42.2: Comparative studies of ICL and Toric ICL for myopia and compound myopic astigmatism

	El- Danasoury et al, ‡	El- Danasoury et al, ‡	El- Danasoury et al, ‡	Sanders et al,[10]	FDA clinical trial,7	Uusitalo et al,[37]	Pienda-Fernandez et al.[38]	Zaldivar et al,5
Dates of surgery	2005 - 2006	2005 - 2006	2005 - 2006	2002-2003	1998 - 2001	1998 - 2000	1998	1993 - 1996
ICL Model	V4	V4	V4 (toric)	V4 (toric)	V4	NA	V3, V4	20202, V1, V2, V3
POPULATION								
Mean age (years)	27	29.5	26	36.4	36.5	39	34.5	34
Eyes operated (eyes)	42	35	68	210	523	38	18	124
Eyes reported (eyes)	34	29	58	186	428	36	18	124
Percent of eyes reported (%)	81	82.9	85.3	88.6	81.8	94.1	100	100
Mean follow up (months)	12	12	12	12	12	13	26.6	11
Preoperative Refraction								
Mean MRSE (D)	-10.50 ± 2.19	-4.69 ± 1.59	-7.07 ± 3.35	-9.36 ± 2.66	-10.05 ± 3.75	-15.1	-15.27 ± 3.47	-13.38 ± 2.23
Range MRSE (D)	-17.25 to -8.38	-8.00 to -2.13	-13.38 to -2.25	-19.50 to -2.38	-20.00 to -3.00	-29.00 to -7.75	-21.25 to -2.75	-18.63 to -8.50
Mean refractive Cylinder (D)	0.73 ± 0.29	0.42 ± 2.6	2.34 ± 0.81	1.93 ± 0.84	NA	NA	1.8 ± 1.30	2.13 ± 1.51
Range refractive cylinder (D)	0.00 to 1.00	0.00 to 1.00	1.25 to 4.75	1.25 to 475	NA	NA	0.50 to 4.00	0.00 to 6.00
Postoperative MRSE								
Mean MRSE (D)	-0.07 ± 0.34	-0.14 ± 0.27	-0.16 ± 0.41	0.05 ± 0.46	-0.50 ± 0.98	-2.00 ± 2.48	-0.62 ± 0.81	-0.78 ± 0.87
Range MRSE (D)	-0.63 to 0.38	-0.75 to 0.25	-1.75 to 1.13	-2.25 to 1.00	-8.00 to 1.13*	-13.00 to 0.13**	-2.75 to 0.75	-3.50 to 1.63
Percent within 0.50 D (%)	79	86.2	84.5	76.9	61.6	71.1	22.2	44
Percent within 1.00 D (%)	97	100	93.1	97.3	84.7	81.6	61.1	69
Percent within 2.00 D (%)	100	100	100	100	96.7	NA	NA	NA
Postoperative Cylinder								
Mean (D)	0.65 ± 0.43	0.43 ± 0.28	0.38 ± 0.66	0.51 ± 0.48	NA	NA	NA	0.96 ± 0.85
Range (D)	0.00 to 1.25	0.0 to 1.25	0.00 to 1.75	0.00 to 3.00	NA	NA	NA	0.00 to 3.75
Baseline SCVA								
20/16 or better (%)	4.8	10.3	6.9	4.8	NA	NA	NA	NA
20/20 or better (%)	73.8	82.8	46.6	83.1	67.7	23.9	NA	5
20/40 or better (%)	97.6	100	96	NA	96.9	63.2	NA	80
Postoperative UCVA								
20/16 or better (%)	11.8	13.8	12.1	NA	NA	NA	NA	NA
20/20 or better (%)	85.3	86	67.2	83.1	60.1	5.3	5.5	2
20/40 or better (%)	100	100	100	NA	92.5	52.6	44.4	68
Postoperative SCVA								
20/16 or better (%)	14.4	20	17	37.6	NA	NA	NA	NA
20/20 or better (%)	94	96	88	96.8	82.4	39.5	NA	19
20/40 or better (%)	100	100	100	NA	98.1	94.7	NA	93
Change in BSCVA								
Loss ≥ 2 or more lines	0	0	0	1.6	0.7	NA	5.6	0.81
Loss 1 line (%)	8.8	6.9	1.7	7.5	5.4	6.2	NA	NA
Unchanged (%)	26.5	48.3	36.1	14.5	44.3	NA	NA	NA
Gain 1 line (%)	47.1	34.5	43.1	57.5	40	31.3	38.8	NA
Gain ≥ 2 or more lines (%)	17.6	10.3	19	18.9	9.6	40.6	NA	36
Complications								
Visually insignificant lens opacities (%)	2.9	0	1.7	2.4	2.1	2.6	5.6	2.42
Visually significant cataract (%)	2.9	0	0	0.5	0.4	2.6	5.6	0
Pupillary block (%)	0	0	0			7.9***	12.5***	4.8
Percent of secondary interventions (total)	2.9	0	5.3	2.4	2.3	13.2	16.7	
Removal (%)	0	0	0	1.6	0	2	0	3.3
Replacement (%)	0	0	0	0.5	1.7	0	0	1.6
Repositioning (%)	0	3.4	0	0	0.7	0	0	0.8
Axis realignment (%)	0	0	5.3	0.5	0	0	0	0
Removal with Cataract extraction (%)	2.9	0	0	0	0.4	5.3	5.6	0
Laser Iridotomies enlargement (%)	0	0	0	0	0	7.9	11.1	0

‡ Ongoing studies
* 9.9 % eyes were not corrected to emmetropia
**31.6 % eyes were not corrected to emmetropia
*** All eyes that developed pupillary block had laser iridotomies before ICL implantation

All patients were rigid contact lens intolerant. Each eye received a myopic toric ICL through a temporal clear corneal incision. At baseline; mean MRSE refraction was -9.62 ± 2.89 D (range; -15.00 to -4.38 D), 12 eyes (52%) eyes could see 20/20 or better with correction. At 12 months (follow-up rate, 87%), MRSE was -0.32 ± 0.52 D (range; -1.50 to 0.13 D), uncorrected visual acuity was 20/40 or better in 20 eyes (90%) and 20/20 or better in 11 eyes (55%); 4 eyes (20%) eyes gained 2 or more lines of spectacle-corrected visual acuity. Due to the nature of the disease, longer follow-up and larger series are needed, however based on our 1 year results we believe that toric ICL implantation is effective, predictable and relatively safe for the correction of compound myopic astigmatism associated with stable keratoconus.

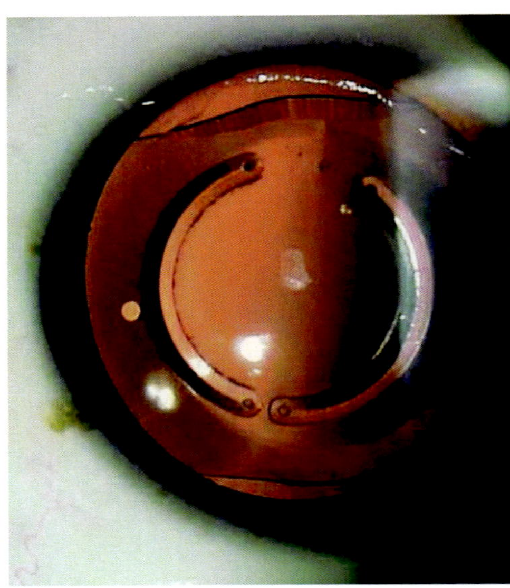

Fig. 42.11: An eye with progressive keratoconus; 2 Ferrara ring segments were implanted to stabilize the ectasia; one year later, a toric ICL was implanted to correct the residual compound myopic astigmatism.

ICL after Corneal ring segments or collagen cross linking in progressive keratoconus

Over the last few years many reports showed the possibility of stabilizing a progressive keratoconus using intracorneal ring segments,[32-33] and corneal collagen cross linking.[34-35] The favorable results published in peer reviewed literature as well as our own unpublished results are encouraging. Implantation of toric ICL after corneal ring segments or cross-linking is possible to correct the residual refractive error (Fig. 42.11) shows an eye with progressive keratoconus that received intracorneal ring segments to stabilize a progressive keratoconus; a toric ICL was implanted one year after the primary procedure to correct residual refractive error.

Toric ICL after corneal grafts

Another important indication for toric ICL is the correction of residual refractive errors after corneal grafting in which keratorefractive techniques are not necessarily good or viable option. Tahzib,[36] described the effective reduction of post-keratoplasty astigmatism in 36 eyes from -7.06 ± 2.01 D preoperatively to -2.0±1.53 D at last follow-up. In a prospective study we evaluated the predictability, efficacy and safety of toric ICL implantation in correcting compound myopic astigmatism after deep anterior lamellar keratoplasty (DALKP); 28 eyes of 28 patients with previous DALKP received toric ICL. All eyes had stable refraction for 6 months after removal of corneal sutures, mean MRSE was -9.4 ± 2.6 D (range; -16.0 to -5.0 D), SCVA of 20/40 or better in all eyes and 20/20 or better in 14 eyes (50%), endothelial cell count more than 2200 cells/mm^2 and anterior chamber depth 2.7 mm or more calculated from the endothelium. One year after surgery, (follow-up rate, 85.7%); MRSE was -0.3 ± 0.5 D, 14 eyes (58.3%) eyes saw 20/20 uncorrected; 6 eyes (25%) gained 2 or more lines of SCVA. No visual threatening complications were observed. ICL and toric ICL can also be implanted in eyes with penetrating corneal graft provided the endothelial cell count is at acceptable level (above 2200 cells/mm^2) and the anterior chamber depth is deep enough (more than 2.7 mm from endothelium).

COMPLICATIONS

Long term follow-up on a large series using the current model of myopic ICL (V4) already established its relative safety,[19] and showed a marked reduction of the rate of complications reported in earlier models.[5,37,38] This dramatic improvement in the safety of ICL shadows our own experience; in our initial series of 100 ICL models V2 and V3 implanted between 1995-1997, we encountered a relatively high incidence of lens opacities (10%) and sizing issues (6%), this made us stop using ICL till the year 2005 when we restarted implanting ICL and toric ICL using the currently available model (V4) and the newly introduced loading and injecting system. Since then we adopted the ICL and toric ICL as our phakic IOLs of choice. In this section we will review the most important complications that we encountered over the last 2 years or were published in the literature.

Improper sizing and poor vaulting

Proper vaulting is critical in ICL surgery as complications reported after ICL implantation resulted largely from improper sizing. Excessive vault may induce peripheral anterior synechiae, pigment dispersion and shallowing of the anterior chamber; also a large ICL may distend the pupil with subsequent glare and halos. A low vault may induce cataract formation. Gonvers et al found no anterior subcapsular cataract when vaulting is >90 µm.[39]

Cataract

The relatively high rate of induced cataract after ICL implantation was a main concern with the earlier models,[40] it decreased significantly after the introduction of the latest model (V4) and the introduction of the loading and injection technique described previously in the methods section. In recent reports where the authors used only the V4 model, the rate of cataract ranges from 0.0 to 2.4%.[7,10,19] A low incidence of late onset cataract was also reported in the US FDA Clinical Trial (0.4%, 2 of 526 eyes).[19] In our hands we had observed a similar low rate of clinically significant cataract after ICL implantation; 2 of 482 eyes (0.41%). Both patients that developed cataract had ICL implantation for high myopia (above 15.00 D) and were older than 45 years of age. This finding supports Lackner and coauthors suggestion that cataract formation is more likely to occur after ICL implantation in patients who are aged > 45 years.[41] In cases where cataract developed after ICL implantation; removal of the ICL and performing a phacoemulsification with IOL implantation resulted in favorable outcome.[7,37,38]

Pupillary block

Peripheral iridectomy or iridotomies are mandatory in ICL surgery; otherwise pupillary block will occur during the early postoperative period. Many surgeons prefer to perform laser iridotomies one or two weeks before the ICL implantation. We prefer surgical iridectomy with a vitreous cutter as described earlier; we did not see any case of pupillary block after surgical iridectomy. Pienda-Fernandez and co-workers reported a relatively high incidence of pupillary block after ICL implantation with laser iridotomies (12.5%), they reported no incidence of pupillary block after they shifted to surgical iridectomies.[38]

Other causes of high intraocular pressure during early postoperative period is retained viscoelastic; Chang and Meau noticed that the most common cause for rise of intraocular pressure in early postoperative period in their series was due to retained viscoelastic; they recommended that the surgeon, at the conclusion of the surgery removes the viscoelastic from the region around the peripheral iridotomies before the other parts of the anterior chamber. This led, in their experience, to a significant decrease in the incidence of transient IOP elevation.[15]

Night glare

Night vision symptoms are less common after ICL implantation compared to anterior chamber lenses. This may be at last partly, due to the relatively larger effective optic diameter of the posterior chamber lenses being closer to the nodal point. Occasionally night glare can be due to peripheral iridectomy; Chang and Meau reported 3 (4.9%) patients with symptoms of glare after initial surgery due to peripheral iridectomies prior to ICL implantation, symptoms persisted only for a short period. Only 1 (1.6%) patient complained of seeing an extra light 6 months after surgery.[15] In their series of 210 eyes Sanders et al reported one patient who complained of a line in his vision from the preoperative laser iridotomies; although the patient insisted upon removal of the ICL, it did not correct for the line in his vision.[7]

Residual refractive error

The excellent predictability and efficacy of ICL and Toric ICL in correcting myopia and compound myopic astigmatism has been proved.[5,7,8,13,20-28] In case of residual refractive errors after ICL implantation, ICL replacement or excimer laser keratorefractive procedure (LASIK or surface ablation) remain valid options. In our practice we perform LASIK as a secondary procedure to correct residual refractive error after ICL implantation (Bioptics). LASIK can be performed as soon as the refractive outcome stabilizes and the wound heals. We usually allow 4 weeks before performing LASIK on an eye who received an ICL. Due to the exceptionally high predictability of the calculation software we did not have to perform a secondary refractive procedure after ICL implantation in more than 400 cases performed in the last 2 years.

Endothelial Damage

Compared to other phakic lenses, posterior chamber lenses are the farthest from the endothelium and the least to induce endothelial cell loss. Apart from the endothelial loss directly related to the surgery, little concerns exist over subsequent endothelial loss after ICL implantation.[10] Pienda-Fernandez and coauthors reported an endothelial cell loss of 4.9% and 6.1% at 6 and 36 months respectively after ICL implantation.[38]

Decrease in Accommodation

Chang and Meau reported a case of 39 years-old man who complained difficulty in reading 1 month after receiving an ICL for high myopia despite having UCVA of J2 at near and a manifest refraction of 0.13 D and an UCVA of 20/25 at distance. This patient elected to have the ICL removed. After removal, the patient did not lose any lines of SCVA nor did he develop any cataract.[15]

Pigment dispersion

Pigment dispersion after ICL implantation has been a concern, in an earlier study, Trindade et al found contact between the iris and implanted ICL in all eyes.[40] However, with the better vaulting design of the V4 model, chances of contact between the iris and IOL have been reduced.[7] According to international reports, the ICL is safe for implantation in eyes with a minimum anterior chamber depth of 2.8 mm. However, the United States Food and Drug Administration (FDA) approved lens use for a minimum anterior chamber depth of 2.7 mm. In Chang and Meau series, 23% of eyes had anterior chamber depth between 2.8 and 3.0 mm, but they did not find any significant pigment dispersion in any eye; in another study of 18 eyes with a minimum anterior chamber depth of 3.0 mm, the same authors found no significant pigment changes in any of the eyes.[15]

Retinal complications

Retinal complications have been reported in high myopic eyes after ICL implantation, these include macular hemorrhage, retinal detachment and progressive dry macular degeneration. The preoperative high myopia and the pre-existing myopic degenerations probably contributed to the eventual hemorrhages and detachment seen in these eyes rather than the ICL surgical procedure.[7,15,19,38] Detailed fundus examination is highly recommended before ICL implantation especially in highly myopic eyes to diagnose and if needed, to treat any pre-existing myopic degenerations prior to ICL implantation.

Future carries promises for improvements including more accurate sizing, more understanding of the ciliary sulcus anatomy, the position of the ICL in relation to ciliary sulcus and zonules, and possible wavefront customized lenses to compensate the pre-existing high order aberrations in highly aberrated eyes.

So far, the excellent predictability and efficacy combined with the very low incidence of post-operative complications and overwhelming patient satisfaction make the ICL and the toric ICL extremely valuable tools for refractive surgeons to address the needs of their patients.

REFERENCES

1. Baikoff GB, Joly P. Comparison of minus power anterior chamber intraocular lenses and myopic epikeratoplasty in phakic eyes. Refract Corneal Surg 1990;6:252-60.
2. Baïkoff G. Phakic anterior chamber intraocular lenses. Int Ophthalmol Clin. 1991;31:75-86.
3. Fechner PU, Worst JGF. A new concave intraocular lens for the correction of high myopia. Eur J Implant Refract Surg 1989;1:41-3.
4. Brauweiler PH, Wehler T, Busin M. High incidence of cataract formation after implantation of a silicone posterior chamber lens in phakic, highly myopic eyes. Ophthamology 1999;106:1651-5.
5. Zaldivar R, Davidorf JM, Oscherow S. Posterior chamber phakic intraocular lens for myopia of -8 to -19 diopters. J Refract Surg 1998;14:294-305.
6. Durrie DS, Lesher MP, Cavanaugh TB, Classification of variable clinical response after photorefractive keratectomy for myopia. J Refract Surg 1995;11:341-7.
7. The Implantable Contact Lens in Treatment of Myopia (ITM) Study Group. U.S. food and drug administration clinical trial of the implantable contact lens for moderate to high myopia. Ophthalmology. 2003;110:255-66.
8. Pesando PM, Ghiringhello MP, Tagliavacche P. Posterior chamber collamer phakic intraocular lens for myopia and hyperopia. J Refract Surg 1999;15:415-23.
9. Sanders DR, Vukich JA; ICL in treatment of myopia (ITM) study group. Incidence of lens opacities and clinically significant cataracts with the implantable contact lens; comparison of two lens designs. J Refract Surg. 2002;18:673-82.
10. Sanders DR, Schneider D, Martin R, Brown D, Dulaney D, Vukich J, Slade S, Schallhorn S. Toric Implantable Collamer Lens for moderate high myopic Astigmatism. Ophthalmology 2007;114:54-61.
11. Marcos S. Aberrations and visual performance following standard laser vision correction. J Refract Surg. 2001;17:S596-601.
12. El Danasoury A, El Maghraby A, Gamali TO. Comparison of iris-fixed Artisan lens implantation with excimer laser insitu keratomileusis in correcting myopia between -9.00 and -19.50 D. Ophthalmology 2002;109:955-64.
13. Gonvers M, Othenin-Girard P, Bonet C, Sickenberg M. Implantable contact lens for moderate to high myopia; short-term follow-up of 2 models. J Catract Refract Surg, 2001;27:380-8.
14. Reuland MS, Reuland AJ, Nishi Y, Auffarth GU. Corneal radii and anterior chamber depth measurements using the IOL-Master Versus the Pentacam. J Refract Surg. 2007;23:368-73.
15. Chang JS, Meau AY. Visian collamer phakic intraocular lens in high myopic Asian eyes. J Refract Surg. 2007;23:17-25.
16. Choi KH, Chung SE, Chung TY, Chung ES. Ultrasound biomicroscopy for determining Visian implantable Contact lens length in Phakic IOL implantation. J Refract Surg; 2007;23:362-7.
17. Pop M, Payette Y, Mansour M. Predicting sulcus size using ocular measurements. J Cataract Refract Surgery. 2001;27:1033-8.
18. Holladay JT. Refractive power calculations for intraocular lenses in the phakic eye. Am J Ophthalmol. 1993;116:63-6.
19. Sanders DR, Doney k, Poco M; ICL In Treatment of Myopia (ITM) Study Group. United States Food and Drug Administration Clinical Trial of The Implantable Collamer Lens (ICL) for moderate to high myopia; three-year follow up. Ophthalmology. 2004;111:1683-92.
20. Martin RG, Gills JP. Evaluating outcomes of cataract surgery In: Sanders DR, Koch DD, eds. An Atlas of Corneal Topography. Thorofare, NJ: SLACK Inc.: 1993:67-8.
21. Arne JL, Lesueur LC Phakic posterior chamber lenses for high myopia: functional and anatomical outcomes. J. Cataract Refract Surg 2000;26:369-74.
22. Menezo JL, Peris-Martinez C, Cisneros A, Martinez-Costa R. Posterior chamber phakic intraocular lenses to correct high myopia: a comparative study between STAAR and Adatormed models.J Refract Surg 2001;17:32-42.
23. Assetto V, Benedetti S, Pesando P. Collamer intraocular contact lens to correct high myopia. J Cataract Refract Surg1996;22:551-6.
24. Fink AM, Gore C, Rosen E. Cataract development after implantation of the Staar Collamer posterior chamber phakic lens. J Cataract Refract Surg 1999;25:278-82.
25. Jimenez-Alfaro I, Benitez del Castillo JM, Garcia-Feijoo J, et al Safety of posterior chamber phakic intraocular lenses for the correction of high myopia. Anterior segment changes after posterior chamber phakic intraocular lens implantation. Ophthalmology 2001;108:90-9.
26. Kaya V, kevser MA, Yilmaz OF. Phakic posterior chamber plate intraocular lenses for high myopia. J Refract surg. 1999;15:580-5.
27. Rosen E. Gore C. Staar Collamer posterior chamber phakic intraocular lens to correct myopia and hyperopia. J Cataract Refract Surg 1998;24:596-606.
28. Sanders Dr, Brown DC, Martin Rg, et al, Implantable contact lens for moderate to high myopia; phase I FDA clinical study with 6 month follow-up J Cataract Refract Surg 1998;24:607-11.
29. Sanders DR, Sarver EJ. Standardized Analyses of correction of astigmatism with the Visian toric phakic implantable collamer lens. J Refract Surg. 2007;23:649-60.

30. Leibowitz HM, Morello S. Keratoconus and noninflammatory thinning disorders in Leibowitz HM, Waring GO: Corneal disorders, clinical diagnosis and management. W.B. Saunders, chap 12, 1998;349-74.
31. Bartels MC. Saxena R. van den Berg TJ. et al. The influence of incision-induced astigmatism and axial lens position on the correction of myopic astigmatism with the Artisan toric phakic intraocular lens, Ophthalmology 2006;113:1110-7.
32. Kymionis G, C. Siganos C, Tsiklis N, Anastasakis A, Yoo S, Pallikaris A, N. Astyrakakis N, Pallikaris I. Long-term Follow-up of Intacs in Keratoconus. Am J Ophthalmol 2003; 143:236-44.
33. Colin J, Cochener B, Savary G, Malet F, Holmes-Higgin D. INTACS Inserts for Treating Keratoconus: One Year Results. Ophthalmology 2001;108:1409-14.
34. Spoerl E, Wollensak G, Seiler T. Increased resistance of crosslinked cornea against enzymatic digestion. Curr Eye Res. 2004 Jul;29(1):35-40.
35. Chan CCK, Sharma M, Boxer Wachler BS. The effect of inferior segment Intacs with and without corneal collagen crosslinking with riboflavin (C3-R) on keratoconus. J Cataract Refract Surg 2007;33:75-80.
36. Tahzib Ng, Cheng YY, Nuijts RM. Three-year follow-up analysis of Artisan toric lens implantation for correction of postkeratoplasty ametropia in phakic and pseudophakic eyes. Ophthalmology 2006;113:976-84.
37. Uusitalo RJ, Aine E, Sen NH, Laatikainen L. Implantable contact lens for high myopia. J Cataract Refract Surg. 2002;28:29-36.
38. Pienda-Fernandez AP, Jaramillo J, Vargas J, Jaramillo M, Jaramilo J, Galindez. Phakic posterior chamber intraocular lens for high myopia. J Cataract Refract Surg 2004;30:2277-83.
39. Gonvers M. Bornet C, Othenin-Girard P. Implantable contact lens for moderate to high myopia: relationship of vaulting to cataract formation. J Cataract Refract Surg. 2003;29:918-24.
40. Trindade F, Pereira F, Cronemberger S. Ultrasound biomicroscopic imaging of posterior chamber phakic intraocular lens. J Refract Surg, 1998;14:497-503.
41. Lackner B, Pieh S, Schmidinger G, Simader C, Franz C, Dejaco-Ruhswurm I, Skorpik C. Long-terms results of implantation of phakic posterior chamber intraocular lens. J Cataract refract Surg. 2004;30:2269-76.

43 Bioptics

JL Guell, M Vazquez

INTRODUCTION

Management of high refractive errors currently includes keratorefractive procedures, clear lens extraction with intraocular lens (IOL) implantation and phakic IOL implantation. Unpredictability, regression, and poor quality of vision under dim illumination conditions are the main limitations with LASIK in this range of correction.[1-2] The loss of accommodation and a greater incidence of postoperative retinal detachment are the major problems related in the literature with lens extraction.[3,4] Respect to the phakic IOL approach, the main concern with anterior chamber lenses is progressive endothelial cell loss. Meanwhile with the posterior chamber designs it is cataractogenesis and pigmentary dispersion.

Strampelli[6,7] designed the first anterior chamber biconcave phakic IOL, but it was Barraquer[8] who popularized this type of lens. Corneal edema, chronic iridocyclitis and hyphema were some of the complications cited as the cause of lens explantation, probably due to poor manufacturing quality at that time.[9] Baikoff et al[10,11] designed a concave phakic IOL to correct high myopia, which has been progressively improved by increasing the optical zone size, lowering the haptic angulation and thinning and treating the optical edge.[12] In 1986, Worst and Fechner developed a biconcave iris-supported phakic IOL (iris claw lens) in order to correct high myopia.[13] Later on, the optical part of the lens was modified creating a convexoconcave model.[14]

Recently, Fyodorov introduced the idea of implanting phakic soft silicone IOLs in the posterior chamber.[15,16] This IOL was modified by Chiron-Adatomed (Munich, Germany) under Fechner's guidance. This author has reported an incidence of cataractogenesis of 18 percent (8 out of 45 eyes).[17] Some of the pathophysiological mechanisms that might explain this effect besides surgical trauma, would be chronic subclinical inflammation,[18] pressure onto the crystalline lens by the posterior chamber IOL itself[19] and interference with the metabolism of the lens.[20] Another complication reported was endothelial damage with corneal edema. Marcon et al discussed several possible hypotheses to explain this endothelial decompensation. He suggested a biochemical origin, mechanical factors or product degradation with liberation of toxic products to the endothelium.[21] Another posterior chamber phakic IOL, strangely called implantable contact lenses, made of a collagen copolymer, Collamer™ (Staar surgical AG) is also being used to correct high myopia[22,23] with promising results.

We decided to work with Artisan™ lens, the last design for the iris claw IOL, due to the following reasons: (i) its location into the eye although in the anterior chamber, far away from the corneal endothelium and obviously avoiding the posterior chamber space, (ii) its location permits it to be made with a larger optical zone than the other phakic IOLs for the same correction range, and (iii) centration over the pupil is dependent on surgeon ability instead of on the relation between the pupil and the angle for the Baikoff style lens or the ciliary sulcus for the posterior chamber phakic IOLs.

As in corneal refractive surgery, phakic IOLs optical zone need to be built smaller as higher is the degree of myopia to be corrected to reduce the peripheral height of the IOL (in the cornea, the goal is to reduce the central ablation depth). This results in a suboptimal visual performance under dim illumination conditions and large pupils, with halos and poor night and low contrast vision.

The bioptics concept was first introduced by Zaldivar et al.[5] The idea appeared because it was not possible to get IOLs with negative power higher than –20.00. So a secondary refractive procedure (LASIK—laser-in-situ keratomileusis) was necessary to correct the residual error.

On the other hand, combined procedures have been tried in order to get an additive effect due to the difficulty in correcting high myopia and/or astigmatism.[24-26] The objective of these combined techniques is to reduce the myopia and/or astigmatism with the first procedure—Artisan™ lens implantation or arcuate keratotomy, correcting the residual error with LASIK, maintaining a minimal 6 mm optical zone in both procedures, as our main goal.

In high myopic candidates for phakic IOL implantation, it is possible to perform at the same time the lamellar cut prior to the IOL implantation avoiding the possible endothelial-IOL touch during the microkeratome pass, or the subluxation into the anterior chamber of a posterior chamber phakic IOL. Once all the sutures have been removed and the residual cylinder has been stable for at least a four-week period, we can adjust the final refraction with LASIK by lifting the flap, as in any other LASIK enhancement, and doing the ablation with the excimer laser. **This approach is what we have called "ARS—adjustable refractive surgery"**.[27]

Using a 5.0 mm optical zone Artisan™ lens alone, it is possible to correct the highest degrees of myopia, but because of the possibility of glare and contrast sensitivity loss, we do not regularly recommend this option.

With the ARS approach it is possible to maintain a real 6.0 mm optical zone due to the additive effect of both procedures, reducing drastically the possibility of glare, night halos and reduced vision at night. At the same time, we increase the predictability of the technique and avoid the risks related to the suction ring and the microkeratome in eyes with a phakic IOL inside. The predictability is higher with this technique because we are correcting low residual ametropia with the second procedure and, as we all know, LASIK predictability in low myopia is very high.[1]

PATIENT SELECTION

Patients submitted for ARS must be older than 28 years, with stable myopia for at least one year, greater than –14.00 D, a normal ophthalmological examination and unsatisfactory correction with spectacles or contact lenses for medical, professional or personal requirements.

Preoperative basic evaluation must include: uncorrected and best-corrected visual acuity, manifest and cycloplegic refraction, slit-lamp microscope examination, applanation tonometry, keratometry (Javal) and indirect ophthalmoscopy.

We recommend to measure the mean subjective response for satisfaction through a scale from 1 to 5, with 1 meaning very poor, 2 poor, 3 moderate, 4 good and 5 excellent. Glare and halos, as well as, other bothering (pain, itching, foreign body sensation) can be scored as very intense, intense, moderate, few and none from 1 to 5, respectively.

The following complementary examinations are performed in all the patients included in our ARS protocol: videokeratography (EyeSys Corneal Analysis System, Houston, Texas), central corneal pachymetry (Accutome, Kremer Corneometer, Broomal, PA, USA), axial length and anterior chamber depth with our ultrasonic biometer

(CompuScan LT Model N° 1000, Storz, St Louis, MO USA), pupil diameter in photopic (2.70 footcandle) and scotopic conditions (pupillometer), endothelial cell count (Topcon SP, 1000 noncontact specular microscope and the Imaginet Analysis System from Topcon) and contrast sensitivity (CSV-1000, Dayton, Ohio).

INDICATIONS FOR ARS (ADJUSTABLE REFRACTIVE SURGERY)

- Patients younger than 35 years old with myopia higher than –15.00 D in whom LASIK will be needed to correct the residual refractive error.
- Very high myopic and hyperopic patients submitted for clear lens or cataract extraction with IOL implantation in whom no residual refractive error is the goal.

CONTRAINDICATIONS FOR ARS

Contraindications for any Refractive Surgery

- Monocular patient (although there are exceptions to be discussed with our patients)
- Progressive and unstable myopia
- Keratoconus, although some surgeons[28] are performing excimer laser surgery in these cases
- Preexisting pathology of anterior segment of the eye
- Active ocular pathology or previous history of eye inflammation (herpes simplex virus keratitis, herpes zoster ophthalmicus, HIV +/AIDS, uveitis)
- Severe dry eye syndrome
- Glaucoma
- Autoimmune and systemic collagen diseases (rheumatoid arthritis, lupus)
- Systemic vasculitis
- Diabetes mellitus (DM) when diabetic retinopathy or other systemic findings are present, suggesting not controlled DM
- Pregnancy
- Subnormal intelligence quotient or highly uncooperative patient.

Contraindications for Artisan™ Lens Implantation

- Anterior chamber depth less than 3 mm
- Endothelial cell count below 2.000 cells/mm^3
- History of retinal detachment in one eye or extensive retinal pathology.

Contraindications for LASIK

- Corneal thickness less than 450 μ.
- Abnormal eyelid closure
- Flat cornea (mean keratometry < 41.00 D). It is of course depending on the degree of myopia to be corrected. We do not recommend that the expected postoperative keratometry (after LASIK) be less than 37 D.

Contraindications for both Procedures

- Incipient lens opacities.
- Pupil diameter higher than 6 mm under standard illumination conditions.

SURGICAL TECHNIQUE

Worst IOL Implantation

The procedure is done under 3 cc of retrobulbar anesthesia (4 cc of a combination of mepivacaine 2 percent—Mepivacina Inj, 2 percent, Braun™, bupivacaine 0.75 percent—Bupivacaina Inj, 0.75 percent, Braun™ and mucopolysaccharidase-Thiomucase, Funk™).

We center the 9.5 mm suction ring of our microkeratome ALK-E (automated corneal shaper (ACS), Chiron Vision, Clairemont, Calif, USA. Serial number 286) on the pupil at the sclerocorneal limbus and the guides and corneal surface are moistened. Once the lamellar flap (160 microns) is obtained, it is folded over the nasal side of the eye (Fig. 43.1) using our LASIK retreatment spatula (ASICO™). After checking the quality of the flap, we clean the interface, replace the flap and dry its border carefully with microsponges.

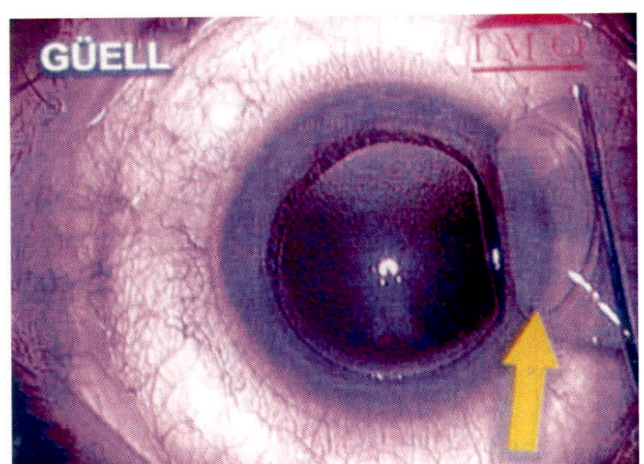

Fig. 43.1: Flap created for LASIK. Arrow indicates the flap which is folded on the nasal side

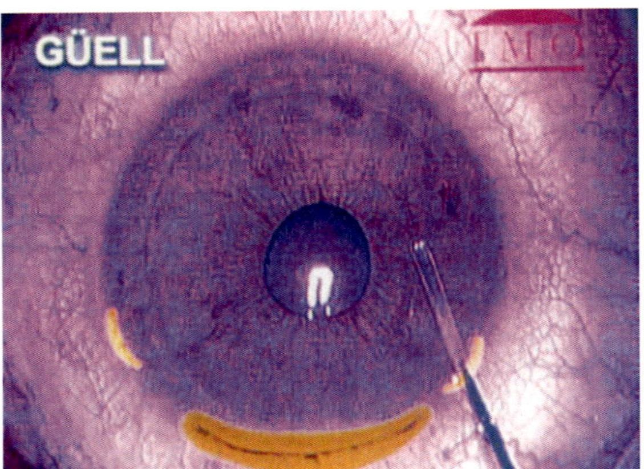

Fig. 43.2: Intracameral injection of acetylcholine. Note the 2 yellow lines on the sides indicating the two paracentesis incisions. The yellow line in the center is the 6.2 mm long posterior corneal incision

After confirm adequate adhesion of the flap border, we initiate the implantation of the Artisan lens.The two-plane 6.2 mm long posterior corneal incision is centered at 12 hours. The first nonpenetrating plane of the incision and two vertical paracentral paracentesis at 10 and 2 o'clock hours are done. After the intracameral injection (Fig. 43.2) of acetylcholine and our standard viscoelastic material (Sodium hyaluronate, Healon™), the second plane of the incision is performed, opening the anterior chamber. The lens is then completely introduced in one step (to avoid any direct or indirect contact between the front part of the IOL and the crystalline lens) and afterwards, under viscoelastic protection, rotated 90° into a horizontal position, from 3 to 9 o'clock hours (Fig. 43.3). The IOL is fixated as J Worst described,[14] with a blunt 30 gauge blended needle grasping, through both paracentesis, the iris into both "claws" (Figs 43.4A and B). The iris is enclavated at the midperiphery, because it is an area with almost no movement during physiological pupil dilation and also is far from the main iris vascularization (J Worst, personal communication). Again, all these maneuvers must be performed under viscoelastic protection. Finally, a peripheral slit iridotomy (Fig. 43.5) at 12 o'clock is performed, the viscoelastic material exchanged (Fig. 43.6) with balanced salt solution (BSS®), and the incision closed with 5 or 6 interrupted 10-0 nylon sutures. We use so many sutures to completely close the incision with the minimal tension. The correct tension of the sutures is checked with our standard qualitative Maloney keratometer (Fig. 43.7).

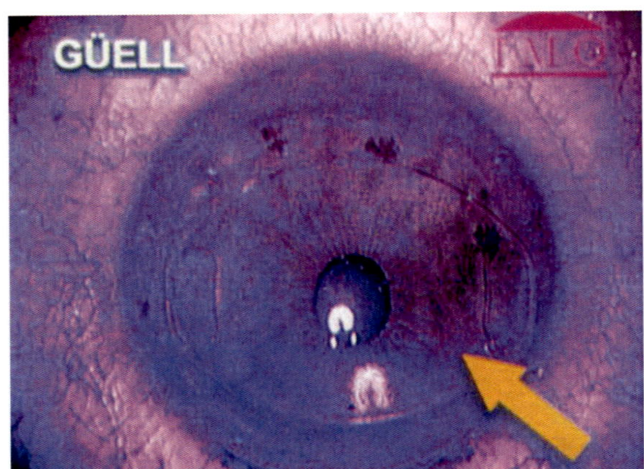

Fig. 43.3: Artisan IOL introduced into the eye

Postoperatively, prednisolone and chloramphenicol ointment are used four times per day during the first 15 days, and then tapered during the next week.

LASIK

Once all the sutures have been removed, between 1 and 3 months after IOL implantation, and the residual cylinder is stable for at least a 4-week period, the second procedure, LASIK, is programmed.

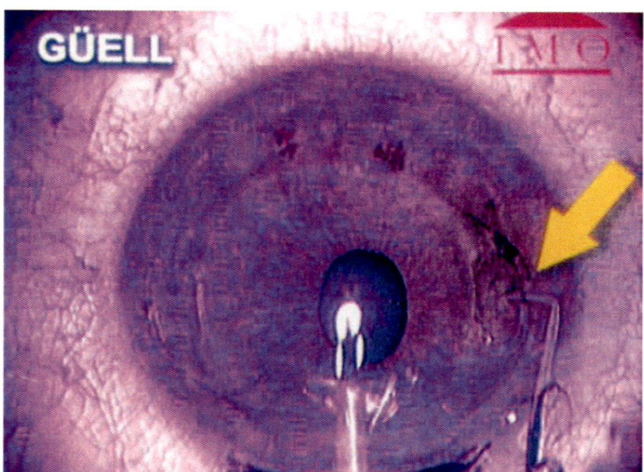

Fig. 43.4A: The claw of the IOL fixed onto the iris. Arrow indicates the fixation

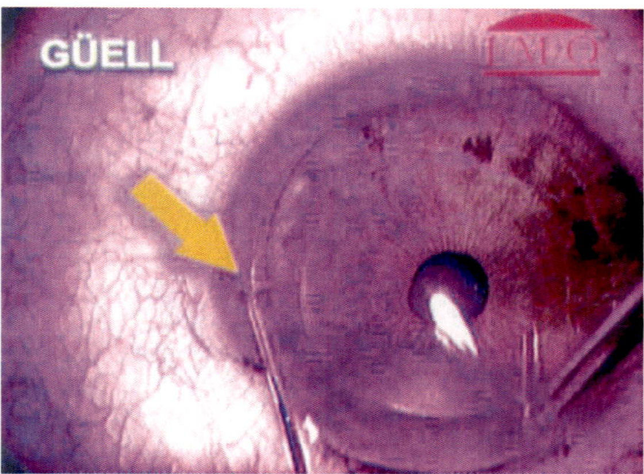

Fig. 43.4B: The other claw in now fixed onto the iris. Arrow indicates the fixation

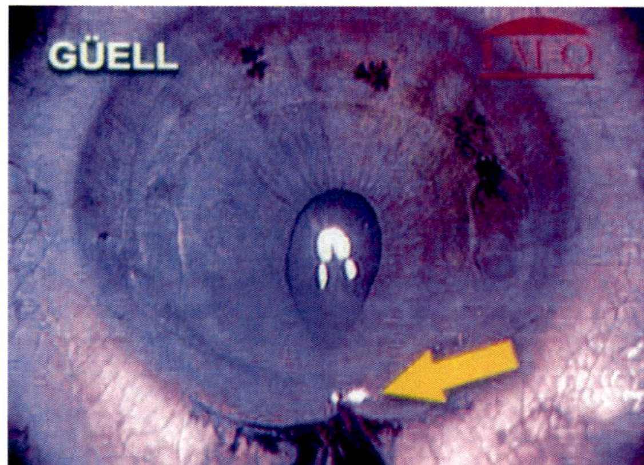

Fig. 43.5: Peripheral iridectomy done

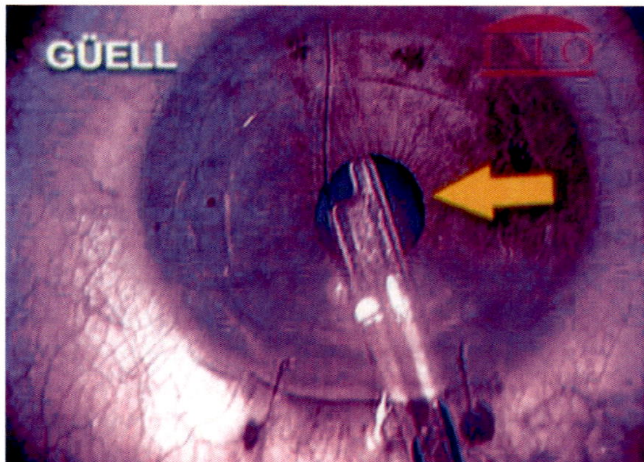

Fig. 43.6: Viscoelastic removed and replaced with balanced salt solution (BSS)

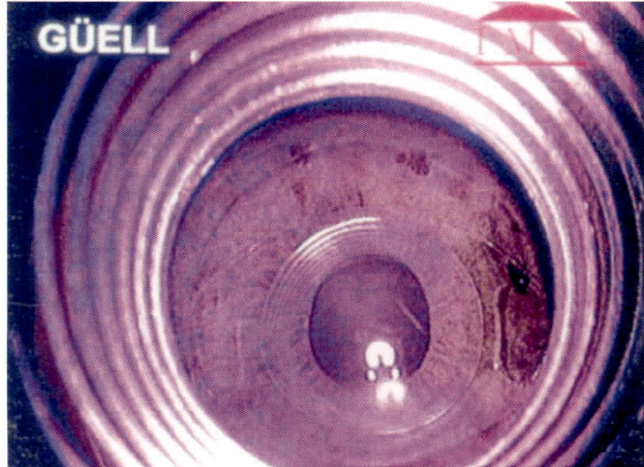

Fig. 43.7: Tension of sutures checked with the Maloney keratometer

A third-generation excimer laser system, the Keracor 117 CT, 50 Hz Planoscan (Chiron Technolas) is used. The software we have been working with is the V 2.67 036 with an optical zone of 6 mm and a peripheral treatment zone from 6 to 8.7 mm.

LASIK is performed under topical anesthesia (Fig. 43.8), as any other LASIK procedure. We lift the flap and keeping the stromal bed without any extrahydration or desiccation during 15/25 seconds, we focus the helium neon aiming beam of the laser on the center of the pupil installing the active Eye Tracker System, then the ablation is performed. After the ablation, we wash the stromal bed with saline solution (Ringer lactate), and the flap is then replaced on its original position and its border carefully dried with microsponges. To confirm adequate adhesion, the peripheral cornea is indented with forceps to check for the presence of striae passing from the periphery into the flap. After the lid speculum is carefully removed, one drop of

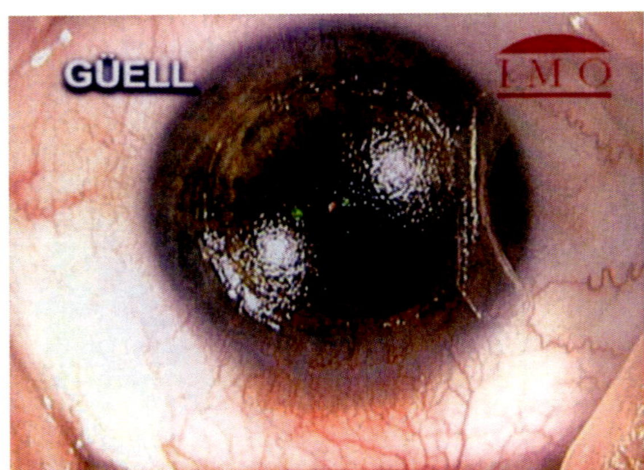

Fig. 43.8: LASIK (excimer laser ablation) is performed

gentamicin and diclofenac are instilled. We recommend oral analgesics if necessary, during the immediate postoperative time, a topical broad-spectrum antibiotic three times per day is prescribed during the first week, and artificial tears for eight weeks.

DATA ANALYSIS

We evaluated 26 eyes of 18 patients (8 male, 10 females) submitted to ARS, with age ranging from 28 to 35 years (31.30 ± 2.20), and a preoperative spherical equivalent refractive error ranging from –16.0 to –23.0 D (mean –18.42 ± 2.73). Patients with or without astigmatism were included.

The preoperative uncorrected visual acuity (UCVA) was lower than 0.063 in all of the eyes (Table 43.1), the mean preoperative best-corrected visual acuity (BCVA) was 0.39 ± 0.16 (range 0.10 to 0.50, contact lens overrefraction).

All the patients were examined the first day, at 1, 3, 6, 12, 18, 24, and 28 months after Artisan™ lens implantation, and a complete ophthalmological examination was performed, as previously described.

RESULTS

Refraction

Mean preoperative spherical equivalent refraction was –18.42 ± 2.73 (–16.00 to –23.50). Mean postoperative spherical equivalent refraction before LASIK was –3.65 ± 1.62 (–1.75 to –6.50) and after LASIK was –0.34 ± 0.51 (1.00 to –1.25) and –0.38 ± 0.65 (1.00 to –1.00) at 1 and 12 months, respectively, remaining stable after a 24 months follow-up.

Twenty-four months postoperatively, all of the eyes were within ± 1.00 D of emmetropia and 21 eyes (80.7%) were within ± 0.50 D.

Mean preoperative spherical component of the refractive error was –17.38 ± 1.83 (–15.00 to –21.00) and decreased to –3.65 ± 1.62 (–1.25 to –4.75) following IOL implantation. Following LASIK it decreased to 0.04 ± 0.72 D (–0.75 to –1.00) and to –0.06 ± 0.66 (–0.50 to –1.50) at 1 and 12 months, remaining stable at the 24 months follow-up.

Mean preoperative astigmatism was –1.35 ± 1.00 D (0 to –4.00). Following IOL implantation, mean postoperative astigmatism was –1.15 ± 0.79 (0 to –3.00). One, 12 and 24 months after LASIK it was –0.59 ± 0.67 (0 to –3.25), –0.66 ± 0.66 (0 to –3.00) and –0.66 ± 0.66 (0 to –3.00), respectively. Sixty-five percent of the eyes were within ±1.00 D of astigmatism before IOL implantation. After LASIK this percentage increases to 84.60 percent at 3 months, and remained unchanged for the rest of the follow-up.

Table 43.1: Preoperative, pre-LASIK and post-LASIK (24 months postoperatively) values of the patients submitted to ARS

	UCVA	*SCVA*	*SE*	*Cylinder*
Preoperative	< 0.063	0.39 ± 0.16	–18.42 ± 2.73	–1.35 ± 1.00
Pre-LASIK	0.11 ± 0.10	0.55 ± 0.16	–3.65 ± 1.62	–1.15 ± 0.79
Post-LASIK	0.51 ± 0.14	0.59 ± 0.17	–0.38 ± 0.65	–0.66 ± 0.66

UCVA—uncorrected visual acuity, BCVA—best-corrected visual acuity (contact lens overrefraction), SCVA—spectacle-corrected visual acuity, and SE—spherical equivalent

Visual Acuity

Pre-LASIK UCVA ranged from < 0.063 to 0.32 (0.11 ± 0.10). One month after LASIK, UCVA ranged from 0.16 to 0.70 (0.50 ± 0.15), from 0.25 to 0.63 (0.51 ± 0.14) and from 0.25 to 0.63 (0.51 ± 0.14) at 12 and 24 months, respectively.

Postoperative spectacle-corrected visual acuity (SCVA) ranged from 0.25 to 1.00 (0.55 ± 0.16) and from 0.25 to 1.00 (0.59 ± 0.17) at 1 and 12 months after LASIK, with no changes at 24 months.

Seventy-seven percent of the eyes (20 eyes) achieved an UCVA of 0.50 (20/40) or better.

No eyes lost a single Snellen line of SCVA, but 30.70 percent of the eyes gained 1 line of SCVA, 15.38 percent gained 2 lines, and 26.90 percent, 3 or more, after LASIK, as the second part of the procedure.

Contrast Sensitivity

No differences between preoperative and postoperative contrast sensitivity values were documented at 3 and 24 months after LASIK, at all spatial frequencies when the CSV-1000 test was used. It must be pointed out again that preoperative values were measured with contact lens overrefraction.

Subjective Response

On a scale from 1 to 5, the mean subjective response for satisfaction was 4.00 (3 to 5), 3.5 (3 to 5) for glare and halos and 4 (3 to 5) for other bothering, at 24 months after LASIK.

Corneal Endothelium

Mean preoperative endothelial cell density was 2782 ± 392 cells/mm^2 (1937 to 3225) (Table 43.2). After 12 months of IOL implantation mean endothelial density slightly decreased to 2765 ± 389 cells/mm^2 (1925 to 3201). Twenty-eight months after IOL implantation, endothelial cell count presented a slight variation (2749 ± 388 cells/mm^2, range 1915 to 3181).

Endothelial cell count (ECC) showed a 0.61 percent mean loss during the first 12 months and a 0.6 percent loss during the next 16 months after IOL implantation.

Table 43.2: Preoperative, 12 and 24 months postoperative endothelial cell count (ECC) of the patients submitted to ARS

	EECC	*Percentage loss*
Preoperative	2782 ± 392	
12 months	2765 ± 389	0.61
24 months	2649 ± 388	0.60

Complications

Major complications were not observed during the follow-up period. Complications related to microkeratome included a free cap 9.2 mm in diameter (one case), a traumatic flap dislocation 1 day after surgery (one case), and a short flap with 8.0 mm in horizontal length (one case). Mild elevation of intraocular pressure (less than 4 mm Hg) was found in 19.23 percent of the cases during the first week after IOL implantation. No cataracts, pupillary block or retinal complications appeared during the follow-up period.

SUMMARY

The primary goal of refractive surgery today is to obtain the smallest residual refractive error with the best quality of vision measured with the contrast sensitivity test and/or through the subjective opinion of the patient. To achieve this goal, combined procedures have been tried in order to get an additive refractive effect increasing predictability and visual quality preservation. Some of them are planned before any surgery is done.[24-26] Others are planned as a secondary refractive procedure to reduce the residual refractive error of the first surgery.[29]

Despite improvement in IOL calculation formulas with cataract surgery, it is not infrequent to find residual refractive defects, usually in highly myopic and hyperopic eyes. The use of corneal refractive surgery to correct smaller defects has been used, as well as IOL exchanges or the insertion of a piggyback IOL in those cases where the refractive defect was significant.

Several corneal refractive surgery techniques have been employed to refine the final refraction after intraocular refractive surgery, such as radial keratotomy (RK), astigmatic keratotomy (AK) and photorefractive keratectomy (PRK).[30-31] LASIK is a good option to correct residual myopia and/or astigmatism whether or not the first performed procedure has been refractive. It is well recognized that LASIK's predictability is better when correcting low to moderate myopia, but decreases in high myopia.[1]

Since March 1994, we have been using LASIK to correct residual ametropia after intraocular surgery with IOL implantation, penetrating keratoplasty, pars plana vitrectomy, PRK, radial and arcuate transverse keratotomy, and phakic IOL implantation.[32] Refractive accuracy with these combined procedures was 95.7 percent ± 6.10 at 6-month follow-up. Seventy-seven percent of the eyes were within ± 1.0 D and 57.4 percent within 0.5 D of emmetropia. This is similar to our LASIK results on virgin eyes.

In correcting high myopia (spherical equivalent higher than –12.00 diopters) it is extremely important to have a minimal 6 or 6.5 mm optical zone for both, corneal ablational procedures and IOLs implantation into a phakic eye.

It is not advisable to work with large optical zones when we are dealing with high myopia. Reasons that might support this statement are—the larger the optical zone the deeper the ablation, and the thicker the periphery of the phakic IOLs which may lead to surrounding tissue damage. This was the rationale for combining a 6 mm optical zone Artisan™ IOL and LASIK with 6.5 mm optical zone ablation for correction of high myopia. Moreover, the fact of doing LASIK as the second procedure to correct residual ametropia increases the predictability of the technique.

ARS avoids risks associated to microkeratome in eyes that contain an IOL. Other advantages are: larger diameter ablation zones, thinner IOLs with lesser peripheral optical aberrations and high predictability in the correction of ametropia outside the range of LASIK or IOLs alone.

The refractive results of our study, combining two techniques were excellent. All of the eyes were within ± 1.00 D of emmetropia and 80.70 percent (21 eyes) were within 0.50 D. These results are better than those of previous studies only implanting the Artisan™ lens.[33,34] Perez-Santonja et al[35] and Krumeich et al[36] have reported a postoperative spherical equivalent refraction within ± 1.00 D in 91 and 95 percent of the eyes, results that resemble more to ours.

Seventy-three percent of the eyes gained one or more lines of their preoperative BCVA. We think it is important to perform contact lens overrefraction to avoid overestimations on visual acuity gain. In this way we can also get a more exact refraction and more appropriate contrast sensitivity testing.

Corneal astigmatism after intraocular surgery was lowered to almost preoperative values after suture removal. In any case, one of the main advantages of the combined procedure is to be able to precisely correct the residual ametropia after the intraocular surgery with LASIK.

Zaldivar et al[5] recommend to perform LASIK following ICL implantation (bioptics) in patients with spherical equivalents of –18.00 D or greater, patients with high levels of preoperative astigmatism (greater than –2.00 D), and patients in whom lens power availability is a problem. In a group of 44 myopes who were corrected with Bioptics, the mean post-ICL/pre-LASIK spherical equivalent and cylinder were –5.05 ± 2.52 and –1.66 ± 1.25 D, respectively. Following LASIK, the mean postoperative spherical equivalent and cylinder were –0.11 ± 0.63 and –0.43 ± 0.61 D, respectively. After LASIK, the spherical equivalent data have been stable for 3 to 6 months (mean follow-up 32 days post-LASIK). Zaldivar et al[5] reported no additional visual significant complications in this group, compared to their "ICL only" counterparts. The maximal optical zone of this posterior chamber IOL is 5 mm (although in the higher correction group, it must be reduced to 4), and our goal is to maintain a 6 mm optical zone in both the lens and LASIK a requirement that is fulfilled by the Artisan™ lens in ARS.

Respect to the corneal endothelium, we observed a slight decrease on cell count (a 0.61% mean loss during the first 12 months and a 0.6% loss during the next 16 months), which might be due to the surgery itself or to the presence of a foreign body in the anterior chamber. The mean endothelial cell loss found in our study is similar to that reported by Krumeich et al[36] but lower than that reported by other authors.[33,37-39] A careful follow-up of this item must be done to determine the stability of the ECC in these patients. From our point of view, the measure of the ECC during the first 5/10 years compared to an age-matched group control will be very important in accepting this surgery for high myopia as a standard. Another critical issue will be to standardize the measurement (contact vs non-contact specular microscopes and area included in the study). The main advantage of ARS is avoidance of endothelial-IOL touch risk during microkeratome cut. In a previous report[24] employing the combined technique (Artisan™ lens implantation plus LASIK) but not ARS, the mean ECC after Artisan™ lens implantation and before LASIK (2629 ± 366) was similar to the ECC after 12 months of the LASIK procedure (2612 ± 347). In spite of these findings, we still feel more comfortable and safe performing the flap before IOL implantation. When we deal with angle-fixated anterior chamber IOLs, endothelial-IOL touch becomes critical and we highly recommend to perform the flap prior to the implantation of the IOL if we are thinking that an enhancement procedure will be necessary in the near future.

Subjectively, the patients were very satisfied with the results, and only two patients presented some visual disturbances at night. In our experience nocturnal halos and an important decrease in the quality of vision under dim illumination conditions appear when the pupil is in a middilated position with any of the other "phakic" IOLs or LASIK alone, when we are dealing with the same range of correction. In our cases, it seems that thanks to the greater optical zone of the 6 mm Artisan™ IOL, these complaints are drastically reduced or completely disappeared, and the final visual acuity was not altered by such phenomena. Here we want to emphasize one important concept—the entrance pupil.[40] If we project the pupil onto the cornea, the size of this projection will be larger as deeper is the anterior. That means that the real optical zone of our correction must be larger as further we are from the pupil level. In other words, a 6 mm optical zone LASIK is probably similar to a 4.8 PMMA (polymethyl methacrylate) optic at the pupil in a standard eye. Applying this concept into the anterior chamber, the effective optical zone will always be smaller in an angle-fixated IOL than in an iris-supported lens, because of the more anterior position of the first one.

Some other complications had been described with these iris-claw style lenses. Decentration is an important point to be considered. Perez-Torregrosa et al[41] using the Imaginet analogical digital system, measured its positioning and found no decentration more than 1 mm in any of the eyes. Fechner et al[42] referred difficulty in centrating the lens initially with severe exudative iritis in three eyes which required repeated incarceration to fixate the IOL. We had no clear decentration, measured at the slit-lamp and we consider that one of the advantages of the Artisan™ lens is the capability of the surgeon to centrate it, factor that becomes critical when we are dealing with descentrated pupils, quite common in high myopes (nasally more frequent).

No postoperative glaucoma has been observed, only a mild transient elevation of intraocular pressure (IOP), which disappeared when corticosteroids were discontinued, in accordance to other series.[35-36,41]

Fechner et al[37,42] reported a high incidence of retinal detachment one month after aphakia Artisan™ lens implantation. Menezo et al[43] reported a high incidence of retinal complications (cystoid macular edema and retinal detachment) in aphakia Artisan™ lens primary implantation when capsular support is absent compared to secondary implantation. We did not observe any retinal complications during the follow-up period in our phakic IOL group.

Other complications not found in our study but cited in the literature related to Artisan™ lens implantation are cystic wounds,[35] Urrets-Zavalia syndrome (fixed, dilated pupil, iris atrophy and secondary glaucoma),[42] giant papillary conjunctivitis,[35] lens opacity,[35] and ischemic optic neuropathy.[44]

The excellent optical results with this combined large optical zone procedure allow us to recommend it. Preservation of accommodation in young patients and high quality of vision under dim illumination conditions, characteristically decreased after LASIK or phakic IOL alone in our very high myopic patients, are advantages to consider when we are evaluating the possible surgical options for these patients. Other advantages are its predictability and safety, due to the avoidance of contact between the endothelium and the IOL during the suction in LASIK. As a matter of fact we evidence a low mean loss in ECC.

ARS concept can be applied to other intraocular surgeries or other phakic IOLs, such as angle-fixated anterior chamber lenses and silicone/collamer posterior chamber lenses. Pressure from suction during LASIK could be more dangerous for high myopic eyes when they are pseudophakic or could dislocate a posterior chamber lens.

Of course, from our point of view, technology will improve and, in the future, materials with higher refractive index or new optics cofiguration will allow us to only use phakic IOLs with 7 or 8 mm optical zone to correct high myopia and hyperopia.

In the mean time, ARS seems to us the best and safest approach.

REFERENCES

1. Güell JL, Muller Ana. Laser in situ keratomileusis (LASIK) for myopia from –7 to –18 diopters. J Refract Surg 1996;12:222-8.
2. Salah T, Waring GO, El Maghraby A, et al. Excimer laser in situ under a corneal flap for myopia of 2 to 20 diopters. Am J Ophthalmol 1996;121:143-55.
3. Gris O, Güell JL, Manero F et al. Clear lens extraction to correct high myopia. J Cataract Refract Surg 1996;22:686-9.
4. Colin J, Robinet A. Clear lensectomy and implantation of lower-power posterior chamber intraocular lens for the correction of high myopia. Ophthalmology 1994;101:107-12.
5. Zaldivar R, Davidorf JM, Oscherow S. The intraocular contact lens. In Buratto L, Brint SF (Eds): LASIK: Principles and Techniques NJ, Slack: Thorofare, 1997;401-13.
6. Strampelli B. Supportabilita di lenti acriliche in camera anteriore nella afachia o nei vizi di refrazione. Annali di Ottomologia o Clinica Oculistica Parma 1954;80:75-82.
7. Strampelli B. Anterior chamber lenses—present technique. Arch Ophthalmol 1961;66:12-7.
8. Barraquer J. Anterior chamber plastic lenses—result of and conclusions from five years' experience. Transac Ophthalmol Soc UK 1959;79:393-424.
9. Drews RC. The Barraquer experience with intraocular lenses—20 years later. Ophthalmology 1982;89:386-93.
10. Baïkoff G, Colin J. Intraocular lenses in phakic eyes. Ophthalmol Clin North Am 1992;5(4):789-95.
11. Baïkoff G. Phakic anterior chamber intraocular lenses. Int Ophthalmol Clin 1991;31:75-86.
12. Baïkoff G, Arne JL, Bokobza Y et al. Angle-fixated anterior chamber phakic intraocular lens for myopia of –7 to –19 diopters. J Refract Surg 1998;14:282-93.
13. Fechner PU, Worst JGF. A new concave intraocular lens for the correction of high myopia. Eur J Implant Refract Surg 1989;1:41-3.
14. Landesz M, Worst JGF, Siertsema JV, et al. Correction of high myopia with the Worst myopia claw intraocular lens. J Refract Surg 1995;11:16-25.
15. Fyodorov SN, Zuew VK, Amavayew VM. Intraocular correction of high myopia with negative posterior chamber lens. Oftalmochirurgia 1991;3:57-8.
16. Fyodorov SN, Zuew VK, Tumanyan NR, et al. Clinical and functional follow-up of minus IOL implantation in high grade myopia. Oftalmochirurgia 1993;2:12-7.
17. Fechner PU, Haigis W, Wichmann W. Posterior chamber myopia lenses in phakic eyes. J Cataract Refract Surg 1996;22:178-82.
18. Perez-Santonja JJ, Iradier MT, Benitez del Castillo JM et al. Chronic subclinical inflammation in phakic eyes with intraocular lenses to correct high myopia. J Cataract Refract Surg 1996;22:183-7.
19. Wiechens B, Winter M, Haigis W et al. Bilateral cataract after phakic posterior chamber top hat-style silicone intraocular lens. J Refract Surg 1997;13:392-7.
20. Kashani A. Phakic posterior chamber intraocular lens for the correction of high myopia (letter). J Refract Surg 1996;12:454-6.
21. Marcon GB, Galan A, Rappo G et al. Edematous decompensation of the cornea after silicone implant of the posterior chamber in a phakic eye. J Fr Ophthalmol 1996;19(2):149-52.

22. Asetto V, Benedetti S, Pesando P. Collamer intraocular contact lens to correct high myopia. J Cataract Refract Surg 1996;22:551-2.
23. Zaldivar R, Davidorf J, Oscherow S. Posterior chamber phakic intraocular lens for myopia of –8 to –19 diopters. J Refract Surg 1998;14:294-305.
24. Gûell JL, Vázquez M, Gris O et al. Combined surgery to correct high myopia—Artisan® lens and laser in situ keratomileusis (LASIK). J Refract Surg (In press).
25. Gûell JL, Vazquez M. ARS (Adjustable Refractive Surgery)—6 mm Artisan® lens plus LASIK for the correction of high myopia. J Refract Surg (In press).
26. Gûell J, Vázquez M, Gris O, et al. Correction of high astigmatism with astigmatic keratotomy and laser in situ keratomileusis (LASIK). J Refract Surg (In press).
27. Gûell JL. The adjustable refractive surgery concept (ARS)—(letter to the editor) J Refract Surg 1998;14:271.
28. Mortensen J, Carlsson K, Ohrstrom A. Excimer laser surgery for keratoconus. J Cataract Surg 1998;24:893-8.
29. Gûell J, Vazquez M. Lasik enhancement following other surgical procedures. In Buratto L, Brint SF (Eds): LASIK: Principles and Techniques. Slack Inc: Thorofare, 1999.
30. Gûell JL, Manero F, Muller A. Transverse keratotomy to correct high corneal astigmatism after cataract surgery. J Cataract Surg 1996;22:331-6.
31. Maloney RK, Chan WK, Steinert R, et al. Summit therapeutic refractive study group—a multicenter trial of photorefractive keratectomy for residual myopia after previous ocular surgery. Ophthalmology 1995;102:1042-52.
32. Gûell J. Lasik enhancement following other surgical procedures. In Buratto L, Brint SF (Eds): LASIK: Principles and Techniques. Slack Inc: Thorofare, 1998.
33. Landesz M, Worst JGF, van Rij. Opaque iris claw lens in a phakic eye to correct acquired diplopia. J Cataract Surg 1997;23:137-8.
34. Menezo JL, Cisneros A, Hueso JR, et al. Long-term results of surgical treatment of high myopia with Worst-Fechner intraocular lenses. J Cataract Refract Surg 1995;25:93-8.
35. Perez-Santonja JJ, Bueno J, Zato MA. Surgical correction of high myopia in phakic eyes with Worst-Fechner myopia lenses. J Refract Surg 1997;13: 268-81.
36. Krumeich JH, Daniel J, Gast R. Closed-system technique for implantation of iris-supported negative-power intraocular lens. J Refract Surg 1996;12:334-40.
37. Fechner PU, Wichmann W. Correction of myopia by implantation of minus optic (Worst iris claw) lenses into the anterior chamber of phakic eyes. Eur J Implant Refract Surg 1993;5:55-9.
38. Menezo JL, Cisneros AL, Cervera M, et al. Iris-claw phakic lens—intermediate and long-term corneal endothelial changes. Eur J Implant Refract Surg 1994;6:195-9.
39. Menezo JL, Aviño JA, Cisneros A, et al. Iris claw phakic intraocular lens for high myopia. J Refract Surg 1997;13:545-55.
40. Uozato H, Guyton DL. Centering corneal surgical procedures. Am J Ophthalmol 1987;103(3 Pt 1):264-75.
41. Perez-Torregrosa VT, Menezo JL, Harto MA. et al. Digital system measurement of decentration of Worst-Fechner iris claw myopia intraocular lens. J refract Surg 1995;11:26-30.
42. Fechner PU, Strobel J, Wicchmann W. Correction of myopia by implantation of a concave Worst-iris claw lens into phakic eyes. Refract Corneal Surg 1991;7:286-98.
43. Menezo JL, Martinez MC, Cisneros AL. Iris-fixated Worst claw versus sulcus-fixated posterior chamber lenses in the absence of capsular support. J Cataract Surg 1996;22:1476-84.
44. Perez-Santonja JJ, Bueno JL, Meza J, et al. Ischemic optic neuropathy after intraocular lens implantation to correct high myopia in a phakic patient. J Cataract Refract Surg 1993; 19:651-4.

SECTION SIX

Complications

44 Flap Complications

Arthur Cummings, Frank Lavery

INTRODUCTION

Complications with the creation of the flap have diminished with the use of the newer microkeratomes. Some of the complications to be discussed would not be very rare, thanks to technological advancements with the new microkeratomes.

COMPLICATIONS

Complications can be divided into intraoperative, early postoperative and late postoperative stages (Table 44.1).

MANAGEMENT OF COMPLICATIONS

Complete Free Flap

The complete free flap would most probably be the most serious and devastating complication for both the surgeon and the patient. It occurs very infrequently and is usually as a result of inadequate suction on the suction ring, a very flat cornea or an adjustable microkeratome that has been set incorrectly. The instant recognition of the problem as well as the appropriate management is of paramount importance. Once the flap has been located and stored safely in a sterile container, the bed needs to be inspected. If the bed is suitable for laser, the treatment can be applied. The flap is then replaced onto the cornea and any of the following procedures can be followed: the flap can be managed in the usual fashion and then once the surgeon is satisfied that it has reattached, the patient can be monitored at regular intervals in the ensuing 6 hours to make sure that the flap remains on the cornea. Bandage contact lenses (soft disposable contact lenses) can be applied to further secure the free flap. Not all surgeons agree that the contact lens enhances the chances of the flap remaining in position, however, and there are some who believe it places the flap at additional risk of

Table 44.1: Types of flap complications

Intraoperative
1. Complete cut
   a. Free flap
   b. Decentered flap
   c. Superficial/too thin/irregular flap
   d. Perforated cap
2. *Incomplete cut*
   a. Under half
   b. Over 3/4

Early postoperative period (within the first hours to days)
1. Dislocated/moved flap
2. Foreign bodies
3. "Sands of the Sahara"
4. Keratitis
5. Microstriae

Late postoperative period (from 2 days to first few weeks)
1. Infection
2. Keratitis
3. Dry eye syndrome
4. Epithelial ingrowth

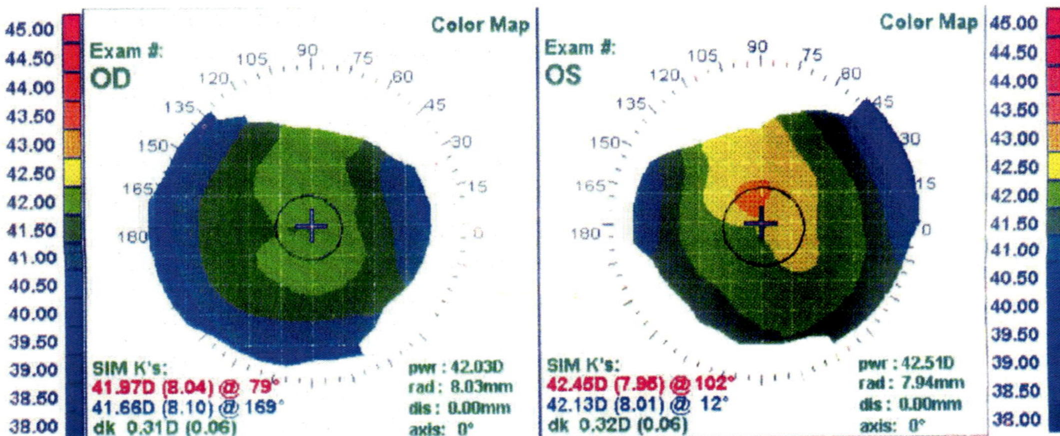

Fig. 44.1: The preoperative corneal topography of both the left and right eyes. The preoperative refraction was –2.25 sph on the right and –2.50/–0.50 axis 76 on the left

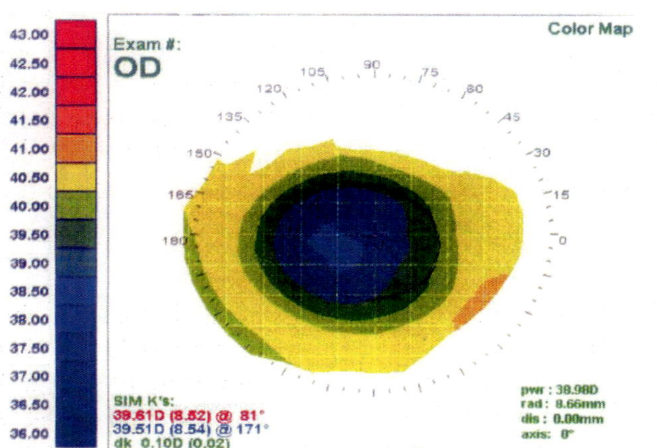

Fig. 44.2: The postoperative corneal topography of the right eye. The right eye looks just as expected on day 1 with 6/6 unaided vision

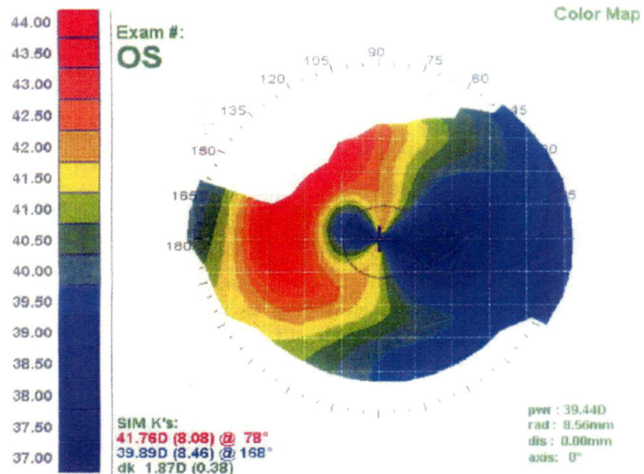

Fig. 44.3: The day 1 postoperative topography of the left eye with very unusual appearance of steepening nasally and flattening temporally. This is due to a free cap created the day before with LASIK, having been placed incorrectly on the eye due to poor reference marks. The flap appeared hazy and the best corrected visual acuity (BCVA) was 6/7.5 with +3.00/–6.00 axis 160

displacing and getting lost. Free flaps have also been secured in position by placing 2 or more 10-0 nylon sutures through the flap into the adjacent superficial cornea. This prevents loss of the cap better than any other procedure, but almost always will cause striae in the flap. Fortunately very few microkeratome cuts have ended up with free flaps so that there is not much data around on the best method to manage this problem. It is also true that most free flap cases do end up with a satisfactory result. It is very important to note that if enhancement surgery is to be performed, then a new flap needs to be fashioned with the microkeratome. The initial cause of the free flap must be borne in mind and all possible precautions should be taken to prevent it from occurring again. Figures 44.1 to 44.5 show a patient who had a free cap and how he was managed.

Some surgeons state that the corneal reference markings are unnecessary. These are essential if one needs to reposition the flap in the correct orientation

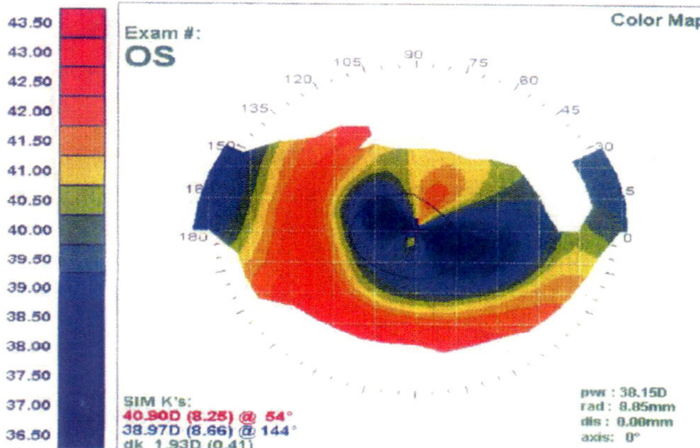

Fig. 44.4: 3 weeks later the flap was removed and rotated through 180 degrees. The corneal topography looks very similar to the previous one and the refraction is also very similar, namely +4.00/–6.00 axis 155. Best corrected vision now 6/12

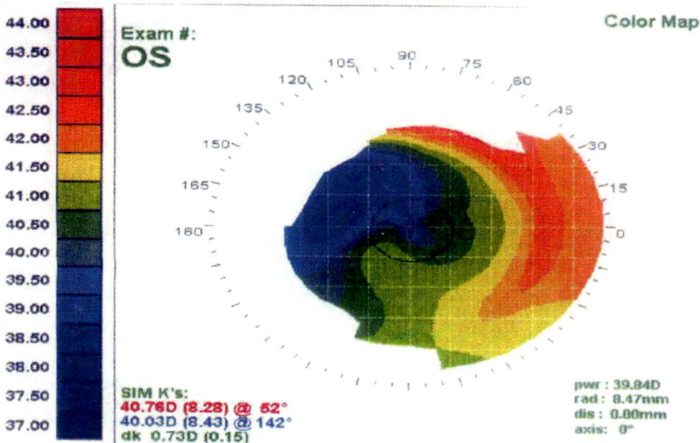

Fig. 44.5: 3 weeks later the flap was again completely removed and the corneal bed was debrided of any epithelium. The flap was replaced and repositioned again to give the most appropriate fit. This topography shows the day 1 appearance after this procedure. The unaided visual acuity was now 6/15- and with a correction of +1.00/–1.25 axis 110 the visual acuity was 6/9+. One week later the refraction was +1.75/–1.25 axis 115 and the visual acuity 6/7.5+2. Four months later the refraction is +0.50/–0.75 axis 5 and the vision is 6/5. Unaided visual acuity is 6/9. The refraction has remained stable at this level for the past 2 years. This case demonstrates the importance of aligning the flap correctly postoperatively and the importance of reference marks especially in the case of a free flap

after a free flap has been made. They are also very useful to correctly align the flap in any case where the surgery has gone perfectly well too. Figure 44.1 illustrates the value of these markings following a case where a free flap occurred. In those rare cases where a free flap eventually loses permanently, the management varies according to the final visual and refractive result. Most postoperative lost cap refractions will be hyperopic in nature. Once the refraction is stable and the cornea clear, laser correction can be done for the manifest refractive error if it is within the range successfully treated with hyperopic photorefractive keratectomy (PRK). A lamellar keratoplasty can also be performed with the donor button being fashioned with a microkeratome off the donor eye. This is placed onto the recipient corneal bed and sutured into position. Once the healing process is complete and the refraction stable, laser-in-situ keratomileusis (LASIK) or PRK can be performed for the residual refractive error. It is very worthwhile remembering that contact lenses can be very useful in some of these patients and that they might be the preferred method of visual rehabilitation where cap problems might be expected again.

Decentered Flap

The decentered flap occurs infrequently because the fact that the suction ring is decentered is usually observed before the microkeratome is activated and the flap cut. If it is noticed that the suction ring is not well centered, the suction is broken by switching off the vacuum and the ring is reapplied. If there is a deep scleral groove all the way round the limbus, it would be better to wait for 30 minutes or until the groove has disappeared and then reapply the suction ring. Decentration can occur after the suction ring has been engaged and accepted to be adequately centered. Once the flap has been cut and the suction ring removed, the decentered flap is noticed then sometimes. In these cases, only one of two options can be followed. Either the decentration is so minimal that the planned ablation zone can still be delivered under the flap, in which case the operation simply proceeds as usual, or, the flap is so decentered that the ablation zone will not be under the flap in its entirety. Then, the decision needs to be made to abort the procedure, wait 6 to 12 weeks for the flap to reattach firmly, and then start from anew. The use of a caliper set to the optical zone to be treated, is of great benefit in assessing whether the area to be lasered lies beneath the area of the flap.

The best way to eliminate decentered flaps would be to apply the suction ring to the eye and applanate it manually, quite firmly, and in your mind's eye, stretching the underlying bulbar conjunctiva posteriorly so that the suction ring is sucking down onto a flat, stretched-out surface rather than a rolled-up surface with excess tissue. Once this manual applanation is deemed to be adequate, the vacuum pump is activated and the suction ring is officially applied.

Thin Flap

Occasionally flaps are created that are thinner than intended. This would occur where the suction on the eye was not adequate and an insufficient protrusion of cornea through the suction ring is achieved. In almost all instances, the laser treatment can still be applied. The thin flap often results in subepithelial corneal scarring. **If the flap is less than 100 microns thick, do not proceed. Replace the flap and wait for 6 to 12 weeks before recutting. If one proceeds, he or she would notice severe subepithelial haze, especially if the correction to be lasered is over 3 D spherical equivalent.**

Perforated Flap

Perforated flap, a rare complication, arises when suction is inadequate and when the corneal curvature is very flat. A doughnut shaped-flap is fashioned with the central area remaining uncut. Obviously it is impossible to laser in this situation and the flap must simply be replaced, and there should be a waiting period of at least 3 months before this is attempted again. Scarring can occur along the margin of the perforation and this can be reduced with the use of cortisone drops.

Incomplete Flaps

Half Cut

The flap is replaced and allowed 3 months to heal at which time, the procedure is approached as any new procedure would be with new refraction, etc.

Three-fourth Cut

Three-fourth cut flap can sometimes still facilitate treatment especially where a cylinder is involved. If the area to be treated can fit onto the exposed area, laser treatment can continue. If the area to be treated cannot fit onto the exposed area, the flap is replaced into position and a 3-month waiting period is entered into again before recutting the flap. **Never try to enlarge the flap by manual dissection.**

Dislocated or Moved Flap

Dislocated or moved flap occurs approximately 0.5 percent of the times. More than 90 percent will displace or move within the first hour after surgery and for this reason, patients should be examined 1 hour postoperatively before being dismissed to ensure that the flap has not moved. The displacement is usually very minimal and the management required is to immediately return to the operating room, lift the flap, stretch it out, make sure that any epithelial tissue is removed from the corneal bed and then the flap is replaced and managed further in the usual way. One hour later the eye is reexamined to ensure that the flap is in position. Flaps can also move if the eye is rubbed or the patient blinks forcefully after the first hour. This has only happened twice in more than 4500 patients, so it is a very rare finding. It is usually observed on the first postoperative day or earlier if the patient complains about any unusual or unexpected symptom afterwards and calls the office before the first day postoperative visit. The treatment is the same as with the earlier dislocation. It should just be noted that epithelial ingrowth or coverage of the exposed corneal bed can be substantial overnight and that the corneal bed and undersurface of the flap must be scrupulously cleaned from epithelial cells so as to minimize the chances of epithelial ingrowth occurring. A small phototherapeutic keratectomy (PTK) may be done over the area of ingrowth to destroy microscopic nests of epithelial cells.

Foreign Bodies

Often foreign bodies like particles of eye make-up, debris from linen sterile drapes, oil globules from the lid margin, etc. can land up beneath the corneal flap. The majority of these are removed when the flap is being replaced after doing the laser treatment, but sometimes tiny particles might still remain. In clinics where there is a 1 hour postoperative examination, these particles are detected very early, and if it is deemed necessary due to the nature, size or position of the particle, they can be removed immediately by returning to the theater, lifting the flap and rinsing away the particle. Where patients are seen the next day for the first time postoperatively, only more serious particles would justify going back to the theater to remove them. Centrally located particles or any particles that might cause visual disturbances or increase the risk of infection, should be removed.

Sands of the Sahara

Sands of the Sahara is used for a condition of sterile nonspecific interlamellar kereratitis. It reflects a situation of considerable confusion as to the etiology. It is noninfectious as in no cases thus far has any culture been positive. There are many possible causes including toxic effects, side effects of medications, sterile inflammations and more nonspecific causes. It is our feeling that it occurs most likely due to the use of nonsteroidal antiinflammatory drops intra- and postoperatively. We have had little experience of this condition, but since abandoning the use of NSAIDs, have not yet seen another case. The treatment is the early detection of the condition and the liberal use of topical steroids used hourly initially and tapered over the next 2 to 3 weeks. **It seems appropriate to recommend that if you have not yet encountered this condition, do not change anything in your intra- and postoperative regimen. If you do encounter the phenomenon on a regular basis, change one variable at a time to try and establish the cause in your specific setting.** This condition may have a variable number of criteria to meet before manifesting. The final outcome is usually good and very few cases proceed to corneal melt or loss of the flap.

Keratitis

Keratitis (noninfective) can occur as a result of reactions to the chemicals used to clean the equipment, the antiseptics used to clean the area around the eye as well as the eye, and it may result from the use of eyedrops to which the patient is sensitive. It often blurs the vision and causes discomfort. Cylinders are also often induced by asymmetrical or paracentral areas of keratitis. The typical appearance is that of punctate superficial keratitis. It responds to topical lubrication with natural tears (preservative-free preferably) and low-dosage cortisone preparations and may sometimes take 6 weeks or even longer to clear up. The condition usually clears up within 2 to 3 weeks however.

Microstriae

Microstriae are very fine vertical, horizontal or obliquely orientated folds or lines within the corneal cap. If they involve the central visual axis and are detracting from the visual acuity, it is advisable to lift the flap and reposition it again. The earlier the folds are detected, the greater the probability that they are resolved by lifting and repositioning the flap. If the folds are only detected during the later visits at the 3-month period, no visual benefit will be detected by lifting the cap and relifting it. It is also interesting to note that some fine microstriae present on day 1 have resolved by the second week. **It appears that microstriae are less of a problem with the down-up keratomes (e.g. Hansatome, Chiron) that create a horizontal hinge than with the conventional microkeratomes that create a nasal vertical hinge.**

Infection

Not much can be said about infection except that it would be a very unwanted complication. This is a problem that is extremely rare. In more than 4500 cases, this problem has not yet been encountered in our practice. The most likely place for the infection to manifest itself would be under the corneal cap. In the event that such an infection occurred, the most appropriate management would include the lifting of the corneal flap, the rinsing or the washing away of the infected material (after taking a pus swab for culture) and then replacing the flap. Antibiotic drops would have been used from directly after the

At the end of each session, prior to storage, the distal 2 to 3 mm of the motor is dipped in 99 percent alcohol and is electrically driven forward and in reverse for 15 seconds. The tip is then wiped with a Merocel spear sponge.

The motor is stored with the drive tip down—this prevents liquids from migrating down into the motor and gear box and will keep the motor clean and running smoothly.

If the motor becomes jammed, the distal 2 to 3 mm of the motor tip is soaked in 99 percent alcohol for up to one hour and is then cleaned as above.

The microkeratome is cleaned by soaking it in alcohol and by washing the gears with Palmolive soap. This keeps them well lubricated and prevents excessive wear and tear of the gears and motor.

Blades are supposed to be for single use only but are often used for 2 eyes of the same patient. Once a blade has been used, it may still be fit to make another safe cut. By inspecting it under the microscope and having considered it fit for further use, it can be sterilized again by soaking it for a minimum of 10 hours in Cidex long life solution. In poorer countries where new blades are at a premium, recleaned and resterilized blades can be used once more if they are found to be still in good condition following microscopic examination.

PEARLS TO ASSIST WITH THE MAKING OF A GOOD FLAP

First apply the suction ring to the eye and applanate it well before the suction is applied. It helps stretch out the bulbar conjunctiva posteriorly as the suction ring is applied to ensure a good applanation and final suction. Check the IOP with the tonometer before proceeding and we always enquire about the vision at this stage. In most cases, it has already darkened in front of the eyes and even blacked out completely. This confirms that the suction ring is adequately applied and ready for the microkeratome pass.

Some surgeons reckon that it is better to have visual feedback on exactly what the microkeratome is doing and to look at the flap being created. Our feeling is that if your faith in the microkeratome is very good and that your complication record suggests that you are experienced with creating flaps, then there is absolutely no advantage in being able to see the flap being fashioned. The possibility exists that the procedure can be unduly interrupted by a surgeon watching the flap being created and thinking that there is a problem, terminating the pass of the microkeratome. This could occur in spite of everything going ahead well.

SUMMARY

In summary, our own studies presented at the European Society of Cataract and Refractory Surgery (ESCRS) meeting in Nice, France in 1998 and a larger study presented in Cambridge, UK in March 1999, show the following: The visual results are not different using the Hansatome or any other microkeratome that has created a good flap. The refractive results are also completely comparable. The ease of use however of the Hansatome and the fact that excellent flaps are created all of the time in our experience thus far, have taken a load off our shoulders and the experience of doing LASIK has changed from a bit of a "hope and see" attitude to one where the result is basically guaranteed.

45 Flap Complications and Mitomycin C

Francesco Carones

INTRODUCTION

Laser in situ keratomileusis (LASIK) is the most common refractive surgery procedure performed worldwide. This procedure involves creation of a disc-shaped corneal lamellar flap, usually hinged to the cornea nasally or superiorly. The lamellar flap can be made with either a mechanical microkeratome, or with a femtosecond laser. Although LASIK is generally safe and effective, surgical complications can occur. The technology improvements made the flap-creation process safer and safer, however the most significant surgical complications involve problems with the lamellar flap. Flap complications have been reported in up to 8% of LASIK procedures when using 1st generation mechanical microkeratomes,[1-3] whereas this figure dramatically reduced to less than 0.2% when using last generation mechanical microkeratomes or femtosecond lasers. Buttonhole flaps, partial flaps, dissected flaps, excessive thin flaps have been become very rare, but still these complications may be associated with loss of best spectacle-corrected visual acuity, contrast sensitivity and visual symptoms. The etiology of visual loss and side effects associated with these types of flap abnormalities is most often the higher order aberrations and irregular astigmatism secondary to scarring and epithelial ingrowth.[4]

FLAP COMPLICATIONS

The optimal technique for the management of flap surgical complications continues to evolve. For buttonhole or partial flaps the two main treatment options involve repeating the microkeratome pass after a period of time (usually longer than two months),[5,6] or ablating the surface over the previously attempted flap.[4,7] There are several disadvantages associated with a second microkeratome pass over a complicated flap. Unless a readily identifiable cause of the initial complication is known and corrected (which is not the case in most of the situations), a second complication can occur. The new cut can intersect with the original flap, leading to potential loss of corneal tissue and significant irregular astigmatism. Moreover, the waiting period that can be associated with significant anisometropia can be a cause of considerable patient anxiety and discomfort, whereas both the surgeon and the patient are generally motivated in managing the complication early in the postoperative period. The use of a femtosecond laser to cut the second flap may reduce risk for both complications and waiting period, though final conclusion on its use in such cases is still debated, and this technology is not widely accessible.

Disadvantages are associated with surface ablation (PRK, LASEK, EpiLASIK) over an irregular and complicated LASIK flap as well. There may be a significant risk for developing subepithelial haze, leading to all the well-known side effects and visual disturbances like best spectacle-corrected visual acuity loss, blurred vision, loss of contrast sensitivity and night-vision disturbances.[8]

Haze formation embodies the excessive wound healing response to the corneal tissue ablation, and is characterized by stromal reaction, keratocyte activation, collagen and amorphous material deposition. Haze has been shown to be aggressive when ablating the corneal surface over a LASIK flap for enhancement purposes,[8] although shallow ablations like those for treating flap striae are less likely to induce stromal reaction.[9] Certain circumstances tend to magnify both haze density and chance of appearance. Among them, the amount of intended correction is probably the most important: the higher, the worse.[10-13] But other factors like ultraviolet light (sun) exposure, delay in reepithelialization, irregularity of the ablation surface, are also implicated in haze formation.

MITOMYCIN C

Treatment of severe haze involves the use of pharmaceuticals applied topically. Corticosteroid produced some controversial results, and are frequently ineffective.[14,15] The second category of drugs employed at this aim are antimetabilites, of which mitomycin C (MMC), 5 fluorouracil, and thio-tepa are those experimented the most. Haze can be removed by a second laser ablation in a therapeutic fashion, but this approach also is often ineffective because laser ablation generated the haze in the first place and may induce haze recurrence. A very effective option to manage intraoperative flap complications involves surface ablation with adjunctive mitomycin C (Fig. 45.1).

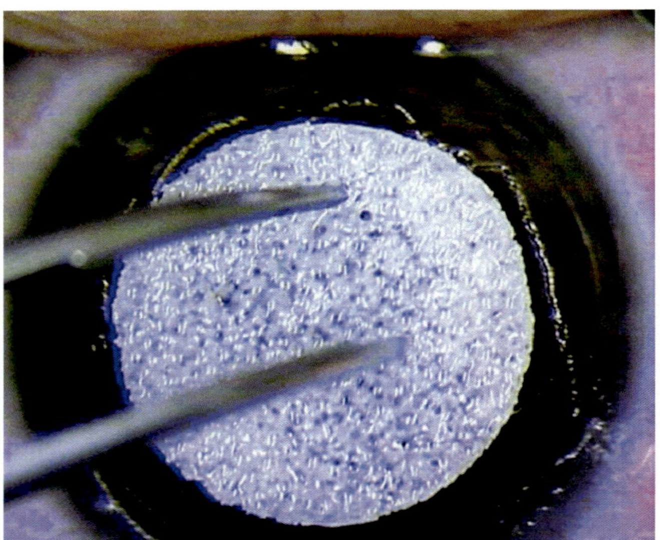

Fig. 45.1: This image shows the microsponge soaked with 0.02% MMC solution, positioned over the corneal stroma, immediately after scraping.

MMC is an antibiotic/chemotherapeutic agent with alkylating properties, which enables it to inhibit DNA synthesis. It is commonly used topically after glaucoma surgery, pterygium excision, in the treatment of conjunctival and corneal intraepithelial neoplasia, and in the treatment of ocular pemphigoid. Rationale to its use relies on its long-term, possibly permanent, cytostatic effect on tissue. More specifically, its use after surface ablation is intended to inhibit subepithelial fibrosis as the result of an abnormal activation or proliferation of stromal keratocytes following laser ablation.[16] This use was originally proposed by Talamo and associates on an experimental model.[17] Haze reduction following mitomycin C administration was also documented by Xu and associates in rabbit eyes.[18] More recently, Majmudar and coworkers reported a successful series of eyes treated using a 0.02% (0.2 mg/ml) mitomycin C solution, to remove haze after PRK and radial keratotomy.[19]

For corneal refractive surgery, MMC is widely used either therapeutically in those eyes already exposed to surface ablation that present significant haze,[20-23] or it can be used in a prophylactic fashion to avoid haze formation in those virgin eyes where the treatment is at risk (the use of MMC appears of particular interest for those eyes with limited stromal thickness, where LASIK is contraindicated. These eyes may benefit from the great accuracy of MMC prophylactic therapy and the application of wide ablation diameters as well).[24-28]

Results achievable with MMC (Figs 45.2 and 45.3) used to avoid further haze formation once the scar is removed are extremely positive. Corneal transparency, once restituted, maintains over time in the vast majority of the cases. The gain in best spectacle-corrected visual acuity is significant in most of the cases, and may mean avoiding more invasive procedures like penetrating keratoplasty. Recurrence of haze is quite rare and in all cases milder than the original onset. Literature assesses haze recurrence around 5-10% of cases, in which in a second approach may be advisable. Also, this therapeutic approach is more likely to be successful when applied on scars not very dated: recent-onset haze is easier to be removed, and recurrence is even less frequent.

Even when used prophylactically, results of surface ablation MMC-assisted are astonishing. MMC does not interfere with re-epithelialization or early wound healing period. Haze rates are extremely low, whenever present, also for high corrections and ablation depths. The accuracy of the procedure is reported as much higher than for surface ablation without the use of MMC, with lower standard deviations. All the published series report a marked trend to overcorrection (in the range 10-15%, according to the laser used and individual nomograms), thus suggesting a programmed undercorrection when using MMC.

Given these very positive results, the association of surface ablation with MMC for the treatment of intraoperative flap complications and performing the excimer laser correction seems very viable. The technique to be adopted has not been widely accepted, given also the wide range of potential complications and their different outcomes. Basically, the two major issues are, the time when to perform the treatment, and the modality for removing the epithelium. In the event a buttonhole or an incomplete flap occurs, the shift to surface ablation may be done immediately, or after a certain healing period. For both options there are advantages and disadvantages. Both the patient and the surgeon would probably prefer to manage and solve flap complications directly at the time when the complication occurs, to speed-up recovery time and manage the potential induced anisometropia. In case of an incomplete flap, it seems more reasonable to shift to surface ablation quite immediately, as the risk of having flap displacement are minimal. When

Fig. 45.2: The image shows a very severe haze (grade 4) that was evident in a patient who was treated for –12.00 D correction by myopic PRK

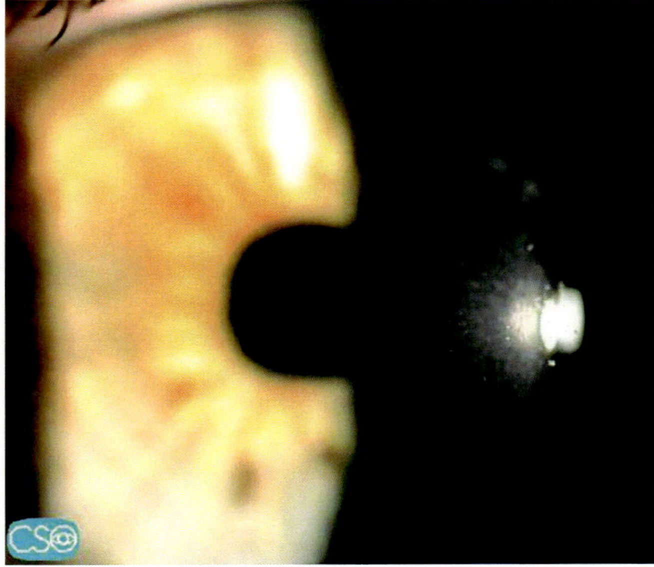

Fig. 45.3: The slit-lamp examination of the eye seven years after treatment showed a transparent cornea, with no haze traces

perforating or damaging the flap, like in case of a buttonhole or a damaged, intersected partial flap, the risk of displacing the remaining flap and/or facilitating epithelial ingrowth suggest to postpone surface ablation for a certain amount of time, as to achieve epithelial healing and some stromal adhesion between the two flap sides. This healing period is not to be as long as to produce stromal reaction, which means that it should not exceed 2-3 weeks from the original attempted procedure. During this period, local corticosteroids to control keratocytes activation are advised. Waiting longer than 2-3 weeks has no advantages in terms of safety of the procedure, but the potential disadvantage of treating a stromal tissue which already has activated keratocytes, with consequent greater risk of aggressive wound healing and haze formation.

The way to remove the epithelium may be influenced by the type of the occurred flap complication. If the flap surface is smooth, the flap is adherent (such as after 2-3 weeks after the attempted surgery), and the flap has not been intersected (like in a buttonhole or a partially damaged flap), all epithelial removal techniques may be safely used. Mechanical scraping should be carefully performed, paying attention to scraping in the direction where the hinge was intended, without applying rotational forces. A diluted 20% alcohol solution applied for 20-25 seconds may be very beneficial in such cases to reduce the adherence between the epithelium and Bowman's membrane, to make the scraping process much more gentle and less aggressive. Brushes look less indicated due to the lower control they have on epithelium removal, and to the torsional movement they apply onto the flap which may determine some shift and/or flap displacement. Laser epithelium removal in a therapeutic fashion seems the technique with less chances of displacing the attempted flap, though a precise way to remove the whole epithelium in a homogeneous way over the entire ablation surface is still difficult to perform, due to the different thickness the epithelium has. The observation of fluorescence during the ablation helps the surgeon in evaluating this process.

For all flap complications where the flap has been intersected, it seems more reasonable to perform transepithelial ablation in a no-touch technique, or at least to extensively use alcohol to assist mechanical epithelium removal. Particular care has to be paid in avoiding to compromise the integrity of the previously flap-intersected junction, to minimize risk of flap displacement, irregularity, and epithelium ingrowth. The stromal surface must be as smooth, regular and continuous as possible for a proper laser ablation.

The ablation strategy may be different in relation to the previous flap complication. When the stromal surface is regular and not involved by the previous attempt to cut the flap (incomplete cut, very thin flap), the attempted correction may be entered as for the original ablation. When the central part of the cornea has been involved by the previous flap complication (buttonhole, intersected flap, flap tear, etc.), it may be necessary to perform some phototherapeutic ablation in relation to the irregularity of the stromal surface. Masking fluids such as hyaluronic acid may be necessary to achieve a smooth and regular surface, where each case is quite unique and it is very difficult to give general indications. Usually, it is much more advisable to perform phototherapeutic keratectomy using very large ablation diameters to regularize the entire corneal surface than performing small ablation zones to remove the irregularity in a localized fashion. The following refractive ablation to correct preexisting error has to be adjusted according to the amount of phototherapeutic ablation performed, in order to avoid overcorrection. Again, it is very difficult to give generic advices, being the refractive effect of phototherapeutic keratectomy very technique-, ablation diameter-, and laser-dependent.

Once the ablation has been performed, MMC has to be applied on the stromal surface to avoid haze formation. There are different techniques to apply MMC. Some surgeons use marking trephine to be filled with MMC solution, most of them use circular sponges soaked with MMC solution. The concentration of MMC in its dilution, and the application time are also controversial. The original studies performed by Majmudar and colleagues suggested a 0.02% (0.2 mg/ml) concentration for a two-minute application time.[19] Most of the published literature assesses this concentration and application time to be effective in avoiding haze formation, and no side effects or complications related to the use of MMC have been reported over a follow-up period longer than 10 years. Shorter application times and lower dosages have been investigated on laboratory animals and on patients for MMC when applied prophylactically to avoid haze formation on virgin eyes, and results were favorable. However, no laboratory studies have been performed to assess the efficacy of MMC in the treatment of flap complications, and no clinical data have been reported. Given this, it seems more reasonable to use the original 0.2 mg/ml (0.02%) concentration for two minutes application time.

CARONES TECHNIQUE

My personal technique involves the use of a circular merocel microsponge, 1.0 mm smaller in diameter than the depithelialized diameter, soaked with a 0.02% (0.2 mg/ml) mitomycin C solution to be placed on top of the stromal surface. This has to be left in place for two minutes. The surface is then irrigated copiously with 20 cc balanced salt solution to remove all MMC particles and remnants. Postoperativley a bandage contact lens is applied and left in place until reepithelialization is complete (usually 4-5 days). During this period, antibiotic drops and non steroidal anti-inflammatory drops are applied four times per day, together with artificial tears. The patient is also prescribed oral narcotics as needed for pain. Once the bandage contact lens is removed, topical fluorometholone drops are applied three times per day for two weeks, and then for twice per day for other two weeks. Artificial tears are administered as needed thereafter.

RESULTS

Reported results of this approach are positive, although there may be some variability in relation to the severity of the original flap complication. Muller and coworkers reported a series of 10 eyes, with postoperative uncorrected visual acuity in the range 20/20 to 20/40 (mean 20/28), and best spectacle-corrected visual acuity in the range 20/20 to 20/25 (mean 20/21).[29] No complications have been reported over a follow-up ranging 8 to 28 months. Similar results have been reported by Taneri and associates in a case series study,[30] and by Chalita and coworkers and Solomon and colleagues in two separate case reports.[31,32]

COMPLICATIONS

The major criticism in the use of MMC after any kind of laser refractive surgery refers to the potential side effects and complications associated to its long-term cytostatic action on tissues, when applied in a topic fashion on the corneal stroma. Several Authors reported corneoscleral melt after MMC application after pterygium excision.[33-35] Also, the long-term integrity of the endothelial layer is supposed to be at risk.

It is worthwhile mentioning that all report referring to corneoscleral melting differ in substance from the approach used after refractive surgery. First, the concentration of MMC was reported to be higher, and for application times longer than the two-minute maximum time it is currently performed when MMC is applied on the corneal stroma. Second, the previous melting reports always involve the conjunctivo-scleral district, which is substantially different from the cornea as regard the tissue structure, vascularization, and origin.

SUMMARY

So far, it is estimated that more than 150.000 procedures have been applied with the use of MMC worldwide, and there are no reports of corneal melting or endothelium toxicity over a 10 year follow-up period. However, the use of MMC has to be very cautious, in order to reduce at minimum these potential risks. The concentration has to be 0.2 mg/ml because higher concentrations determined the previously reported complications while lower concentrations may be not as effective in such challenging cases. The application time should never exceed two minutes, and studies are undergoing for evaluation of the efficacy at shorter application times. After MMC application, it is suggested to wash the corneal surface and the entire conjunctival sac quite abundantly using balanced salt solution, in order to avoid the interaction of MMC both with the epithelial stem cells and the conjunctiva. The use of MMC according to these rules has been proven safe and effective.

REFERENCES

1. Stulting RD, Carr JD, Thompson KP, et al. Complications of Laser in Situ Keratomileusis for the correction of myopia. Ophthalmology 1999;106:13-20.
2. Lin RT, Maloney RK. Flap complications associated with lamellar refractive surgery. Am J Ophthalmol 1999;127:129-36.
3. Tham VM, Maloney RK. Microkeratome complications of laser in situ keratomileusis. Ophthalmology 2000;107:920-24.
4. Kapadia MS, Wilson SE. Transepithelial photorefractive keratectomy for treatment of thin flaps or caps after complicated laser in situ keratomileusis. Am J Ophthalmol 1998; 126:827-29.
5. Farah SG, Azar DT, Gurdal C, et al. Laser in situ keratomileusis: literature review of a developing technique. J Cataract Refract Surg 1998;24:989-1006.
6. Holland SP, Srivannaboon S, Reinstein DZ. Avoiding serious complications of laser assisted in situ keratomileusis and photorefractive keratectomy. Ophthalmology 2000;107:640-52.
7. Jain VK, Abell TG, Bond WI, et al. Immediate transepithelial photorefractive keratectomy for treatment of laser in situ keratomileusis flap complications. J Refract Surg 2002; 18:109-12.
8. Carones F, Vigo L, Carones AV. Evaluation of photorefractive keratectomy retreatments after regressed miopi laser in situ keratomileusis. Ophthalmology 2001;108:1732-37.
9. Ashrafzadeh A, Steinert RF. Results of photorerapeutic keratectomy in the management of flap striae after LASIK before and after developing a standardized protocol: long-term follow-up of an estended patient population. Ophthalmology 2007;114:1118-23.
10. McCarthy CA, Aldred GF, Taylor HR. Comparison of results of excimer laser correction of all degrees of myopia at 12 months postoperatively. Am J Ophthalmol 1996;121:372-83.
11. Krueger RR, Talamo JH, McDonald MB, et al. Clinical analysis of excimer laser photorefractive keratectomy using a multiple zone technique for severe myopia. Am J Ophthalmol 1995;119:263-74.
12. Sher NA, Hardten DR, Fundingsland B, et al. 193-Nm excimer photorefractive keratectomy in high myopia. Ophthalmology 1994;101:1575-82.
13. Carson CA, Taylor HR. Excimer laser treatment for high and extreme myopia. Arch Ophthalmol 1995;113:431-6.
14. Gartry D, Kerr Muir MG, Lohmann CP, Marshall J. The effect of topical corticosteroids on refractive outcome and corneal haze after photorefractive keratectomy. Arch Ophthalmol 1992;110:944-52.
15. Carones F, Brancato R, Venturi E, Scialdone A, Bertuzzi A, Tavola A. Efficacy of corticosteroids in reversing regression after myopic photorefractive keratectomy. Refract Corneal Surg 1993;9(suppl):S52-6.
16. Shipper I, Suppelt C, Gebbers JO. Mitomycin C reduces scar formation after excimer laser (193 nm) photorefractive keratectomy in rabbits. Eye 1997;11:649-55.
17. Talamo JH, Gollamudi S, Green RW, et al. Modulation of corneal wound healing after excimer laser keratomileusis using topical mitomycin C and steroids. Arch Ophthalmol 1991;109:1141-6.
18. Xu H, Liu S, Xia X, et al. Mitomycin C reduces haze formation in rabbits after excimer laser photorefractive keratectomy. J Refract Surg 2001;17:342-9.
19. Majmudar P, Forstrot L, Dennis R, et al. Topical mitomycin-C for subepithelial fibrosis after refractive corneal surgery. Ophthalmology 2000;107:89-94.
20. Vigo L, Scandola E, Carones F. Scraping and mitomycin C to treat haze and regression after photorefractive keratectomy for myopia. J Refract Surg 2003;19:449-54.
21. Porges Y, Ben-Haim O, Hirsh A, et al. Phototherapeutic keratectomy with mitomycin C for corneal haze following photorefractive keratectomy for myopia. J Refract Surg 2003;19:40-43.
22. Winkler von Mohrenfelds C, Hermann W, Gabler B, et al. Topical mitomycin C for the prophylaxis of recurrent haze after excimer laser photorefractive keratectomy. Klin Monatsbl Augenheilkd. 2001;218:763-7.
23. Raviv T, Majmudar PA, Dennis RF, et al. Mitomycin-C for post-PRK corneal haze. J Cataract Refract Surg 2000; 26:1105-6.
24. Carones F, Vigo L, Scandola E, et al. Evaluation of the prophylactic use of mitomycin-C to inhibit haze formation after photorefractive keratectomy. J Cataract Refract Surg. 2002;28:2088-95.
25. Lacayo GO, Majmudar PA. How and when to use mitomycin-C in refractive surgery. Curr Opin Ophthalmol 2005;16:256-9.
26. Gambato C, Ghirlando A, Moretto E, et al. Mitomycin C modulation of corneal wound healing after photorefractive keratectomy in highly myopic eyes. Ophthalmology 2005;112:208-18.
27. Hashemi H, Taheri SM, Fotouhi A, et al. Evaluation of the prophylactic use of mitomycin-C to inhibit haze formation after photorefractive keratectomy in high myopia: a prospective clinical study. BMC Ophthalmol 2004;14;1:12.
28. Lee DH, Chung HS, Jeon YC, et al. Photorefractive keratectomy with intraoperative mitomycin-C application. J Cataract Refract Surg 2005;31:2293-8.
29. Muller LT, Candal EM, Epstein RJ, et al. Transepithelial phototherapeutic keratectomy/photorefractive keratectomy with adjunctive mitomycin-C for complicated LASIK flaps. J Cataract Refract Surg 2005;31:291-6.
30. Taneri S, Koch JM, Melki SA, et al. Mitomycin-C assisted photorefractive keratectomy in the treatment of buttonholed laser in situ keratomileusis flaps associated with epithelial ingrowth. J Cataract Refract Surg 2005;31:2026-30.

31. Chalita MR, Roth AS, Krueger RR. Wavefront-guided surface ablation with prophylactic use of mitomycin C after a buttonhole laser in situ keratomileusis flap. J refract Surg 2004;20:176-81.
32. Solomon R, Donnenfeld ED, Perry HD. Photorefractive keratectomy with mitomycin C for the management of a LASIK flap complication following penetrating keratoplasty. Cornea 2004;23:403-05.
33. Rubinfeld RS, Pfister RR, Stein RM, et al. Serious complications of topical mitomycin-C after pterygium surgery. Ophthalmology 1992;99:1647-54.
34. Fujitani A, Hayasaka S, Shibuya Y, Noda S. Corneoscleral ulceration and corneal perforation after pterygium excision and topical mitomycin C therapy. Ophthalmologica 1993;207:162-4.
35. Dougherty PJ, Hardten DR, Lindstrom RL. Corneoscleral melt after pterygium surgery using a single intraoperative application of mitomycin-C. Cornea 1996;15:537-40.

Post-LASIK Iatrogenic Ectasia

Melania Cigales, Jairo Hoyos-Chacón, Jairo E Hoyos

INTRODUCTION

Iatrogenic ectasia may manifest months or years after LASIK surgery in the form of topographic steepening causing progressive myopia together with irregular astigmatism and loss of visual acuity. With an incidence ranging between 0.12 and 0.8% according to the different series in the literature,[1-4] post-LASIK ectasia is an uncommon, but potentially visually disabling complication.

The source of the ectasia may be a subclinical keratoconus that goes undetected during the pre-operative examination and is then decompensated as a result of induced corneal thinning. There are cases where there is no prior corneal disorder and ectasia results from excess corneal thinning during surgery. Although ectasia has been described since the early implementation of lamellar techniques for refractive surgery,[5] in recent years, limits to surgical corneal thickness have become more stringent and important advances have been made in pre-operative diagnostic tools used for detecting diseased corneas that may tend themselves to this complication. We will analyze risk factors and treatments for post-LASIK iatrogenic corneal ectasia.

SUBCLINICAL KERATOCONUS

Corneal ectasic degenerations (Fig. 46.1) such as keratoconus and pellucid marginal degeneration are caused by corneal thinning leading to progressive corneal steepening, progressive myopia, irregular astigmatism and, eventually, reduced visual acuity.

In the initial phases, ectasic degenerations usually show a normal biomicroscopic appearance with the only symptom being a visual defect that cannot be properly corrected with spectacles. Topography is usually the examination of choice for detecting early curvature changes (Fig. 46.2). Pachymetry may also be used for measuring corneal thinning, long before it can be seen under the slit lamp; however, because of significant variability among normal subjects, it is an elusive diagnosis. Since the early years of refractive surgery, ectasic degenerations of the cornea have been known to be a counterindication for surgery, but the challenge lies in the ability to arrive at a clear diagnosis. It has been reported[6] that close to 6% of patients coming for refractive surgery are rejected because of a forme frustre keartoconus that might result in post-LASIK corneal ectasia. In 1946, Amsler[7] offered one of the initial descriptions of forme frustre keratoconus (FFKC). Since then, many more diagnostic tools have been developed and much knowledge has been gained for diagnosing this desease.

The preoperative examination provides information that may suggest the presence of a forme frustre keratoconus as a risk factor for post-LASIK iatrogenic ectasia.

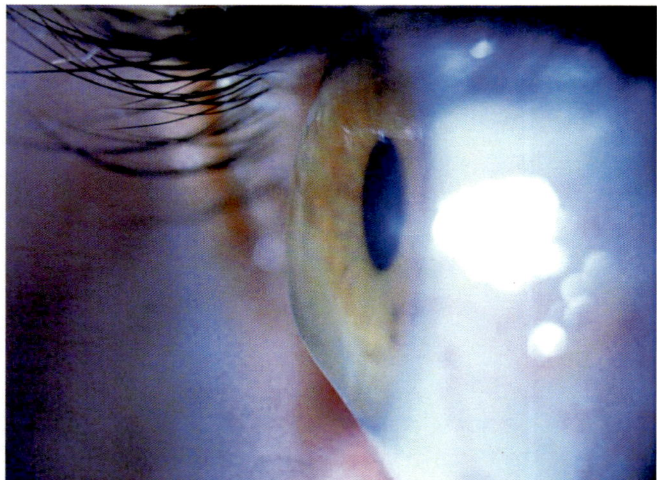

Fig. 46.1: Corneal ectasic degeneration

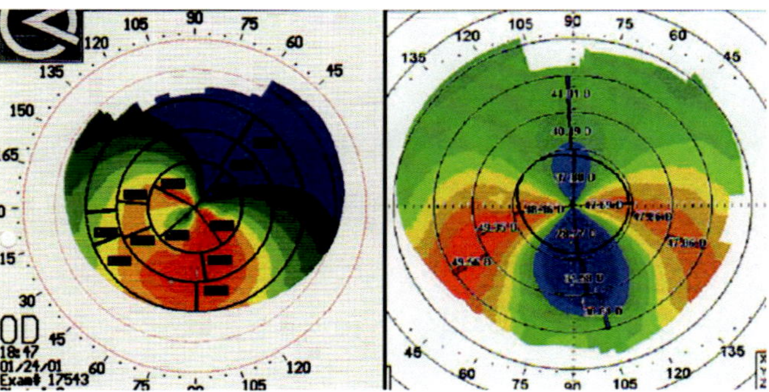

Fig. 46.2: Topographic images of keratoconus (left) and pellucid marginal degeneration (right)

Clinical History

Etiological factors associated with keratoconus are also predisposing factors for post-LASIK ectasia. Keratoconus is usually idiopathic and is not associated with race or sex, although there is a group of cases that follow an inheritance pattern, and there are descriptions of keratoconus associated with atopia.[8] Even in the absence of atopia, the incidence of keratoconus has been found to be greater in patients with chronic persistent eye-rubbing.[9] Hence the need to ask patients interested in refractive surgery about potential family history of keratoconus or a personal history of atopia or chronic eye-rubbing, considering the higher risk of postoperative corneal ectasia.

Refraction

While current technological breakthroughs have led to sophisticated diagnostic systems for detecting early signs of keraconus, we must not forget the important information derived from the basic ophthalmological examination. For instance, even in very early stages of keratoconus, it is possible to see the scissor reflex on retinoscopy or the oil droplet sign through a dilated pupil with back-illumination.[10] Moreover, keratoconus must be suspected in those cases where 20/20 vision is not attained with best refraction and there is no logical explanation for this usually mild form of amblyopia.

Anterior Corneal Curvature

The best system to study anterior corneal curvature is computer-assisted topographic analysis of videokeratoscopic images. When there is an established keratoconus, the topographic image provides a clear diagnosis (see Figure 46.2). But topography may also reveal subtle signs, not diagnostic of keratoconus by themselves but, when added together in the same patient, especially if associated with other findings, may lead to the diagnosis of FFKC.

The most common suspicious topographic findings on the anterior curvature include: [2,11,12]

1. Corneal curvature greater than 47 D.
2. Asymmetry between inferior and superior curvatures (I-S), where the inferior curvature is 1.4 D greater than the superior curvature (Fig. 46.3).
3. Skew of steepest radial axes (SRAX) greater than 20° in corneas with astigmatism greater than 1.5 D (Fig. 46.4).
4. Difference in central corneal power between fellow eyes greater than 1 D.
5. Distance between the apex and the center of the cornea greater than 1 mm.

The combination of different quantitative topographic indices including central diopter value (central K), simulated keratometry (Sim K), inferior-superior asymmetries (I-S), nasal-temporal asymmetry and skewed radial axis value (SRAX), may help with the early diagnosis of keratoconus.[13] There are new programs for topographic detection of keratoconus using quantitative measurements,

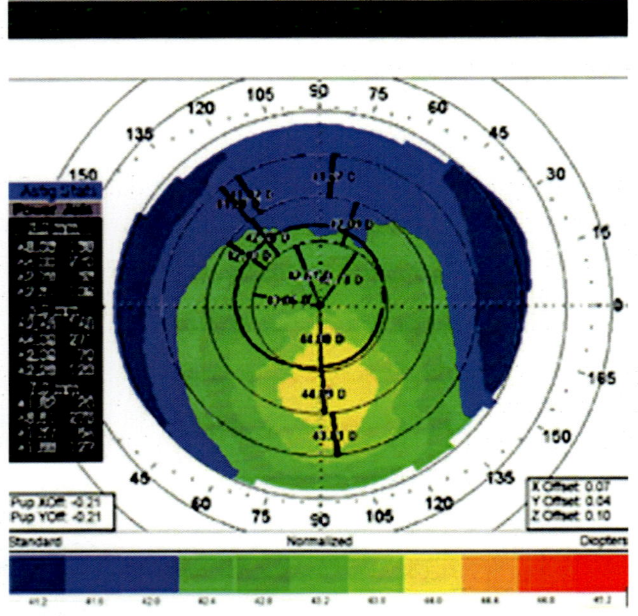

Fig. 46.3: Asymmetry between the inferior and superior curvatures, with a difference greater than 1.4 D

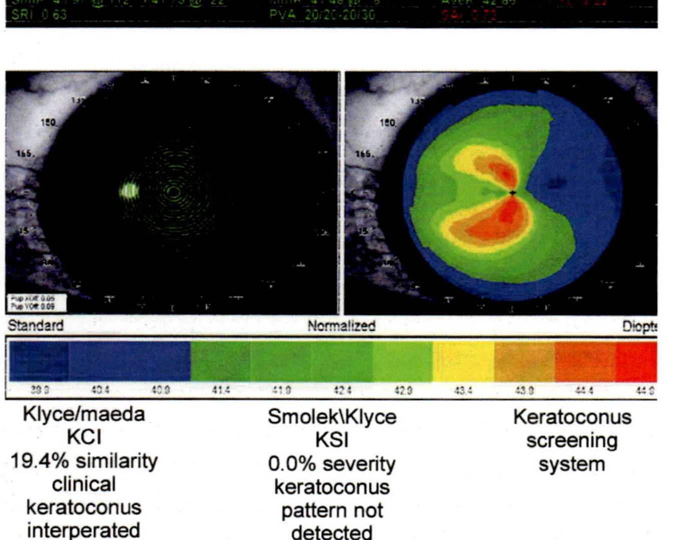

Fig. 46.4: Angulation of radial axes (SRAX = skewed radial axis) in a cornea with normal curvature (Sim 43.97/41.75) and 2.22 D cylinder. The keratoconus screening system using clinical keratoconus interpreted Klyce/Maeda (KCI) shows a 19.4% similarity

including the Rabinowitz, Klyce/Maeda o Smolek/Klyce methods. Using these software packages for analyzing suspicious topographic readings it is possible to recognize early signs or keratoconus and FFKC.

Faced with an irregular or suspicious topographic image, it is mandatory to rule out contact lens-induced corneal warpage.[14] Contact lens-induced topographical abnormalities of the cornea include central irregular astigmatism, loss of radial symmetry, reversal of the normal topographic pattern of progressive flattening of corneal contour from the center to the periphery, and keratoconus-like images (Fig. 46.5).[15] Contact lens wear should be discontinued before refractive surgery and should any topographic signs of corneal warpage be observed, they must be followed until they normalize.[16] In the event topographic signs do not normalize, a forme frustre keratoconus must be suspected and surgery must be discouraged.

Posterior Corneal Elevation

The topographer has become an indispensable diagnostic system in corneal refractive surgery. At first, Placid ring-based topographers offered the possibility of analizing the anterior surface of the cornea almost to its full extent. Elevation topographers that measure the height of different points on the cornea in relation to a perfect sphere came about years later. One of the first elevation topographers was the PAR System[17] that analyzed the elevation

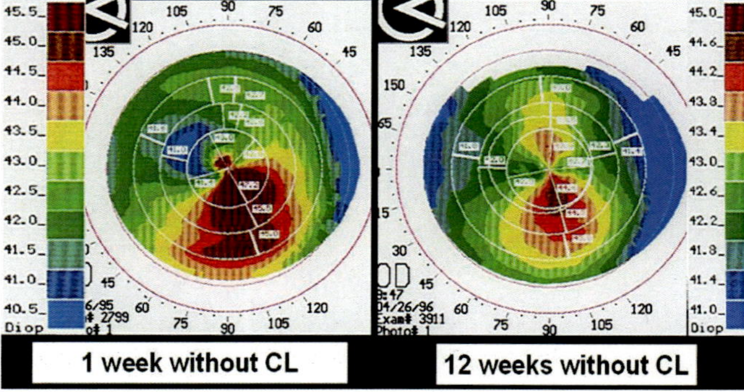

Fig. 46.5: Corneal warpage in a 26-year-old female, RGP contact lens wear (CL wearer for 10 years, 14 hours/day), with a topographic keratoconus-like image

of the anterior surface of the cornea by means of a grid projection. But the advent of the Orbscan (Bausch & Lomb, Rochester NY)[18] (Fig. 46.6) based on a slit scan created a whole new concept in corneal analysis – the study of the posterior surface. In keratoconus posterior surface abnormalities may be present, even before significant changes are seen on the anterior surface, and keratoconus is suspected

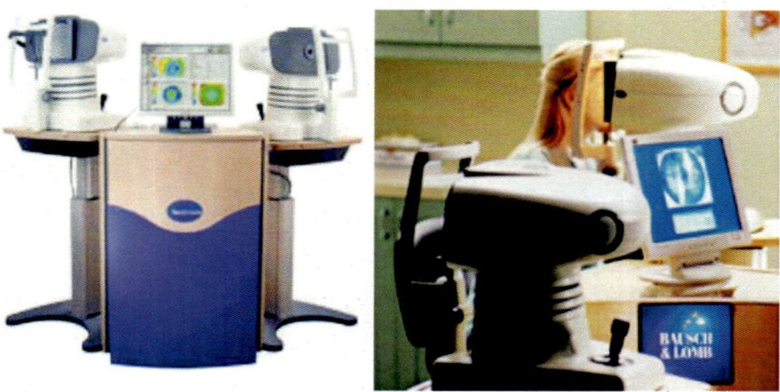

Fig. 46.6: Orbscan (Bausch & Lomb, Rochester NY).

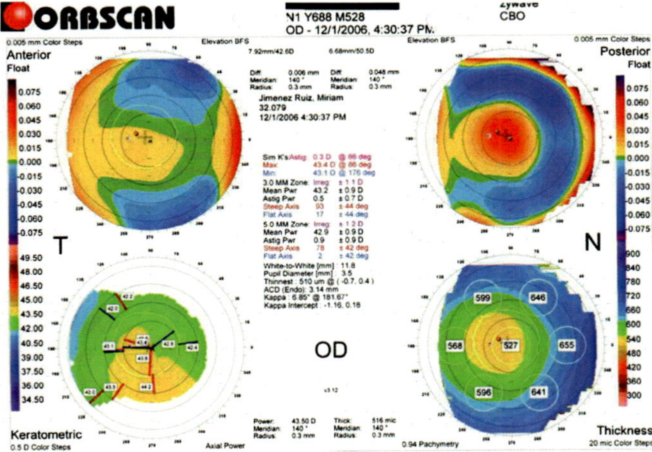

Fig. 46.7: Orbscan topography in a forme frustre keratoconus. The curvature map (bottom left) shows I-S asymmetry with a posterior surface elevation (top right) of 48 microns; the pachymetric map (bottom right) shows apical eccentricity. This patient was refused for refractive surgery with a –1.5 D of refraction and 20/15 of BCVA.

in cases with a posterior surface elevation greater than 40 µm as measured by the Orbscan (Fig. 46.7).[19] New technologies have been developed in recent years for the study of the posterior surface of the cornea, including the Pentacam HR (Oculus Inc, Lynnwood WA) (Fig. 46.8), that uses a rotating Scheimpflug camera and appears to offer more accurate results.[20] In tests performed with the Pentacam, keratoconus is suspected with posterior surface elevations greater than 25 µm (Fig. 46.9).[21] Future studies will determine whether the Pentacam underestimates the posterior vault or if the Orbscan overestimates this height.

Pre-operative Pachymetry

Most surgeons advice against corneal refractive surgery when the central corneal thickness is less than 480 microns. Today, even central thicknesses of less than 500 microns may be a risk factor for post-LASIK iatrogenic ectasia.[22] A thin cornea in a patient seeking refractive surgery poses two problems. First, the corneal thickness may be insufficient for correcting ametropia and still respecting the

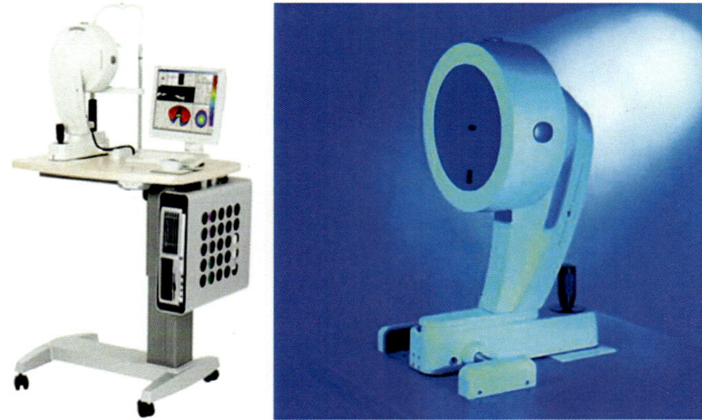

Fig. 46.8: Pentacam (Oculus Inc, Lynnwood WA)

limits of corneal thickness in order to avoid iatrogenic ectasia. Second, a thin cornea may be due to a previous subclinical ectasic disease (keratoconus or pellucid marginal degeneration), and refractive surgery may induce a decompensation. Progressive corneal thinning is common to all ectasic degenerations of the cornea. In keratoconus, corneal thinning is usually central or inferior paracentral, and in pellucid degeneration it is inferiorly located 1-2 mm from the limbus.

It is normally assumed that the thinnest portion of the cornea, used as reference for the surgical calculations, is at the center. When the finest point

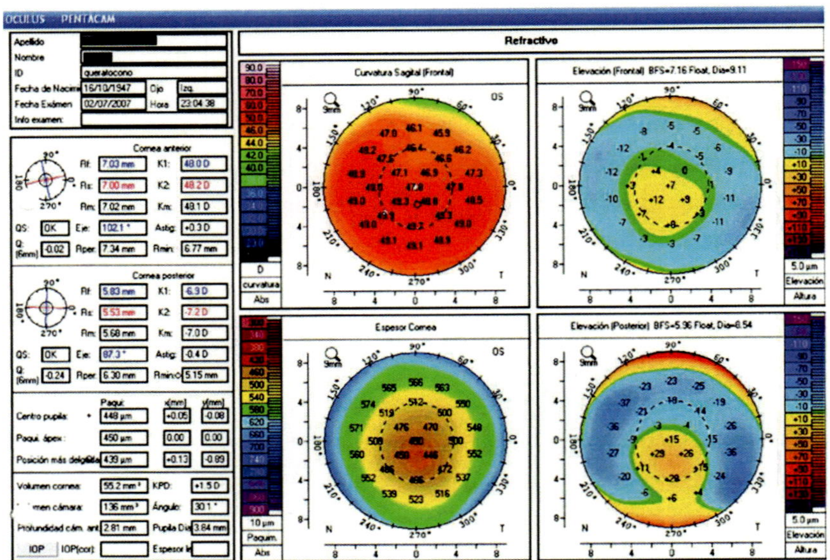

Fig. 46.9: Pentacam topography in a case of forme frustre keratoconus. The curvature map (top left) shows a curvature greater than 47 D with I-S asymmetry and a posterior surface elevation (bottom right) of 29 microns; the pachymetric map (bottom left) shows a thin, 450-micron cornea with apical eccentricity. The option of refractive surgery was abandoned in this case with a low refraction (-1.5 -1.25 x 100°) and BCVA of 20/15

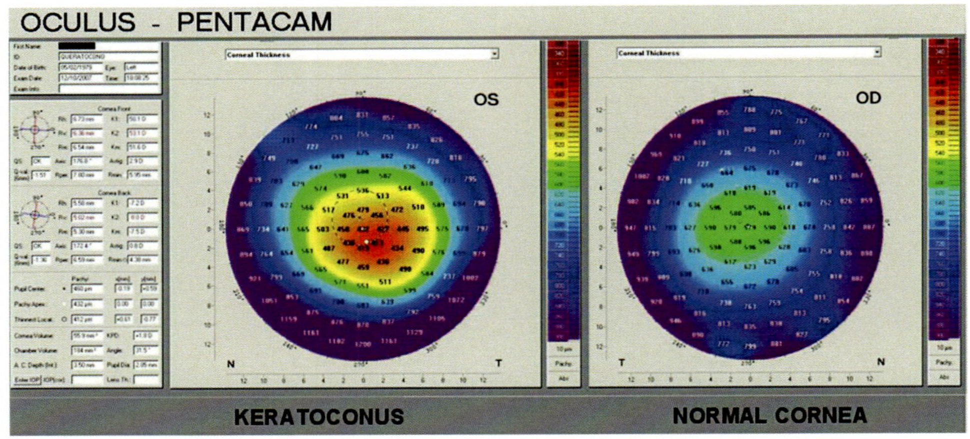

Fig. 46.10: Pachymetric map of keratoconus with a thin cornea and a displacement of the thinnest point towards the inferior temporal area. A normal pachymetric map is shown on the right

of the cornea is not central and, moreover, when it coincides with the steepest anterior curvature and the greatest elevation of the posterior surface, a forme frustre keratoconus must be suspected (Fig. 46.10).[19-20] For this reason, aside from determining central corneal thickness during the preoperative examination, a pachymetric map of the entire cornea must be obtained. Ultrasound pachymetry is the most accurate method for measuring corneal thickness, but it is not useful for obtaining a pachymetric map. Although the Orbscan and the Pentacam provide slightly higher corneal thicknesses than those measured by ultrasound, they offer valuable information in the form of a pachymetric map that can help detect FFKC.[23]

Corneal Hysteresis

Corneal Hysteresis is a new parameter used to describe the biomechanical strength or elasticity of the cornea. This concept is based on the Ocular Response Analyzer technology - ORA (Fig. 46.11), and uses a rapid air pulse on the cornea. Due to its biomechanical properties, the cornea offers resistance to the air pulse causing a delay in its inward and outward flattening motion and creating two different values. Corneal Hysteresis (CH) is the difference between these two pressure values and it measures the properties of the corneal tissues as a result of the cornea's elastic depression. CH is low in keratoconus and, theoretically, normal corneas with CH values lower than the mean may be at a higher risk of developing post-LASIK ectasia.[24]

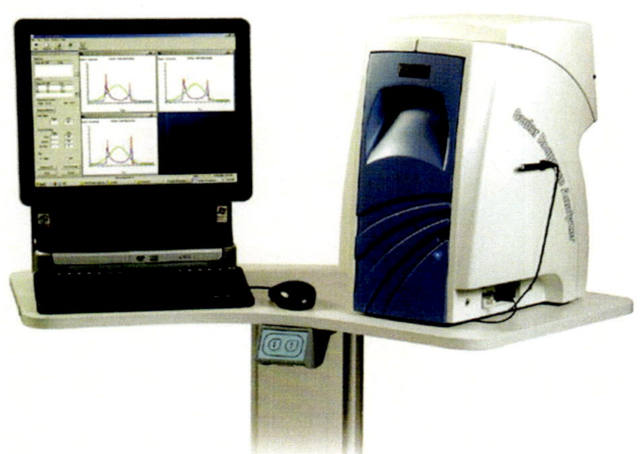

Fig. 46.11: Ocular Response Analyzer (ORA; Reichert Ophthalmic Instruments, New York, USA), for measuring corneal hysteresis (CH)

Post-LASIK Ectasia in FFKC

Patients who are candidates for LASIK surgery must be worked up rigorously and carefully in order to avoid iatrogenic ectasia. Most of the reported cases[25,26] had preoperative topographic and/or clinical evidence of forme frustre keratoconus (FFKC), frank keratoconus or pellucid marginal degeneration. There is a growing amount of data on FFKC explaining many post-LASIK ectasias. When faced with an unexplained ectasia, it is important to revisit the preoperative topography in search for any missed signs of subclinical keratoconus (Figs 46.12 and 46.13). Table 46.1 shows a list of factors that may lead to the suspicion of subclinical keratoconus.

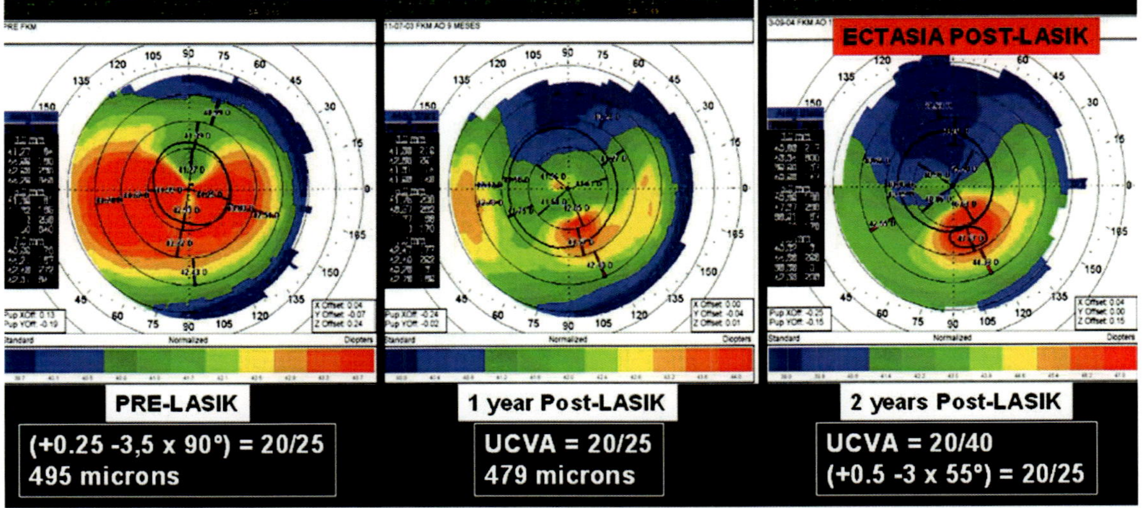

Fig. 46.12: Post-LASIK ectasia in a 24-year-old male with high astigmatism against the rule and a slightly thinned-out cornea. Two years into the postoperative period, the patient came back complaining of reduced vision, and ectasia was diagnosed. Examining the preoperative topography we can see that the steep astigmatic axis is slightly inferior, there is I-S asymmetry and the cornea is slightly thin in what is a condition consistent with forme frustre keratoconus

Table 46.1: Factors for suspected subclinical keratoconus

- Family history of keratoconus
- Personal history of atopia or chronic eye-rubbing
- Retinoscopic scissor reflex and oil droplet sign
- Unexplained mild amblyopia
- Anterior corneal curvature >47 D
- I-S asymmetry with inferior steepening >1,4 D
- Skew of steepest radial axes (SRAX) greater than 20° in astigmatism >1,5 D
- Difference in central corneal power between fellow eyes >1 D
- Apex-to-central corneal distance greater than 1 mm
- Elevation of the posterior corneal surface >40 μm (Orbscan) or >25 μm (Pentacam)
- Thin cornea < 500 μm
- Eccentric location of the thinnest corneal point coinciding with the steepest point and the point of highest posterior surface elevation
- Reduced corneal hysteresis

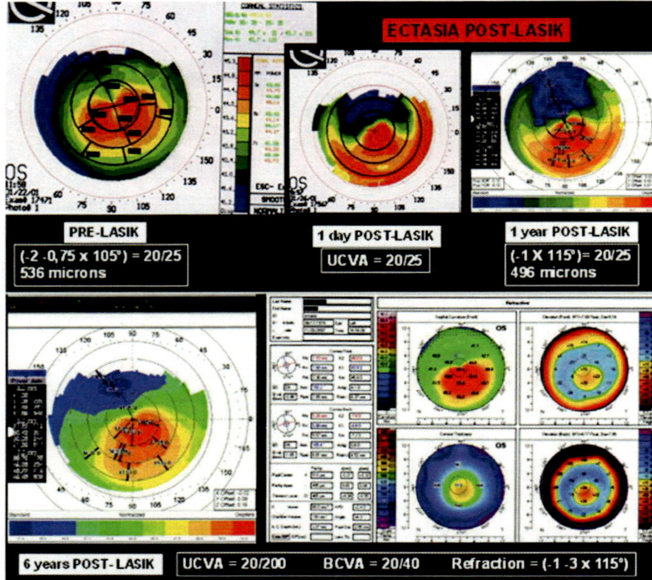

Fig. 46.13: Twenty-six year-old low myopic male patient with topographic signs of ectasia on the first postoperative day, despite good visual acuity. The patient maintained good visual acuity for 6 years. At that point, he came back complaining of diminished vision, and frank ectasia was diagnosed. The patient had a history of ocular allergy and a mild unexplained amblyopia had been found before surgery (only 20/25 with a refractive error of –2 –0.75 x 105°). Examining the preoperative topography, there is an I-S asymmetry despite a 44 D corneal curvature and a central pachymetry of 536 microns

CORNEAL THICKNESS LIMITS

In the absence of prior corneal disease, ectasia may occur when corneal thickness limits are exceeded during surgery. The residual stromal bed (Fig. 46.14) is considered one of the most important thickness limits ever since JI Barraquer, in his early lamellar techniques, determined that 250 microns must remain behind the ablation in order to avoid iatrogenic ectasia.[5] Several studies report[1,27] that the amount of residual corneal thickness after ablation is critical to the development of post-LASIK ectasia and suggest that the 250 μm limit is safe. In 1996, the US Food and Drug Administration approved a residual stromal bed of 250 μm for LASIK.[28] In the event preoperative surgery planning suggests that the residual stromal bed might be less than 250 μm, PRK or phakic IOL must be recommended. In recent years, and as a result of the growing number of reported ectasias, some authors prefer to increase the limit to 300 microns.[3] Others argue that the residual bed is not a magic number and that what is really important is to leave at least 50-55% of the corneal thickness behind the ablation.[22] In any event, a very deep ablation implies a risk factor. The causes

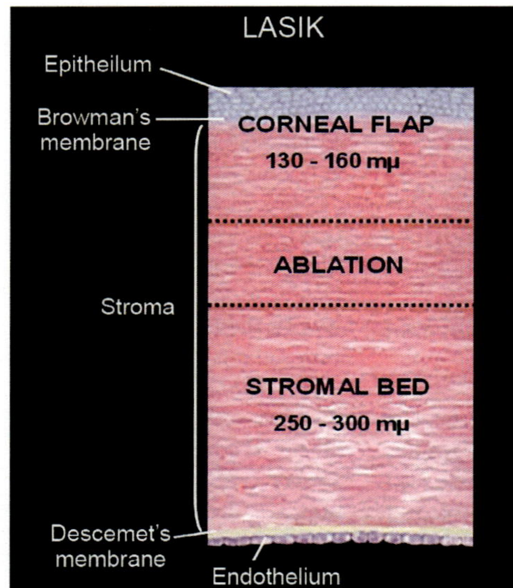

Fig. 46.14: The thickness of the LASIK flap is 130-160 microns and includes epithelium, Bowman's membrane and anterior stroma. A stromal bed of at least 250-300 microns must remain under the ablation in order to avoid ectasia

for insufficient residual bed are thick flaps or excessive ablations.

Thick Flap

It is widely accepted by LASIK surgeons that the ideal flap thickness is 130-160 µm. However, the current trend is towards finer flaps of approximately 100 µm, in order to leave behind a maximum residual bed, thus reducing the risk of keratectasia. Flap thickness is determined by the microkeratome head or plate. However, several pachymetric studies[29] have indicated a high degree of variability in the thicknesses achieved. This variability is associated with corneal K readings, corneal exposure, blade condition and vibration speed, intraocular pressure when cutting, and blade quality.[30] Blade quality varies considerably and that is why it is crucial to check and calibrate the blade in order to set the GAP (Fig. 46.15). The GAP is the distance between the blade and plate, and correlates with the thickness of the keratectomy.[31] By calibrating the blades before using them it is possible to predict flap thickness more accurately in order to select the most appropriate blade for each case.

Some surgeons[26] without checking during surgery, assume that the flap is of the correct thickness, something that may explain some ectasias reported as unexplained. Given the great variability in flap thickness, it is incumbent upon us to perform intraoperative measurements in order to determine the thickness obtained. In the event the flap is found to be too thick, we are required either to modify the optic zone of the ablation in order to maintain a sufficiently thick residual bed, or to abort the procedure. Subtraction ultrasonic pachymetry can provide quite an accurate estimate of flap thickness. This method measures corneal thickness in the center of the pupil after lifting the flap and subtracting this

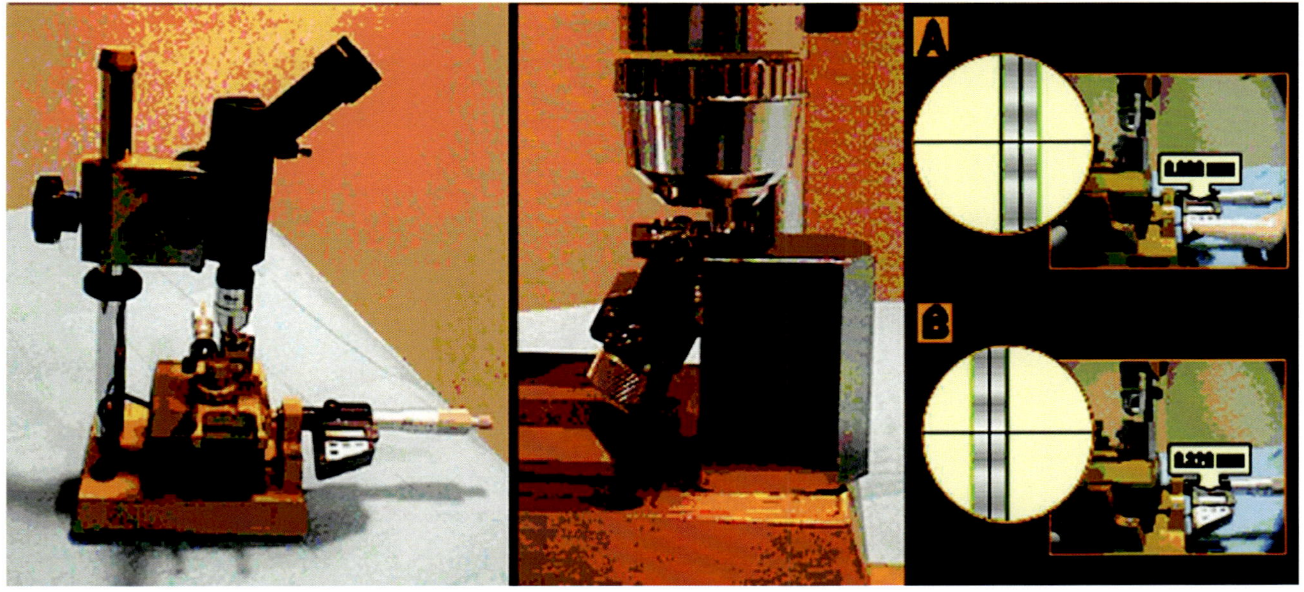

Fig. 46.15: GAP measurement (the distance between the blade and plate correlates with the thickness of the keratectomy). The Magnum Diamond Micron-scope, designed to calibrate the RK knife, is useful for checking and calibrating the microkeratome blade. The microkeratome head, set up with the blade and a 160 µm plate, is placed under the microscope in a vertical position using a specially designed metal holder: (A) Using the microscope's controls, the vertical line on the eye-piece is aligned with the front end of the blade in the image, and the micrometer's digital marker is set at zero; (B) Next, the same line is aligned with the end of the blade in the image and the digital micrometer indicates the measurement in microns. The image observed through the microscope corresponds to the blade and its mirror image, hence the need to divide it by two in order to obtain the blade GAP. In the picture, the micrometer indicates 320 µm and, therefore, the blade GAP is 160 µm

value from the value of the pre-operative pachymetry.

It appears that the newer technologies for creating the flap – like the femtosecond laser – result in greater reproducibility of the flap, thus reducing the risk of iatrogenic ectasias due to exceedingly thick flaps.[32] However, it is fair to say that the femtosecond laser is not free of complications, not to mention its high cost.[33]

Large Ablation

Although in the early years of LASIK surgery people undertook to perform high myopic corrections, poor visual results obtained in some cases and the rapid development of phakic IOLs led to the narrowing of the range of LASIK corrections. Recent studies have suggested that performing LASIK above -8 D is a risk factor for ectasia.[2,22] It has been speculated that the reason why ectasia develops is because the residual stromal bed is inadequate for sustaining the structural integrity of the cornea.[34] A review of the literature points to a higher incidence of post-LASIK iatrogenic ectasia in high corrections where large ablations are performed. However, there are retrospective studies of large series of LASIK in high myopia showing good stability in time when ablation diameters are decreased so as to ensure maximal preservation of the stromal bed thickness.[2,35] Notwithstanding good results, these studies conclude that high myopia has been considered a risk factor for post-LASIK ectasia, although adherence to proper screening and intraoperative pachymetry data appear to decrease the risk. Cases have been reported of ablations greater than 200 µm that went on to develop progressive ectasia, even after having preserved a 250 µm residual bed.[36] In our practice, we tend to leave a residual bed greater than 250 µm and we try to end with a total corneal thickness greater than 400 µm and not to perform ablations greater than 150 µm.

Retreatments

We must be particularly careful with post-LASIK retreatments and be fully aware of corneal thickness limits in order not to be surprised by the development of ectasia after retreating a small residual defect. Before choosing to retreat after LASIK we must ascertain refractive and topographic stability in order to establish the differential diagnosis between undercorrection and regression. Regression is usually the first symptom of ectasia, and a new ablation may accelerate the process. Moreover, it is important to know the available stromal bed and perform intra-operative pachymetry after lifting the flap, in the event that information is not available as part of the clinical history. There are reports[37] of greater corneal stability and a lower risk of ectasia when retreatment of small post-LASIK undercorrections is performed on the stromal surface of the flap. However, it is important to remember that the goal of refractive surgery, regardless of its modality, is not ametropia but greater independence from optical correction. Right patient selection is paramount in order to avoid the need for retreatments and the associated risk of ectasia.

KERATECTASIA TREATMENTS

The treatment for post-LASIK ectasia depends on the stage of the disease and the patient's needs and attitude. We can often suspect subclinical ectasia or post-LASIK ectasic progression when the patient experiences refractive regression with topographic steepening, while still maintainig best corrected visual acuity with spectacles. At that stage, we may suspect a mild regression or early ectasia. External pressure applied on a thin cornea may trigger post-LASIK ectasia, as is the case of patients with chronic persistent eye-rubbing.[9] Patients with keratectasia must be made aware of the importance of not rubbing their eyes if they are to avoid rapid progression of the disease. There is even a report on bilateral ectasia resulting from ocular compression by the air-bag in a car accident.[38] Likewise, the effect of the internal intra-ocular pressure (IOP) on the thin cornea may cause topographic steepening and even transient ectasia when it rises above normal.[39] It has also been shown that when IOP is lowered with medications, even in normotensive patients, there is greater topographic corneal flattening (Fig. 46.16). Treatment with *ocular pressure-lowering medications* is indicated when the first signs of refractive regression and topographic steepening are observed, beside their use as initial treatment for post-LASIK ectasia.[40] Hipotensive drugs stabilize surgically-induced corneal flattening and they even revert small regressions and topographic steepenings. The risk of ectasia could be reduced by maintaining a low IOP in LASIK patients, particularly those undergoing high corrections. In our experience, we have found that it is useful to prescribe topical beta-blockers in post-LASIK regressions with topographic steepening, which is not the case with the use of prostaglandin analogues.

On the other hand, visual acuity is compromised in cases of established ectasia. In very early stages, aside from prescribing ocular pressure-lowering agents, we also prescribe contact lenses or spectacles in order to restore visual acuity. Spectacles do not correct irregular astigmatism, a common finding in this complication, which explains why they do not provide good visual rehabilitation. As a result, the treatment of choice is *contact lense* fitting.[41] Early on, soft contact lenses may be appropriate, particular in central ectasia. However, in more advanced stages, or in cases of paracentral ectasia, the resilient soft contact lens cannot compensate irregular astigmatism and, therefore, a rigid gas permeable contact (RGP) lens is required. RGP lenses allow for an optically regular surface and good visual acuity.[41] Hard-soft combination lenses (a rigid center with a soft annular ring) or piggy-back (a rigid lens placed onto a soft) may be helpful when a RGP lens cannot be tolerated because of discomfort or staining.[42] But contact lens fitting usually is not a satisfactory treatment for patients who elected to undergo surgery in order not to be dependent on their optical correction. Moreover, contact lenses do not prevent the visual deterioration or the progression of the ectasia. In advanced stages there is often intolerance to contact lenses and results tend to be poor.

Penetrating keratoplasty, where the ectasic cornea is replaced with a healthy cornea, would constitute definitive treatment (Fig. 46.17). However, keratoplasty is not free of complications and visual results are not always as expected. For this reason, it is recommended in very advanced stages when

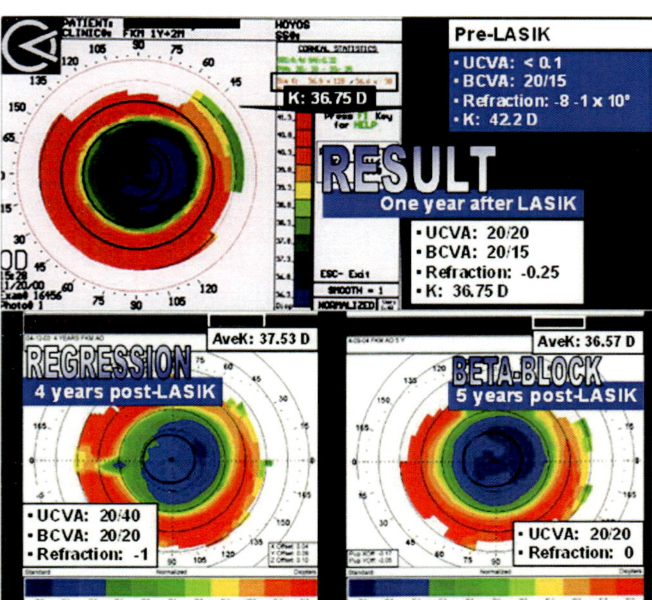

Fig. 46.16: Intermediate myopic patient who presented with refractive regression of –1 D and topographic steepening (from 36.75 D to 37.53 D) 4 years after LASIK. The use of topical beta-blockers for lowering intraocular pressure reduced the refractive error and the topographic steepening (from 37.53 D to 36.57 D), stabilizing the cornea

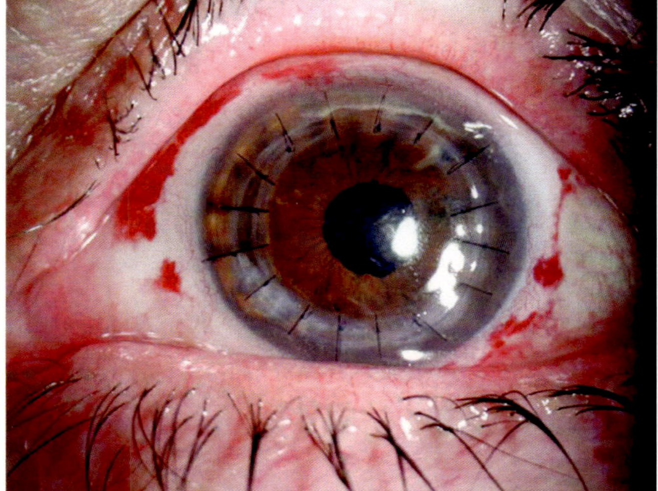

Fig. 46.17: Penetrating keratoplasty after *in situ* keratomileusis

visual results with other forms of treatment are not satisfactory. New treatment options that improve the visual prognosis for these patients have emerged in recent years for not very advanced cases of ectasia. These include crosslinking and intracorneal rings, designed to improve and stabilize the cornea, thus delaying progression and the eventual indication for keratoplasty.[40] On the other hand, the development of lamellar keratoplasty techniques has improved outcomes and prognosis with this procedure when it becomes necessary.[43]

Riboflavin-UVA Crosslinking

Riboflavin and ultraviolet-A (UVA) crosslinking of corneal collagen increases the biomechanical stability of the cornea by inducing additional crosslinking between or within collagen fibers.[44] This treatment produces hardening of the cornea and can arrest, and in some cases partially reverse, the progression of iatrogenic keratectasia after LASIK.[45] The treatment consists of removing the corneal epithelium over the central 8 mm of the cornea and applying riboflavin as photoactivator for approximately 30 minutes (until the aqueous stains yellow from the effect of riboflavin). The cornea is then exposed to a 365 nm UVA light source for 30 minutes while instilling riboflavin at the same time (Fig. 46.18).

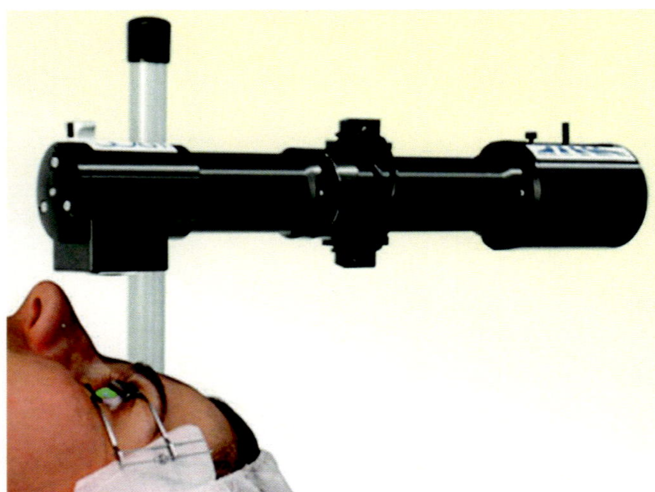

Fig. 46.18: Crosslinking (PESCHKE Meditrade GmbH, Huenenberg—Switzerland)

Pachymetry is crucial in selecting patients, given that this procedure is counterindicated in corneas of less than 400 microns in thickness because it may induce endothelial damage.[46]

Intracorneal Rings

Intra-corneal rings are semicircular PMMA segments placed in the mid periphery of the ectasic cornea in order to flatten the central cornea and re-center the corneal apex (Fig. 46.19). These effects result in refractive improvement because of a lowering of myopia and astigmatism, and also in improvement of visual acuity as a result of the regularization of the corneal surface.[47,48] Considering that ectasia is progressive, the rings are not definitive, but they help improve visual acuity and stabilize the cornea, thus delaying the need for keratoplasty by many years.[49]

There are two types of intracorneal ring segments on the market:

- *Ferrara Ring™* segments (Mediphacos Inc, Belo Horizonte, Brazil): 160° arc length, triangular shape, thicknesses ranging between 150 and 350 microns (50 µm increments); and curvature radius of 4,4 inner and 5,6 mm outer diameters.
- *Intacts™* micro-thin inserts (Addition Technologies LLC, Fremont, CA, USA): 150° arc length, hexagonal cross section, thicknesses ranging between 250 and 450 microns (50 µm increments) and curvature radius of 6,8 inner and 8,1 mm outer diameters.

Results with both implants are similar, but the higher curvature radius of the Intacts reduce ring show and glare, whereas the smaller radius of the Ferrara Ring appears to increase the applanation

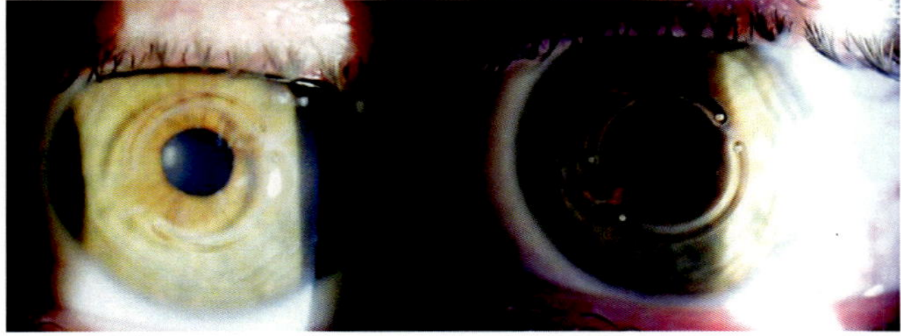

Fig. 46.19: Intracorneal rings in keratectasia

effect, since it is closer to the central cornea.[47,48] The ring-induced effect is directly proportional to the thickness of the ring and inversely proportional to its curvature radius. The larger the thickness and the smaller the diameter of the ring, the higher the induced effect. It is also possible to insert 2 rings, one in the steeper hemicornea and a second mirror ring, either of equal thickness or asymmetrical (the thicker in the steeper hemicornea), or to implant a single ring[51] in the steeper hemicornea. The indication depends on the degree and type of ectasia.

The rings may be inserted deep in the corneal stroma through a corneal tunnel. One of the challenges with this technique is the manual shaping of the corneal tunnel, especially in LASIK patients, considering the potential of entering the interphase during dissection and creating a shallow tunnel. Using the femtosecond laser to make the tunnel renders the technique much easier and does not change the results.[52]

Lamellar Keratoplasty

Long-term graft survival rates and endothelial cell counts after penetrating keratoplasty continue to drop for many years after surgery, clearly showing the disadvantage of unnecessary replacement of healthy endothelium in anterior stromal disorders. Recent developments in anterior lamellar keratoplasty enable targeted replacement of corneal stroma without replacement of endothelium, and include procedures such as deep anterior lamellar keratoplasty, and microkeratome or laser-assisted anterior lamellar surgery.[43]

- The *deep anterior lamellar keratoplasty (DALK)* technique is based on surgical manipulation that allows visualization of the lamellar dissection depth using a posterior approach to reach the predescemetic space. Techniques that use air and ophthalmic viscosurgical devices to directly expose Descemet's membrane have dramatically reduced surgery time. The anterior 80% of the central corneal stroma is replaced by a donor button without Descemet's membrane, and sutured in place.[53,54]
- The development of new artificial chamber models such as automated lamellar therapeutic keratoplasty (ALTK) SystemÒ, Moria, have provided simplicity, precision and accuracy to the *microkeratome-assisted anterior lamellar keratoplasty* (Fig. 46.20).[55] The ALTK system requires a donor cornea with a scleral rim to guarantee proper vacuum during the microkeratome cut. The microkeratome is used to cut partial-thickness sections through the anterior surface of the donor and host corneas. The donor disc is placed on the recipient bed with interrupted sutures (Fig. 46.21).[56]
- *Excimer laser-assisted anterior lamellar keratoplasty* is using to augment thin corneas as corneal ectasia after LASIK. A donor stromal button approximately 350 µm thick received a 100 µm excimer laser ablation on the endothelium. The remaining cornea (epithelium, Bowman's membrane, and stroma) is punched with a 7.5 or 7.7 mm trephine. After transepithelial ablation of the host cornea to 200 µm thickness, the corneal button is sutured with interrupted sutures.[57]

These new forms of surgery are viable alternatives to conventional penetrating keratoplasty

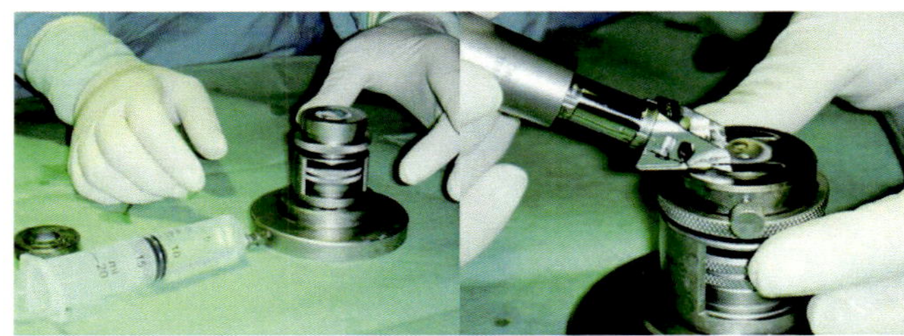

Fig. 46.20: Cutting the donor cornea with the LSK-One microkeratome and the artificial anterior chamber, AAC, Moria (*Courtesy:* Dr. MT Iradier)

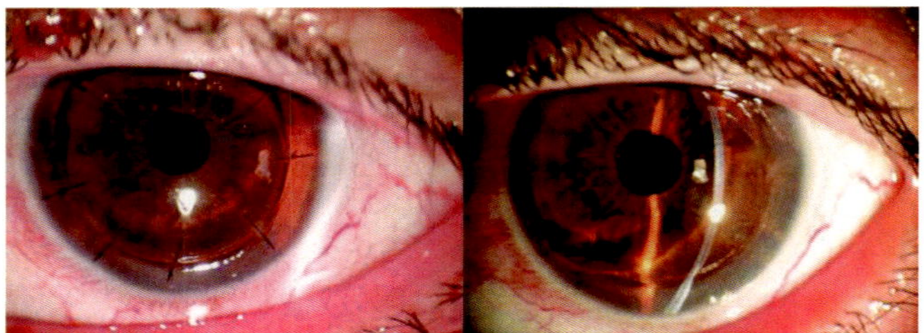

Fig. 46.21: Anterior lamellar keratoplasty in a case of post-LASIK ectasia (*Courtesy:* Dr. MT Iradier)

and bring added safety profiles for long-term visual rehabilitation and restoration of tectonic integrity in corneal ectasia.

REFERENCES

1. Pallikaris IG, Kymionis GD, Astyrakakis NI. Corneal ectasia induced by laser in situ keratomileusis. J Cataract Refract Surg 2001;27(11):1796-802.
2. Condon PI, O'Keefe M, Binder PS. Long-term results of laser in situ keratomileusis for high myopia: risk for ectasia. J Cataract Refract Surg 2007;33(4):583-90.
3. Reinstein DZ, Srivannaboon S, Archer TJ, Silverman RH, Sutton H, Coleman DJ. Probability model of the inaccuracy of residual stromal thickness prediction to reduce the risk of ectasia after LASIK part II: quantifying population risk. J Refract Surg 2006;22(9):861-70.
4. Rad AS, Jabbarvand M, Saifi N. Progressive keratectasia after laser in situ keratomileusis. J Refract Surg 2004;20(5 Suppl):S718-22.
5. Barraquer JI. Complicaciones postoperatorias profilaxis y tratamiento. En: Cirugía refractiva de la cornea. Instituto Barraquer de America, Bogota (Colombia) 1989; 449-50.
6. Nesburn AB, Bahri S, Salz J, Rabinowitz YS, Maguen E, Hofbauer J, Berlin M, Macy JI. Keratoconus detected by videokeratography in candidates for photorefractive keratectomy. J Refract Surg 1995;11(3):194-201.
7. Amsler M. Keratocône classique et keratocône frustre, arguments unitaires. Ophthalmologica 1946;11:96-101.
8. Rabinowitz JS. Keratoconus. Surv Ophthalmol 1998; 42:297-319.
9. Ioannidis AS, Speedwell L, Nischal KK. Unilateral keratoconus in a child with chronic and persistent eye rubbing. Am J Ophthalmol 2005;139(2):356-7.
10. Barraquer RI, De Toledo MC, Torres E. Alteraciones corneales ectasicas. En: Distrofias y degeneraciones corneales. Espaxs Publicaciones Medicas, Bercelona 2004;271.
11. Abad JC, Rubinfeld RS, Del Valle M, Belin MW, Kurstin JM. Vertical D: a novel topographic pattern in some keratoconus suspects. Ophthalmology. 2007;114(5):1020-6.
12. Rabinowitz YS. Videokeratographic indices to aid in screening for keratoconus. J Refract Surg 1995;11:371-9.
13. Seiler T, Quurke AW. Iatrogenic keratectasia after LASIK in a case of forme fruste keratoconus. J Cataract Refract Surg 1998;24(7):1007-9.
14. Lebow KA, Grohe RM. Differentiating contact lens induced warpage from true keratoconus using corneal topography. CLAO J 1999;25(2):114-22.
15. Wilson SE, Lin DT, Klyce SD, Reidy JJ, Insler MS. Topographic changes in contact lens-induced corneal warpage. Ophthalmology. 1990;97(6):734-44.
16. Wang X, McCulley JP, Bowman RW, Cavanagh HD. Time to resolution of contact lens-induced corneal warpage prior to refractive surgery. CLAO J 2002;28(4):169-71.
17. Belin MW, Zloty P. Accuracy of the PAR corneal topography system with spatial misalignment. CLAO J 1993;19(1):64-8.
18. Auffarth GU, Wang L, Volcker HE. Keratoconus evaluation using the Orbscan topography system. J Cataract Refract Surg 2000;26(2):222-8.
19. Rao SN, Raviv T, Majmudar PA, Epstein RJ. Role of Orbscan II in screening keratoconus suspects before refractive corneal surgery. Ophthalmology 2002;109(9):1642-6.
20. Ho JD, Tsai CY, Tsai RJ, Kuo LL, Tsai IL, Liou SW. Validity of the keratometric index: evaluation by the Pentacam rotating Scheimpflug camera. J Cataract Refract Surg 2008;34(1):137-45.
21. Quisling S, Sjoberg S, Zimmerman B, Goins K, Sutphin J. Comparison of Pentacam and Orbscan IIz on posterior curvature topography measurements in keratoconus eyes. Ophthalmology 2006;113(9):1629-32.
22. Binder PS. Analysis of ectasia after laser in situ keratomileusis: risk factors. J Cataract Refract Surg 2007;33(9): 1530-8.
23. Kim SW, Byun YJ, Kim EK, Kim TI. Central corneal thickness measurements in unoperated eyes and eyes after PRK for myopia using Pentacam, Orbscan II, and ultrasonic pachymetry. J Refract Surg 2007;23(9):888-94.
24. Shah S, Laiquzzaman M, Bhojwani R, Mantry S, Cunliffe I. Assessment of the biomechanical properties of the cornea with the ocular response analyzer in normal and keratoconic eyes. Invest Ophthalmol Vis Sci 2007;48(7):3026-31.
25. Rao SN, Epstein RJ. Early onset ectasia following laser in situ keratomileusis: case report and literature review. J Refract Surg 2002;18(2):177-84.
26. Amoils SP, Deist MB, Gous P, Amoils PM. Iatrogenic keratectasia after laser in situ keratomileusis for less than -4.0 to -7.0 diopters of myopia. J Cataract Refract Surg 2000; 26(7):967-77.
27. Seiler T, Koufala K, Richter G. Iatrogenic keratectasia after laser in situ keratomileusis. J Refract Surg 2002;18(2):177-84.
28. Ophthalmic Devices Advisory Panel, Food and Drug Administration. Checklist of information usually submitted in an investigational device exemption (IDE) application for refractive surgery lasers. J Refract Surg 1997;13:579-88.
29. Giledi O, Daya SM. Unexpected flap thickness in laser in situ keratomileusis. J Cataract Refract Surg 1998;14(3):312-7.
30. Buratto L, Brint S, Ferrari M. Surgical instrument. In Buratto L, Brint S (Eds): LASIK: Principles and Techniques. Thorofare, NJ, SLAK Inc 1998; 35-68.
31. Cigales M, Hoyos JE. J. Thin flaps and buttonholes. In Buratto L, Brint S (Eds): Custom LASIK: Surgical Techniques and Complications. Thorofare, NJ, SLAK Inc 2003; 224-5.
32. Kim JH, Lee D, Rhee KI. Flap thickness reproducibility in laser in situ keratomileusis with a femtosecond laser: optical coherence tomography measurement. J Cataract Refract Surg 2008;34(1):132-6.
33. Netto MV, Mohan RR, Medeiros FW, Dupps WJ Jr, Sinha S, Krueger RR, Stapleton WM, Rayborn M, Suto C, Wilson SE. Femtosecond laser and microkeratome corneal flaps: comparison of stromal wound healing and inflammation. J Refract Surg 2007;23(7):667-76.
34. Spadea L, Palmieri G, Mosca L, Fasciani R, Balestrazzi E. Latrogenic keratectasia following laser in situ keratomileusis. J Refract Surg 2002;18(4):475-80.
35. Alio JL, Muftuoglu O, Ortiz D, Perez-Santonja JJ, Artola A, Ayala MJ, Garcia MJ, de Luna GC. Ten-year follow-up of laser in situ keratomileusis for myopia of up to -10 diopters. Am J Ophthalmol 2008;145(1):46-54.

36. Spadea L, Palmieri G, Mosca L, Fasciani R, Balestrazzi E. Iatrogenic keratectasia following laser in situ keratomileusis. J Refract Surg. 2002 Jul-Aug;18(4):475-80.
37. Maldonado MJ, Nieto JC, Diez-Cuenca M, Pinero DP. Posterior corneal curvature changes after undersurface ablation of the flap and in-the-bed LASIK retreatment. Ophthalmology 2006;113(7):1125-33.
38. Mearza AA, Koufaki FN, Aslanides IM. Airbag induced corneal ectasia. Cont Lens Anterior Eye 2007; Oct 25.
39. Toshino A, Uno T, Ohashi Y, Maeda N, Oshika T. Transient keratectasia caused by intraocular pressure elevation after laser in situ keratomileusis. J Cataract Refract Surg 2005; 31(1):202-4.
40. Randleman JB. Post-laser in-situ keratomileusis ectasia: current understanding and future directions. Curr Opin Ophthalmol 2006;17(4):406-12.
41. Eggink FA, Beekhuis WH. Contact lens fitting in a patient with keratectasia after laser in situ keratomileusis. J Cataract Refract Surg 2001;27(7):1119-23.
42. O'donnell C, Welham L, Doyle S. Contact lens management of keratectasia after laser in situ keratomileusis for myopia. Eye Contact Lens 2004;30(3):144-6.
43. Tan DT, Por YM. Current treatment options for corneal ectasia. Curr Opin Ophthalmol 2007;18(4):284-9.
44. Wollensak G, Spoerl E, Seiler T. Riboflavin/ultraviolet-a-induced collagen crosslinking for the treatment of keratoconus. Am J Ophthalmol 2003;135(5):620-7.
45. Hafezi F, Kanellopoulos J, Wiltfang R, Seiler T. Corneal collagen crosslinking with riboflavin and ultraviolet A to treat induced keratectasia after laser in situ keratomileusis. J Cataract Refract Surg 2007;33(12):2035-40.
46. Wollensak G. Crosslinking treatment of progressive keratoconus: new hope. Curr Opin Ophthalmol 2006;17(4):356-60.
47. Lovisolo CF, Fleming JF. Intracorneal ring segments for iatrogenic keratectasia after laser in situ keratomileusis or photorefractive keratectomy. J Refract Surg 2002;18(5):535-41.
48. Kymionis GD, Siganos CS, Kounis G, Astyrakakis N, Kalyvianaki MI, Pallikaris IG. Management of post-LASIK corneal ectasia with Intacs inserts: one-year results. Arch Ophthalmol. 2003;121(3):322-6.
49. Kymionis GD, Tsiklis NS, Pallikaris AI, Kounis G, Diakonis VF, Astyrakakis N, Siganos CS. Long-term follow-up of Intacs for post-LASIK corneal ectasia. Ophthalmology 2006;113(11):1909-17
50. Sharma M, Boxer Wachler BS. Comparison of single-segment and double-segment Intacs for keratoconus and post-LASIK ectasia. Am J Ophthalmol. 2006;141(5):891-5.
51. Pokroy R, Levinger S, Hirsh A. Single Intacs segment for post-laser in situ keratomileusis keratectasia. J Cataract Refract Surg 2004;30(8):1685-95.
52. Carrasquillo KG, Rand J, Talamo JH. Intacs for keratoconus and post-LASIK ectasia: mechanical versus femtosecond laser-assisted channel creation. Cornea 2007;26(8):956-62.
53. Villarrubia A, Perez-Santonja JJ, Palacin E, Rodriguez-Ausin P P, Hidalgo A. Deep anterior lamellar keratoplasty in post-laser in situ keratomileusis keratectasia. J Cataract Refract Surg 2007;33(5):773-8.
54. Shimmura S, Tsubota K. Deep anterior lamellar keratoplasty. Curr Opin Ophthalmol 2006;17(4):349-55.
55. Behrens A, Dolorico A, Kara DT, Novick LH, McDonnell PJ, Chao LC, Wellik SR, Chuck RS. Precision and accuracy of an artificial chamber system in obtaining corneal lenticules for lamellar keratoplasty. J Cataract Refract Surg 2001; 27(10):1679-87.
56. Busin M, Zambianchi L, Arffa RC. Microkeratome-Assisted lamellar keratoplasty for the surgical treatment of keratoconus. Ophthalmology 2005;112(6):987-97.
57. Bilgihan K, Ozdek SC, Sari A, Hasanreisoglu B. Excimer laser-assisted anterior lamellar keratoplasty for keratoconus, corneal problems after laser in situ keratomileusis, and corneal stromal opacities. J Cataract Refract Surg 2006; 32(8): 1264-9.

47 Diffuse Lamellar Keratitis

Jaime Javaloy, Vanessa Pongo, Jorge L Alió

INTRODUCTION

Diffuse lamellar keratitis is a multietiologic syndrome characterized by an inflammatory reaction confined to the interface of eyes operated by LASIK surgery which appears during the first week after surgery.[1-3]

In 1998, Smith and Maloney published 13 cases belonging to 12 patients who presented diffuse multifocal infiltrates between the 2nd and 6th day after LASIK limited at the interface without anterior or posterior extension and accompanied with pain, photophobia, red eye and tearing. All cases disappeared without sequels after being treated with antibiotics or fluormetholone (Fig. 47.1).[1]

Several terms had been used for this entity: "Sahara's Sands Syndrome (SSS)" due to the granulated and undulated pattern, "PostLASIK Interface's Keratitis (PLIK)", "Non Specific and Diffuse Interstitial Keratitis (NSDIK)" and "Diffuse Intralamellar Keratitis (DIK)". However, DLK is the most employed term when referring this disease.[2]

The reported prevalence of DLK varies in different papers with values ranging between 0.4 percent and 2 percent.[4,6]

In this chapter we will overview this topic considering the physiopathology, treatment and prophylactic measures of DLK and our experience when managing this entity.

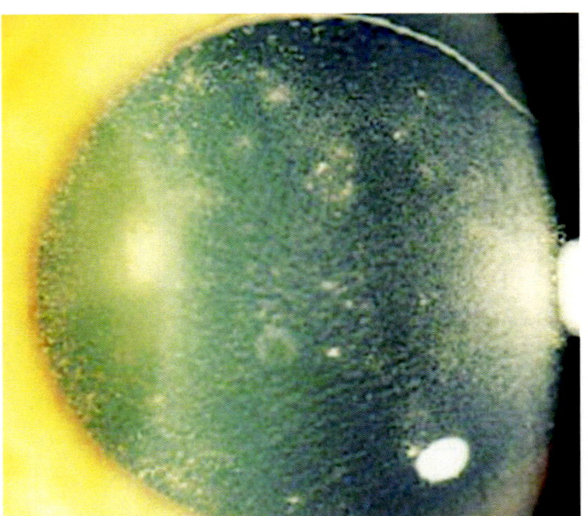

Fig. 47.1: DLK 2 day postlasik[1]

ETIOLOGY

There have been many factors involved in the genesis of DLK, bacterial endotoxin being one of the most demonstrated agents in different clinical and experimental studies.[3-5,7]

The main related causes of DLK are:

Outer Agents

Metallic particles were initially related with the origin of the syndrome, but later studies did not confirm any inflammatory reaction around these kinds of particles when they were inserted at the interface of operated rabbits. On the other hand, the authors of this paper suggest a more possible implication of plastic particles.[8]

The presence of rests of detergents as palmolive ultra 100 percent, klenzyme 100 percent or sterilizing substances as glutaraldehyde in the instruments, either lubricant oils in the blade of microkeratome have been proposed.[2,3,6,10]

Associated Conditions

It has been described a greater risk of DLK for atopic patient, even under antihistaminic treatment.[11]

Meibomial secretions and exotoxins of S. aureus present in patients suffering chronic blepharitis have been associated to DLK, because the powerful of these toxins to promote lymphocyte T activation and inflammatory response. For such reasons strict cleaning of the edge of the lids must be recommended before surgery.[10,12]

Epithelial Defects

A strong association between DLK and intraoperative epithelial defect has been reported, with increases in the risk of suffering the disease among 13 and 24 times regarding eyes with undamaged epithelium.[3,13,14]

Endotoxin

Many studies have been carried out in models of animals and has reported cases of DLK cluster associated definitely with a bacterial endotoxin.[7]

Holland concluded that clusters DLK are related to endotoxin releases of biofilms gram negative in sterilization reservoirs, the endotoxins can survive short sterilization cycles of steam sterilizers as Burkholderia pickettii[4] (Fig. 47.2).

Asano Kato et al examine at immunohistochemical level the corneal reaction, after deposition of lipolysaccharides LPS released by gram negative bacteria in the interface made in rabbit eyes. They found high infiltration of neutrophils and IL8. The inmunoreactivity for IL8 was observed only in corneas with sever inflammation.[16]

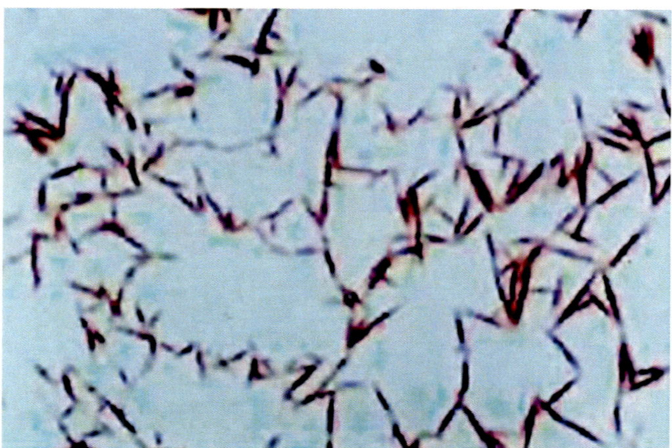

Fig. 47.2: Burkholderia pickettii aislated of a reservoirs[4]

Villarubia et al reported 188 cases of DLK isolated from the reservoirs and silicone tubes connected to the autoclave Sphingomona paucimobilis y Burkholderia pickettii both belong to the same family of aerobic gram negative bacilli, catalase positive and nonfermentative.[5]

Others

We reported the case of a patient with DLK after LASIK with intralase and presented corneal melting and hypermetropic change. The patient was treated with steroids. We decided to alter the parameters used in the intralase to make a reduction in the levels of energy to prevent some new cases[15] (Fig. 47.3).

CLASSIFICATION

- Linebarger et al (1999), proposed four stages of clinical classification taking into account the severity and location of the lamellar interface inflammation[2] (Fig. 47.4).[2]

  Stage 1: Presence of white granular infiltrates in the periphery of the flap outside the visual axis. The frequency of this form is 1 in 25-50 cases.

  Stage 2: Visual axis is affected. The frequency is 1 in 200 cases.

  Stage 3: Infiltrate appeared more condensed in the visual axis, this is often associated with a decline in visual acuity by 1or 2 lines. The frequency is 1 in 500 cases.

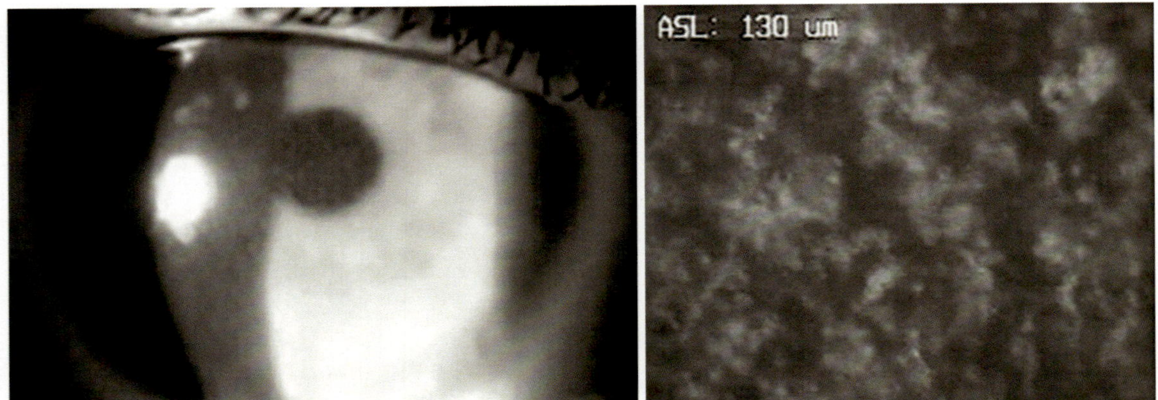

Fig. 47.3: Patient of our center with infiltrate in cornea central and confocal microscopical examination after surgery[15]

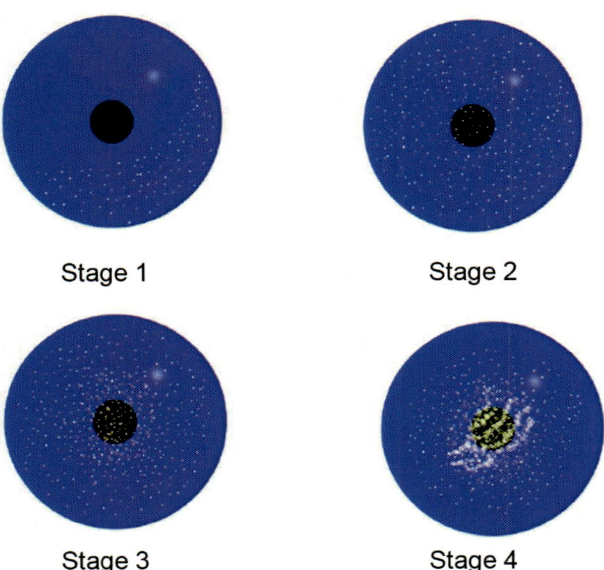

Fig. 47.4: Classification proposed by Linebarger[2]

Stage 4: Severe lamellar keratitis with stromal melting due to release collagenases results in stromal volume loss and a hyperopic shift. The incidence is approximately 1 in 5000 cases.

- Jonson and coauthors proposed a new classification (2000) based on the extent of centripetal migration of inflammatory cells and if the occurrence is sporadic or cluster.[3]

Type I It was designated as center sparing and subdivided into:
IA Sporadic
IB Cluster
An association between epithelial defects and DLK especially type I appears to exist.

Type II Involves the visual axis and subdivided into:
IIA Sporadic
IIB Cluster
The occurrence of clusters is an important factor when managing DLK. Type IIB is associated with a greater risk of visual loss and it is strongly associated to endotoxins.[3]

- Bühren and coauthors proposed stage 4 classification based on confocal microscopy in relation to the findings under slit-lamp. With this technology we can study the resulting inflammatory activity[17] (Fig. 47.5) (Table 47.1).

DIFFERENTIALS DIAGNOSIS

Epithelial Ingrowth

When Smith and Maloney published the first report, they recommended to differ DLK from epithelial ingrowth.[1]

Table 47.1: Characteristic features based on slit-lamp and confocal microscopy

DLK stage	*Slitlamp characteristics*	*Confocal microscopio characteristics*
1	Infiltrate in the periphery, sparing the center	Granulocytes and monocytes in the anterior stroma and the flap interface
2	Infiltrate involves the center	Granulocytes and monocytes in the anterior stroma and the interface involvement of the central cornea, spindle shaped structures mostly in dense infiltrates
3	Infiltrate more condensed at the corneal center	Accumulation of decayed inflammatory cells in the flap interface, spindle shaped structures
4	Folds, stromal opacity	No inflammatory cells detectable, microfolds and activated keratocytes at the interface.

Epithelial ingrowth become apparent weeks after the surgery and usually without pain. The opacity often appears as a colection of small, discrete white cysts at the flap edge.

Central Flap Necrosis

Recently Hainline y col (2007) published 9 cases of central flap necrosis, after LASIK with microkeratome and femtosecond laser. Central lamellar flap necrosis to differ from DLK at the location of stromal inflammation is not in the flap interface rather in the flap anterior stroma. Treatment with corticosteroids seemed to have little effect on the outcomes. The irrigation under the flap was associated in some cases with a decrease in inflammation. It usually causes a temporary hyperopic shift which regresses in most patients.[18]

During the evolution of this disease, we can see the "Mercedes-Benz sign" (Fig. 47.6) which was named by Marc Mullie Y Gordon Belazy, where inflammatary product lines are formed at various angles within the area of the flap, this disease is present without pain.

Therefore, the authors concluded that the central necrosis of the flap appears to be a separate entity from DLK, presumably due to other causes as of rests of detergents used as cidex and it does not appear to have profound visual morbidity although it can lead to some visual loss.

TREATMENT

For stage 1 and 2 as Linebarger recommended the administration of topical steroids as prednisolone acetate 1 percent hourly and dexamethasone 1 percent ointment at night, with a control at 24 and 48 hours to assess improvements or progression of the disease and subsequently decreased frequency of application.

In case of stage irrigation of the bed and the undersurface of the flap with balanced salt solution BSS with the target of removing remnants of

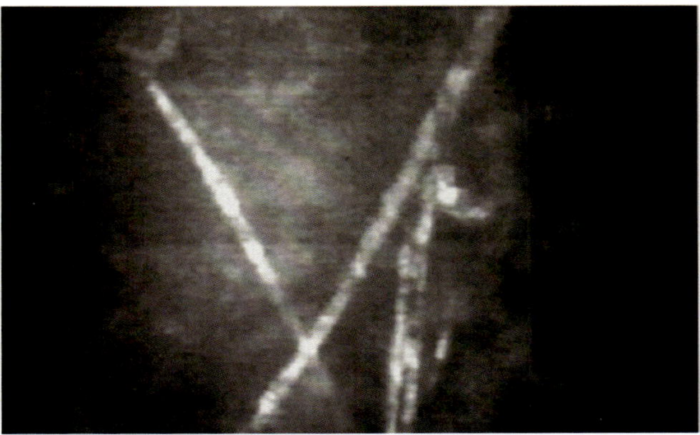
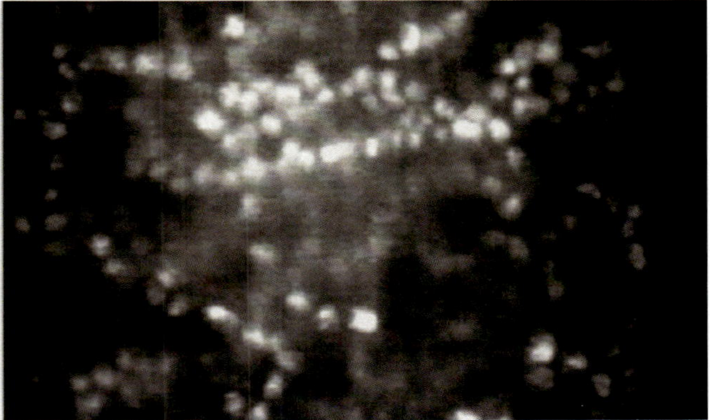

Fig. 47.5: Stage 2 under confocal microscopy to the left spindle shaped bodies and to the right clusters of granulocytes in the interface[17]

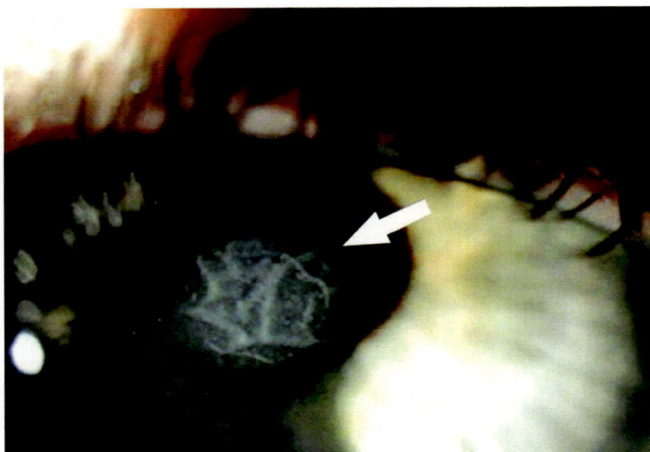

Fig. 47.6: Mercedes Benz sign[18]

inflammatory cells and lifting the flap is recommended. The irrigation of flap must be done gently, an aggressive intervention is not recommended to avoid generating more response Inflammatory Worsening trends. This treatment with the application of topical steroids is indicated.[3,5]

Some authors suggest in stage 4 the irrigation and lifting the flap, but we share the view that in a case like this it is better to only treat with drugs due the possibility of an increase in the loss of stromal volume. Continuous and intensive treatment with topical steroids have led to the end best corrected visual acuity of even 20/25.[5] Hoffman and Fine standardized as a treatment for stage 3 the use of topical and systemic corticosteroids indicating Prednisolone between 40 to 80 mg per day reducing doses as improvement to 20 to 30 mg/day, they do not recommend treating the flap.[21]

RECOMMENDATIONS

Due to the identification of Endotoxins as one of the main etiological factors of DLK, different sterilization protocols allows us a better control and reduction of the incidence of DLK.[4-7,9,19,20]

Yuhan demonstrated with the implementation of new cleaning and sterilization protocols of instrumental and draining the reservoirs after every surgical day reduce the incidence from a 11 to 2 percent. Holland reports similar decreases.[4,6]

Endotoxins survive short sterilization cycles of steam sterilizers, they can resist temperatures of 120 centigrade grades for up to 1 hour periods. The use of contaminated instruments during surgery could introduce endotoxin in interface, thus initiating a sterile keratitis in susceptible individuals.[6]

Therefore, we recommend:

1. A cleaning and sterilization of instruments without scanting in economic investment or time.
2. After the cleaning of instruments with brush and appropriate enzymatic detergents with neutral pH and not corrosive as DAROSCOPE, should be rinsed with distilled water, then proceed with drying and compressed later on to pack and to take to STATIM with an appropriate chemical control.
3. Regarding the STATIM, a daily control should be made at the end of each surgical session. The reservoirs should be evacuated and mechanically scrubed and then filled with isopropyl alcohol 70 percent for one hour, and finally dried with air. A strict biological control is very important to determine possible colonies. All the instruments should enter the cassette accompanied by a chemical control strip.
4. A biological control is also recommended for the long cycle sterilization in the autoclave.
5. We recommended to change it when it is necessary and according to biological controls, the silicone tubes between the reservoirs and the autoclave.

All these measures has been adopted by our center with the purpose of diminishing maximum DLK incidence.[4-7,9,19,20]

Finally, after reviewing the possible causes it is recommended to carry out surgeries in an atraumatic manner, in order to avoid epithelial defects which can cause the appearance of such conditions.

CONCLUSIONS

DLK is a multietiological condition. Therefore, all investigations or reports will contribute to a better understanding of this pathology. The surgeons should try to minimize the risks for its occurrence based on our recommended atraumatic procedure and to work with the appropriate sterilization measures.

REFERENCES

1. Smith RJ, Maloney RK. Diffuse lamellar keratitis. A new syndrome in lamellar refractive surgery. Ophthalmology. 1998;105(9):1721-6.
2. Linebarger EJ, Hardten DR, Lindstrom R. Diffuse lamellar keratitis: diagnosis and management. J Cataract Refract Surg 2000;26(7):1072-7.
3. Johnson JD, Harissi-Dagher M, Pineda R, Yoo S, Azar DT. Diffuse lamellar keratitis: incidence, associations, outcomes, and a new classification system. J Cataract Refract Surg 2001;27(10):1560-6.
4. Holland SP, Mathias RG, Morck DW, Chiu J, Slade SG. Diffuse lamellar keratitis related to endotoxins released from sterilizer reservoir biofilms. Ophthalmology 2000; 107(7):1227-33; discussion 1233-4.
5. Villarrubia A, Palacín E, Gómez del Río M, Martínez P. Description, etiology, and prevention of an outbreak of diffuse lamellar keratitis after LASIK. J Refract Surg 2007;23(5):482-6.
6. Yuhan KR, Nguyen L, Wachler BS. Role of instrument cleaning and maintenance in the development of diffuse lamellar keratitis. Ophthalmology 2002;109(2):400-3.
7. Peters NT, Iskander NG, Anderson Penno EE, Woods DE, Moore RA, Gimbel HV. Diffuse lamellar keratitis: isolation of endotoxin and demonstration of the inflammatory potential in a rabbit laser in situ keratomileusis model. J Cataract Refract Surg 2001;27(6):917-23.
8. Bissen-Miyajima H, Minami K, Miyake-Kashima M, Taira Y, Nakamura M. Observation of the corneal flap interface with metal particles in a rabbit model. J Cataract Refract Surg 2005;31(7):1409-13.
9. American Society of Cataract and Refractive Surgery; American Society of Ophthalmic Registered Nurses. Recommended practices for cleaning and sterilizing intraocular surgical instruments. J Cataract Refract Surg. 2007;33(6):1095-100.
10. Holzer MP, Solomon KD, Vroman DT, Vargas LG, Sandoval HP, Kasper TJ, et al. Diffuse lamellar keratitis: evaluation of etiology, histopathologic findings, and clinical implications in an experimental animal model. J Cataract Refract Surg 2003;29(3):542-9.
11. Boorstein SM, Henk HJ, Elner VM. Atopy: a patient-specific risk factor for diffuse lamellar keratitis. Ophthalmology 2003;110(1):131-7.
12. Fogla R, Rao SK, Padmanabhan P. Diffuse lamellar keratitis: are meibomian secretions responsible? J Cataract Refract Surg 2001;27(4):493-5.
13. Shah MN, Misra M, Wihelmus KR, Koch DD. Diffuse lamellar keratitis associated with epithelial defects after laser in situ keratomileusis. J Cataract Refract Surg 2000;26(9):1312-8.
14. Sachdev N, McGhee CN, Craig JP, Weed KH, McGhee JJ. Epithelial defect, diffuse lamellar keratitis, and epithelial ingrowth following post-LASIK epithelial toxicity. J Cataract Refract Surg 2002;28(8):1463-6.
15. Javaloy J, Artola A, Vidal MT, Muñoz G, de Rojas V, Alió JL. Severe diffuse lamellar keratitis after femtosecond lamellar keratectomy. Br J Ophthalmol 2007;91(5):699.
16. Asano-Kato N, Toda I, Shimmura S, Noda-Tsuruya T, Fukagawa K, Yoshinaga M, Matsukawa A, et al. Detection of neutrophils and possible involvement of interleukin-8 in diffuse lamellar keratitis after laser in situ keratomileusis. J Cataract Refract Surg 2003;29(10):1996-2000.
17. Bühren J, Baumeister M, Cichocki M, Kohnen T. Confocal microscopic characteristics of stage 1 to 4 diffuse lamellar keratitis after laser in situ keratomileusis. J Cataract Refract Surg 2002;28(8):1390-9.
18. Hainline BC, Price MO, Choi DM, Price FW Jr. Central flap necrosis after LASIK with microkeratome and femtosecond laser created flaps. J Refract Surg 2007;23(3): 233-42.
19. Whitby JL, Hitchins VM. Endotoxin levels in steam and reservoirs of table-top steam sterilizers. J Refract Surg. 2002;18(1):51-7.
20. Bigham M, Enns CL, Holland SP, Buxton J, Patrick D, Marion S, et al. Diffuse lamellar keratitis complicating laser in situ keratomileusis. J Cataract Refract Surg 2005;31(12):2340-4.
21. Hoffman RS, Fine IH, Packer M. Incidence and outcomes of lasik with diffuse lamellar keratitis treated with topical and oral corticosteroids. J Cataract Refract Surg 2003; 29(3):451-6.

48 Diffuse Lamellar Keratitis: Making the Correct Diagnosis and Preventing Treatment Errors

Ronald J Smith

DEFINITION AND DESCRIPTION

Diffuse lamellar keratitis (DLK) is a syndrome of cellular inflammation within the cornea in patients who have undergone LASIK or other forms of lamellar corneal surgery. It was also called Sands of the Sahara Syndrome by the visual imagery evoked by the appearance on slit lamp examination.[1] I chose the name diffuse lamellar keratitis with Robert Maloney in order to highlight the three most important clinical signs of the condition.[2] The syndrome is characterized by fine inflammatory infiltrates diffusely scattered in the interface between the surgically created stromal flap and the underlying corneal stromal bed. Early cases can be detected by looking for the fine infiltrates near the flap edge using the scleral scatter technique of slit lamp examination or using the contrast against the darkness at the pupil margin (Fig. 48.1). There is little or no conjunctival inflammation and no discharge. The ocular surface is intact. Typically there is no epithelial defect, or if one occurred during surgery, it has already healed. There is no anterior chamber reaction nor endothelial keratic precipitates. The inflammation respects the boundaries of the flap without posterior extension into the bed nor anterior extension into the flap, nor extension peripherally beyond the flap margin.

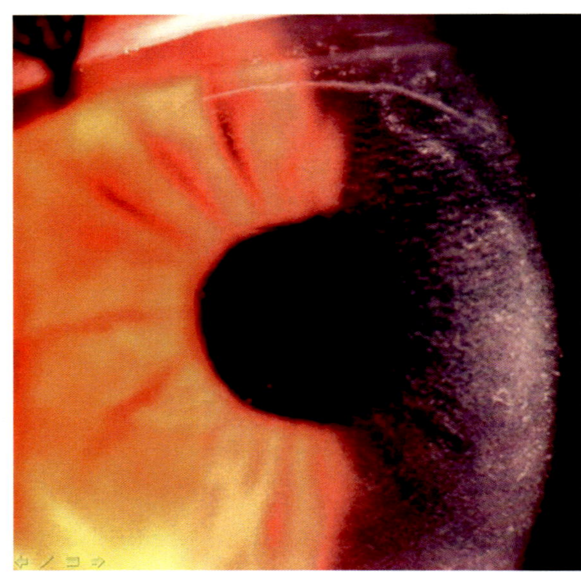

Fig. 48.1: DLK in a 44 yo M 3 days after LASIK (performed in 1995 when astigmatic keratotomy, AK, was performed under the flap to correct astigmatism). Fine granular punctate infiltrates are diffusely scattered in the lamellar interface. Smith RJ, Maloney RK. Diffuse Lamellar Keratitis: A new syndrome in lamellar refractive surgery. Ophthalmology 1998; 105:1721-1726

The case in (Fig. 48.2) illustrates both the diffuse scattering of inflammatory cells best seen along the pupil margin and the localization of the infiltrates to the lamellar interface. The patient was a 33 yrs M with anisometropic amblyopia in the right eye who underwent LASIK in 1995. A preoperative refraction of –9.50+2.00 × 080 corrected his vision to 20/40. His refraction in the left eye was –1.50+2.00. × 180 with an acuity of 20/15. The postoperative regimen at the time included topical antibiotics (ofloxacin qid) but did not include corticosteroids. On the first postop day, there were no infiltrates. The patient presented the next day with eye pain and diffuse infiltrates (Fig. 48.2). The epithelial surface was intact. The infiltrates were confined to the lamellar interface with neither anterior, nor posterior, nor peripheral extension. An astigmatic keratotomy incision which had been performed under LASIK flap was relatively spared. There were no keratic precipitates, and there was no anterior chamber reaction.

Linebarger and coworkers published a clinical staging system to describe the severity of DLK.[3] Stage 1 is defined as a diffuse scattering of fine infiltrates in the periphery of the flap interface outside of the visual axis. In Stage 2, the diffuse interface infiltrates are also seen within the visual axis involving the center of the flap interface. In Stage 3, there is some clumping of the interface infiltrates in addition to the diffuse infiltrates involving the visual axis. In stage 4 there is an increased density of the interface infiltrates forming several roughly parallel curves which may appear like waves.

Within stage 4 DLK, they also described a rare syndrome of central haze extending into the stromal bed, flattening with hyperopia and deep stromal folds which persist long after the infiltrates are gone. This syndrome probably represents a sequelae of DLK or an unrelated comorbidity following surgery, but should not be called DLK, since the three primary characteristics of diffuse lamellar keratitis are absent or not prominent as the syndrome of haze, hyperopia and folds. Figure 48.3 is a composite of the slit-lamp photograph and topography of the condition showing the flattening and folds. The appearance, management and probably the mechanism of the syndrome of central haze, hyperopia and folds are so different from diffuse lamellar keratitis that a different name should be used. The syndrome has been called central focal interface opacity,[4] central flap necrosis,[5] and central toxic keratopathy (CTK).[6] In this chapter, the triad of central haze, hyperopia and folds will be referred to as central toxic keratopathy.

SOURCES OF DIAGNOSTIC ERROR

DLK is an acute inflammatory condition which occurs within the first day after lamellar corneal surgery or after an injury in a patient who previously had lamellar corneal surgery. The differential diagnosis for DLK is listed in Table 48.1. The most devastating complications of diagnostic errors regarding DLK are to miss infectious

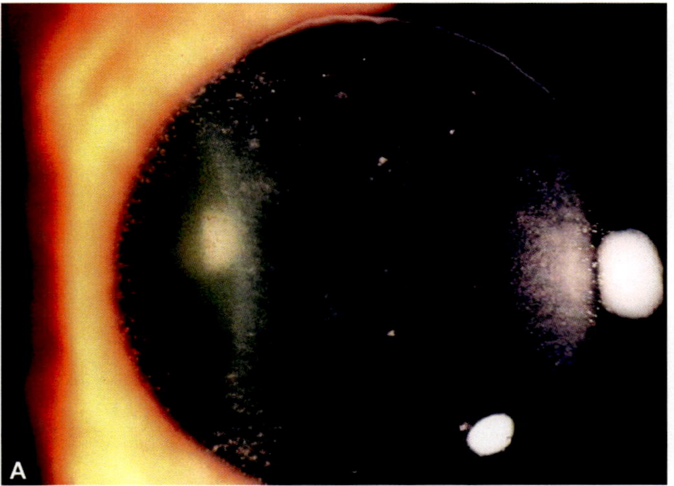

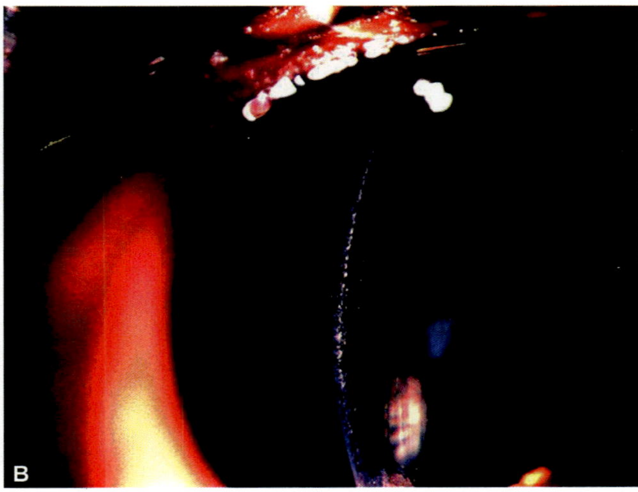

Fig. 48.2: DLK in a 33 years M 2 days after LASIK (combined with AK under the flap) (A) Fine infiltrates are diffusely scattered through the interface and best seen at the pupillary margin (B) Slit-lamp exam localizes the pathology to the flap interface. Smith RJ, Maloney RK. Diffuse Lamellar Keratitis: A new syndrome in lamellar refractive surgery. Ophthalmology 1998; 105:1721-1726

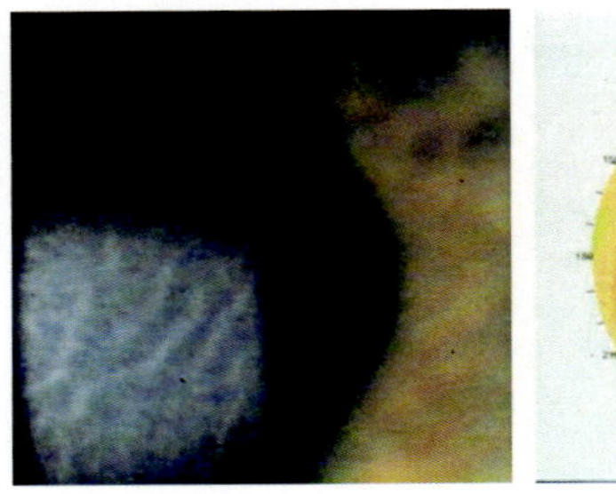

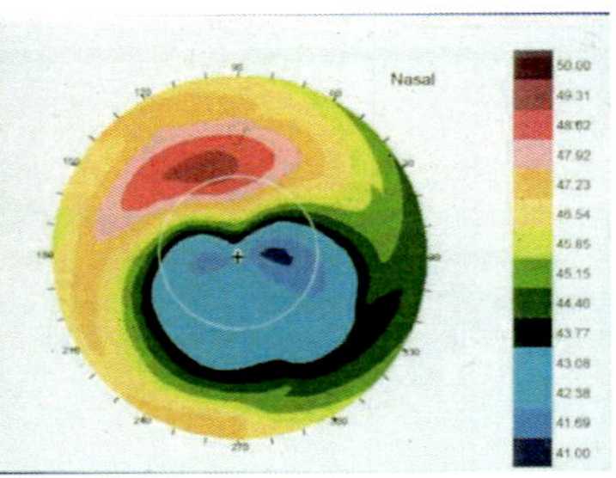

Fig. 48.3: Central haze, hyperopia and folds. Central Toxic Keratopathy after DLK. Corneal flattening with hyperopia on topography and central haze and folds on slit lamp exam. Corneal stromal healing takes the course of months to years like PRK haze. Courtesy of Dr. David R. Hardten and Dr. Richard Lindstrom

keratitis, leading to corneal ulceration with scarring or perforation, or to treat patients with inappropriately long courses of corticosteroid causing subsequent visual field loss from corticosteroid induced glaucoma.

In the first day or two following surgery or injury, acute infectious keratitis, superficial punctate keratopathy, and interface debris are in the differential diagnosis. Over subsequent days to weeks, mycobacterial keratitis, fungal keratitis, central toxic keratopathy, interface fluid, and epithelial ingrowth should also be considered.

Acute infectious keratitis must be differentiated from DLK. In contrast to DLK, a case of post LASIK infectious keratitis is shown in Figure 48.4.[7] There is prominent conjunctival hyperemia and discharge. The tear film breaks up over a rough irregular epithelial defect overlying a prominent, dense, focal infiltrate which extends anteriorly to the surface, posteriorly into the stromal bed and may extend peripherally beyond the flap edge. The infiltrate does not respect the boundaries of the interface. In the case depicted, a keratotomy incision from prior RK was also involved (Fig. 48.4). An anterior chamber reaction is present. Keratic precipitates on the endothelium, and a hypopyon may also be present. Management for infectious keratitis includes intensive topical antibiotics, flap lift, culture and interface irrigation with antibiotics. Management strategies for infectious keratitis following LASIK are presented in this textbook by Amar Agarwal in his chapter *Post-LASIK Infections*.

Table 48.1: Differential Diagnosis for Diffuse Lamellar Keratitis

1. Acute infectious keratitis
2. Superficial punctate keratitis
3. Interface debris
   a. Meibomian gland secretions
   b. Metallic or other foreign bodies
4. Mycobacterial or fungal keratitis
5. Central toxic keratopathy
6. Interface fluid
7. Epithelial ingrowth

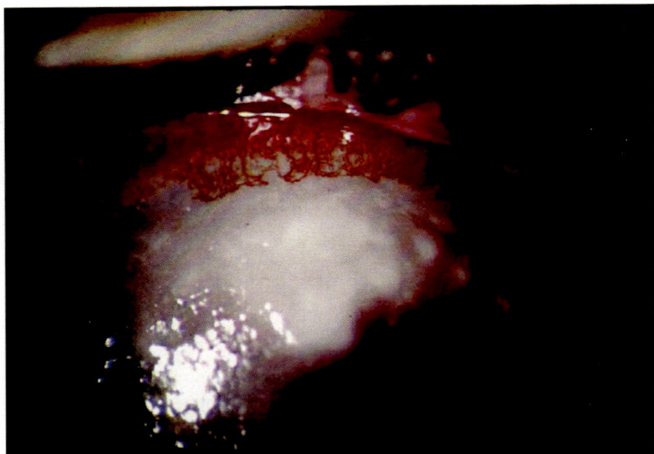

Fig. 48.4: *Staph. aureus* infection after LASIK. Dominant focus with extension anteriorly, posteriorly and peripherally. The infiltrate does not respect the flap margins. Redness and irritation were present on the first postoperative day, and fluffy white infiltrates appeared on the second day after LASIK. (Photographed 2 weeks postoperatively) Hovanesian JA, Faktorovich EG, Hoffbauer JD, Shah SS, Maloney RK. Bilateral bacterial keratitis after laser in situ keratomileusis in a patient with human immunodeficiency virus infection. Arch Ophthalmol. 1999 Jul;117(7):968-70

The diffuse pattern of superficial punctate keratopathy may resemble the pattern of DLK, but a drop of topical fluorescein should localize the pathology of punctate keratopathy to the surface and not the interface. Punctate keratopathy responds to dry eye management.

Meibomian secretions deposited along the interface can be distinguished from DLK by a history of intraoperative findings of oily tear secretion during the procedure and by postoperative slit lamp appearance of a well demarcated area of focal or frothy translucent debris in the interface.

Metallic foreign bodies, for example from a microkeratome blade, can be distinguished by their bright reflectivity. They are usually well tolerated.

Epithelial ingrowth may also present as opacities in the interface most concentrated toward the flap edge several days to weeks after LASIK. It can be thought of as a fistulous tract growing in from the flap edge. The time frame of epithelial ingrowth is usually slower than DLK. In a case series of 43 eyes with epithelial ingrowth, by Wang and Maloney, the ingrowth was detected at 1 month in 78 percent cases and in 2 months in 11 percent, and in 1 patient the ingrowth was not apparent until 5 months postoperatively. It first may appear as clear ovoids of variable sizes which then become increasingly opaque without inflammation. In advance of the pearly ovoid opacities, a faint demarcation line is present which reveals the full extent of the ingrowth (Fig. 48.5). Surgical removal of the ingrowth is indicated if it is approaching the visual axis, inducing astigmatism or glare, or if it is causing surface irritation or necrosis.[8]

Infectious keratitis from mycobacterial or fungal organisms may present a few weeks after LASIK.[9-11] A history of an intensive course of corticosteroids is often reported, and may well be promoting or accelerating the condition. The interface may have diffusely scattered fine infiltrates, but there will also be a dominant focus or multiple foci. The focal infiltrates may be soft and globular or rough and granular (Figs 48.6 and 48.7).

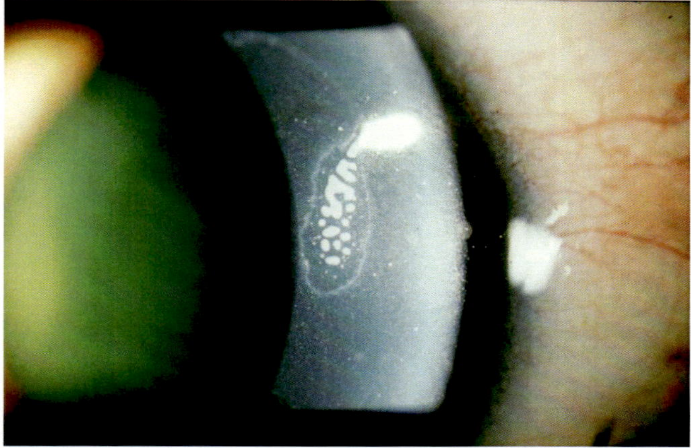

Fig. 48.5: Epithelial ingrowth from the flap edge. A demarcation line is seen at the edge of the ingrowth. In this eye, epithelial pearls are also prominently visible. Wang MY, Maloney RK. Epithelial ingrowth after laser in situ keratomileusis. Am J Ophthalmol. 2000 Jun;129(6):746-51

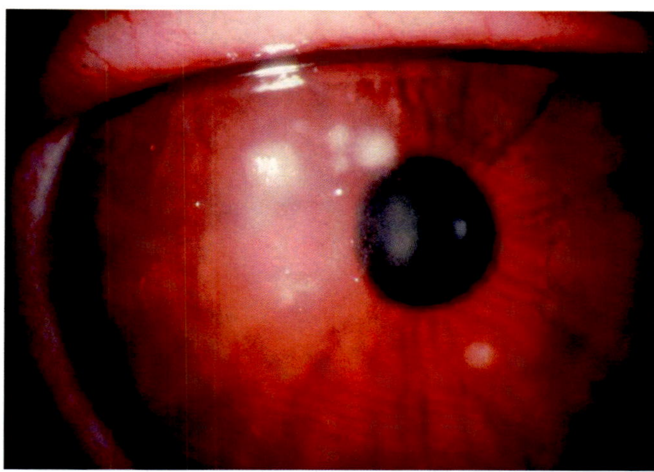

Fig. 48.6: Mycobacterial keratitis 20 days after LASIK. Focal round corneal opacities at the interface. History was positive for intense topical and oral prednisone for DLK during the first postoperative week, and the patient was on a corticosteroid taper at the time of presentation. Chandra NS, Torres MF, Winthrop KL, Bruckner DA, Heidemann DG, Calvet HM, Yakrus M, Mondino BJ, Holland GN. Cluster of *Mycobacterium chelonae* keratitis cases following laser in-situ keratomileusis. Am J Ophthalmol. 2001 Dec;132(6):819-30

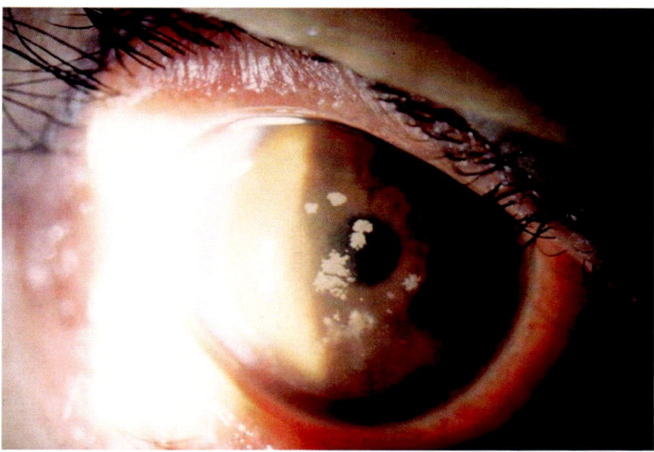

Fig. 48.7: Multiple focal intrastromal infiltrates 49 days after LASIK. The patient was receiving a long course of topical corticosteroids and already had undergone a flap lift with antibiotic and corticosteroid irrigation of the interface 3 weeks earlier. A 1 mm diameter flap perforation in the inferior mid peripheral cornea and epithelial ingrowth were also present. Ultimately required flap removal and cultures grew *Mycobacterium fortuitum*. Seo KY, Lee JB, Lee K, Kim MJ, Choi KR, Kim EK. Non-tuberculous mycobacterial keratitis at the interface after laser in situ keratomileusis. J Refract Surg. 2002 Jan-Feb;18(1):81-5

Central toxic keratopathy is a rare complication of LASIK presenting as a triad of central stromal haze, deep stromal folds and flattening with hyperopia (Fig. 48.8). The largest and most detailed clinical description of the condition has been published by Sonmez and Maloney. The condition presents 3-9 days after LASIK and is usually preceded by DLK, but persists for months after the infiltrates are gone. The central haze and folds extend posteriorly into the stromal bed. The pathology is not confined to the interface. The haze and scarring are most prominent in the area of greatest laser treatment which led them to postulate that the etiology is related to the laser-corneal interaction. After several months to a year or more, the haze clears and the refraction stabilizes-sometimes achieving the patient's refractive goal after a long period of hyperopia. In others, the refraction is stable and amenable to further laser treatment. If flap folds persist and are causing irregular astigmatism along with negative fluorescein staining, the flap can be lifted and smoothened after the haze has subsided. Lindstrom found that the patients who had the best outcomes were those who refused early surgical intervention. He had 3 patients whose haze cleared, and hyperopia and irregular astigmatism resolved over the course of several years in a manner similar to patients with PRK haze.[12] Importantly, the condition does not respond to corticosteroid treatment, and a pitfall of misdiagnosis is long term corticosteroids causing steroid induced glaucoma.

Steroid induced glaucoma can usually be detected by measuring an elevation of intraocular pressure (IOP) on standard Goldman applanation, but in the after LASIK setting, aqueous may be forced through the cornea and accumulate in the interface causing a spuriously low pressure reading. Tonometry no longer measures the intraocular pressure but the pressure within the fluid filled thin walled cystic interface cavity. Galal and coworkers have reported the diagnostic dilemma of the fluid filled space appearing as corneal clouding which may be mistaken for DLK.[13] The opacity is a diffuse haze rather than a fine scattering of infiltrates (Fig. 48.9). A cursory exam may miss the presence of the cystic space, but Hamilton and coauthors have published useful signs for identifying the interface fluid condition; corneal steepening on topography or increased keratometry, myopic regression, and microcysts at the flap edge (Fig. 48.10).[14] The IOP elevation can be detected if the pressure is measured outside of the margins of the flap.

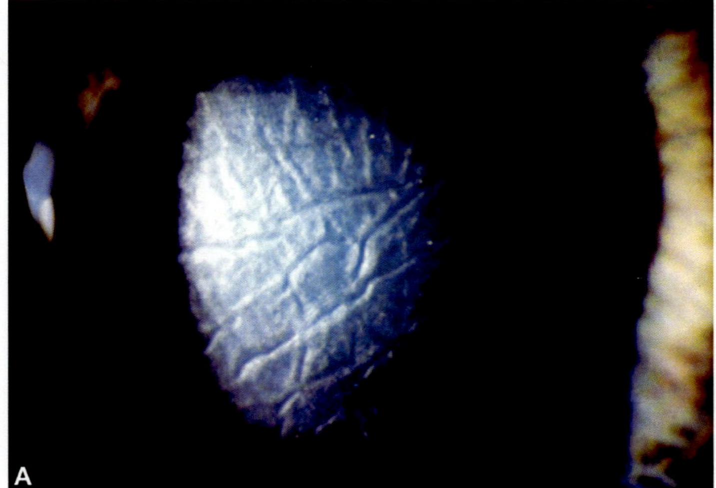

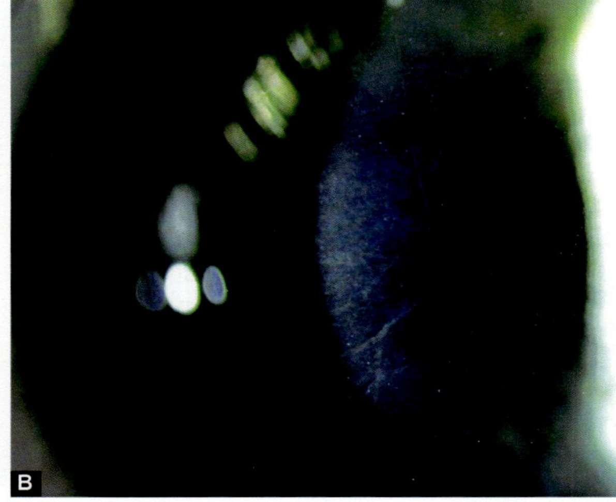

Fig. 48.8: Central Toxic Keratopathy (A) Central Toxic Keratopathy 2 months after LASIK for moderate myopia. Severe central stromal opacification extending posterioly from the interface halfway to the endothelium is present. Striae also extend into the posterior stromal bed (B) Eventual clearing with time. Sonmez B, Maloney RK: Central Toxic Keratopathy: Description of a Syndrome in Laser Refractive Surgery. Am J. Ophthalmol 2007; 143:420-427

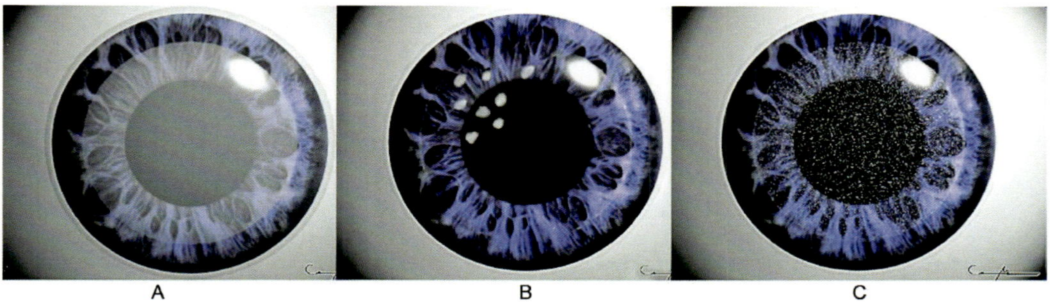

Fig. 48.9: Diagram of the haze of interface fluid syndrome (A) compared with the foci of infectious keratitis (B) compared with the fine scattering of infiltrates of DLK (C). Galal A, Artola A, Belda J, Rodriguez-Prats J, Claramonte P, Sánchez A, Ruiz-Moreno O, Merayo J, Alió J. Interface corneal edema secondary to steroid-induced elevation of intraocular pressure simulating diffuse lamellar keratitis. J Refract Surg. 2006 May;22(5):441-7

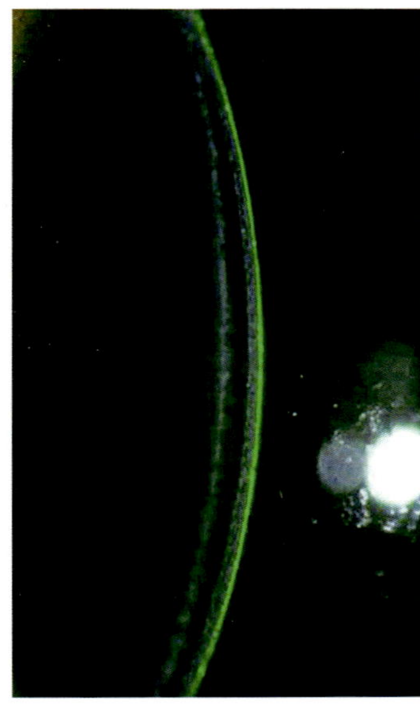

Fig. 48.10: Interface fluid in a patient on a long course of intense topical and oral corticosteroids. Photographed 7 weeks after LASIK while patient was on corticosteroids. Standard Goldmann applanation measured 01mm Hg, but Tono-pen peripherally measured 40 mmHg. One week later, after stopping corticosteroids and starting glaucoma medications, the peripheral IOP dropped to 10 mm Hg, the interface fluid had nearly resolved, and the vision improved. Glaucomatous field loss remained. Hamilton DR, Manche EE, Rich LF, Maloney RK. Steroid-induced glaucoma after laser in situ keratomileusis associated with interface fluid. Ophthalmology. 2002 Apr;109(4):659-65

Steroid induced glaucoma has been evaluated post LASIK by confocal microscopy and is found not to be associated with any collection of inflammatory cells and therefore it should not be described as pressure induced keratitis.[15,16] The mainstay of treatment is to stop the corticosteroid.

In the late postoperative period diffuse lamellar keratitis itself can occur or reoccur if the flap is lifted or otherwise traumatized. Three of our first cases followed enhancement surgery and two followed removal of epithelial ingrowth procedures. DLK has also been reported after traumatic corneal abrasion long after the initial LASIK procedure.[17]

MECHANISM AND CAUSES OF DIFFUSE LAMELLAR KERATITIS

Diffuse lamellar keratitis is a noninfectious inflammation that can be induced by one or a combination of inflammatory agents. Bacterial endotoxin, high femtosecond laser energy, high excimer laser treatment, epithelial defects, powder on gloves, oils from gloves, povidone iodine, meibomian gland secretions each alone or in combination have been implicated. Bacterial endotoxin causes epidemic outbreaks DLK.[18,19] When action is taken to reduce or eliminate the bacterial endotoxin, the rate declines. On a sporadic level, intraoperative epithelial defects are the most common cause for DLK.

Initial assessment of DLK's mechanism was hampered by the diffuse nature and normal course of the condition which precludes obtaining specimens from a typical case of diffuse lamellar keratitis. When tissue can be obtained clinically, for example if the infiltrate becomes dense and focal, i.e. no longer diffuse and lamellar, the diagnosis may be questioned, and the pathology may not be representative of DLK. Animal models, confocal microscopy, tearfilm analysis, and epidemiology in addition to clinical examination have improved the understanding of DLK.

Endotoxin is a potent inflammatory agent that has been useful in developing animal models for corneal inflammation, and has recently been implicated in toxic anterior segment syndrome in cataract surgery. The ability of heat stable bacterial endotoxin to incite a vigorous inflammatory response has been observed years before the advent of LASIK. In 1977 Mondino et al demonstrated that intracorneal injection of bacterial endotoxin into rabbit corneas stimulates the alternative complement pathway leading to a rapid polymorphonuclear neutrophil response that presents within the first few days after the initial insult.[20] Holzer and coworkers have developed an elegant model for DLK that involves applying endotoxin to the interface of surgically created corneal flaps in rabbits to reliably cause DLK. Direct histopathology and immunohistopathology studies have confirmed that the predominant cells within the interface in DLK are indeed neutrophils and that corticosteroids significantly reduce the incidence of DLK while NSAIDS do not.[21] Esquenazi also found that the infiltrates histologically were comprised of granulocytes and monocytes and that an antagonist of platelet-activating factor (PAF) decreased the incidence and severity of DLK suggesting that PAF may be an important mediator for the condition.[22] Asano-Kato also found the infiltrate to be composed of granulocytes-mainly neutrophils and identified interleukin (IL) 8 as a mediator.[23]

A novel approach to study the mechanism for DLK in patients was described by Asano-Kato who studied tear film cytology and found that the tears of a patient with DLK contained numerous neutrophils whereas the control of a normal LASIK patient did not.[24] Javaloy and coworkers performed confocal microscopy on a case of stage 3 DLK 1 week after femtosecond laser LASIK and detected cells confined within the interface that had the confocal findings of granulocytes.[25] Buhren J et al in 2001 reported the findings of 2 cases of DLK, one after a relift enhancement and the other after primary LASIK, and compared them to a normal post LASIK control.[26] Cells were found in the interface that had the confocal characteristics of granulocytes and monocytes. Based on overwhelming evidence, diffuse lamellar keratitis (DLK) can be definitively described--true to its name--as a condition involving inflammatory cells within the lamellar interface.

PREVENTION OF DIFFUSE LAMELLAR KERATITIS

Postoperative prophylactic topical corticosteroids, usually four times per day, during the first few days can help prevent DLK. The most useful measure to prevent epidemic DLK has been attention to the sterilization system and instrument cleaning protocol. Standing fluids enable bacteria to proliferate and leave a heat stable endotoxin biofilm before being sterilized. Holland et al described the findings of an indepth investigation of a DLK outbreak that occurred in their center between October 1998 and January 1999. They studied microbial cultures for bacteria, limulas assay for endotoxin and electron microscopy for biofilm, and all were positive. Cultures of the sterilizer reservoir grew *Burkholderia picketti*. Endotoxin was found on the ultrasonic instrument cleaner, the surgical instruments at the end of the sterilization cycle, in the distilled water, and on the ocular surface of a patient with DLK. Biofilm was detected in the sterilizer. They controlled the outbreak by instituting a protocol that involved draining the sterilizer at the end of each surgical day and using mechanical scrubbing and 70 percent isopropyl alcohol in the sterilizer at the end of each surgical day and allowing it to evaporate. Boiling water treatments were then performed in the morning before and at the end of each surgical day. They found that if they inoculated a clean sterile sterilizer with the bacteria, biofilm would redevelop and cultures would again become positive within 6-11 days. Their findings give strong evidence that epidemics of DLK can be caused by bacterial endotoxin released from gram negative bacterial biofilms in sterilizer reservoirs which survive short cycle steam sterilization, and the toxin incites a polymorphonuclear (PMN) inflammatory reaction in susceptible individuals resulting in DLK.

A more simple change in protocol was effective in controlling an outbreak reported by Yuhan in which the only changes in protocol were to switch the distilled water in plastic surgical bowls after each patient instead of at the end of each day, secondly to replace the plastic surgical bowls at the end of each day instead of at the end of each week and thirdly to eliminate the use of ultrasonic cleaning of the keratome head. There was no change in maintenance of the autoclave reservoir, and the autoclave was refilled with distilled water when the water level was low or empty as during the outbreak.

More recently Villarrubia and coworkers controlled an outbreak at their center by instituting the following changes in their protocol.[27] Sterile water instead of distilled water was used to clean instruments prior to placing them in the sterilizer. Sterile water instead of distilled water was used in the sterilizer reservoir, and the instruments were steam sterilized between each patient instead of daily. Chemical sterilization of the instruments in peracetic acid bath between patients was discontinued. At the end of each surgical day, the reservoir was drained, and any residual fluid was removed by aspiration or by using a wet-dry vacuum. Also at the end of the surgical day, the instruments were cleaned with sterile water and air dried using compressed air and left in a dry autoclave cassette until the following surgical day. At the beginning of the next surgical day, the reservoir was filled with sterile water and the instruments were sterilized. Their findings highlight the importance of air drying the microkeratome head and surgical instruments, draining the reservoir of the steam sterilizer, and aspirating the sterile water at the end of each surgical session.

While the femtosecond LASIK flap eliminates the need for sterilizing the microkeratome, a sterile flap lifting instrument like the Seibel Intralasik Flap lifter and a sterile irrigating cannula are used for each case, and thus attention to cleaning protocols remains important for centers with femtosecond lasers as well. The femtosecond laser, for example, the IntraLase (IntraLase Corp. Irvine, CA) can itself cause DLK (Fig. 48.11). Javaloy and coworkers in a prospective masked study of 200 eyes of 100 consecutive patients comparing Moria microkeratome LASIK to IntraLase femtosecond LASIK found DLK in 16 percent of eyes in the Intralase laser group and none in the microkeratome group. When they subsequently reduced the side cut energy from 1.6 mJ to 1.2 mJ, their incidence of DLK decreased to 3.5 percent. A 15 kHz femtosecond was used in the study, instead of 60 kHz which is now available. Optimizing the energy parameters for the femtosecond laser can help prevent DLK.

Intraoperative epithelial defects are a major cause of spontaneous cases of DLK. The incidence of DLK in patients with epithelial defects may exceed 50%.[28] Preventing epithelial defects would be the ideal solution, but that may not be possible. Preoperative screening for epithelial basement membrane dystrophy (with maps, dots or fingerprints) can help identify those at risk for an epithelial defect. Patients with epithelial basement membrane dystrophy or recurrent corneal erosions are not good candidates

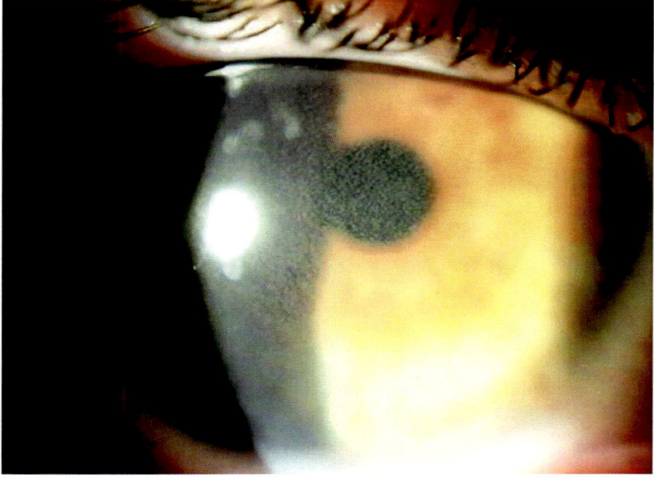

Fig. 48.11: DLK after IntraLase LASIK. Photograph courtesy of Dr. Jaime Javoloy and Dr Jorge Alió.

for LASIK but may be considered for surface laser treatment (PRK). For patients with minimal or equivocal findings of epithelial basement membrane dystrophy, the provocative test described by Anthony Aldave can help make the diagnosis. Topical anesthetic is instilled. The test involves gently pressing a Weck cell sponge on the suspicious part of the corneal surface. If an abrasion or a slough is created the patient is at risk for an intraoperative epithelial defect and is not a good candidate for LASIK. (The patient also needs to be treated for the abrasion created during the test.) If an intraoperative epithelial defect does occur during the LASIK procedure, then prophylactic steroids should be instituted at a more frequent dosing regimen, for example, prednisolone 1 percent every 1-2 hours while awake. Other preventative measures include covering Meibomian gland orifices, avoiding getting povidone iodine under the flap, and to irrigating the interface after laser treatment.

TREATMENT OF DIFFUSE LAMELLAR KERATITIS

A short course of strong topical corticosteroids like prednisolone acetate 1 percent every 1-2 hours while awake with close observation is indicated. Usually topical corticosteroids are sufficient. Adding oral corticosteroids in severe cases has also been effective.[29] The disease should start to improve within a day or two. When the density of inflammatory infiltrates has significantly decreased, then taper off the corticosteroids. If the infiltrates are worsening despite treatment, then reconsider the possibility of an infectious etiology and lift the flap, culture for bacteria, mycobacteria and fungus, irrigate the interface and increase the frequency of topical antibiotics. While the cultures are pending, the patient can usually be continued on the short course of corticosteroid. If fungal or mycobacterial keratitis is high on the differential, however, then corticosteroid should be stopped. It's worth noting that most of the patients in the initial report on DLK had resolution of DLK even without use of corticosteroid. DLK is not a chronic condition. Corticosteroid treatment should last no more than a couple of weeks.

SUMMARY

DLK is an acute cellular inflammatory response to one or a combination of agents following LASIK or other forms of lamellar corneal surgery and usually improves promptly with a short course of corticosteroids. If the condition is not resolving, the flap should be lifted, the infiltrate cultured and then irrigated. Long courses of corticosteroids are not indicated and put the patient at risk for infection, interface fluid and steroid induced glaucoma.

REFERENCES

1. Maddox R, Hatsis A. Sands of the Sahara syndrome [poster]. Presented at the ASCRS annual meeting, San Diego, CA, USA, April 1998.
2. Smith RJ, Maloney RK. Diffuse Lamellar Keratitis: A new syndrome in lamellar refractive surgery. Ophthalmology 1998;105:1721-6.
3. Linebarger EJ, Hardten DR, Lindstrom RL. Diffuse lamellar keratitis: diagnosis and management. J Cataract Refract Surg 2000;26(7):1072-7.
4. Fraenkel GE, Cohen PR, Sutton GL, Lawless MA, Rogers CM. Central focal interface opacity after laser in situ keratomileusis. J Refract Surg 1998;14(5):571-6.
5. Hainline BC, Price MO, Choi DM, Price FW Jr. Central flap necrosis after LASIK with microkeratome and femtosecond laser created flaps. J Refract Surg 2007; 23(3):233-42.
6. Sonmez B, Maloney RK. Central Toxic Keratopathy: Description of a Syndrome in Laser Refractive Surgery. Am J Ophthalmol 2007;143:420-7.
7. Hovanesian JA, Faktorovich EG, Hoffbauer JD, Shah SS, Maloney RK. Bilateral bacterial keratitis after laser in situ keratomileusis in a patient with human immunodeficiency virus infection. Arch Ophthalmol 1999; 117(7):968-70.
8. Wang MY, Maloney RK. Epithelial ingrowth after laser in situ keratomileusis. Am J Ophthalmol 2000;129(6):746-51.
9. Chandra NS, Torres MF, Winthrop KL, Bruckner DA, Heidemann DG, Calvet HM, et al. Cluster of Mycobacterium chelonae keratitis cases following laser in-situ keratomileusis. Am J Ophthalmol 2001;132(6):819-30.
10. Seo KY, Lee JB, Lee K, Kim MJ, Choi KR, Kim EK. Nontuberculous mycobacterial keratitis at the interface after laser in situ keratomileusis. J Refract Surg 2002;18(1):81-5.

11. Peng Q, Holzer MP, Kaufer PH, Apple DJ, Solomon KD. Interface fungal infection after laser in situ keratomileusis presenting as diffuse lamellar keratitis. A clinicopathological report. J Cataract Refract Surg 2002;28(8):1400.
12. Lindstrom RL. In: Belville JK, Smith RJ (Eds): LASIK Techniques: Pearls and Pitfalls. Slack Inc. Thorofare, NJ, 2004;92.
13. Galal A, Artola A, Belda J, Rodriguez-Prats J, Claramonte P, Sánchez A, et al. Interface corneal edema secondary to steroid-induced elevation of intraocular pressure simulating diffuse lamellar keratitis. J Refract Surg 2006;22(5):441-7.
14. Hamilton DR, Manche EE, Rich LF, Maloney RK. Steroid-induced glaucoma after laser in situ keratomileusis associated with interface fluid. Ophthalmology 2002; 109(4):659-65.
15. Cheng AC, Law RW, Young AL, Lam DS. In vivo confocal microscopic findings in patients with steroid-induced glaucoma after LASIK. Ophthalmology 2004; 111(4):768-74.
16. Kurian M, Shetty R, Shetty BK, Devi SA. In vivo confocal microscopic findings of interlamellar stromal keratopathy induced by elevated intraocular pressure. J Cataract Refract Surg 2006;32(9):1563-6.
17. Haw WW, Manche EE. Late onset diffuse lamellar keratitis associated with an epithelial defect in six eyes. J Refract Surg 2000;16(6):744-8.
18. Yuhan KR, Nguyen L, Wachler BS. Role of instrument cleaning and maintenance in the development of diffuse lamellar keratitis. Ophthalmology 2002;109(2):400-3.
19. Holland SP, Mathias RG, Morck DW, Chiu J, Slade SG. Diffuse lamellar keratitis related to endotoxins released from sterilizer reservoir biofilms. Ophthalmology 2000; 107(7):1227-33.
20. Mondino BJ, Rabin BS, Kessler E, Gallo J, Brown SI. Corneal rings with gram-negative bacteria. Arch Ophthalmol 1977;95(12):2222-5.
21. Holzer MP, Solomon KD, Vroman DT, Vargas LG, Sandoval HP, Kasper TJ, et al. Diffuse lamellar keratitis: evaluation of etiology, histopathologic findings, and clinical implications in an experimental animal model. J Cataract Refract Surg 2003;29(3):542-9.
22. Esquenazi S, He J, Bazan HE, Bazan NG. Prevention of experimental diffuse lamellar keratitis using a novel platelet-activating factor receptor antagonist. J Cataract Refract Surg 2004;30(4):884-91.
23. Asano-Kato N, Toda I, Shimmura S, Noda-Tsuruya T, Fukagawa K, Yoshinaga M, et al. Detection of neutrophils and possible involvement of interleukin-8 in diffuse lamellar keratitis after laser in situ keratomileusis. J Cataract Refract Surg 2003;29(10):1996-2000.
24. Asano-Kato N, Toda I, Fukumoto T, Asai H, Tsubota K. Detection of neutrophils in late-onset interface inflammation associated with flap injury after laser in situ keratomileusis. Cornea 2004;23(3):306-10.
25. Javaloy J, Vidal MT, Abdelrahman AM, Artola A, Alió JL. Confocal microscopy comparison of intralase femtosecond laser and Moria M2 microkeratome in LASIK. J Refract Surg 2007;23(2):178-87.
26. Bühren J, Baumeister M, Kohnen T. Diffuse lamellar keratitis after laser in situ keratomileusis imaged by confocal microscopy. Ophthalmology 2001;108(6):1075-81.
27. Villarrubia A, Palacín E, Gómez del Río M, Martínez P. Description, etiology, and prevention of an outbreak of diffuse lamellar keratitis after LASIK. J Refract Surg 2007; 23(5):482-6.
28. Shah MN, Misra M, Wihelmus KR, Koch DD. Diffuse lamellar keratitis associated with epithelial defects after laser in situ keratomileusis. J Cataract Refract Surg 2000; 26(9):1312-8.
29. Manche EE. In: Belville JK, Smith RJ (Eds): LASIK Techniques: Pearls and Pitfalls. Slack Inc. Thorofare, NJ, 2004;134.

49 Decentered Ablation

Helen Boerman, Tracy Swartz, Ming Wang

INTRODUCTION

Clinically significant decentered excimer ablations result in symptoms such as glare, shadows, dim lighting disturbances, distortion, and monocular diplopia, as well as loss of best-corrected visual acuity due to irregular astigmatism. Decentration can be a corollary of poor fixation due to poor patient instruction, anxiety, over-sedation, or blurry vision due to high refractive error, or the exposed stromal bed causing difficulty seeing the laser's target. It can also result from improper stabilization of the eye with a Thornton ring during excimer ablation.

Centration over the entrance pupil center has been accepted as the standard for many years and still remains the recommendation for many laser systems. However, variations in pupil size can affect the location of the entrance pupil center. Therefore, centration by this technique is not the most reliable estimation of the visual axis.[1] This has led to the use of the coaxially sighted corneal light reflex for more accurate centration during refractive procedures. This reflex represents the corneal intercept of a line from the point of fixation to the center of corneal curvature.

In addition, hyperopic ablations may result in more clinically significant symptoms than myopic ablations following equal magnitude refractive treatments.[1,2] The functional optical zone in hyperopic treatments is smaller, emphasizing any possible decentration of the ablation zone. This is further accentuated by a greater average angle kappa in hyperopes as compared to myopes.[1]

Proper centration of ablation requires careful preoperative and intraoperative instructions, especially with regard to the fixation target. It is important to keep both eyes open, preparing patients with regards to sounds and smells that may startle them. The head and body must remain still during surgery.[3-6] The advent of modern laser tracking systems, iris registration software, and wavefront-guided excimer laser technology has significantly reduced the incidence of decentration.[6, 7]

CLINICAL DEFINITION

The following clinical signs and symptoms often present in patients with a decentered ablation: (1) decentration of the ablation zone on corneal topography, (2) increased higher order aberrations as measured using wavefront aberrometry, predominantly coma, (3) the appearance of a tail on point spread functions , (4) reduced best spectacle-corrected visual acuity which improves only with gas permeable lenses, (5) a cylinder measurement on autorefraction and wavefront that differs from manifest refraction, and (6) a history of reduced vision immediately following surgery that fails to improve with time.

Topographic Decentration

To evaluate decentration on corneal topography, both axial curvature and elevation maps are useful. The axial map provides the refractive result of ablation, i.e. the optical zone. A large corneal curvature gradient between treated and untreated cornea, such as that resulting from a highly myopic correction, creates a smaller optical zone, increasing the refractive effect of the decentration.[8] Curvature maps indicate surface shape using the axial radius of curvature, or the distance along the normal from the surface to the optic axis.[9] Once a radius is determined, it is converted to a dioptric value using a paraxial keratometry formula, resulting in error for more peripheral points.

In contrast, elevation maps using an appropriate reference surface describe subtle variations in surface geometry and are valuable when true topography is required.[9] Therefore, elevation maps are far more valuable in both diagnosing and treating corneal decentration, and in monitoring surface changes.

Wavefront Aberrations

The growing application of wavefront aberrometry demonstrates increased higher order aberrations in patients following keratorefractive surgery, specifically those with decentered ablations. Mrochen et al[10] found that subclinical decentrations less than 1 mm significantly increase wavefront aberrations, deteriorating the optical quality of the retinal image. All Zernike coefficients increased postoperatively, with coma being the predominant higher order aberration. Decentrations as small as 0.2 mm increased wavefront aberrations; however, those less than 0.5 mm are considered clinically insignificant.

Wavefront aberrometers offer a variety of displays describing aberrations, including Point Spread Functions (PSF) and Snellen letter appearance simulations. Examples of a wavefront map, simulated Snellen letters, and point spread function with increased coma of a patient with a decentration are shown in Figures 49.1 to 49.3.

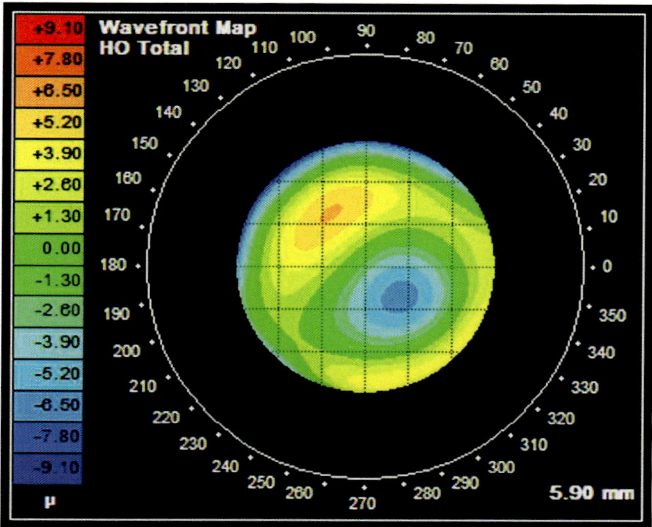

Fig. 49.1: Wavefront map in a patient with increased coma

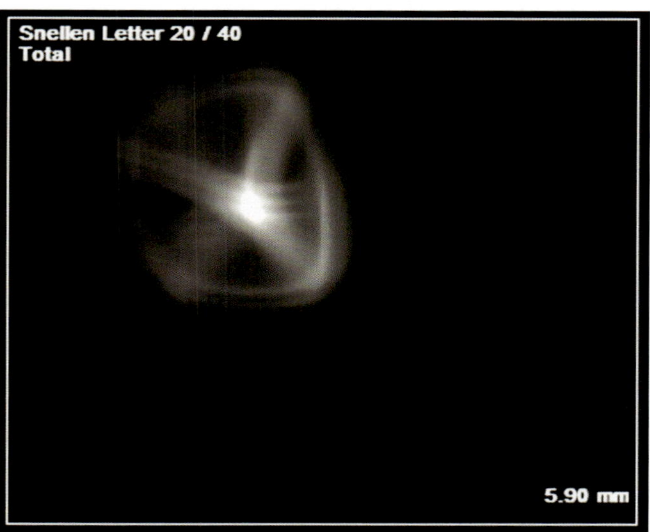

Fig. 49.2: Simulated 20/40 Snellen letter "E" in a patient with increased coma

MANAGEMENT OF DECENTERED ABLATION

While the diagnosis of decentration is fairly straightforward, reducing or eliminating symptoms associated with decentration can be difficult. The most frequently used non-surgical method involves gas permeable lenses, which restore visual quality by optically reshaping the anterior cornea surface.

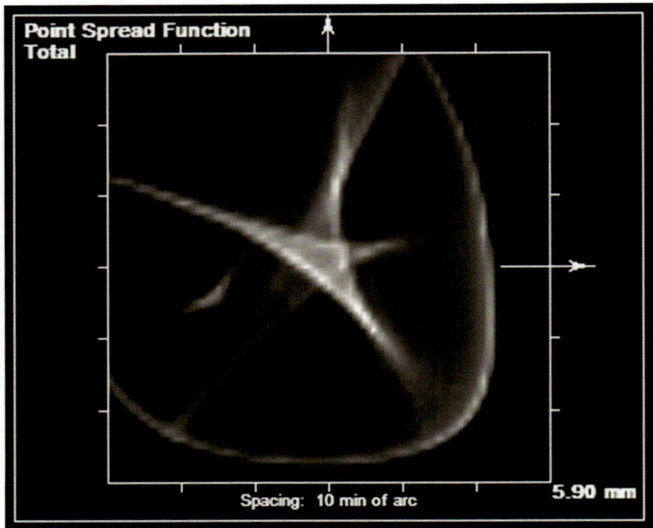

Fig. 49.3: Point spread function in a patient with increased coma

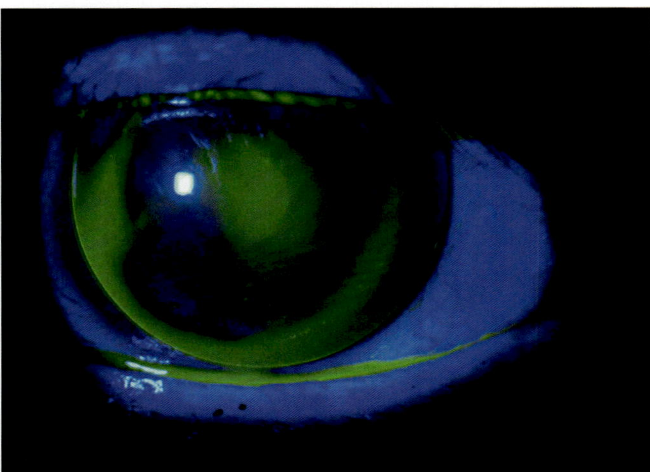

Fig. 49.4: Rose K Irregular Corneal (BLANCHARD CONTACT LENS INC, Manchester, New Hampshire) design on a patient with irregular astigmatism resulting from a decentered ablation. Note the asymmetry in the fluorescein pattern. The patient was 20/100 best corrected in spectacles, and 20/20 with this lens

Comparing BSCVA to the visual acuity obtained with a gas perm (GP) lens may provide the prognosis of visual success. Unfortunately, achieving fitting success can be difficult, often requiring novel lens types such as reverse geometry or specialty aspheric designs. An example of such a gas perm fitting is shown in Figure 49.4. Even in cases when the vision significantly improves, failures result due to poor comfort and limited wearing time. Most patients are not receptive to returning to contact lenses after investing time and money in refractive surgery.

We typically address any tear film instability or deficiency by aggressive ocular surface lubrication. Punctal plugs and topical 0.05 percent cyclosporin (Allergan, Irvine, CA) both work well to smooth the irregular surface and decrease visual symptoms. Treatment of meibomian gland disease using oral doxycycline or topical Azacite (Inspire Pharmaceuticals, Durham, NC) may be used to stabilize the tear film, possibly increasing the Snellen acuity and decreasing the aberrations such that the patient appreciates visual improvement without further surgery.

Surgical Correction of Decentered Ablation

Several options for surgical correction of decentered ablations exist with variable results. PTK[10] and purposeful decentered ablation in the opposite direction of the initial treatment[11] have been proposed but such techniques are not widely used. Correction of decentration using wavefront-driven treatment, Custom Corneal Ablation Pattern treatment, and topography-guided treatment are more likely to be used in patients suffering vision loss following keratorefractive surgery.

Wavefront-guided Treatment

Custom wavefront treatments have been used to address the visual effects of a previous refractive surgery, including decentered ablation.[12-15] Topographical abnormalities translate into wavefront aberrations, which can be addressed with wavefront-guided treatment. While severely irregular corneas may not be adequately measured using wavefront aberrometry, when data can be captured, it has been found to improve vision.[16-19]

In case I, a patient presented after undergoing LASIK followed by an enhancement and epithelial cleaning in her hometown. Uncorrected vision was 20/70, which corrected to 20/20 with a refraction of $-1.75 + 0.50 \times 128$. Topography and aberrometry

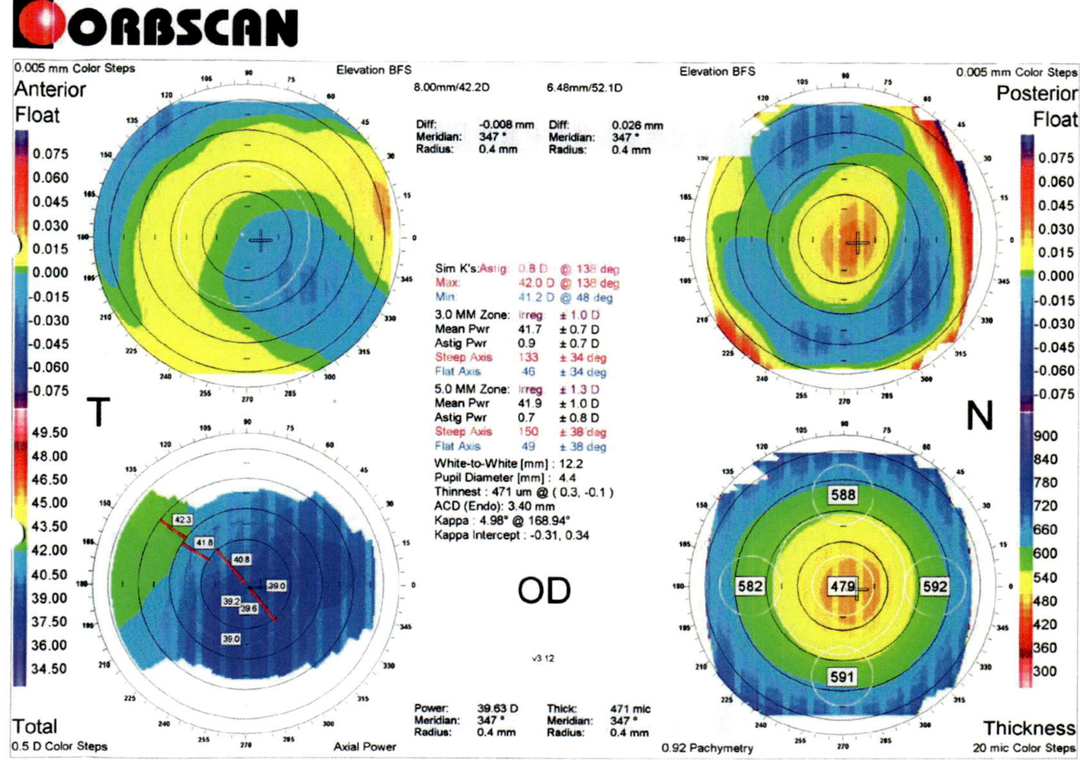

Fig. 49.5: Preoperative topographical map showing superior decentration

are shown in Figures 49.5 and 49.6. Gas permeable over-refraction yielded 20/20 vision with significant improvement in subjective visual quality. WaveScan-guided (AMO, Santa Ana, CA) PRK using ablation was performed, and the patient reported improved visual quality the following day. Later, she reported although the vision was better than prior to custom treatment, shadows persisted. Postoperative aberrometry is shown in Figure 49.7. Note that while the refractive error was greatly reduced, the RMS value did not significantly improve.

Topography-guided Treatment

Topography-guided options are limited to Custom-CAP (Carl Zeiss Humphrey, Jeno, Germany) treatments in the United States. Use of Custom-Cap has been shown to be effective in correcting decentered ablation.[20-22] It enables the surgeon to create a customized excimer laser ablation pattern to reduce areas of topographic irregularity on the anterior corneal surface via computerized simulations. Creation of plans directing the excimer laser beam size, shape, depth, and location to match the corresponding irregularity on the computerized corneal topography elevation map results in a more regular corneal shape. The laser beam varies in diameter from 0.6 to 6.5 mm, and can be centered or offset in any direction from the visual axis. The required VisionPro software (Carl Zeiss Humphrey, Jeno, Germany) allows the programming of up to 20 different sequential ablations.

In case II, utilized this technology to correct a decentered ablation in a patient with a history of previous LASIK to correct myopia. She was best corrected to 20/40 and complained of shadows and distorted vision. Her preoperative topography is shown in Figure 49.8. The VisionPro software ablation plan is shown in Figure 49.9. Following

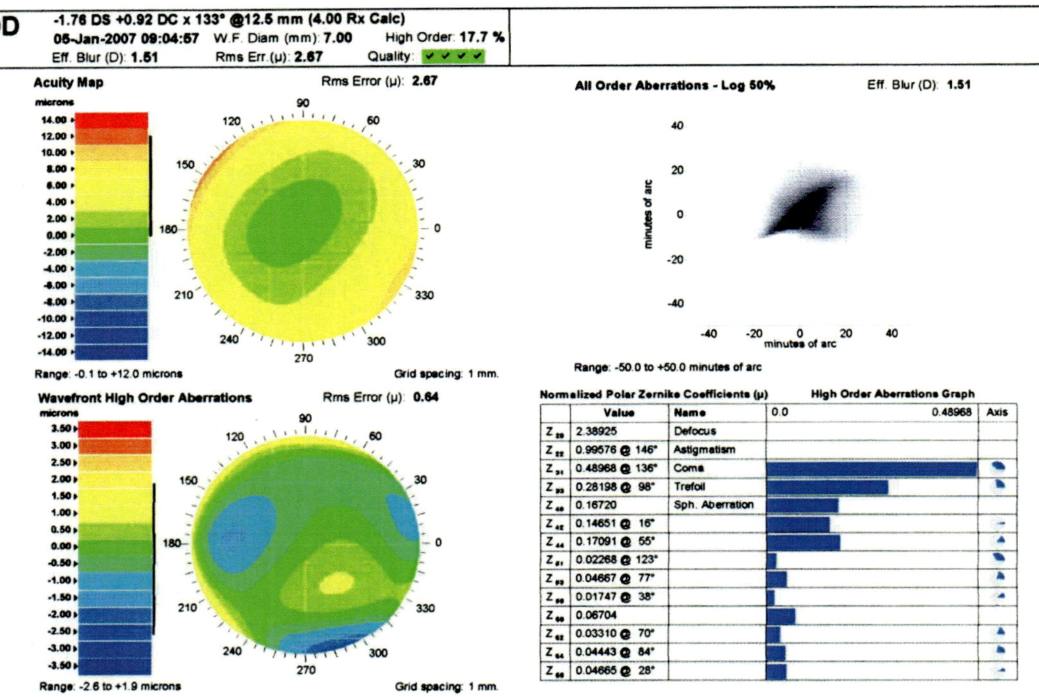

	Value	Name	0.0 … 0.48968	Axis
Z_{20}	2.38925	Defocus		
Z_{22}	0.99576 @ 146°	Astigmatism		
Z_{31}	0.48968 @ 136°	Coma		
Z_{33}	0.28198 @ 98°	Trefoil		
Z_{40}	0.16720	Sph. Aberration		
Z_{42}	0.14651 @ 16°			
Z_{44}	0.17091 @ 55°			
Z_{51}	0.02268 @ 123°			
Z_{53}	0.04667 @ 77°			
Z_{55}	0.01747 @ 38°			
Z_{60}	0.06704			
Z_{62}	0.03310 @ 70°			
Z_{64}	0.04443 @ 84°			
Z_{66}	0.04665 @ 28°			

Fig. 49.6: Preoperative WaveScan aberrometry maps showing coma, as expected with a decentered ablation

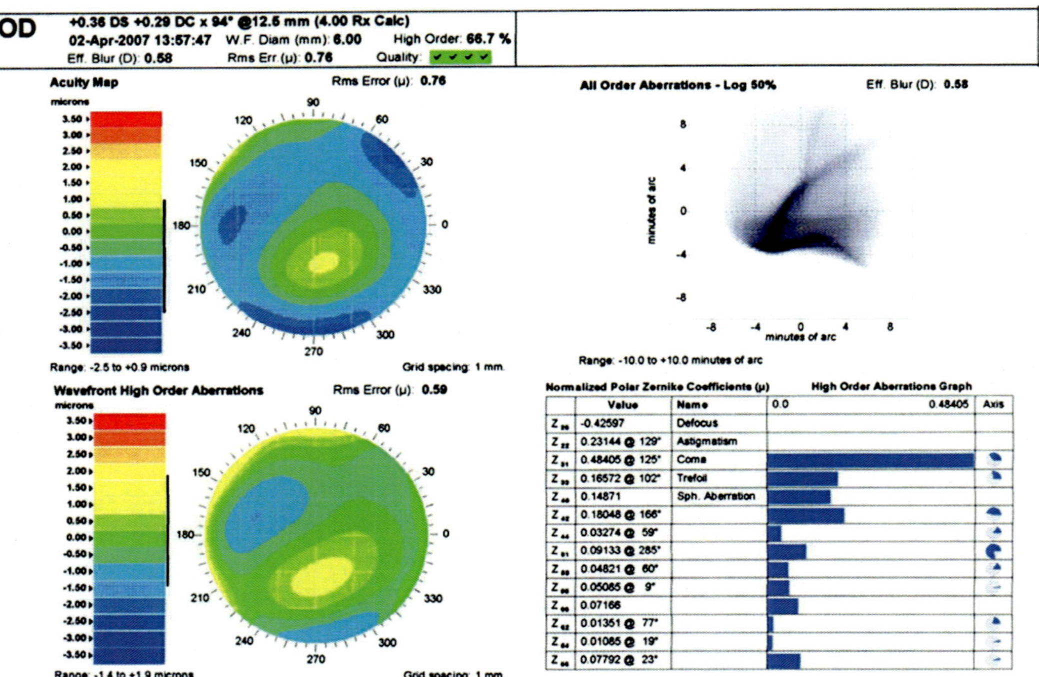

	Value	Name	0.0 … 0.48405	Axis
Z_{20}	-0.42597	Defocus		
Z_{22}	0.23144 @ 129°	Astigmatism		
Z_{31}	0.48405 @ 125°	Coma		
Z_{33}	0.16572 @ 102°	Trefoil		
Z_{40}	0.14871	Sph. Aberration		
Z_{42}	0.18048 @ 166°			
Z_{44}	0.03274 @ 59°			
Z_{51}	0.09133 @ 285°			
Z_{53}	0.04821 @ 60°			
Z_{55}	0.05065 @ 9°			
Z_{60}	0.07166			
Z_{62}	0.01351 @ 77°			
Z_{64}	0.01085 @ 19°			
Z_{66}	0.07792 @ 23°			

Fig. 49.7: Postoperative WaveScan aberrometry maps. Note the RMS values for higher order aberrations did not significantly improve

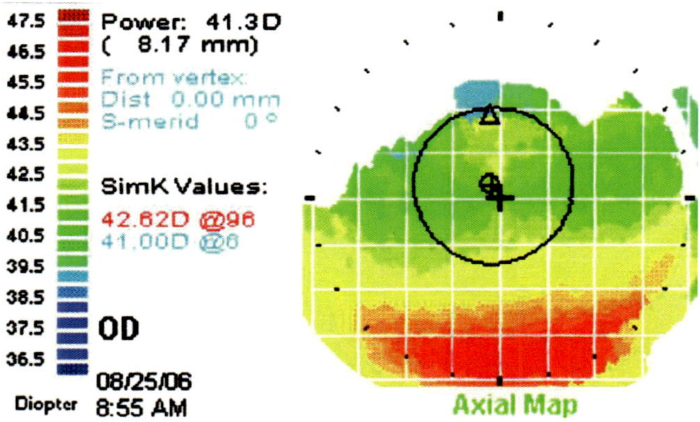

Fig. 49.8: Preoperative topographic map in a patient with a decentered ablation

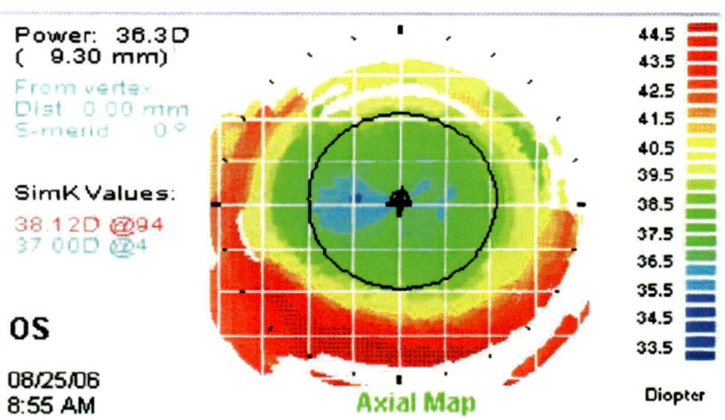

Fig. 49.10: The topographical maps following Custom-CAP treatment show a significantly improved topographical regularity

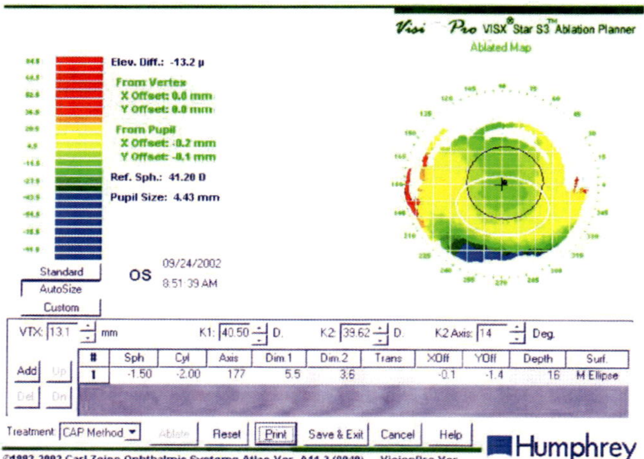

Fig. 49.9: Custom-CAP ablation plan parameters are displayed numerically, with the simulated result of the planned ablation pictured in the ablated map, for the patient in Figure 49.8

treatment, her best corrected vision improved to 20/25 and the post-operative topography showed improved regularity (Fig. 49.10).

Topography-guided treatment of decentration may be advantageous compared to wavefront, which addresses topographical irregularities secondarily. Decentration is a topographical phenomenon, which is directly corrected using topographically-driven treatments. Because the ablation is derived from corneal topography data directly, restoration of the natural aspheric shape of the cornea is possible. Topographical treatments may incorporate tissue saving algorithms, important in patients with limited stromal bed thickness. Published reports find topography-guided treatment to be effective, improving UCVA, BSCVA and the regularity of the corneal surface.[23-27] However, residual refractive error, under-correction of topographic abnormalities and regression have been reported.[12,28,29]

In case III, illustrates the efficacy of the MEL80 with TOSCA software (Asclepion-Meditec, Jena, Germany) and the CRS-Master (Carl Ziess Meditech, Jena, Germany). This system includes algorithms to correct decentrations and enlarge small optical zones.[30] The CRS-Master features improved control of sphere and cylinder while correcting topographical irregularities. The system incorporates corneal anterior surface wavefront information derived from topography, and whole-eye optical data to determine the refraction of the front surface and the ablation required to remove the irregularities independent of the refractive change.[31] This patient presented with a history of RK rather than LASIK, reporting stable vision for the first 12 years, with progressive hyperopia and reduced visual quality more recently. Her refraction was +3.75-1.00 x 165, which corrected her vision to 20/20. Topography is shown in Figure 49.11. Surgery was performed with a target of plano, with the intention of improving the corneal surface regularity. PRK was performed with an optical zone of 7.00 mm. Six months later, the patient was 20/32 uncorrected, and +1.00-0.75 x 85 improved her

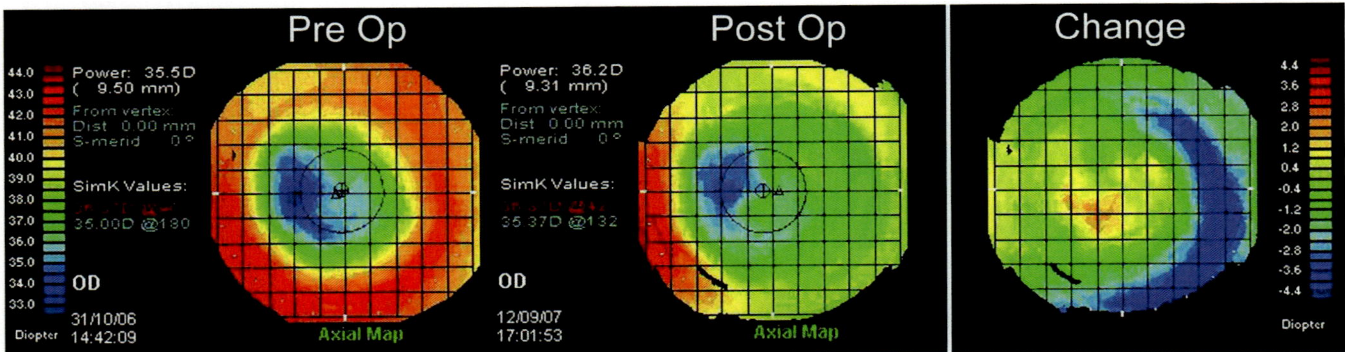

Fig. 49.11: Topography maps for Case III, a patient with a decentered optical zone following RK corrected with the Mel80 and CRS-master (Carl Zeiss Meditech, Jena, Germany) (*Courtesy:* Dan Reinstein, MD and Tim Archer)

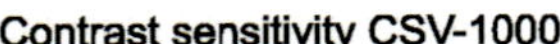

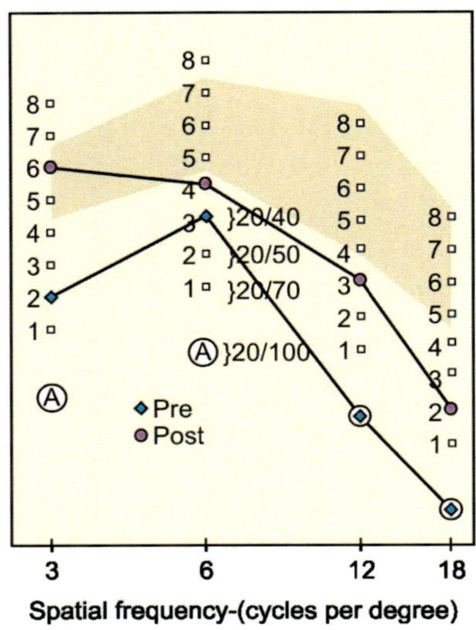

Fig. 49.12: Contrast sensitivity testing before (blue) and after (red) PRK custom treatment to correct the decentrated optical zone (*Courtesy:* Dan Reinstein, MD and Tim Archer)

vision to 20/16. Figure 49.12 shows the improvement in contrast sensitivity.

Two systems incorporate pupil size, topographic elevation data, and refractive status with surgical recreation of the morphological axis. The morphological axis is defined as the axis of corneal symmetry approximating the best match between the axis of ideal shape and that of the current form of the cornea. Following a decentration, the visual axis shifts in am attempt to correct the induced visual effect of the decentration. Any measurement taken using the patient's fixation, such as autorefraction, wavefront aberrometry, and placido topography, will then measured along the incorrect axis. This is the reason decentration is difficulty to correct using wavefront aberrometry measurements, and why conventional treatments often increase rather than improve the decentration.

Ablation software combines pupil, refractive and corneal elevation information, creating topographically-driven ablations with tissue saving algorithms. The two systems are the Corneal Interactive Programmed Topographic Ablation (CIPTA) (Ligi, Taranto, Italy) and AstraScan (LaserSight, Orlando, FL). The following two cases illustrate the two systems.

In case IV, demonstrates a successful treatment using CIPTA. A patient presented with a decentered ablation following LASIK, which manifested as 2.10 D of astigmatism. Preoperative topography and pachymetry maps are shown in Figures 49.13 and 49.14. Incorporation of the pupillometer data, topography, and refraction is illustrated in Figure 49.15A which displays the imported topographic map and the ideal shape with restoration of the morphological axis. The ablation plan is shown in Figure 49.15B, which details the corrective ablation (right) and the predicted elevation topography (left). The actual resulting topography and pachymetry maps are shown in Figures 49.16 and 49.17, demonstrating improved centration and decreased pachymetry.

In case V, illustrates a case of decentration corrected using AstraScan. Figure 49.18 shows a

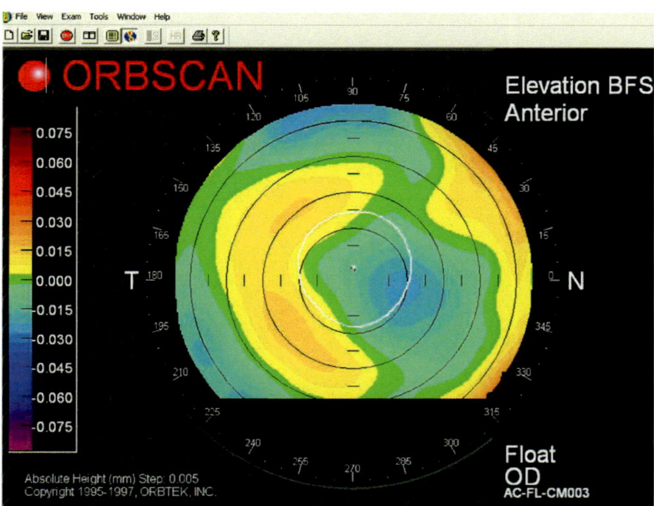

Fig. 49.13: Preoperative topography map for a patient with a decentered ablation following LASIK. (*Courtesy:* Chuck Stewart, OD and Ligi, Taranto, Italy)

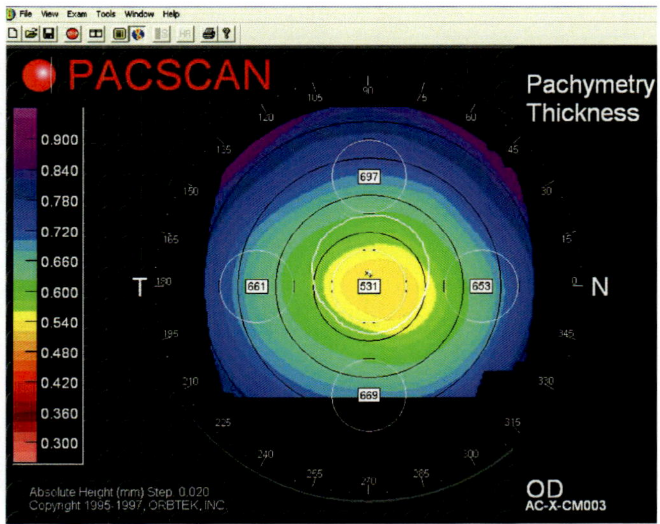

Fig. 49.14: Preoperative pachymetry map for the patient in Figure 49.13 (*Courtesy:* Chuck Stewart, OD and Ligi, Taranto, Italy)

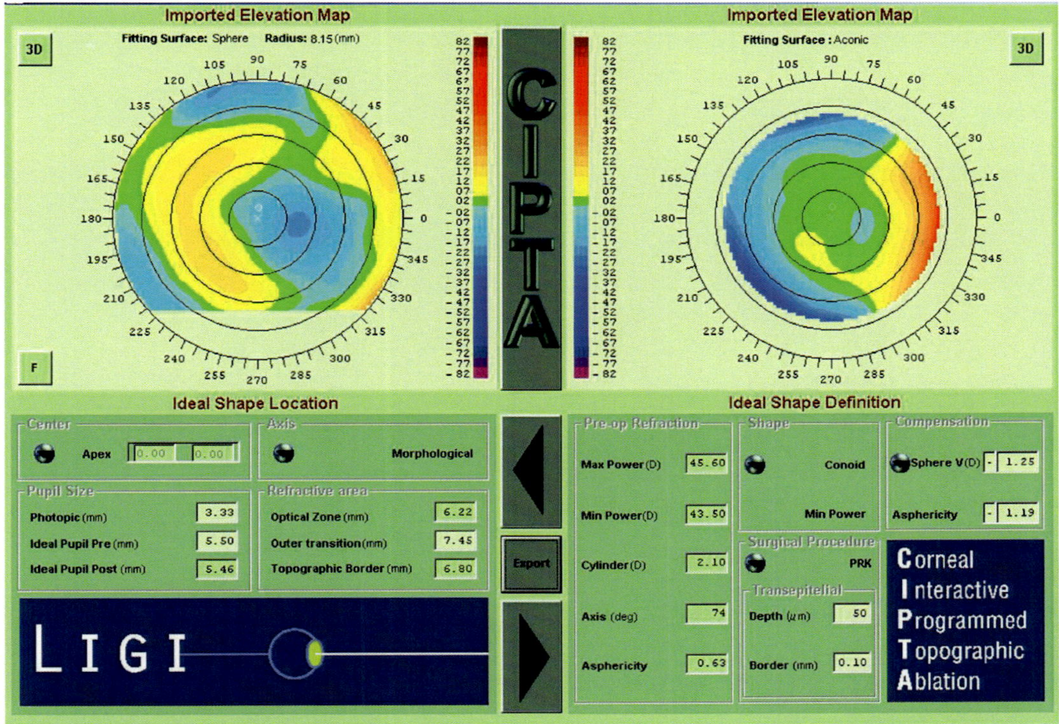

Fig. 49.15A: CIPTA software planning imports the elevation data (upper left) and creates the ideal corneal surface with reference to the morphological axis (upper right) (*Courtesy:* Chuck Stewart, OD and Ligi, Taranto, Italy)

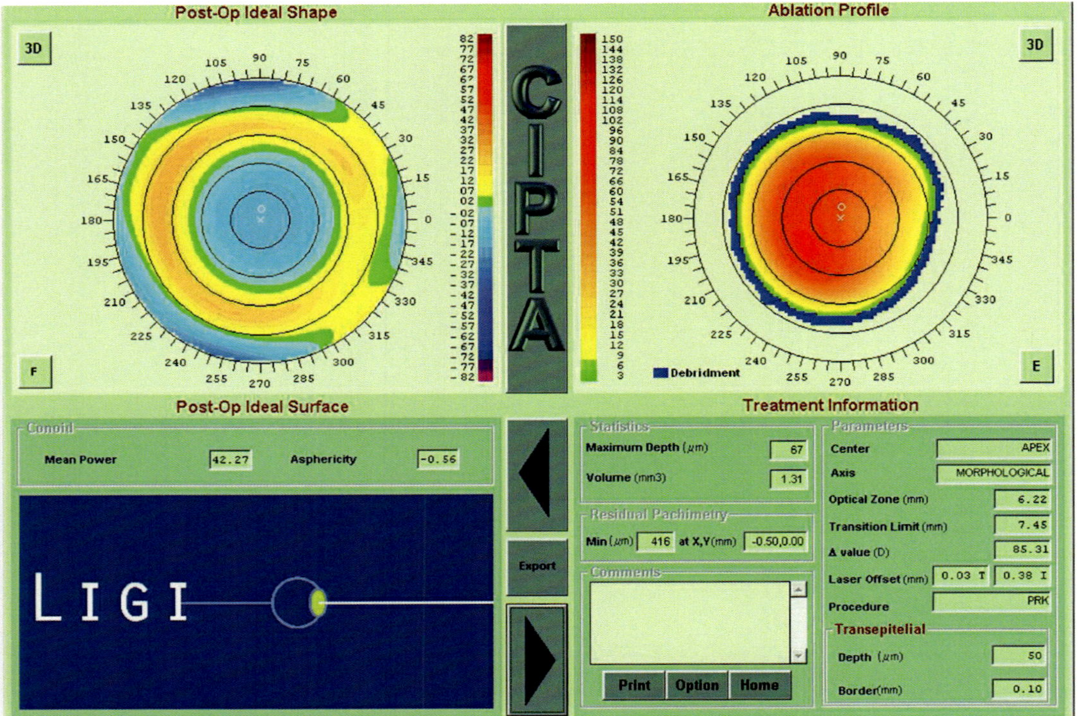

Fig. 49.15B: CIPTA software creates the ablation profile (upper right) to create the simulated elevation map (upper left) (*Courtesy:* Chuck Stewart, OD and Ligi, Taranto, Italy)

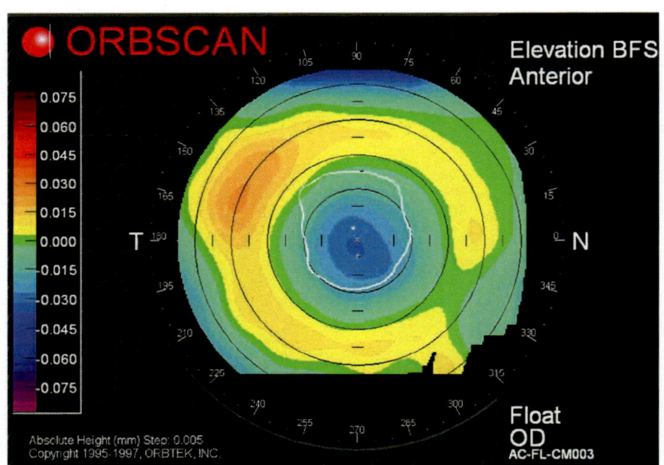

Fig. 49.16: Actual elevation map following CIPTA treatment. (*Courtesy:* of Chuck Stewart, OD and Ligi, Taranto, Italy)

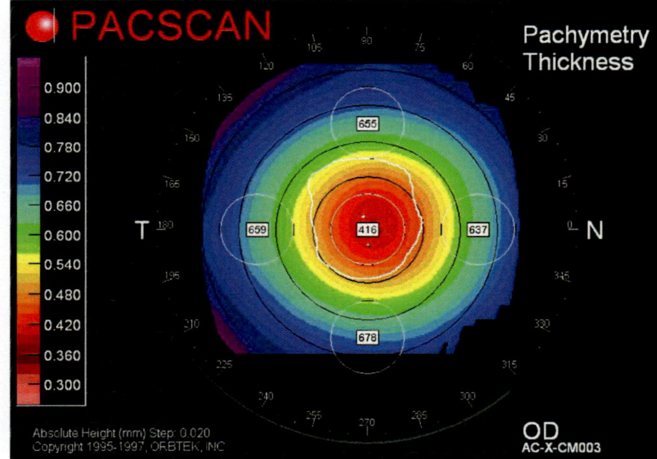

Fig. 49.17: Actual postoperative pachymetry map following CIPTA treatment. (*Courtesy:* Chuck Stewart, OD and Ligi, Taranto, Italy)

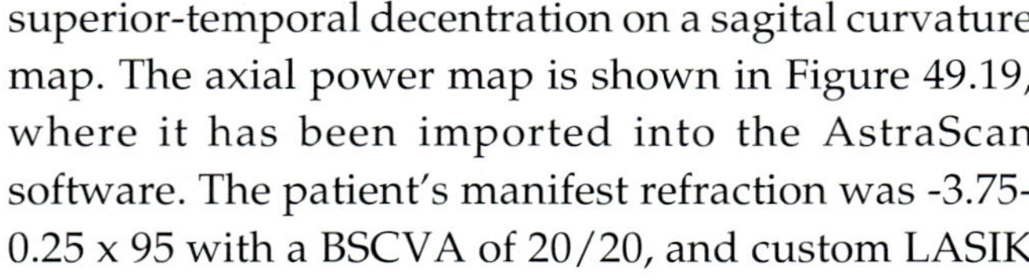

superior-temporal decentration on a sagital curvature map. The axial power map is shown in Figure 49.19, where it has been imported into the AstraScan software. The patient's manifest refraction was -3.75-0.25 x 95 with a BSCVA of 20/20, and custom LASIK surgery was planned to correct the decentration and address the refractive error. Figure 49.20 illustrates the planned ablation profile. Note that the pre-enhancement elevation (lower left), when using the optimized post-enhancement corneal vertex as the

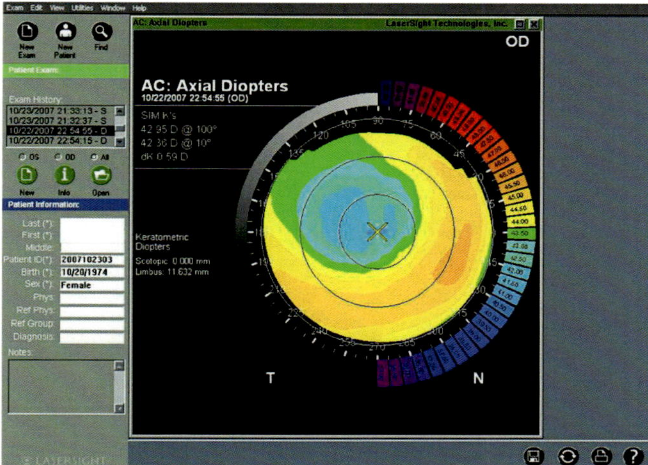

Fig. 49.18: Preenhancement axial curvature map, showing significant decentration of the ablation supero-temporally. (*Courtesy:* Dr. Bing Liu, General Air Force Hospital)

reference axis, shows the same elevated pattern as the enhancement ablation profile (upper right). In this example, the optimized axis is offset of 0.035 mm temporally, and 0.044 mm superiorly from the pre-enhancement corneal vertex axis. Figure 49.21 shows the post-enhancement axial power map showing the decentration has been completely corrected. Figure 49.22 shows the pre- (left) and post-operative (right) elevation maps. The difference map can be seen in Figure 49.23.

CONCLUSION

When a patient with a history of refractive surgery presents with loss of best-corrected visual acuity and expresses symptoms of glare, night vision difficulty, and monocular diplopia, decentered ablation needs to be ruled out. Understanding of elevation topography, and aberrometry is crucial for the diagnosis. Modern surgical options are presently evolving and gaining success in addressing this complication to improve visual quality in post-refractive eyes.

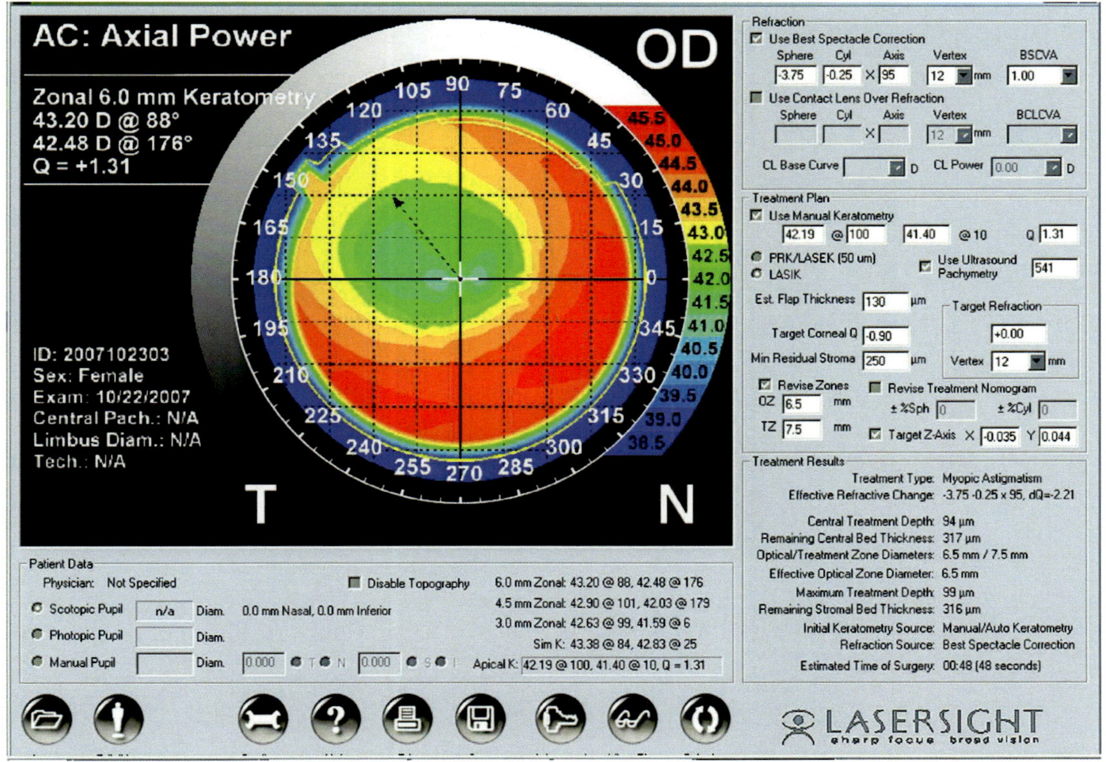

Fig. 49.19: AstraPro 2.2Z Custom Planning Software User Interface where the imported power map, pachymetry, keratometry, refractive information, and ablation plan are displayed (*Courtesy:* Dr. Bing Liu, General Air Force Hospital)

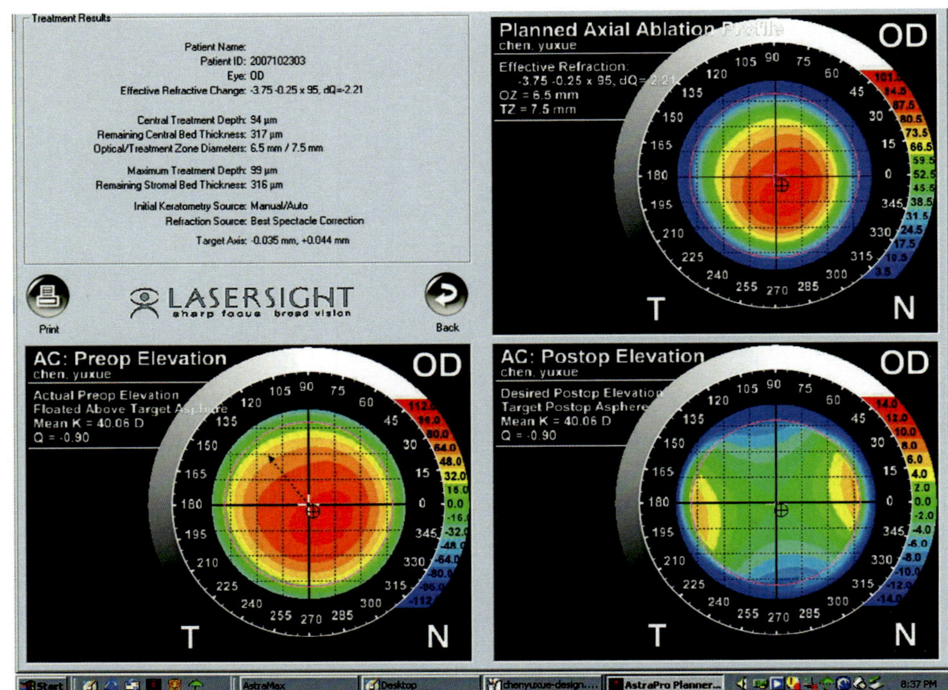

Fig. 49.20: AstraPro 2.2Z planned enhancement ablation profile (upper right), pre-enhancement elevation with the target A-axis optimized (lower left) and predicted post-operative elevation map (lower right). Note that the pre-enhancement elevation shows the same elevated pattern as the enhancement ablation profile when using the optimized post-enhancement corneal vertex as the reference axis. In this example, the optimized axis is offset 0.035 mm temporally, and 0.044 mm superiorly from the pre-enhancement corneal vertex axis (*Courtesy:* Dr. Bing Liu, General Air Force Hospital)

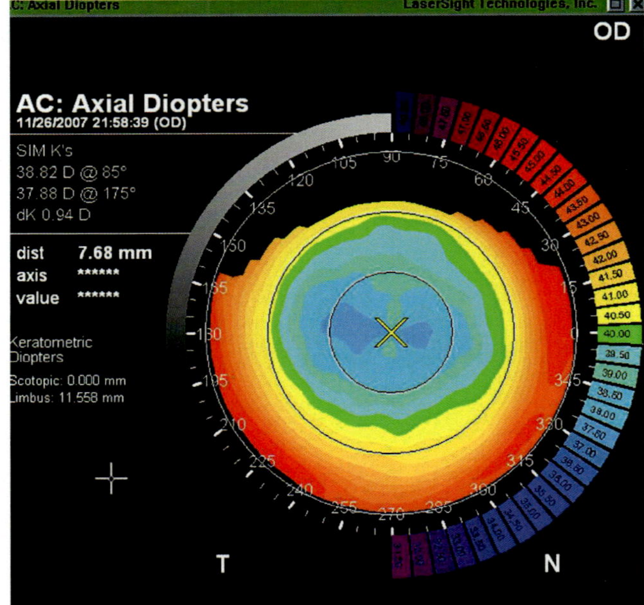

Fig. 49.21: Post-enhancement axial curvature map showing the decentration has been completely corrected (*Courtesy:* Dr. Bing Liu, General Air Force Hospital)

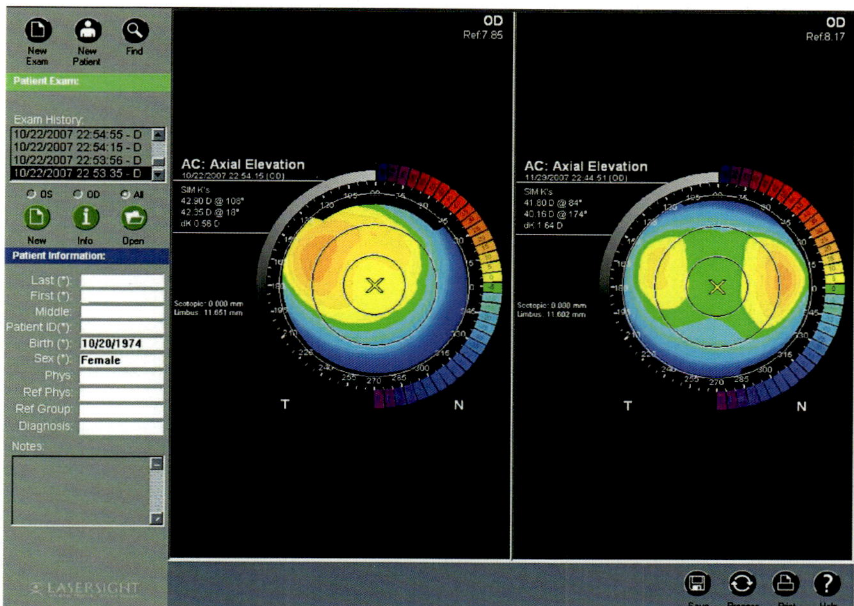

Fig. 49.22: Pre-enhancement and post-enhancement axial elevation map. Note that when the vertex normal is not changed (as in this figure), the elevation map of the decentered ablation shows elevation where the cornea was actually ablated for a myopic treatment. This is because the area becomes flatter. Compare this map to the lower left corner of Fig. 49.20, where the corneal-vertex normal is optimized (Target Z axis). Using the optimized axis gives an elevated area where no adequate ablation was applied, consistent with the optimized enhancement ablation profile as indicated in Fig. 49.20, upper right. (*Courtesy:* Dr Bing Liu, General Air Force Hospital)

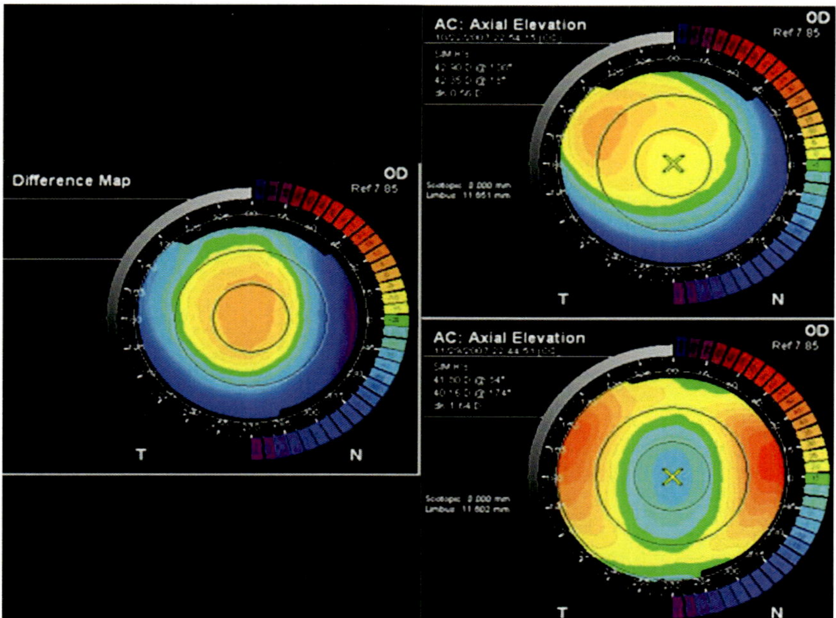

Fig. 49.23: Pre-enhancement and post-enhancement axial elevation difference map, showing pre-enhancement elevation (upper right), post-enhancement elevation (lower right) and elevation difference (left), using a reference sphere of 7.85 mm (*Courtesy:* Dr Bing Liu, General Air Force Hospital)

REFERENCES

1. Chan CC, Boxer Wachler BS. Centration analysis of ablation over the coaxial corneal light reflex for hyperopic LASIK. J Cataract Refract Surg 2006;22:467-71.
2. Amano S, Nanba A, Hamada N, et al. Corneal irregular astigmatism after hyperopic laser in situ keratomileusis. Cornea 2005;24(7):789-92.
3. Gimbel, Howard V. Refractive Surgery: A Manual of Principles and Practice. SLACK Incorporated, 2000;75-8, 114.
4. Mulhern M, Foley-Nolan A, O'Keefe M, Condon P. Topographic analysis of ablation centration after excimer laser photorefractive keratectomy and laser in situ keratomileusis for high myopia. J Cataract Refract Surg 1997; 23:488-94.
5. Schalhorn SC, Amesbury EC, Tanzer DJ. Avoidance, recognition, and management of LASIK complications. Am J Ophthalmol 2006;141(4):733-9.
6. Randleman JB, Etiology and clinical presentations of irregular astigmatism after keratorefractive surgery. In Irregular Astigmatism: Diagnosis and Treatment. Wang MX (Ed). SLACK Incorporated, 2008;73-5.
7. Ou JI, Manche EE. Topographic centration of ablation after LASIK for myopia using the CustomVue VISX S4 excimer laser. J Cataract Refract Surg 2007;23:193-7.
8. Vinciguerra P, Camesasca FI. Decentration after refractive surgery. J Refract Surg 2001;17 (2 Suppl):S190-1.
9. Salmon TO, Horner DG. Comparison of elevation, curvature, and power descriptors for corneal topographic mapping. Optom Vis Sci 1995;72(11):800-8.
10. Rachid MD, Yoo SH, Azar DT. Phototherapeutic keratectomy for decentration and central islands after photorefractive keratectomy. Ophthalmology 2001;108:545-52.
11. Lafond G, Bonnet S, Solomon L. Treatment of previous decentered excimer laser ablation with combined myopic and hyperopic ablations. J Refract Surg 2004; 20:139-48.
12. Carones F, Vigo L, Scandola E. Wavefront-guided treatment of symptomatic eyes using the LADAR6000 excimer laser. J Refract Surg 2006;22(9):S983-9.
13. Kanellopoulos AJ, Pe LH. Wavefront-guided enhancements using the wavelight excimer laser in symptomatic eyes previously treated with LASIK. J Refract Surg 2006; 22(4):345-9.
14. Mrochen M, Krueger RR, Bueeler M, Seiler T. Aberration-sensing and wavefront-guided laser in situ keratomileusis: management of decentered ablation. J Refract Surg 2002;18(4):418-29.
15. AliÃ J, Galal A, MontalbÃjn R, Piñero D. Corneal wavefront-guided LASIK retreatments for correction of highly aberrated corneas following refractive surgery. J Refract Surg 2007;23(8):760-73.
16. Salz JJ. Wavefront-guided treatment for previous laser *in situ* keratomileusis and photorefractive keratectomy: case reports. J Refract Surg 2003;19(6):S697-702.
17. Schwartz GS, Park DH, Lane SS. CustomCornea wavefront retreatment after conventional laser *in situ* keratomileusis. J Cataract Refract Surg 2005;31(8):1502-5.
18. Montague AA, Manche EE. CustomVue laser *in situ* keratomileusis treatment after previous keratorefractive surgery. J Cataract Refract Surg 2006;32(5):795-8.
19. Lin DY, Manche EE. Custom-contoured ablation pattern method for the treatment of decentered laser ablations. J Cataract Refract Surg 2004;30(8):1675-84.
20. Tamayo Fernandez GE, Serrano MG. Early clinical experience using custom excimer laser ablations to treat irregular astigmatism. J Cataract Refract Surg 2000; 26(10):1442-50.
21. Tamayo F, Serrano MG. Treating Irregular Astigmatism and Keratoconus with the VISX C-CAP Method. Int Ophthalmol Clin 2003 Summer;43(3):103-10.
22. Alessio G, Boscia F, La Tegola MG, Sborgia C. Corneal Interactive Programmed Topographic Ablation Customized Keratectomy for Correction of Postkeratoplasty Astigmatism. Opthalmology 2001;108:2029-37.
23. Stojanovic A, Suput D. Strategic planning in topography-guided ablation of irregular astigmatism after laser refractive surgery. J Refract Surg 2005;21(4):369-76.
24. Toda I, Yamamoto T, Ito M, Hori-Komai Y, Tsubota K. Topography-guided ablation for treatment of patients with irregular astigmatism. J Refract Surg 2007; 23(2):118-25.
25. Pedrotti E, Sbabo A, Marchini G. Customized transepithelial photorefractive keratectomy for iatrogenic ametropia after penetrating or deep lamellar keratoplasty. J Cataract Refract Surg 2006;32(8):1288-91.
26. Mularoni A, Laffi GL, Bassein L, Tassinari G. Two-step LASIK with topography-guided ablation to correct astigmatism after penetrating keratoplasty. J Refract Surg 2006;22(1):67-74.
27. Seitz B, Langenbucher A, Kus MED MER, Harrer M. Experimental correction of irregular corneal astigmatism using topography-based flying-spot-mode excimer laser photoablation. Am J Ophtalmol 1998;125:252-6.
28. Alessio G, Boscia F, La Tegola MG, Sborgia C. Topography-driven Excimer Laser for the Retreatment of Decentralized Myopic Photorefractive Keratectomy. Opthalmology 2001;108:1695-1703.
29. Kymionis GD, Panagopoulou SI, Aslanides IM, Plainis S, Astyrakakis N, Pallikaris IG. Topographically supported customized ablation for the management of decentered laser *in situ* keratomileusis. Am J Ophthalmol 2004;137(5):806-11.
30. Reinstein DZ, Archer TJ, Gobbe M. Topography Guided Ablation with the Carl Zeiss Meditec MEL80 and CRS Master. In Irregular Astigmatism: Diagnosis and Treatment. Ming Wang, (Ed). Slack, Inc, Thoroughfare, NJ. 2007.
31. Stojanoviæ A, Jankov MR. Regularizing the cornea – the concept of an ideal corneal surface (iVIS Suite approach to the treatment of irregular astigmatism). In Corneal Topography in the Wavefront Era. Wang MX, (Ed). Slack, Thoroughfare, NJ, 2007.

50 Femtosecond Laser-associated Complications

Payman Haft, George Kymionis, William W Culbertson, Sonia Yoo

INTRODUCTION

Recently, corneal flap creation by the femtosecond laser has emerged as a new option in LASIK. The femtosecond laser applies patterned pulses of ultrashort wavelength energy at many intrastromal points at a predetermined depth. Each laser pulse generates a small amount of micro-plasma without affecting anterior tissues, which results in an interface of microscopic gas bubbles and flap interface creation.

Femtosecond-laser assisted flap creation has rapidly been gaining popularity. This technology offers many advantages over the microkeratome, including improved uniformity of the flap, better predictability of the flap thickness, and above all, increased safety of the procedure. Furthermore, flap creation by the femtosecond laser has been shown to be safe and to produce similar outcomes compared to the microkeratome in terms of high-contrast visual acuity, manifest refractive error, contrast sensitivity, and patient preference.

Flap creation by the femtosecond laser is more predictable and reliable than traditional microkeratomes.[1-3] There are, however, potential problems with the femtosecond laser, including complications associated with femtosecond corneal flap creation such as suction loss, vertical gas epithelial break through, anterior chamber gas bubbles and opaque bubble layer (OBL), transient light sensitive syndrome, diffuse lamellar keratitis, macular hemorrhage and irregular or decentered flaps.

Femtosecond-laser associated complications related to refractive surgery can more accurately be organized into direct and indirect complications. A recent retrospective review by Yoo et al[4] of 4772 eyes at one academic center with Intralase-assisted LASIK performed showed a 1.3% rate of total complications. The rate of direct laser-associated complications was 0.9%, and the rate of indirect complications was 0.42%. Some of the more common direct complications of the femtosecond laser include suction loss, epithelial breaks, gas bubbles in the anterior chamber, transient light sensitivity, and irregular flaps.

SUCTION LOSS

Suction loss may occur during laser flap creation, which can lead to an incomplete flap. Retreatment to complete the flap may be problematic, because original plane of cutting may not be found and a second interface may be created. Also, a thin, buttonholed, or irregular flap may be created.

Improper technique in applying the suction ring to the eye can cause loss of suction. A study examining risk factors for loss of suction in microkeratome-assisted LASIK found other risk factors for inadequate fixation, including narrow palpebral fissures, flat corneas, and young age.[16] Narrower palpebral fissures leave limited room to effectively apply the suction apparatus to the eye. Younger patients may have stiffer lids that do not open as easily with a lid speculum. Conjunctival chemosis at the limbus may also interfere with the suction ring, not allowing adequate suction to build. Conjunctival massage can be used to push fluid away from the limbus in the case of conjunctival edema from repeated suction attempts. In addition, a conjunctival incision can be used to drain fluid and lessen edema. Sometimes, delaying the procedure for a few hours to few days may be needed for the edema to resolve.[17]

Binder reported suction loss in six eyes out of 1000 cases.[1] In a retrospective study of 4772 eyes after Femtosecond-LASIK in Bascom Palmer Eye Institute, the rate of suction loss was 0.06%.[4] A second pass successfully managed incomplete flaps resulted in flaps as planned. All the procedures were completed, and the operative eyes that were followed up for at least 6 months had excellent visual and refractive results.

EPITHELIAL BREAKS

Epithelial breakthrough during femtosecond laser flap creation has been reported and studied very recently; there have been only a few cases reported in the literature of this type of complication. Srinivasan and Herzig[5] first reported a case of subepithelial gas breakthrough during flap creation for LASIK. They proposed that thin flaps, or a focal break in Bowman's membrane may contribute to vertical gas breakthrough. Seider et al[6] reported 4 cases of epithelial breakthrough in 2922 IntraLase-assisted LASIK procedures (0.14%). Three out of the four cases reported in this study had corneal stromal scars, which the authors felt contributed to the condition. Two out of three cases with corneal scars had epithelial breaks occur during flap lifting. One case had epithelial gas breakthrough during IntraLase flap creation. Subsequent follow up data from the same institution reported 8/4772 eyes with this type of complication (0.17%). It was proposed that for gas breakthrough, a focal area of altered epithelium and thinned stroma in the area of scarring created a low-resistance pathway that allowed the gas bubbles to escape toward the surface, instead of through the typical lamellar plane. For epithelial breaks during flap lifting (after the femtosecond laser assisted flap was created), it has been proposed that stromal scarring may trap gas bubbles and not allow advancement through the flap interface to allow completion of the flap. In addition, during flap lifting itself, stromal fibrosis may anchor the flap to the underlying bed and induce breakthrough and flap tears. For these reasons, femtosecond laser flap creation should be done with caution in patients with corneal scars. If possible, increasing flap thickness may allow the creation of a flap interface more posterior to the scars. If scars are widespread and visualization of anterior chamber structures is difficult, femtosecond laser flap creation should be avoided.

ANTERIOR CHAMBER GAS BUBBLES

Gas bubbles in the anterior chamber (Fig. 50.1) are an increasingly recognized potential complication of the femtosecond laser. Obscuration of anterior chamber structures (i.e. iris and pupil) with bubbles can result in faulty laser pupil tracking and iris registration, which can affect excimer laser ablation. Lifshitz et al[7] reported a case in a 48 year-old woman undergoing wavefront-guided LASIK for myopia.

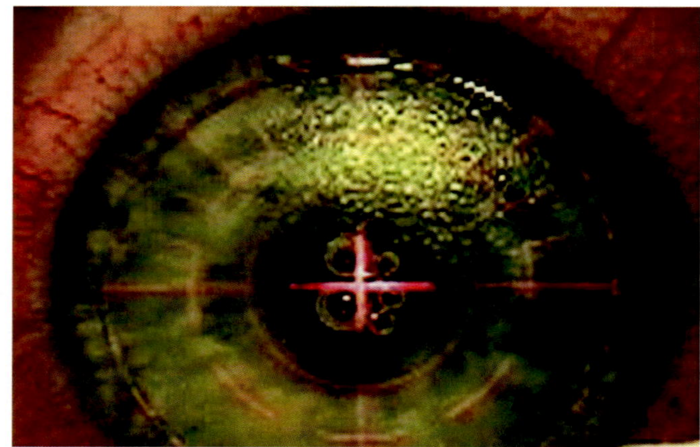

Fig. 50.1: Gas bubbles in the anterior chamber obscuring the patient's view of the laser fixation light

Bubbles were noted in the anterior chamber, which disappeared after 30 minutes. After the procedure, uncorrected visual acuity was 20/25 in both eyes; and specular microscopy showed normal corneal endothelial findings. Srinivasan and Rootman[8] later reported anterior chamber bubble formation in a 30-year-old man underwent customized wavefront-guided LASIK for myopia. The case was uncomplicated and uneventful, and no bubbles were seen the next day. In the Yoo et al series,[4] 8/4772 eyes (0.17%) had anterior chamber bubbles, all of which interfered with laser pupil tracking and iris registration. Overall, anterior chamber bubbles seem to be by themselves harmless and transient, but they can affect the excimer laser ablation, rendering the procedure problematic or impossible when they are present.

OPAQUE BUBBLE LAYER (OBL)

This complication is the formation of gas bubbles in the corneal lamellae during the flap creation (Fig. 50.2). During the photodisruptive cutting process, high pressure bubbles located in the interlamellar spaces of the cornea may create an opaque bubble layer. These opacities could interfere with flap interface quality or excimer laser ablation. In order to eliminate this complication, surgeons should adjust femtosecond laser settings (such as pocket creation) or applanation technique (docking technique). In a recent study, Kaiserman et al[9] found that there was a predisposition for higher rate of OBL in thicker corneas and small flap diameters. In cases with excessive OBL, postponing the treatment may be preferred in order to allow the absorption/elimination of these bubbles.

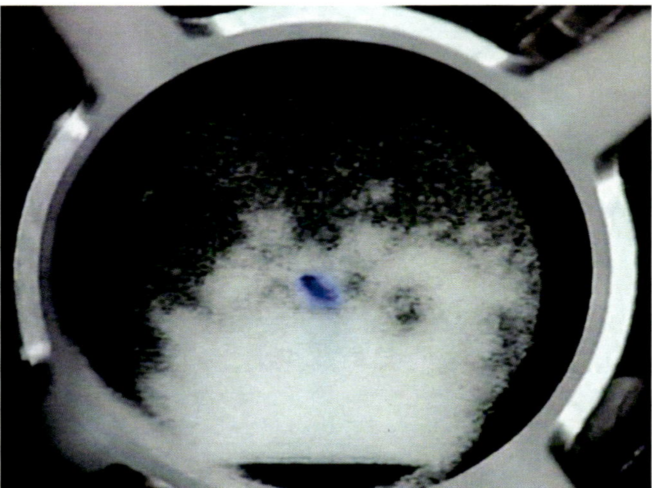

Fig. 50.2: Gas bubbles deep to the interface in the anterior stromal bed ("deep OBL")

TRANSIENT LIGHT SENSITIVITY SYNDROME

The term transient light-sensitivity syndrome (TLSS) has been used to describe a clinical condition characterized by unusual photosensitivity with normal visual acuity several weeks after otherwise uneventful LASIK with the femtosecond laser that typically responds to topical treatment with topical steroids or cyclosporin. Stonecipher et al[10] reported a 1.1% rate of this complication (5667 total cases). All of these patients were treated with prednisolone acetate drops, whereas 1 surgeon also used cyclosporine 0.05% ophthalmic solution. Patients noted improvement of symptoms within 1 week of treatment. Munoz et al[11] also reported on TLSS after femtosecond laser-assisted LASIK. They reported a 1.3% incidence of TLSS, which decreased with aggressive use of postoperative topical steroids. Yoo et al[4] reported 12 eyes (0.25%) with transient light sensitivity.

IRREGULAR FLAP

An irregular or decentered flap may also occur. Irregular flaps can result from loss of suction. Patients with deep set eyes or small corneas, or eyes with conjunctival edema, can result in inadequate contact with the suction apparatus. Avoidance of cutting the flap when the IOP is low (low suction) is an important precaution. Pressures of 80 mm Hg or more may be required for safe flap creation. Steep corneas and buttonhole flap formation were more of a problem with microkeratome-assisted flap creation, due to buckling of the cornea at the applanation head, as well as proposed increased corneal resistance with upward movement of the cutting blade.[17]

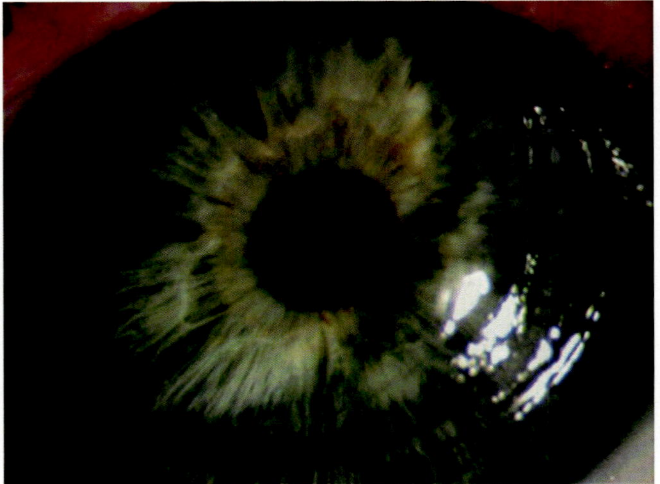

Fig. 50.3: Flap torn during attempt to forcefully dissect flap with spatula

With these types of complications, the safest management may be to reposition the flap and aborting the procedure (Fig. 50.3). A deeper flap can typically be recut about 3 months later. In the Yoo retrospective study of Femtosecond LASIK by Yoo et al,[4] this complication was found in only one eye. Despite that, the procedure was completed uneventfully.

DIFFUSE LAMELLAR KERATITIS (DLK)

Diffuse lamellar keratitis (DLK, sands of the Sahara, SOS) is a syndrome that can result in diffuse haze of the interface.[12] This usually occurs from postoperative day 1-6 and can cause decreased vision after refractive procedures (Fig. 50.4). It is a noninfectious condition in which white blood cells infiltrate the space between the flap and the stromal bed shortly after laser in-situ keratomileusis (LASIK). This complication can also appear months or even years after LASIK and is associated with other conditions, such as trauma, epithelial abrasions or iritis. Diffuse lamellar keratitis is typically associated with moderate foreign-body sensation and decreased visual acuity, and it usually resolves without sequelae with appropriate treatment. Treatment includes topical steroids, oral steroids (in more severe cases), and lifting of the flap and irrigating the stromal bed with balanced salt solution. Binder[13] reported moderate DLK in the first 20 eyes in a series of 103 eyes (19.4%) operated on with the IntraLase 6 kHz femtosecond laser. Javaloy et al[14] reported stage 1-3 DLK in 17 of 100 eyes (17%) using a 15 kHz femtosecond laser. Gil-Cazorla et al[15] reported 5 cases of stage 2-3 DLK in 1000 eyes with the IntraLase 15 khz laser. The lower incidence of DLK in the IntraLase group in the Gil-Cazorla et al study may be explained by the more intense anti-inflammatory therapy (8 times daily in the femtosecond group instead of 4 times daily) during the first postoperative week. In the study by Yoo et al,[4] 20 eyes (0.42%) developed post-LASIK diffuse lamellar keratitis (DLK, stage 1-2). All patients had clinically evident DLK on postoperative day 1, and all were treated with an intensive course of steroids. No surgical intervention was needed (e.g. flap lift). At one year follow-up, all patients were emmetropic without loss of BCVA.

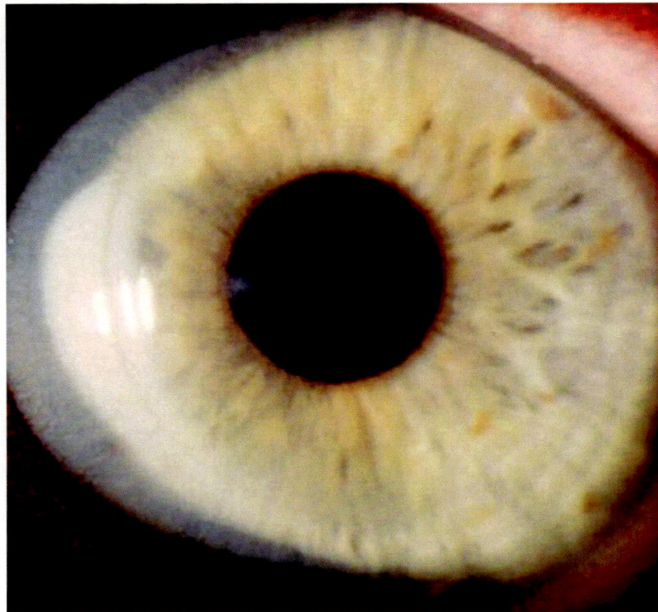

Fig. 50.4: Diffuse lamellar keratitis

SUMMARY

In conclusion, even though the application of femtosecond technology in refractive surgery does not completely eliminate LASIK complications, there is a significantly lower incidence of Femtosecond LASIK complications in comparison with microkeratomes (which are estimated approximately 5%). Further improvements in femtosecond laser technology could further enhance LASIK outcomes.

REFERENCES

1. Binder PS. One thousand consecutive IntraLase laser in sitů keratomileusis flaps. J Cataract Refract Surg. 2006 Jun;32(6): 962-9.
2. Stulting RD, Carr JD, Thompson KP, et al. Complications of laser in situ keratomileusis for the correction of myopia. Ophthalmology 1999;106:13–20.
3. Gimbel HV, Penno EE, van Westenbrugge JA, et al. Incidence and management of intraoperative and early postoperative complications in 1000 consecutive laser in situ keratomileusis cases. Ophthalmology 1998;105:1839–47.
4. Yoo SH, Kymionis GD, Ide T, Haft P, Deobhakta A, Seider M. LASIK Complications with IntraLase Femtosecond Laser. Presented at the 2007 American Academy of Ophthalmology Annual Meeting, Refractive Surgery Subspecialty Day.
5. Srinivasan S, Herzig S. Sub-epithelial gas breakthrough during femtosecond laser flap creation for LASIK. Br J Ophthalmol 2007; 91(10):1373.
6. Seider MI, Ide T, Kymionis GD, Culbertson WW, O'Brien TP, Yoo SH. Epithelial Breakthrough: A Complication During IntraLase Flap Creation for Laser In Situ Keratomileusis.
7. Lifshitz T, Levy J, Klemperer I, Levinger S. Anterior chamber gas bubbles after corneal flap creation with a femtosecond laser. J Cataract Refract Surg 2005;31(11): 2227-9.
8. Srinivasan S, Rootman DS. Anterior chamber gas bubble formation during femtosecond laser flap creation for LASIK. J Refract Surg 2007;23(8):828-30.
9. Kaiserman I, Maresky H, Bahar I,Rootman DS. Incidence, possible risk factors, and potential effects of an opaque bubble layer created by a femtosecond laser J Cataract Refract Surg 2008; 34:417–423
10. Stonecipher KG, Dishler JG, Ignacio TS, et al. Transient light sensitivity after femtosecond laser flap creation: clinical findings and management. J Cataract Refract Surg 2006;32: 91-94.
11. Muñoz G, Albarrán-Diego C, Sakla HF, Javaloy J, Alió JL. Transient light-sensitivity syndrome after laser in situ keratomileusis with the femtosecond laser. Incidence and prevention. J Cataract Refract Surg 2006;32(12):2075-9.
12. Smith RJ, Maloney RK. Diffuse lamellar keratitis; a new syndrome in lamellar refractive surgery. Ophthalmology 1998;105:1721-6.
13. Binder PS. Flap dimensions created with the IntraLase FS laser. J Cataract Refract Surg 2004;30:26-32.
14. Javaloy J, Vidal MT, Abdelrahman AM, Artola A, Alio JL. Confocal microscopy comparison of IntraLase femtosecond laser and Moria M2 microkeratome in LASIK. J Refract Surg 2007;23: 178-87.
15. Gil-Cazorla R, Teus MA, de Benito-Llopis L, Fuentes I. Incidence of diffuse lamellar keratitis after laser in situ keratomileusis associated with the IntraLase 15 kHz femtosecond laser and Moria M2 microkeratome. J Cataract Refract Surg 2008;34(1):28-31.
16. Asano-Kato N, Toda I, Hori-Komai Y, Takano Y, Tsubota K. Risk factors for insufficient fixation of microkeratome during laser in situ keratmileusis. J Refract Surg 2002;18(1):47-50.
17. Melki SA, Azar DT. LASIK complications: etiology, management, and prevention. Surv Ophthalmol 2001;46(2):95-116. Review.

51 Vitreoretinal Complications of Refractive Surgery

Steve Charles, Adam M Katz, Kent Zocchi

INTRODUCTION

Refractive surgery has grown at a phenomenal pace during the 1990s fueled by new techniques and technology, medical economics, marketing, and an explosion of interest in self-image. The incredible growth of cosmetics, fashion, exercise equipment and services, and plastic surgery are indicators of this trend. Many people couple the wearing of glasses with their self-image and relate glasses to difficulty in finding partners, careers, and social acceptance. Refractive procedures are almost invariably paid for by the patient rather than a third party. The typical surgical candidate is in the third or fourth decade of life and therefore has many years to live with the outcome of refractive surgery. Most refractive surgery candidates live active lives, play multiple sports, and have visually demanding occupations. Cataract and refractive surgeons have worked very hard to improve predictability and promote a patient-friendly approach with the promise of rapid return to full, *normal* function. Print and electronic advertising, patient seminars, videos, physician preoperative counseling and educational brochures infrequently mention vitreoretinal complications. The candidates typically have excellent vision with glasses and/or contacts. The psychodynamics created by this environment often lead to litigation if the patient is not satisfied with the outcome, especially in the United States.

The purpose of this chapter is to explore the potential and proven vitreoretinal complications of refractive surgery. The authors are vitreoretinal surgeons and have no bias for, or against, refractive surgery. Vitreoretinal surgeons are increasingly being asked to "clear" patients for refractive surgery. This process creates moral obligation to the patient and may cause contributory legal responsibility for the consultant. It is impossible to "clear" a patient for surgery and "guarantee" that no vitreoretinal complication will occur.

Temporal association between events implies, but does not prove causality. A retinal detachment or macular hemorrhage occurring hours after any refractive procedure would "prove" causality to the patient, jury, and the general public even if the temporal association was mere coincidence. It is well known that myopic patients have a higher incidence of retinal breaks, detachment and choroidal neovascular membranes than the emmetropic population. It is often thought that this is a mechanical, acquired, phenomenon based on the notion that the eye grows longer, stretching the retina and making it thinner. This primitive explanation is unwarranted and is as ridiculous as saying "all tall people must be thin". High myopes without peripheral retinal degenerations have much lower detachment rates than emmetropic patients with peripheral retinal degenerations. It is better to think of peripheral retinal degenerations as being genetically linked to myopia and the primary factor in retinal detachment. It is not known if a longer eye is prone to retinal detachment because of length alone.

PREOPERATIVE EXAMINATION

It is unknown what examination methods are required, when a refractive surgery candidate is referred to a retinal consultant before surgery. Is indirect ophthalmoscopy sufficient or are 360-degree scleral depression and/or 3-mirror contact lens necessary? In view of the notion of "clearing" patients for refractive surgery, it behooves the retinal consultant to perform a very careful examination while explaining to the patient that "clearing" or a "guarantee" is impossible.

PROPHYLAXIS OF RETINAL BREAKS AND DEGENERATIONS

The efficacy of laser or cryopexy prophylaxis in preventing retinal breaks and detachment in the event of subsequent refractive procedures has not been shown. The majority of retinal breaks in retinal detachment failure cases are immediately posterior to areas of cryopexy raising questions about the concept of "making a new ora serratta". Which breaks should be treated is not known:

- Should all breaks be treated or only symptomatic breaks?
- Should only breaks outside lattice be treated or those inside lattice as well?
- Should lattice without breaks be treated?
- Should peripheral retinal degenerations other than lattice be treated.
- Should "atrophic" breaks be treated?
- Does location matter?
- Does family history of retinal detachment matter?
- Does eye length matter?

There is significant controversy about whether extensive peripheral retinopexy is effective in preventing retinal detachment in giant break, proliferative vitreoretinopathy (PVR), and clear-lens extraction patients.

SOURCES OF INFORMATION FOR THIS CHAPTER

The worldwide web via a variety of metasearch engines was used to search for publications citing vitreoretinal complications of refractive surgery. The Journal of the American Society of Cataract and Refractive Surgery, Archives of Ophthalmology, Retina, Ophthalmology, Survey of Ophthalmology, Ophthalmology Times, American Journal of Ophthalmology and Ocular Surgery News were included in the search. Many leaders in refractive surgery were contacted by phone call with a request for publications, case reports, or other information relating refractive surgery and vitreoretinal complications. A request for information was posted on the members-only Vitreous Society Website and many responses were received.

THEORETICAL MECHANISMS RESULTING IN RETINAL BREAKS AND DETACHMENT

Anterior Chamber Shallowing

Anterior movement of lens and anterior vitreous causes "traction" forces on peripheral retina which, in turn, may lead to retinal breaks. Microperforation is a significant cause of anterior chamber shallowing during radial keratotomy, astigmatic keratotomy, the microkeratome step in LASIK, or the placement of intrastromal rings (Fig. 51.1). Pachymetry, depth adjustments on diamond knives, better microkeratome technology and other precautions have reduced, but not eliminated, microperforation.

Clear-lens extraction causes intraoperative anterior shallowing and anterior movement of the lens and vitreous in *all* cases (Fig. 51.2). Many point out that an IOL may prevent anterior displacement of the vitreous, but this is true *only* in the postoperative period. There are many cases of retinal detachment after clear-lens extraction and many experts feel that this procedure is never indicated. Clear-lens extraction is probably contraindicated in the young, axial myopia (>29 mm), and in eyes with peripheral chorioretinal degenerations.

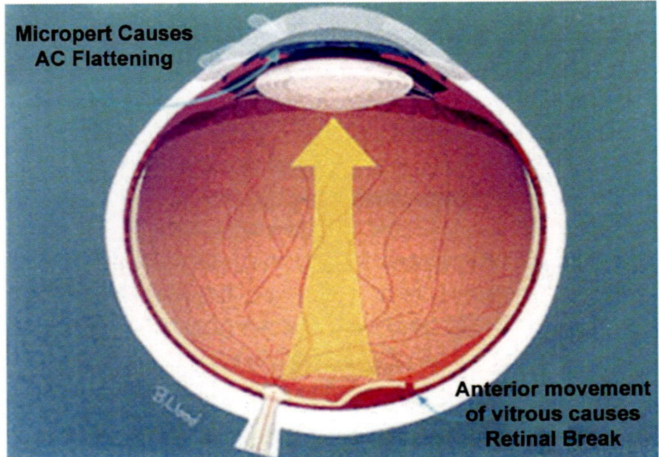

Fig. 51.1: Microperforation of the cornea can lead to anterior chamber shallowing. This allows anterior movement of the vitreous, with resulting retinal breaks at areas of high vitreoretinal adherence

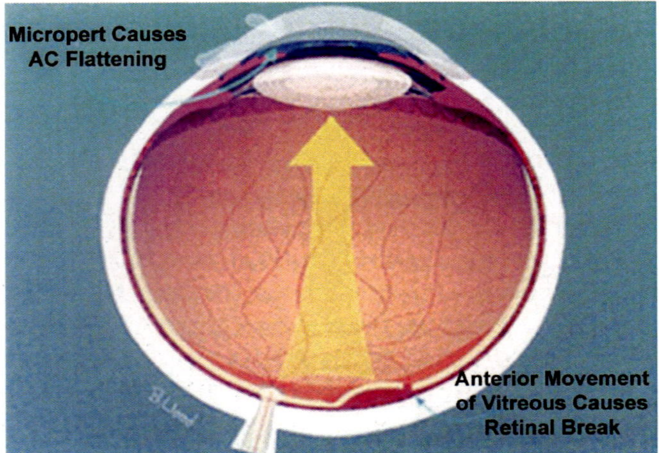

Fig. 51.2: Lens displacement during clear-lens extraction causes movement of the vitreous and subsequent traction on peripheral retina

Phakic IOLs for high myopia are assumed by many surgeons to have no risk of retinal detachment but again this is untrue because of the obligatory intraoperative shallowing of the anterior chamber. One of the authors (SC) was referred a case of bilateral inoperable retinal detachment from Russia occurring soon after phakic IOL implantation in a young male. Both eyes had inoperable retinal detachments and went on to become phthisical. There are less articles on this subject and it is likely that the incidence is less than in clear-lens extraction cases.

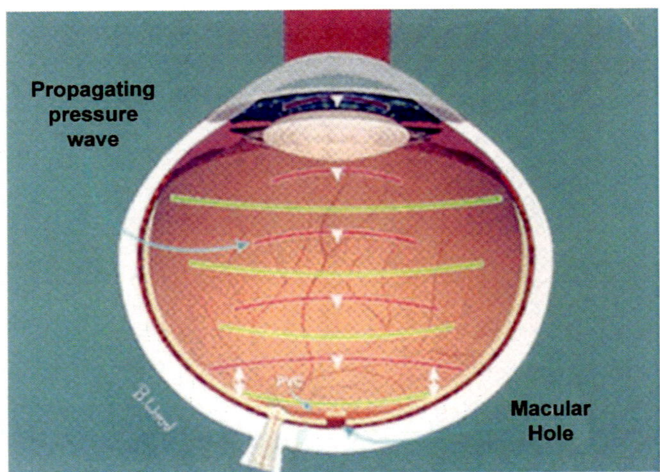

Fig. 51.3: Propagating pressure waves from laser-tissue interaction may lead to pulsatile movement of the posterior vitreous cortex, causing macular hole formation

Acoustic Effects

Laser-tissue interaction causes acoustic pressure waves to propagate through the vitreous theoretically causing retinal breaks (Fig. 51.3). The concave surface of the ocular interior can focus the acoustic energy, significantly increasing local acoustic damage. Photorefractive keratectomy (PRK) and laser-in-situ-keratomileusis (LASIK) produce high-energy acoustic waves, which have the potential of producing significant forces on the vitreous and retina. One of the authors (SC) has seen a patient that developed a macular hole instantaneously *during* a YAG (yttrium-aluminum-garnet) laser capsulotomy. A careful and experienced surgeon used normal power settings and a low number of pulses and the patient had a normal pretreatment macula. It is probable that an acoustic pressure wave pulled in a pulsatile fashion on posterior vitreous cortex attached to the macula.

There is a striking paucity of articles on vitreoretinal complications of LASIK and PRK. Many anecdotal case reports were obtained from experts in the field and retinal consultants. The incidence of vitreoretinal complication appears to be rather low in the few series published. A low incidence may, however, be explained by lack of awareness, observer bias, short follow-up intervals, lack of a control group, and poor study design.

Macular Hemorrhage

Macular hemorrhage secondary to choroidal neovascular membranes occurs in myopic patients that have not undergone refractive surgery. It has been reported (Blair) that age-related macular degeneration (AMD) patients have an increased incidence of submacular hemorrhage immediately after cataract surgery. It is thought that pre-existing neovascular membranes are caused to bleed by the obligatory lowering of IOP that occurs during lens removal and IOL placement. This mechanism is similar to the pathogenesis of suprachoroidal hemorrhage during or after cataract surgery. It is probable that the same mechanism could occur in any refractive procedure that transiently lowers the IOP. An optimist would assume that any membrane that bled would have done so without surgery. Many choroidal neovascular membranes have a self-limited course in myopic patients and never hemorrhage. It should be assumed that some patients will develop a submacular hemorrhage as a result of refractive surgery that otherwise would have stabilized without bleeding. These patients would have a worse visual outcome than a patient without bleeding.

A careful history and examination with Amsler's chart should be taken preoperatively to determine if the patient has suspicious changes or clinical evidence of a choroidal neovascular membrane. Any suspicious changes indicate the need for fluorescein angiography. Any active, untreatable membranes should be observed until inactive before any refractive procedure is performed.

Nerve Fiber Layer Damage

Nerve fiber layer damage can be caused by increased IOP during suction cup usage before LASIK. An upcoming paper demonstrates reduction of this effect by the use of Brimonidine in a randomized, controlled clinical trial.

Endophthalmitis

Endophthalmitis can occur anytime an incision is made into the eye. There are few reports of endophthalmitis after refractive surgery, but the results can be devastating in at least 50 percent of the patients. Few patients are informed about this potential complication before surgery is performed.

Dislocated Phakic Intraocular Lenses

The authors received a recent case report of (a posterior dislocation of a plate haptic Staar IOL into the vitreous cavity discovered on postoperative day 1 after LASIK) dislocated phakic IOLs immediately after LASIK. Acoustic effects most likely caused this complication, but suction cup use could play a role as well.

SUMMARY

It is apparent that clear-lens extraction causes a relatively high incidence of retinal detachment. Microperforation and phakic IOL insertion have a lesser but significant incidence of retinal detachment, while uncomplicated LASIK and PRK have the lowest incidence. Referring to the incidence of complications as "low" is a value judgement based on our much larger experience with management of diseases that result in loss of vision if no treatment is undertaken. Only a well-informed patient can determine the acceptable risk for a procedure performed for convenience or vanity, rather than a vision-threatening disorder. Careful preoperative examination of the retina and prophylaxis is essential, but offers no guarantee that retinal breaks/detachment will not occur. Careful examination of the macula is essential for these patients. Greater emphasis on vitreoretinal complications should result in better-informed doctors and patients as well as better strategies.

SECTION SEVEN

Miscellaneous

52 Conductive Keratoplasty

Scott G Hauswirth, Elizabeth A Davis

INTRODUCTION TO CONDUCTIVE KERATOPLASTY

History

Several methods of changing corneal curvature to alter the refractive properties of the eye exist, including excimer laser surgery, non-excimer laser surgery, incisional surgery, and corneal ring implants. Conductive keratoplasty is a method of reshaping the corneal curvature to correct for hyperopia, hyperopic astigmatism, and to induce myopia to assist in presbyopia. It was developed on the same foundations as radial keratometry and laser thermal keratoplasty, and incorporates central ideas from both procedures. Radial keratotomy began in Russia in the 1960s when it was found that relaxing incisions performed in a radial pattern on the cornea would flatten the corneal curvature, shifting patients toward hyperopia. Any refractive procedure which flattens the cornea will shift the patient towards hyperopia. Steepening the central cornea then should induce a shift towards myopia.

Thermokeratoplasty used to correct refractive error was used by Fyodorov in 1981.[1] A nickel-chromium probe heated to 600 degrees Fahrenheit was inserted into the corneal stroma to a depth of 95 percent. A radial pattern was used to induce collagen contraction in a circumferential fashion for treatment of spherical hyperopia. It was initially met with reasonable results; however long-term clinical usefulness was marred by regression. Rowsey attempted to use radiofrequency energy in the same fashion. However it was clinically unsuccessful due to rapid regression.[2-3]

Lasers were then applied to the thermokeratoplasty principles to achieve a more desirable effect. Laser thermokeratoplasty (LTK) uses a Holmium-YAG laser at a wavelength of 2.06 μm to create lesions in concentric rings on the cornea and around the pupil. The energy of the laser heats the corneal tissue to a sufficient level to cause contraction of the collagen fibrils in the stroma. Clinical studies using the Holmium-YAG laser were promising. However the long-term results showed high levels of regression.[4] This seemed to be due to the limitation of energy absorption into the deeper layers of tissue. In LTK, absorption of the laser energy is limited by water in the tissues creating greater energy absorption at the surface than deeper in the stroma. This cone-shaped energy absorption profile has a limit to corneal penetration of approximately 60 percent of the stromal depth, below which little to no collagen shrinking occurs. This is at least partly responsible for the increased amount of regression noted in LTK patients.

Conductive keratoplasty builds upon the foundation of these surgeries by applying similar principles under a more controlled setting to achieve correction of hyperopia, astigmatism, and presbyopia (Fig. 52.1).

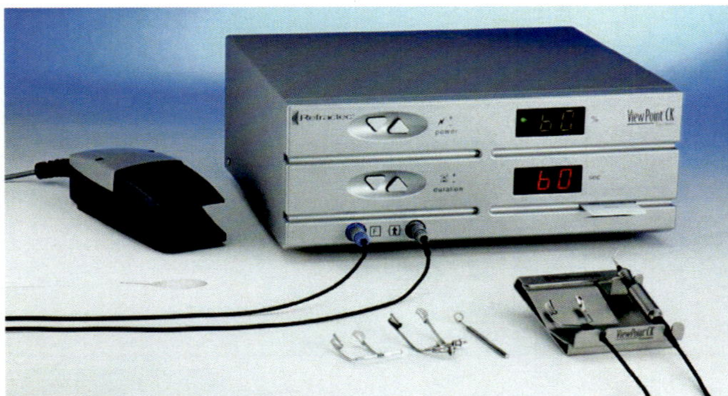

Fig. 52.1: Refractec ViewPoint system

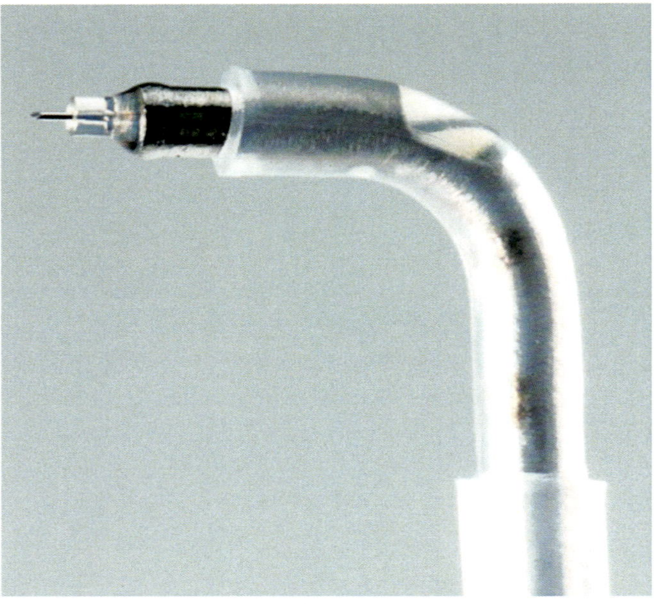

Fig. 52.2: Conductive keratoplasty probe tip

Mechanism of action

The CK probe is 450 microns long and 90 microns wide (Fig. 52.2), and emits high monopolar radiofrequency energy into the surrounding stromal tissue. Energy is released by the probe beginning at the tip of the probe and progressing upwards along the shaft. The probe itself is not hot—it releases electrical energy which is then converted to heat by the electrochemical properties of the surrounding tissue, chiefly by resistance. The conversion of the typical spiral, triple-stranded helix formation of collagen into the contracted form is called denaturation. The corneal stroma is composed of primarily collagen, which begins to contract at approximately 60 degrees C. Between 75 to 80 degrees, collagen experiences maximum shrinkage. Beyond 85 degrees however, it begins to convert to an amorphous form called gelatin. The even energy distribution along the probe along with the relatively homogenous level of resistance in the tissues causes a contraction of the surrounding collagen in a cylindrical pattern, with an average maximum depth of tissue contraction to approximately 80 percent of stromal depth and extending laterally outwards from the probe to about 125 um.[5]

Tissue healing studies in CK have encountered several changes in tissue postoperatively. Histology, confocal light microscopy, immunofluorescence, and transmission electron microscopy reveal the following changes. Epithelial basal cell hypertrophy occurs at the level of Bowman's membrane as well as basal cell elongation at the edge of the break in Bowman's from probe insertion. This elongation serves to fill in the gap left by the probe. A hypercellular fibrotic scar with increased keratocyte presence is found in the anterior stroma to a depth of 50 to 75 um.[6] Below this, a hypocellular primitive scar forms down to nearly the level of Descemet's membrane. The scar serves to fix the striae more permanently, changing the corneal curvature for a longer period of time. Confocal microscopy confirms the presence of these striae up to 12 months postoperatively following CK, indicating a long lasting effect.

Morphologic changes in the human cornea following conductive keratoplasty were studied by Dr. Noumidi.[7] Six human corneas of patients undergoing corneal transplant underwent three CK spot treatments at the 6mm optical zone, and then subsequent penetrating keratoplasty at different postoperative intervals. Corneal buttons were examined with light and electron microscopy.

Twenty-four hours after treatment, morphologic changes to the most anterior structures were minor, the most notable being accumulation of fluid in the anterior portion of Bowman's membrane. The epithelium was only mildly disrupted. Microfolds were seen in the area of the basement membrane. The corneal stroma 24 hours following CK shows crumpled layers of collagen, with some loss of keratocytes. Descemets membrane exhibits no folds, breaks, or cracks. In a study by Guimaraes, 2 of 6 cases were noted to have some endothelial cell loss.[8] However, this is not consistent among other published studies.

Each CK spot creates contraction of the collagen, creating a depression at that particular site. Adjacent spots form striae between them, creating a band of tightening, and a linear area of depression. When the spots are circumferential in the entire cornea, the tightening forces in the periphery create a steepening effect on the central cornea, increasing the corneal curvature. The deeper the degree of depression and the smaller the optical zone, the greater the increase in central curvature.

Traditionally, surgeons' preferences were to use heavy pressure to insert the device tip into the cornea, which resulted in compression and distortion of the corneal tissues, and lessening the effect of the procedure. Proposal of less aggressive means of insertion was made by Milne, termed "Light Touch" CK.[9] The newer OptiPoint device helps to minimize overcompression and ensures correct depth of penetration, accurate placement of the probe, correct angle of approach, and correct spacing of CK spots on the radial axis. This has the potential advantage of decreasing regression as well as increasing the effect of CK.

Indications and patient selection

Patient selection for conductive keratoplasty is similar to that for other refractive procedures with a few exceptions. As with other forms of refractive surgery, candidates should be out of contact lenses for a minimum of 2 weeks for soft lens wearers, and minimum of 3 weeks for rigid gas permeable or hard lens wearers. Refraction, including cycloplegic refraction, should be stable for a minimum of one year (within +/- 0.50DS). There should be no corneal pathology, including anterior basement membrane dystrophy, history of herpetic keratitis, or interstitial keratitis. As with other forms of refractive surgery, dry eye candidates or those with aggressive blepharitis or meibomitis should be treated and stabilized first for optimal results. Conductive keratoplasty candidates should have pachymetry readings of at least 560 microns at the 6-mm zone to avoid full thickness penetration by the probe.

Candidates for surgery should have hyperopia up to +5.00D, with astigmatism less than 1.00 D. For monovision correction for presbyopia, the ideal profile of a presbyopic patient is between 40-58 years of age, -0.75 to +1.00D of spherical refraction, with all of the above physical characteristics.

For astigmatism, generally the correction is viable up to +3.00D of cylinder.

Keratoconus or other keratectasia present interesting challenges and may also be treated with conductive keratoplasty to increase corneal regularity. In addition, it has been used with good results in treating residual refractive error from other refractive procedures, such as LASIK or PRK.[10] Some surgeons have started using it adjunctively as well in an intraoperative setting to supplement refractive lensectomy to reduce postoperative astigmatism.

Method and Technique

Prior to surgery, selection of number of spots and respective optical zones (Fig. 52.3) are selected. Initially, the surgeon may use the nomogram provided by Refractec (Table 52.1). However, surgeons are encouraged to modify the nomogram according to their outcomes.

Table 52.1: LightTouch CK nomogram

Correction	*6mm OZ*	*7mm OZ*	*8mm OZ*
+0.75 to +1.25D	—	—	8 spots
+1.75 to +2.00D	—	8 spots	—
+2.00 to +2.25D	8 spots	—	—
+2.25 to +2.75D	—	8 spots	8 spots
+3.00 to +3.50D	8 spots	8 spots	—

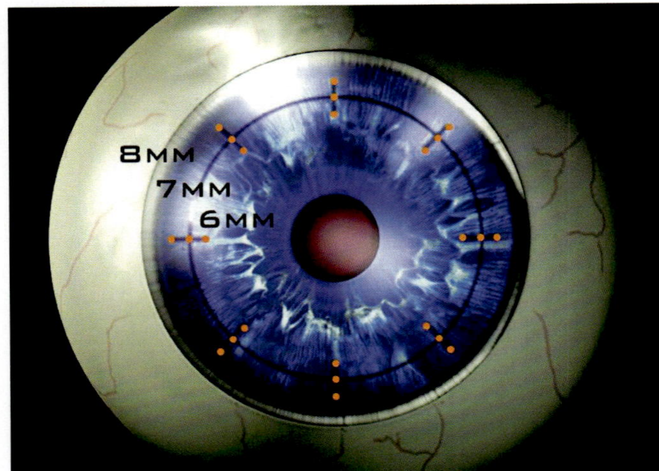

Fig. 52.3: Optical zone diagram

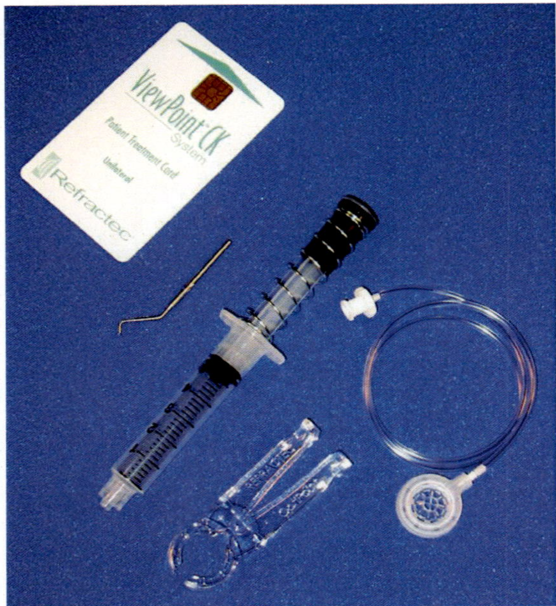

Fig. 52.4: Photo of OptiPoint kit

The patient is managed in much the same way as a pre-excimer laser surgery patient, in terms of perioperative preparation. Due to the compact nature of the CK device, it can easily be used in a laser suite rather than using a fully-equipped operating room.

1. Inspect the NearVision CK(trademark) package to ensure it is untampered and sealed. Do not use if seal has been broken.
2. Assemble the OptiPoint template (Fig. 52.4).

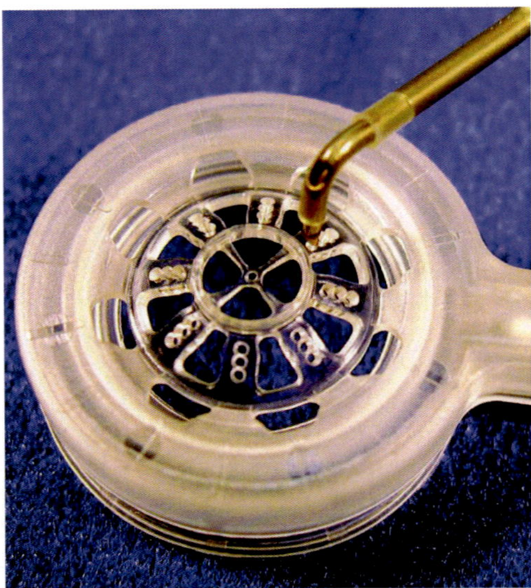

Fig. 52.5: Photo of OptiPoint stencil with probe

3. Position the patient under the laser microscope and prep the eye with topical anesthetic. The eyelids may be prepped with povidone-iodine solution, depending on surgeon preference.
4. Insert the grounded lid speculum into the superior and inferior conjunctival fornices. Check to make sure the palpebral fissure width will accommodate the OptiPoint device (Fig. 52.5).
5. Administer one drop of sterile saline solution to the eye. Allow the limbus to remain moist enough to ensure adequate suction of the OptiPoint device. Mark the center of the cornea with a Sinskey hook.
6. Depress and hold the syringe inward to the 2ml volume mark on the syringe.
7. Align the center hole of the OptiPoint device with the mark on the center of the cornea. Apply firm downward pressure to the device onto the cornea. Release the vacuum on syringe – the OptiPoint device should be secured onto the cornea. If suction breaks, reposition syringe for vacuum and retry.
8. Once the device engages and the eye is fixated, lightly mark the cornea between the wings of the device using a gentian violet marking pen. This assists in eliminating rotational error, and with repositioning if needed.

9. Insert the probe into the guideholes provided on the OptiPoint stencil (Fig. 52.5). The cuff at the superior end of the probe limits depth of insertion by coming into contact with the OptiPoint device.
10. At the completion of the procedure, depress and hold the syringe to release suction.
11. Remove the lid speculum and administer topical medications.

For astigmatic CK correction, the surgeon must place additional spots along the axis of the flattest meridian to account for desired tightening, generally at the 7mm or 8mm optical zones.[11]

Postoperative care

Postoperative medications include a topical steroidal anti-inflammatory agent, a topical non-steroidal anti-inflammatory, and a broad spectrum topical antibiotic. The author's preference is to use the medications each four times per day for one to two weeks. Copious lubrication is advised using artificial tears. Some surgeons prefer to use a bandage contact lens for the first 24 hours to improve patient comfort, although there is usually not a great deal of discomfort after the procedure.

Typical follow-up visits may vary according to surgeon preference, however all patients should be seen on day one postoperatively.

On the first postoperative day, examination includes visual acuity and biomicroscopy. The CK spots seen under the biomicroscope are seen as white patches with a pinpoint break in Bowman's membrane anteriorly, with an overlying epithelial defect and a cylindrical leukoma extending down deep into the stroma.(Fig. 52.6) Striae may be seen radiating out from the spots, and oftentimes may be noted stretching between adjacent CK spots in a circumferential fashion. This denotes the "belt-tightening" which is hallmark for a successful steepening of the central corneal curvature. If a bandage contact lens is used it may be removed on the first postoperative day.

The patient should avoid eye rubbing, and be careful about avoiding splashing water in the eyes.

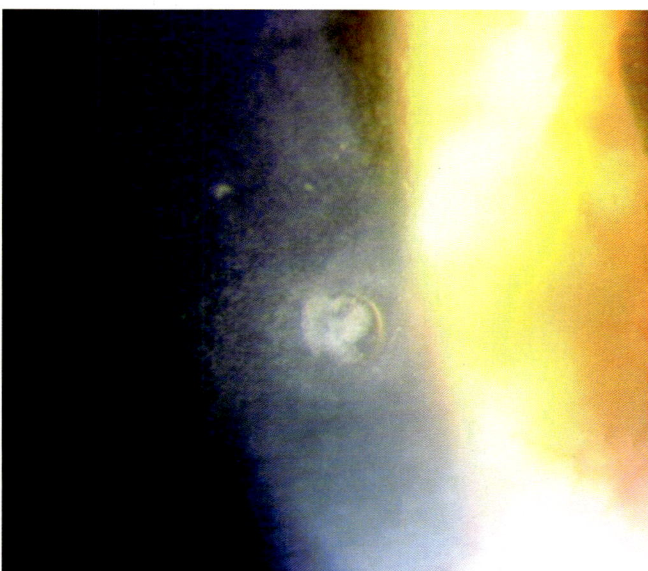

Fig. 52.6: CK spot, one day postoperative

Activities such as swimming or use of hot tubs should be avoided for two weeks following surgery.

One month postoperative tests include visual acuity, manifest refraction, corneal topography, biomicroscopy, and tonometry. Leukomas are still present, and while breaks in Bowman's membrane are still visible, they are completely re-epithelialized. Striae are still present. Some mild irregularity may still be noted on topography, although this varies according to the degree of hyperopic shift desired.

Typical follow-up schedule continues at 3, 6, and 12 months postoperatively.

An important consideration for the post-conductive keratoplasty patient concerns the effect on intraocular pressure measurements by the procedure. A study involving 32 eyes in 18 patients undergoing CK examined these effects.[12] Variables such as device used for measuring IOP (Goldman tonometry) as well as the examiner were held constant. All patients had within +/-0.75D of correction by similar format. A 1.56mmHg drop in IOP was measured which was statistically significant. Due to the small number of patients, and lack of understanding of the mechanism, further studies are warranted.

US FDA TRIALS AND RESULTS

Hyperopia

The US FDA granted approval of the Viewpoint CK System (Refractec, Irvine, CA) for the treatment of low to moderate hyperopia in April of 2002. Initial data used by the FDA included one-year results of a two-year prospective study on 401 eyes from a 13 center, multisite study involving 20 surgeons across the United States. Patient selection criteria included hyperopia ranging from +0.75D to +3.00D with astigmatism of equal to or less than +0.75D; peripheral pachymetry readings of no less than 560 microns at the 6mm optical zone; best corrected visual acuity of 20/40 or greater. Exclusionary criteria included concurrent ocular disease, corneal abnormalities, unstable refractive error, and prior refractive surgery.

No intraoperative complications or adverse events were reported for any of the surgeries.

Postoperative examinations were performed at days 1 and 7, and at months 1,3,6,9, 12, and 24.

At the 12 month visit, UCVA was 20/20 or better in 87 of 171 eyes. Near UCVA increased by an average of 6 Jaeger lines. Mean residual spherical equivalent was within +/-0.50D of plano in 99 of 171 eyes. 156 eyes were within +/-1.00D of plano, and 169/171 were within +/-2.00D of plano.[13] Contrast sensitivity with and without glare was also examined, and at 12 months, no statistically significant difference was found.

At the 12 month visit, only 0.50 percent (1 eye) lost 2 lines of BCVA, and 0.50 percent gained greater than 2.00D of cylinder.

Presbyopia

Treatment of presbyopia with conductive keratoplasty was performed in a prospective, consecutive series with data out to six months by McDonald et al.[14] 176 eyes of 143 patients were enrolled into the clinical trial with monovision providing increased near vision. All patients had prior success in monovision with contact lenses. Eligibility for study included maximum preoperative hyperopic refractive error of +2.00D or less with less than 0.75D of cylinder. Six month results showed 47/73 individuals with UCVA at near of J2 or better, 56/73 with J3 or better, and 65/73 had J5 or better. 72 percent of patients reported extreme or marked improvement in their near vision at 6 months. 76 percent reported being very satisfied with the procedure.

Results out to three years were reported in nine of ten patients by Stahl.[15] Patients were treated with standard pressure technique (as opposed to LightTouch), using monovision in the non-dominant eye. Mean age was 51+/-3.1 years. All but one patient received 16 spot treatment, with all but one target refraction of -1.25DS. As with other forms of hyperopic non-excimer correction, long-term stability over the three year period was assessed. At three years, 22 percent of eyes were within 0.25D of intended refraction, 44 percent were within 0.50D, and 78 percent were within 0.75D. The untreated eyes refractive drift was assessed at +0.26D shift over the three year period. In the CK treated eyes, the drift was +0.25D from year one to year three, indicating excellent refractive stability even with the older technique.

Astigmatism

Correction of hyperopic astigmatism was performed with follow-up to two years by Naoumidi, et al.[11] 47 eyes of 34 patients were examined, with preoperative hyperopic astigmatism up to +3.50D. Preoperative MRSE was +2.11 +/-0.88D. This was reduced to -0.52 +/- 0.73D at twelve months, and held to -0.50 +/- 0.77D at two years. 37 percent of patients reported 20/20 vision or better.

Results using the OptiPoint Device

Between Sept of 2006 to March 2007, 50 procedures were performed using the CK OptiPoint device with follow-up to six months (Durrie, unpublished data). The six month results showed zero percent of patients with 1.00D of induced cylinder.

COMPLICATIONS

Due to the relatively non-invasive nature of conductive keratoplasty, complications tend to be less frequent and less severe than compared to incisional procedures or excimer laser procedures. With careful patient selection and proper use of technique, many complications can be avoided.

Irregular Astigmatism

Irregular astigmatism is possible following conductive keratoplasty, and is the most common complication encountered with the procedure.

Shape changes in the cornea induced by conductive keratoplasty were examined in 19 eyes over a 12 month follow-up period.[16] Preoperative spherical hyperopia ranged from +0.75 to +3.25 D with astigmatism <0.75 D. Twelve months postoperatively, mean asphericity increased +0.044+/-0.24 D (P>.05), mean cylinder increased 0.19+/-0.36 D (P<.05), mean regular astigmatism increased 0.25+/-0.49 D (P>.05), and mean irregular astigmatism decreased 0.01+/–0.13 D (P>.05). Conductive keratoplasty induced a slight regular astigmatism in some eyes, which reportedly decreased over time. The increase in mean corneal asphericity indicated possible induction of central and peripheral cornea changes, however presence of lower amounts of irregular astigmatism postoperatively seem to indicate this may be more of a temporary phenomenon.

Infection

Infection of the site of entry of the CK probe is rare. Although theoretically it may occur, particularly in individuals who have delayed healing of the overlying epithelium, the incidence of infection or abscess formation following CK has not been reported in medical literature.

Epithelial Defects

Persistent epithelial defects overlying the CK sites may occur. Damage to the basement membrane via the probe and heat damage in the most anterior layers of the stroma may lead to epithelial sloughing at the CK sites. These may be problematic from a patient comfort standpoint, as well as increasing the risk for infection.

Over/Undercorrection

Over or undercorrection may occur due to changes in corneal shape during the healing response. Of the two, undercorrection is far more common, with a frequency of between 5 to 8 percent of cases.[17] Error is most likely due to incorrect placement of the probe, insertion which is not perpendicular to the corneal surface, or overcompression of the corneal tissues. These variables are minimized by using the newer OptiPoint device, which reportedly lowers regression and increases accuracy in initial studies. No data containing refractive outcomes has been published in peer-reviewed literature to this date. However, the author's experience with this device has been promising.

Regression

Regression has been problematic with all previous forms of thermal-based keratoplasty, including hot needle and LTK. Results with CK have been more predictable and have shown better longevity than previous techniques, likely due to better consistency in heating of collagen, and deeper penetration into the corneal stroma, both of which assist in a sustained effect. Further modification of technique through innovations such as LightTouch and OptiPoint may provide additional stability. According to a long term study by Lin, et al, using the traditional method for CK, only 34 percent of patients were outside +/-0.50D of intended correction at the two year mark.[18] An increasing number of studies are being performed examining the data pool for patients now approaching 5 years and longer.

Endothelial Damage

While it has been postulated that it is possible to induce endothelial damage from CK, the US FDA clinical trials showed no clinically or statistically significant changes in the mean endothelial cell count.[19] Preoperative data was collected from the in central, midperipheral (3 mm OZ), or peripheral (6 mm OZ) zones and compared to measurements taken at 3, 6, and 12 month postoperative visits. Examination with confocal microscopy also seem to confirm that when patients are selected carefully using corneal thickness measurements of 560 microns at the 6 mm optical zone, no endothelial damage occurs.

ADVANTAGES OVER OTHER PROCEDURES

Conductive keratoplasty has a number of advantages over other refractive procedures. Compared to LASIK or other excimer laser surgeries, surgical invasiveness is much more focal, and thus avoids causing broad tissue changes, including those affecting corneal neuropathies and progressive ectasia.

Dry Eye

It is well documented that LASIK, PRK, and other ablative refractive procedures cause dry eye, presumably by decreased nerve conduction through the severing of the primary nerve bundles in the cornea. Conductive keratoplasty offers an advantage in that only a small percentage of patients may have a decrease in their tear production, as no major nerve centers are damaged during the procedure.

Contrast Sensitivity

Unlike in excimer laser refractive surgery, the central cornea is untouched during CK. It has been documented that the changes in central corneal structure initiated by excimer laser surgery (particularly PRK) cause a decrease in contrast sensitivity.[20-21] Studies with wavefront guided systems, or thin flap techniques seem to be less conclusive.[22-23] By avoiding tissue modification in the central cornea, decreased contrast sensitivity is also minimized.[11,24]

Little Risk of Infection

Although the probe is inserted deep into the corneal tissue, there is very little risk of infectious keratitis for several reasons. The insertion sites are quite small– the probe is only 90 microns in width, so the epithelium usually heals quite rapidly. Heat generated during the procedure in the stromal tissue immediately surrounding the probe tip will likely destroy many microbes which may be carried into the cornea. Deep abscess formation is extremely rare.

No Ectasia

Because no tissue is removed, there is no risk of iatrogenic keratectasia. Careful patient selection regarding good ocular health and corneal thickness of 560 microns at the 6 mm zone is optimal. Therapeutic CK may be done on patients with existing ectasia, to attempt to create a more regular surface.

Large Optical Zone

The largest optical zone which can be used during CK is 8.0 mm, but in clinical practice this is dependent on the amount of hyperopia correction desired. For smaller corrections, a zone of up to 7.0 mm can be used. For larger corrections, spots must be placed in the 6.0 mm zone.

Little Risk of Loss of BCVA

Conductive keratoplasty does not alter the structure of the central corneal tissue. This leaves little risk for loss of BCVA. There are reported cases of induced irregular astigmatism in some patients.

OTHER USES OF CONDUCTIVE KERATOPLASTY

Conductive keratoplasty, while primarily devised to correct refractive error in healthy corneas, has also been used as a means of improving regularity in ectatic or irregular corneas. Currently this is considered off-label use for the device, however studies have shown promise and therapeutic benefits with relatively low risk.

Successful use of the procedure in keratoconus was demonstrated by Alio et al, using three patients.[25] Improvement was noted in topography and corneal regularity following CK.

Iatrogenic ectasia has been problematic for surgeons using excimer laser techniques such as LASIK or PRK. [26] While not common, not all cases of post-excimer keratectasia seem to have well-defined pathology preoperatively. Conductive keratoplasty may be useful in reshaping the ectatic cornea, similar to the method used in keratoconus.

DISCUSSION

While the bulk of refractive procedures to correct ametropia are done with excimer laser surgery, conductive keratoplasty provides distinct advantages over other procedures in the presbyopic, hyperopic, and hyperopic astigmatic population. The advent of the new OptiPoint device and the techniques learned over the first few years of clinical practice have assisted in honing the technique and improving outcomes. Good results have been shown in the FDA trials as well as in other published data, over increasingly longer periods of time. In addition, the flexibility of the CK system for use in treating irregular corneas is gaining popularity, and will continue to serve as an important tool for improving regularity in conditions such as keratoconus and iatrogenic ectasia.

REFERENCES

1. Caster AI. The Fyodorov technique of hyperopia correction by thermal coagulation: a preliminary report. J Refract Surg 1988;4:105-8.
2. Rowsey JJ, Doss JD. Preliminary report of Los Alamos keratoplasty techniques. Ophthalmology 1981;88:755-60.
3. Neumann A, Sanders D, Raanan M, et al. Hyperopic thermokeratoplasty: Clinical evaluation. J Cataract Refract Surg 1991;17:830-8.
4. Koch D, Kohnen T, McDonnell P, et al. Hyperopia correction by non-contact holmium:YAG laser thermal keratoplasty. US Phase IIA Clinical study with 2-year follow up. Ophthalmology 1997;104:1938-47.
5. Choi B, Kim J, Welch AJ, Pearce JA. Dynamic Impedance Measurements During Radio-Frequency Heating of Cornea. IEEE Trans Biomed Engin 2002;49(12):1610-16.
6. Dawson DG, Edelhauser HF, Grossniklaus HE. Long-term histopathologic findings in human corneal wounds after refractive surgical procedures. Am Jour Ophthal 2005;139(1): 168-78.
7. Naoumidi TL, Pallikaris IG, Nauomidi II, Astyrakakis NI. Conductive keratoplasty: histological study of human corneas. Am J Ophthalmol 2005;140(6):984-92.
8. Guimaraes MR, Guimaraes RQ, Castro RD. Radio frequency to correct hyperopia and astigmatism: short term histopathology of six human corneas: symposium on Cataract, IOL, and Refractive Surgery. San Diego, CA. 1995; Best papers of sessions edition:31-5.
9. Milne, R. Light Touch Conductive Keratoplasty. In Panelli R, Pascucci SE (Eds): Conductive Keratoplasty: A Primer. 2005 Slack inc., Thorofare, NJ. Ch 8;pp79-84.
10. Alio JL, Claramonte PJ, Caliz A, Ramzy MI. Corneal modeling of keratoconus by conductive keratoplasty. J Cataract Refract Surg 2005;31(1):190-7.
11. Naoumidi TL, Kounis GA, Astyrakakis NI, Tsatsaronis DN, Pallikaris IG. Two-year follow-up of conductive keratoplasty for treatment of hyperopic astigmatism. J Cataract Refract Surg 2006;32(5):732-41.
12. Kymionis G, Naoumidi T, Aslanides I, et al. Intraocular pressure measurements after conductive keratoplasty. J Refract Surg 2005;21:171-5.
13. Asbell PA, Maloney RK, Davidorf J, Hersh P, McDonald M, Manche E. Conductive Keratoplasty Study Group. Conductive Keratoplasty for the Correction of Hyperopia. Tr Am Ophth Soc 2001;99:79-87.
14. McDonald MB, Durrie D, Asbell P, Maloney R, Nichamin L. Treatment of presbyopia with conductive keratoplasty: Six-month results of the 1-year USFDA clinical trial. Cornea. 2004;23(7):661-8.
15. Stahl JE. Conductive keratoplasty for presbyopia: 3-year results. J Refract Surg 2007;23:905-10.
16. Haji SA, Brocks DC, Fahim MM, Asbel PA. Videokeratography in conductive keratoplasty. J Refract Surg 2004; 20(4):329-36.
17. Pascucci SE. Complications Management. In Pinelli R, Pascucci SE (Eds): Conductive Keratoplasty: A Primer. 2005 Slack inc., Thorofare, NJ. Ch 9;pp 87-93.
18. Lin DY, Manche EE. Two-year results of conductive keratoplasty for the correction of low to moderate hyperopia. J Cataract Refract Surg 2003;29(12):2339-50.
19. McDonald MB, Hersh PS, Manchee EE, Maloney RK, Davidorf J, Sabry M. Conductive Keratoplasty United States Investigators Group. Conductive keratoplasty for the correction of low to moderate hyperopia: U.S. clinical trial 1-year results on 355 eyes. Ophthalmology 2002;109(11):1978-89; discussion 1989-90.
20. Sakata N, Tokunaga T, Miyata K, Oshika T. Changes in contrast sensitivity function and higher order aberration by conventional myopic photorefractive keratectomy. Jpn J Ophthalmol 2007;51(5):347-52.
21. Montes-Mico R, Espana E, Menezo JL. Mesopic contrast sensitivity function after laser in situ keratomileusis. J Refract Surg 2003;19(3):353-6.
22. Tuan KM, Liang J. Improved contrast sensitivity and visual acuity after wavefront-guided laser in situ keratomileusis: in-depth statistical analysis. J Cataract Refract Surg 2006;32(2):215-20.
23. Cobo-Soriano R, Calvo MA, Beltran J, Llovet FL, Baviera J. Thin flap laser in situ keratomileusis: analysis of contrast sensitivity, visual, and refractive outcomes. J Cataract Refract Surg 2005 ;31(7):1357-65.
24. Pallikaris IG, Naoumidi TL, Astryakakis NL. Long-term results of conductive keratoplasty for low to moderate hyperopia. J Cataract Refract Surg 2005;31(8):1520-9.
25. Alio JL, Claramonte PJ, Caliz A, Ramzy ML. Corneal modeling of keratoectasias by conductive keratoplasty. J Cataract Refract Surg 2005;31(1):190-7.
26. Rabinowitz YS. Ectasia after laser in situ keratomileusis. Curr Opin Ophthalmol 2006;17(5):421-6.

53 Intacs™: Refractive Correction with an Intracorneal Device

Terry E Burris, Debby Holmes-Higgin

Introduction

Intracorneal ring technology has shown rapid development in the past twelve years, and clinical results are confirming outstanding results for the correction of low to moderate refractive myopias. The Intrastromal Corneal Ring Segments (ICRS® or Intacs®) are currently undergoing rigorous investigation in FDA regulated clinical trials in the U.S. Results to date indicate the surgical procedure is safe and easily performed, visual results are excellent, and the device provides stable and predictable correction postoperatively. Enhancements can be easily performed by device exchange, and Intacs can be removed, reversing the refractive effect. Intacs are available in Europe and Canada for clinical use, and are anticipated to be FDA approved in the near future in the U.S.

HISTORY

The intrastromal ring concept was proposed by A. E. Reynolds in 1978. The device was to be placed in the corneal periphery through a single, peripheral radial incision. Central corneal curvature could be either flattened or steepened, respectively, by constricting or expanding the ring. As a refractive surgical device, the proposed benefits included surgical preservation of the central cornea, elimination of wound healing as a determinant of surgical outcome, rapid vision improvement, and capability to adjust or even reverse the procedure to expand patient options.

Later theoretical and animal study work on this device continued with funding from KeraVision, Inc. (Fremont, CA)[1] to confirm its feasibility. Human eye bank eye studies by Burris and associates[2] showed that ring thickness produced corneal flattening, which eliminated the need to constrict or expand the device. The current product, the intrastromal corneal ring segments (ICRS®), or Intacs™ corneal ring segments, is designed to correct low to moderate myopia by modulation of device thickness. Intacs have been approved for clinical use in Europe and Canada and FDA regulated clinical trials are currently being completed in the U.S.

Initial Clinical Studies

Non-functional human eye studies of a full circle ring implant, the ICR® (Intrastromal Corneal Ring), were conducted in 1991 in Brazil and U.S.[3,4] This 360° implant was made of polymethyl methacrylate (PMMA) and had an inner diameter of 6.8 mm, and outer diameter of 8.1 mm. The ICR was placed into a 360° intrastromal channel fashioned at two-thirds corneal depth, via a two millimeter radial incision. These studies demonstrated that the ICR could be easily implanted and safely tolerated by the cornea, achieve consistent corneal flattening, and with removal result in return of original corneal curvature.

The ICR was placed in the first ten human sighted eyes in 1991.[5] The most recently reported results (4 year) indicated that uncorrected visual acuity was 20/40 or better in nine eyes, eight eyes were within ±1.00 D of their intended correction as determined by manifest spherical equivalent refraction, and refractive effect was stable over time. One patient had the ICR removed at postoperative Month 6.

Phase II ICR clinical trials in the U.S. were begun in 1993 under the direction of David Schanzlin, MD. These studies, conducted with either a radial or circumferential incision, further confirmed that the ICR was well tolerated in the cornea with predictable, stable optical correction of myopic eyes. Recently reported results indicated that, of sixty-six patients who had reached postoperative Month 12 at the reporting period, 85% had uncorrected visual acuity of 20/40 or better.[6]

Current US Clinical Studies

The original 360° ICR was modified to consist of two 150° PMMA arc segments (ICRS) in order to facilitate the surgical procedure and avoid potential incision related complications. Each device segment is inserted into its respective semi-circular shaped intrastromal channel made through a single 1.8 mm radial incision located in the superior cornea near the limbus. An Intacs in situ is presented in Fig. 53.1. Original thicknesses of the Intacs for the U.S. Phase II and III clinical studies were 0.25, 0.30, 0.35, 0.40 and 0.45 mm; an additional thickness of 0.21 mm was added for the Phase III trial. U.S. clinical trials are currently ongoing and nearing completion.

SURGICAL PROCEDURE

The surgical procedure is illustrated in stepwise fashion by Fig. 53.2.[6] Patient preparation and Intacs placement are performed under topical anesthesia using techniques similar to LASIK.

The corneal geometric center is marked and peripheral corneal thickness is measured by

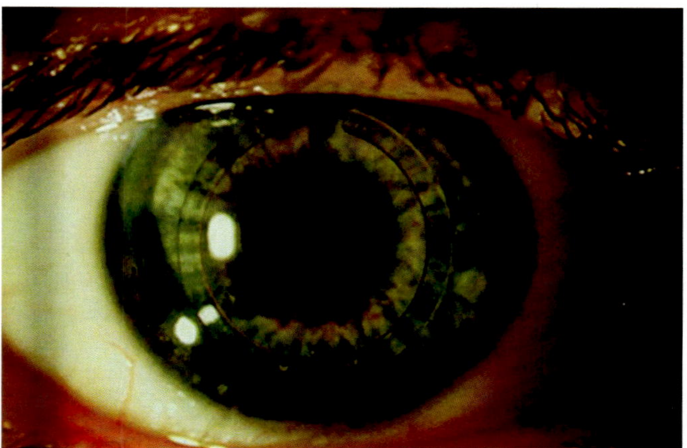

Fig. 53.1: The Intacs refractive device placed in situ

ultrasonic pachymetry over the planned incision site, typically at the 12:00 meridian. A diamond knife is set to 68% of the peripheral corneal thickness and is used to create a 1.8 mm incision allowing introduction of the lamellar dissecting instruments (KeraVision, Inc., Fremont, CA). A pocket spreader (modified Suarez spreader) is used to initiate the lamellar dissection in both a clockwise and counterclockwise direction. A vacuum centering guide is applied to the globe, and the clockwise or counterclockwise stromal separator is introduced through the incision and rotated 180° to 190° to create a midperipheral semi-circular channel. The separator is rotated out of the channel, and the other separator is used to fashion the opposing half channel. The vacuum centering guide is removed. One of two Intacs is irrigated with BSS, inserted and rotated into either the clockwise or counterclockwise channel, and finely placed with a Sinskey hook. Its mate is similarly rotated into its respective portion of the channel. A single 10-0 or 11-0 nylon suture (optional) is placed to ensure closure of the incision edges, drops of topical antibiotic/corticosteroid combination are applied and an eye shield taped into place for the immediate postoperative period.

Postoperative discomfort is managed with a topical non-steroidal anti-inflammatory agent such as Voltaren®. An antibiotic steroid combination drop, such Tobradex®, is used four times a day for one week, and can then be tapered rapidly over the following week. The nylon suture, if placed, is

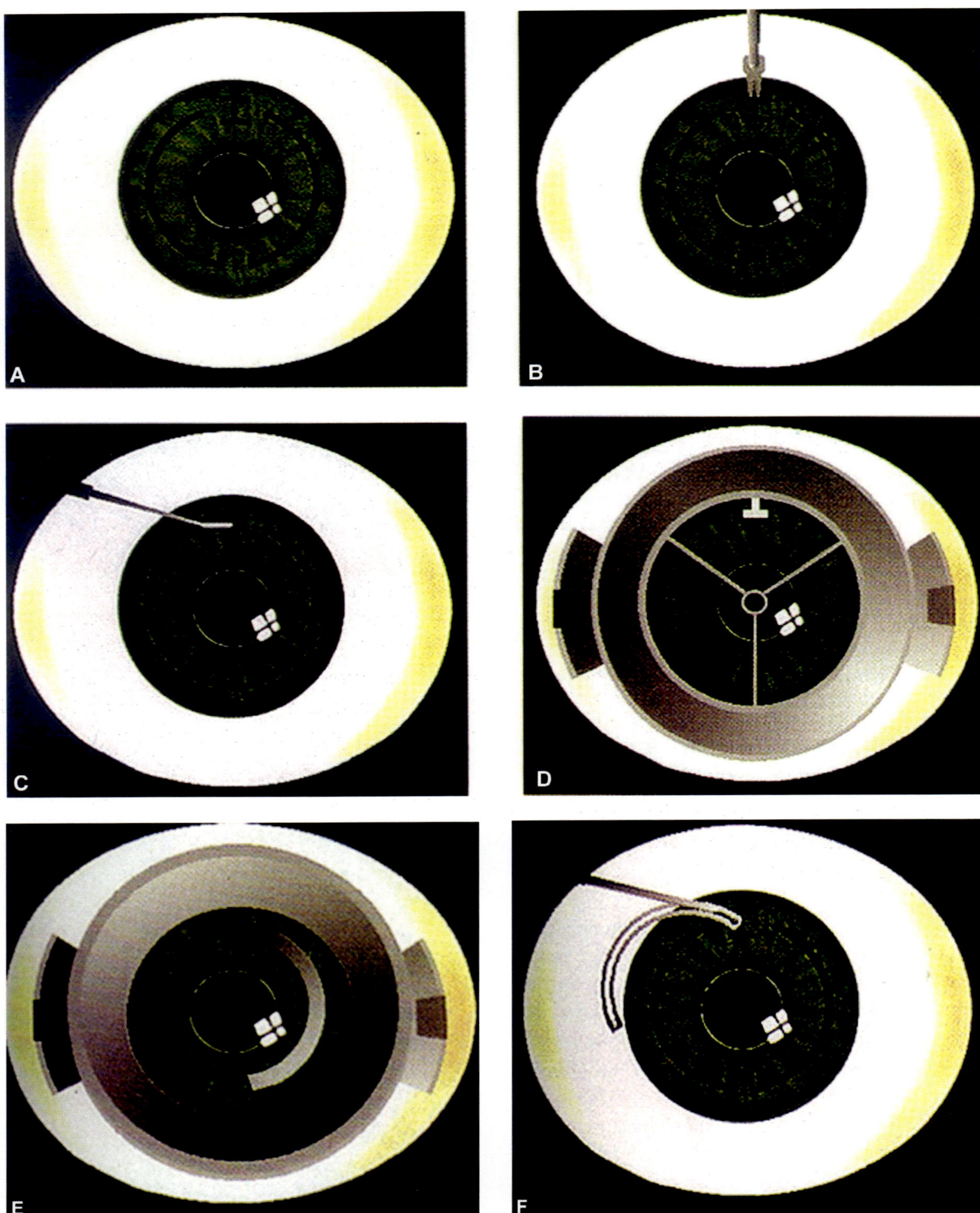

Fig. 53.2A to F: Surgical procedure for placement of the Intacs: **A.** Incision and placement for Intacs marked **B.** Radial incision (~1.8 mm) made **C.** Pocket created as a requisite for stromal separation and Intacs placement **D.** Vacuum centering guide used to facilitate stromal separation **E.** Stromal separation in the clockwise direction **F.** Intacs segment inserted

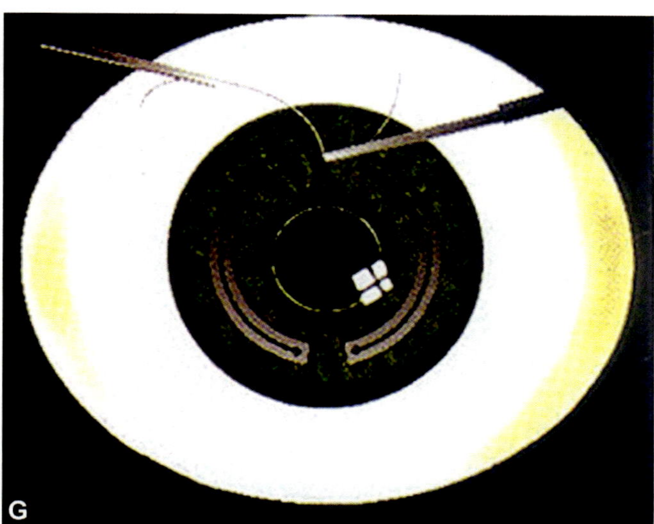

Fig. 53.2G: Incision closed

removed when loose, or by two weeks postoperatively. Any suture removal should be covered with antibiotic three to four times a day for four days after the removal. The patients should be examined about one week after cessation of antibiotic to ensure no late infections have occurred.

CLINICAL OUTCOMES

Visual Results

Month 12 postoperative results for the Phase II and III U.S. Intacs clinical trial cohort surveyed for the FDA pre-market approval (PMA) application were recently reported for three Intacs thickness.[7-8] Nominal predicted correction was –1.30 diopters for the 0.25 mm Intacs, –2.00 diopters for the 0.30 mm Intacs and –2.70 diopters for the 0.35 mm Intacs. Uncorrected visual acuity in 97% of patients (total n=410) was 20/40 or better (Fig. 53.3). Ninety-nine percent of patients (409/410) had preserved best spectacle-corrected visual acuity at postoperative Month 12 (Fig. 53.4). One eye lost eleven ETDRS letters (about two lines) at postoperative Month 12, but had visual acuity (both uncorrected and best spectacle-corrected) of 20/20.

Perioperative Observations and Complications

Perioperative observations with the Intacs are most representative of current surgical techniques reported for the FDA PMA cohort of 410 eyes.[7,8] Mild subconjunctival hemorrhages are seen at surgery from manipulating the conjunctiva with surgical instruments. Adverse intraoperative complications for this clinical study cohort included one posterior corneal perforation into the anterior chamber, due to a deviation in surgical procedure, three anterior corneal surface perforations, due to superficial dissection of the intrastromal channel, and one case of subconjunctival chemosis, resulting from an allergic response to the surgical scrub. In

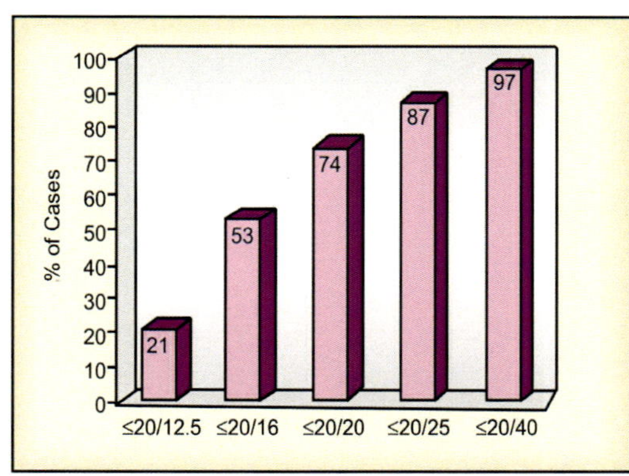

Fig. 53.3: Uncorrected visual acuity at postoperative Month 12 with the Intacs

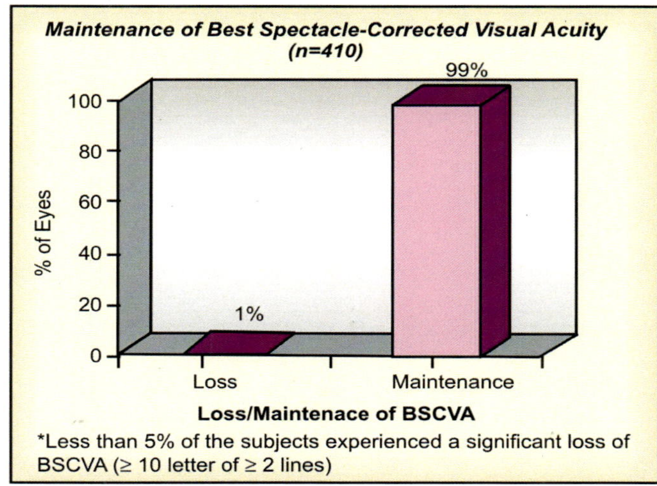

Fig. 53.4: Best spectacle-corrected visual acuity at postoperative Month 12 with the Intacs

all five cases the Intacs were not placed at the time the event occurred, although two of these patients subsequently had Intacs successfully placed in contralateral eyes. Best spectacle-corrected visual acuity for patients experiencing intraoperative complications have returned to baseline, or improved, compared to preoperative values.

Postoperative Observations

Epithelial wound closure over the incision occurred for 96% of patients by Day 7 after receiving Intacs. All eyes had completely healed by Day 14. Small epithelial inclusion cysts were noted in 37.6% of patients at some point postoperatively, and appeared well embedded in the stroma with no fluorescein staining; these remained in only 7% of eyes at postoperative one year.

At Month 3, other clinically insignificant findings included mild channel haze, as well as tiny refractile deposits in the lamellar channel, and hazy cloudy deposits in the segment positioning holes, and/or at the ends of the segments in most patients (Fig. 53.5). The location of the haze correlates with the zone of blunt lamellar stromal dissection, which is slightly larger than the width of the Intacs. Small

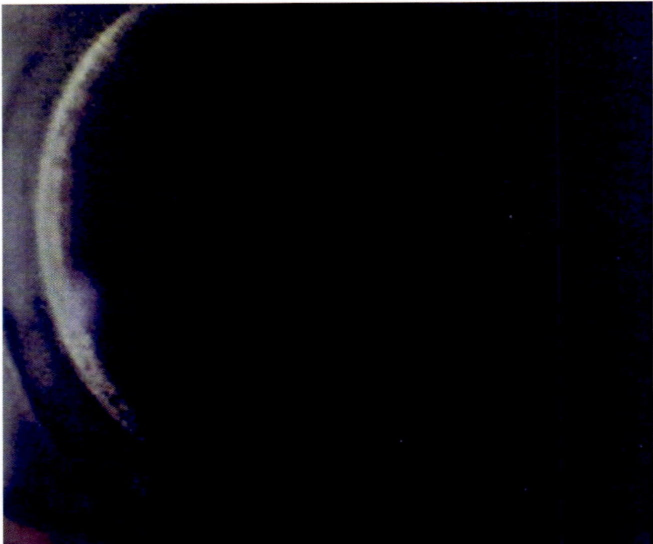

Fig. 53.5: Mild channel haze and tiny refractile deposits in the lamellar channel are normal postoperative findings with the Intacs device

amorphous chalky deposits develop adjacent to the ICRS in many patients. These increase for several months in many patients and tend to disappear by two years postoperatively. Haze and deposits have never been observed to extend outside the channel either peripherally or toward the visual axis for any patient.

Eight patients (8%) had corneal sensation losses of 20 mm or greater (Cochet-Bonnet aesthesiometry) at Month 3, and no patient had total loss of corneal sensation. This effect appears to be transient and principally limited to the central three millimeters of the cornea. No patient demonstrated signs of neurotrophic keratitis, such as punctate keratitis, filaments, epithelial breakdown or trophic ulceration. Subsequent study shows corneal sensation to be returning in all patients.

Postoperative adverse event occurred in 5/454 (1%) of the enrolled patient eyes in the PMA cohort. These included one incident of infectious keratitis, one incident of shallow segment placement, and two incidents of anterior chamber perforation during surgery. All adverse event patient eyes had a best spectacle-corrected visual acuity of 20/20 or better at their last reported exam and none of them has experienced a permanent loss.

Twenty patients experienced induced astigmatism of greater than or equal to 1.0 D based on manifest refraction (Month 3). This is believed to be related to incisional healing effects and possibly due to suture tightness at surgery. Corneal topography in these cases confirm a typical with-the-rule induced cylinder effect originating from the area of the incision site at 12:00. In spite of the induced cylinder, nineteen of the twenty patients maintained uncorrected visual acuity of 20/40 or better. By Month 12, 15/410 patients (3.7%) had greater than one diopter of induced refractive astigmatism. Three patients (0.7%) experienced greater than one and a half diopters of induced astigmatism. All three of these patients had uncorrected visual acuity of 20/25 and best spectacle-corrected visual acuity of 20/16 or better.

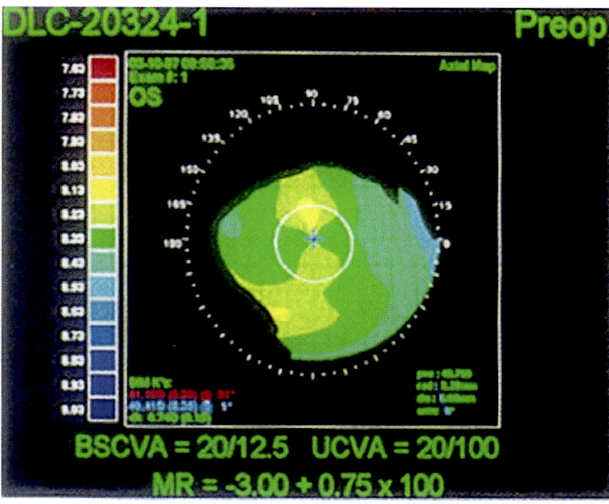

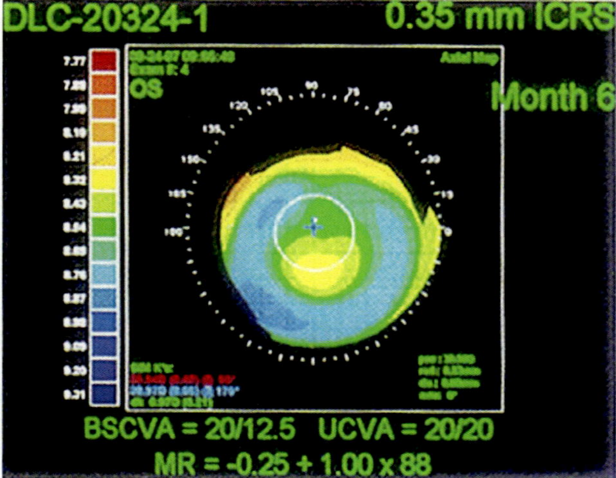

Fig. 53.6: Color axial topography maps representing normal corneal topography before and after the Intacs refractive procedure

Corneal Topography

Corneal topography observations confirm that central corneal flattening increases incrementally with greater thickness Intacs.[2] In addition, postoperative corneal shape remains prolately aspheric, a potentially unique optical characteristic of the Intacs compared to other refractive correction procedures.[2,9-12] Color axial maps representing typical anterior corneal surface topography, preoperatively and with a 0.35 mm Intacs, are presented in Figure 53.6. These maps qualitatively illustrate the topographic flattening which occurs with Intacts. Preoperative prolate asphericity is accentuated with Intacs, but does not appear to be related to standard clinical visual performance measures including best spectacle-corrected visual acuity and contrast sensitivity.[10-12]

Radius of curvature flattening profiles, adapted from methodology reported for previous corneal topography investigation,[13] were used to quantify induced topographic corneal flattening with each Intacs thickness. Flattening across the zero to six millimeter diameter optical zones was determined by subtracting the average postoperative axial radius of curvature values for each zone from respective preoperative values. Profiles have been designed to visually simulate mean axisymmetrical corneal curvature change; the zero millimeter zone mean value is placed at the center of each profile and each successive mean zone value is shown redundantly to each side. These profiles graphically illustrate average central and pericentral corneal flattening, in addition to showing trends of topographic change between the corneal diameter millimeter zones. Radius of curvature difference profiles indicated that flattening with Intacs was prolately aspheric; relatively more flattening occurred pericentrally than centrally (Fig. 53.7). Confidence intervals (95%) suggested that the average radius of curvature change was significantly different between Intacs thicknesses for most millimeter diameter optical zones.

Anterior corneal surface topography with the Intacs has been typified. Color axial topography maps from eyes in the Phase III FDA clinical trial were classified by predominant qualitative pattern by two masked observers according to pre-specified topography classifications and guidelines.[14] The classification scheme was developed primarily from previously published works[15-20] and included the following prolate patterns: spherical (SPH), non-toric prolate asphere (PAS), symmetrically toric (STO), asymmetrically toric (ATO), multizonal (MZA), or non-central prolate asphere and unclassifiable (UNC). Preoperative and postoperative Month

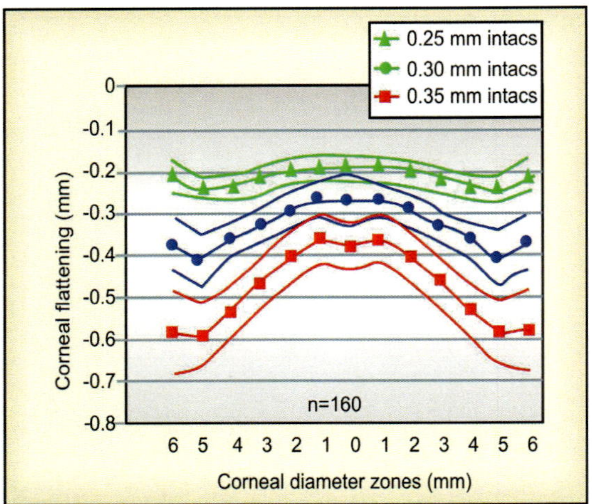

Fig. 53.7: Mean (with 95% confidence intervals) radius of curvature flattening profiles for three different thickness Intacs

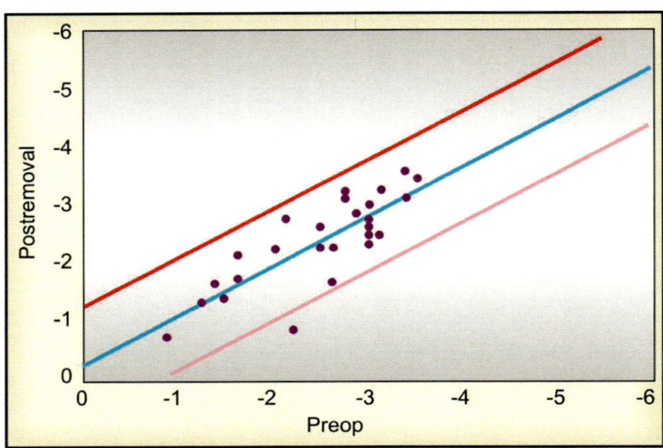

Fig. 53.8: Manifest refraction spherical equivalent preoperatively and after removal (Month 3) of the Intacs for individual eyes

6 corneas with the Intacs approximated patterns published for normal eyes, with a few exceptions.[15]

Reversibility of Refractive Effect After Intacs Removal

A unique characteristic of the Intacs refractive surgical procedure is its potential reversibility. Recently reported results for 449 eyes indicated that Intacs have been removed from 31 eyes (6.9%) with no apparent residual refractive effect.[8,21] Reasons for Intacs removal included dissatisfaction with correction achieved (12 eyes), dissatisfaction relating to glare and/or halos (16 eyes), bacterial infection (1 eye), and personal reasons (2 eyes). Manifest refraction spherical equivalent at Month 3 after Intacs removal returned to within one diopter of preoperative value for most eyes (Fig. 53.8). Corneal topography analyses supported these refractive results.[22] Color axial trend maps for a sample eye clearly demonstrate the return of corneal curvature to approximate baseline levels after removal of the Intacs (Fig. 53.9).

Refinement of Refractive Effect with Intacs Exchange

Several patients have undergone Intacs exchange to treat over-or undercorrection. These brief procedures were easy to perform and preliminary reports indicate a good response.[8]

Safety Assurance and Further Indications

All U.S. FDA safety and efficacy endpoints have been reached for the 0.25, 0.30 and 0.35 mm Intacs and FDA market approval is expected soon in the United States. Intracorneal ring technology demonstrates a promising new technique for rapid, predictable vision correction with no removal of corneal tissue or surgical violation of the central cornea. At postoperative Month 12, uncorrected visual acuity is stable and best spectacle-corrected visual acuity is maintained. Preliminary Intacs exchange data show enhancements to be easily performed and efficacious. Finally, Intacs are removable and the optical effect is reversible, making this technique uniquely appealing to patients who want to preserve future corrective options.

The effective range of treatment with the current Intacs design will likely apply to myopias up to five diopters, although newer permutations may have other refractive applications (i.e. astigmatism concurrent with myopia, hyperopia,). Astigmatism is not currently being corrected with the Intacs in U.S. clinical trials, although prototype device designs[23,24] and early patient results from Brazil have been reported.

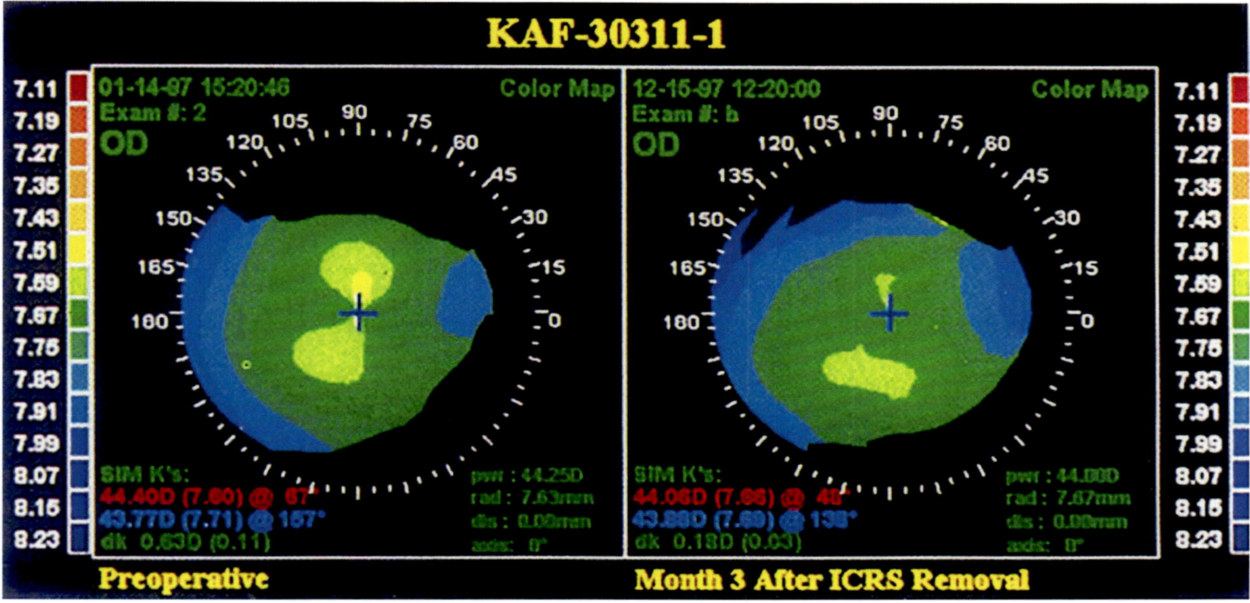

Fig. 53.9: Color axial corneal topography trend map for a case, preoperatively and after removal of the Intacs

Complications of the U.S. Intacts procedure to date have been few and easily managed. Importantly, there have been no complications resulting in permanent loss of uncorrected or best spectacle-corrected visual acuity. Transient loss of corneal sensation is consistent with that seen in cataract surgery, incisional keratotomy and ablation procedures.[25-29] In all cases where the Intacs were removed, the refractive effect has been shown to be reversible.

The unique topography of the Intacs, showing maintenance of prolate corneal asphericity, has theoretical optical advantages that may be further exploited in the future.[9] One of our surgical refractive goals should be to minimize induced optical anomalies such as spherical aberration, which can degrade contrast sensitivity and image quality. Further studies of intracorneal implant technology and correlation with clinical outcomes will help refine our understanding of ocular optical principles as they apply to refractive surgery. Intacs have been approved for commercial use in the European Union, and may soon join the U.S. refractive armamentarium for correction of low to moderate myopia.

FEMTOSECOND LASER

Intacs can also be implanted after the channel is made with the femtosecond laser.

REFERENCES

1. Fleming JR, Reynolds AI, Kilmer L, Burris TE, Abbott RL, Schanzlin DJ. The intrastromal corneal ring: Two cases in rabbits. J Refract Surg 1987;3:227-32.
2. Burris TE, Baker PC, Ayer CT, Loomas BE, Mathis ML, Silvestrini TA. Flattening of central corneal curvature with intrastromal corneal rings of increasing thickness: an eye-bank eye study. J Cataract Refract Surg 1993; 19(suppl):182-7.
3. Nosé W, Neves RA, Schanzlin DJ, Belfort R. Intrastromal corneal ring—one-year results of first implants in humans: a preliminary nonfunctional eye study. Refract and Corneal Surg 1993;9:452-8.
4. Assil KK, Barrett AM, Fouraker BD, Schanzlin DJ. For the Intrastromal Corneal Ring Study Group. One-year result of the intrastromal corneal ring in nonfunctional human eyes. Arch Ophthalmol 1995;113:159-67.
5. Nosé W, Neves RA, Burris TE, Schanzlin DJ, Belfort R, Jr. Intrastromal corneal ring: 12-month sighted myopic eyes. J Refract Surg 1996;12(1):20-8.
6. Schanzlin DJ, Asbell, PA, Burris TE, Durrie DS. The ICRS: Phase II results for the correction of myopia. Ophthalmology 1997;104(7):1067-78.
7. Waring GO III, Abbott RL, Asbell PA, Assil KK, Burris TE, Durrie DS, et al. One-year outcomes of Intrastromal

Corneal Ring Segments for the correction of –1.0 to –3.5 diopters of myopia. In American Academy of Ophthalmology Meeting, New Orleans, LA, 1998.
8. Waring GO III, Abbott RL, Asbell PA, Assil KK, Burris TE, Durrie DS, et al. One-year outcomes of Intrastromal Corneal Ring Segments for the correction of –1.0 to –3.5 diopters of myopia. Submitted for publication, Ophthalmology, 1998.
9. Burris TE, Holmes-Higgin DK, Silvestrini TA, Scholl JA, Proudfoot RA, Baker PC. Corneal asphericity in eye bank eye implanted with the intrastromal corneal ring. J Refract Surg 1997;13(6):556-67.
10. Holmes-Higgin, DK, Baker, PC, Burris, TE, Silvestrini, TA. Characterization of the aspheric corneal surface in ICRSÒ (Intrastromal Corneal Ring Segments) Patients. IOVS 1998;39(4):S74.
11. Holmes-Higgin DK, Baker PC, Burris TE, Silvestrini TA. Characterization of the aspheric corneal surface with the ICRS® (Intrastromal Corneal Ring Segments). Accepted for publication, J Refract Surg 1999.
12. Holmes-Higgin DK, Burris TE, Silvestrini TA, Baker PC, Torres AR and the Phase III ICRS Study Group. Topographic corneal asphericity and visual outcome with the ICRS® (Intrastromal Corneal Ring Segments). In Pre-AAO International Society of Refractive Surgery Meeting. New Orleans, LA, 1998.
13. Waring GO, Hannush SB, Bogan SJ, Maloney RK. Classification of corneal topography with videokeratography. In: Schanzlin DS, Rubins B (Eds): Corneal Topography. New York, NY:Springer Verlag; 1992;47-73.
14. Burris TE, Holmes-Higgin DK, Asbell PA, Durrie DS, Schanzlin DJ. Month 3 corneal topography analysis of patients with the ICRS (Intrastromal Corneal Ring Segments). In American Academy of Ophthalmology Meeting, Atlanta, GE, 1996.
15. Bogan SJ, Waring GO, Ibrahim O, Drews C, Curtis L. Classification of normal corneal topography based on computer assisted videokeratography. Arch Ophthalmol 1990;108:945-9.
16. Lin DTC, Sutton HF, Berman M. Corneal topography following excimer photorefractive keratectomy for myopia. J Cataract Refract Surg 1993;19(Suppl):149-54.
17. Lin DTC. Corneal topographic analysis after excimer photorefractive keratectomy. Ophthalmology 1994; 101(8):1432-9.
18. Young JA, Siegel IM. Three dimensional digital subtraction modeling of corneal topography. J Refract Surg 1995;11:188-93.
19. Hersh PS, Schwartz-Goldstein BH, and the PRK study group. Corneal topography of Phase III excimer laser photorefractive keratectomy. Ophthalmology 1995; 102:963-78.
20. Levin S, Carson CA, Garrett SK, Taylor HR. Prevalence of central islands after excimer laser refractive surgery. J Cataract Refract Surg 1995;21:21-6.
21. Burris TE, Holmes-Higgin DK, Abbot RL, Asbell PA, Durrie DS, Verity SM and Schanzlin, DJ. Corneal topography after removal of the ICRS. IOVS 39(4):S74.
22. Burris TE, Abbott RL, Asbell PA, Assil KK, Durrie DS, Fouraker BD, et al. Reversibility of refractive effect after removal of the ICRS. In Pre-AAO International Society of Refractive Surgery Meeting. New Orleans, LA, 1998.
23. Holmes-Higgin DK, Burris TE, Silvestrini TA, Scholl JA, Proudfoot RA. Evaluation of topographic corneal astigmatism change in eye bank eyes with variable thickness ICRÒ prototypes. IOVS 1996;37(3):S66.
24. Burris TE, Holmes-Higgin DK, Silvestrini TA, Scholl JA, Proudfoot RA. Preliminary eye bank eye topography studies with toric ICR prototypes developed to reduce astigmatism. IOVS 1996;37(3):S66.
25. Belfort R Jr, Nose W, Neves R, Burris TE, Silvestrini TA, Schanzlin DJ. Intra Corneal Implants. In World Congress on the Cornea IV Meeting, Orlando, FL, 1996.
26. Shivitz IA, Arrowsmith PN. Corneal sensitivity after radial keratotomy. Ophthalmology 1988;95:827-32.
27. Campos M, Hertzog L, Garbus JJ, McDonnell PJ. Corneal sensitivity after photorefractive keratectomy. Am J Ophthalmol 1992;114:51-4.
28. John T. Corneal sensation after small incision, sutureless, one-handed phacoemulsification. J Cataract Refract Surg 1995;21:425-8.
29. Mathers WD, Jester JV, Lemp MA. Return of human corneal sensitivity after penetrating keratoplasty. Arch Ophthalmol 1988;106:210-11.

54 Surgical Reversal of Presbyopia

Gene W Zdenek, Jack C Griffis, III

INTRODUCTION

One cannot begin to explain the cause of presbyopia and its subsequent treatment without first understanding the actual mechanism of accommodation. Ever since 1677 when Descartes first observed the ability of the human eye to focus on objects at different distances in a visual field, the mechanism has fascinated and eluded physiologists and optical physicists.

COMPARING THE THEORIES OF ACCOMMODATION

It was not until 1855 when Hermann von Helmholtz learned that the central portion of the human lens thickened during accommodation and the mechanism of accommodation was theorized. From this observation, he concluded that contraction of the circular ciliary muscle produces relaxation of zonules, which reduces the tension on the zonule and allows the lens to increase its convexity. This mechanism of accommodation is an active contraction of the ciliary muscle that passively allows the change in the shape of the lens.

Helmholtz hypothesized that presbyopia is caused by the hardening of the lens with age. Decrease in flexibility of the lens and the loss in elasticity of the lens capsule that occur with aging, progressively hinders the focusing mechanism. As such, presbyopia, the progressive loss of accommodation with age, was attributed to sclerosis of the lens.

In 1970, the American ophthalmologist DJ Coleman developed a hydraulic model of accommodation, based on the mutual action of humor aqueous and humor vitreous. Coleman proposes that the lens, zonule, and anterior vitreous comprise a diaphragm between the anterior and vitreous chambers of the eye. According to Coleman, this construct behaves in a manner analogous to a hydraulic suspension bridge, or catenary. In addition, the tone of the extraocular muscles changed during accommodation, without producing any detectable impact. The conclusion was drawn that, the vitreous humor, under the mechanical action exerted by the extra ocular muscles on the eyeball, would affect in turn the tension of the hyaloid membrane and lens zonules, thus resulting in accommodation.

In 1992, Ronald A Schachar, MD, proposed an alternative hypothesis. He suggests that presbyopia is a result of a decrease in distance between the ciliary muscles and lens equator. It is known that lens tissue continues to grow over the lifetime of an individual (0.02 mm equatorial diameter/year), while sclera stops growing at approximately age 13. Therefore, there is a linear decrease in the distance between the ciliary muscles and the lens over time. Ciliary muscles are smooth with striations, and thus, the amount of tension they can develop is directly related to the degree to which they are stretched. Over time, the amplitude of accommodation is reduced because the distance between the lens and the muscles is decreased, resulting in presbyopia.

To date, the underlying cause of presbyopia, loss of accommodation, is generally not agreed upon in the medical community. Elucidation of the mechanism remains controversial and multiple theories for accommodative loss have been proposed and gained prominence over the past few decades. However, all mechanisms predominantly fall into one of two schools of thought:

1. *Lenticular theories* are broadly based on age-related changes in properties of the lens, including the lens substance, the lens capsule, or the zonular fibers. These theories stem not only from purported changes in the elasticity of the tissues but also from continued growth and changes in the thickness and the curvature of the lens with age. Helmholtz's lenticular theory of the loss of accommodation is the most widely accepted.
2. *Extralenticular theories* consider age-related changes in the accommodative structures outside of the lens, capsule, and zonules. These factors include anatomical, morphological, and physiological changes in the ciliary muscle, connective tissue, and choroid.

The Helmholtz Theory

For the past 150 years, Helmholtz's lenticular theory of the loss of accommodation has been the accepted basis for the underlying physiological mechanisms that lead to presbyopia. Helmholtz hypothesized that presbyopia is caused by the hardening of the lens with age. According to Helmholtz, as the ciliary body contracts for accommodation, it constricts inwardly, relaxing the zonules and allowing the crystalline lens to become more convex for near point focus. The relaxation of the zonules causes the lens to "round up" and bring the near objects into focus more easily. With aging, the decrease in flexibility of the lens and the loss in elasticity of the lens capsule progressively hinders the ability of the lens to change shape, resulting in the amplitude of accommodation in response to the relaxation of the zonules.

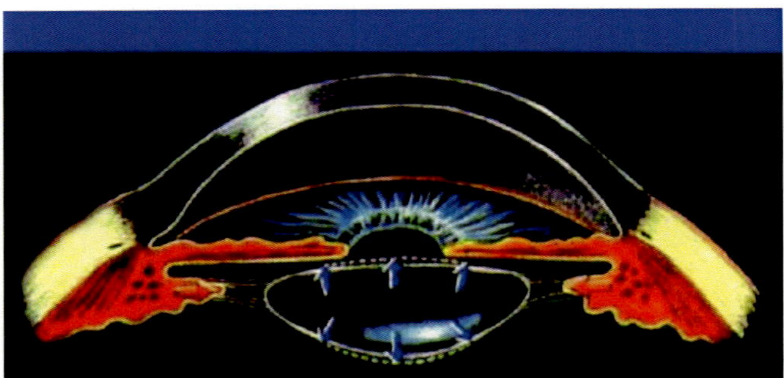

Fig. 54.1: Line drawing depicting the Helmholtz theory

Although generally accepted, Helmholtz's theory cannot fully explain the mechanism by which the lens alters its shape, nor can it fully explain the reason or means by which aging uniformly affects accommodation across the population. The first and most compelling contradiction to Helmholtz's theory occurs when trying to apply the theory in order to make a deformable lens, similar to the young human crystalline lens that can change optical power by approximately 10 diopters. According to Helmholtz's theory, a small outward equatorial displacement of a deformable lens should produce a decrease in central optical power (Fig. 54.1). In fact, a small outward equatorial displacement produces a large increase in the central optical power of a deformable lens.

Spherical aberration is a common optical occurrence in all lenses. Based on optical physics spherical aberration increases when the central and peripheral curvatures of a given lens become steeper. The Helmholtz theory contends that both the central and peripheral lens convexity will uniformly increase during accommodation. In other words, the convexity of the entire lens during accommodation should steepen becoming more uniform. The spherical aberration of a lens can be decreased if its convex surface is aspherical. There is more convexity to the central portion of the lens than there is to the peripheral portion of the lens. It has been clinically and experimentally shown that during accommodation the human crystalline lens demonstrates less spherical aberration. Optical physics, however, states that this can only occur if the convexity of the lens is becoming less uniformly convex, i.e. the convexity of the center of the lens is increasing while the convexity of the periphery is decreasing. This is one of the major inconsistencies in the Helmholtz theory.

There is yet another perplexing problem with the theory of accommodation as explained by the Helmholtz theory. This has been so baffling to physiologists and optical physicists that it has been named the "lens paradox". Because the lens tissue is ectoderm, it continues to grow and its diameter increases approximately 20 microns per year. As the crystalline lens grows in diameter, the optical power should increase. Therefore, emmetropes should progressively become myopic with presbyopia. During accommodation and gradually with age, there is a decrease in tension of the zonules according to Helmholtz. If this decrease in tension does occur, it should have two effects. First, the lens should passively accommodate, which would mean myopia would occur with presbyopia. Secondly, gravity should have more of an effect on the larger, heavier lens. In fact, our clinical experience with presbyopia is that patients become hyperopic.

An additonal observation that is inconsistent with Helmholtz's theory is the effect of gravity on the lens during accommodation. In accordance with the Helmholtz theory, gravitational forces should displace the lens during accommodation. The reason for this belief is that with contraction of the ciliary muscle (causing a relaxation of the zonules) the lens should then be less stable in the eye and therefore should be able to shift with gravity. Experiments by Dr. Ron Schachar in 1994 clearly show that there is no effect of gravity on the young accommodating crystalline lens. Curiously, in 1998, when a 76-year-old presbyopic John Glenn re-entered outer space, no change in his spectacle correction was required. There was clearly no shift in the lens position of his crystalline lens in a weightless environment, further validating Dr. Schachar's findings.

A very reasonable deduction from the Helmholtz theory is that if there were an anterior disinsertion of the ciliary muscle, the eye should automatically lose accommodation and become myopic. To verify this corollary, an experiment was conducted in which the anterior ciliary muscle of primates was disinserted. There was a loss of accommodation, but with the result of hyperopia as opposed to the anticipated myopia.

If the lens was in fact preventing accommodation because of sclerosis, then theoretically the circular muscle fibers, which are largely responsible for accommodation, should atrophy. Histological examination of the circular muscle fibers by Tamm et al, clearly shows that just the opposite occurs.

With the Helmholtz theory in mind, the majority of the ophthalmology community's belief has been that presbyopia is caused by sclerosis or stiffening of the lens, preventing it from passively becoming more spherical. The disease of presbyopia, which occurs as a result of the decline in the amplitude of accommodation, is a process that occurs with stunning predictability throughout life for generations and is independent of genetics, environmental pressures, race or culture (Fig. 54.2). A simple question must be

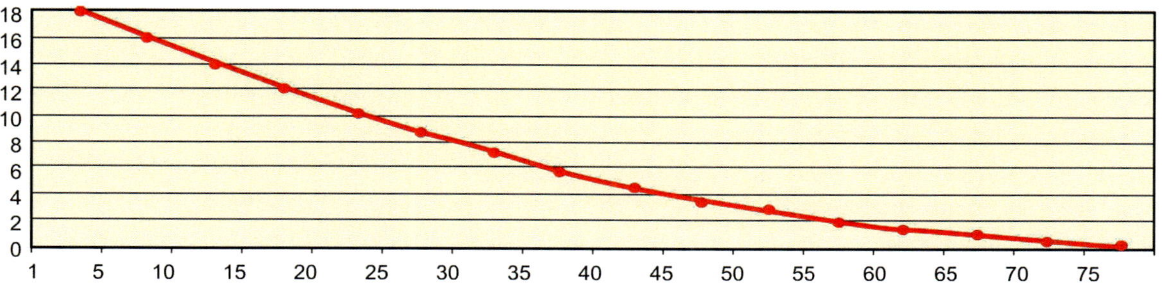

Fig. 54.2: Age-related loss of accommodation graph: The close relationship presbyopia has to age, contradicts the Helmholtz theory

asked: What disease known to man exists that can be predicted in 100 percent of the population within one and a half years of a given age?

It is these compelling discrepancies and inconsistencies in the Helmholtz theory that have driven ophthalmologists to challenge and explore these paradoxical questions.

The Coleman Theory

To explain the deficiencies or inconsistencies in Helmholtz theory of accommodation and to further refine the definition and cause of presbyopia, both Coleman and Schachar began their long journeys to develop new theories for the mechanism of accommodation. Each theory is based on extralenticular factors.

Coleman assumes that the lens, together with the zonule fibers, forms a diaphragm which is held in a catenary shape due to the pressure difference between the aqueous and vitreous humor of the eye. By theory, when the ciliary muscles contract to accommodate the lens, pressure is increased in the vitreous compartment. Simultaneously, pressure in the anterior chamber is decreased due to the expansion of the trabecular meshwork and opening of the canal of Schlemm which occurs with ciliary body contraction (refer to Flocks and Zweng reference as per Coleman's thesis). According to Coleman, a pressure gradient is thus established between the two chambers resulting in a posterior flattening of the lens and, anteriorly, in a steeper radius of curvature in the center of the lens in conjunction with a slight flattening at the periphery.

Coleman further suggests that the anterior capsule and the zonules form a hammock-shaped surface that can be predicted mathematically based on the circumference of the ciliary body (Müeller's muscle). Much like the pylons of a suspension bridge he says, the ciliary body dictates the shape of the catenary. Thus he believes the accommodated state appears to be supported by the fluid volume differential with very little energy expenditure.

Coleman's hypothesis has been tested by comparing a mechanical model of accommodation with in vivo measurements of lens geometry changes during accommodation (measurements included ultrasound, MRI, and optical techniques).

However, recent examinations of this process have been reported using finite element models. Heiner Martin et al, used an axisymmetric static finite element model of the lens based upon literature data for geometry, material properties and loads. They calculated the refractive power of the lens for two different ages groups (29 and 45 years). Contrary to Coleman's theory, their results suggest that the application of a pressure to the posterior lens surface would not yield an increase in refractive power change during accommodation. They concluded that a simulation in accordance with the Coleman theory would not yield physiological values of refractive power change.

The Schachar Theory

To explain the deficiencies or inconsistencies in Helmholtz and Coleman theories of accommodation and to further refine the definition and cause of presbyopia, Schachar proposed a new theory for the mechanism of accommodation. His extralenticular theory states that the human crystalline lens is under increased tension equatorially during accommodation as opposed to decreased tension. He suggested that it is the anterior radial muscle fibers of the ciliary muscle that arch towards the sclera during accommodation. This explains why the anterior radial muscle fibers atrophy following presbyopia. This arching increases the tension on the equatorial zonules, leaving the anterior and posterior zonules more relaxed. The anterior and posterior zonules are allowed to relax, because the posterior longitudinal and posterior radial muscle fibers move anteriorly. Schachar's theory claims the tension that the equatorial zonules place on the equator of the human crystalline lens produces a central steepening along with a peripheral flattening of the lens during accommodation (Fig. 54.3).

This theory explains why spherical aberration decreases during accommodation. Schachar demonstrates this central steepening and peripheral flattening of a deformable biconvex lens when he pulls on the

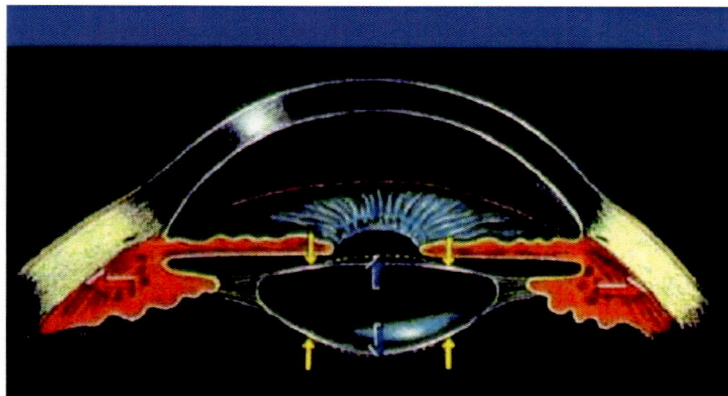

Fig. 54.3: Line drawing depicting the Schachar's theory

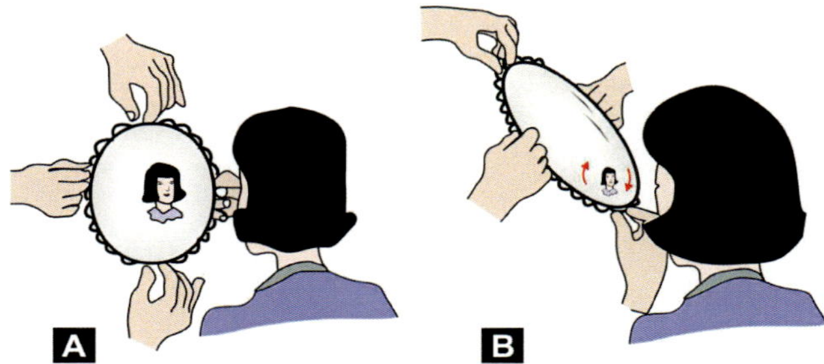

Fig. 54.4: Line drawings of Mylar balloon with patient: (A) Look at your reflection in the *center* of an air-filled Mylar balloon. (B) Note that your reflection in the center of the balloon minifies when the balloon's equator is stretched. This demonstrates clearly that the center of the balloon is steepening with the equatorial stretching

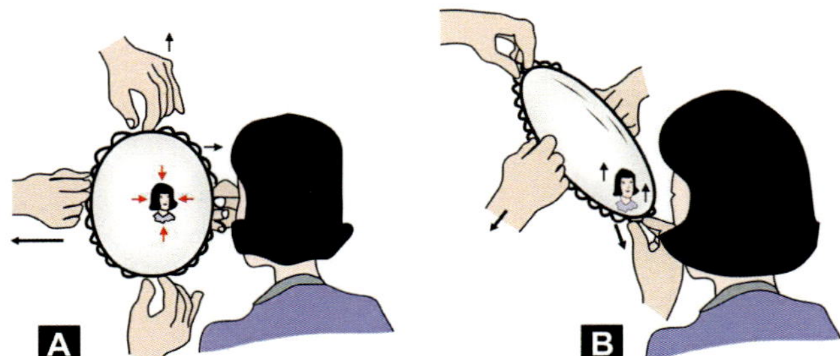

Fig. 54.5: Line drawings of Mylar balloon: (A) Look at your reflection in the *periphery* of the same Mylar balloon. (B) Note that your reflection in the periphery of the balloon enlarges when the balloon's equator is stretched. This demonstrates that the periphery of the balloon is flattening while the center is steepening when the balloon's equator is stretched (*Courtesy:* R Schachar)

equator of a biconvex air-filled Mylar balloon (Figs 54.4 and 54.5). The reflections of a person's face in the Mylar balloon reflect the evidence that there is central steepening and peripheral flattening of this convex surface.

It is interesting to compare the mechanisms that are proposed by the Helmholtz theory of accommodation to what we, as surgeons know about changes of the cornea after surgery. The Helmholtz theory states that if the zonules are put on tension, the center and periphery of the lens flattens. Ever since ophthalmologists began suturing cataract incisions, we have unknowingly been observing and using Schachar's theory of lens deformation. If Helmholtz were correct, a tight 12 o'clock suture on a cataract incision should cause central and peripheral corneal flattening in that meridian. This has not been clinically demonstrated. When sutures are placed too tightly in a surgical incision, both slit-lamp and topographical examinations reveal flattening of the peripheral cornea and adjacent sclera, as Schachar's theory suggests. The central portion of the cornea becomes steeper in that meridian. With a tight stitch at 12 o'clock, astigmatism occurs "with-the-rule (WTR)". This is a potential clinical verification of Schachar's theory.

When a spherical object is pulled or has increased tension circumferentially, the central portion of the spherical object becomes steeper, and the peripheral portions of the spherical object become flatter. Assuming the Schachar theory adequately explains the onset of presbyopia, we can begin to examine the many possibilities for reversing presbyopia, and three methods become theoretically apparent.

- Stopping the growth of the crystalline lens (20 microns/year)
- Shrinking the length of the equatorial zonules in order to increase their tension
- Increasing the ciliolenticular space between the ciliary muscle and the equator of the lens. This would then indirectly increase the tension on the equatorial zonules by putting them on stretch.

Any one or combination of these three mechanisms should lead to the reversal or prevention of presbyopia. Due to technological limitations, surgeons are neither able to stop the growth of the lens, nor shrink the equatorial zonules. For these reasons, the only currently plausible reversal of presbyopia is an expansion of the space between the ciliary muscle and the equator of the crystalline lens. This is known as scleral expansion.

Radial sclerotomies to produce scleral expansion were first described by Schachar. It has recently been popularized by a multicenter study headed by Spencer Thornton. It appears that early results of radial sclerotomy (either by diamond knife or excimer laser) yield less than 3 diopters of restored accommodation and the effect decreases with time, often within months. This is still an area of active research and supports Schachar's theory of accommodation. However, the most successful technique for surgical reversal of presbyopia (formerly SRP—renamed Scleral Spacing Procedure, or SSP, as part of ongoing FDA clinical trials) is scleral expansion. This technique involves re-establishing the physiological space between the lens equator and the ciliary muscle. Once the anterior ciliary muscle fibers are stretched, accommodation begins immediately and improves over several months as the muscles regain their strength. Phase I and Phase II of the FDA study for scleral expansion clearly showed an increased ability to read in the presbyopic age group.

HISTORY AND DEVELOPMENT OF THE SCLERAL EXPANSION BAND

Between 1971 and 1998, various attempts at developing a mechanism for expanding the ciliolenticular space were investigated. This includes evaluating the basic theory through testing on animal and cadaver eyes with trials of radial and zig-zag scleral incisions. The procedure produced slight amounts of increased accommodation (0.50 to 1.50 diopters). This surgically acquired accommodation was determined to regress at a faster rate than associated with physiological aging. The faster rate of regression was most likely related to scleral healing and contraction of fibers. This led to the assumption that a permanent structure must remain in place to maintain the increased ciliolenticular space.

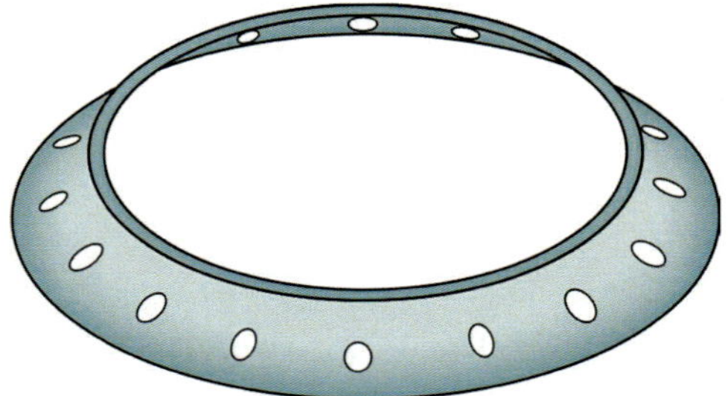

Fig. 54.6: Circumferential scleral expansion band (SEB)

In Monterrey Mexico, Schachar, Jose de la Garza Viejo and Antonio Garza performed the first scleral expansion surgeries using hand-made polymethylmethacrylate (PMMA) encircling scleral expansion bands (SEBs). The bands had 16 equally spaced holes placed centrally in the 2 mm wide bands (Fig. 54.6). A fornix based 360-degree peritomy was used. The band was sutured to the sclera using 6-0 Mersilene sutures. A total of six eyes in six presbyopic patients underwent the surgery.

Postoperatively, the six patients had results ranging from 5.8 to 11.1 D of accommodation. However, the suture eroded through the fornix based conjunctival flaps. As a result, the SEBs were removed from one to three months postoperatively. Subsequently, the SEBs were injection molded to insure all exterior surfaces were smooth and to reduce postoperative trauma. A special order 6-0 clear Prolene suture from Ethicon was developed to attach the SEB to the sclera.

Multiple presbyopic patients had SEB surgery under the auspices of an institutional review board (IRB) in Houston by Warren D Cross, MD. All patients experienced improvement in accommodation ranging from 1.5 to 12 D. All patients underwent a 6 mm 360-degrees limbus based peritomy. Using a specially developed caliper, scleral diameters were measured allowing the multiple sized bands to be custom fitted to the globe. The SEB was attached using a continuous running Prolene suture with a knot buried under the band. The conjunctiva was meticulously closed using a horizontal running mattress suture.

Five bands were removed within three days because of an acute increase in intraocular pressure

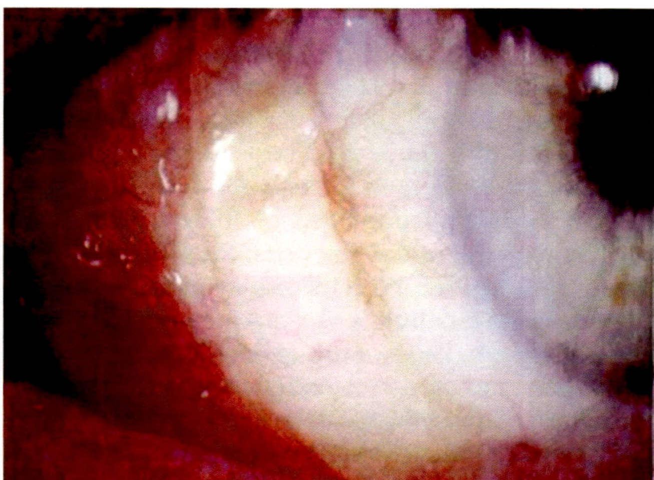

Fig. 54.7: Close-up of scleral band, six years postoperative (*Courtesy:* Warren Cross)

(IOP) secondary to tight sutures. Additional bands were removed over the next 14 months because of conjunctival erosion secondary to knot placement. One band was removed before cataract surgery in a patient who developed bilateral posterior subcapsular cataracts (not related to the unilateral band application). The first two original patients continued to have their bands in place 6 years postoperatively. The effect on accommodation decreased with age but was still measurable. Both are cosmetically acceptable. The first patient (SH) age 59, six years postoperatively had at least 1.75 D of accommodation, requiring +0.25 add over distance correction to read J1 at 40 cm. The world's second patient (KH) age 48 at six years postoperative read J1 at 40 cm without an add (Fig. 54.7). Both patients had normal IOPs.

Over the following years, multiple SEB prototypes were developed and tested by Schachar, Cross and Richard Yee in an attempt to avoid the use of sutures. Prototypes used steel and titanium SEBs with adjustable clips that were micro-machined by IBM. The concept was that the size of the band could be adjusted like the clips of a hatband. The metal SEB prototypes could not be safely passed around the eye even when viscoelastics, mineral oil or special surfactants were used. As a result, the metal SEB prototypes were abandoned.

Due to these difficulties, a SEB prototype was developed consisting of four individual PMMA sections instead of an encircling band. Each section of the SEB was passed through scleral belt loops (sutureless), overlapped and then fused while on the eye using a specially designed micro-sized ultrasonic fusing device. The ultrasonic fusing device had a 2 mm square tip. The individual sections were overlapped and placed between a footplate and the ultrasonic fusing tip. Using hand pressure, the ultrasound was applied to produce fusion of each section. The band could now be custom fitted to the size of the globe and no sutures were needed to attach the band to the sclera.

In Monterrey Mexico; Viejo, Cross and Yee performed the first SEB surgery passing the four individual sections of the band through 4 sclera belt loops using the individual overlapping sections and the hand driven 2 mm tip ultrasonic device. As a result, the patient obtained approximately six diopters of accommodation. These results were independently verified by Larry Lothringer. However, the ultrasonically welded joints in the band were found to be too rough and, ultimately, the band was removed because of recurrent conjunctival erosion problems.

At the University of Texas Medical Branch, Houston, under the auspices of an IRB, Yee with Cross performed SEB surgery on six patients using individual segments which were overlapped and fused with the ultrasonic device. The fusion sites were smoothed with a special diamond and carbide dental drill. The four belt loops were placed along the 6:00, 9:00, 12:00, and 3:00 meridians. However, the fusion sites remained insufficiently smooth and five patients requested removal of their SEBs due to chronic redness and discomfort. The patient with the remaining band continues to do well and has good accommodation. Three additional patients had SEBs but the belt loops were made thicker, i.e. the scleral dissection was deeper. The three patients developed anterior segment ischemia and the bands were immediately removed. None of these patients lost vision or had a change in their refraction.

Ultimately, the SEB segments were modified to have a tongue and groove junction. The ultrasonic hand piece was modified to have a 1 mm, air pressure controlled tip in order to insure a constant force during the fusion process. The time and force applied during the fusion process was automatically controlled. The smoothing device was further refined and all scleral belt loops were made along the 45° meridians. All patients receiving the new system had an increase in their amplitude of accommodation, but in some of the patients there was still a problem with conjunctival erosion. There were also occasional episodes of anterior segment ischemia requiring removal of the SEB. As a result of this unacceptable risk of anterior segment ischemia, a new approach to scleral expansion was developed.

INTRODUCTION OF THE [SEGMENTED] SCLERAL IMPLANT

In an attempt to prevent the anterior segment ischemic syndrome problems and to simplify and decrease instrumentation cost a new prototype was developed. The new design consisted of four individual PMMA segments, which were not connected to each other. The segments were placed in scleral belt loops along the 45° meridians. Initial segments were 7 mm long and 1.2 mm wide. The segments were inserted into 2 mm wide and 5 mm long scleral belt loops. The increased technical ease of the surgery and the postoperative accommodation results were excellent. However, these segments were found to be too long and continued to show signs of sector anterior ischemia. As a result, the scleral belt loops were narrowed to 900 microns wide and 4.0 mm in length with initial clinical success.

Further dimensional modifications to the scleral implants were introduced in order to increase the amplitude of accommodation and enhance implant long-term stability (Fig. 54.8). Improved surgical instruments for the creation of scleral belt loops and placement of implants were developed and implemented. As a result of successful preclinical evaluation of the modified scleral implants (version 3, see Fig. 54.8), US FDA Clinical trials began Phase I studies in six academic programs.

Clinical Results of these Various Implant Designs Produced the Following Early Results

Postoperative follow-up at 6 months was reported for all but one patient enrolled in the Phase I clinical trial.

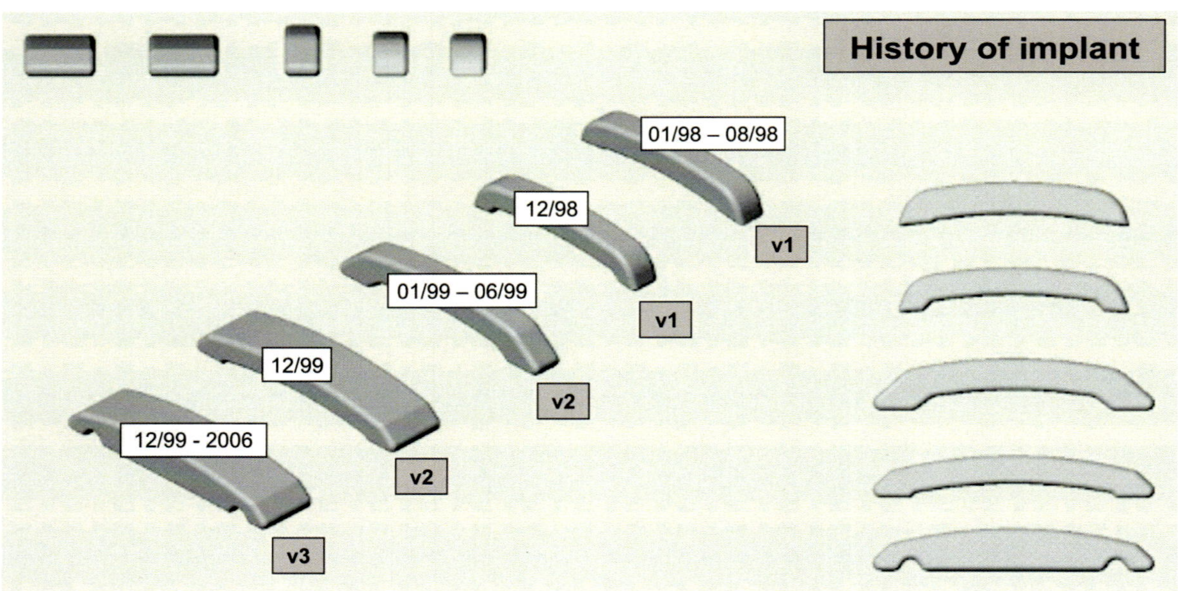

Fig. 54.8: Evolution of [segmented] scleral implants

Accommodative amplitude was measured monocularly using a near point "push" technique from both a 70 cm and 30 cm starting point. An increase in accommodative amplitude of surgical eyes by +1.7 diopters (σ = 1.5 diopters) and +1.5 diopters (σ = 1.2 diopters) at these two testing distances, respectively, was noted ($p < 0.0001$). Correspondingly, near visual acuities at 40 cm, 30 cm and 20 cm each improved in the operated eye by approximately 3 lines ($p < 0.0001$) at 6 months. This improvement seemed to mirror changes in accommodative amplitude during this period.

Changes in spherical equivalent, axial length and central keratometry readings were not statistically significant. There were no reports of anterior segment ischemia or malignant glaucoma. Adverse effects were limited to a transient elevation of intraocular pressure in one patient and misalignment of individual implants due to inadequate scleral tunnel formation in three patients. Only one implant was replaced.

The results from the Phase I clinical trial provided sufficient evidence of safety and effectiveness and supported expansion of the clinical trial into Phase II and, ultimately, Phase III. The majority of patients experienced an improvement in near visual acuity, and all but one of the complication and adverse events resolved without sequelae. Improvements to the quality and reproducibility of the scleral tunnel formation and implant placement were implemented to improve the long-term efficacy of the procedure, and led to the development of the *PresVIEW*™ System and *PresVIEW*™ Scleral Implants (PSI's).

SURGICAL REVERSAL OF PRESBYOPIA (SCLERAL SPACING PROCEDURE—SSP)

Patient Selection

The ideal candidate is between 40 and 70 years of age with minimal distance refractive error. If patients are in need of refractive surgery, it is recommended that they have their distance vision corrected first followed by SSP approximately 4 to 6 months later. Generally, it is preferable to performed LASIK before the SSP. A proper add should be determined for near vision. The proper add is to a larger extent determined by the person's age. Age 40 to 45 generally requires a +1.00. Age 50 to 55 generally requires a +2.00 and age 60 to 65 generally requires a +2.50 to +3.00.

It is recommended that the preoperative evaluation of the patient include the following:

1. Distance visual acuity with correction in place.
2. Visual acuity at 40 cm, 30 cm, and 20 cm using the Sloan method.
3. Visual acuity starting at 70 cm and bringing the eye chart closer until the smallest line starts to blur. *Note:* this test gives you the baseline diopters of accommodation. The formula to measure this is 1/distance in centimeters × 100 (i.e. if the patient is able to read the line clearly up to 50 cm, the formula applied would be 1/50 × 100 = 2.00 D of accommodation).
4. Axial length measurement and corneal topography.
5. Scleral thickness 3.5 mm posterior to the angle as verified via B-scan (with appropriate tissue velocity correction factors—refer to applicable diagnostic imaging literature).

Step 3 listed above is also important in the postoperative evaluation to measure the amount of accommodation gained. When repeating this step postoperatively, it is important that the patient use the same line he was able to see preoperatively (even if it was only 20/200). Have the eye chart brought in toward the patient as before to find the gain in accommodation. To illustrate (continuing from the example in step 3): if the patient is able to clearly see the same line on the eye chart when brought up as close as 20 cm, this would result in 5.00 D of accommodation. These measurements are obviously more subjective than objective, though objective means of evaluating the gain in accommodation may be soon available.

The results in step 4 should not be affected as a result of the surgery. Corneal topography may show induced astigmatism immediately postoperatively. In all cases, this astigmatism is temporary, and typically resolves within 1-3 months.

Patients who are more than +1.00 hyperopic may not attain enough accommodation to satisfy their near vision needs. Depending on the expectations of your patient, this may or may not be satisfactory. Since the procedure is performed with the intention of giving as much accommodation as is physiologically possible, the variability lies within the patient's own anatomy as well as the surgeon's skill.

SSP may be considered an optional, cosmetic procedure with the same inherent issues. Therefore, it may not be for everyone. Patients need to be aware of the need to exercise and work at strengthening the muscle for several months after the procedure to gain optimum effects. The SSP patient's eyes will be quite red for a few weeks following the surgery as sub-conjunctival thrombus is slowly eliminated. Post-operative expectations given prior to the procedure are extremely important. When taking the patient's history, the physician should note the following contraindications:

- Insulin-dependent diabetes mellitus
- Severe hypertension
- Blood dyscrasias
- Chronic or recurrent uveitis or other recurrent anterior or posterior segment inflammation
- Previous eye surgery (including cataract, corneal transplant, glaucoma filtering surgeries, retinal detachment repair, etc)
- Patients on anticoagulant therapy, such as Heparin or Coumadin
- Sjörgren's syndrome
- Chronic systemic disease (i.e. sub-acute lupus erythematosus, Crohn's disease, collagen vascular disease, rheumatoid arthritis, etc)
- Scleral thickness less than 530 microns as measured 3.5 mm posterior to the angle.

Scleral thickness is important as the *PresVIEW™* System utilizes an automated scleratome designed to produce scleral tunnels at a repeatable depth of 400 microns. (PresVIEW™ is the trademark held by ReFocus Group, who is currently funding the FDA Study now in Phase III) It has been theorized that the optimum depth of the lamellar scleral tunnel is between 2/3 and 3/4 the full scleral thickness. As such, scleral thicknesses of less than 530 microns might result in sub-optimal outcomes. In addition, the scleral bed that remains intact between the incision and the choroidal space provides a boundary in the event of scleral erosion (though no instances of this have ever been reported).

Current Surgical Techniques

There are 6 basic steps, not including preoperative anesthesia, to the scleral spacing procedure (SSP) for surgical reversal of presbyopia.

1. Meridian marking
2. Opening the conjunctiva
3. Scleral marking
4. Lamellar scleral tunnel formation
5. Implant placement
6. Conjunctival closure.

Each of these steps with appropriate clinical pearls will be discussed in detail. After appropriate positioning of the patient in the supine position, the operative site is prepped and draped in the usual sterile fashion. Although the trend seems to be a bilateral procedure, there are occasions where a single eye may be operated on. If doing a bilateral case, I usually operate on the dominant eye first. If there is a reason not to progress on to the second eye, the dominant eye should attain better results.

This procedure may safely be performed under local and topical anesthesia. The addition of light sedatives is beneficial to the comfort and wellbeing of the patient. If the surgeon feels more secure with the assistance of an anesthesiologist, he should remember the benefits of minimal sedation, to allow them to incorporate the patient's assistance by looking in various directions during the surgery. This will allow better exposure of the four quadrants of the eye being operated on.

The only anesthesia that I now use in all my cases is 4 percent xylocaine (AstraZeneca, Waltham, MA) placed on a pledget and applied to each quadrant prior to performing surgery on that quadrant. Alphagan eye drops administered 15 to 30 minutes prior to beginning the procedure helps decrease operative bleeding. Light sedation may be achieved in a couple of different ways.

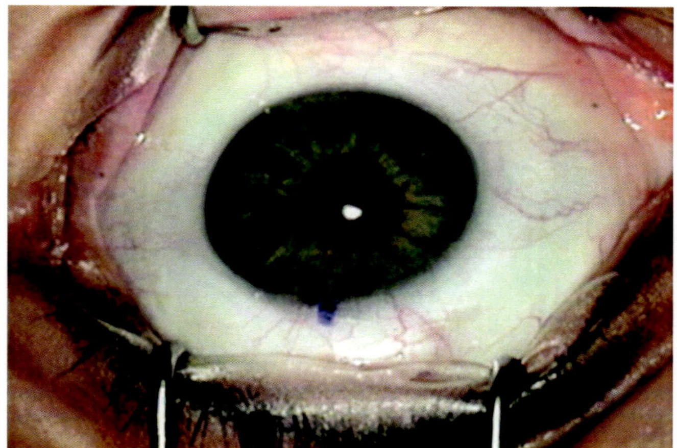

Fig. 54.9: 12 o'clock marking while patient upright

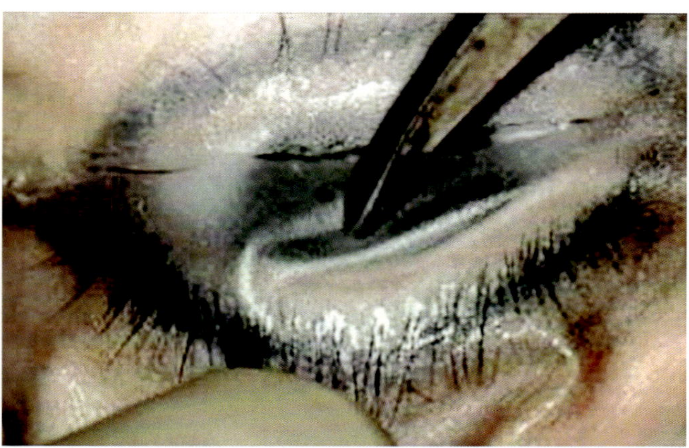

Fig. 54.10: Lid draping and exposure

Lorazepam 1 to 2 mg or diazepam 10 to 20 mg may be given preoperatively about an hour before the procedure is started. Letting the patient know in advance what he or she can expect are during the surgical procedure (and why they are not being put to sleep) will greatly enhance their ability to cooperate. General anesthesia and its inherent risks are not indicated because of the effectiveness of topical anesthesia. In addition, local injectable anesthesia should be avoided due to conjunctival swelling and reactive hyperemia. I have tried many different topical/local anesthesia techniques and found the aforementioned the most successful.

After the instillation of 0.5 percent proparacaine, the patient should have his or her eyes marked with a skin scribe or marking pen at the 12 o'clock position (Fig. 54.9) while remaining upright. It is documented that up to 10 to 15 degrees of torsion or eye movement can occur when the patient is in a supine position as compared to the upright position. If this mark is not placed accurately, the implants may be off by as much as 20 degrees. This inaccuracy in positioning may be sufficient to compromise the anterior circulation of the eye. Anterior segment ischemia is a potential complication of improper implant positioning.

The lid and surrounding area should be scrubbed using betadine and alcohol wipes prior to draping. When draping the eye, it is important to capture the lashes such that they remain outside the surgical area. The drape is then slit to expose the eye, and cut at the 12 o'clock positions to allow for easier placement of the lid speculum (Fig. 54.10).

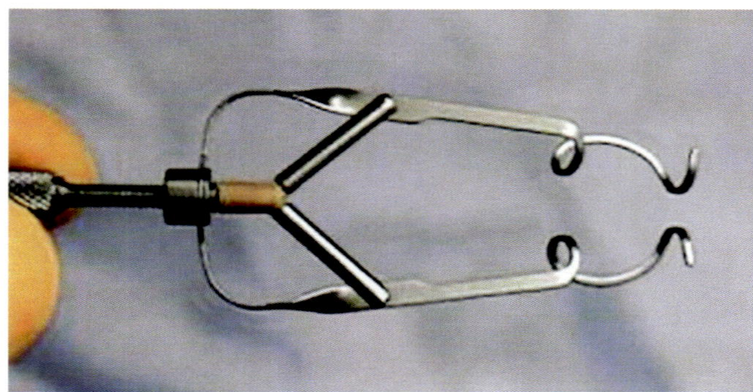

Fig. 54.11: Eyelid speculum

Meridian Marking

An eyelid speculum is used to open the eye for maximum exposure (Fig. 54.11). With the proparacaine administered, the precision calipers (Fig. 54.12) are set to 6.0 mm and the corneal center is determined using a four point interpolation procedure. One point of the caliper is inked for marking, and the other point placed at the edge of the limbus. The inked point of the caliper is used to mark the cornea center based upon the 6.0 mm distance. This process is repeated for the 3, 6, 9 and 12 o'clock positions. The corneal center is determined to be the point central to all four marks (Figs 54.13 and 54.14).

The meridian marker (Fig. 54.15) is inked and used to mark the 45-degree meridians (Fig. 54.16). The point of the central locating feature of the marker

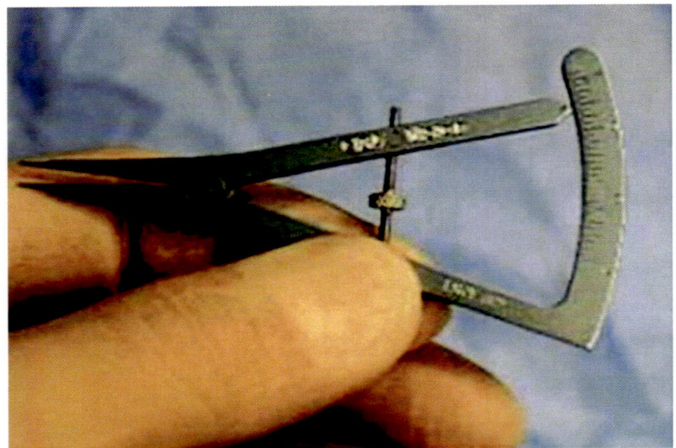

Fig. 54.12: Precision caliper

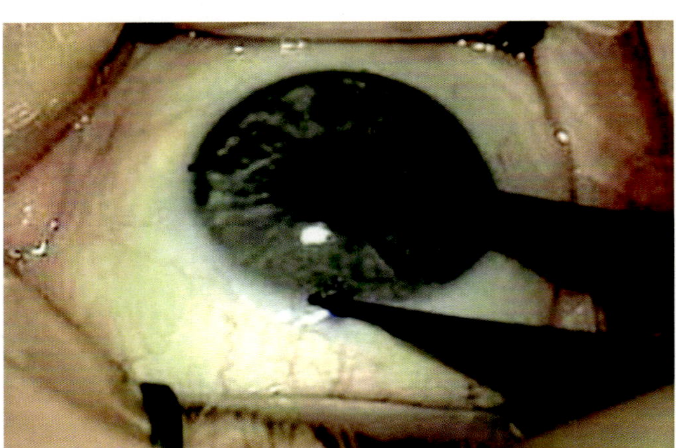

Fig. 54.13: Corneal center marks

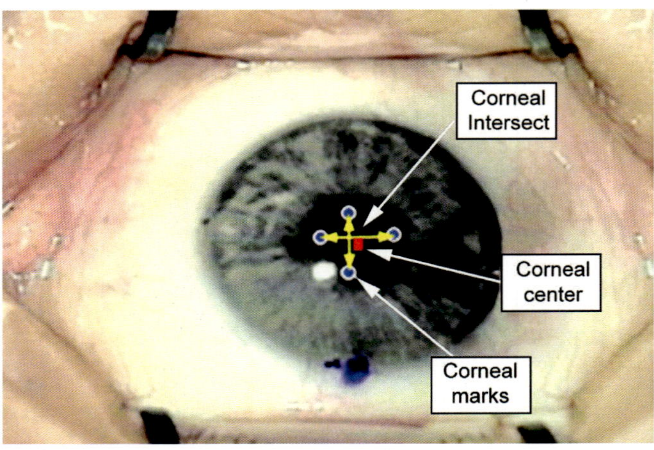

Fig. 54.14: Corneal center interpolation

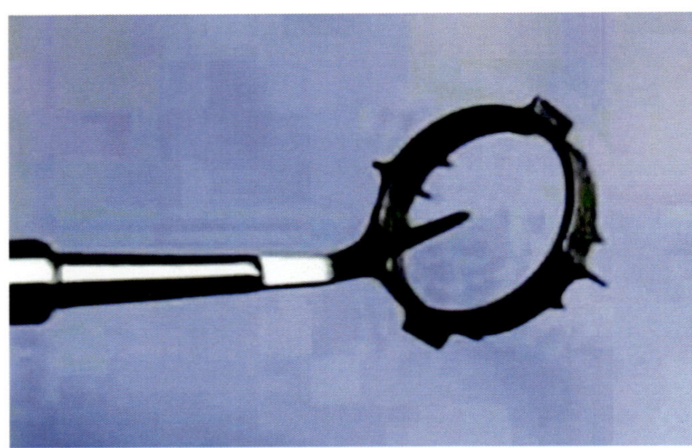

Fig. 54.15: Meridian marker

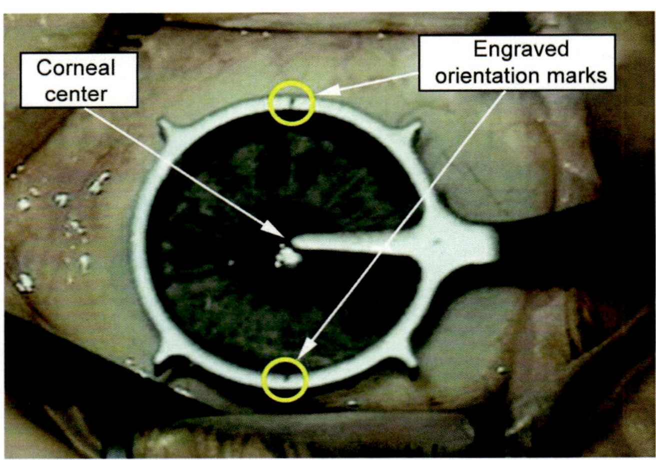

Fig. 54.16: Meridian marker positioning on cornea

should be placed at the corneal center and either one of the two engraved marks oriented with the 12 o'clock position. This will ensure that the marks are delivered accurately at the oblique meridians. The marks will not necessarily be made directly onto the limbus. Most likely they will be about 0.5-1.0 mm posterior. Their purpose is to delineate the axis for the placement of the lamellar scleral tunnel, and not the limbus location (Fig. 54.17).

You may need to re-ink any of the marks that you feel may fade by the time you are ready to use them. Also remember that you are going to be creating a flap in the conjunctiva and you want your marks to be visible. This may necessitate remarking closer to

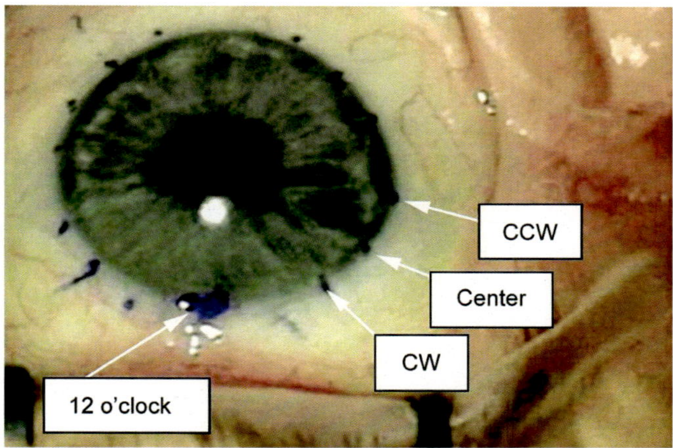

Fig. 54.17: Meridian marks

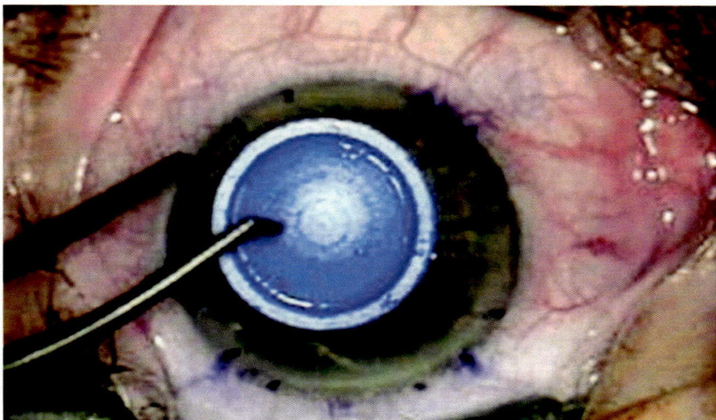

Fig. 54.18: Corneal shield in place

the limbus. What you should see after successfully completing the marking is twelve separate spots in groups of three. They are centered on the 45-degree meridians. Straddling those will be two marks that are 4 mm apart (the length of the belt loop). A corneal shield can then placed on the cornea with viscoelastic or viscous artificial tear (Fig. 54.18). This shield is placed after the quadrant marks have been made to insure stable ink markings, which could be interfered with by the viscous fluid.

Opening the Conjunctiva

When using the PresVIEW™ System automated scleratome, the method of exposure is to make a 360-degree peritomy with relaxing incisions using pointed tipped scissors at the 3 and 9 o'clock positions (Fig. 54.19). The Tenon's capsule can be pulled back using

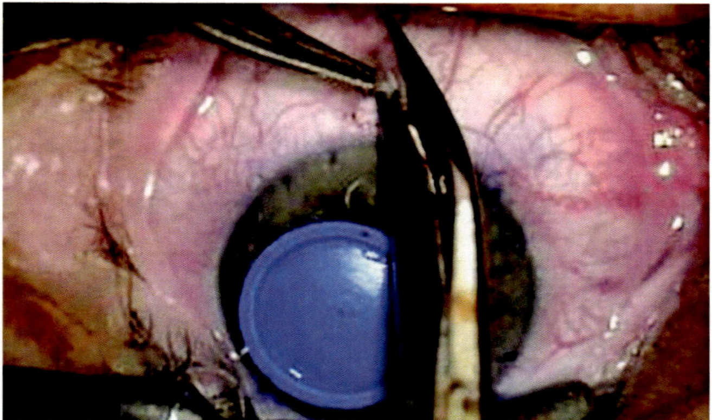

Fig. 54.19: Conjunctival relaxing incision

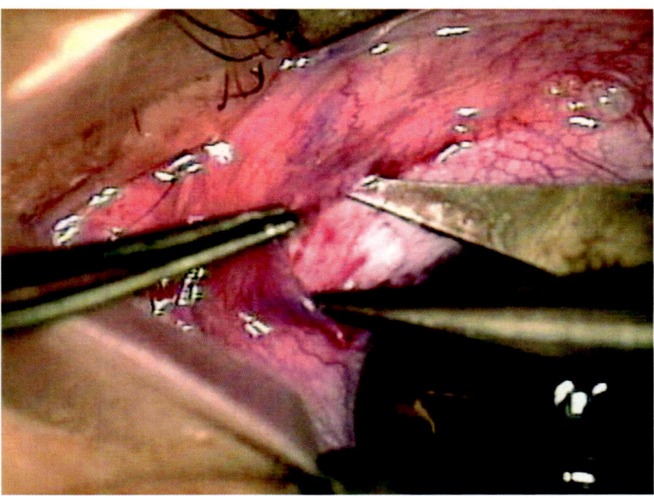

Fig. 54.20: Push back of Tenon's capsule with blunt scissors

blunt tipped scissors as well as completing the peritomy (Fig. 54.20).

I recommend performing surgery on the inferior quadrants first for the following reasons. The time to perform the surgery will be longer than the anesthetic's (Xylocaine) effect. After the topical anesthetic wears off, in many patients there is a reactive hyperemia and/or a post anesthesia hyperesthesia. These conditions make further anesthesia more difficult to attain. While anesthetizing the superior quadrants, the anesthetic pools in the lower quadrants. By the time the surgeon approaches the lower quadrants, they have already gone through the cycle of anesthesia, as mentioned above. When deciding between the inferior nasal or temporal quadrants, choose the quadrant with the least amount of bleeding to operate on first. By the time you approach the second quadrant, natural homeostasis should have occurred.

Scleral Marking

After proper exposure, the next step is marking for the scleral tunnels. Using a proprietary method, Refocus Group has determined a range of distances for creation of the lamellar scleral tunnel posterior to the meridian marks based upon the following assumptions:

1. The transverse scleral sphere of the globe varies little between myopic or hyperopic eyes; or between male and female eyes.
2. The variations in distance from the anterior surface of the cornea to the lens equator in an emmetropic eye are mostly due to variations in the depth of the lens.

In addition, adoption of these ranges to a myopic or hyperopic eye can also be made based upon the following:

1. The majority of variation in the depth of the anterior chamber in myopic and hyperopic eyes is due to the changing shape of the cornea.
2. The relative position of the anatomy from the iris to the posterior lens remains relatively constant and similar to an emmetropic eye.

Based upon an A-scan of the patient sagittal lens depth, Refocus Group has calculated distances for marking the posterior position for fixating the *PresVIEW*™ System Scleratome. This mark is made using a precision "1-step" marker (Fig. 54.21) by inking the underside (more explanation?) as follows:

- Sagittal lens depth less than 4.10 mm—use "short marker"
- Sagittal lens depth 4.11 mm to 4.89 mm—use "medium marker"
- Sagittal lens depth more than 4.90 mm—use "long marker".

The anterior (non-inked) points of the marker are positioned on the meridian marks. The posterior line and point are pressed firmly and perpendicular to the scleral surface to produce a lasting mark (Figs 54.22 and 23) to provide reference points for placement of the *PresVIEW*™ System Scleratome.

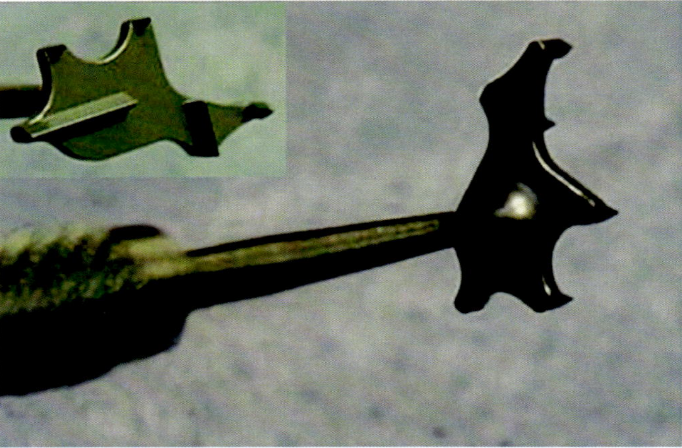

Fig. 54.21: Precision "1-step" marker for scleratome positioning

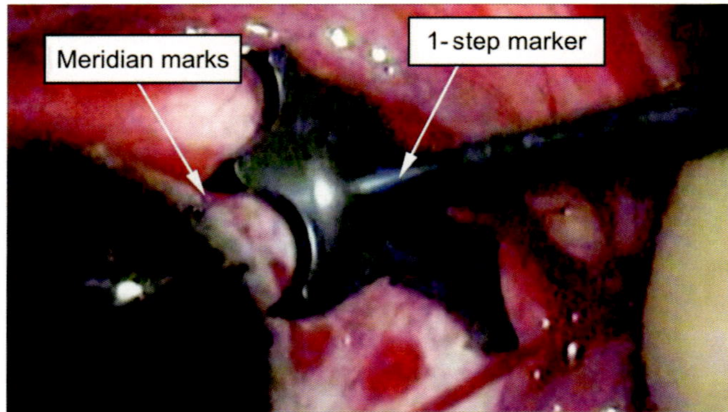

Fig. 54.22

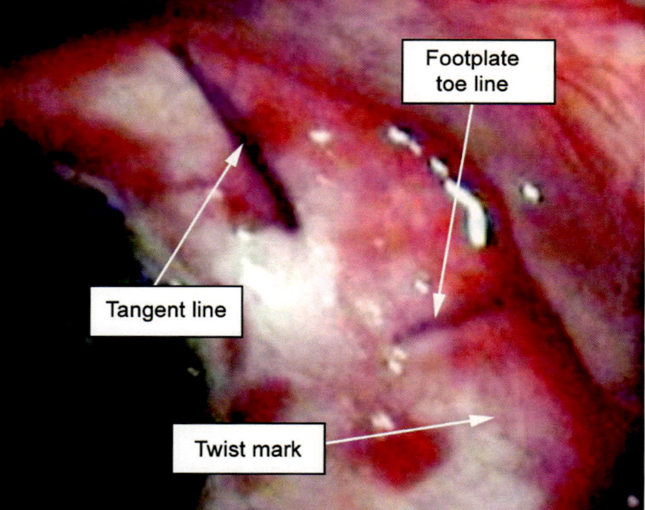

Fig. 54.23

Figs 54.22 and 54.23: Posterior positioning marks using the "1-step" marker

Lamellar Scleral Tunnel Formation

The *PresVIEW*™ System Scleratome should be prepared beforehand according to the *PresVIEW*™ System Instructions for Use (Fig. 54.24). The blade is handled using the blade loading tool (Fig. 54.25) to remove the blade safely from the case (Fig. 54.26) and to align and fix the blade to the *PresVIEW*™ System Scleratome hand piece (Fig. 54.27). The footplate and blade guard should already be attached to the hand piece with the blade guard closed over the new blade prior to use (Fig. 54.28). The blade guard ensures unhindered blade motion through the sclera, as loose tissue and thrombus can infiltrate the blade connection to the hand piece and reduce the efficiency of the blade travel, comparatively between the first tunnel and the last tunnel. The blade should be lubricated before the creation of each tunnel by activating the scleratome while suspending the hand piece assembly in a bowl of sterile saline. Care should be taken when performing this operation, as the fixation features on

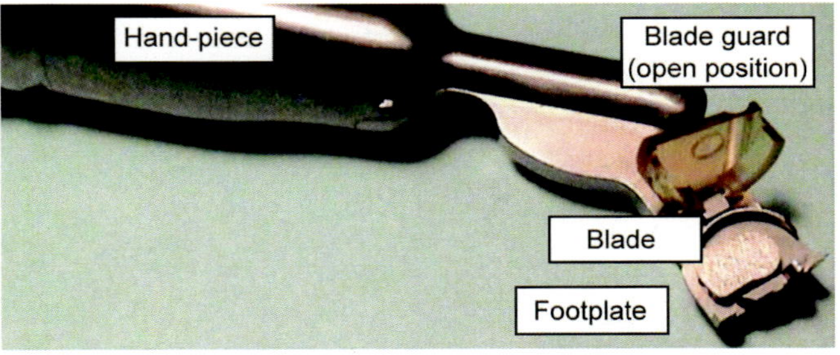

Fig. 54.24: *PresVIEW*™ scleratome hand piece with blade guard open

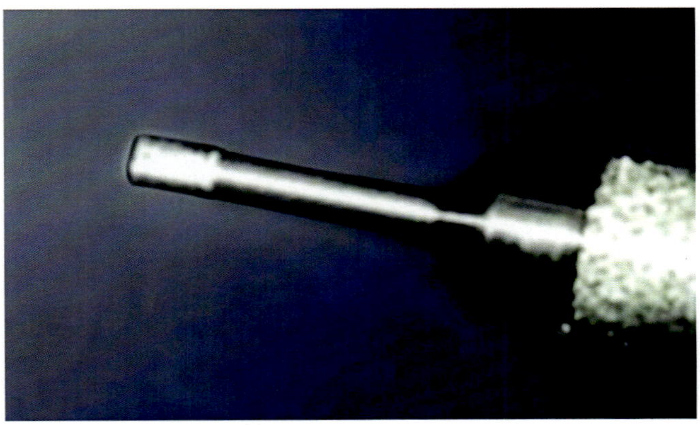

Fig. 54.25: Blade loading tool

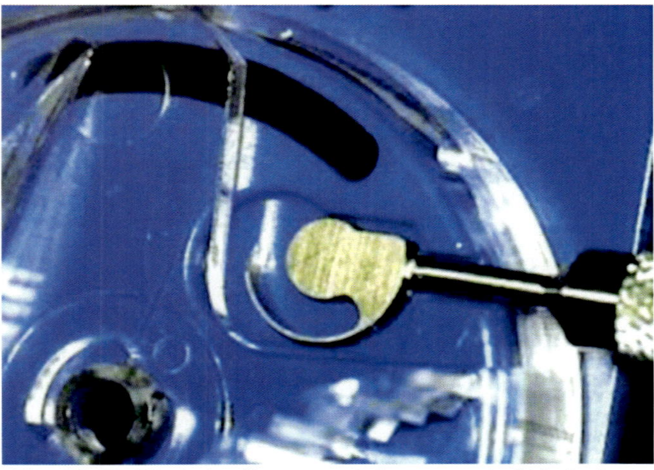

Fig. 54.26: Blade loading wrench for removal of blade from protective case

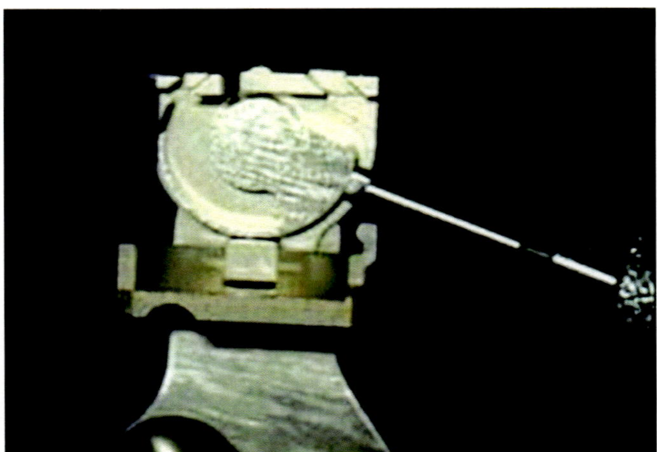

Fig. 54.27: Blade loading onto *PresVIEW*™ scleratome hand piece

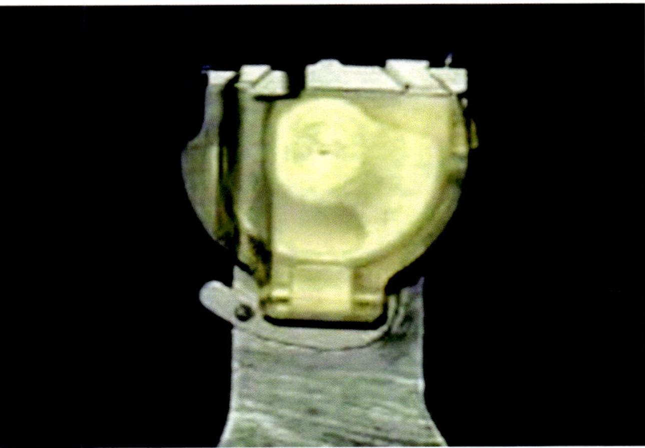

Fig. 54.28: Blade loaded and blade guard replaced

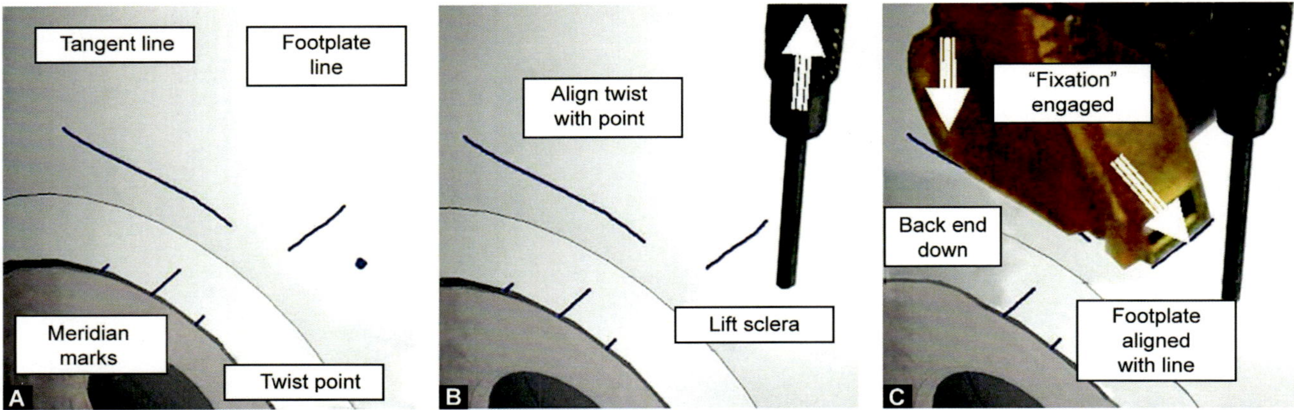

Figs 54.29A to C: *PresVIEW*™ scleratome footplate placement

the Scleratome footplate are delicate and can become damaged during handling.

The technique that I prefer in creating the lamellar scleral tunnels is as follows: The forward fixation features on the "toe" of the *PresVIEW*™ Scleratome footplate are aligned with the radial mark made in the sclera clockwise and posterior to the twist pick mark (Figs 54.29A to C). The points of the fixation features should be engaged into the sclera followed by maneuvering of the hand piece flush with the surface of the sclera. The anterior side of the footplate should be aligned with the anterior edge parallel to the tangent line. It is important to push back the conjunctiva with a cellulose spear to, once again, absorb moisture and prevent interference between the sclera surface and the underside of the *PresVIEW*™ Scleratome footplate. It is important to ensure that the "heel" of the footplate is flush with the scleral surface so that the blade path is uninterrupted and produces a smooth tunnel.

Fixation of the *PresVIEW*™ Scleratome footplate is achieved using a twist fixation instrument (Fig. 54.30) and the forward fixation features of the footplate. The twist is placed at the toe of the footplate, perpendicular to the sclera and oriented with the forward twist mark (Fig. 54.31). Fixation is achieved by turning the twist clockwise approximately 180 degrees. This will engage the bottom features of the twist into the sclera, and prevent shifting of the footplate during blade passage.

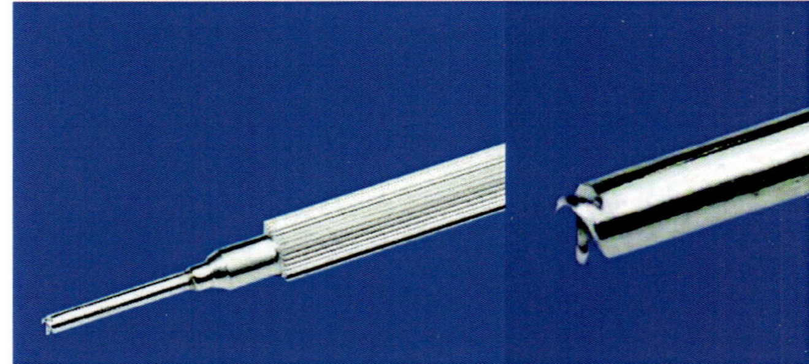

Fig. 54.30: Twist fixation instrument

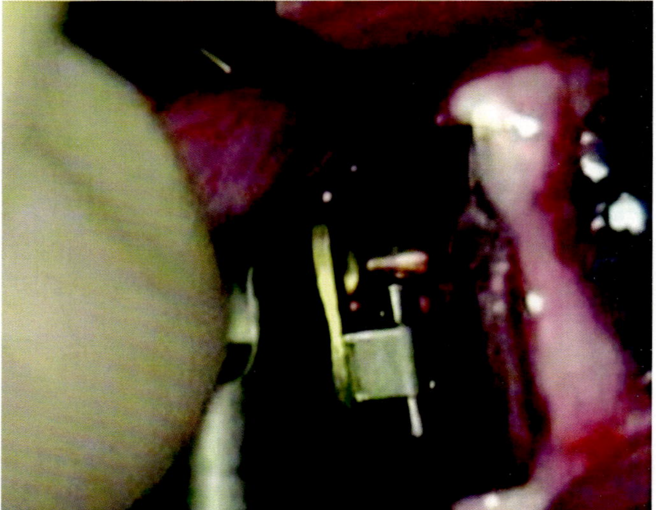

Fig. 54.31: Twist fixation instrument secured to sclera and engaged with footplate

Activation of the *PresVIEW*™ Scleratome is achieved via a foot pedal (Fig. 54.32). Constant pressure on the black activation pad of the pedal is required

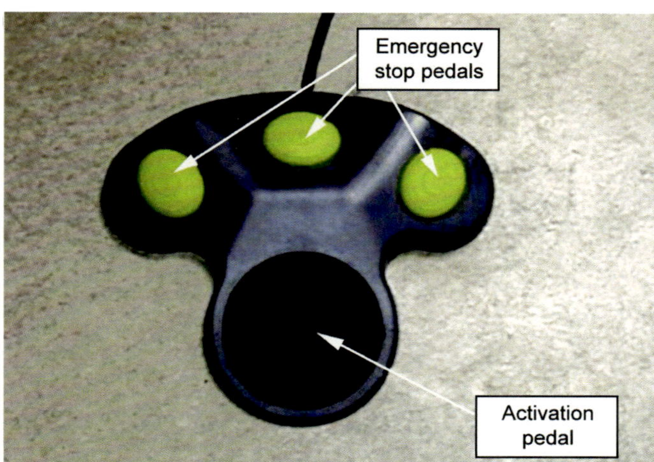

Fig. 54.32: *PresVIEW*™ scleratome controller foot pedal

to ensure the blade completes the entire incision and return circuit. The control box for the *PresVIEW*™ System Scleratome will beep during the incision cycle; short beeps during incision, long beeps during retraction. Once the blade circuit is complete, the twist can be removed via counter clockwise turn and the footplate lifted from the sclera surface (heel first, then toe).

It is my preference to complete all four lamellar scleral tunnels before placing the first *PresVIEW*™ Scleral Implant. Since use of the hand piece can sometimes cause a reduction in ocular pressure over time, making all four tunnels while the eye is still firm ensures the highest quality tunnels—start to finish. In addition, the amount of pressure exerted by the surgeon when using the hand piece is the primary source of discomfort for the patient during the procedure, and varies patient-to-patient as well as surgeon-to-surgeon. By completing all four tunnels sequentially, the time period through which the patient must experience this discomfort will be minimized.

After completion, each tunnel must be assessed for adequacy. This is important, as tunnel length may vary depending on globe firmness and footplate fixation during blade circuit. Each lamellar scleral tunnel requires the insertion of a tapered measuring spatula that provides immediate visual feedback on tunnel quality (Fig. 54.33). The spatula has gold engraved marks across the mid-section that indicates tunnel length between 3.50 and 4.00 mm in length. The *PresVIEW*™ System Scleratome produces tunnels that generally range between 3.50 and 4.25 mm in length. The optimal LST (lamellar scleral tunnel) length is 4.00 mm. Tunnels less than 3.5 mm in length require extension via a manual sclerotomy using a lamellar diamond blade. Tunnels in excess of 4.50 mm can result in an increased risk of subluxation of the implant. Reduction in tunnel length using the vertical diamond blade is recommended.

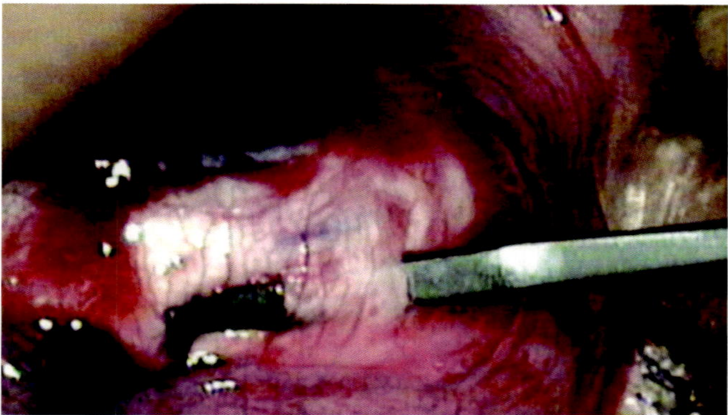

Fig. 54.33: Tapered spatula placed across scleral tunnel

Implant Placement

The most efficient way to proceed to the next step of implant insertion is by maintaining globe fixation, especially if good fixation is already established. The assistant will then hand the implant loaded in the implant forceps to the surgeon (Figs 54.34 and 54.35). It is important to decide at this point whether the implant should be placed upside down and then rotated or placed directly right side up through the belt loop. The following consideration should be made in making this decision.

If there is any difficulty in forming the lamellar scleral tunnel, whether being excessively deep (as a function of the percentage incision depth versus pre-operative scleral thickness) or needing to change the length of the tunnel using a lamellar diamond blade, one should opt for putting the implant in upside down. It is important to understand that when inserting the implant, if it is placed right side up, the

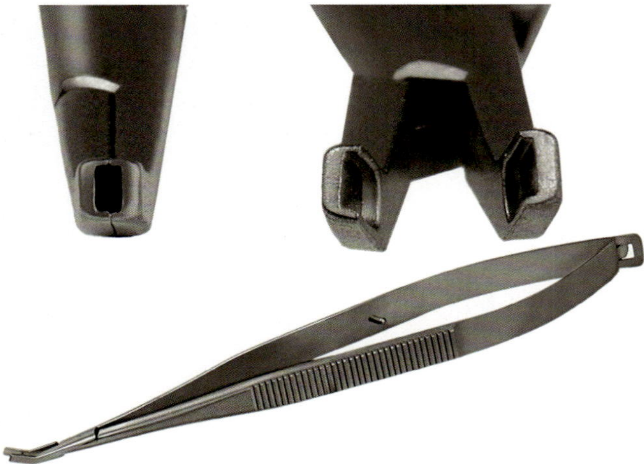

Fig. 54.34: Implant forceps

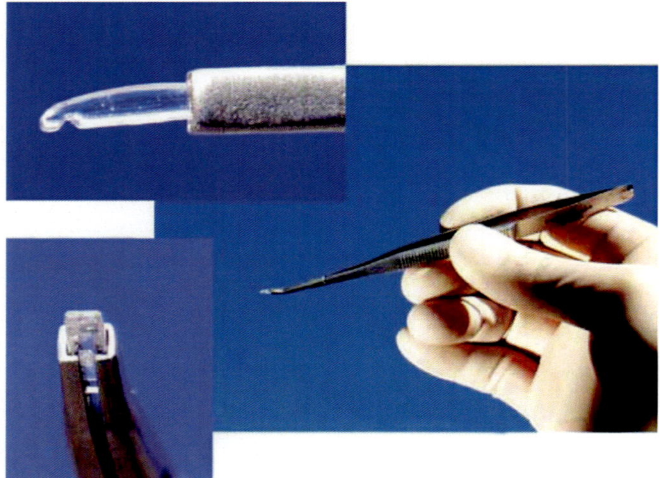

Fig. 54.35: Implant forceps loaded with implant (right side up)

leading nose of the implant has a tendency to want to project inwardly or toward the inner globe. This is due not only to the shape of the implant, but also because the tight scleral tunnel pushes down constantly on the implant as it is being inserted. This is consistent with the design intent of the implant "lifting" the sclera anterior to the implantation site.

Due to this natural tendency, and if the surgeon is overly aggressive in manipulating the implant across a tight tunnel, the implant may penetrate the underlying sclera and enter the suprachoroidal space. Though extremely rare, even I have had this occur in my own hands. The few documented occurrences of this event have not resulted in serious side effects. I am personally aware of two implants that were inadvertently placed into this supra-choroidal space and were left there with no significant sequelae.

When inserting the implant right side up, it is easier to place the implant within the entrance point first. In order to get the insertion of the implant started, it has to be delivered at about a 45-degree angle and inserted into the lamellar scleral tunnel blade entrance side. This angle is maintained until the underside notch of the implant is reached (which is 0.75 mm from the end of the implant). Once the tip portion of the implant is fully within the tunnel, the channel forceps should be angled up enough to prevent the tip of the implant from rubbing the sclera at the base of the tunnel. Once this angle is maneuvered, the implant can be fully advanced through the tunnel.

This maneuver will prevent the leading edge of the implant from damaging the scleral bed beneath or penetrating due to tearing this portion of sclera. Of equal importance is the hand that is holding the fixation device. As the implant is being placed, the fixation device held in the other hand applies an equal counter pressure – i.e. as the implant is being inserted into the tunnel, the fixation device is pushed toward the implant. This slightly "puckers" the lamellar scleral tunnel exit, provided appropriate scleral depression of the fixation device is applied. The exit site of the tunnel will then fish mouth and allow an easier exit of the leading edge of the implant being placed.

If fixation is lost during this counter pressure maneuver, the surgeon can try re-fixating or even change to a different fixating device. Likewise, if the surgeon is using the twist pick, it is important to remember to apply the appropriate rotational force in order to maintain fixation on the sclera. By not applying this rotational force, the surgeon may inadvertently rotate the twist pick and fixation will be lost. Another key point on using the twist pick is that the surgeon must rotate the twist pick at least 180 degrees in order to achieve good scleral fixation.

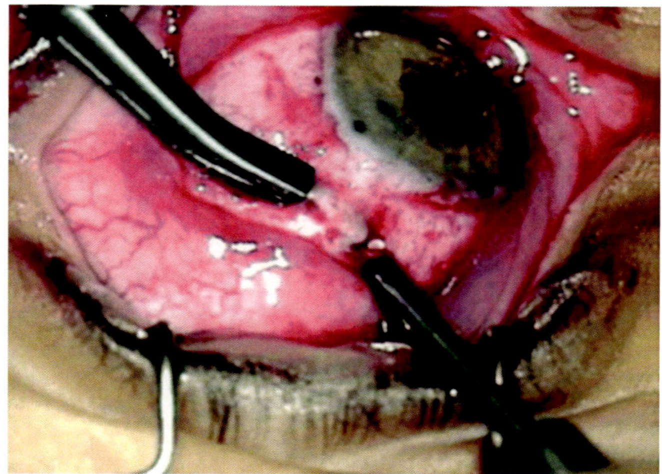

Fig. 54.36: Implant placement in scleral tunnel using forceps and twist fixation

The lamellar scleral tunnel should be very tight, and it is often at this point just prior to the implant exiting the tunnel that a lot of pressure needs to be exerted (Fig. 54.36). Sometimes a slight wiggling of the implant will help and may be called for if the surgeon feels that the implant cannot be exited. Otherwise, the implant can be removed and inserted from the other direction or inserted upside down. Once the implant is inserted from the exit site, and as it approaches the original entrance to the tunnel, its advancement from the LST will be much easier. This is due to the fact that the tunnel has been stretched by the first attempt of the implant insertion. If the fit of the implant is too tight, the tapered spatula can be reinserted into the tunnel and used to temporarily "stretch" the sclera for a better fit.

When the implant is nearly ready to exit, the surgeon can use the tapered spatula to both depress the sclera and form a ramp for the implant to exit. If the spatula is placed parallel to the LST, only very mild counter-traction can be applied safely. If too much pressure is applied, the spatula will unexpectedly slip into the suprachoriodal space. For this reason I place the spatula parallel to the exit incision and perpendicular to the tunnel. This will then allow the surgeon to exert as much counter-pressure as is necessary.

The advantage of placing the implant upside down is that the leading edge of the implant does not have a tendency to "submarine" into the supra-choroidal space, but rather it hugs the undersurface of the LST and allows for an easier exit. The disadvantage of upside-down insertion is that the LST is slightly stretched by rotating the implant back into its upright position. The "submarine" effect of the implant can occur when inserted from either the entrance or exit side of the tunnel.

If during the tunnel formation there was a need for extending or reducing the incision length using the diamond blade, consider inserting the implant upside down. This implant insertion approach will avoid blind pockets (due to manual extension in tunnel length) or scleral flaps (due to manual reduction in tunnel length). When inserting the implant upside-down, the position of the implant has to be greater than a 45-degree angle toward the entrance point of the sclerotomy in order to get the tip of the implant into the LST. If difficulty is still encountered prior to implant exiting, counter pressure is needed in order to push the implant through the tunnel exit. It should be noted here that no viscoelastic or other lubricating material should be used to help the implant slide through the sclera, because whatever allows the implant to slide in easily will also allow the implant to slide out easily. To prevent post-operative subluxation, none of these lubricants should be considered. In addition, any viscoelastic agent underneath the conjunctiva causes a prolonged swelling and conjunctival edema and will prevent early adhesion of Tenon's and conjunctiva to the surface of the tunnel, which will help secure the implant in place. We learned this from experience, which again emphasizes the reason that I encourage surgeons to refrain from making any changes until they are more comfortable with the procedure. Once the upside-down implant has exited and has equal portions extending out of both ends of the LST, the implant is now ready to be rotated.

When rotating the implant, the surgeon should position his or her wrist and hand in a way that anticipates the 180 degree rotation and will allow this movement to be made in a single, smooth step. Often, due to poor exposure or other difficulties, this cannot be achieved, so 0.12 forceps can be used at the other end of the implant. Once the implant is rotated halfway, the other forceps can be used to grab the opposite end of the implant and complete the rotation. If the implant is not extended evenly on either side of the LST, the edge of the implant that is least prominent should be the one that is grasped by the forceps for rotation. The reason for this is that, as the surgeon rotates with the forceps, it has a tendency to pull out the implant. If the surgeon were to grab the edge of the implant that was more exposed, the other end may fall back into the tunnel. When using the channeled forceps, the implant can be rotated as soon as the leading edge of the implant has exited the LST.

Currently, I find it preferable to insert the implants upside-down followed by rotation. Once the implant is in position, one has to make sure it is symmetrically exiting on either side of the tunnel (Fig. 54.37). This is particularly important, because the notches on the underside of the implant should be aligned with the entry and exit points of the tunnel. This is the reason for the precise 3.50 to 4.00 mm width of the engravings on the tapered spatula for visual verification of tunnel length. By ensuring that the channels under the implant are on or just past both edges of the sclera, it encourages the sclera to ride up into the notch and prevent the implant from subluxating.

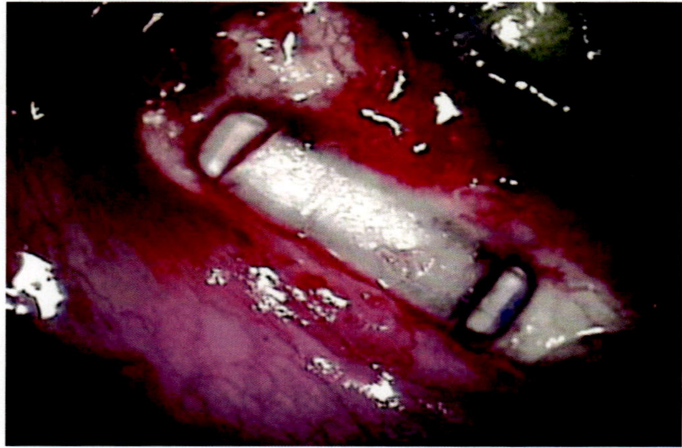

Fig. 54.37: Implant spacing across lamellar scleral tunnel

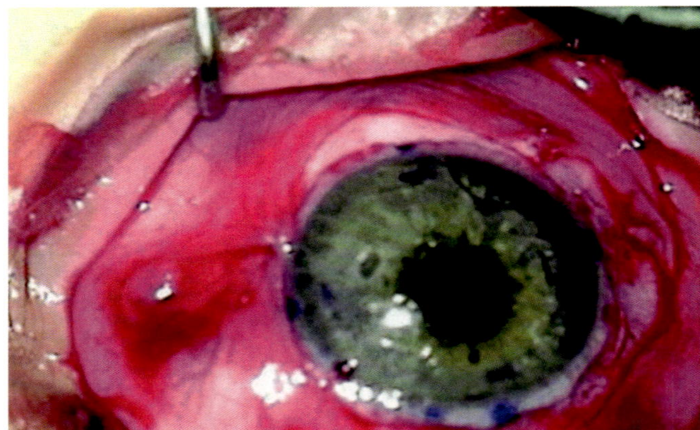

Fig. 54.38: Closing the conjunctiva

Closing the Conjunctiva

After all implants are in position, the surgical site should be thoroughly flushed clear of thrombus, followed by the conjunctiva pulled over the implants and back towards the original conjunctival relaxing incisions. The two corners of the conjunctiva at each relaxing incision are then identified and a single 10-0 nylon suture is placed at the 3 and 9 o'clock positions. The suture should be tied in a buried knot fashion, taking a scleral bite at the limbal interface to prevent the migration of conjunctiva (Fig. 54.38).

If the conjunctiva is stretched or torn prior to placing the 10-0 nylon in the sclera, one should pull the conjunctiva and make sure the extreme aspects do provide sufficient coverage. This coverage should mean that the conjunctiva should be within 1.0 to 1.5 mm of its original insertion. If it is not, the suture bite should take a little extra-conjunctiva and pull it towards the 6 or 12 o'clock position in order to pull it tighter. Only a single suture is necessary for each relaxing incision, and it has provided adequate coverage in all of my cases to date.

POSTOPERATIVE CARE

Pharmaceutical Regimen

Based on the surgeon's experience and anticipated speed of surgery, at some time during the final implant, the staff is instructed to start the 250 cc of 20 percent mannitol IV. At the conclusion of the case, the pupil should be observed and if it is dilated or asymmetrical, 1 percent pilocarpine should be given to assure the pupil is round and symmetrical. If there is any oblique shape to the pupil, pilocarpine should be applied and the patient observed closely until the pupil is round.

The patient's eyes are patched only if there is a corneal abrasion. Otherwise, no patching is necessary. For the most part, the postoperative pain usually only requires extra strength acetaminophen, but there have been a few patients that have had more serious pain. Of course, if there is any corneal abrasion, I would recommend against putting on a collagen shield or contact lens, because this could migrate underneath the conjunctiva and prevent it from sealing down around the implant. Postoperative eyedrops include antibiotic Ciloxan (Alcon, Fort Worth, Tex) and usually Flarex (Allergan, Irvine, CA) or another mild steroid is sufficient. For cases of marked inflammation postoperatively, one can change to a prednisone acetate 1 percent or even add Voltaren (CIBA Vision, Duluth, GA). This is very rare, however, and most of the patients tolerate the postoperative irritation.

Rehabilitation

SSP patients must undergo rehabilitative eye exercises to ensure optimal results. The ciliary muscle of these presbyopes has not been used for a number of years and requires physical therapy. Before the exercises are started the quality and quantity of the tear film must be evaluated. During the first few weeks, the conjunctiva is swollen over the implants. This prevents the eyelids from spreading the tear film adequately and artificial tears are necessary. Tears should be used every two hours and a bland ointment at bedtime. Sometimes punctal plugs are also necessary.

The accommodative exercise is called the push-up/push-out technique. The patient is given a reading card and told to hold it at 10 cm from their eyes. They are instructed to focus on the smallest line they can see and then concentrate without squinting, and notice if they can see any letters on the next smaller line. This exercise is repeated as the patient slowly moves the near card away from their eyes while keeping the smaller line in focus until the near card is at arm's length. Then instruct the patient to bring the near card slowly back up to 10 cm from his or her eyes while trying to keep the same line in focus. Once the card is 10 cm from their eyes, they should be instructed to try and see the next smaller line. This exercise should be done 6 to 8 times in each eye, 4 to 5 times a day.

Potential Complications

The surgical reversal of presbyopia is a delicate and precise procedure. It is important to keep in mind that each operated eye represents, essentially, four cases (because of the four implants being inserted). In addition to the primary objective of reversing presbyopia, one of the major advantages of this procedure is its safety and reversibility. However, if the procedure is not approached as a surgical procedure, then problems can arise. Though this procedure has the advantage of affecting neither distance vision nor refractive error, the patient or surgeon should not take this procedure lightly.

The only three major complications reported with this procedure have been a single case of endophthalmitis and two cases of anterior segment ischemia in over 300 surgeries (or 1,200 implantations). Since this procedure, or any procedure, is not risk free, the surgeon and surgical team should approach this just as they would any intraocular procedure. It inadvertently can become an intraocular procedure if the implants are inserted too deeply and penetrate into the suprachoroidal space. Vitreous can be lost in these situations, but loss is minimal and easily tamponaded by the implant. The barrier of the intact eye has been compromised; therefore, infection is possible. With good sterile technique, endophthalmitis should not occur. It is important to remember that SSP is not a LASIK procedure; which is generally approached in a clean manner. SSP is a procedure that should be treated as an intraocular procedure, and adherence to aseptic technique is of utmost importance. The current FDA presbyopia clinical trials require the surgeon to conduct all surgeries in an ambulatory surgical center (ASC).

RESEARCH AND ONGOING IMPROVEMENTS

The best method for correlating long-term clinical efficacy of the scleral spacing procedure to actual clinical outcomes would be to objectively measure implant location, intrascleral, posterior to the crystalline lens equator. This has not been possible until just recently. With the development of infrared optical coherence tomography in the 1310 nanometer wavelength, imaging of the implants is now possible. Previous attempts at visualizing the implants intrascleral have met with limited success.

The Visante™ OCT (optical coherence tomography) obtained FDA clearance on September 30th, 2005 as a non-contact, high resolution tomographic and biomicroscopic device indicated for in vivo imaging and measurement of ocular structures in the anterior segment. The advantage to utilizing this instrument as an alternative to ultrasonic biomicroscopy (UBM) in diagnostic imaging is that images of ocular structures can be obtained with the OCT without the need for ocular anesthesia and water bath. In addition, the Visante™ OCT utilizes infrared imaging technology with a wavelength of 1310 nanometers which readily penetrates the *PresVIEW*™ Scleral Implant material (PMMA) without the image scatter inherent with ultrasound energy. The OCT scanning speed is approximately 4,000 axial scans per second with a resolution accuracy of 10 microns.

Lessons Learned and Long-term Efficacy

As such, clear and distinct images of the implant intrascleral can be obtained (Fig. 54.39); making the OCT capable of providing postoperative follow-up of study patients. This provides the opportunity to objectively evaluate implant placement intra-scleral and determine the effect of implant location in relation to clinical efficacy. Significant effort has been undertaken to collect and analyze the data with interesting results. Of greatest importance is the long-term stability of the implant; or the lack of occurence of "subluxation".

Verification of implant state was obtained in a large quantity of patients using the OCT (approximately 88 eyes as of November, 2007) and assessed for subluxation, orientation, etc, as applicable. Each measurement was analyzed from the OCT images, including:

- Lens depth and thickness
- Sclera and conjunctiva thickness anterior to implant for each of four implants
- Scleral thickness under implant for each measurement for each of four implants
- Thickness of tissue over implant for each measurement for each of four implants
- Distance from top-side anterior edge of each of four implants to angle
- Distance from bottom-side anterior edge of each of four implants to angle.

Of greatest importance was the discovery of the impact that subluxation had on the clinical outcomes (Fig. 54.40). This is especially important, as it provides substantial evidence to support the Schachar theory of accommodation. In particular, it was discovered that:

- All 4 implants stable = 84 percent of the patients achieve distance corrected near visual acuities (DCNVA) of 20/40 or better.

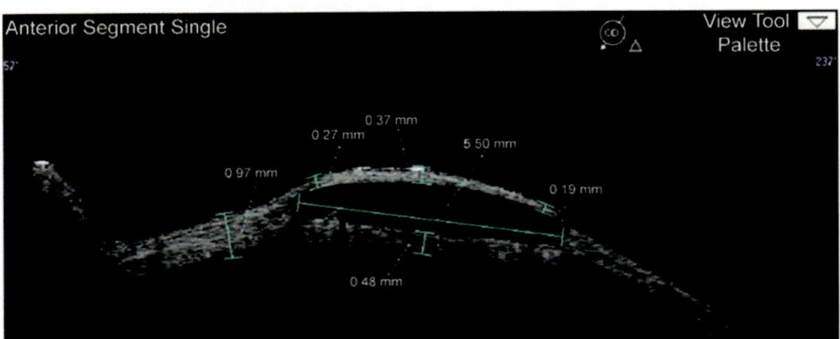

Fig. 54.39: PresVIEW™ scleral implant image using Visante™ OCT

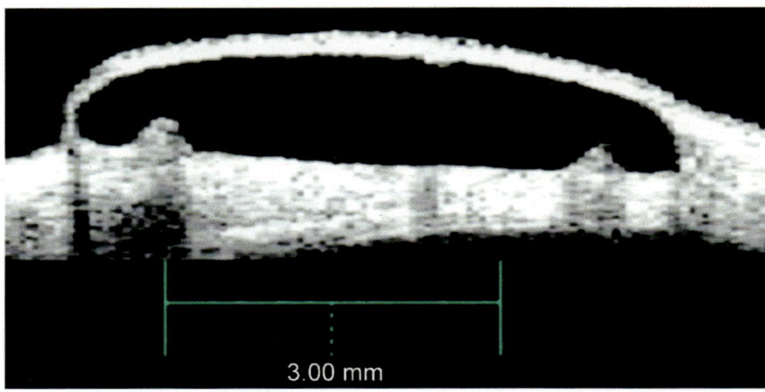

Fig. 54.40: Subluxed presVIEW™ scleral implant image

- If even 1 implant is subluxed = only 45 percent patients achieve DCNVA 20/40 or better.
- 2 implants subluxed = only 36 percent patients achieve DCNVA 20/40 or better.
- 3+ implants subluxed = only 12 percent patients achieve DCNVA 20/40 or better.

Interestingly enough, patients return either to or close to their best distance corrected near visual acuity upon repositioning of their subluxed implants. As such, Refocus Group has undertaken further design improvements of the *PresVIEW*™ Scleral Implant to reduce the likelihood of postoperative subluxation. This involves a two part design that "locks" across the scleral tunnel and prevents implant shifting due to either eye rubbing or scleral tunnel loosening postoperatively. Once the main body is placed across the tunnel, a mid-body section is locked into place, completing the implant placement.

A significant number of patients have now been enrolled in the Refocus Group's international clinical trial with outstanding results. As of (date/implant design?)October, 2007, over 46 eyes have been implanted without postoperative subluxation. Refocus Group intends to begin enrolling patients in their ongoing Phase III US FDA clinical trial using the improved system once they receive approval for their IDE supplement. An image showing implant stability using the Visante™ OCT system is shown in Figure 54.41.

Advancements in the Surgical Procedure

This design improvement also includes incorporating a means to deliver the implants with greater ease and less risk of the "submarine effect" described in the surgical techniques section. This improved method utilizes a shuttle and "feeder tube" to allow the implant to be pulled across the lamellar scleral tunnel without the pushing or prodding required for the current implant (Figs 54.42 and 54.43). Recent international clinical training has shown that the use of the new implantation procedure can reduce surgical time to less than 15 minutes per eye.

Further improvements related to ease and accuracy of the surgical procedure have been undertaken.

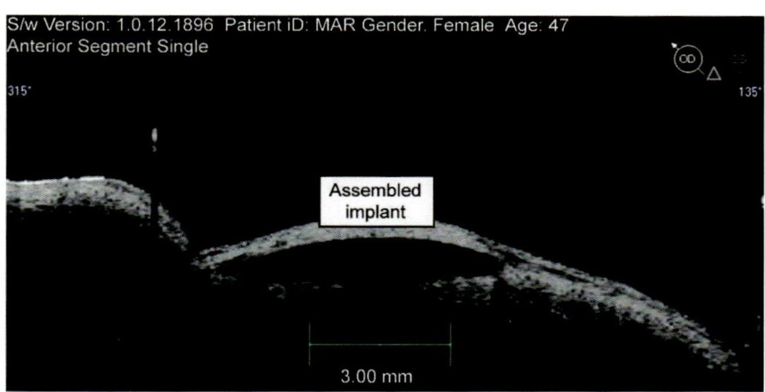

Fig. 54.41: "Anti-subluxating" presVIEW™ scleral implant image using the Visante™ OCT

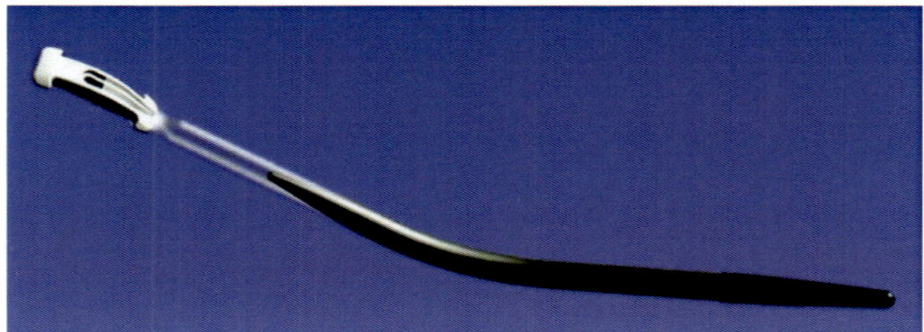

Fig. 54.42: "Shuttle" delivery of the new *PresVIEW*™ scleral implant

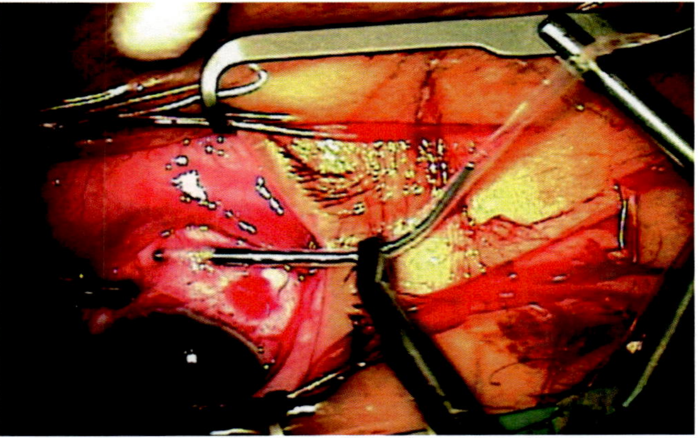

Fig. 54.43: "Shuttle" delivery of the new *PresVIEW*™ scleral implant—in vivo

Reproducibility of the lamellar scleral tunnel using the PresVIEW™ System Scleratome is of primary importance. Once the tunnel has been made, implant location both in depth and relative location to the ciliary body is fixed. Suboptimal placement will, ultimately, lead to suboptimal results. Ocular fixation is difficult with the current system and relies on the use of a "twist pick" fixation element. This twist can be unreliable, and can "slip". This slippage allows the scleratome to move during blade advancement and

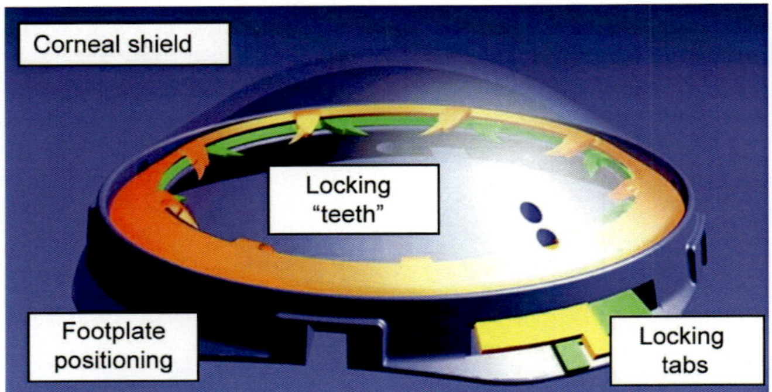

Fig. 54.44: Ocular fixation device for the improved *PresVIEW™* system

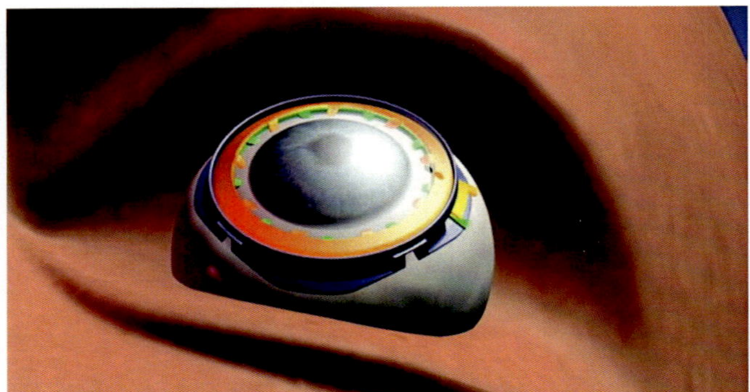

Fig. 54.46: Ocular fixation device placed and locked on the globe

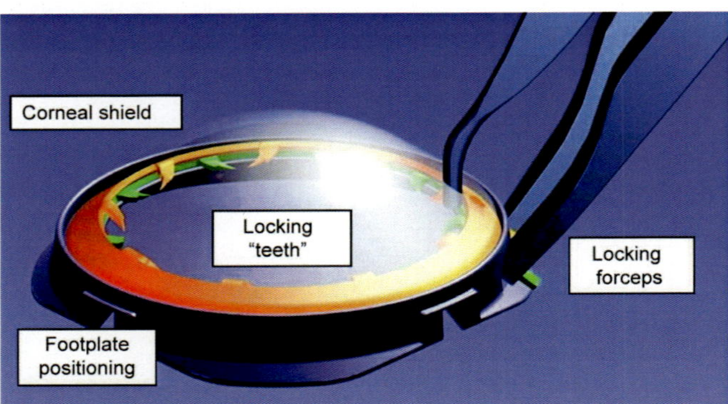

Fig. 54.45: Ocular fixation device with locking forceps to close "teeth"

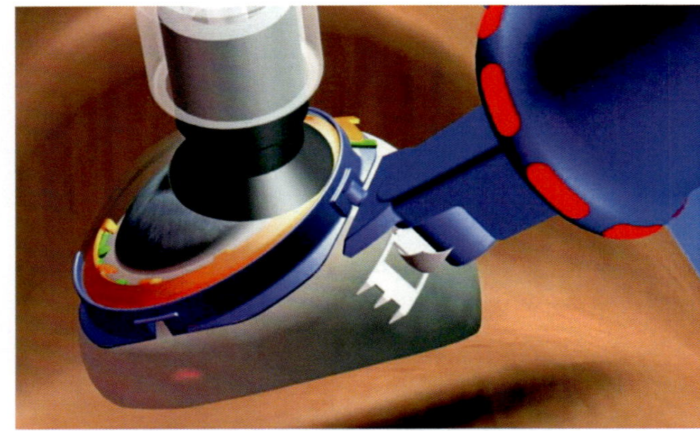

Fig. 54.47: Ocular fixation device with suction manipulator and showing 2nd generation scleratome and footplate "Docked" to the device

can result in the creation of the LST in a suboptimal location or short. As such, Refocus Group has developed a system for "locking" the globe and providing for physical stops for the scleratome relative to the corneal center (Figs 54.44 to 54.46). This fixation device is similar to the suction rings utilized in LASIK surgery, but without the damaging effects of long-term increased IOP due to the vacuum. The Refocus Group device utilizes tiny metal fixation elements circumferentially placed around the limbus to provide the fixation. A manipulation device utilizing suction fixes to the clear plastic corneal shield.

A second generation PresVIEW™ System Scleratome and footplate have also been developed that "dock" to the ocular fixation device. This new footplate provides improved stability for the device once docked to the fixation device, and produces the same consistent lamellar scleral tunnels as the current system, but with a lower profile and improved ergonomics (Fig. 54.47).

These system improvements, when combined with the latest "anti-subluxating" implant and shuttle implantation techniques, should further reduce surgical time to less than 10 minutes per eye (Figs 54.48 to 54.50). The two-part implant design is shown in the images more clearly than the in vivo images presented in the preceding section, and represent the ease of implantation associated with improved ocular manipulation and control.

Quantitative Assessment of Accommodation

The second diagnostic technology having significant potential for improving the long-term efficacy of scleral spacing as well as proving out the clinical

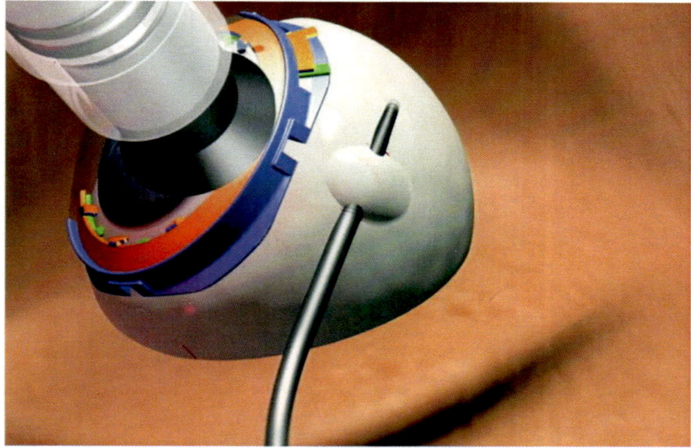

Fig. 54.48: Placement of shuttle through lamellar scleral tunnel

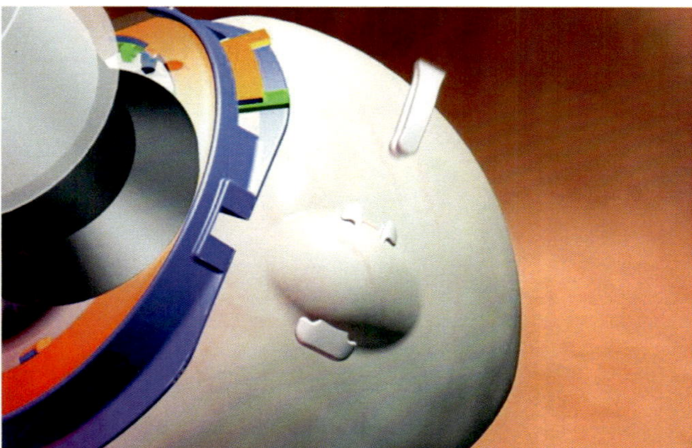

Fig. 54.49: Assembly of two-part "anti-subluxating" *PresVIEW*™ scleral implant

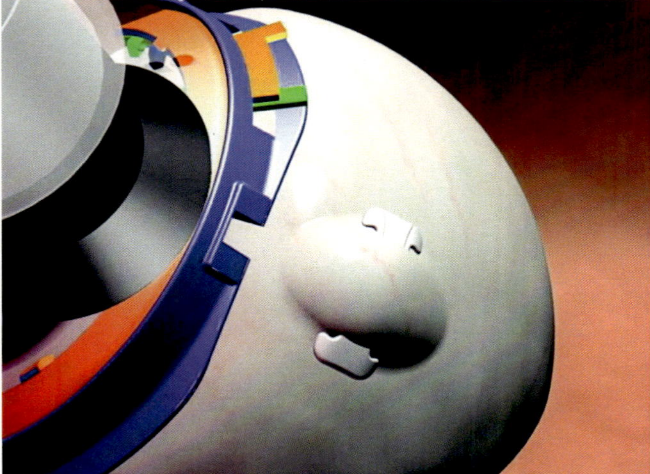

Fig. 54.50: Assembled "anti-subluxating" *PresVIEW*™ scleral implant

mechanism by which scleral spacing truly introduces net accommodative improvement is the latest improvement to the iTrace Dynamic Laser Refractor from Tracey™ Technologies. The Schachar theory behind the effect of scleral spacing revolves around the central steepening of the crystalline lens. This theory also correlates well with the understanding that near visual acuity is best assessed with bright lighting conditions.

Assuming that pupil contraction in bright environments does improve near vision, small pupil diameter dynamic laser refraction would be more capable of measuring these small diopter improvements in near visual acuity under the assumption that central steepening is the primary mechanism by which scleral spacing operates. The latest iTrace Dynamic Laser Refractor is capable of auto refraction with pupil diameters as small as 2 mm. Current auto refractors generally operate best when pupil diameters are 4 mm or greater. A recent international patient having received the "anti-subluxating" PresVIEW™ Scleral Implants is shown in Figure 54.51. Additional SSP patients have been evaluated using the iTrace Dynamic Laser Refractor with similar results.

SUMMARY OF SSP

It is apparent that there are many flaws in the Helmholtz and Coleman theories of accommodation. This is best exemplified by the fact that researchers have been unable to duplicate a variable-focus single lens system similar to the human crystalline lens or that finite element analysis of the catenary approach have been unsuccessful at supporting the assumption of changes to accommodative amplitude. Furthermore, Helmholtz theory fails to have widespread applications to other scientific phenomena. In contrast Schachar's theory not only has produced a variable-focus single element lens, but also has widespread applications to many different scientific disciplines. For example, the mechanism by which the human crystalline lens deforms during accommodation is similar in mechanism to the counterintuitive shape changes of the earth's tides, the shape change of a

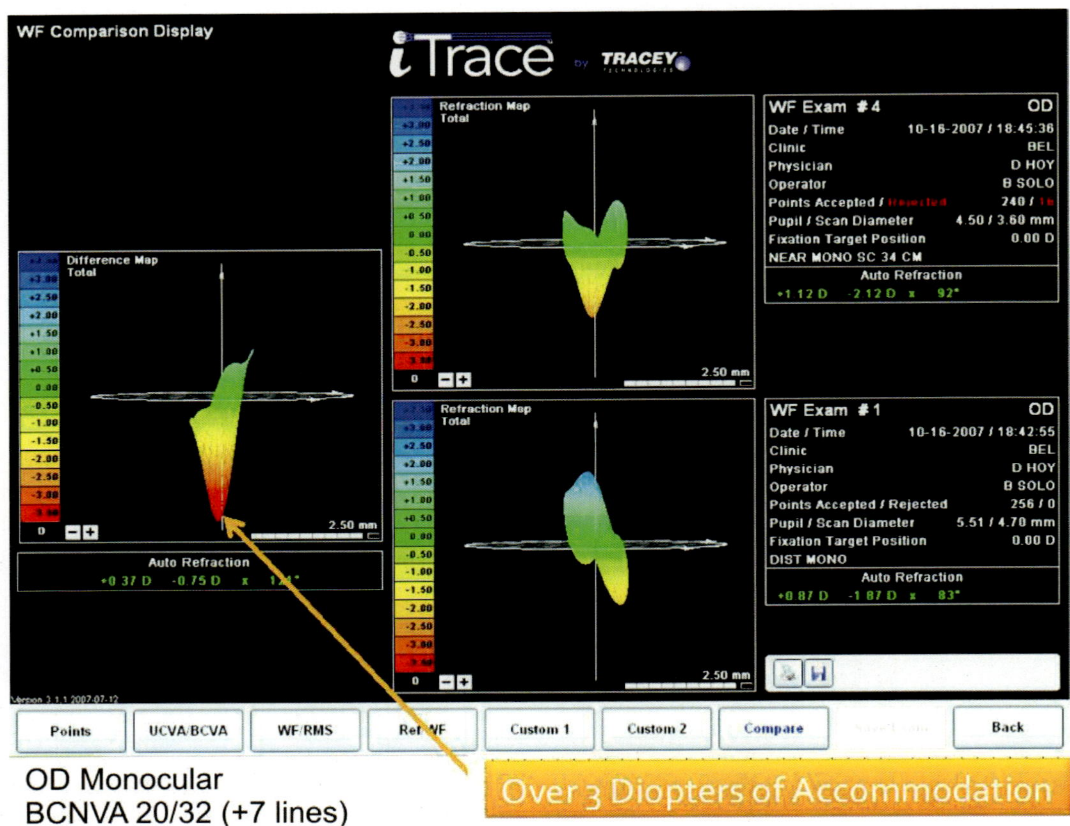

Fig. 54.51: Example of central lens steepening as shown using the iTrace device and with a 2 mm pupil diameter

drop of magnetic fluid within a magnetic field, and the similar but mysterious shape of many spiral galaxies that demonstrate central steepening and peripheral flattening. What is truly amazing is the impact that Schachar's theory will have on the camera industry, defense industry (focusing on targets), optical computers and astronomy.

The visual correction revolution that we are currently in appears to be complete. Given the concept that presbyopia is a surgically correctable condition, the last major hurdle in refractive surgery has been overcome. While not everyone in the world needs glasses to see at distance, 100 percent of the population over the age of 40 will eventually need correction for presbyopia. The global impact of this immense population will be a driving force for the continued research and development of this procedure.

FURTHER READING

1. Agarwal MS. Agar: Presbyopia, a Surgical Textbook. Slack Publishing, 2002.
2. Atchison DA. Accommodation and presbyopia. Ophthalmic Physiol Opt 1995;15(4):255-72[Medline].
3. Belville J Kevin, Smith Ronald J. Presbyopia Surgery, Pearls and Pitfalls. Slack Publishing, 2006.
4. Brown N. The Shape of the lens equator. Exp Eye Res 1974;19(6):571-6[Medline].
5. Coleman DJ, Fish SK. Presbyopia, accommodation, and the mature catenary. Ophthalmology 2001;108(9):1544-51.
6. Coleman DJ. On the Hydraulic suspension theory of accommodation. Trans Am Ophthalmology Soc 1986;84:846-68.
7. Coleman DJ. Unified model for the accommodative mechanism. Am J Ophthalmology 1970;69:1063-79.
8. Coulombre JL, Coulombre AJ. Lens Development. IV. Size, Shape, and Orientation. Invest Ophthalmol 1969; 8(3):251-7[Medline].
9. Duke-Elder S, Wybar KC. The Anatomy of the Visual System. In: Duke-Elder S (Ed): System of Ophthalmology, London: Henry Kimpton 1961;2:80-1.

10. Farnsworth PN, Shyne SE. Anterior Zonular Shifts with Age. Exp Eye Res 1979;28(3):291-7[Medline].
11. Fitch RC. Procedural Effects on the Manifest Human Amplitude of Refraction. Amer J Optometry Arch Amer Acad Optometry 1971;7:918-26.
12. Flocks M, Zweng HC. Studies on the mode of action of pilocarpine On aqueous outflow. Am J Ophthalmol 1957;44:380-7.
13. Fukasaku H. Silicone Expansion Plug Implant Surgery for Presbyopia. In: Am Soc of Cataract Refractive Surg Symposium. Boston, Ma: 2000.
14. Fukasaku H. Surgical Correction of Presbyopia. Presented at: ASCRS Meeting; April 1999; Seattle, WA.
15. Glasser A, Campbell MCW. Presbyopia and the Optical Changes in the Human Crystalline Lens with Age. Vision Res 1998;38:209-29.
16. Glasser A, Kaufman PL. The mechanism of accommodation in primates. Ophthalmology 1999;106:863-72.
17. Heiner Martin, Rudolf Guthoff, Thom Terwee, Klaus-Peter Schmitz. Comparison of the Accommodation Theories of Coleman and of Helmholtz by Finite Element Simulations. Vision Research 2005;45(22):2910-5.
18. Koretz JF, Cook CA, Kaufman PL. Accommodation and presbyopia in the human eye. Changes in the anterior segment and crystalline lens with focus. Invest Ophthalmol Vis Sci 1997;38:569-78.
19. Lim SJ, Kang SJ, Kim HB. Analysis of zonular-free zone and lens size in relation to axial length of eye with age. J Cataract Refract Surg 1998;24(3):390-6[Medlline].
20. Marshall J, Beaconsfield M, Rothery S. The anatomy and development of the human lens and zonules. Trans Ophthalmol Soc U K 1982;102 Pt 3:423-40[Medline].
21. Rafferty NS. Lens morphology. In Maisel H (Ed): The Ocular Lens. New York: Dekker, 1985;2-6.
22. Schachar RA, Anderson DA. The Mechanism of ciliary muscle function. Ann Ophthalmol 1995;27:126-32.
23. Schachar RA, Cudmore DP, Black TD, et al. Paradoxical optical power increase of a deformable lens by equatorial stretching. Ann Ophthalmol 1998;30:10-8.
24. Schachar RA. Cause and treatment of presbyopia with a method for increasing the amplitude of accommodation. Ann Ophthalmol 1992;24(12):445-7, 452[Medline].
25. Schachar RA. Histology of the ciliary muscle-zonular connections. Ann Ophthalmol 1996;28:70-9.
26. Schachar RA. The scleral expansion band procedure for the treatment of ocular hypertension and primary open angle glaucoma. Ann Ophthalmol 2000;32:87-9.
27. Schachar RA. The scleral expansion band procedure for the treatment of ocular hypertension and primary open angle glaucoma. Ann Ophthalmol 2000;32:87-9.
28. Strenk SA, Semmlow JL, Strenk LM. Age-related changes in human ciliary muscle and lens: a magnetic resonance imaging study. Invest Ophthalmol Vis Sci 1999;40(6): 1162-9[Medline].
29. Taylor VL, al-Ghoul KJ, Lane CW, et al. Morphology of the normal human lens. Invest Ophthalmology Vis Sci 1996;37:1396-410.
30. von Helmholtz H. Uber Die Akkommodation Des Auges. Albrecht Von Graefe Arch Opthalmology 1855;1:1-89.

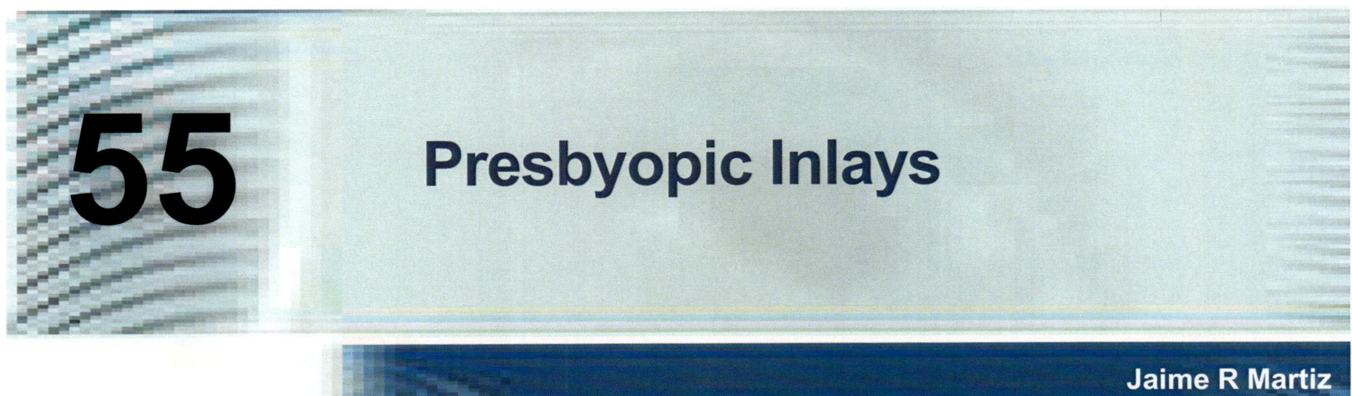

55 Presbyopic Inlays

Jaime R Martiz

INTRODUCTION

Presbyopia, age related loss in accommodative amplitude, is a common problem for people over the age of 40 to 45 (Table 55.1). Several possible explanations for the development of Presbyopia have been proposed. The most common explanation is that an age related reduction in the ability of the crystalline lens to accommodate develops over time. This may be caused by either age related "hardening"of the crystalline lens itself or by changes in the lens capsule. Some propose that Presbyopia may be caused by age related reduction in the ciliary muscle leading to reduced accommodation amplitude. This theory is not supported by more recent studies in monkey's eyes where ciliary muscle's function has not been shown to be reduced with age.

Regardless of the causing mechanism, Presbyopia interferes with near vision. When left uncorrected it may cause a reduction in productivity when performing close-up work, reading for pleasure, and participation in certain sports. The debilitating effect of Presbyopia needs to be corrected for the subject to regain near vision functionality (Table 55.2).

Table 55.1: Presbyopic IOL, cataracts and refractive lens exchange

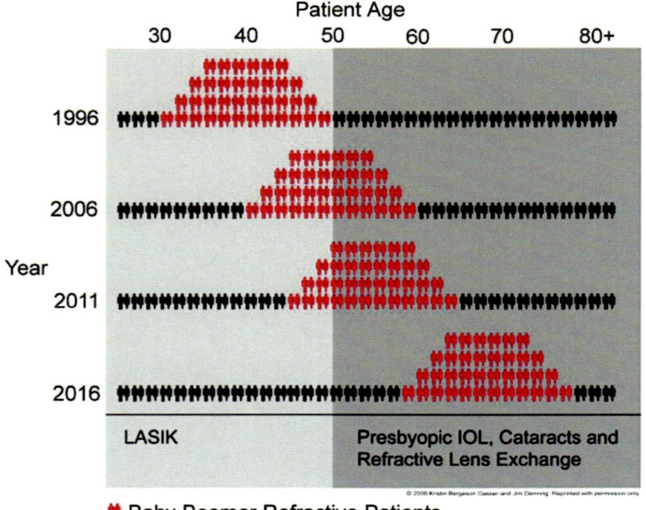

PRESBYOPIA

A variety of optical devices are currently being used to help correct Presbyopia. These include "reading glasses", bifocal glasses, contact lenses and intraocular lenses, as well as a variety of surgical corneal techniques aimed at "steepening" the center of the cornea (Table 55.3). None of the systems currently

Table 55.2: Presbyopia decision making

- Baseline refractive error
- Previous surgery
- Vocation
- Recreational pursuits
- Age
- Pupil size
- Iris color

Table 55.3: Non spectable treatment of presbyopia
• Monovision contact lenses
• Corneal surgery (monovision and multifocal)
• Surface laser surgery (PRK, LASEK)
• LASIK
• Conductive keratoplasty
• Synthetic procedures

available is totally satisfactory to the majority of presbyopic subjects.

An outpatient surgical system that would be proven safe and clinically effective in correcting Presbyopia and allow people to regain their near vision without depending on external optical devices may become the treatment of choice for presbyopic subjects and their ophthalmologists.

CORNEAL INLAYS

Corneal inlay treatment is still experimental as of mid 2008, but clinical studies are progressing and seems encouraging. This method treats Presbyopia by inserting a very tiny lens into the central cornea. This procedure is less invasive than LASIK, intraocular lens surgery including cataract removal and/or clear lens insertion.

The current inlays products are designed to surgically insert a small sized lens with or without positive refractive power in the corneal stroma at a point that is exactly in front of the center of the pupil. With the Inlays implanted, the cornea becomes bifocal, hyperprolate shape or pinhole depending on the product.

TYPES OF INLAYS

Currently, three different corneal inlays are being developed: the AcuFocusä/Bausch & Lomb ACI 7000, (Irvine, California), the Invue™ intracorneal Inlay (Biovision, Switzerland) and the PresbyLens® (ReVision Optics, Lake Forest, California) Table 55.4. The corneal inlays are somewhat very similar to each other in diameter. All of them are under investigation and are designed to be implanted in the non-dominant eye, but the problem is biocompatibility, they got all the advantages and fewer disadvantages of other technologies (Table 55.5). All of them can use a femtosecond laser to create the flap, tunnel or pocket to increase precision and safety.

Table 55.5: Potential complications
• Displacement
• Bioincompatibility- haze, corneal melt
• Discoloration
• Glare and Halos
• Under/over correction
• Loss of BSCV
• All risk associated with flap creation

Acufocus

The ACI 7000 is a small diameter aperture optic and the furthest along in U.S. clinical trials. It increases the depth of focus by using pinhole optics; it has a 1.6 mm center aperture with a 3.6 mm surround and numerous little holes for nutritional purpose flow, and about 10 mm thickness (Fig. 55.1). Peripheral rays are obscured and the central rays pass unaffected and doesn't change corneal power but depth of focus. It generates improved near vision of about 1.5 D add, and does it with no measurable loss of distance vision. Placed on the non-dominant eye, a corneal flap is cut as in standard LASIK, the inlay is placed on the stromal bed, and the flap is then replaced (Fig. 55.2). Placement of the inlay is important as well as any of

Table 55.4: Current inlays under investigation

	Diameter	*Thickness*	*Material*	*Optics*
Revision	1.5 mm	10-35 μm	Copolymer	Steepening
Biovision	3.0 mm	20 μm	Hydrogel	Annular add
Acufocus	3.8 mm	10 μm	PVDN Kynar^{tm}	F22 depth focus

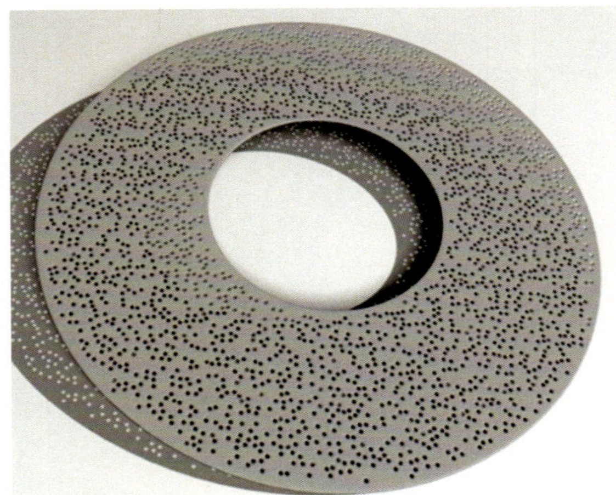

Fig. 55.1: ACI 7000 is a small diameter aperture optic using a pinhole optic, 1.6 mm center and 3.6 mm surround, numerous little holes and 10 μm thickness

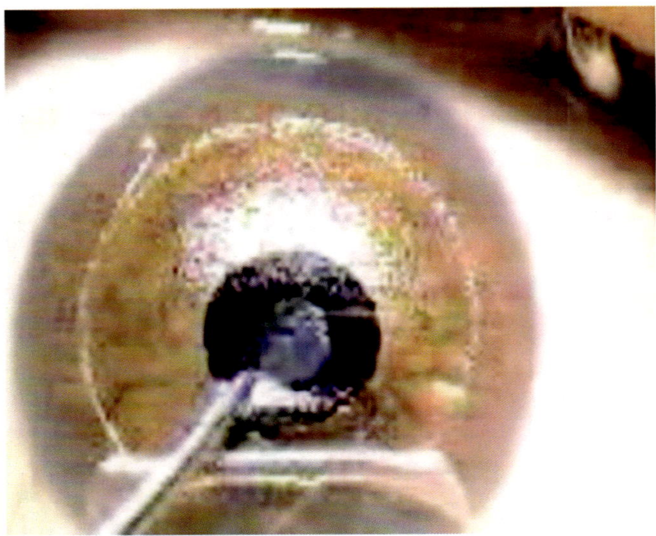

Fig. 55.2: Acufocus/Bausch & Lomb ACI 7000, placed on the non-dominant eye, a corneal flap is cut as in standard LASIK, the inlay is placed on the stromal bed

the other products. Most patients have a little loss of quality of night vision and would not want this in both eyes.

Biovision Invue

The Biovision Invue^{TM} inlay is a hydrogel-based; the surgeon positions the lens in a tunnel in the center of the cornea. Centration is easy, and if necessary, the lens can be removed (Fig. 55.3). This lens is a good choice for the regular emmetropic presbyopic whose cornea is of proper power for distance and who doesn't have more than a 0.75 D of astigmatism. It's the same concept as the multifocal IOLs, but it's creating a multifocal cornea. It's giving really good near acuity with a small loss of distance, about 1-2 lines, in current trials in Europe, Mexico and South America. Because the inlay creates a multifocal cornea, it does have the potential side effects of multifocal optics, just as the IOLs do. The Inlay is a 3 mm total diameter, and 1.8 mm center diameter with no power. There's a ring of add around that, anywhere from 1.2 D to 5 D. The international trial results in Europe and South America have been excellent. There's quick recovery; patients don't have to wait to get the results; the average is about 3 weeks. There's been little night glare reported but Confocal images look similar to normal stroma (Figs 55.4 and 55.5). The inlay is implanted in a tunnel at 250 microns mid-stroma (Fig. 55.6). There's a special microkeratome that creates the 3.5 mm tunnel to implant the 3 mm lens, the implants are 20 microns thick, making them very well tolerated.

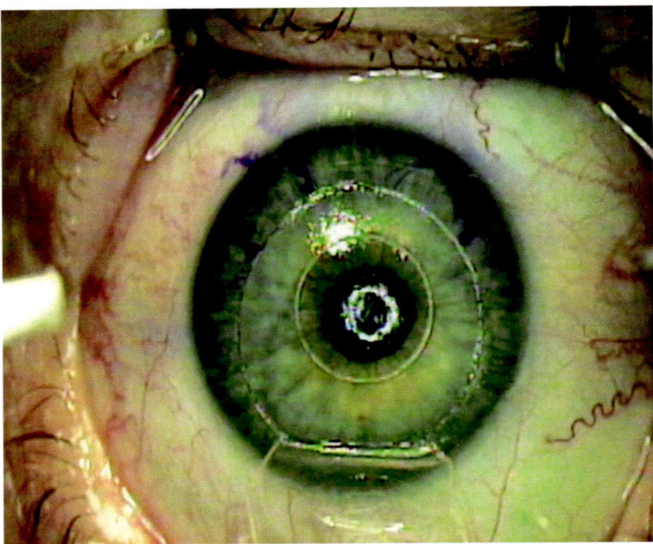

Fig. 55.3: The Biovision Invue^{TM} is a hydrogel-based, the surgeon positions the lens in a tunnel in the center of the cornea

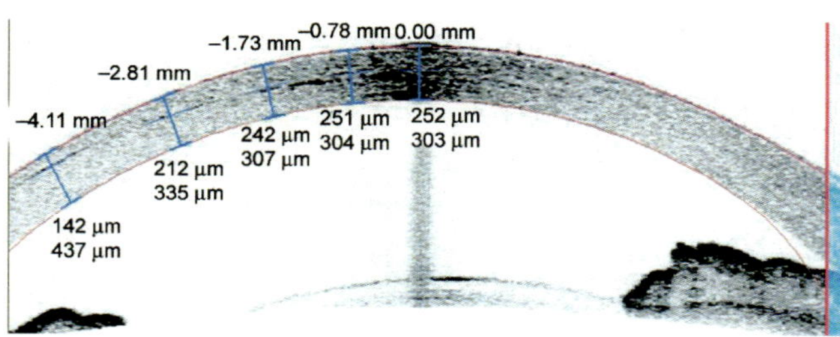

Fig. 55.4: The Biovision Invue™ inlay is implanted in a tunnel at 250 microns mid-stroma

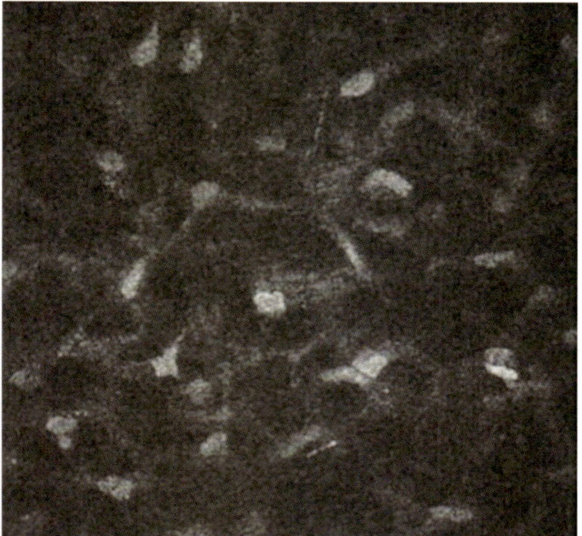

Fig. 55.5: Normal Confocal stroma

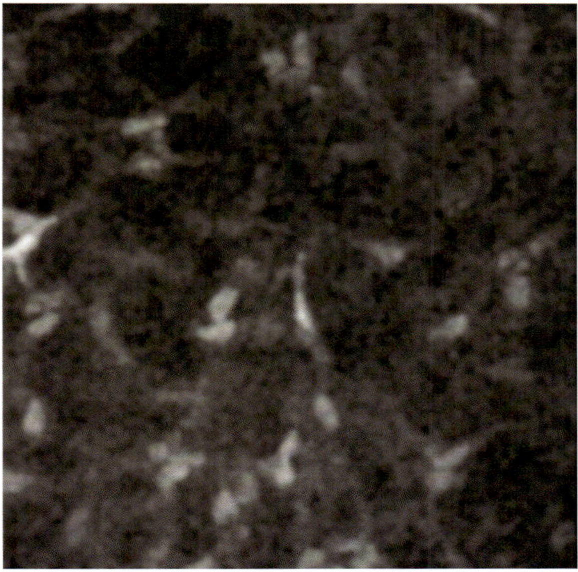

Fig. 55.6: Inlay Confocal stroma

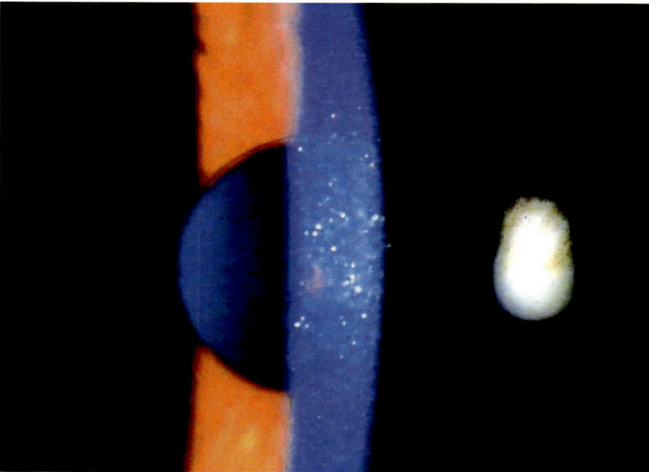

Fig. 55.7: After implantation of the Invue™ lens, the patient is able to enjoy both effective distance and near vision. On distance gaze the bifocal cornea will be producing two images at the macular level

The central part of the cornea where the lens is implanted provides the near vision correction and the peripheral unaltered part of the cornea does not effect the distance vision.

After implantation of the Invue™ lens, the patient is able to enjoy both effective distance and near vision. On distance gaze the bifocal cornea produce two images at the macular level. The rays of light coming from a distant object refract on the areas of the cornea that surround the small central lens and will be sharply focused on the macula. This will produce a sharp image of the distant object. The light rays coming from a distant object but going through the centrally implanted Invue™ lens is out of focus at the macular plane. This blurry image will be ignored by the visual system (Figs 55.8A and B).

Presbylens

ReVision Optics PresbyLens®: The PresbyLens, developed by ReVision Optics (formerly IntraLens), is made from a proprietary micro-porous hydrogel material called Nutrapore®, the PresbyLens is composed of 78 percent water, with the same refractive index as the human cornea. It is also the first bio-engineered intracorneal implant to be used for keratophakia. This lens is used to change the

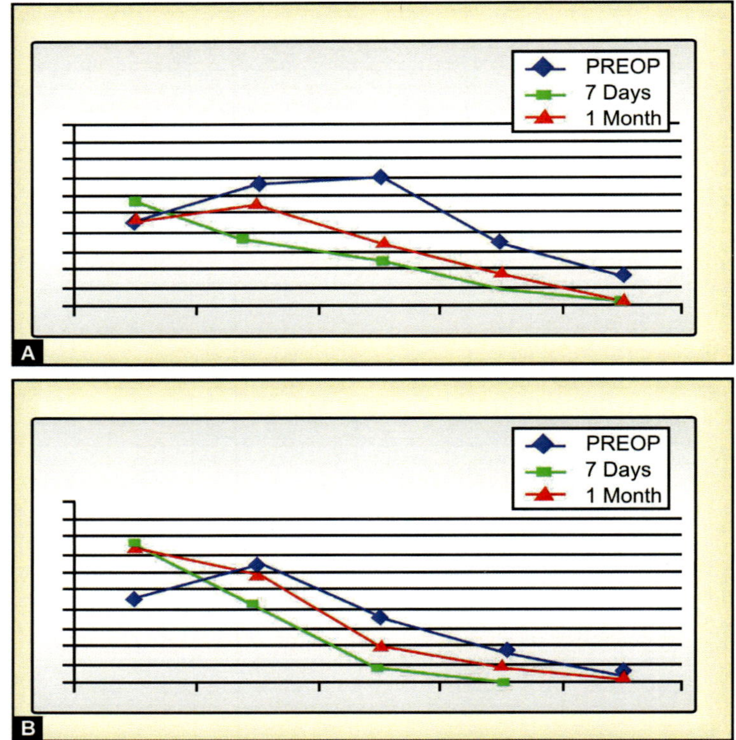

Figs 55.8A and B: Scotopic vision preoperative and postoperative inlay implantation

anterior curvature of the cornea when placed under a LASIK flap. One and 1.5 millimeters in diameter, the Presbylens is an intracorneal implant designed to provide a central near add zone and a paracentral intermediate zone, which allows the remaining cornea to be used for distance vision. The lens is placed in the patient's nondominant eye, and can be combined with LASIK, with bilateral plano vision as the objective. Currently ReVision Optics is operating clinical trials at several international sites to evaluate Presbylens for Presbyopia correction. Clinical trials are also underway in the US to determine this lens' efficacy in hyperopia up to +6 D. The nice thing of any of these procedures is that they're reversible and exchangeable.

SUMMARY

Intracorneal inlays are potentially safe, simple and minimally invasive procedures that present a new solution for presbyopes in all ranges – including the emmetropic patient. Research data continues to suggest that inlay technology offers promising results and high patient satisfaction, by preserving distance vision and enhancing near vision.

56 Use of Platelet-rich Plasma in Ophthalmology and Refractive Surgery

Jorge L Alio, Silvia Pastor

INTRODUCTION

Laser Assisted *In Situ* Keratomileusis (LASIK)

Successful refractive eye surgery can help to reduce common vision disorders such as myopia, hyperopia and astigmatism. The most common refractive methods use **excimer lasers** to reshape curvature of the cornea. An excimer laser is a form of ultraviolet (UV) chemical laser and is short for 'excited dimer'. An excimer laser typically uses a combination of an inert gas such as argon and a reactive gas, such as fluorine or chlorine. Upon electrical stimulation a dimer is created in an energized state giving rise to laser light in the UV range.[1]

The **UV light** from an excimer laser is well absorbed by biological matter and organic compounds. The excimer laser has the sufficient energy to disrupt the molecular bonds of the surface tissue, which effectively disintegrates into the air in a tightly controlled manner through **ablation** rather than burning. These lasers act removing exceptionally fine layers of surface material with almost no heating or change to the remainder of the material which is left intact. These properties make excimer lasers well suited to perform delicate surgeries such as the eye surgery, known as **Laser *In Situ* Keratomileusis** (LASIK).

During this procedure, the surgeon uses a microkeratome to cut a flap of the corneal tissue (usually with a thickness of 100-180 microns). The flap is lifted keeping it bound to the eye through a hinge and the stroma is exposed. The targeted tissue, a certain amount of stroma, is then removed with an excimer laser. The flap is then placed back to its normal position.

Platelet-rich Plasma

Platelet-rich Plasma (PRP) is a component of whole blood that contains concentrated amounts of platelets and growth factors. Fresh platelet-rich Plasma is obtained by apheresis of total blood drawn into sodium citrate tubes (no coagulation takes place) and prepared simply by spinning the tube in a centrifuge, under specific conditions of temperature, speed and time, until the blood cells fall to the bottom of the tube (Figs 56.1A and B). Preparation of the product is carried out under optimal sterile conditions to ensure low-risk of foreign infection. Some platelets and growth factors remain in the upper yellow faction (Platelet-poor Plasma, PPP), and the highest concentration of platelets remains in the middle fraction along with white blood cells and growth factors (Platelet-rich Plasma, PRP).

PRP is usually applied as a clot by adding calcium chloride[2] which induces activation of the platelets. Raising the temperature to 37°C enhances the platelet-rich plasma to precipitate or clot.[3,4]

PRP has been used clinically for over a decade as a complement to tissue regeneration procedures[5]

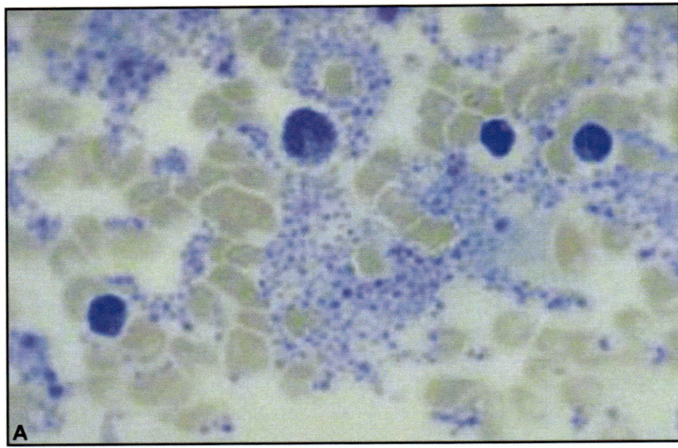

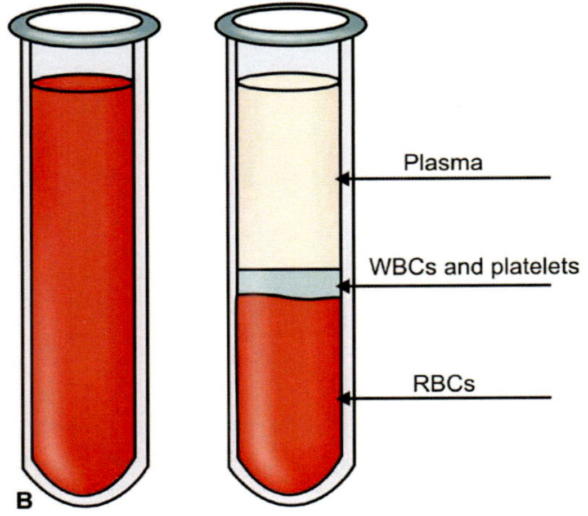

Figs 56.1A and B: (A) PRP under the microscope, (B) blood fractions after centrifugation of total unclotted blood

in specialties such as oral and maxillofacial surgery,[6,7] reconstructive surgery,[7] orthopedics,[8] cardiovascular surgery,[9] and plastic surgery.[2,10] Dental implant surgery with guided bone regeneration is one situation in which an autologous platelet-rich clot has been shown to accelerate ossification after tooth extraction and/or around titanium implants, with marked reductions in the time required for implant stabilization and an improved success rate.[11,12] Orthopedic surgery, muscle and/or tendon repair, reversal of skin ulcers, hole repair in eye surgery, and cosmetic surgery are other situations in which autologous platelets have shown to accelerate healing.[5] Concentrated platelet preparations are also used to induce bone regeneration when prosthetic devices are to be implanted[13] in maxillofacial and implant surgery and also in traumatology, combined with hydroxyapatite, autologous bone, and other biomaterials.[14-16]

Platelet-rich plasma is the only available product that contains high levels of many growth factors.[17] These growth factors are maintained in precisely the same ratios found in circulating blood in the body. Although recombinant products are available, these products are usually synthetic derivatives of a single growth factor. Fibrin glue is another product available for the physician that has been used previously in eye surgery.[18,19] However, the fibrin glues currently on the market do not contain any growth factors and are virally inactivated derivatives of blood components drawn from other donors. Epidermal growth factors have been well characterized as wound-healing agents;[20,21] also, nerve growth factors, insulin growth factors, fibroblast growth factors,[22–25] and, more recently, fetal umbilical cord blood[26] are gaining interest in the ophthalmic community. The use of growth factor preparations released from platelet concentrates after thrombin stimulation also has been reported recently. Human corneal epithelial cells have been tested *in vitro* for cell growth, migration, and differentiation in response to these factors; they have shown a dramatic effect on cell growth, with acceptable migration and differentiation.[27]

Platelets are known for their healing abilities on epithelial and internal wounds. They adhere to the damaged endothelium and start a healing reaction, releasing numerous cytokines and growth factors. Fibrinogen is transformed into fibrin, providing the structural support of the healed wound.[27] α-granules in these platelets liberate many growth factors, biological mediators that promote cell proliferation by binding to specific cell surface receptors.[28,29] Platelet-derived angiogenesis factor, platelet-derived growth factors (PDGF), platelet factor IV, platelet-derived epidermal growth factor and transforming growth factor-β (TGF-β) are some of the factors described to date.[30-32] Each of them has been reported to accelerate different aspects of wound healing.[29,33] PDGF attracts and induces mitosis of fibroblasts along with TGF-β, resulting in collagen build-up.

Since 2004, 100 percent autologous PRP has been successfully applied in ophthalmology by us with great success, either as eye drops or as a clot on corneal ulcers, dry eye and Ocular Surface Syndrome (OSS) cases based on the properties of PRP acting on the re-epithelization processes and wound healing. In the following pages we shall review the results obtained with the use of PRP in these different clinical situations.

DORMANT CORNEAL ULCERS

An ulcer is defined as a break in skin or mucous membrane with loss of surface tissue, disintegration and necrosis of epithelial tissue, and often pus. Corneal ulcers are generally an acute and sight-threatening disorder needing of quick and aggressive management. Usually the term ulcer is used to describe an infectious keratitis of bacterial ethiology; however, this is not always the case.

Corneal ulcers may have different ethiologies that can be classified as infectious and non-infectious. Infectious ulcers include those caused by external microbial pathogens including bacteria (*Pseudomonas aeruginosa*), viruses (*Herpes simplex Type I*), fungi (*Fusarium sp*) and amoebae (*Acanthamoeba sp*). Non-infectious ulcers may occur secondarily to neuro-trophic disease, immunologic disease, trauma or toxicity. For both cases, the ulcer develops with a series of cellular and chemical reactions resulting in immune-mediated inflammation at the level of the corneal stroma that includes leukocyte migration and infiltration and necrosis of adjacent tissue.

Corneal wound healing is mediated by many proteins that are inducers of corneal cell migration, proliferation, and differentiation; these proteins include growth factors (GF): epithelial GF (EGF), fibroblast GF (FGF), and platelet GF (PDGF), among others. These GF may make their entrance by infiltrating through the tear film. Platelets are great suppliers of these proteins and are known for their ability to heal epithelial and internal wounds. This is why, treatment with PRP is effective on dormant corneal ulcers unresponsive to conventional treatment.

Study on Patients with Corneal Ulcers Treated with PRP

In a study published by us, a total of 40 eyes of 38 patients (22 female, 16 male) with dormant corneal ulcers who had not responded to previous conventional treatment and had shown no improvement for at least 15 days were consecutively enrolled. Subjects underwent a complete ophthalmic examination, including best-corrected visual acuity (VA) measurements, biomicroscopy, anterior segment photography, and corneal fluorescein staining before and after treatment with autologous platelet-rich plasma. In the ocular examination, particular attention was paid to ulcer diameter, conjunctival appearance (edematous, non -edematous), inflammation, conjunctival or ciliary hyperemia (intensive, medium, low, or absent), discharge, tear secretion, pain, and discomfort (defined as present or absent). Patients were assigned to 2 groups according to the type of ulcer and method to apply autologous platelet-rich plasma: group I, 26 eyes with chronic corneal ulceration treated by instillation of platelet-rich plasma (12 neurotrophic, 9 herpetic, and 5 inmunological ulcers), and group II, 14 eyes treated surgically by a clot of platelet-rich plasma combined with amniotic membrane transplantation (AMT) in perforated eyes or eyes with a high-risk of perforation due to deep chronic corneal ulcers.

Amniotic membrane transplantation is indicated for patients with perforated eyes or eyes with a high-risk of perforation.[34] A clot of autologous platelet-rich plasma is placed under the amniotic membrane to seal the impending or actual corneal perforation and to increase the therapeutic effect of the amniotic membrane. The fragments of amniotic membrane to be used as grafts are preserved at –80°C in a glycerol solution and are flattened onto nitrocellulose paper with the epithelium side up.[35-37] Surgery with autologous platelet-rich plasma and AMT therapy consists of wound debridement, excision and removal of devitalized tissue, and application of amniotic membrane to the wound site with the epithelial side up. All patients are anesthetized using a retrobulbar block. Several drops of 1:1000 adrenaline (epinephrine) are applied initially to the ocular surface to prevent excessive bleeding. After thawing at room temperature, the amniotic membrane is removed from its storage medium, peeled from the nitrocellulose backing paper, and placed over the cornea with the basal membrane side facing up. The membrane is sutured into place with a continuous 10-0 nylon suture to the conjunctiva, and a running suture is applied so that the membrane tightly adheres to the entire corneal surface. Topical neomycin/polymyxin B/dexamethasone suspension is instilled, and the eye is closed with a temporary tarsorrhaphy.

An independent observer followed up each case taking notes of the patient's evolution, including a photographic report at each visit. Follow-up visits included an interview with the patient assessing the presence or absence of pain or discomfort. Biomicroscopic examination included a description of the level of either ciliary or conjunctival hyperemia, discharge, or conjunctival edema.

Primary outcome measures were the reduction in size or depth of the corneal ulcer and improvement in best-corrected vision. Secondary outcome measures were reduction of pain or discomfort, decrease in conjunctival or ciliary hyperemia, or conjunctival edema if present. A Kaplan–Meier survival test was used for statistical analyses.

Results of the Study on Chronic Corneal Ulcers

Evident improvement in the corneal ulcer, following the criteria mentioned above, was observed in 38 of the 40 eyes (95%) after 3 to 45 days (mean, 15±12) (Fig. 56.2A). Complete re-epithelialization with no ulcer staining as observed with fluorescein was achieved in 20 of these 38 eyes (53%); 18 improved significantly (47%) and 2 eyes showed no change (5%). None of the eyes suffered a relapse during a follow-up period of 9.10±5.48 months. In both groups, the clinical condition improved with respect to pain, inflammation, and healing of the ulcerative process. Far vision improved up to 12 lines in the best case. Excluding the 2 eyes that showed no change, 60.5 percent of eyes gained VA, with 34 percent of eyes gaining 1 to 3 lines, 16 percent gaining 4 to 5 lines, and 10.5 percent gaining ≥ 6 lines. Photophobia and ocular discomfort were absent in 85.7 percent of cases and substantially diminished in the remaining 14.3 percent. In 4 eyes (13%), a relapsing epithelial defect, defined as observation of a new epithelial defect located at the level of the previous ulcer with positive fluorescein staining under slit-lamp examination, occurred after 6 months to 1 year. These eyes were treated successfully by keratoplasty; 2 of them were from group I (eyes treated by instillation of autologous platelet-rich plasma) and 2 from group II (a clot of autologous platelet-rich plasma and AMT). Penetrating or lamellar keratoplasty was performed with no inflammation or active ulcer in these cases.

Group I

Thirteen eyes healed (50%), 11 improved significantly (42%), and 2 showed no change (8%) (Fig. 56.2B). No eye had a recurrence during a follow-up period of 6.3 ± 4.2 months. Thirty-one percent of eyes gained 1 to 3 lines of VA; 15 percent, 4 to 5; and 12 percent, ≥ 6. Forty-two percent did not improve at all. Vision improved up to 12 lines in the best case. The reduction in inflammation occurred by 1 to 2 weeks, with a decrease in ocular pain.

Group II

Ten eyes healed (71%) and 4 eyes improved significantly (29%) (Fig. 56.2C). None of them had a recurrence during a follow-up period of 11.1 ± 3.2 months. Thirty-six percent of the eyes gained 1 to 3 lines of VA; 14 percent, 4 to 5; and 7 percent, ≥ 6. Forty-three percent did not improve. Vision improved up to 11 lines in the best case.

Conclusions of the Study on Chronic Corneal Ulcers

Amniotic membrane has been used as a strategy for limbal stem cell grafting and treatment of corneal ulcerations and has been applied for more than 5 years with success.[36-38] Kruse et al suggest that amniotic membrane epithelial cells are not viable

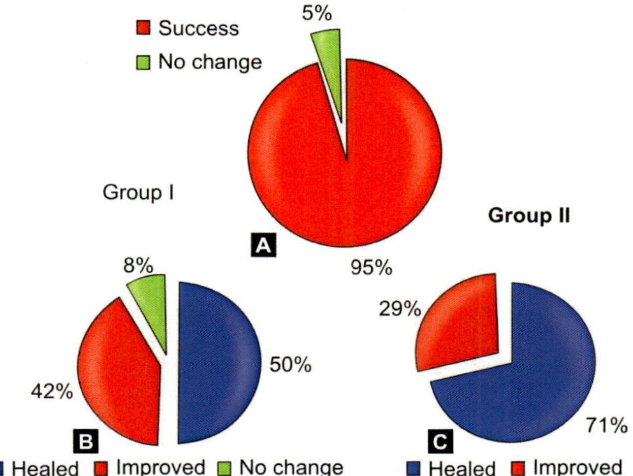

Figs 56.2: Success rate and level of reepithelialization. (A) Percentage of success of re-epithelialization in all groups combined, (B) Percentage of patients from group I, treated by instillation of platelet-rich plasma, who totally healed, improved, or showed no change, (C) Percentage of patients from group II, treated surgically by a clot of platelet-rich plasma in combination with amniotic membrane transplantation, who healed or improved after treatment

after the glycerol method of preservation, and it is unclear whether the growth factors survive cryopreservation and whether such preservation devitalizes not just amniotic epithelial cells but also stromal cells.[39] Based on this report, Prof. Alio and colleagues applied the clot of autologous platelet-rich plasma in combination with AMT to improve the concentration of the growth factors. Very fast wound healing was observed in the 9 corneal perforations treated by amniotic membrane application in combination with a PRP clot containing autologous growth factors. Whether the healing effect of the PRP in combination with AMT was higher than using AMT alone cannot be ascertained in this study, as previous reports on the subject offer different results depending on disease severity and the degree of previous inflammation.[36,40-42] Differences in the use of AMT, temporary tarsorrhaphy, and associated treatments preclude any comparison of these series of studies with previous reports on the subject. However, theoretically, PRP combined with AMT should further promote corneal wound-healing processes and further decrease inflammation due its intrinsic characteristics. To the best of our knowledge, this is the first study in which the use of autologous PRP topically and surgically, as a clot, is reported in the treatment of chronic corneal ulcers. In the platelet-rich plasma preparation used in the present study, the platelets are intact and can adhere to the ocular surface and improve the biochemical and biological mechanism. In summary, this report shows that PRP improved photophobia, pain, and inflammation; facilitated re-epithelialization, promoting corneal wound healing and improving clinical conditions; and resulted in improved vision in the majority of the patients included in the study. Autologous PRP is shown to be a reliable and efficient procedure to restore the corneal epithelial surface in patients with dormant corneal ulcers (Figs 56.3A and B).

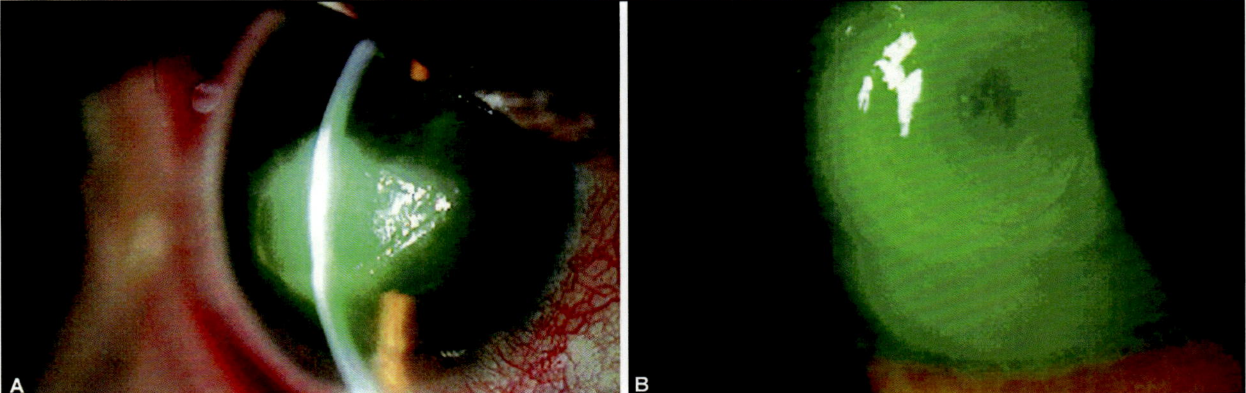

Figs 56.3A and B: Neurotrophic ulcer (A) Pretreatment appearance of a right eye with a neurotrophic ulcer. B, After treatment with Amniotic Membrane Transplantation (AMT) and autologous platelet-rich plasma clot for 2 months

DRY EYE

Dry eye is an ocular surface disease that can be caused by several factors and has different degrees of severity. Some patients experience mild symptoms that can be effectively treated with artificial tears. Others develop severer complications from keratoconjunctivitis sicca. The consequences are mainly inflammatory but the patients are also exposed to other risks like infection, epithelial metaplasia, glandular dysfunction and neurotrophic damage. Tear secretion depends on different ocular structures that include the cornea, conjunctiva, meibomian glands, goblet cells and ocular glands in combination with the tear film. All these components are interrelated to each other by neural, hormonal and chemical feedback mechanisms.[43-45] Alteration of any of these components may affect this complex system and change its functionality. Some studies have shown that dry eye is often associated with a low-grade inflammatory condition of the ocular surface with production of pro-inflammatory cytokines, and a status of activation of T cells in the lacrimal glands and conjunctiva either with or without Sjögren's syndrome.[45,46] These alterations can result in an excess of mucus production inducing the formation of mucin filaments, and the reduction of tear volume may decrease the natural antimicrobial defences of the eye and cause allergic reactions. Nerve fibers can also be affected by dry eye when associated with ocular inflammation, which can affect the stimulatory process of lacrimal secretion. Dry eye symptoms usually correlate with the severity of the disease but, according to recent reports, when accompanied by inflammation, they may cause a downregulation of sensory receptors leading to a decrease in symptoms while milder conditions may cause the opposite effect.

Platelet-rich plasma (PRP) obtained from total unclotted blood is very rich in platelets and growth factors. Only recently has PRP been brought to the ophthalmology field[47,48] showing very promising results. With all its know properties, PRP could help to improve ocular surface regeneration in cases of micropunctate keratitis, decrease inflammation, accelerate and stimulate wound healing processes and may also have a lubricant effect.

Results of a pilot study which reports for the first time, the effectiveness of the use of topical eye drops of autologous PRP in treating patients suffering from significant dry eye symptoms is next described.

Study on Dry Eye Patients Treated with PRP

18 patients (15 women, 3 men, 36 eyes), with a mean age of 50±13 years, affected with moderate to severe dry eye syndrome and classified by the triple classification of Madrid[49] were included in this study. All showed punctate keratitis, were highly symptomatic and showed severe ocular surface dysfunction. Previous treatments were stopped 48h before starting the PRP treatment, and there was a follow-up period of 1 month in all cases (Figs 56.4A and B).

All patients were showing relevant symptoms with punctate keratitis, fluorescein staining on at least 50 percent of the corneal surface and clinical signs of ocular surface inflammation.

Disappearance of subjective symptoms after treatment; increase in visual acuity; tear meniscus height and tear breakup time (BUT); decrease in inflammation and fluorescein staining and improvement of impression cytology were measured.

Patients suffering from different degrees of dry eye symptoms, treated with topical eyedrops of autologous PRP where evaluated by the ophthalmologist by a subjective questionnaire, and the patients gave their impressions about the status of their eyes previously and after treatment. Itching, dryness and foreign body sensation were evaluated. Tear BUT test was performed after mixing the tear fluid with a fluorescein dye in a stripe applicator (Haag-Streit, Köniz, Switzerland) applied with an impregnated paper to the cornea for a few seconds. After the application of the dye and a few blinks, the cornea was observed through a slit-lamp biomicroscope. The time between the last blink and the appearance of the first dark spot was considered to be the BUT. Five measurements were taken and the mean value was calculated. BUT values between 10 and 15 seconds are considered to be normal in our institution and others for this examination.[50,51] Conjunctival impression cytology was performed by using a special cellulose-acetate membrane (Supor 200, Sigma) in small pieces pressed onto the bulbar and tarsal conjunctiva obtaining a thin layer of conjunctival tissue that was fixed and stained by PAS-Giemsa and visualized through the light microscope. We evaluated the goblet cell densities (Fig. 56.5). Normal levels on the superior bulbar conjunctiva were considered to be over 400 cells/mm^2 and those on the inferior bulbar conjunctiva over 600 cells/mm^2. A final score for squamous metaplasia was given according to Nelson's classification.[50,52]

The tear meniscus is located between the ocular surface, lid margin and air. The distance from the lid margin to the boundary between the ocular surface and the edge of the tear is the tear height. This value was measured using a slit-lamp. For the evaluation of patients with dry eye on this study, we defined four levels: increased, normal, low and absent.[53] Visual Acuity was measured by Snellen charts on a conventional projecting screen. The slit-lamp was also used to evaluate bulbar conjunctival hyperemia, and values were given to evaluate the different grades: 0 = no hyperemia, 1 = slight regional hyperemia, 2 = diffuse or marked regional hyperemia and 3 = diffuse episcleral or scleral hyperemia.[54] Superficial punctate keratopathy was evaluated by fluorescein staining, and the following scale was used for evaluation: grade 1 = isolated, a few spots on the third inferior segment of the cornea; grade 2 = affects around half the cornea; grade 3 = affects 50-75 percent of the cornea; grade 4 = affects the whole area of the cornea.

PRP was given topically as eye drops (4-6 times a day per eye) to patients suffering from moderate to severe dry eye symptoms. Patients were monitored for improvement every week. For the purpose of this study only data after 1 month of treatment were used.

Statistics for impression cytology were calculated on 12 patients using Student's t test, and values of $p < 0.05$ were considered to be statistically significant.

Results of the Study on Severe Dry Eye

Eighteen patients (36 eyes, 15 females and 3 males) were evaluated in this pilot study for the different parameters mentioned. Twelve patients were suffering from moderate dry eye and 6 patients suffered from severe dry eye symptoms related to Sjögren's syndrome or Stevens-Johnson disease. There was a significant subjective improvement in patients treated with PRP. Eighty-nine percent of the patients (16 out of 18) experienced a relevant improvement or full disappearance of subjective symptoms after 1 month of treatment. Three patients improved very significantly and 13 improved significantly. Only 2 patients did not experience any improvement, and none of the patients got worse during the observation period. Twenty-eight percent of the patients (5 out of 18) experienced an improvement of 1 line or more of best corrected vision. In no cases was visual acuity loss documented. Fifty-six percent of cases improved the tear meniscus height from low to normal while 44 percent of the patients did not experience any change. Tear BUT fifty percent of the patients improved their BUT on 2 seconds. The other 50 percent remained without changes. Of those patients suffering from conjunctival inflammation (7 out of 18), 86 percent (6 out of 7) had a significant improvement in slit-lamp appearance. Superficial Punctate Keratitis fluorescein staining improved significantly in 72 percent of the cases (13 out of 18); 28 percent of the patients did not show any changes. None of them got worse.

Twelve patients were analyzed for impression cytology. The number of goblet cells on the superior and inferior bulbar conjunctiva was quantified before and after 1 month of PRP treatment. The patients were suffering from moderate to severe dry eye. Statistical analysis was performed using Student's t test and p values were calculated.

Conclusions of the Dry Eye Study

Dry eye is a disorder of the tear film[55-57] caused by disturbances in the composition and quantity of tears, which can be caused by different factors.[50,52,53-58] Generally, aqueous deficiency or excessive evaporation are two of the main reasons for developing dry eye symptoms. Sjögren's

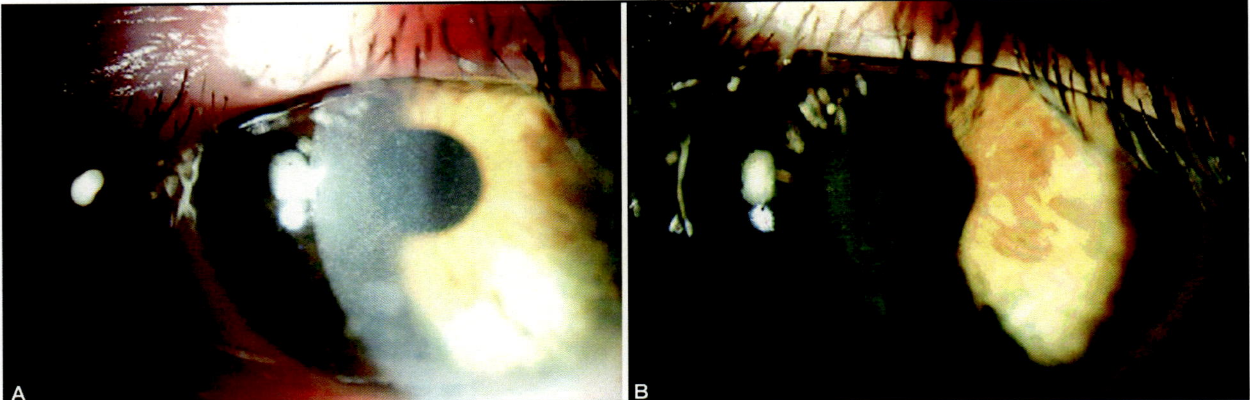

Figs 56.4A and B: Results of PRP treatment on a patient with dry eye on both eyes. A, Epithelial punctate keratitis associated with tear film instability. B, Corneal surface improvement after 1 month of treatment with PRP

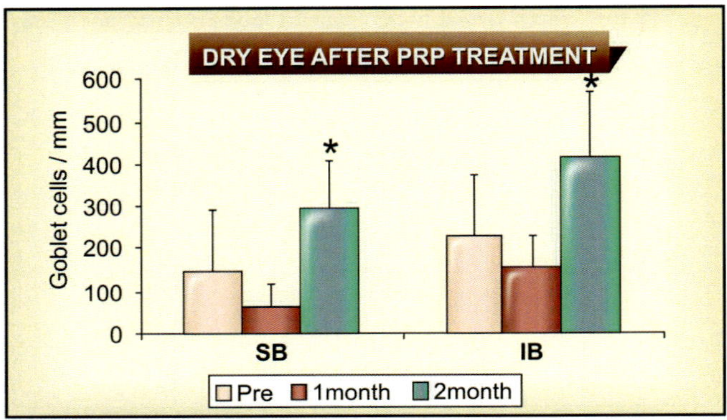

Fig. 56.5: Goblet cell densities on the superior and inferior bulbar conjunctiva of patients suffering from different degrees of dry eye after 1 and 2 months of treatment with PRP. The p value for superior bulbar (SB) cell density was 0.004 and the p value for inferior bulbar (IB) cell density was 0.005, after 2 months of treatment, when comparing with pre-treatment. Hence, significant changes were observed (*)

syndrome or lacrimal gland diseases affect tear production showing a partial or absolute deficiency of the aqueous phase of the tear film. This can lead, in some cases, to an association between aqueous deficiency and secondary infection such as bacterial conjunctivitis or keratitis. Stevens-Johnson syndrome or blepharitis also induce dry eye and are related to mucus deficiency due to decreased quantity and quality of surface mucus that may lead to impaired surface wetting of the epithelial interface, associated with decreased tear stability.

Lid surface abnormalities, which make the blinking process difficult, can also induce a desquamation process due to the lack of wetting of the cornea and conjunctiva. Irregular ocular surface topography, the use of contact lenses or low humidity are also important factors that may lead to decreased tear stability contributing to dry eye symptoms. Inflammation of the lacrimal gland is of main importance in the pathogenesis of dry eye due to ocular surface damage. Some research groups have identified proinflammatory cytokines such as γ-interferon and activated T cells in the lacrimal glands of patients affected with dry eye;[45] such is the case in Sjögren's syndrome.[43,44,46,59-61] In clinical trials, patients with dry eye symptoms seemed to respond advantageously to treatment with corticosteroids.[62,63] Androgens could also be related to dry eye pathology, according to some studies, by regulating the homeostasis of tear secretion.[64] These results are supported by the fact that women on hormone replacement therapy, with increasing estrogen levels, have an increased rate of dry eye incidence.[65,66] In Sjögren's syndrome, a rare autoimmune disorder in which mononuclear inflammatory cells invade the lacrimal and salivary glands, dryness by decreasing tear production is the main feature which is due to an exocrine dysfunction. It affects up to 1 percent of the population and is sex biased towards women, with a predominance of approximately 1:9. Dry eye is the main symptom, with foreign body sensation, inability to wear contact lenses and photophobia as the main signs. Due to the different types of dry eye that can be observed as a result of the alteration of different aspects in the control of tear management (e.g. aqueous tear deficiency, lipid tear deficiency, delayed tear clearance in blepharitis), a very specific diagnosis is difficult to obtain, hence treatment is not always 100 percent successful. Autologous PRP contains high levels of platelets and growth factors. It is a preservative-free biological product obtained directly from the patient's own blood; in this sense, when the preparation of the product has been done following all sterile procedures, the risks of contamination are minimal and so are the problems of infection. Regarding side effects, none have been observed yet, even in some patients with a follow-up of up to 6 months. Topical steroids have also been proved to relieve symptoms rapidly but their long-term usage may result in side effects such as an increased risk of infection, intraocular pressure elevation and cataract formation.[63] The preservative component present in these steroid solutions can also affect the bonds between epithelial cells of the cornea inducing punctate keratopathy that may develop into a corneal ulcer. PRP does not contain any preservatives so these risks are not considered.

OCULAR SURFACE SYNDROME POST-LASIK (OSS POST-LASIK)

Laser *in situ* keratomileusis (LASIK), although highly successful,[67] has a common side effect—ocular surface syndrome. This complex multifactorial entity distresses patients and physicians, and is characterized by the following symptoms: dry eye, micropunctate keratitis, decreased and unstable tear film, and decreased best spectacle-corrected visual acuity (BSCVA) and visual quality. Ocular surface syndrome has a neurotrophic etiology, is long lasting, and is difficult to treat. A main function of the ocular nerves often damaged during LASIK is the regulation of secretion activities of the lacrimal and meibomian glands. Their damage causes neurotrophic epitheliopathy and affects tear composition.[68] All lipidic, aqueous and mucus components of tears are involved in the quality of the tear film, and any alteration can affect the ocular surface. When there is a deficiency present on the aqueous phase of the tear film, the risk of infection by pathogens increases. A decrease in the quantity or quality of the mucus associated with goblet cells of the conjunctiva decreases tear stability. The same is observed when alteration of the lipid composition of tears affects the tears' evaporation control.[69] An abnormal lid surface function and epitheliopathy may also affect the ocular surface. Finally, an alteration of the normal microvilli on the ocular surface may present difficulties in the adherence of the tear film to the epithelial surface.[50]

Platelet-rich plasma has a lubricating effect and has been effective in regenerating the ocular surface in cases of micropunctate keratitis, decreasing inflammation in patients suffering from dry eye,[50] and stimulating wound-healing processes in dormant corneal ulcers.[70] This pilot study reports the results obtained from patients treated with topical eye drops of autologous platelet-rich plasma for ocular surface syndrome following LASIK.

Study on Patients Suffering form Ocular Surface Syndrome (OSS) after LASIK Treated with PRP

Twenty-six eyes of 13 myopic patients (9 women and 4 men), aged 30 to 60 years, who underwent Laser *in situ* keratomileusis (LASIK) for myopia of –2.00 to –7.50 diopters (D) and were affected postoperatively by severe to moderate dry eye syndrome (according to the Triple Classification of Madrid)[49] for > 6 months were included in this prospective study.

All surgeries were performed using a mechanical microkeratome (Moria M2, disposable head; Moria, Paris, France). A 9.5 mm flap was created with a superior hinge of 3.5 to 4 mm. Flaps were tentatively programmed to be 130 µm thick based on an intended flap thickness of 160 µm.[71] LASIK was performed using the Esiris excimer laser (Schwind, Kleinostheim, Germany).

Informed consent of the patients was obtained before the initiation of the study and patient recruitment. Patients presented with highly symptomatic punctate keratitis and moderate to severe ocular surface dysfunction. Patients were treated with 6 topical eye drops per day of autologous PRP. Previous treatments were stopped 48 hours prior to receiving the autologous plasma. Six of 13 patients suffered from moderate ocular surface dysfunction symptoms prior to treatment, and 7 showed severe symptoms. Best spectacle-corrected visual acuity decreased from 1 to 4 lines. All patients were positive for fluorescein staining and showed a tear break-up time between 4 and 9 seconds. Follow-up was performed following the same postoperative protocol for 1 month. Main outcome measures included subjective symptom disappearance, increased visual acuity, increased tear meniscus and tear break-up time, decreased inflammation and fluorescein staining, and improvement in impression cytology. All tests were performed ≥ 12 hours after the last topical instillation of PRP. The Triple Classification of Madrid was used to qualify and quantify the postoperative recovery.[49]

Results of the Study on OSS Post-LASIK

Patients were asked to complete a questionnaire that measured subjective symptoms, such as foreign body sensation, eye redness, burning, itching, tearing, and photophobia. Answers were graded from 1 to 4, and a global evaluation of subjective symptoms was determined, which included excellent, good, minimum, no improvement, and worse. Six (46%) of 13 patients experienced excellent improvement, and 5 (38%) experienced good improvement. One (8%) patient experienced minimal improvement and 1 (8%) other showed no improvement. No patients experienced a worsening of symptoms. Best spectacle-corrected visual acuity increased 1 line in 10 (38%) of 26 eyes, 2 lines in 4 (15%) eyes, 3 lines in 2 (8%) eyes, and 4 lines in 2 (8%) eyes. Eight (31%) eyes experienced no gain. Fluorescein staining analysis showed complete fluorescein disappearance in 18 (69%) out of 26 eyes. Six (23%) eyes presented isolated positive staining, and 2 (8%) eyes showed 25% surface staining. All fluorescein staining results at follow-up were better or the same compared to those observed prior to the treatment (Figs 54.6A and B). Tear break-up time increased > 2 seconds in 12 (46%) of 26 eyes. Fourteen (54%) eyes showed a 0 to 2 second tear break-up time increase. Twelve (92%) of 13 patients demonstrated excellent tolerance to PRP. Only 1 (8%) patient developed intolerance after 4 weeks.

Conclusion of the Study on OSS Post-LASIK

Dry eye symptoms are common after LASIK as a result of corneal nerve damage during flap performance and alteration of the tear film volume and composition.[50] Autologous PRP adds a new tool for ocular surface syndrome treatment after LASIK. As

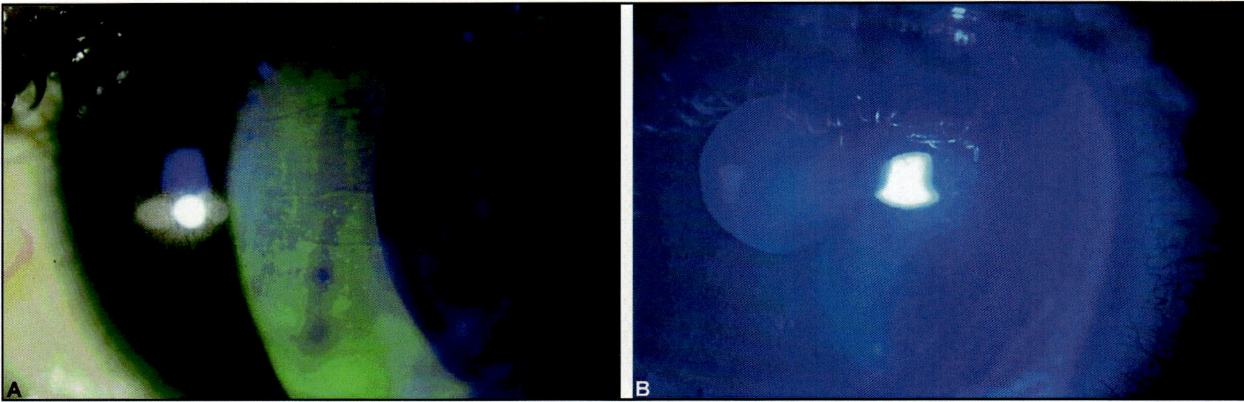

Figs 54.6A and B: Fluorescein staining shows the clinical improvement of a patient's left eye with ocular surface syndrome after LASIK on both eyes. (A) Before treatment with PRP, punctate epithelial erosions were observable. (B) After 1 month of treatment, improvement was noticeable. A transparent cornea could be seen in both eyes

autologous serum is rich in vitamins and growth factors, PRP is also rich in platelets that, in the presence of calcium, are activated to provide a prolonged release of growth factors, thus increasing the endurance of their effects with fewer applications. In this study, patients were instructed to handle the product with extreme cleanliness and to replace what remained after 7 days with a fresh, new vial kept at –20ºC to maintain its qualities and avoid additional risk of contamination. Platelet-rich plasma for the treatment of ocular surface syndrome seems promising and may present a new alternative treatment for these difficult cases.

PRP may also improve the regeneration of sub-basal corneal nerves, damaged during LASIK procedure and important mediators on corneal sensitivity and normal tear secretion. A new study will be started shortly by our group to study the regeneration of the sub-basal corneal nerves and corneal sensitivity on patients after LASIK procedure and treated with PRP. Through confocal microscopy and corneal esthesiometry, we expect to observe a faster recovery of corneal sensitivity and sub-basal nerves on those patients treated with PRP compared to control patients.

CONCLUSIONS ON THE USE OF PRP IN OPHTHALMOLOGY AND IN REFRACTIVE SURGERY

Platelets are known for their role in hemostasis, with which they help in preventing blood loss at sites of vascular injury. To do this, they adhere, aggregate, and form a procoagulant surface, leading to thrombin generation and fibrin formation. Platelets also release substances that promote tissue repair and influence the reactivity of vascular and other blood cells in angiogenesis and inflammation. Growth factors are released from the α-granules of the platelets.[3,72-74] They contain storage pools of growth factors, including platelet-derived growth factors, TGF-β, epithelial growth factors, fibroblast growth factors, insulin-like growth factor I, and vascular endothelial growth factors, as well as cytokines, including proteins such as PF4 and CD40L. Chemokines and newly synthesized active metabolites are also released.[17] The fact that platelets secrete growth factors and active metabolites means that their applied use can have a positive influence in clinical situations requiring rapid healing and tissue regeneration[9]. Their administration as a fibrin clot or fibrin glue provides an adhesive support that can confine secretion to a chosen site.[19] As concentrated platelets contain huge reservoirs of growth and wound-healing factors, they may represent a significant therapeutic tool in chronic corneal ulcerative processes, dry eye and OSS post-LASIK.

On the other hand, 100 percent autologous serum has been used previously in some of the patients suffering from dry eye as a combined therapy with PRP. Still, there is a slight difference: considering that the main difference between PRP and serum is the presence of platelets in the former and, due to this fact, there is a prolonged release of growth factors, PRP should be considered the product of choice in cases of dormant corneal ulcers and severe dry eye where the presence of growth factors acting for longer periods of time is more beneficial. With these results, it seems that PRP is doing a great job in regenerating the affected surface of the cornea by means of growth factors and their regenerating properties.

Future studies will be directed towards the molecular mechanism by which PRP could help to promote corneal regeneration, will clarify our understanding of the effects of this autologous biological substance and unravel other potential clinical applications for ocular surface disorders.

REFERENCES

1. International Union of Pure and Applied Chemistry. "excimer laser". Compendium of Chemical Terminology Internet edition.
2. Man D, Plosker H, Winland-Brown JE. The use of autologous platelet-rich plasma (platelet gel) and autologous platelet-poor plasma (fibrin glue) in cosmetic surgery. Plast Reconstr Surg 2001;107:229-37.
3. Anitua E, Andia I, Ardanza B, et al. Autologous platelets as a source of proteins for healing and tissue regeneration. Thromb Haemost 2004;91:4-15.

4. Sclafani AP, Romo T III, Ukrainsky G, et al. Modulation of wound response and soft tissue ingrowth in synthetic and allogeneic implants with platelet concentrate. Arch Facial Plast Surg 2005;7:163-9.
5. Yazawa M, Ogata H, Nakajima T, et al. Basic studies on the clinical applications of platelet-rich plasma. Cell Transplant 2003;12:509-18.
6. Sammartino G, Tia M, Marenzi G, et al. Use of autologous platelet-rich plasma (platelet-rich plasma) in periodontal defect treatment after extraction of impacted mandibular third molars. J Oral Maxillofac Surg 2005;63:766-70.
7. Choi BH, Im CJ, Huh JY, et al. Effect of platelet-rich plasma on bone regeneration in autogenous bone graft. Int J Oral Maxillofac Surg 2004;33:56-9.
8. Marx RE. Platelet-rich plasma (platelet-rich plasma): what is platelet-rich plasma and what is not platelet-rich plasma? Implant Dent 2001;10:225-8.
9. Englert SJ, Estep TH, Ellis-Stoll CC. Autologous platelet gel applications during cardiovascular surgery: effect on wound healing. J Extra Corpor Technol 2005;37:148-52.
10. Bhanot S, Alex JC. Current applications of platelet gels in facial plastic surgery. Facial Plast Surg 2002;18:27-33.
11. Roldan JC, Jepsen S, Schmidt C, et al. Sinus floor augmentation with simultaneous placement of dental implants in the presence of platelet-rich plasma or recombinant human bone morphogenetic protein-7. Clin Oral Implants Res 2004;15:716-23.
12. Garg AK, Gargenese D, Peace I. Using platelet-rich plasma to develop an autologous membrane for growth factor delivery in dental implant therapy. Dent Implantol Update 2000;11:41-4.
13. Mazor Z, Peleg M, Garg AK, Luboshitz J. Platelet-rich plasma for bone graft enhancement in sinus floor augmentation with simultaneous implant placement: patient series study. Implant Dent 2004;13:65-72.
14. Velich N, Nemeth Z, Hrabak K, et al. Repair of bony defect with combination biomaterials. J Craniofac Surg 2004;15:11-5.
15. Siebrecht MA, De Rooij PP, Arm DM, et al. Platelet concentrate increases bone ingrowth into porous hydroxyapatite. Orthopedics 2002;25:169-72.
16. Lieberman JR, Daluiski A, Einhorn TA. The role of growth factors in the repair of bone: biology and clinical applications. J Bone Joint Surg Am 2002;84-A:1032-44.
17. Frechette JP, Martineau I, Gagnon G. Platelet-rich plasmas: growth factor content and roles in wound healing. J Dent Res 2005;84:434-9.
18. Thorn JJ, Sorensen H, Weis-Fogh U, Andersen M. Autologous fibrin glue with growth factors in reconstructive maxillofacial surgery. Int J Oral Maxillofac Surg 2004;33:95-100.
19. Alio JL, Mulet E, Sakla HF, Gobbi F. Efficacy of synthetic and biological bioadhesives in scleral tunnel phacoemulsification in eyes with high myopia. J Cataract Refract Surg 1998;24:983-8.
20. Brown GL, Nanney LB, Griffen J, et al. Enhancement of wound healing by topical treatment with epidermal growth factor. N Engl J Med 1989;321:76-9.
21. Tripathi RC, Raja SC, Tripathi BJ. Prospects for epidermal growth factor in the management of corneal disorders. Surv Ophthalmol 1990;34:457-62.
22. Matsumoto Y, Dogru M, Goto E, et al. Autologous serum application in the treatment of neurotrophic keratopathy. Ophthalmology 2004;111:1115-20.
23. Nakamura M, Kawahara M, Morishige N, et al. Promotion of corneal epithelial wound healing in diabetic rats by the combination of a substance P-derived peptide (FGLM-NH2) and insulin-like growth factor-1. Diabetologia 2003;46:839-42.
24. Hoppenreijs VP, Pels E, Vrensen GF, Treffers WF. Basic fibroblast growth factor stimulates corneal endothelial cell growth and endothelial wound healing of human corneas. Invest Ophthalmol Vis Sci 1994;35:931-44.
25. Klenkler B, Sheardown H. Growth factors in the anterior segment: role in tissue maintenance, wound healing and ocular pathology. Exp Eye Res 2004;79:677-88.
26. Vajpayee RB, Mukerji N, Tandon R, et al. Evaluation of umbilical cord serum therapy for persistent corneal epithelial defects. Br J Ophthalmol 2003;87:1312-6.
27. Hartwig D, Harloff S, Liu L, et al. Epitheliotrophic capacity of a growth factor preparation produced from platelet concentrates on corneal epithelial cells: a potential agent for the treatment of ocular surface defects? Transfusion 2004;44:1724-31.
28. Knighton DR, Ciresi K, Fiegel VD, Schumerth S, Butler E, Cerra F: Stimulation of repair in chronic, nonhealing, cutaneous ulcers using platelet-derived wound healing formula. Surg Gynecol Obstet 1990; 170: 56-69.
29. Ernesto C. Growth factors and their potential clinical value. J Clin Endocrinol Metab 1992; 75: 1-4.
30. Knighton DR, Hunt TK, Thakral KK, Goodson WH. Role of platelet and fibrin in the healing sequence: an *in vivo* study of angiogenesis and collagen synthesis. Ann Surg 1982; 196: 379-388.
31. Ross R, Glomset J, Kariya B, Harker L. A platelet-dependent serum factor that stimulates the proliferation of arterial smooth muscle cells *in vitro*. Proc Natl Acad Sci USA 1974;71:1207-10.
32. Antoniades HN, Scher CD, Stiles CD. Purification of human platelet-derived growth factor. Proc Natl Acad Sci USA 1979; 76:1809-13.
33. Lynch SE, Colvin RB, Antoniades HN. Growth factors in wound healing: single and synergistic effects on partial thickness porcine skin wounds. J Clin Invest 1989; 84:640-46.
34. Alió JL, Abad M, Scorsetti DH. Preparation, indications and results of human amniotic membrane transplantation for ocular surface disorders. Expert Rev Med Devices 2005;2:153-60.
35. Kenyon KR. Amniotic membrane: mother's own remedy for ocular surface disease. Cornea 2005;24:639-42.

36. Lee SH, Tseng SC. Amniotic membrane transplantation for persistent epithelial defects with ulceration. Am J Ophthalmol 1997;123:303-12.
37. Azuara-Blanco A, Pillai CT, Dua HS. Amniotic membrane transplantation for ocular surface reconstruction. Br J Ophthalmol 1999;83:399-402.
38. Hick S, Demers PE, Brunette I, et al. Amniotic membrane transplantation and fibrin glue in the management of corneal ulcers and perforations: a review of 33 cases. Cornea 2005;24:369-77.
39. Kruse FE, Joussen AM, Rohrschneider K, et al. Cryopreserved human amniotic membrane for ocular surface reconstruction. Graefes Arch Clin Exp Ophthalmol 2000;238:68-75.
40. Kruse FE, Rohrschneider K, Volker HE. Multilayer amniotic membrane transplantation for reconstruction of deep corneal ulcers. Ophthalmology 1999;106:1504-10, discussion 1511.
41. Prabhasawat P, Tesavibul N, Komolsuradej W. Single and multilayer amniotic membrane transplantation for persistent corneal epithelial defects with and without stromal thinning and perforation. Br J Ophthalmol 2001;85:1455-63.
42. Letko E, Stechschulte SU, Kenyon KR, et al. Amniotic membrane inlay and overlay grafting for corneal epithelial defects and stromal ulcers. Arch Ophthalmol 2001;119:659-63.
43. Stern ME, Beuerman RW, Fox RI, Gao J, Mircheff AK, Pflugfelder SC. The pathology of dry eye: the interaction between the ocular surface and lacrimal glands. Cornea 1998;17:584-89.
44. Mathers WD. Why the eye becomes dry: a cornea and lacrimal gland feedback model. CLAO J 2000;26:159-65.
45. Pflugfelder SC, Wilhelmus KR, Osato MS, Matoba AY, Font RL. The autoimmune nature of aqueous tear deficiency. Ophthalmology 1986; 93: 1513-7.
46. Pepose JS, Akata RF, Pflugfelder SC, Voigt W. Mononuclear cell phenotypes and immunoglobulin gene rearrangements in lacrimal gland biopsies from patients with Sjögren's syndrome. Ophthalmology 1990; 97: 1599-1605.
47. Alio JL, Abad M, Artola A, Rodriguez-Prats JL, Pastor S, Ruiz-Colecha J. Use of autologous platelet-rich plasma in the treatment of dormant corneal ulcers. Ophthalmology 2007;114:1286-93.
48. Alio JL, Pastor S, Ruiz-Colecha J, Rodriguez A, Artola A. Treatment of ocular surface syndrome after LASIK with autologous platelet-rich plasma. J Refract Surg 2007;23:617-19.
49. Murube J, Benitez del Castillo JM, Chenzhuo L, Berta A, Rolando M. The Madrid triple classification of dry eye. Arch Soc Esp Oftalmol 2003;78:587-93.
50. Alió JL, Feinbaum C. Management of dry eye (ocular surface syndrome, OSS) after refractive surgery. In Garg A, Sheppard JD, Donnenfeld ED, Meyer D, Mehta CK (Eds): Clinical Diagnosis and Management of Dry Eye and Ocular Surface Disorders (Xero-Dacryology). New Delhi, Jaypee Brothers 2006;198-226.
51. Cho P, Brown B. Review of the tear break-up time and a closer look at the tear break-up time of Hong Kong Chinese. Optom Vis Sci 1993;70:30-8.
52. Nelson JD, Wright JC. Conjunctival goblet cell densities in ocular surface disease. Arch Ophthalmol 1984;102: 1049-51.
53. Mainstone JC, Bruce AS, Golding TR. Tear meniscus measurement in the diagnosis of dry eye. Curr Eye Res 1996;15:653-61.
54. McMonnies CW, Chapman-Davies A. Assessment of conjunctival hyperemia in contact lens wearers. Am J Optom Physiol Opt 1987;64:246-50.
55. Baudouin C. The pathology of dry eye. Surv Ophthalmol 2001;45:211-20.
56. McDonald JE. Surface phenomena of the tear film. Am J Ophthalmol 1969;67:56-64.
57. Lemp MA. Report of the National Eye Institute/ Industry Workshop on Clinical Trials in Dry Eyes. CLAO J 1995; 21:221-32.
58. Foulks GN. What is dry eye and what does it mean to the contact lens wearer? Eye Contact Lens 2003;29:96-100.
59. Foulks GN. The evolving treatment of dry eye. Ophthalmol Clin North Am 2003;16:29-35.
60. Samarkos M, Moutsopoulos HM. Recent advances in the management of ocular complications of Sjögren's syndrome. Curr Allergy Asthma Rep 2005;5:327-32.
61. Mahoney EJ. Sjögren's disease. Otolaryngol Clin North Am 2003;36:733-45.
62. Marsh P, Pflugfelder SC. Topical nonpreserved methylprednisolone therapy for keratoconjunctivitis sicca in Sjögren syndrome. Ophthalmology 1999;106:811-6.
63. Yang CQ, Sun W, Gu YS. A clinical study of the efficacy of topical corticosteroids on dry eye. J Zhejiang Univ Sci B 2006;7:675-8.
64. Sullivan DA, Wickham LA, Rocha EM, Kelleher RS, da Silveira LA, Toda I. Influence of gender, sex steroid hormones, and the hypothalamic-pituitary axis on the structure and function of the lacrimal gland. Adv Exp Med Biol 1998;438:11-42.
65. Schaumberg DA, Buring JE, Sullivan DA, Dana MR. Hormone replacement therapy and dry eye syndrome. JAMA 2001;286:2114-9.
66. Barney NP. Can hormone replacement therapy cause dry eye? Arch Ophthalmol 2002;120:641-2.
67. De Paiva CS, Chen Z, Koch DD, Hamill MB, Manuel FK, Hassan SS, et al. The incidence and risk factors for developing dry eye after myopic LASIK. Am J Ophthalmol 2006;141:438-45.
68. Wilson SE, Ambrosio R. Laser *in situ* keratomileusis-induced neurotrophic epitheliopathy. Am J Ophthalmol 2001;132:405-6.
69. Holly FJ. Physical chemistry of the normal and disordered tear film. Transactions of the Ophthal-

mological Society of the United Kingdom 1985;104:374-80.
70. Alio JL, Colecha JR, Pastor S, Rodriguez A, Artola A. Symptomatic Dry Eye Treatment with Autologous Platelet-Rich Plasma. Ophthalmic Res 2007;39:124-9.
71. Javaloy J, Vidal MT, Ruiz-Moreno JM, Alio JL. Confocal microscopy of disposable and nondisposable heads for the Moria M2 microkeratome. J Refract Surg 2006;22:28-33.
72. Stassen JM, Arnout J, Deckmyn H. The hemostatic system. Curr Med Chem 2004;11:2245-60.
73. Klinger MH, Jelkmann W. Role of blood platelets in infection and inflammation. J Interferon Cytokine Res 2002;22:913-22.
74. Boehlen F, Clemetson KJ. Platelet chemokines and their receptors: what is their relevance to platelet storage and transfusion practice? Transfus Med 2001;11:403-17.

57 General Medicine Diseases and Refractive Surgery

Guillermo Simón-Castellví, Sarabel Simón-Castellví, José María Simón-Castellví, Cristina Simón-Castellví, José María Simón-Tor

The correct approach to a patient in need of refractive surgery begins with detailed medical history and careful physical and ophthalmologic examination. The medical interview collects information of patient's psychological (e.g. depression, future patient's compliance), emotional (e.g. reasons and motivation for refractive surgery) and medical state (ocular and general complaints, physiologic aspects, past and present diseases, laboratory findings, allergies, medications, etc.) of the patient. In medicine, preventing disease is more important than treating it *("primum non nocere")*, and this first interview is essential in screening potentially "dangerous" patients (e.g. Is the medical history significant for AIDS, diabetes or arterial hypertension?) and to improve future patient's compliance by means of building a good patient-doctor relationship.

To be a good candidate for vision correction surgery, patient must meet the physical, health and age criteria for the particular surgery (laser in situ keratomileusis LASIK, laser epithelial keratomileusis LASEK, photorefractive keratomileusis PRK, clear lens exchange, epikeratoplasty-epikeratophakia, laser thermal keratoplasty LTK, astigmatic keratotomies, implantable contact lenses-phakic intraocular lenses, conductive keratoplasty CK to treat presbyopia).

The refractive candidate must fully understand the procedure and be aware of the risks and possible side effects. Limitations for refractive surgery can be ophthalmologic and general. Medical history is important in estimating patient's suitability for surgery: all refractive procedures have ocular, physical, health and age criteria.

In this chapter, after some basic ocular considerations, authors briefly review important aspects - sometimes undervalued of internal medicine, of the outmost importance to avoid problems and complications with the refractive patient.

CONTACT LENSES AND REFRACTIVE SURGERY

Contact lenses can temporarily change the shape of the eye by applying pressure to the cornea. To acquire the best measurements we ask contact lens wearers to remove the contacts for a period of time before the eye exam that varies depending upon which type of lens is worn.

Soft Lenses

Patient should stop wearing contacts for at least **10 days** prior to refraction and the dilated exam.

Toric Lenses

Patient should stop wearing contacts for at least **14 days** prior to refraction and the dilated exam.

Extended Wear Contacts

Patient should stop wearing contacts for at least **30 days** prior to refraction and the dilated exam.

Gas Permeable Lenses

Patient should stop wearing contacts for at least **30-90 days** prior to refraction and the dilated exam. We always perform periodical corneal topographies to ascertain the disappearance of corneal warpage.

Corneal Mold Lenses

Patient should stop wearing contacts for at least **90 days** prior to refraction and the dilated exam. We always perform monthly periodical corneal topographies to ascertain the disappearance of corneal warpage.

To make sure that no corneal change in shape is present, we always perform a corneal topography and a corneal computerized pachymetry the same day of surgery, prior to surgery.

AGE CRITERIA FOR REFRACTIVE SURGERY

Unlike everywhere stated, our candidates include patients over 21 with a stable refraction. We believe that at 18, the myopic eye has not yet finished optical development: most patients' refraction still varies up to 23-24 years, and in some patients, refraction varies during the whole life.

A SPECIAL SITUATION: REFRACTIVE SURGERY IN CHILDREN (PEDIATRICS)

While refractive surgery in adults is mostly a kind of cosmetic surgery to avoid the use of glasses or contact lenses, in some children it has to be considered a therapeutic option in some special cases. Recently, refractive laser surgery has shown to be a good last-resort technique in children who have failed with traditional treatment approaches like highly anisometropic children unable to wear glasses, patching or contact lenses.[1,2] Potential indications for excimer laser procedures in children include accommodative esotropia, bilateral high ametropia, and severe anisometropia (Table 57.1) (Figs 57.1 and 57.2).

When appropriate case selection is applied (e.g. collaborative children), refractive laser surgery can be effectively used with good refractive and visual results, despite the fact that children's refraction will change over time as the child grows: the goal in pediatric cases is to reduce or avoid the risk of severe amblyopia. In most cases, children's vision is maintained or increased. Pediatric candidates to refractive surgery need a special intensive preoperative training of the complete surgical procedure.

Refractive surgery (LASIK or LASEK) in children with high bilateral myopia will improve vision and stereopsis allowing for a better psychological and social status with other children and their families.

Refractive surgery with laser in children has an increased risk of complications during surgery, and therefore a fast and high frequency tracking laser system will be preferred. This will compensate for undesired ocular movements. LASIK or LASEK will be preferred since they induce less postoperative haze than standard PRK. It is not rare that a second laser treatment is necessary to achieve the optimal refractive target.

In the postoperative period it is of the utmost importance to avoid eye grubbing with the use of protective shields or goggles or by means of having the hands tied together.

Table 57.1: Ocular limitations to refractive surgery: special considerations
Absolute contraindications for refractive surgery
Contraindication is related to the activity of the disease: once the disease is over, refractive surgery can be reconsidered with special preventive measures.
Active ocular infection
Viral (e.g. adenoviral keratoconjunctivitis, herpes simplex keratitis)
Bacterial (bacterial conjunctivitis)
Active periocular infection
Chalazia
Blepharitis
Corneal dystrophies and degenerations, corneal scarring
Keratoconus (Implantation of intrastromal corneal ring segments (i.e., INTACS™) to refractively treat this condition is under clinical investigation with promising results)
Recurrent corneal erosion
Advanced glaucoma (*)

(*) Special considerations may apply, please, read further in this chapter

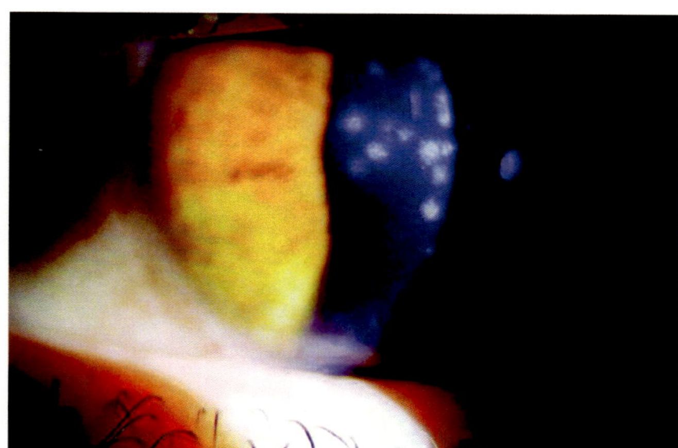

Fig. 57.1: Due to the excellent defence systems of the eye, acute bacterial conjunctivitis is uncommon, but it is still the most common eye disease. In most cases self-limited and benign. Some viral conjunctivitis may become infected by bacteria (rare). An active ocular infection (viral or bacterial) is a temporary absolute contraindication: once the disease is over with appropriate treatment, refractive surgery can be reconsidered with special preventive measures. Subepithelial infiltrates develop 5-12 days after the initial symptoms of an acute viral conjunctivitis. Their presence suggests an infection by adenovirus serotypes 8 and 19. Picture shows dense infiltrates that were decreasing visual acuity and causing glare symptoms. They contraindicate refractive surgery. Adenoviral corneal opacities can persist for a few weeks to months (and may become permanent): they can be seen even after resolution of the acute symptoms. The use of mild topical steroids helps to slowly reduce the degree of the opacity (topical fluorometholone at tapering doses). Early infiltrates may induce topographic changes: wait for complete recovery until performing corneal refractive surgery. The use of topical gancyclovir gel (every 5 hours, for 10 days) has shown to effectively reduce the duration of the acute phase of adenoviral keratoconjunctivitis, and therefore reduce the risk and duration of subepithelial corneal infiltrates in the post-acute phase of the disease

RETINAL DEGENERATIONS AND RETINAL BREAKS

If present, retinal degenerations and retinal breaks must be addressed at least 40 days before surgery. Peripheral retinal examination should be performed once a year in every adult patient, and is mandatory in patients in search for refractive surgery. We perform argon laser photocoagulation (or photocoagulation with a 532 nm laser) of any retinal tears or dangerous degenerations, and complete the treatment with a 360° peripheral laser barrier to reduce the risk of retinal detachment in relation to ocular surgery. Once the laser spots achieve a correct pigmentation (this does not happen until 30-40 days after laser photocoagulation), refractive surgery can be safely performed accepted that the patient knows the risks of surgery.

We perform peripheral 360° laser photocoagulation (in 3 rows of impacts) in every patient (symptomatic or not) with familiar history of retinal detachment, or when peripheral dangerous degenerations are observed.

RETINAL DETACHMENT

We do not refractively treat patients with history of retinal detachment, unless they have cataract. In such patients, careful fundus examination is performed with a preventive 360° peripheral laser photocoagulation 30-40 days before cataract surgery (phacoemulsification will be preferred). The preventive laser treatment is performed even in the eye that did not have retinal detachment ("retinal detachment is a bilateral condition").

MACULAR DISEASE

We do not refractively treat patients with history of macular disease. Optical Coherence Tomography (OCT scan) of the macula is becoming increasingly popular for macular screening in refractive patients: its regular use helps diagnosing macular defects that are quite common in myopic patients. It is not strange to diagnose some macular defect (vitreoretinal traction, RPE defects, macular retinoschisis) in young patients in seek for refractive surgery that would otherwise been diagnosed as normal.

If available, we strongly suggest routine OCT scanning of the macula prior to any refractive surgery (Figs 57.3A and B).

AMBLYOPIA

Some patients in search for refractive surgery have the wrong idea that amblyopia will be corrected with laser surgery: this is completely false. Severe amblyopia, once established, cannot be cured: this happens around age 6-7. Later on, when the patient

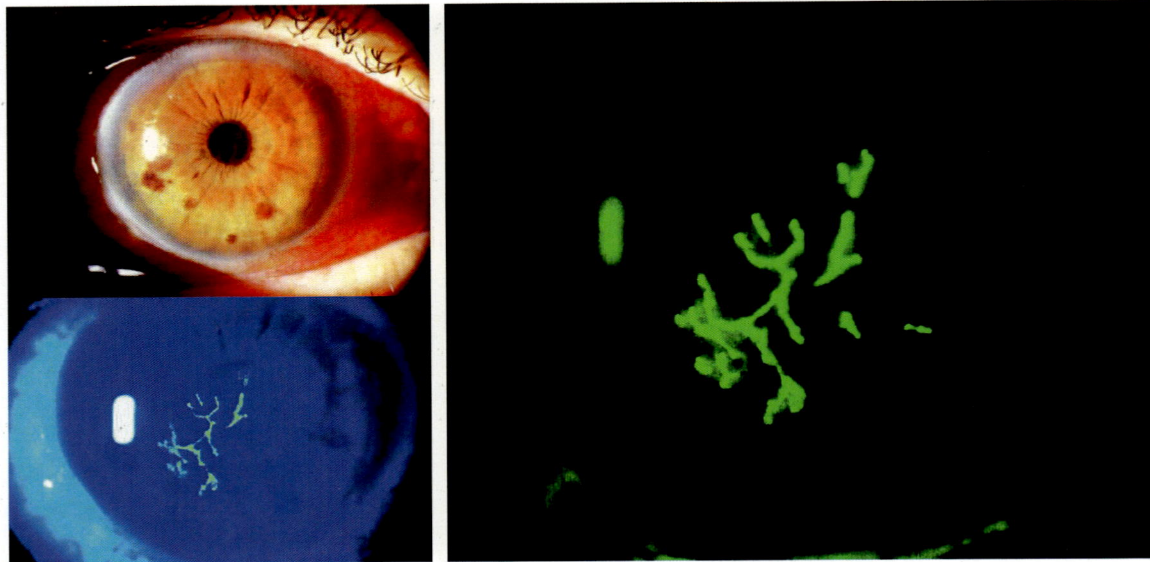

Fig. 57.2: Laser in situ keratomileusis can be safe in patients with a history of ocular herpes; we have seen no recurrences during the follow-up period. Nevertheless, candidates should be selected with caution: we do not perform surgery in eyes in which the herpes has not been inactive for at least 1 year before surgery. We discard patients with recurrent herpes and stromal disease. We perform periodic topography and pachymetry maps, and always check for normal corneal sensitivity. In such patients we always perform perioperative systemic antiviral prophylaxis with oral famcyclovir 750 mg, once a day, starting 4-5 days before surgery. Prophylactic treatment is discontinued 2-3 days after surgery. (Picture courtesy of Pablo Gili, MD)

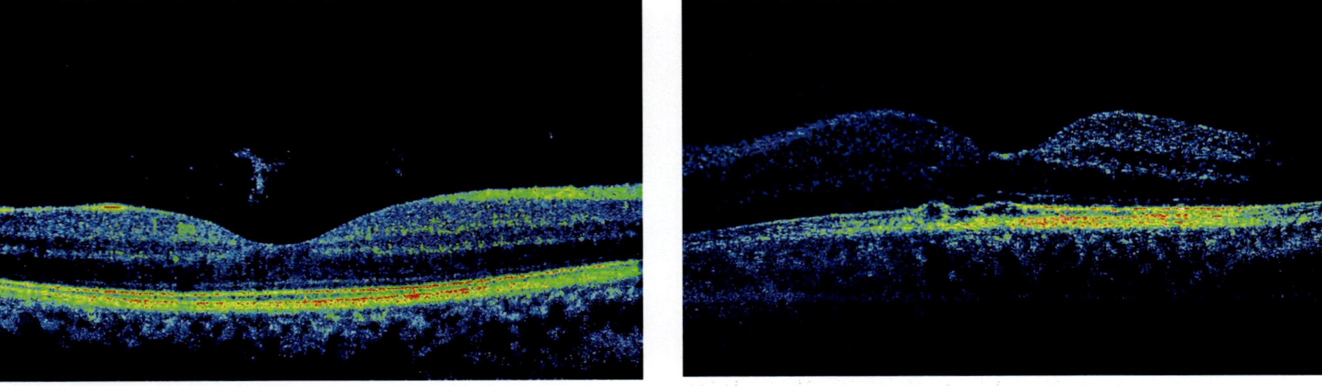

Figs 57.3 and B: (A) As optical coherence tomography becomes popular and available, we suggest routine OCT scanning of the macula before refractive procedures. In most cases, OCT will prove a normal macula, (the picture shows a normal macula with pre-macular vitreous bodies). (B) In other cases, OCT will prove macular anomalies (like retinal pigmentary epithelium detachments or ruptures, shown), that not necessarily contraindicate surgery, but of which the patient should be aware of before surgery

becomes an adult, no refractive treatment will give a normal vision to a true amblyopic eye.

There is only a case where refractive surgery can help: patients with high astigmatism unable to see 20/20 with contacts or glasses, but with a reasonable visual acuity, can greatly benefit from refractive surgery, and in some cases their visual acuity improves a few months after surgery.

GLAUCOMA

Prior to keratorefractive surgery, most techniques will give an acceptably accurate value of intraocular pressure (IOP): pneumotonometer is great for screening, while Goldmann applanation contact tonometry is the golden standard (accepting its limitations). Any other instrument can be used and checked against Goldmann's values. Getting a real and accurate intraocular pressure after a corneal refractive procedure is not easy. **Goldmann's applanation tonometry** depends on specific standards of the cornea, like corneal rigidity and thickness (supposed to be around 520 microns).

Since most postoperative corneas measure less than what they are supposed to measure, we find that normal IOPs are found to be low IOP's after corneal surgery. Central corneal thickness significantly affects IOP readings obtained by applanation tonometry according to the Goldmann principle. Getting an accurate measurement of IOP is not easy in keratorefractive patients: thin flat corneas measured with the Goldmann applanation tonometer or an air puff tonometer will produce false low IOP readings.

The hand-held **Tono-Pen® XL** (Medtronic Ophthalmics, Jacksonville FLO, USA) tonometer may provide an easy method of IOP evaluation after refractive surgery. Unlike Goldmann Applanation Tonometer, the Tono-Pen XL uses MacKay-Marg tonometry with a micro-strain gauge transducer that generates changes in the voltage relative to changes in pressure. It only uses a 1.5-mm diameter head as compared to the 3.03 mm diameter of the Goldmann's tonometer, making it to be less affected by corneal surface and curvature changes, and therefore being more accurate than the Goldmann's tonometer. You can use it outside the central cornea and away from the effects of keratorefractive surgery.

The **PASCAL® Dynamic Contour Tonometer** (Ziemer Ophthalmology, Port, Switzerland) is a slit-lamp mounted digital contact tonometer. It numerically measures both intraocular pressure (IOP) and ocular pulse amplitude (OPA) upon touching the cornea for a few seconds (its main drawback). It dynamically measures IOP pulses. It is supposed not to be influenced by corneal thickness and other biomechanical characteristics of the cornea, giving accurate IOP measurements in post refractive patients and keratoconic eyes. A disposable silicone tip cover can be used to prevent infections and reduce the likelihood of corneal abrasion (it needs a few seconds of corneal contact to give accurate measurements). It is slowly gaining acceptance amongst ophthalmologists as the reference tonometer in post refractive surgery patients.

We can't rely on just one test to diagnose or monitor the progression of glaucoma. We always test refractive patients for glaucoma and acquire as many measurements (intraocular pressure, visual field testing, optic disk imaging, pachymetry) to have a reference baseline pool of data for the future. A myopic patient is more prone to suffer glaucoma, and therefore it is essential to collect these data that will be probably needed in the future (Fig. 57.4).

New diagnostic equipment like optical coherence tomography (OCT) and the instrument called GDx™ (CarlZeiss Meditec, Inc., Oberkochen, Germany) supply useful information about the retinal nerve fiber layer (RNFL). The Heidelberg Retinal Tomograph (latest version HRT-III), from Heidelberg Engineering GmbH, Heidelberg, Germany, details the optic nerve head (ONH), and interpolates different nerve fiber layer values.

When doing **nerve fiber analysis**, we should not forget that LASIK flattens the central corneal curvature when performed for myopia but steepens it when performed to correct hyperopia. This change in curvature directly affects the accuracy of equipment that assumes a normal corneal curvature. Some software updates try to reduce or minimize the effect of corneal curvature (either anterior and/or sometimes posterior corneal curvature) on the measured nerve fiber layer values.

The **scanning laser polarimeter GDx™** uses a confocal scanning laser and an ophthalmoscope together with an integrated polarimeter to evaluate the thickness of the RNFL. By means of analysing the birefringent properties of the retinal ganglion cells' axons, the GDx™ can deduce the thickness of the retinal nerve fiber layer. The lower the thickness, the greater the damage to the retinal nerve fiber layer (which correlates with a worse visual field damage). Nevertheless, when a patient undergoes corneal refractive surgery like LASIK or PRK, the change in corneal curvature alters the polarization properties or the cornea, thus affecting an internal compensator of the instrument which goal is to obtain measurements independently of the crystalline lens (like cataracts) and corneal inherent polarization. After refractive surgery procedures, practitioner must consider the potential for "false positives" when using GDx™. For example, after LASIK, we tend to obtain thinner RNFL measurements, indicating missing nerve tissue that–being normal-can appear to be glaucomatous. Unlike GDX™, some nerve fiber analyzers, such as Talia Technology's Retinal Thickness Analyzed (RTA™, Talia Technology Ltd, Israel) and the various Optical Coherence Tomographers (OCT) available don't rely on polarimetry, and are therefore not so influenced by post-surgical changes in the cornea. These instruments are affected by corneal curvature values and changes in the refractive status of the eye (differences between pre and post-surgical measurements can be found).

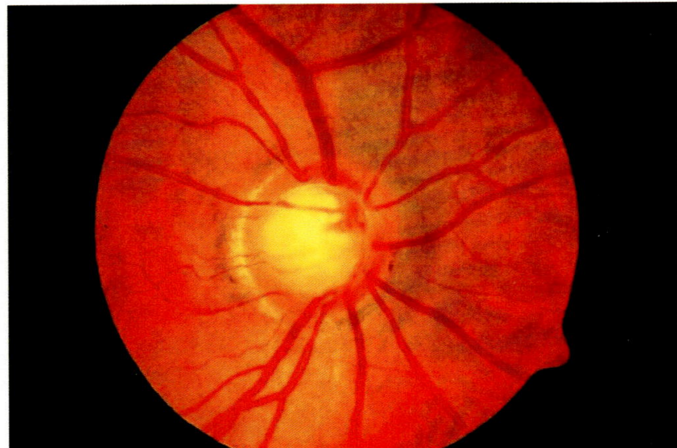

Fig. 57.4: Patients with severe (advanced or terminal) glaucoma should not have LASIK because the intraocular pressure (IOP) of the eye is raised during the procedure, and this could achieve in a paracentral or central scotoma in the visual field. We do not perform refractive surgery (other than cataract surgery) in glaucomatous patients that underwent a filtrating procedure

VISUAL FIELD TESTING AND REFRACTIVE SURGERY

Visual field testing can be affected in complicated refractive surgery cases in which corneal haze or scarring interferes with the transmission of the light stimuli to the retinal ganglion cells. In such cases, the results of these tests are not fully reliable, with false positives and false negatives. In uncomplicated cases, visual field testing remains an invaluable method for assessing progression of glaucomatous damage assuming its own limitations in myopic patients.

When we use the Zeiss-Humphrey Frequency Doubling Technology (FDT) that screens the patient for contrast sensitivity defects, we should remember that corneal refractive surgery (LASIK; PRK; LASEK) shapes the cornea in an oblate manner and that decreases the contrast sensitivity function (CSF), leading to a misdiagnose of glaucoma. The way to check for this problem is to measure pre and early post surgical baseline contrast sensitivity function to determine whether the FDT is reliable or not in each patient.

Cup/disk ratio remains unchanged after refractive surgery (Fig. 57.4). Nevertheless, severe surgical and/or post surgical complications leading to corneal opacification may have a negative impact in the visibility of the optic nerve head. High astigmatism or decentered ablations may change the aspect of the optic disk, thus increasing the asymmetry of the C/D ratio.

Systemic Limitations for Refractive Surgery: Special Considerations

Most surgical procedures cannot be safely performed if the patient has a history of autoimmune diseases (like collagenopathies, rheumatoid arthritis, systemic lupus erythematosus, dermatomyositis, psoriasis, Behcet's disease, Crohn's disease, histocytosis or multiple sclerosis). Most autoimmune diseases are listed in the US Food and Drug Administration (FDA) as contraindications for LASIK due to concerns about potentially damaging effect of wound healing. The American Academy of Ophthalmology (AAO), lists in its guidelines relative and absolute contraindications to laser-assisted in-situ keratomileusis (LASIK) and considers connective tissue or autoimmune diseases and systemic immunosuppresion as **relative** contraindications and only uncontrolled diseases and uncontrolled ocular allergy as **absolute** contraindications.

Some diseases, like **Ehlers-Danlos syndrome** (cutis laxa with laxity of joints) still remain absolute contraindications for corneal refractive procedures. While the molecular basis of this syndrome is heterogeneous, there are three fundamental mechanisms of disease known to produce Ehlers-Danlos syndrome: deficiency of collagen processing enzymes, dominant-negative effects of mutant collagen α-chains, and haploinsufficiency. These mechanisms compromise the strength of the connective tissue complex, and often the collagen fibril itself. This abnormal collagen strength contraindicates laser refractive surgery, as the risk of post-surgical ectasia is presumed higher and the risk of devastating intra-operative complication like globe rupture is possible. Apart from angioid streaks, strabismus or retinal detachment Ehlers-Danlos patients may present limbus to limbus thin corneas, keratoglobus, keratoconus, cornea plana, and corneal opacities: the cornea is very fragile (fragilitas oculi in Ehlers-Danlos syndrome type VI, or kyphoscoliosis) and the risk of keloid formation is extremely high. Indeed, abnormal bleeding may cause extreme difficulty with any surgical procedure.

Recent studies and personal communications suggest that the absolute exclusion from refractive surgery of all patients with certain systemic, collagen or autoimmune diseases needs to be reassessed: performing refractive procedures on such patients may not be as risky as once thought.

One of the most exciting articles recently published is a study by Cobo-Soriano R et al,[3] members of a Spanish group with huge experience in the refractive field, that shows no statistical differences in complications after refractive surgery between patients with controlled systemic diseases (including autoimmune and collagen diseases, diabetes mellitus, psoriasis, intestinal inflammatory diseases, and history of keloid formation) (Figs 57.5 to 57.8) and those without systemic disease. This observational retrospective case-control study clarifies some controversies in a large group of patients with different systemic diseases, and suggests that surgeons should keep an open mind about LASIK in most systemic diseases with proper patient selection. Regarding functional outcome, Cobo-Soriano R et al[3] find a worse refractive outcome in the collagen vascular diseases group when compared with the control group. They publish what has been in our minds for years: that LASIK can be performed effectively and safely in selected patients with stable and controlled systemic diseases. They conclude that the absolute exclusion of certain systemic contraindications should be reconsidered.

Nevertheless, every case has to be considered and evaluated specifically: careful preoperative evaluation holds the key to identifying appropriate candidates. When cornea is intact, LASIK is the safest refractive technique in risky patients. Avoid PRK and other superficial techniques that suppose a higher degree of inflammation.

Mirowitz EH,[4] published a case report of a 42-year-old woman with **systemic mastocytosis** and moderate myopia and astigmatism that underwent bilateral LASIK. Five days after surgery, she suffered a diffuse lamellar keratopathy (DLK) 1+ that was treated successfully with prednisolone acetate. The patient achieved a stable visual acuity of 20/20 in each eye unaided. Three years after surgery, the patient continues to use olopatadine. Mirowitz concludes that because of the rare nature of systemic mastocytosis and the anaphalactoid mechanism of release of mast cells, it may be difficult to assess the risk of undergoing LASIK. He suggests the use of an antihistamine and mast cell stabilizer, as used in this case, since it may have a beneficial effect.

There are special considerations for autoimmune disorders or collagen disease patients who undergo cataract, clear lens exchange or refractive surgery:

1. Write a proper informed consent.
2. Consider LASIK as your first refractive option: PRK creates a large epithelial defect that may predispose the cornea to ulceration.
3. Profit from periods of calm of the disease, specially in treatment pauses or when the disease is stable.
4. Make sure that biologic constants are stable when you perform surgery.
5. Carefully check for infectious concomitant diseases.
6. Give antiherpetic oral prophylaxis prior to surgery and a few days after surgery (ocular herpes can be devastating in such cases) (Fig. 57.2).
7. Corneal melting tends to occur mainly in elderly autoimmune patients, and almost exclusively in those with extra-articular disease. LASIK is relatively safe in rheumatoid arthritis patients that only manifest in the joints. Modern immune response modulators such as etanercept (a class of medications called tumor-necrosis factor –TNF- inhibitors) may help to stabilize rheumatoid arthritis, thus making viable the practice of a refractive procedure. Etanercept is used alone or in combination with other medications to reduce the pain and swelling associated with rheumatoid arthritis, juvenile rheumatoid arthritis, and psoriatic arthritis.

Cyclosporine 0.05 percent ophthalmic emulsion (Restasis®, Allergan Inc.) may help against corneal melting. This use is not currently approved by the FDA, although 0.1 percent cyclosporine eye drops have been successfully used in Europe for years to manage corneal graft rejection and other corneal inflammatory conditions.

DIABETES AND REFRACTIVE SURGERY

Diabetes is becoming increasingly prevalent in the United States of America and Europe. The American Diabetes Association classifies diabetes in 4 main groups: Type I diabetes mellitus (insulin dependent), Type II diabetes mellitus (non-insulin dependent), gestational diabetes mellitus (GDM) and other specific types of diabetes mellitus (mainly genetical diseases or syndromes) (Fig. 57.6).

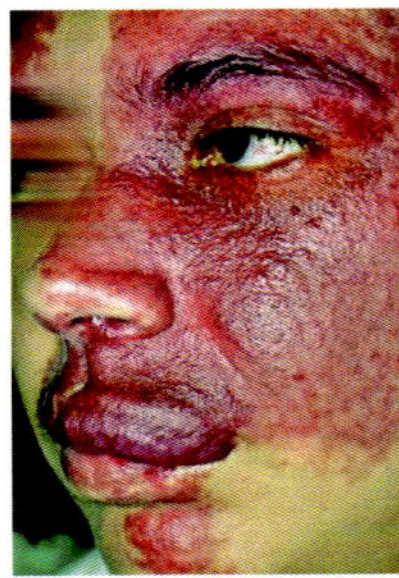
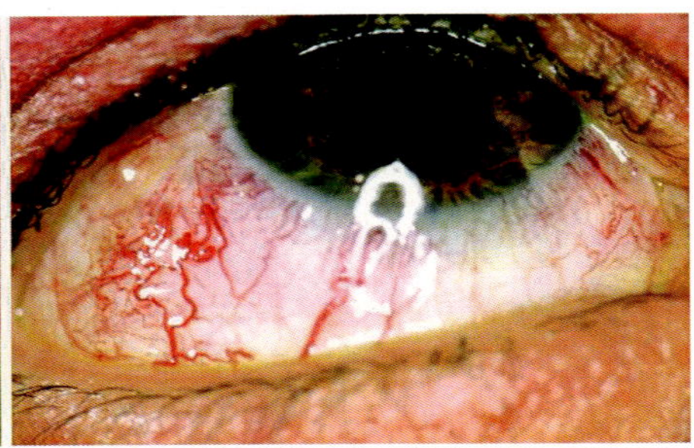

Fig. 57.5: Dilated episcleral vessels in Stürge-Weber-Dimitri syndrome (encephalotrigeminal angiomatosis). Stürge-Weber syndrome is a rare neurological disorder present at birth, characterized by a birthmark (usually on the face) known as a port-wine stain caused by an overabundance of capillaries around the trigeminal nerve beneath the surface of the face, and neurologic problems due to loss of nerve cells and calcification of tissue in the cerebral cortex of the brain on the same side of the body as the birthmark (angiomatosis of the central nervous system). Note the large facial port-wine purple stain on the forehead and upper eyelid of one side of the face: when superior lid is affected, ocular complications are probable (e.g. angiomatous glaucoma). Note the angioma and hypertrophia of the ipsilateral lip. We do not perform refractive procedures in such patients: most neurological syndromes present at birth are contraindications for elective refractive procedures

Type I is the most prevalent type of diabetes among children and young adults, and is characterized by acute onset of the symptoms and insulin dependence.

Type II is the most prevalent form of diabetes, affects older patients and is characterized by insidious development of symptoms, and is not dependent on insulin for survival. Some Type II patients may develop a Type I diabetes picture.

Ocular complications of diabetes mellitus include decreased tear production, III, IV and VI nerve palsies (extraocular muscle dysfunction), corneal abrasions, diabetic retinopathy with or without macular edema, rubeosis iridis and neovascular glaucoma, premature cataract and fluctuating refractive errors (suspect macular edema).

Diabetic patients may benefit from advances in medical therapy (e.g. insulin pump, oral anti-diabetic agents) and ophthalmical treatments (e.g.

photocoagulation, anti-Vascular Endothelial Growth Factor monoclonal antibodies like ranibizumab), but they clearly remain at risk for surgical complications, future decline in quality of life and life expectancy.

Diabetic patients can be considered candidates for cataract, clear lens exchange, and refractive surgery.

There are special considerations for diabetic patients who undergo cataract or clear lens exchange surgery:

1. About one third of diabetic patients with preexisting diabetic retinopathy show further progression of the disease.[5] If possible, diabetic retinopathy should be properly addressed prior to surgery.
2. Macular edema can persist and even worsen following intraocular surgery, specially if posterior capsule is broken during surgery. The advent of highly effective anti-VEGF therapy, greatly reduces the risk of permanent vision loss after intraocular surgery in diabetic patients.
3. Diabetic patients have increased risk of intraocular inflammation with fibrin reaction[6] and or macular thickening. Ideally, intraocular surgery should take place before the patient develops significant diabetic retinopathy, and with the patient under strict glucose levels control.
4. Prefer acrylic hydrophobic intraocular lenses (IOL). Perform intensive anterior and posterior capsule polishing during surgery to reduce the risk of future posterior Nd-YAG laser capsulotomies that may worsen retinal state and macular edema.
5. Consider that healing time is longer in diabetic patients, and therefore the smaller the incision the better.

Although diabetes was once considered a contraindication for refractive surgery, there is an increasing demand of diabetic patients for refractive procedures. We believe that the appropriateness of refractive surgery in diabetic patients really depends on how well controlled the disease is, and on previous retinal-macular state. Before refractive and cataract surgery, we perform OCT and fluorescein angiography in every patient to completely assess the real retinal condition of the patient: fundus examination alone may not be enough to rule out minor cases of diabetic retinopathy.

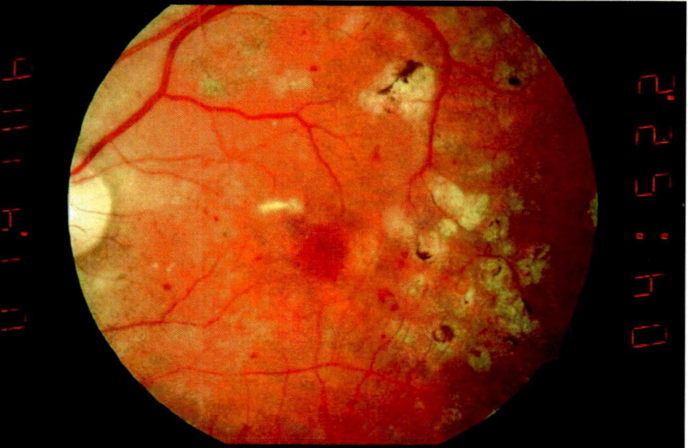

Fig. 57.6: An advanced diabetic patient that underwent panretinal photocoagulation and has diabetic macular edema is not a good candidate for a refractive procedure that will probably worsen its macular or retinal condition

A spanish study by Cobo-Soriano et al[3] showed no statistical differences in complications after refractive surgery between patients with controlled systemic diseases (including diabetes and other diseases) and those without systemic disease. The same results are supported by Halkiadakis et al,[7] although they document less predictable refractive outcomes in patients with controlled diabetes.

There are special considerations for diabetic patients who undergo refractive surgery:

1. Refractive surgery is contraindicated in patients with bad glucose control, macular edema or proliferative retinopathy.[8]
2. Patients with diabetes are at increased risk for punctate keratopathy, recurrent corneal erosions and persistent epithelial defects.[9] Diabetes increases the healing time of any surgical procedure. Therefore intensive lubrication must be provided to reduce dry eye sensation and the risk of eye rubbing.
3. Patients with uncontrolled diabetes are at increased risk for interface epithelialisation and corneal neovascularisation in case of postoperative complications like infection of the interface in LASIK or sustained corneal inflammation.

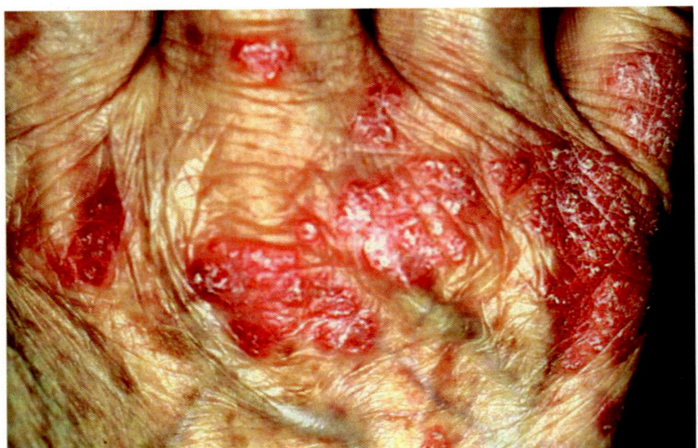

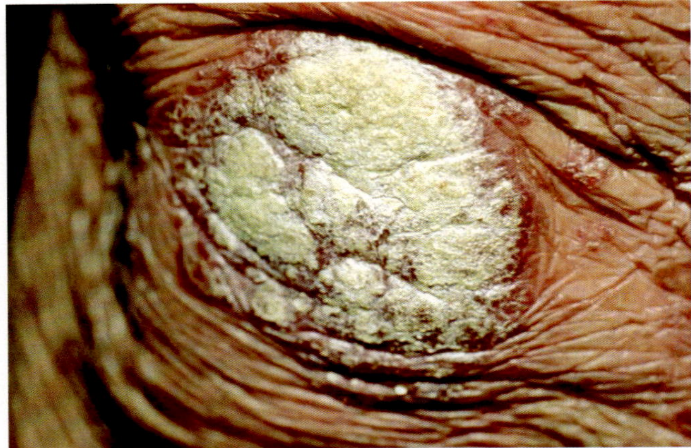

Figs 57.7A and B: Plaque psoriasis is the most common form of psoriasis, a non-contagious inflammatory skin disorder, probably an autoimmune disease, where an excess of T-cell activity is found. Skin is primarily affected, but about 10 percent of the patients develop psoriatic arthritis. Ocular signs occur in about 10 percent of the patients: blepharitis, unspecific conjunctivitis, punctate keratitis, episcleritis, anterior uveitis with arthritis and complications of psoriasis treatment (retinoids and psoralens-UVA) may compromise the result of any refractive procedure. At the moment these lines are written, there is reduced experience in refractive surgery in psoriasis patients, although in recent studies there have been no complications or reactivation of the disease

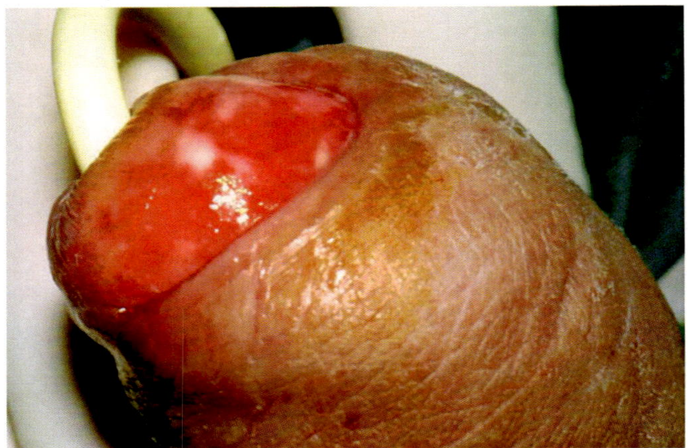

Fig. 57.8: Reiter's disease was originally described as a triad of arthritis, conjunctivitis and urethritis. Urethritis may result in meatal stenosis with urinary retention. Arthirtis is clearly induced by an infection and most patients share HLA-B27 typing. Ocular disease is very common and ranges from transient asymptomatic conjunctivitis to an aggressive recurrent non-granulomatous anterior iridocyclitis that is occasionally refractory to treatment and may cause blindness. At the moment these lines are written, there is reduced experience in refractive surgery in Reiter's disease patients, although in recent studies there has been no complication or reactivation of the disease. Severe recurrent anterior segment inflammation results in cataract formation and occasionally glaucoma: for all these reasons we still contraindicate refractive surgery in patients with Reiter's disease

4. Diabetic patients have less predictable refractive outcomes due to the refractive shifts caused by varying glucose levels, and the varying degree of macular edema caused by sudden glucose level falls.

OCULAR ROSACEA

Rosacea is a common dermatologic condition that affects mainly midfacial region (Figs 57.9A and B). It is characterized by facial flushing and different clinical signs like erythema, facial telangiectasia, coarseness of skin, and inflammatory papulopustular eruption resembling acne, as well as a variety of ocular findings (we refer to them as ocular rosacea) such as blepharitis, keratoconjunctivitis sicca and atopic keratoconjunctivitis. The diagnosis of rosacea is a clinical diagnosis: ocular manifestations may precede the cutaneous signs by years.

Rosacea patients suffer from blepharitis, chronic ocular itching and severe dry eyes: they are not the best candidates for refractive surgery. Wound healing in ocular rosacea is delayed, and dry eye may result in postoperative corneal complications. Nevertheless, in case of need, ocular condition can be treated in order to achieve a reasonable ocular surface status to allow refractive surgery. Even after management, having refractive surgery with ocular rosacea may not be wise because of the possibility of reoccurring outbreaks, and the risk of corneal **neovascularisation**. In such cases we perform refractive surgery of one eye at a time, with a special informed consent.

For the rosacea patients, we recommend strict lid hygiene with antiseptic hydrating gels (e.g. Lepharite®, Laboratorios Thea, Barcelona, Spain), preoperative oral doxycycline, and intensive ocular lubrication with a 0.4 percent sodium hyaluronate solution (Aquoral®, Laboratorio Esteve, Barcelona, Spain), 5 or 6 times-a-day. Five days before surgery, we add topical fluorometholone and an azithromycin ophthalmic solution 1 percent (AzaSite®, Inspire Pharmaceuticals, Durham, NC, USA) four-time-a-day application. Especial antibiotic protection and corneal lubrication for a few months after surgery are recommended. The use of long-term low dose topical fluorometholone reduces the risk of corneal new vessels.

Tetracyclines are traditionally used as antibiotics, they also have important anti-inflammatory properties. They are very useful (Doxycycline, DCI) in treating acne rosacea dry eye during a few months, prior to refractive surgery. They should not be used in pregnant women or when an allergy has been described (in case of allergy to tetracyclines, topical azithromycin will be preferred). The use of a three day treatment with oral azithromycin (500 mg, once-a-day, three days) to be repeated after a week is a valid alternative when tetracyclines cannot be used.

Seborrheic dermatitis and acne rosacea are very silimar diseases: they both involve inflammation of the sebaceous glands. Acne rosacea also involves a vascular component causing flushing, broken blood vessels and rinophyma. In seborrheic dermatitis we observe the presence of greasy flaking in the forehead, nose and around the mouth, crusts, scales, itching and occasionally burning, and may also be found on the scalp, ears and torso. It does not usually involve red bumps as in acne rosacea. The two conditions are very often seen together: the approach of both before refractive surgery is very similar.

Seborrhea and rosacea can both cause LASIK complications (e.g. dry eye, diffuse lamellar keratitis) but under the right circumstances, after treatment, those who suffer with either or both conditions may, safely have PRK or LASIK surgery.

MENSTRUATION, PREGNANCY AND NURSING

During the woman's menstrual cycle some corneal changes occur in parallel with hormonal changes;[10-12] similar changes can be seen during pregnancy and nursing. Changes in corneal curvature (steepening

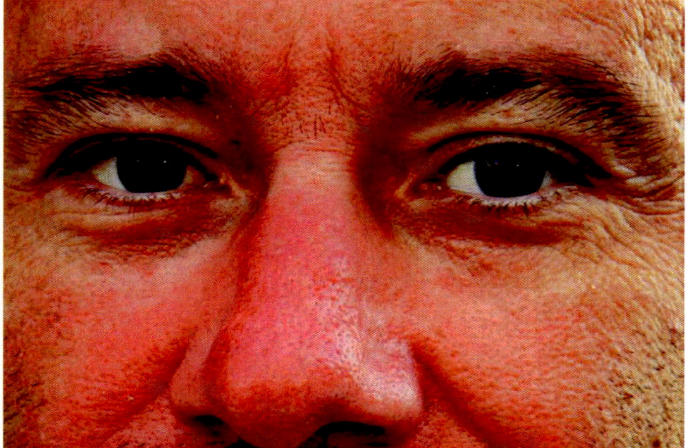

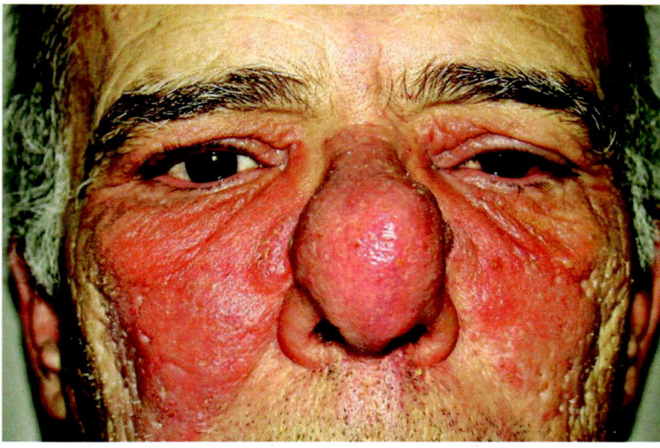

Figs 57.9A and B: (A) Ocular rosacea in a young patient in seek for refractive surgery: facial erythema, blepharitis, severe conjunctivitis sicca and atopic keratoconjunctivitis are classical signs that may be underdiagnosed when they are mild at presentation. Before refractive surgery, medical history should include dermatological aspects to early detect dermatological and autoimmune patients. (B) Older people may also suffer severe rosacea with rhinophyma: an adequate perioperative care with antiseptic lid cleansing and preoperative antibiotic drops will help avoiding complications after cataract surgery

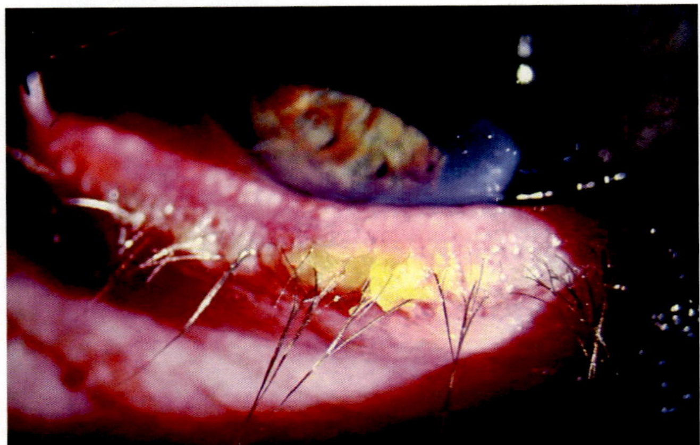

Fig. 57.10: Severe blepharitis must be addressed prior to refractive surgery, and every possible measure taken to avoid post-operative infection. Crusts act as a reservoir for pathogen microorganisms

occurs at the beginning of the cycle), thickness (minimal thickness before ovulation, and maximal thickness at the beginning or end of the menstrual cycle) and sensitivity (decreased corneal sensitivity just before and during the ovulation) during the woman's menstrual cycle have been detected; they are attributed to endocrine influences. If possible, choose the final period of the menstrual cycle to perform refractive surgery.

Candidates for any refractive surgery procedure should not have refractive surgery if pregnant or nursing, or expecting to become pregnant or breast-feeder within six months of refractive surgery.

During pregnancy and nursing, a large number of hormonal, metabolic, immunologic, hematologic, and cardiovascular changes do occur.

Common ocular changes (Fig. 57.10) that may interfere with refractive surgery are reversible after delivery and after nursing, and include: changes in tear composition (increased grease and lysozyme, dry eye symptoms) with mild corneal edema, changes in conjunctival vessels (granular circulation and spasms), reversible increased corneal curvature and corneal thickness, decreased corneal sensitivity, reduced intraocular pressure, lens accommodation changes, unclear visual field changes, candida endophthalmitis, and central serous chorioretinopathy. Some systemic changes or complications of pregnancy, not to mention psychological changes, may interfere with refractive surgery: pregnancy induced hypertension, pseudotumor cerebri, pituitary tumors or vascular occlusive disorders (retinal artery occlusion, retinal vein occlusion, disseminated intravascular coagulopathy, amniotic fluid embolism, thrombotic thrombocytopenic purpura, central venous thrombosis). Pregnancy may also aggravate preexisting ocular disorders like keratoconus, retinitis pigmentosa, diabetic retinopathy, macular edema, optic disc edema, ocular manifestations of Graves disease, uveitis, tumors (uveal melanomas).

Hormones produced during pregnancy and lactation will cause most women's refractive state to fluctuate (sometimes dramatically), with or without refractive surgery. Refraction taken during these fluctuations will be inappropriate. If fluctuation occurs during the recovery period, surgeon will be unable to determine whether this fluctuation is due to pregnancy or surgery.

As a general rule we do not perform refractive surgery at least six months after delivery, or three months after nursing is ended.

Another important consideration is that drugs used in the postoperative period (antibiotics and steroids) or in case of complications may be dangerous to the embryo or fetus, or may pass to the infant through lactation. Little is known about the risk of using ophthalmic medications in pregnant and nursing women.

In general, when eye drops are needed, we instruct pregnant and nursing women using ophthalmic topical medication to achieve digital punctal occlusion at least for 5 minutes after drop instillation. Reversible punctal occlusion with plugs can be performed in uncooperative women. We also prescribe the lowest effective dose of medication, and try to use the drugs with the lowest fetal risk factor (e.g. erythromycin has a B risk factor and will be preferred over chloramphenicol, that has a C risk factor).

HUMAN IMMUNODEFFICIENCY VIRUS DISEASE (HIV DISEASE) ACQUIRED IMMUNODEFFICIENCY SYNDROME (AIDS)

The term AIDS (Acquired Immunodefficiency Syndrome) refers to a constellation of diseases or syndromes characterized by a severe immune dysfunction due to the infection by a virus designed as HIV (Human Immunodefficiency Virus), in which the clinical importance of CD4+ T-Lymphocytes count. It is not our goal to describe general aspects of the diseases related to HIV infection (opportunistic infections or malignancies), and we will only refer to some clinically relevant ophthalmic aspects of AIDS.

Infectious ocular manifestations[13,14] include herpes zoster ophthalmicus (suspect HIV infection in front of a young patient with zoster ophthalmicus), cytomegalovirus retinitis, toxoplasmic retinitis, acute retinal necrosis, HIV retinitis, syphilitic retinitis, and other less common infections like mycobacterial or *Pneumocystis carinii*.

Non-infectious ocular manifestations include periocular or conjunctival Kaposi sarcoma, a Sjögren-like dry eye (20% of the patients), subconjunctival hemorrhages, non-infectious peripheral corneal ulcerations and diverse neuro-ophthalmic disorders (e.g. papilledema, visual-field defects).

Advances in combination pharmacotherapy (where available) have resulted in dramatic improvements in survival and quality of living. AIDS patients do not seek for refractive surgery: they have more important problems to solve. But it is increasingly common, as survival rates of HIV infected patients grow, that HIV infected patients without AIDS manifestations or with minor manifestations ask for refractive procedures to improve their standards of living. Furthermore, HIV/AIDS can impact on ocular surface, and patients become less tolerant to contact lenses.

A good CD4+ cell count is essential to reduce the risk of postoperative complications. When T-cell count is low, the patient is at high risk for herpes and other infectious complications: in such cases oral prophylactic anti-herpetic regime (e.g. Famciclovir, 750 mg/24h × 7 days before surgery) is advisable. The excimer laser, and anxiety before surgery can activate herpes, as commonly seen in laser aesthetic surgery (laser skin rejuvenation). If there is history of herpes in the eye, it is better not to do laser.

HIV alone is not a contraindication to LASIK or other refractive procedures. But in case of infectious complications, they are harder to treat.

Although no cases of AIDS or Creutzfeld-Jacob disease are known or have spread from instrument contamination, we strongly believe that it is not sufficient to use a new blade for each patient and autoclave the microkeratome: furthermore, it is logistically not practical for a busy refractive practice to centrally sterilize the keratome.

Fortunately, this is no longer a problem since the advent of single-use disposable microkeratomes (like the Moria™ One Use-Plus 130 and 90, Moria, Antony, France–Europe). These disposable single use keratomes have the increased advantage of the transparent plastic ring that makes centration easy and allows the surgeon to visualize the cornea and the blade action through the ring.

The use of a disposable keratome is mandatory in terms of ethics when the patient is suspected or known to suffer a transmissible infection or a disease like Human Immunodefficiency Virus related disease (AIDS). When treating HIV patients, prefer single-use sterile instruments if available.

In all cases of corneal refractive surgery the use of non-recycled disposable microkeratomes gives less chance of diffuse lamellar keratitis or pathogen/prion transmission from contaminated instruments.

When necessary, sterilize your reusable instruments with a special antivirus solution/soap, rinse thoroughly with sterile distilled water, and sterilize twice either with plasma (special plasma autoclaves) or autoclave with the dedicated anti prion cycle (longer cycle at higher temperature) that almost any modern autoclaves do provide. HIV is fragile, but all preventive measures are welcome. In the future, we believe that the use of a femtosecond laser to create the flap for LASIK in HIV patients will prove to be advantageous.

In any case, when doing LASIK, LASEK or PRK, it is advisable to schedule the HIV patient at the end of the surgery session, since virus particles can spread throughout the operating theater: intensive filtered aspiration with smoke evacuator of the particles and intensive scrubbing of the bed with a special antiviral cleansing solution/soap should be done. Special filtering masks (or double mask) are advisable, in order to prevent surgeon, assistants and technicians from viral particle inhalation.

Since most HIV patients have **dry eye**, it is of the outmost importance to provide intensive ocular lubrication with the least toxic products (e.g. hourly instillation of **0.18-0.4% sodium hyaluronate** solution). Most of our patients have a high degree of satisfaction and feel very comfortable with the use of sodium hyaluronate solution.

Since HIV+ patients are more susceptible to infection, in the post-operative care, we add intensive antibiotic prophylaxis. A special informed consent is advisable in HIV + patients.

MENTAL RETARDATION

Traditionally, contraindications of refractive surgery include mental retardation. But children with cerebral palsy, mental retardation and other neurological problems often have poor or extremely poor eyesight, which interferes with every aspect of their daily lives: they have a kind of visual autism. Most times these are kids who are legally blind and whom everyone has given up.

Refractive surgery can be performed on children with cerebral palsy, Down syndrome and neuro-behavioral disorders such as autism. In such cases, most surgeons perform laser-assisted subepithelial keratectomy, or LASEK, in which the cornea is reshaped without a surgical flap: this is safer for children, who will inevitably rub their eyes after surgery. In addition, the LASEK technique is able to correct much higher degrees of myopia, or nearsightedness, than the LASIK technique that we commonly use on adults.

For patients with high refractive errors beyond the range of laser correction, we can use other surgical techniques like implantation of phakic intraocular lens (ICL), or phacoemulsification with clear lens extraction and intraocular lens implantation

Since these patients are mostly uncooperative and do not communicate well, most measurements must be done with non-invasive methods, and most times under general anesthesia just before performing surgery. Hand-held pachymeters and biometers are of great help and ease of use inside the operating theater. In such patients, most times there is a lack or precision of measurements, but the patients still benefit from refractive surgery.

Despite the increased post-surgical risks, it is not difficult to obtain parents' permission to perform refractive surgery in children with often no alternative (they cannot or will not wear glasses or contacts). In most cases refractive surgery in mentally impaired children greatly improves the overall development of the child.

Refractive errors are common in **Down syndrome** and they should be detected during screening evaluations (Fig. 57.11). Refractive surgery can be performed in some collaborative patients: first discard the presence of stenotic nasolacrimal ducts, blepharitis and conjunctivitis, which occur frequently. Keratoconus occurs more frequently in adolescents or adults than in the typical child: therefore, topographic screening for keratoconus is essential.

THYROID-ASSOCIATED OPHTHALMOPATHY (GRAVES' DISEASE)

Although Graves' disease most commonly presents around the fourth and fifth decades, it is not strange to discover minor dysthyroidism problems in myopic females around the fourth decade of life in search for refractive surgery (Figs 57.12 and 57.13).

Ophthalmic manifestation of thyroid-associated ophthalmopathy are variable, and are mostly due to hyperthyroidism: upper lid retraction, progressive exophthalmia, progressive lagophthalmos with dry eye disease, chemosis and lid edema, limitation of eye movements, eye injection and exposure keratitis.

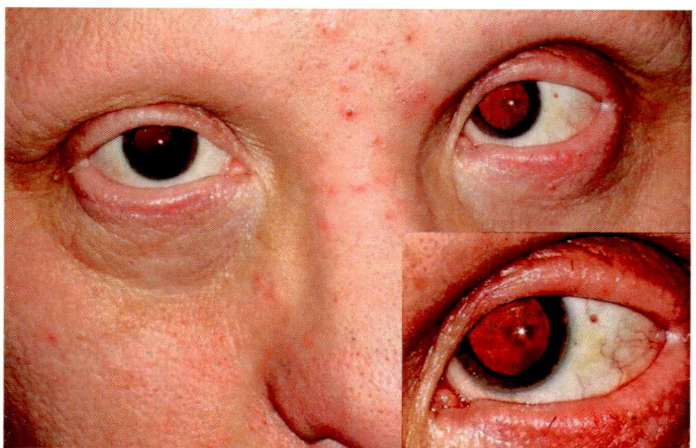

Fig. 57.11: Early in their lives, Down's syndrome patients present some degree of congenital or acquired cataract that rapidly worsens with time. It is essential to rule out the presence of lens opacities with pupil dilation prior to performing refractive surgery. Notice lens opacities in the ocular red reflex of his left eye in an adult Down syndrome in search for refractive surgery. Complete absence of hair (atrichia) and strabismus can also be noted. The patient was not operated, and we decided to wait for a refractive cataract surgery

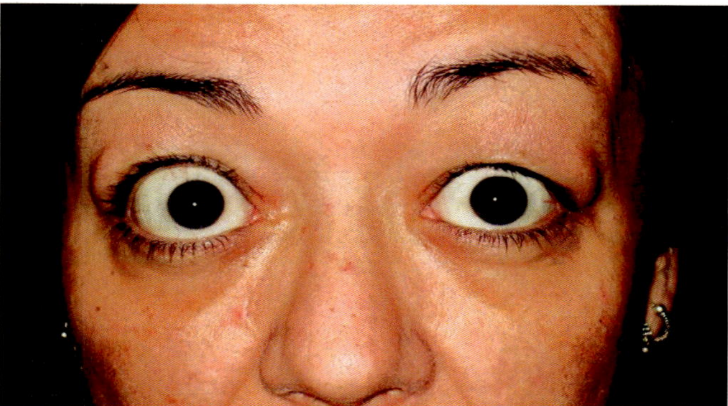

Fig. 57.12: A mid-aged lady in search for refractive surgery was suspected to suffer a thyroid disease because of her aspect and her sensation of lid puffiness and oscillating tired vision. Thyroid hormones were found normal at first, but changed to abnormal three months later, when hyperthyroidism was clearly observed and proven by serum levels of thyroid hormones. In case of doubt, careful checking for a suspected disease may avoid misdiagnoses and possible complications. In doubt, wait and see ...

Patients with thyroid eye disease may have an elevated eye pressure either in primary ocular position or in upgaze. Visual loss is an important but rare complication of Graves' disease and may be due to either optic neuropathy (with or without glaucoma) or due to severe corneal ulceration. Because of its insidious onset, visual loss may be late diagnosed: patients suspected to suffer from thyroid disease should be carefully checked for defects in color vision, afferent pupillary defects and visual field defects. Optic nerve aspect should be periodically checked for hemorrhages and edema.

Refraction and visual acuity is unstable in most cases, and some patients refer accommodation problems. After laser refractive surgery, the follow-up of glaucoma is very difficult in such patients, mostly myopic, with a variable degree of neuropathy and an advanced crystalline lens opacification: visual fields are not reliable and intraocular pressure is difficult to measure.

For all the above-mentioned reasons, we do not operate thyroid-affected patients, unless they suffer minor degrees of Graves' disease without ophthalmopathy (Graves' disease may present with or without ophthalmopathy) and are completely visually stable. We do never operate patients with Graves' orbitopathy. The patient signs a special informed consent that informs of the increased risk of complications (e.g. dry eye, post-surgical diplopia).

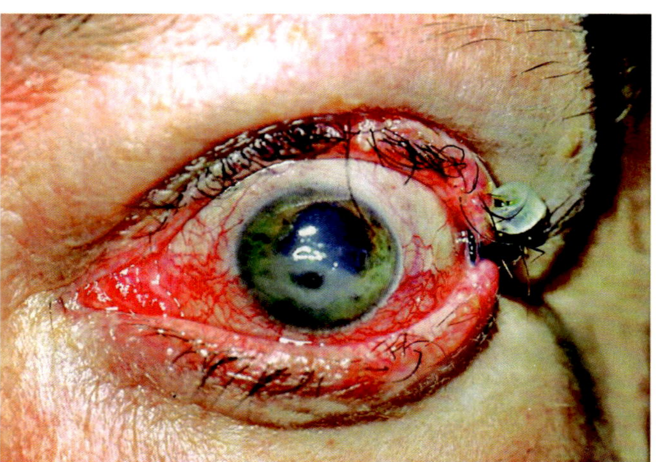

Fig. 57.13: Advanced cases of thyroid disease with severe exophthalmia and corneal ulceration will benefit of lateral tarsorraphy until stabilization of the patient or orbital decompression (if needed). For obvious reasons they remain absolute contraindication for refractive surgery

In case of refractive surgery, in such patients, an adequate intensive corneal lubrication with preservative-free eye drops becomes essential.

REFERENCES

1. Astle WF, Fawcett SL, Huang P, Alewenah O, Ingram A. Long term outcomes of photorefractive keratectomy and laser- assisted subepithelial keratectomy in children. J Cataract Refract Surg 2008;34:411-6.
2. Paysse EA. Refractive Surgery in Children: Is It Ready for Prime Time? The John Pratt-Johnson Annual Lecture. Amer. Orthoptic Jrnl 2007;57(1):79-88; doi:10.3368/aoj.57.1.79.
3. Cobo-Soriano R, Beltran J, Baviera J. LASIK outcomes in patients with underlying systemic contraindications: a preliminary study. Ophthalmology 2006;113(7):1118.el-8.
4. Mirowitz EH. Laser-assisted intrastromal keratomileusis in a patient with systemic mastocytosis. Optometry 2008;79(2):95-7.
5. Mathis A, Pago-Mathis V, Dumas S, et al. Retinal complications of cataract surgery. J Fr Ophtalmol 2000;23(1):88-95. In French, with English summary.
6. Simón-Castellví G, Simón-Castellví JM, Simón-Castellví S, Simón-Tor JM. Uvéite fibrineuse après la chirurgie de la cataracte avec implant de lentille intraoculaire. Ophtalmol 1994;8(3):235-240. In French, with English summary.
7. Halkiadakis I, Belfair N, Gimbel HV. Laser in situ keratomileusis in patients with diabetes. J Cataract Refract Surg 2005;31(10):1895-8.
8. Chandbari H, Ahmadeih H. Aggravation of proliferative diabetic retiopathy after LASIK. J Cataract Refract Surg 2003;29(11):2232-3.
9. Fraunfelder FW, Rich LF. LASIK complications in diabetes mellitus. Cornea 2002;21(3):246-8.
10. Giuffré G, Di Rosa L, Fiorino F, et al. Variations in central corneal thickness during the menstrual cycle in women. Cornea 2007;26(2):144-6.
11. Kiely PM, Carney LG, Smith G. Menstrual cycle variations of corneal topography and thickness. Am J Optom and Physiol Optics 1983;60(10):822-9.
12. Oliver KM, Walsh G, Tomlinson A, et al. Effect of the menstrual cycle on corneal curvature. Ophthal Physiol Opt. 1996;16(6):46773.
13. Rodriguez MP, Garsía S, Balado P, et al. Manifestaciones oculares externas en el paciente infectado por virus de la immunodeficiencia humana (External ocular manifestations in patients with human immunodeficiency virus infection). Arch Soc Esp Oftalmol 1996;70:5-12. In Spanish, with English summary.
14. Medina LC, Gómez T, Rodriguez P et al. Manifestaciones oculares en la meningitis criptocócica en pacientes con SIDA (Ocular manifestations in cryptococcal meningitis in patients with AIDS). Arch Soc Esp Oftalmol 1996;70:85-94. In Spanish, with English summary.

Index

O

P

R

S

T

U

V

W

Z